Medical Language

TERMINOLOGY IN CONTEXT

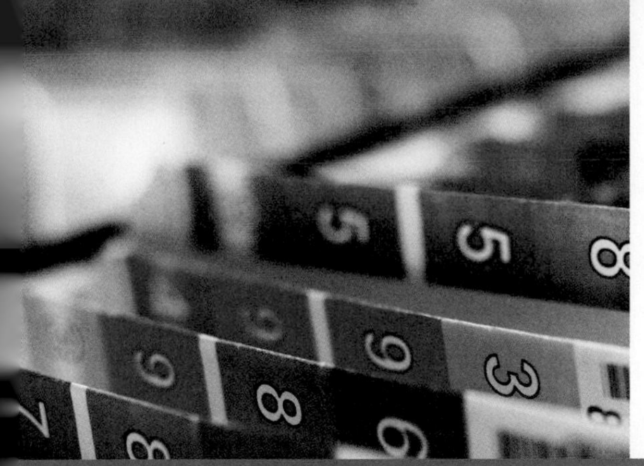

Medical Language

TERMINOLOGY IN CONTEXT

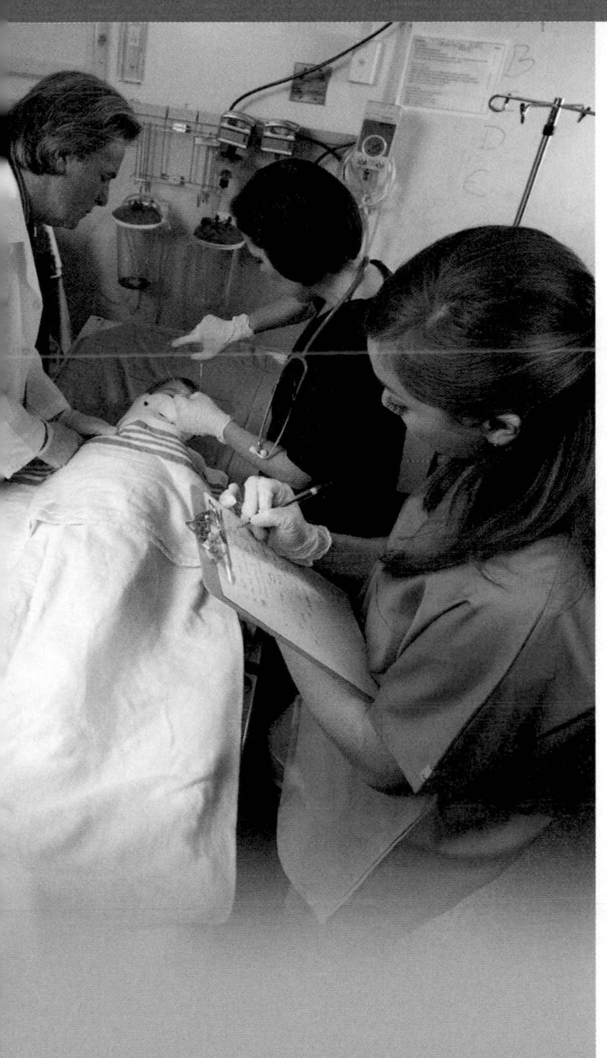

Melodie Hull, RPN, MEd, MSc, BA, TESOL, PID

Nursing Faculty
College of the Rockies
Cranbrook, BC
and
Nursing and Health Faculty
Open Learning Division
Thompson Rivers University
Kamloops, BC
and
President
Clayton International Consulting and Educational Services
Cranbrook, BC

F.A. Davis Company • Philadelphia

F. A. Davis Company
1915 Arch Street
Philadelphia, PA 19103
www.fadavis.com

Printed in the United States of America

Last digit indicates print number: 10 9 8 7 6 5 4 3 2 1

Senior Acquisitions Editor: Quincy McDonald
Manager of Content Development: George W. Lang
Developmental Editor: Vicki Wilt
Art and Design Manager: Carolyn O'Brien

Library of Congress Cataloging-in-Publication Data

Hull, Melodie.
Medical language : terminology in context / Melodie Hull.
p. ; cm.
Includes index.
ISBN 978-0-8036-2683-6
I. Title.
[DNLM: 1. Terminology as Topic—Problems and Exercises. W 18.2]

610.1'4—dc23

2012050504

This book is dedicated to my mother,
Beryl Marguerite (Loeppky) Hull,
who passed away suddenly at Christmas
during this book's development.
My mother was brilliant; she had a quick wit and an intellect that will be sorely missed. How she enjoyed watching this book unfold and trying to guess my next moves! She had studied Latin when she was young, and she loved the opportunity to see it appear in my work and to coach me on it.
Mom followed this manuscript through to the end of Unit 3. How I wish she could see it now.

Foreword

This work is unusual, and that is what drew me into it. When I was approached by the author—whom I had a prior professional relationship with—to provide collaboration for a small piece of this work, I was intrigued by the possibility of learning in such a new and unusual way. I agreed to work with her for the sheer joy of being at the beginning of a great thing.

The 30 years that I have spent in the health-care field have all involved continuing education and ongoing learning. From learning how to function at the bedside to creating materials for new learning by others, each year has included some form of education. These years have been spent with my head down in textbooks that were created in the same mold as all of the textbooks that I have ever studied. This period of education has stretched from the very early 1960s to the present day. Never have I encountered a textbook that has engaged me in the way that this book has.

As we have learned to learn through repetition and ongoing review, we have often forgotten that, in health care, the need is to engage with the person, the patient, the client. The need to be reminded of this is paramount throughout the health-care field. The manner in which the material is presented in this book in no way follows the current prescribed educational mold. It breaks all of the rules, and it engages the learner in a way that is focused on the person. The author continually reaffirms the idea that health care is not about a different vocabulary but rather about people.

The chapters of this book open up the lives of ordinary people to the learners in a way that will draw the learners in and help them to embrace the very idea of learning. The book is engaging and honest while at the same time being factual and correct. Most of all, it is totally unique in its approach. As an educator, manager, and nurse, I believe that this method of teaching and learning for the field of health care is the beginning of a great movement forward.

Laura Sherret, RN, BSN

Preface

Welcome

Congratulations on choosing *Medical Language: Terminology in Context,* a unique, progressive alternative to the teaching and learning of medical terminology. The approach that you will find in this text makes use of the latest and most authoritative information that we have regarding how adults learn and retain language skills. This is a book that **promotes language acquisition.** It is written from the philosophical stance that medical terminology and medical language form an advanced and career-specific subset of the English language and that the best way to actively learn this language is through experiencing it as it is found in clinical scenarios.

This book is based in the context of real-world health care. The study of medical terminology is embedded in context across a broad spectrum of careers and patient care, including the assessment of health, diagnosis, treatment, disease, illness, and injury. Learners walk hand in hand with health and allied health professionals as they care for five specific patients. Each chapter begins with and then follows the patient care of one of the five main characters: one child, two adults, and two older adults who have all been in the same motor vehicle accident. A premature baby is eventually added into the mix.

Another unique feature of this book is that medical language and medical terminology are differentiated. Medical terminology includes those technical, specific, standardized, and precise words, terms, and phrases that are used in medicine, the health sciences, anatomy, physiology, pharmacology, and so on. Alternatively, medical language consists of words, phrases, jargon, acronyms, abbreviations, terms, and expressions that are used less formally to communicate about a patient's status, to confer with peers, and to be sure that meaning is understood during interactions with patients. Health and allied health professionals use a blend of these two vocabularies (lexis). The recognition and use of this career-specific body of language leads to effective and meaningful communication among care providers and their colleagues.

Purpose and Audience

The single most important goal of this book is health literacy, which refers to the degree to which learners are able to obtain, process, and understand basic health information, processes, and procedures and to communicate effectively within this genre. Medical terminology provides that foundation. Terms are presented within the contexts of human anatomy, physiology, pathology, wellness, patient experiences, and so on, so that they may be fully learned rather than simply remembered. The primary learning goal is achieved when learners are able to transfer what is learned into fluent and accurate communication within the appropriate contexts and when language acquisition and competency are demonstrated through use. In this regard, language acquisition is both functional and communicative.

A second learning goal of this book is that of helping learners to develop knowledge of and insight into various health careers. The culture of the health and allied health professions is embedded in the language that is used by the members of those professions. Written and oral competencies in the necessary language provide a means of entry and a point of access for newcomers into the culture of the workplace and into the ranks of the interdisciplinary health-care team. Through contextual learning, this book provides an opportunity for learners to acculturate into the health and allied health professions and to achieve a professional identity. Competency in career-specific language signals to other members of the group that you are one of them.

This is a book for adult learners who are seeking careers that require knowledge of and skills that involve medical terminology and medical language. It is written from that pedagogical stance of adult learning theory for which there is a plethora of evidence to suggest that adult learners not only require but demand relevance in their learning materials. This approach also appreciates that adult learners are often working to support themselves and their families and that they have envisioned their learning needs and outcomes before enrolling in a course such as medical terminology. To that end, the author appreciates the need for the relevance and usefulness of time spent in a classroom or a virtual classroom or performing homework or self-study exercises; this appreciation has been incorporated into the design of the materials.

This textbook is suitable for learners who are fluent in English to at least a 10th-grade reading level.

Approach

This is a language book. The text incorporates the development of language-learning skills, which include reading, writing, speaking, and listening. It teaches word recognition, word knowledge (i.e., composition and construction), and word memory. It offers a multitude of opportunities to use new vocabulary in meaningful contexts to promote language acquisition. This is accomplished by developing the ability to communicate with the use of medical terminology in the contexts of health, health-care, and allied health careers.

Pedagogically, *Medical Language: Terminology in Context* takes a lexical approach to language acquisition by developing the learner's proficiency with words, word parts, and word combinations. This is enhanced through the exploration of the target vocabulary that is used in health and allied health care, and it includes the development of structural skills for word, phrase, and sentence composition as well. When new terms are presented, they are defined, described, and then used in a meaningful contextual manner. Lexically based learning activities provide opportunities that facilitate the recognition of how language is used: where, when, and in what context.

Contextual learning (corpus linguistics) supports language acquisition. Vocabulary is presented in real-world contexts through patient updates, discussions, and dialogues. Adult learners can relate to the material as it reflects on their own wealth of experience and knowledge related to both health and illness. The approach teaches through example how language and terminology in context are used across these broad concepts, as well as across the life span. In doing so, it also sheds light on grammatical features that are common in medical language. These include the career-specific use of jargon (institutionalized utterances), acronyms, and so on.

Organization of the Text

This text is based on principles of cumulative learning. Learners are exposed to increasing levels of difficulty; they are asked to critically think about what is learned; to reflect on new knowledge and skills, as well as those from previous learning; and then to apply that information in meaningful ways. In other words, the repetition and recycling of activities help to keep words, expressions, and knowledge related to core topics in health care and medicine *alive* for the learner as they proceed through the book. In turn, this establishes those concepts as part of the learner's developing repertoire.

Units

The book is organized into four units:

- Unit One: Introduction
- Unit Two: The Language of Assessment
- Unit Three: The Language of Treatment
- Unit Four: The Language of Reparative, Restorative, and Rehabilitative Care

Concepts

Four key concepts are used to organize the material in this text, and they are threaded into each chapter:

1. The knowledge of terminology and career-specific language;
2. The knowledge of health, illness, anatomy, physiology, assessment, treatment, and care to develop professional knowledge for the field of work (i.e., health care);

3. The integration of new knowledge into professional communication; and
4. An understanding of patient-centered care.

Chapter format

Each chapter progresses from simple to complex and follows a series of repetitive stages or cycles that reinforce learning. To promote successful language acquisition, each time that new terminology is presented, a series of exercises follow that allow the learner to explore that terminology. These exercises are used to discover how the terms are formed (i.e., their word parts, origins, and meanings), and opportunities are provided to use these new terms in a wide variety of learning activities and exercises.

Components and features

Medical Language: Terminology in Context focuses on building vocabulary for the purpose of communication in health-care and health science settings with professional colleagues, patients, and their families or significant others.

Components that promote learning include the following:

- Exceptional illustrations and diagrams
- Clinical and medical examples that enhance learning
- A variety of exercises that require the immediate use of new terms and knowledge
- Exercises that require critical thinking about words and their contexts
- Exercises that require reflection on what has been presented to draw meaning from it
- Chapter review exercises
- Instructional tables
- Informative tables
- Clinical algorithms and pathways
- Exposure to and practice with a variety of documentation

Features include the following:

- Patient scenarios and updates
- Dialogues
- Career Spotlights
- Right Word or Wrong Word?
- Critical Thinking exercises
- Free Writing exercises
- Memory Magic
- Eponyms
- Focus Points
- Word Building
- Pronunciation Practice

Ancillary Support

Medical Language: Terminology in Context comes with an extensive array of supplementary support for both the student and the instructor. All of the supplementary materials for this text are easily accessed online, and they fit hand in glove with the material in the textbook.

The Medical Language Lab

Included with every new copy of *Medical Language: Terminology in Context* is access to the ultimate online medical terminology resource for students. The Medical Language Lab is a rich learning environment that makes use of proven language development methods to help students become effective users of medical language. To access the Medical Language Lab, students can simply go to http://www.medicallanguagelab.com and register using the personal identification number provided with each new copy of the book.

Each lesson in the Medical Language Lab teaches the student how to critically listen for important terms, how to respond to others with the use of medical terminology, and how to generate his or her own writing and speech that are rich in terminology. By following the activities in each lesson, students graduate from simple memorization to becoming stronger users of medical language.

In addition to critical listening, response, and generation exercises for each lesson, students are supplied with a wide variety of practice activities that will help them to solidify their recall of key terms from the chapter, as well as audio glossary features during which students can hear words pronounced and used properly in context.

Each activity in the Medical Language Lab has been designed to work seamlessly with *Medical Language: Terminology in Context* and crafted with content that is specific to the textbook. Every chapter in *Medical Language: Terminology in Context* has a corresponding lesson in the Medical Language Lab, so students can be confident that every activity in the Medical Language Lab is relevant and useful for helping them to understand the content of the textbook.

Instructors will benefit from a powerful yet easy-to-understand instructor's page that allows them to decide which chapters and activities will be available to their students. Instructors also control how student scores are reported to them: either through the native Medical Language Lab grade book or through their own Blackboard, Angel, Moodle, or SCORM-compliant course management solution.

Davis*Plus* online instructor resources

Instructors can access a wealth of instructional support at the textbook's Davis*Plus* page. These instructional support materials, which are password protected for safety, provide new and experienced instructors with additional resources to help make the teaching of medical terminology easier and more effective. These materials include the following:

- An electronic test bank with ExamView Pro test-generating software
- PowerPoint presentations for each chapter
- A searchable image bank
- A printable Instructor's Guide
- Resources in Blackboard, Angel, Moodle, and SCORM formats

Electronic test bank

This edition offers a powerful ExamView Pro test-generating program that allows you to create custom-made or randomly generated tests in a printable or online format from a test bank of more than 1,200 test items.

PowerPoint presentations

Bring the book to life in the classroom with the accompanying Lecture Note PowerPoint presentations. Each chapter has an outline-based presentation that consists of a chapter overview, the main functions of the body system, and selected pathology, vocabulary, and procedures. Full-color illustrations from the book and in-class assessment activities are included.

Image bank

The image bank contains all of the illustrations from the textbook. It is fully searchable, and it allows users to zoom in and out and to display a JPG image of an illustration that can be copied into a Microsoft Word document or a PowerPoint presentation.

Instructor's Guide

The Instructor's Guide provides instructors with specific guidance regarding how to organize, pace, and succeed in medical terminology instruction using *Medical Language: Terminology in Context.* Specific resources include the following:

- *Sample syllabi.* Suggested syllabi are provided to help instructors plan courses of various lengths with the use of *Medical Language: Terminology in Context.*
- *Student- and instructor-directed activities.* These comprehensive teaching aids offer an assortment of activities for each chapter that addresses a body system. Instructors can use these activities as course requirements or as supplemental material. In addition, they can assign activities as individual or collaborative projects. For group projects, peer evaluation forms are included.

A Message to Students

Medical Language: Terminology in Context has been written with you, the adult learner, in mind.

It is a language book: you will be learning a new language that is an advanced subset of English. To do so, you will follow five patients as they journey through the health-care system after a motor vehicle accident. The text is written in the context of real-world health-care situations to make it easy to relate to and remember. Exercises in each and every chapter have been included so that new material, terminology, and knowledge can be used as soon as possible. This consolidates your learning. The book progresses from simple to complex as it presents information and new vocabulary.

The chapters have been designed to do the following:

- Provide opportunities for reading, writing, listening, and speaking
- Build a vocabulary that includes foundational medical terminology and that expands to include career-specific language
- Provide opportunities for the practical application of new vocabulary, word building, and word-recognition skills
- Build a foundation in medical terminology and language that is readily transferable to other health situations and employment settings
- Introduce different health-care careers

In addition to the material in the book, you will also find the same progressive, context-based approach in the accompanying Medical Language Lab at www.medicallanguagelab.com. In the Medical Language Lab, you will hear the scenarios from the book come to life through a variety of audio-based activities. With the combination of the text and the Medical Language Lab, you will be immersed in the exciting and dynamic world of health care, and you will be able to see the important role that effective medical language plays in patient care.

Consultants

Robin Brou Hatheway, RN, MSN
Nursing Faculty
Southeastern Louisiana University
Baton Rouge, LA

Roberta May Jokanovich, RN, BScN, MPA
Nursing Faculty
Kwantlen Polytechnic University
Surrey, BC, Canada
and
Langara College
Vancouver, BC, Canada

Dr. Laxman Kumar, DDS
Oral and Maxillofacial Surgeon
External Consultant
School of Oral Health Sciences
University of Technology
Kingston, Jamaica

Karen Lund, PhD (Pathology and Lab Med)
Visiting Faculty Chair, Health Sciences
International University of Business, Agriculture and Technology
Dhaka, Bangladesh

Laura Sherret, RN, BSN
Patient Care Coordinator OBS/Maternity
East Kootenay Regional Hospital
Cranbrook, BC, Canada

Reviewers

Susan E. Ault, RN, BSN
Clinical Instructor
Medical Assistant Program
Ross Medical Education Center
Niles, OH

Renee T. Burwell, ASN, BSN, MSEd, EdD
Coordinator of Health Science Programs
Administration Department
Charlotte Technical Center
Port Charlotte, FL

Deresa L. Claybrook, MS, RHIT
President of Positive Resource Health Care Industry Consultants and Adjunct Professor
Oklahoma City Community College
Moore, OK

Donna Crapanzano, MPH, RPAC
Clinical Assistant Professor
Stony Brook University
Stony Brook, NY

Catherine C. Dawson, MPA, OTR/L
Assistant Professor
Allied Health/Occupation Therapy
Tuskegee University
Tuskegee, AL

Heather M. Kies, MHA, PBT(ASCP)
Assistant Professor
Health and Natural Sciences
Medical Assisting Program
Goodwin College
East Hartford, CT

Douglas Kilts, RN, ANP, MBA, MPA, MS, CEN
Assistant Professor
Nursing
Borough of Manhattan Community College
New York, NY

Diana Lee-Greene, RMA(AMT), MT(ASCP), MBA
Medical Assisting Program Faculty, Coordinator
Health Occupations
Columbia Gorge Community College
The Dalles, OR

Candace Newton, PID
Medical Terminology/Medical Assisting and Unit Clerk Instructor
Surrey, BC, Canada

Brigitte Niedzwiecki, RN, MSN
Program Director and Instructor
Medical Assistant Department
Chippewa Valley Technical College
Eau Claire, WI

Martha Olson, RN, BSN, MS
Associate Nursing Professor
Nursing
Iowa Lakes Community College
Emmetsburg, IA

Carmen Price, BS, MS
Manager and Adjunct Instructor
Health Sciences and Public Health
Hennepin Technical College
Brooklyn Park, MN

Maureen C. Schakett, MA, CCC-SLP
Adjunct Professor
Health Professions
Oklahoma City Community College
Nichols Hills, OK

Janice Vermiglio-Smith, RN, MS, PhD
Division Chair
Health Career
Central Arizona College
Apache Junction, AZ

Doris Wagner, PhD
Business Division
Jefferson Community College
Cortland, NY

Acknowledgments

The opportunity to write this book came to me as a very pleasant surprise. I was honored to have been asked to submit a proposal, and I was pleased beyond words to have had that proposal accepted. For this, I am forever grateful to Quincy McDonald, Senior Acquisitions Editor, at F.A. Davis. Quincy and I were a match from the beginning. We are both highly creative, innovative, and forward thinking. I thank him immensely for allowing me creative license in the writing of this text and for sharing my vision of what it could become. I also thank Quincy for his ongoing guidance and support to keep me focused and moving toward the end goal.

I cannot even begin to sufficiently express my gratitude to my Developmental Editor, Vicki Wilt, but I'd like to try. Within a very short time, Vicki and I had a way of working together, as well as a way of sharing, questioning, collaborating, and caring that has been an absolute pleasure. Vicki is a highly skilled and knowledgeable editor and a true professional. I don't know what I would have done without her. For example, in those instances when I got lost in the enormity of the subject matter, Vicki would be able to refocus me, to ask just the right questions, to make just the right corrections, and to get us back on track. Vicki is an excellent teammate, and I am pleased to now have Vicki as my friend as well.

Thanks go out to George Lang, Manager of Content Development at F.A. Davis, for understanding my approach to the subject of medical terminology and for using that to design a textbook full of color, photos, features, and excitement that will entice the reader to move thoughtfully and eagerly from page to page.

I'd also like to acknowledge the skillful work of Stephanie A. Rukowicz, Associate Developmental Editor at F.A. Davis, who has been so helpful with regard to guiding me through the journey of creating audio ancillaries for this book.

A special acknowledgment of thanks is extended to Amy Simpson of Graphic World for her immense patience, guidance and support through the final editing and proofing of this textbook.

Last but certainly not least, I must acknowledge my husband, Steven. Without his love, patience, and absolute faith that I could accomplish this task, the journey to its fruition would have been so much more challenging. In support, Steven did a myriad of lovely things for me during this time. He surprised me with tea or supper (many of each, actually), made sure I wasn't disturbed when immersed in writing, massaged the knots out of my upper back and neck after long periods of typing, and snuck little sweets and snacks into the house for me to *discover* when I finally took a break. These are but a few examples of his care and consideration, and I love him for them and for so many other reasons.

Contents in Brief

Contents

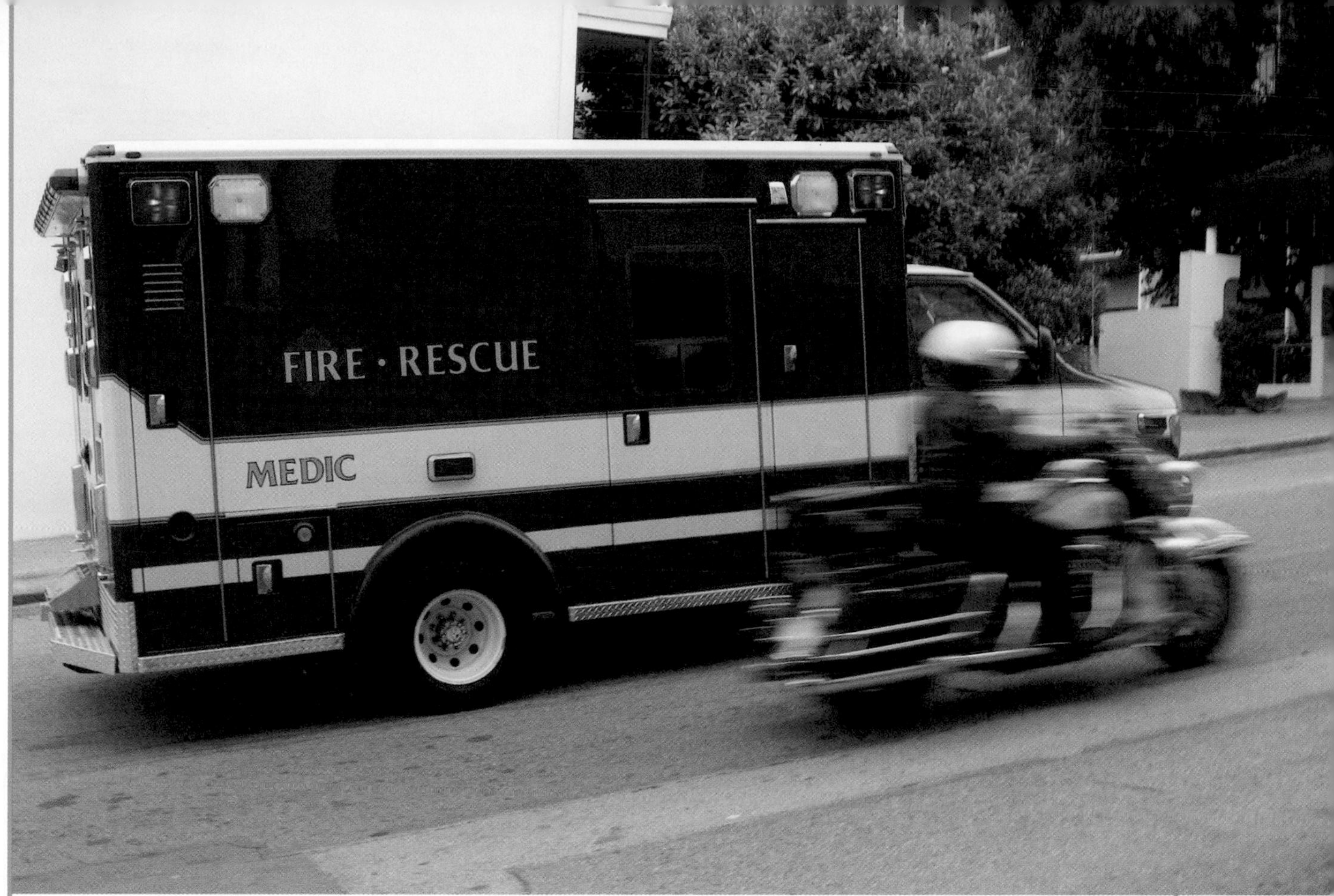

UNIT ONE
Introduction

CHAPTER ONE

Context and Word Structure: The Keys to Learning Language

Focus: Prefixes, Suffixes, Root Words, and Combining Forms

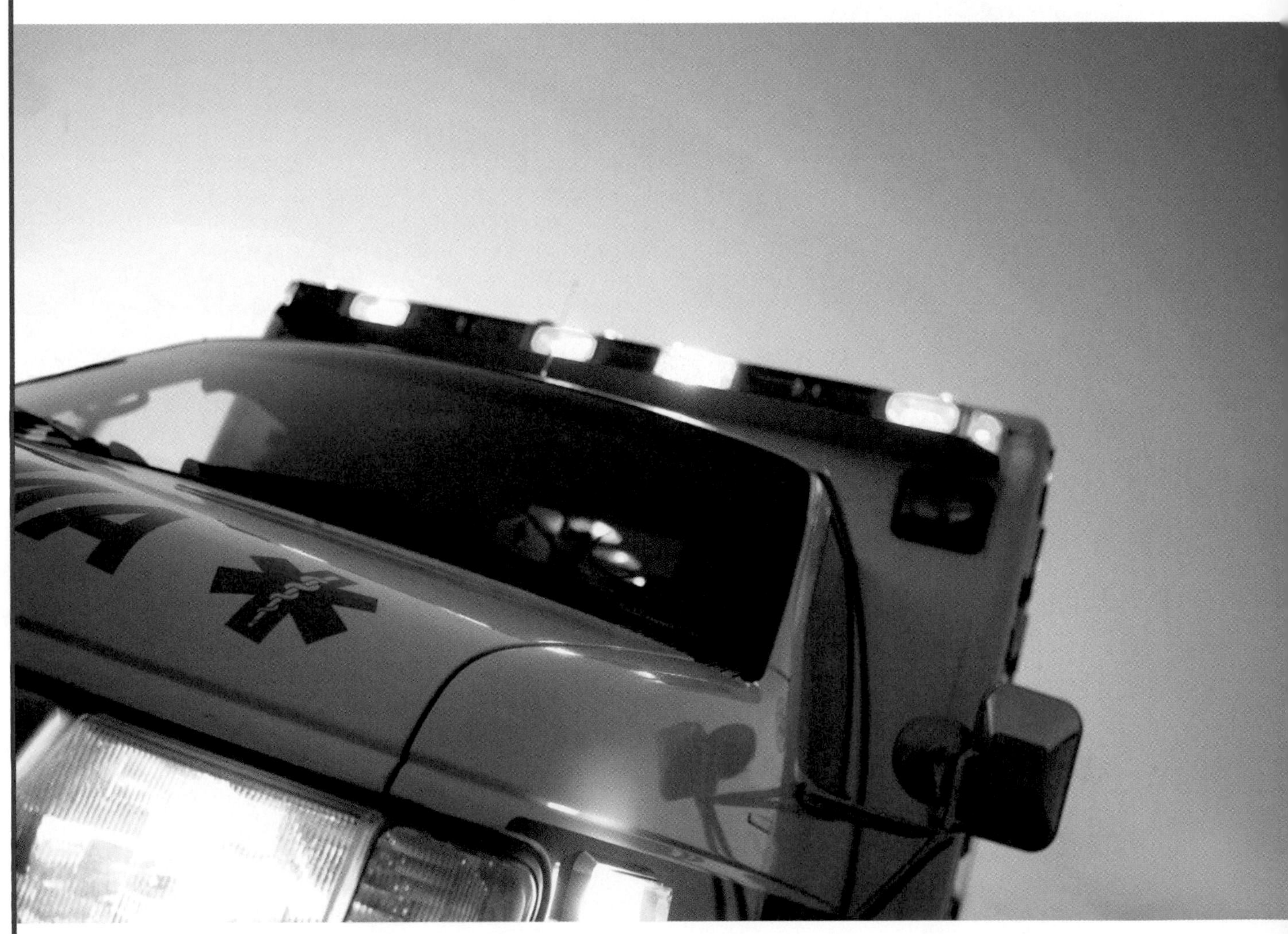

Patient Update

"Rescue 112, what is your 10-20?"

"Rescue 112. Two minutes out."

"Rescue 112. Confirmed. Rescue 155 and 152 on scene. Proceed to white truck, South Sheridan Road, up on curb. Two victims, male and female. Male unconscious. Additional transport en route. Police on scene."

"Confirmed. Rescue 112 out."

"Rescue 112 on scene," reported EMT Stanley into his radio to the Emergency Medical Dispatcher.

"10-4, confirmed. Rescue 112 on scene MVA, intersection of South Sheridan Road and Shawnee Boulevard. Time 11:05. Rescue 121, what is your ETA to the scene?" responds the Emergency Medical Dispatcher.

"Rescue 121 ETA en route; 4 minutes out" came the reply, but it was too late for Stanley and his partner EMT Raybuck to hear, because they were already out of the ambulance. Stanley grabbed the backboard and binders, Raybuck grabbed the emergency kit, and they ran toward the white one-ton truck that had obviously run into a wooden power pole. They scanned the scene. Firefighters and police were on hand, keeping bystanders away. No power lines were down, but they'd heard Dispatch say that city workers were en route to secure the power pole, which was leaning slightly at an angle. Rescue Units 155 and 152 were attending to the victims of the second vehicle involved in the crash, which was on the other side of the intersection.

A police officer joined Stanley and Raybuck as they ran to assist the injured individuals. She updated them on the situation. "Two victims here. Male, unconscious, nonresponsive, and still in the vehicle. Didn't want to move him till you got here. Looks like multiple fractures. Bleeding from the face. Female outside of vehicle, apparently the passenger. Officer with her. Witnesses say she got out of the truck by herself and then passed out. She's alert now. Pregnant. Maybe her water broke. Bleeding from her leg. We've got three victims in the car on the other side of the intersection. We've got EMT and officers there, waiting for the next bus to arrive for transport."

"Raybuck, check the female," directed Stanley as he headed for the truck, where another police officer was attending.

As Stanley and the police officer approached the male victim, the officer said, "Unresponsive. Probably out for at least 10 minutes now. Wife says his name is Gil, Gil Loeppky."* While he listened to the officer, Stanley began trauma assessment, starting with the ABCs. He moved on to neuro, speaking aloud as he did so, "pupils sluggish but reactive" he noted and then continued the assessment. "Raybuck, status report," he called.

"Alert. Oriented. Deep laceration; bleeding controlled. Possible fracture to hand. May be going into labor. I've called for transport to General," Raybuck replied.

"I need you here, then," said Stanley. "Bring the board. Get the stretcher, STAT. Officer, give us a hand. Let's get a collar on him first, then get him out of the vehicle." In the background, they heard sirens and knew that ambulances had arrived. "This guy's going to Trauma. Can't be sure if he's spinal or neuro. Resps and rates are okay. Facial hematoma. Maybe hit the windshield and dashboard. Hope that's it. Watch the back when we move him. Raybuck, we'll need the binders."

Moving quickly, Raybuck had arrived back with the stretcher, and he placed the backboard on top. "New crew here. Taking care of the woman now. I filled them in on the run," he reported to Stanley. "They're heading out now." He turned his concentration to the patient at hand.

The patient suddenly groaned loudly as they began to move him. "Fractured femur," Stanley observed aloud, as they laid the patient carefully on the stretcher. While Stanley ran another quick neurological and vital sign assessment, his partner completed the head-to-toe review. "Still out. Responsive to pain," commented Stanley.

"No evidence of internal injury," Raybuck reported. "Let's get the head block in place and get him in the bus; get a line started to KVO. O_2, also. You want to splint that femur?" His partner shook his head "no."

*Pronounced *lep-key*.

Stanley reached for his radio. "Dispatch, we're stabilizing and en route to Trauma. Please notify. Possible head injury in an unconscious male patient, vitals okay, fractured femur; facial laceration and hematoma," he reported.

"Dispatch. Confirmed. Rescue 112 en route to Trauma Center, ETA 15 minutes. Will notify of incoming."

"10-4, Dispatch, we'll take it from here. Out," concluded Stanley.

Reflective Questions

Reflect on the story that you've just read.

1. Did you understand all of the medical terms and jargon involved?

   ____

2. Did you understand the medical abbreviations that were used to identify personnel?

   ____

3. Were you able to understand some unfamiliar terms simply by reading them in the context of the sentence, paragraph, or story? Which ones?

   ____

For audio exercises, visit **http://www.MedicalLanguageLab.com.** 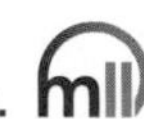

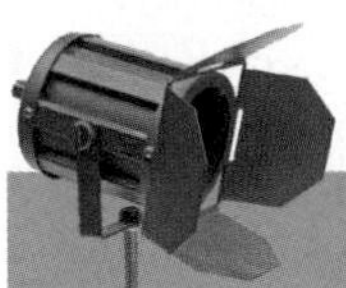

CAREER SPOTLIGHT: Emergency Medical Dispatch

The *emergency medical dispatcher* (EMD) is often referred to simply as "Dispatch" by emergency service personnel. As a professional telecommunicator, the EMD is responsible for answering emergency telephone calls from the public, ascertaining the needs of these individuals, determining the severity of the situation, providing assistance or instructions to callers over the phone, and then assigning and dispatching the appropriate emergency service personnel to respond to the emergency. The EMD continues his or her involvement in the emergency until emergency medical services personnel arrive on the scene and the EMD's services are no longer needed. In some situations, the EMD coordinates the transfer of patients to the hospital and dialogues with the receiving facility until the patient arrives.

Introduction

As you were reading the scenario that opened this chapter, you likely encountered a lot of unfamiliar words. However, you probably got a fairly good idea of what the emergency personnel were talking about by paying attention to the **context**, which is given by the clues in the story. Learning in context is the natural way of learning language. When you were a child, you learned new words by noticing how the people around you used those words in their speech and writing. Learning words in context also helped you to remember the words later and to apply them in similar situations.

In this book, you will learn medical language in context as you follow the stories of five patients who have been injured in a traffic accident. As the patients progress through the stages of diagnosis, treatment, and rehabilitation, you will learn the terminology and other special language used by medical professionals at each stage.

Before you get started, it will help to learn or review a few things about how words in general—and medical terminology in particular—are built from roots, prefixes, and suffixes.

Learning Objectives

After reading Chapter 1, you will be able to do the following:

- Recognize word parts in standard medical terms derived from early Greek and Latin.
- Identify word parts: roots, prefixes, suffixes, and combining vowels.
- Analyze words by dividing them into their basic word parts.
- Determine word meanings by constructing and deconstructing the words' component parts.

What Is Medical Terminology?

Medical terminology includes all of the specialized vocabulary that medical professionals use to identify human anatomy (structures) and physiology (functions), as well as words that indicate location, direction, planes of the body, medical status, and instructions for administering medication.

Medical terminology also includes *eponyms,* which will be important to learn in the health-care field. An eponym is a word that is created from the name of a person. A medical eponym is created by naming a disease, a test, or another facet of medicine for the person who discovered it, suffered from it, or in some other way contributed to it by way of a legacy. Although it is impossible to learn all medical eponyms from just one book, examples of some of the more common ones will appear throughout this text.

Eponyms:

Lou Gehrig's disease was named for a famous American baseball player of the 1920s and 1930s. He acquired and subsequently died of the disease amyotrophic lateral sclerosis (ALS). Gehrig's struggles with the disease and the positive attention that he brought to the importance of research and treatment led many people to refer to amyotrophic lateral sclerosis (ALS) as *Lou Gehrig's disease.*

Alzheimer's disease was named for Alois Alzheimer, a German psychiatrist and neurologist who identified this degenerative, terminal disease of the brain around the turn of the 20th century. This disease is part of the family of dementias, and it has retained Dr. Alzheimer's name to honor his contributions to science and medicine in its regard.

Salmonella was named after the veterinarian Dr. D. E. Salmon. Although salmonella is commonly known as an illness, it more accurately describes a genus of bacteria. During the early 20th century, Dr. Salmon's assistant discovered the genus, but it was named in honor of the doctor.

Etymology: The Origins of Medical Terminology

The history of a word is called its *etymology.* Medical terms generally derive from the early Greek and Latin languages. They include word parts that are well recognized in health care in large parts of the world, particularly in countries or among people whose own languages had similar origins or were at one time (many hundreds of years ago) part of the Greek or Roman empires. For example, these types of medical words appear in the English, French, Spanish, Portuguese, and German languages. The countries in which these languages are spoken, in turn, influenced the languages of other nations when they, too, went through an age of empire; that's why you may very well hear a medical term that you recognize spoken in the Bangla language of Bangladesh or in Swahili in certain parts of Africa. To illustrate the long and rich history of the development of medical terminology, in this book, you will find references to the original meanings of many medical word parts. It is hoped that you will find this information interesting and relevant to your studies.

Take a look at Table 1-1 to see how influential the early Greek and Latin languages have been on the languages of the world.

TABLE 1-1: Common Word Parts Derived from Greek and Latin

Word Part	Origin	Examples
hyper- A prefix meaning *over, above,* or *excessive*	From the Greek word *hyper*	hyperactive (English) hyperactive (French) hiperaktif (Turkish) hyperacteif (Dutch)
hydro- A prefix meaning *water*	From the Greek word *hydor*	hydraulic (English) hydraulisk (Danish) hidraulico (Spanish) hidrolik (Turkish)
-ology A suffix meaning *study*	From the Greek suffix *-ology*	biology (English) biológiában (Hungarian) biologia (Italian) bioloģija (Latvian)
contra- A prefix meaning *opposite* or *against*	From the Latin prefix *contra-*	contraindicated (English) contraindicat (Catalan) kontraindikováno (Czech) kontraindikasi (Indonesian)
semi- A prefix meaning *half*	From the Latin prefix *semi-*	semicircle (English) semicircle (Icelandic) semicerchio (Italian) semicírculo (Portuguese)

How Is Medical Terminology Constructed?

Medical terminology is constructed systematically. These terms are often a combination of prefixes (at the beginning of words), roots (generally in the middle of words), and suffixes (at the end of words). Although not all medical terms are the result of combining Latin or Greek word parts, many are. Learning these word parts and acquiring the ability to combine them in meaningful ways will help you to recognize and understand new combinations when you encounter them in the workplace. You will be able to work through unfamiliar terms by analyzing their parts.

Let's begin. For now, don't worry about remembering all of the material presented in the following readings and exercises. This medical language will reappear and be reinforced for you throughout the rest of this book. What is important here is that you become familiar with the components of medical words and appreciate how these parts can be combined. First, let's review how words are generally constructed in English.

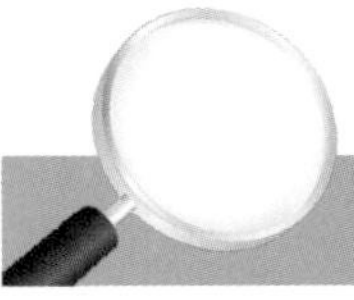

FOCUS POINT: Labeling Word Parts

Not all medical dictionaries or medical terminology reference books are the same when it comes to labeling word parts as roots, prefixes, and suffixes. These differences in labeling word parts will not affect your ability to succeed with medical terminology as it is taught in this book. Remember that your goal is to recognize the words, learn their meanings, and use the terminology correctly. Labeling word parts as roots, prefixes, and suffixes is not a priority.

Root words

A **root word** contains the core meaning of a word. It is the word's foundation. You can form new words from this foundation by adding a prefix, a suffix, or another root word. Root words are also called *word stems* or *root elements.*

How can you recognize a root word?

Root words are word parts that can stand alone as words on their own. You can expand a root word and change its meaning by adding a prefix before the word or a suffix after the word. For example, you can expand the root word *part* to form *partial, impartial, partially, partly, depart,* and *parted.*

Free Writing

Answer the following questions without looking at the Answer Key first.

Consider the word *houseboat.*

1. What root word(s) do you see in this word? ______________________
2. Can you expand the word *house* without combining it with another word? If so, write the new words here. ______________________
3. Can you expand the word *boat* without combining it with another word? If so, do so now. ______________________
4. Review what you have just written. Was your answer to question 1 correct, or have you changed your mind? ______________________
5. Think about what you have just learned. Explain it in your own words. ______________________

Refer to Table 1-2 for examples of common root words that can be combined with other word parts.

Master roots

Master roots cannot stand alone as words in English, but they still form the foundation, or basic meaning, of a larger word. Master roots are generally—but not always—found in the middle of a word. See Table 1-3 for some examples.

Medical roots

In medical terminology, too, root words and master roots are most often—but not always—found in the middle of a word, and they usually identify a body part or an action. Recognizing the root of a medical term takes practice.

Table 1-4 introduces you to some common medical roots. Read them, and study their meanings. You don't need to memorize them at the moment. Again, the goal right now is only to familiarize yourself with these word parts. You will have many opportunities to see them again in upcoming exercises and to work with them in subsequent chapters. Consider this an introduction.

TABLE 1-2: Expanding Root Words to Form New Words

Root Word	Add Another Root or a Prefix or Suffix	New Word
tail	bone (root word)	tailbone (compound word consisting of two root words)
hand	-ful (suffix)	handful
appear	dis- (prefix)	disappear

TABLE 1-3: Words Formed from Master Roots

Master Root	Words Formed from Root	Master Root	Words Formed from Root
nat (meaning *to be born*)	un**nat**ural super**nat**ural **nat**ive **nat**ionality	aud (meaning *to hear*)	**aud**ible **aud**iotape **aud**itorium
cept (meaning *to hold or to take*)	ac**cept** con**cept** con**cept**ion inter**cept** inter**cept**ion	man/manu (meaning *hand or by hand*)	**manu**facture **manu**al **manu**script **man**ipulate **man**icure
cog (meaning *to think*)	re**cog**nize **cog**nizant		

TABLE 1-4: Common Medical Roots

Medical Root	Meaning	Medical Root	Meaning
aud(i)	hear	hepat(o)	liver
auto	self	man/u	manual
bio	life	meter	measure
card(i, io)	heart	myo	muscle
cerebr(o)	brain	neuro	nerves
contra	against	nephro	kidneys
cyst(o)	cell	orbi(t, to)	circular or around the eye
dors(a, o)	back	ology*	the study of
derm(a, o)	skin	oste(o)	bones
duct	lead	ped(i, o)	child
encephal(o)	brain	pneumo	lungs
enter(o)	intestine	script	write
esophag(o)	throat, gullet	sphere	ball
fract	break	thyr/o	thyroid
gastr(i, o)	stomach	ur(o)	urinary
glyco	sugar	vac	empty
graph	write, record	ven(i, o)	blood, veins
hem(o, ato)	blood		

*This root is sometimes labeled as a suffix in other books. What is most important to you, the learner, is to know what the word part means.

Let's Practice

Refer to Table 1-4 to complete this exercise.

Read the following statements made by health-care providers.

Next, identify words in each statement that contain one or more medical roots. Write each root and its meaning.

Finally, check your answers with your instructor or by using the Answer Key. (See pages 875-972.)

1. Nurse Roberta: "Mr. Johnson was admitted last night with pneumonia. He's on antibiotics by intravenous."

   ____

2. Doctor Major: "We're looking at an esophageal hemorrhage."

   ____

3. EMT Stanley: "We're incoming with possible multiple fractures, particularly in the orbitonasal and femoral areas."

   ____

4. Medical Intern Marilyn: "I believe the patient is experiencing a myocardial infarction, Doctor." ____________________

5. Pharmacy Technician Sergio: "You are quite right, nurse. That medication is contraindicated with the meds that your patient is currently on and could contribute to nephrotic difficulties."

   ____

There are many more medical roots than you've just seen in Table 1-4, and it is impossible to remember all of them. What might help you learn them, however, is to put them in groups that have some relevance to your health-care career. For example, you might find that learning medical root words can best be managed by placing them in categories such as body systems, body parts, or career-specific terms. As you work through this textbook, you will be exposed to more and more medical roots by virture of the patient-care scenarios. As you encounter these new roots, you can make your own reference tables. The following tables demonstrate different ways that you might organize these terms as you learn them.

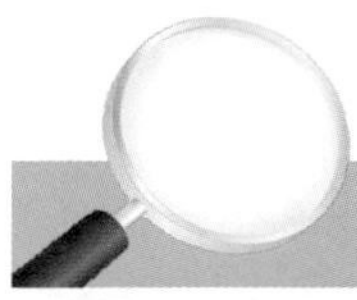

FOCUS POINT: Terminology in Context

As you work through this book, new medical terms will be frequently introduced in a health-care context. You will be taught medical roots and their combined forms through the language of body systems as they apply to ongoing case studies. (Please remember that the learning of anatomy and physiology is not the goal of this text.)

Break It Down

Now that we've explored root words and medical roots, try to find the roots in the following words that are used in health care. You might do this alone or in a classroom setting with your peers. When you finish, check your answers against the Answer Key.

TABLE 1-5: Medical Roots Organized by Body Systems

Body System	Medical Roots	Body System	Medical Roots
Circulatory	card(i, io) hem(o, ato)	Nervous	neuro encephalo cerebr
Respiratory	pneumo pleuro		
Digestive	gastr/i, o	Urinary	ur nephro ren/o
Reproductive	gynec		
Muscular	myo	Integumentary	cyt(o) derm(a, o)
Skeletal	oste/o arthr	Endocrine	adreno

TABLE 1-6: Medical Roots Organized by Body Parts

Body Part	Medical Root	Body Part	Medical Root
Head	cran	Kidney	nephro
Heart	cardio	Stomach	gastr
Lung	pneumo	Liver	hep
Intestine	ileu		

TABLE 1-7: Medical Roots Organized by Career Focus

Career	Roots
Radiology	oste(o), pneumo, arthr, dors(a,o), fract, graph
Laboratory Sciences	cyst(o), ren/o, hem(o, ato)

Circle each root word or medical root in the italicized words. (Be careful. You will see some compound words made up of two root words that have been combined.)

1. Mr. Loeppky was in a car accident. Although he is unconscious, he indicates that there is pain in his *thighbone* by moaning when it is moved.
2. Bob broke his *collarbone* in a car accident.
3. Little Chantal *fractured* her wrist.
4. Franklin has pains in his stomach that won't go away. He is likely suffering from *gastritis.*
5. Mrs. Watson has *pneumonia* and is having trouble breathing.

Combining vowels

Combining vowels are often needed to connect a medical root with a prefix or suffix to form a medical term. Because of their importance, whenever you see a list of medical roots, you will also see one or two vowels listed after each root. These combining vowels usually follow a slash mark (/) or appear in parentheses like this: (o) .

Inserting a vowel makes the pronunciation of medical terms easier when the root ends in a consonant. For example, a record of the electrical activity of the brain is called an *electroencephalogram.* The components of this word are *electr + o + encephal + o + gram.*

Combining forms of medical words

The combination of a medical root and a vowel produces a **combining form**. Although the combining vowel is usually an *o,* it may be any vowel. See the Word Building Formula for examples.

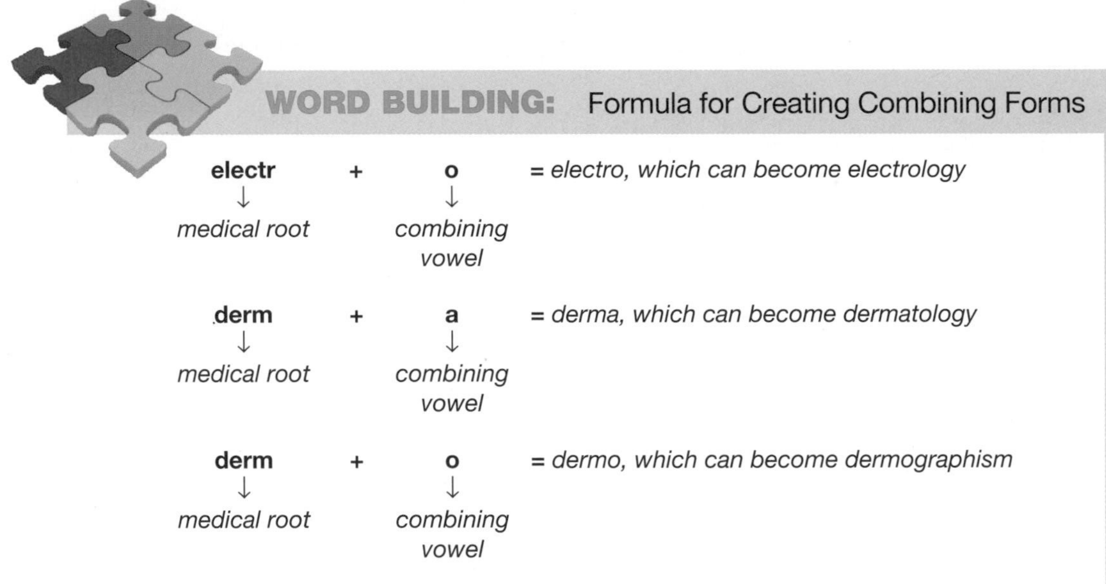

As you can see from the Word Building examples, the concept of creating combining forms applies to medical roots derived from Greek or Latin. This does not necessarily apply, however, to other words in medical language. For example, many English medical words are combined without the use of a combining vowel: *collarbone, backbone,* and *stomachache.*

Let's Practice

Identify the combining vowel in the italicized medical term, and then write it in the blank space provided. Try to do this exercise alone. Complete it and review it before checking your answers with your instructor or the Answer Key.

1. Mrs. Watson has *pneumonia* and is having trouble breathing. ____________
2. Henry has *hemophilia.* ____________
3. Mr. Blakemore has to see the *urologist.* ____________

4. Mrs. Blakemore has severe eczema and wants to see a *dermatologist.* ___________________

5. Kenny has an *auditory* impairment. ___________________

Prefixes

Prefixes are descriptive, and they expand the meaning of a root word. They sit at the beginning of words. Although they cannot generally stand alone as a complete word, they do have meaning.

How can you recognize a prefix?

A **prefix** is a word part; it is made up of a syllable or syllables that appear at the beginning of many words. Prefixes can be grouped according to their descriptive function.

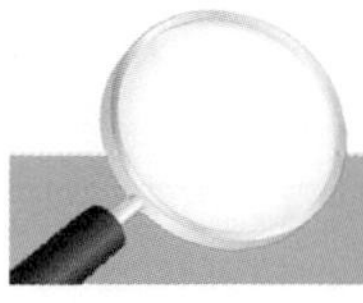

FOCUS POINT: The Disappearing Hyphen

Notice that a hyphen is shown at the end of each prefix in this book. This hyphen alerts you to the fact that prefixes appear at the beginning of a word. However, when the full word is written, the hyphen usually disappears. There is no set rule for when to include a hyphen in a word with a prefix. You will learn individual examples as you proceed through this book.

Common prefixes

A quick review of some common prefixes will help you to recall them. Take a look at Table 1-8.

Medical prefixes

In medical terms, prefixes generally alert you to size, shape, color, or status. They prepare the reader for the rest of the word by describing something about it. Tables 1-9 through 1-15 illustrate the common functions of medical prefixes. For example, prefixes that refer to color appear in Table 1-9, and those that refer to time appear in Table 1-15. In Chapter 2 and throughout the rest of this book, you will learn even more medical prefixes.

TABLE 1-8: Common Prefixes

Prefix	Meaning	Medical Examples	Prefix	Meaning	Medical Examples
anti-	against	antidepressant	over-	above or excessive	overweight
auto-	self	automatic	pre-	before	premarital
co-	with	cooperate	re-	again or back	reconstruct
dis-	not, the opposite of	disregard	semi-	partial or half	semisoft
ex-	out of, former	exfoliate	sub-	under	sublingual
im-	not	immobile	un-	not	unusual
inter-	between	interdisciplinary	under-	under or beneath the surface	underbelly
mid-	middle	midway	uni-	one	unipolar
mis-	wrongly	misinterpret			
non-	not	noncompliant			

TABLE 1-9: Medical Prefixes That Describe Color

Prefix	Meaning	Prefix	Meaning
chlor/chloro-	green	rub/e/o-	red,
cyano-	blue	rubr-	blood red
leuco/leuko-	white	sang/ui-	

TABLE 1-10: Medical Prefixes That Describe Size

Prefix	Meaning	Prefix	Meaning
macr/o-	long or large	micr/o-	small

TABLE 1-11: Medical Prefixes That Describe Amount and Quantity

Prefix	Meaning	Prefix	Meaning
demi- hemi- semi-	one half	multi- poly-	many
equi-	equal, same		

TABLE 1-12: Medical Prefixes That Describe Direction, Place, or Location

Prefix	Meaning	Prefix	Meaning
ab/s-	away from	in-	not, in
ex-	out, off, without; outside of	intra-	within
e-	out of, out from		

TABLE 1-13: Medical Prefixes That Describe Relationships

Prefix	Meaning	Prefix	Meaning
anti- contra-	opposing, against	sym- syn- zyg/o/us-	joined, together, with, alongside
circum- peri-	surrounding, around	trans-	across, through, over
epi-	on, upon, in addition		

TABLE 1-14: Medical Prefixes That Describe Function or Characteristics

Prefix	Meaning	Prefix	Meaning
a-	lacking, without, negation	heter/o-	different, other
an-		hom/eo/o-	alike, same, unchanged
aer/i/o-	air	hyper-	above, extreme, excessive
ambul-	walk	hypo-	under, decreased, below

TABLE 1-15: Medical Prefixes That Refer to Time

Prefix	Meaning	Prefix	Meaning
ante-	before, prior	pre-	ahead of, before, anterior
arch/e/i-	original, first, beginning	primi-	first
noct/i/o-	night	tard-	late, tardy, slow
post- postero-	after	terti-	third

Break It Down

Read each sentence. Write the prefix found in each italicized word, and then write the meaning of that prefix. Work alone or with another student. The answers can be found in the Answer Key when you have completed the exercise.

1. Jamison fractured his clavicle (collarbone) and finds it very difficult to *abduct* his right arm.
   Prefix: ____________________ Meaning: ____________________
2. At the hospital, Mr. Loeppky will require a *preliminary* consult with a radiologist before his physician can make a diagnosis related to his head injury.
   Prefix: ____________________ Meaning: ____________________
3. The patient has had surgery. The dressing covering the wound appears *sanguineous*.
   Prefix: ____________________ Meaning: ____________________
4. Adolescents have a tendency to be *nocturnal*. They rarely go to bed early.
   Prefix: ____________________ Meaning: ____________________
5. The baby was born *prematurely*.
   Prefix: ____________________ Meaning: ____________________
6. When deprived of sufficient oxygen, *cyanosis* is easily seen on a person's lips.
   Prefix: ____________________ Meaning: ____________________
7. *Microbiologists* study tiny organisms that are invisible to the naked eye.
   Prefix: ____________________ Meaning: ____________________

Prefixes change the meaning

Prefixes can change the meaning of a word in important ways. In the study of medical language, it is *extremely* important to understand this so that you use prefixes accurately in your communication as a medical professional. Using the correct prefix is sometimes literally a matter of life and death for your patient. See Table 1-16 for examples of how significantly a prefix can change the meaning of a medical term.

TABLE 1-16: How Prefixes Change Word Meanings

BEGIN with a Prefix	ADD a Root Word	COMBINE to Create a New Word
im- (not)	balance (stable, healthy relationship among contrasting or interacting forces)	imbalance (relationship that is not stable or healthy)
in- (not)	visible (can be seen) operable (surgery can be performed)	invisible (cannot be seen) inoperable (surgery cannot be performed)
ab- (away from or removed from)	normal (usual, routine or healthy)	abnormal (away from or not the usual, not routine or not healthy)
dis- (to separate or take apart)	orientation (person's awareness of where he or she is in time and space)	disorientation (person's lack of awareness of where he or she is in time and space)
ir- (not)	regular	irregular (not regular [i.e., an irregular heartbeat])
micro- (small, very small)	biology (the study of all life and living things)	microbiology (the study of the smallest elements of life)
dys- (painful or difficult)	urea (urine)	dysuria (painful urination or difficulty voiding urine)

Build a Word

Review Tables 1-8 through 1-16, and then read the following sentences. A prefix is missing from a medical term in each sentence. Consider the context or overall meaning of the sentence, and then fill in the blank with the correct prefix.

1. When the fire alarm rings, you must _________ vacuate all of the patients from the building.
2. Mr. Williams suffers from _________ glycemia. Sometimes his blood sugar levels are too low.
3. The paramedic started an _________ venous on his patient while en route to the emergency department.
4. Mr. Robinson is _________ ventilating. He can't catch his breath.
5. The new patient is a 35-year-old _________ sexual male with a wife and two children.
6. The lab reports an abnormal finding in her _________ cyte count. The number of white blood cells is reportedly lower than normal.
7. Frances has an _________ dermal rash. It's quite visible.
8. Many parasites have _________ biotic relationships with their hosts. They live in close proximity to each other and often interact.

Mix and Match: Prefixes

Combine each prefix in the left column with a term in the right column to form a new word. Write the new words below, and then explain the meaning of each new term in your own words.

	PREFIX	TERM
1.	hyper-	typical
2.	pre-	glycemia
3.	a-	operative
4.	poly-	jointed
5.	micro-	conscious
6.	dis-	organism
7.	semi-	partum
8.	post-	uria

1. Word: ______________________________
   Meaning: ______________________________
2. Word: ______________________________
   Meaning: ______________________________
3. Word: ______________________________
   Meaning: ______________________________
4. Word: ______________________________
   Meaning: ______________________________
5. Word: ______________________________
   Meaning: ______________________________
6. Word: ______________________________
   Meaning: ______________________________
7. Word: ______________________________
   Meaning: ______________________________
8. Word: ______________________________
   Meaning: ______________________________

Antonyms

Do you recall learning about antonyms when you were in grade school? **Antonyms** are words that are opposite in meaning, such as *good* and *bad* or *happy* and *sad.* Many antonyms are created by adding a prefix to a root word.

Common antonyms

In the context of medicine, let's review some of the more common antonyms that you will come across. Complete the following exercise to test your recall of these common words.

Fill In the Blanks

Fill in the blank with the most accurate antonym that you can think of. Try to work on your own.

1. Mr. Loeppky isn't conscious; he's ______________________________.
2. Darlene is sighted, but Darren is ______________________________.
3. Erin is mobile, but Eric is ______________________________.
4. Frances is well, but Frank is ______________________________.
5. Gary has a limp handshake, while Greg's is ______________________________.
6. Henri's bandages are tight, but Hank's are ______________________________.
7. Ilona clenches her jaw when she is nervous, but Ian's jaw remains ______________.
8. Jake has a muscle contraction in his right hand from an old injury, but Jane has full muscle ______________________________.
9. Kevin says his kids bring him joy most of the time, but sometimes they bring him ______________________________.
10. Dr. Levine begins the surgery by opening the abdominal cavity and ends it by ______________________________ the cavity.

Medical antonyms

You have already learned some prefixes that mean *not* or *the opposite of.* You can add one of these prefixes to a medical term to create a term with the opposite meaning. Negative prefixes alter the meaning of a term to change the word from positive to negative, to indicate that something that was present is now absent, or to change the location of something.

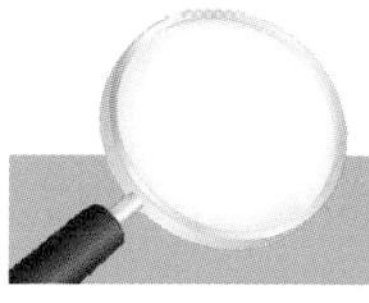

FOCUS POINT: *In-* or *Im-*?

Change the prefix *in-* to *im-* before words that begin with the letters *b, m,* or *p.*

Build a Word

Add a negative prefix to each italicized word to create a word with the opposite meaning. Use the choices provided.

a- anti- dis- in- im- mis- non- un-

1. Marnie is *mobile* and able to walk for miles and miles without rest.
   Mr. Loeppky is ________________ and unable to walk.
2. Nathan doesn't believe that all *bacterial* cells are harmful.
   Norm does believe this and thus uses ________________ soap.
3. Olga's behavior is *typical* of a 2-year-old.
   Orem's behavior is ________________ of a 10-year-old.

4. Pablo is calm now because he is *medicated.*
   Pat is agitated because he is still ________________.
5. Queenie says that she has a glass of wine every day for *medicinal* purposes.
   Quentin says wine is ________________.
6. Rupert has no difficulty with his *equilibrium.*
   Rae suffers from ________________.
7. Samantha is *able* to feed and dress herself without assistance from care staff.
   Sam is ________________ to do so.
8. Trent was able to *mobilize* his left ankle with the help of early intervention from a physiotherapist.
   In preparation for knee surgery, Taylor was advised that the surgeon would ________________ his knee to restrict all movement for a period of 1 week.
9. Ulysses is *compliant* with taking his medications as prescribed.
   Uriah doesn't like the side effects of his medications and is ________________ with regard to taking them.
10. Veronica *diagnosed* her patient with Parkinson's disease.
    Vangeline ________________ her patient with the same illness.

Read Aloud

Go back over the exercise that you've just completed. Try to say the words you've written out loud; this can help you to decide if the antonyms you've written *sound* correct. Check your answers with the Answer Key.

Let's Practice

Continue working with antonyms. In this exercise, turn a negative into a positive by removing the prefix from the word in italicized type. Write the new word in the blank.

1. An *imbalance* in electrolytes in the body can lead to a sense of confusion, cramps, and dizziness.
   A ________________ between oxygen, nitrogen, and carbon dioxide is necessary to sustain life.
2. An *incomplete* fracture of a bone is called a *stress fracture.* The entire bone is not broken.
   A ________________ fracture is one in which the bone is broken into two or more pieces.
3. The tumor is malignant, metastasized, and therefore *inoperable.*
   The surgeons will explore the abdomen before deciding whether the tumor is ________________.
4. The surgeons decided that the bullet is *nonresectable* at this time. They cannot remove it.
   The foreign body found in the patient's abdomen is ________________.
5. Dr. Blavenstock was able to *dislodge* the pea in young Jimmy's nose.
   The patient presented in the Emergency department with a fish bone ________________ in his esophagus.

Suffixes

Suffixes are word parts that are added to the end of a root word to change its meaning or its part of speech. The English word *suffix* is derived from a Latin word that means *to attach one thing to the end or below another thing.*

How can you recognize a suffix?

A **suffix** is added to the end of a word. To determine where the suffix begins, try to find the root first. Suffixes appear frequently in our daily communication, and you very likely studied them in grade school. Common suffixes are widely used in medical language, too.

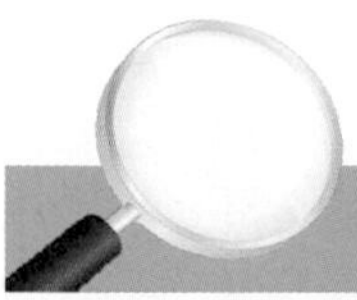

FOCUS POINT: Suffixes with Hyphens

When you see suffixes listed in tables, notice that they appear with a hyphen before them. This is just a quick signal to alert you that a suffix is added to the end of a word. When the full word is written, the hyphen will almost always disappear.

Common suffixes

Take some time now to refresh your memory regarding common suffixes and their meanings. Table 1-17 identifies some of the most common suffixes and applies them to parts of speech (verbs, adverbs, adjectives, and nouns). Notice that the examples in the table can all be applied in medical contexts.

TABLE 1-17: Suffixes for Different Parts of Speech

Suffixes for Verbs	Meaning or Function [used to show tense or to form verbs]	Examples
-ed	past tense	dilat**ed**, examin**ed**
-fy -ify	forms a verb meaning *to make or to cause to become*	pur**ify**, humid**ify**, lique**fy**
-ing	present participle of a verb; happening now	bleed**ing**, sneez**ing**
Suffixes for Adverbs	**Meaning or Function: (added to adjectives to form adverbs (words that modify verbs)**	**Examples**
-ly	describing how something occurs	competent**ly**, surgical**ly**
Suffixes for Adjectives	**Meaning or Function: added to nouns or verbs to form adjectives (words that describe nouns)**	**Examples**
-able -ible	describes a capacity: what can be done or accomplished	cap**able**, endur**able**
-al -ial	refers to a characteristic	person**al**, famil**ial**
-ic	having a characteristic or property of	asthmat**ic**, psychiatr**ic**
-en	made of; consisting of	rott**en**, silk**en**, wood**en**
-ful	full of, able to be	harm**ful**, pain**ful**, use**ful**
-t/ive	having the nature or tendency of	pallia**tive**, talka**tive**
-y	having the quality of, apt or inclined to	risk**y**, blood**y**, runn**y**, wheez**y**
-less	without	child**less**, home**less**
-ous	having the quality of	bulb**ous**, nause**ous**
Suffixes for Superlatives	**Meaning or Function: changes an adjective or adverb to show rank**	**Examples**
-er	compares two persons or things	great**er**, long**er**
-est	compares three or more persons or things	sick**est**, weak**est**

Continued

TABLE 1-17: Suffixes for Different Parts of Speech—cont'd

Suffixes for Nouns	Meaning or Function: form plurals or amounts; added to verbs and adjectives to form nouns	Examples
-s -es	more than one	infant**s**, gas**es**
-er	the person who is doing something	examin**er**, practition**er**
-ful	identifies an amount	cup**ful**, teaspoon**ful**
-i/ty	identifies a quality or condition	san**ity**, fragil**ity**
-ment	the end result of an action	excre**ment**, induce**ment**
-t/ion	the state resulting from an action	dila**tion**, muta**tion**
-ness	the state of or condition of	full**ness**, empti**ness**
-y	identifies an action or result	surger**y**, remed**y**

Medical suffixes

A suffix is added to a medical root or a combining form to modify its meaning and to change its part of speech. Suffixes can begin with consonants or vowels. Follow these rules when adding a suffix to a medical root or a combining form:

- When the suffix begins with a *consonant* and the root has a combining vowel, simply add the suffix.
- When the suffix begins with a *vowel* and the root has a combining vowel, drop the combining vowel of the root before adding the suffix.

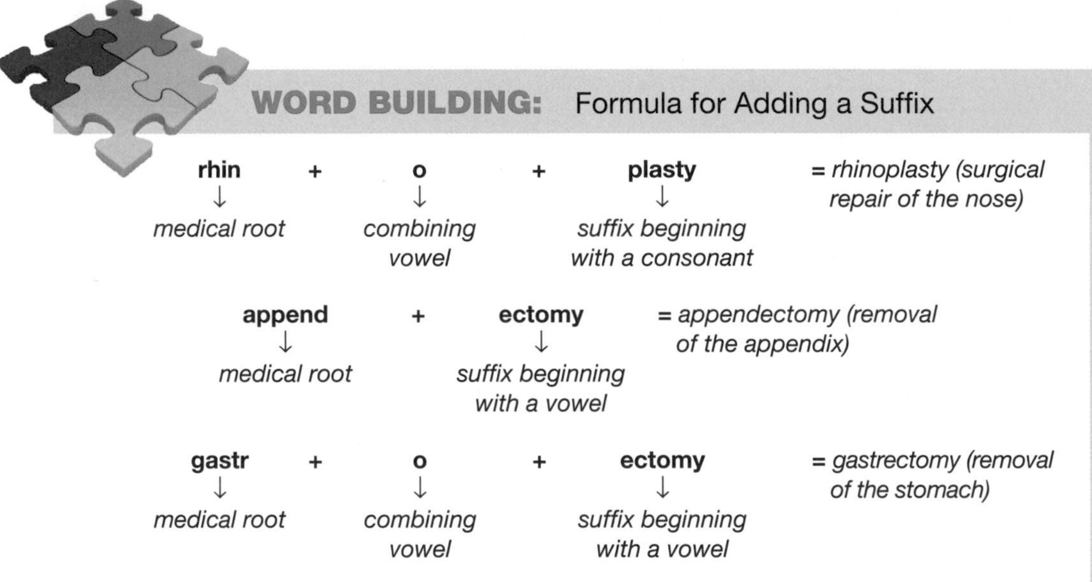

Medical suffixes can be organized by their purpose or function. This type of organization is very helpful when you are trying to learn terms that are not common to your everyday word usage. Tables 1-18 through 1-23 present some commonly used medical suffixes that are organized by how they are most often used. These are just a few of the many suffixes that you will be using in your health-care career. The tables demonstrate how suffixes are combined with medical roots or their combining forms to create different medical terms from the same roots.

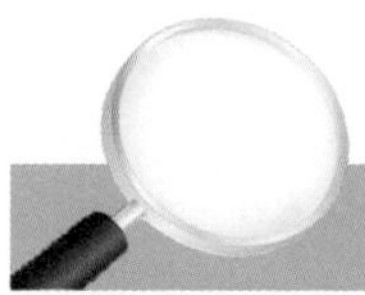

FOCUS POINT: Don't Panic!

You don't have to memorize all of theses suffixes now. Like the other word parts that you have studied in this chapter, the suffixes will reappear in later units of this book, where you will learn how they are used on the job by medical professionals. For example, Unit 2 highlights the language of diagnostics and assessment, Unit 3 explores treatments and procedures (including surgical language), and Unit 4 introduces the language of recovery and rehabilitation. In each of these units, you will learn about the suffixes, prefixes, and roots specific to the topics at hand.

TABLE 1-18: Suffixes for Nouns That Name Pathologies (illnesses or signs and symptoms of illness)

BEGIN with a Root or Combining Form	ADD a Medical Suffix That Refers to Pathology (Disease)	COMBINE to Create a New Word That Explains a Pathology
root +	suffix =	new noun
neur/o (root meaning *nerve, brain, or mind*)	-algia (pain)	neuralgia = nerve pain
my/a (root meaning *muscle*)	-asthenia (loss of strength)	myasthenia = loss of muscle strength
inert (root meaning *not active*)	-ia (referring to a condition that is usually but not always abnormal)	inertia = condition of sluggishness or lack of activity such as sleep inertia
botul (combining form of *botulinum*, a neurotoxin)	-ism (state or condition)	botulism = type of food poisoning that can cause paralysis and even death
tonsil (root word referring to the oval mass of lymph tissue in the pharynx of the mouth)	-itis (inflammation)	tonsillitis = inflammation of the tonsils
sarc (combining form meaning *flesh*)	-oma (tumor)	sarcoma = malignant type of tumor of the flesh or connective tissue of the body
halit (combining form of *halitus*, meaning *breath*)	-osis (condition, disease, or increase)	halitosis = offensive or bad breath
neur/o (root meaning *nerve*)	-pathy (disease of suffering)	neuropathy = disease or disorder of the nerves or neural pathways

TABLE 1-19: Suffixes for Nouns That Name Diagnostic or Surgical Procedures

BEGIN with a Medical Root or Combining Form	ADD a Medical Suffix That Describes a Type of Diagnostic or Surgical Procedure	COMBINE to Create a New Word
root +	suffix =	new noun
amnio (combining form of root *amnion*, meaning *the thin, transparent sac holding a fetus in utero*)	-centesis (puncture or aspirate)	amniocentesis = diagnostic test performed to remove fluid from the amniotic sac to determine a fetus's health
arthr(o) (combining form meaning *joint*)	-desis (binding)	arthrodesis = fusion or joining of two bones

Continued

TABLE 1-19: Suffixes for Nouns That Name Diagnostic or Surgical Procedures—cont'd

BEGIN with a Medical Root or Combining Form	ADD a Medical Suffix That Describes a Type of Diagnostic or Surgical Procedure	COMBINE to Create a New Word
append (combining form of root *appendix*)	-ectomy (to remove)	appendectomy = surgical removal of the appendix
son(o) (combining form meaning *sound*)	-gram (photographic or pictorial representation)	sonogram = ultrasound picture of the internal body
radi(o) (combining form of root *radiation*)	-graphy (field or science of taking photographs or creating, developing, and interpreting pictorial representations)	radiography = field or science of x-ray photography
bio (combining form meaning *life*)	-opsy (view of something)	biopsy = procedure that removes living tissue for examination
lob (combining form of the word *lobe,* meaning *a well-defined part of an organ*)	-otomy (cutting)	lobotomy = surgical cut in a lobe
jejun(o) (combining form of *jejunum,* the second portion of the small intestine)	-ostomy (creating an opening or mouth)	jejunostomy = surgical creation of an opening into and from the jejunum to the outside of the body
fluor(o) (root meaning *luminous* or *fluorescent*)	-scope (to view)	fluoroscope = specialized instrument used for viewing an x-ray immediately on a screen
end(o) (root meaning *within or inside*)	-scopy (field or science of viewing and interpreting same)	endoscopy = process of viewing the interior of the body using an endoscope

TABLE 1-20: Suffixes for Nouns That Name Health Professionals or Fields of Medicine

BEGIN with a Medical Root Word in Its Combining Form	ADD a Medical Suffix That Means *A Person Who*	COMBINE to Create a New Word
root +	suffix =	new noun
physic/o (body) pedi/atr (child) obstetr/i (pregnancy, childbirth) clini (medical practice)	-ian → -ician →	physician = medical doctor pediatrician = doctor specializing in children's health obstetrician = doctor specializing in pregnancy and the birth of children clinician = health professional working directly with patients or clients
optham/olog (eye) card/iolog (heart)	-ist →	ophthalmologist = physician specializing in the health and functioning of the eyes and vision cardiologist = physician or surgeon specializing in the health and functioning of the heart
pod (foot) psych (brain, mind)	-iatry →	podiatry = field of medicine dealing with the treatment of the feet psychiatry = field of medicine dealing with the treatment of the mind and the brain
gynec (woman, female)	-ologist →	gynecologist = doctor who assesses, diagnoses, and treats diseases and conditions of the female reproductive organs

TABLE 1-21: Suffixes That Create Adjectives (Note that all of these suffixes mean *belonging to or referring to.*)

BEGIN with a Medical Term (Noun)	EXTRACT the Combining Form	ADD a Medical Suffix That Creates Adjectives	COMBINE to Create an Adjective
noun	combining form +	suffix =	adjective
ilium (a bone that is part of the pelvis)	ili/o	-ac	iliac Example: iliac fossa (the concave shape of the iliac bones)
ileum (the lower portion of the small intestines)	ile/o	-ac -al	ileac ileal Example: ileal conduit (a method of surgically diverting urinary flow)
nasus (nose)	nas/o	-al	nasal Example: nasal congestion
nausea (a wavelike sensation that may lead to vomiting)	nause/a	-ous	nauseous Example: a nauseous feeling
thorax (chest or chest wall)	thorac-	-ic	thoracic Example: thoracic surgery
scapula (shoulder blade)	scapula/o	-ar	scapular Example: scapular lesion
card (heart)	cardi/io	-ic -ial	cardial, cardiac Example: cardiac arrest
aud (hearing)	audi/it	-ory	auditory Example: auditory hallucinations
colon (the large intestine)	col/o- colon- colono-	-scopy -scope -ic	colonoscopy, colonic, colonoscope Example: colonoscopy exam

TABLE 1-22: Medical Suffixes That Change Verbs into Nouns

BEGIN with the Combining Form of a Word or Root That Can Function as a Verb	ADD a Medical Suffix	COMBINE to Create a Noun
combining form of verb +	suffix =	noun
auto(m)	-ation	automation
cre(o)	-ation	creation
contain	-ment	containment
acknowledge	-ment	acknowledgement

TABLE 1-23: Medical Suffixes That Can Have More Than One Meaning

Suffix	Meanings	Suffix	Meanings
-ate	• action • use • possession • having the form of	-gram	• record • weight
-blast	• newly created cell • immature cell • embryonic cell • germ cell	-ive	• nature of • quality of
-ectasis	• dilation • dilatation • distension • stretching	-lysis	• separation • breakdown • loosening • dissolution • destruction
-gen	• formation • produce	-penia	• lack of • decreased level of
		-rrhea	• flow • discharge

Mix and Match: Suffixes with Roots

It's your turn now. Combine each root in the left column with a suffix in the right column to form a new word. Write the new words below, and then explain the meaning of each new term in your own words. You might want to check your answers with your instructor or another student before looking at the Answer Key. Seeking feedback from others is an excellent way to enhance your own learning.

	ROOT	SUFFIX
1.	gynec	-itis
2.	orbit	-gen
3.	tonsil	-ectomy
4.	append	-oma
5.	carcin + o	-gram
6.	son + o	-therapy
7.	aud	-al
8.	chem + o	-ible
9.	phys	-ician
10.	sarc	-ology

1. Word: ______________________
   Meaning: ______________________
2. Word: ______________________
   Meaning: ______________________
3. Word: ______________________
   Meaning: ______________________
4. Word: ______________________
   Meaning: ______________________
5. Word: ______________________
   Meaning: ______________________
6. Word: ______________________
   Meaning: ______________________

7. Word: ______________________________
   Meaning: ______________________________
8. Word: ______________________________
   Meaning: ______________________________
9. Word: ______________________________
   Meaning: ______________________________
10. Word: ______________________________
    Meaning: ______________________________

Break It Down

Read the following sentences to yourself or a partner. Circle the suffixes in the words that are used to describe each medical condition. Check your answers.

1. Bob dislocated his shoulder as a result of a skiing accident over the weekend. The shoulder is painful, and Bob cannot move his right arm or upper body very well.
2. Angela suffers from a neuropathy. She has a lot of generalized nerve pain.
3. Billie suffered from a sore, infected throat off and on over many years. Finally, at age 12, he had a tonsillectomy. Now, this health situation has been resolved.
4. Mrs. Henderson has just been diagnosed with anemia. According to the lab reports, her vitamin B_{12} count is very low.
5. The College of Physicians and Surgeons can provide a list of oncologists who are registered in your state or province.

Free Writing

Add a medical suffix to each root below, and then use the new word—along with the words in parentheses—to write a sentence. You may need to add a few of your own words to make the sentence logical. When you are done, check your answers.

EXAMPLE: radiolog_______
(Brenda, Diagnostic Imaging, x-rays)
Sentence: Brenda is a radiologist who takes x-rays in Diagnostic Imaging.

1. dermat ______________________________
   (skin, red, itchy, rash, swollen) ______________________________
2. physic ______________________________
   (clinic, examined, patient) ______________________________
3. my ______________________________
   (Brendan, pain, difficult, walking, legs) ______________________________
4. amnio ______________________________
   (pregnant, determine, health, fetus) ______________________________
5. melan ______________________________
   (work outdoors, ultraviolet rays, cancer, skin) ______________________________
6. gastro ______________________________
   (look inside, stomach) ______________________________
7. audit ______________________________
   (hallucinations, patient, hearing) ______________________________
8. colono ______________________________
   (doctor, view, patient, bowel) ______________________________
9. pediatr ______________________________
   (doctor, children) ______________________________

Let's Practice

For each meaning, write one or more suffixes that can add that meaning to a word. List as many suffixes as you can. Try not to refer to the Answer Key or to any of the tables in this chapter until you have completed this exercise. Challenge yourself.

1. Meaning: disease or medical condition ______________________
2. Meaning: an action or process ______________________
3. Meaning: already occurred; past tense ______________________
4. Meaning: in comparison to ______________________
5. Meaning: pain ______________________
6. Meaning: to puncture and then aspirate (extract liquid) ______________________
7. Meaning: a type of health care professional ______________________
8. Meaning: viewing or looking ______________________
9. Meaning: stretching or dilation ______________________

Singular and plural suffixes

For the most part, you have been studying singular suffixes. Now, begin to work with plural suffixes. A plural suffix is an ending that is added to indicate more than one of something. Of course, we all know how to add an *-s* or *-es* to English words to form plurals. Plural suffixes for medical terms are more complicated, especially for terms that derive from Greek and Latin. There are a number of rules that apply that you will, in this case, have to memorize. Study Table 1-24 to prepare for some practice exercises.

TABLE 1-24: Singular and Plural Suffixes

Singular Suffix	Rule to Create Plural Form of Suffix	Example: From Singular to Plural
-a	-ae 1. Keep the *a.* 2. Add an *e.*	petechia → petechi**ae**
-ax	-aces 1. Drop the *x.* 2. Replace with *ces.*	thorax → thor**aces**
-en	-ina 1. Drop the *en.* 2. Replace with *ina.*	semen → sem**ina**
-ex -ix	-ices 1. Drop the *ix* or *ex.* 2. Replace with *ices.*	cortex → cort**ices** appendix → append**ices**
-is	-es 1. Drop the *is.* 2. Replace with *es.*	diagnosis → diagnos**es** metastasis → metastas**es**
-ma	-mata 1. Keep the *ma.* 2. Add *ta.*	trauma → trau**mata** sarcoma → sarco**mata**
-on -um	-a 1. Drop the *on* or *um.* 2. Replace with *a.*	phenomenon → phenomen**a** ammoni**um** → ammoni**a** datum → dat**a**
-um	-ia 1. Drop the *um.* 2. Replace with *ia.*	clostridium → clostrid**ia**
-us	-i 1. Drop the *us.* 2. Replace with *i.*	nucleus → nucle**i** alveolus → alveol**i**
-us	-era 1. Drop the *us.* 2. Replace with *era.*	viscus → visc**era**

TABLE 1-24: Singular and Plural Suffixes—cont'd

Singular Suffix	Rule to Create Plural Form of Suffix	Example: From Singular to Plural
-x	-nges 1. Drop the *x*. 2. Replace with *ges*.	phalanx → phala**nges** larynx → lary**nges**
-x	-ces 1. Drop the *x*. 2. Replace with *ces*.	crux → cru**ces** matrix → matri**ces**
-y	-ies 1. Drop the *y*. 2. Replace with *ies*.	biopsy → biops**ies** deformity → deformit**ies**

Let's Practice

Write the plural form of each medical term. Simply follow the rules in Table 1-24. It is not important to know the meanings of these words right now; that information will come later.

1. trauma ______
2. pelvis ______
3. lumen ______
4. embolus ______
5. vertebra ______
6. bacterium ______
7. diverticulum ______
8. viscus ______
9. index ______
10. appendix ______
11. thorax ______
12. prognosis ______
13. diagnosis ______
14. neurosis ______
15. specialist ______
16. specialty ______
17. urologist ______
18. science ______
19. pharmacokinetic ______
20. pharynx ______

Homonyms and homographs

Homonyms are words that sound alike but that have different meanings, such as *ate* and *eight*. **Homographs** are words that are spelled alike but that have different meanings and, often, different pronunciations: for example, "The nurse *wound* the bandage around the *wound*."

There are many medical terms that sound alike or that have similar spellings. Identifying the correct word and meaning on the job is of critical importance. In this book, these troublesome words are highlighted in a regular feature called "Right Word or Wrong Word?" The goal of this feature is to alert you to pay close attention to the context in which you find these words so that you will be able to discern which word you are reading, writing, or hearing.

You have already encountered some of these troublesome words in Chapter 1. Have you noticed them? Try the "Right Word or Wrong Word?" activities that accompany this chapter.

Right Word or Wrong Word: *Ileo* or *Ilio*?

These two word parts sound the same; thus, they are homonyms. The combining form of the root word *ileum* is *ileo,* and it refers to the lower portion of the small intestines. To what does the root *ilium* and its combining form *ilio* refer? When you are satisfied that you have the correct answer, check your answers in the Answer Key.

Right Word or Wrong Word: *Dilation* or *Dilatation*?

Be careful: these two words are not spelled or pronounced the same, but they look very similar. Which word means *the process of expanding or widening?* When you are satisfied that you know, check your answers in the Answer Key.

Right Word or Wrong Word: *Diagnose, Diagnosis,* or *Diagnoses*?

These three words sound very similar, but they mean somewhat different things.

diagnosis or *diagnoses:* Which word means more than one?

diagnoses: Is it a verb or a noun?

CHAPTER SUMMARY

Chapter 1 has introduced medical language and medical terminology in the context of various health-care professions. It is a foundational chapter that provides the core elements of word structure and composition. The chapter highlighted root words, medical roots, combining forms, prefixes, and suffixes through examples and practice exercises. Acquiring this knowledge gives you the building blocks that you will need as you learn more medical language and terminology in subsequent chapters of this book.

See How Much You've Learned

For audio exercises, visit **http://www.MedicalLanguageLab.com.** 

Chapter 1 has introduced you to some medical abbreviations. These have been organized into a study table here for quick reference. Some of them you will recognize immediately, and some will reappear throughout the following chapters with more explanation and application.

TABLE 1-25: Medical Abbreviations

Medical Abbreviation	Full Term	Medical Abbreviation	Full Term
MVA	Motor vehicle accident	KVO	Keep vein open
ETA	Estimated time of arrival	O_2	Oxygen
EMT	Emergency medical technician		

Key Terms

antonyms	**homographs**	**prefix**
combining forms	**homonyms**	**root word**
context	**medical terminology**	**suffix**

CHAPTER REVIEW

What Do You Know?

Answer the following questions.

1. In most cases, what do medical roots identify?

____

2. What four characteristics do medical prefixes usually describe?

____

3. List three types of nouns you can create by adding a medical suffix.

____

Break It Down

Break these words into their component parts of prefix-root-suffix, as applicable. Name each element.

1. gynecology ____________________
2. postoperative ____________________
3. antiepileptic ____________________
4. contraindicated ____________________
5. hematuria ____________________
6. thyroidectomy ____________________
7. pneumothorax ____________________
8. polyunsaturated ____________________
9. cerebrospinal ____________________
10. hyperirritability ____________________

Translate the Terminology

Use your new skills to decipher medical language. On the line provided, explain what is being said to the best of your ability. Try to do so without the use of a medical dictionary. You may, of course, look back through this chapter for help.

1. Radiologist to physician: "The patient has a *midline fracture* of the *scapula*."

____

2. Dental assistant to dentist: "Mrs. Blundell is afraid of dentists and is *hyperventilating*."

____

3. Paramedic to emergency department staff: "We have a 41-year-old male in *respiratory* distress."

____

4. Doctor to nurse in emergency department: "We have a blunt force *trauma* to the abdomen with internal *hemorrhaging*."

____

5. Medical equipment sales rep to optometrist: "I'd like to show you our new 2013 *optometer*."

____

Define the Root

Fill in the blanks with the meaning of each medical root.

1. hem(o) ______
2. glyc(o) ______
3. pod ______
4. arthr(o) ______
5. my(o) ______

Name the Root

Read the definition, and then write the correct root.

1. A medical root word meaning *not active:* ______
2. A medical root word naming an oval mass of lymph tissue in the pharynx of the mouth: ______
3. A medical root beginning with the letter *o* that means *bones* or *skeletal*: ______
4. A medical root describing a system related to eating: ______
5. A medical root meaning *life*: ______

Define the Prefix

Write the meaning of each prefix.

1. ante- ______
2. pre- ______
3. macro- ______
4. equi- ______
5. ex- ______

Critical Thinking

Think critically (deeply) about each question, and then relate it to your experience with suffixes.

1. Zoology is one of these. What is it? ______
2. These are medical specialists who treat disorders that involve the creation and elimination of fluid wastes from the body. Who are they? ______
3. If you are often nervous or are preoccupied with feelings of guilt, self-esteem, and how others regard you, a psychiatrist might diagnose you as having a ______.
4. This word can name a body part or a section at the back of a textbook. What is it? ______
5. You have many of these in your back, and you have just learned how to make the plural form of the word that names them. What are they? ______
6. Today, it is very popular to buy soap that rids the skin of these, but not all of them are actually harmful to the body. What are they? ______
7. Unless you are a doctor, you may not have the legal right to make these. What are they? ______
8. In the diagnostic imaging department of your local hospital, pictures of broken bones are usually taken by professionals in what specialty? ______

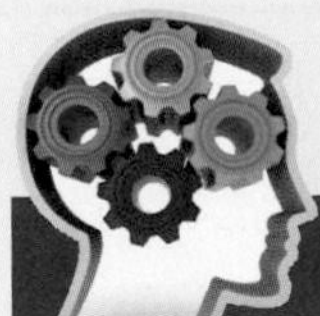

MEMORY MAGIC

Are you wondering how in the world you will ever remember so many new terms? Try this simple exercise to help:

Obtain some 3 × 5-inch colored index cards, or use three different colors of felt-tipped pens to differentiate your cards.

Use one color of index card or pen for medical roots. Write down 9 or 10 roots and their combining forms that you would like to remember at this stage of your studies, and write a brief definition for each. (Write fairly large, and include maybe three or four roots per card.)

Keep these cards with you for at least 24 hours. Keep them in your pocket, your purse, or somewhere very close at hand. Pull them out frequently, and read them or simply look at them for at least 30 seconds each time.

After 24 hours, test yourself. See how many roots and combining forms you can list without looking at your index cards.

Congratulate yourself!

Now, repeat the process for prefixes, using a different color of index card or pen. When you succeed at that, follow the same process using yet another color of card or pen for 10 of your favorite suffixes.

Keep These Cards.
They will Come in Handy
For the Rest of This Book.

CHAPTER TWO

Naming and Describing: Medical Language for the Body

Focus: Anatomy, Physiology, and Position

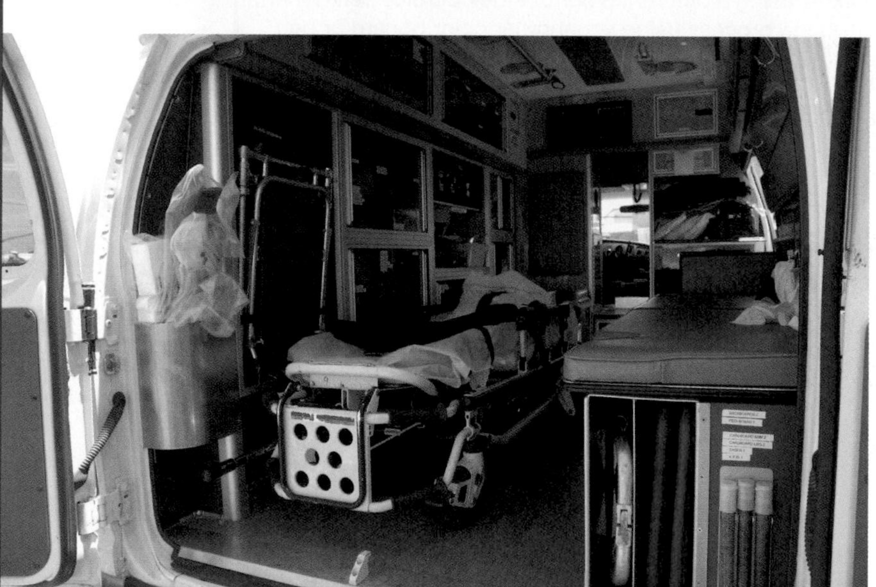

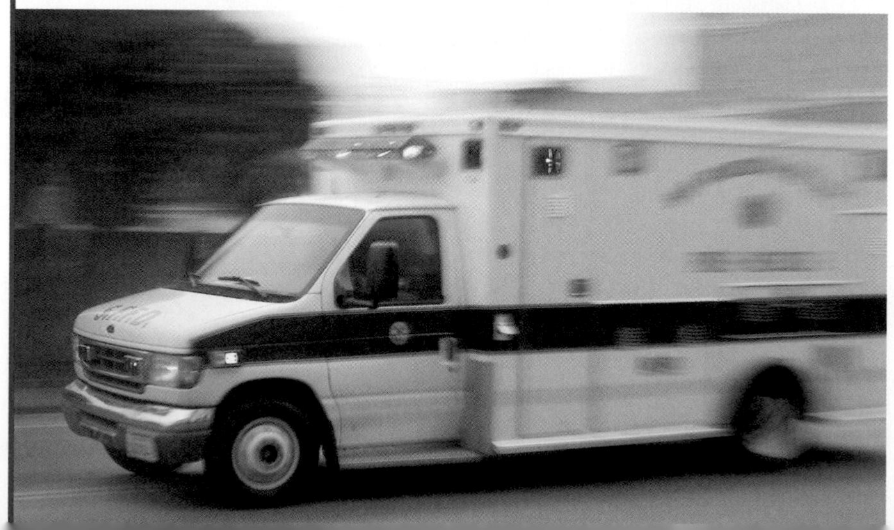

Patient Update

The intersection at the corner of Shawnee Boulevard and South Sheridan Road was chaos. Two vehicles—one a car and the other a delivery truck—had collided. Police, fire and rescue units, and ambulances were on the scene. Police were securing the perimeter to keep onlookers and reporters from interfering while the emergency medical personnel attended to the accident victims. Traffic was blocked on all sides of the intersection (EMT), and a couple of police officers were rerouting it away from the scene.

Near the car, an elderly woman was pacing back and forth in the company of an emergency medical technician. The older woman was wringing her hands, and she seemed to be muttering to herself. EMT Shondra Wallis was speaking calmly and softly, trying to convince the woman to sit down. It was near noon, and the temperature on this sunny June day was increasingly hot. Even so, the EMT offered to drape a blanket over the woman's shoulders. "Here, put this on. I don't want you going into shock," she said quietly to the woman. It was brushed away. "What's your name?"

"Stevie-Rose," the woman replied. "Stevie-Rose Davis."

"Well, Ms. Davis, you've been in an accident, and you need to sit down and let me take care of you. My name's Shondra, and I am an emergency medical technician with the fire department here." Ms. Davis did not respond and instead stared out into the intersection and at the commotion there. The EMT was able to do a preliminary assessment of Ms. Davis while this occurred; she noted no obvious external injuries but did notice that the woman was very pale. Because Ms. Davis was ambulant, EMT Wallis touched her elbow and gently began to direct her toward a grassy spot on the median of Shawnee Boulevard. EMT Wallis then assisted Ms. Davis into a sitting position under a tree. "Ms. Davis, do you have any pain anywhere? Are you hurt?" inquired EMT Wallis as she began a more comprehensive assessment for signs and symptoms of trauma.

"What's that, dear? Pain? No, I don't think so. What makes you ask me that?" Ms. Davis replied. Then she swayed momentarily and raised a hand to her head.

"Are you all right?" EMT Wallis interjected as she reached out to steady Ms. Davis.

"Yes, yes, I'm okay. Just a little lightheaded. Must be the heat," replied the elderly lady, now looking at Wallis directly. The EMT took the opportunity to quickly evaluate Ms. Davis's pupils for size and response to light as part of a neurological assessment. The woman's eyes were dilated, and this concerned the EMT. While Wallis was using the penlight, the patient reached out to move it away from her eyes. As she did so, Wallis noted a fine tremor in the woman's arm and hand, and she also noticed some disfigurement of the woman's fingers.

"Ms. Davis, did you bump your head?" EMT Wallis inquired.

"I don't know, Miss. Did I?"

"I'm going to examine your head, Ms. Davis. I'm just going to touch your scalp and your cheekbones and so on. I need to determine if you hit your head during the accident," advised the EMT. Wallis proceeded to palpate the cranium and cervical spine of her patient while kneeling beside her. She then gently examined the bones of the patient's face, proceeding from the proximal point of the nose at the brow line and working outward from there for bilateral assessment. She paused for a moment to palpate the patient's temporal pulses. She then continued the head examination by palpating the mandible and then moving her fingers downward to assess the clavicle. The patient was cooperative during this assessment and gave no evidence of pain or discomfort.

"Now I need to take your pulse and check your arms and legs for any cuts or abrasions, Ms. Davis." EMT Wallis continued her assessment bilaterally, beginning on the left side of her patient and then moving to the right, assessing the upper body before the lower, one side at a time. Although Ms. Davis' radial pulse was somewhat rapid, she showed no signs of cardiovascular impairment at the moment.

"Ms. Davis, I see that you have some fine tremors in your hands, and the knuckles of your fingers are quite prominent. Do you have arthritis?" asked Wallis, returning now to her previous observations. "Do you usually have fine tremors?"

"What? What are you asking me?" The elderly woman seemed distracted and confused. She was chewing just a little at her bottom lip.

"Ms. Davis, do you have arthritis in your hands?" Ms. Davis nodded yes. "Your hands are trembling a bit. Is that normal for you, too?" To this, the patient shook her head no. EMT Wallis suspected that the fine tremors might be related to shock. She completed her assessment of the patient's upper body and moved distally to begin an integumentary, circulatory, and musculoskeletal assessment of the woman's lower extremities. Finding no major injuries, she said, "Ms. Davis, we need to go now, over there to my truck. Do you see it? There, the fire and rescue unit over there. That's my rig. It's like a mini ambulance. I'd like you to walk over there with me, and we can take you to the hospital for further assessment. Can you walk with me?"

"Yes, I can walk if you help me up. I seem to be a bit lightheaded. Do you know why that is?" Ms. Davis asked in a puzzled voice. "I'm not usually so dizzy. I wonder if I had breakfast today. Do you know if I had breakfast today?" she asked as the EMT helped her to her feet.

"No ma'am, I can't say. Ms. Davis, you've been in a car accident, and I think you might be feeling a bit confused right now. I'm going to take you to the hospital to see a doctor and get a full checkup." They began to walk together toward Wallis's unit. Wallis wanted to get the woman on a stretcher and give her some oxygen; she hoped that this would improve Ms. Davis's color and her ability to cope with the shock of the accident. She wanted to take Ms. Davis's blood pressure, too. Wallis would do this while she waited for her partner, EMT-Paramedic Russell, to come back from helping someone who was still in the accident vehicle.

As they proceeded, Wallis observed an EMT from Rescue Unit 155 nearby, talking softly to an elderly man who was sitting on the back step of his unit. He was taking the man's blood pressure. Wallis was just close enough to hear the EMT say, "Sir, let me help you up into the van. Sir, you need to come up into the van so that I can check you over. I'll help you." The patient did not move. He stared at his feet and clasped his hands.

"You okay there, Manuel?" Wallis called to her colleague.

"Yup, I just can't seem to convince him to let me assess him," replied the EMT. "We'll be okay. You?"

"We're okay," EMT Wallis replied, looking over her shoulder at Manuel and his patient. Then she looked at her own patient. "Ms. Davis, do you know that man over there?" she asked, pointing to the elderly man she'd been observing.

"Yes, dear, that's my husband, Zane." She paused a moment and added, "I wonder what he's doing here." Ms. Davis then continued on toward EMT Wallis' rescue unit without looking back at him again.

Suddenly, a third ambulance arrived, which created a raucous noise of sirens. Crew members jumped out and dashed over to the car to join the emergency medical team that was attending to someone who was apparently still in the vehicle. From where she stood, EMT Wallis could see that they were lifting what appeared to be a child out of the back seat and onto a stretcher. She heard loud groaning, the voice of a child.

"Ms. Davis, who was in the car with you today?"

"In the car? Why, I don't know," said Ms. Davis. "Was I in a car? Where was I going?" she asked confusedly.

"Ms. Davis, you've been in a car accident. I'm taking you to the hospital now to get you checked out. You were in the car with your husband. Who was in the backseat, Ms. Davis?"

"Oh, that would be Clay. He's our grandson, you know."

Reflective Questions

Reflect on the story that you've just read.

1. How many emergency medical personnel are in this scene? Can you name them by their professional titles?

   ____

2. Ms. Stevie-Rose Davis seems confused. What is she confused about?

   ____

3. What terminology and other medical language did you notice in the scenario? Find at least five examples.

   ____

4. Which medical terms did you understand from the story context? Which do you need more information about to fully understand?

   ____

For audio exercises, visit **http://www.MedicalLanguageLab.com.** 

Introduction

The opening scenario for this chapter introduced you to a patient named Stevie-Rose Davis, an elderly woman who has been injured in a traffic accident. As EMT Wallis began assessing Ms. Davis's condition at the accident scene, she used different kinds of medical language to name and describe what she observed of the patient's condition.

Chapter 2 will help you to learn basic medical language for naming and describing parts of the body, thereby expanding your ability to recognize and interpret the language of health-care professionals. It will introduce anatomical terms for body organs and systems, as well as terms for locations, sites, and directions on the body.

Learning Objectives

After reading Chapter 2, you will be able to do the following:

- Identify the basic anatomy of the body.
- Describe the physiology of the body.
- Locate specific points on and planes of the body.
- Explain the movements and positions of the body.
- Use medical and health-care descriptors to communicate.

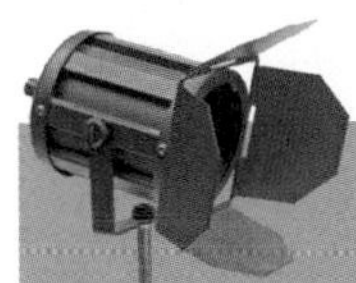

CAREER SPOTLIGHT: Emergency Medical Technicians and Paramedics

The designation *emergency medical technician* (EMT) applies to trained medical responders who offer immediate aid to victims of accidents and other emergency health situations. EMTs are trained to accurately assess and treat, and they are skilled in lifesaving procedures. EMTs work primarily at the scene of the crisis, although they continue to care for the affected individuals while transporting them to a hospital or another medical facility, if needed. Upon arrival, they report about their patients' conditions to the attending physician and staff, and they often remain in the emergency room with their patients to provide assistance until the treatment team is able to take over fully.

An *EMT-Basic* certificate is the most common form of certification for this allied health professional. This first responder can provide first aid, deliver babies, apply splints, treat allergic reactions, and manage cardiovascular and respiratory emergencies, among other things. Alternatively, an *EMT-Paramedic* can respond to, assess, and treat all of these conditions and more. The EMT-Paramedic has a larger scope of practice. This technician can work beyond the patient's skin. This means that he or she can give injections, insert catheters and tubes, start intravenous lines, give medications, and use and interpret a number of monitors and pieces of equipment. An EMT-Paramedic has considerably more training than an EMT-Basic. Emergency response teams are usually made up of one EMT-Basic and one EMT-Paramedic. These individuals are referred to as "the EMT" and "the paramedic," respectively.

EMTs are required to be licensed by state or federal law.

Right Word or Wrong Word: *Rescue Unit* or *Ambulance*?

Do you know what the difference is between a rescue unit and an ambulance? Can these terms be used interchangeably? Perhaps you can guess from what you've just read.

Think about this, and perhaps mull it over with a friend or colleague. When you're ready, check the answer in the Answer Key.

The ability to name and describe is essential in health care. Whether you are a medical transcriptionist or a frontline worker, you will be required to listen to descriptions of events and medical conditions delivered by participants in a health-care situation. If you are a frontline worker and thus a health-care provider, you will be expected to do even more. *You* must describe things in such a way that the person listening to you or reading your reports will get a clear and accurate picture of what you observe. For starters, you need to be able to name and describe the parts of the body and how they function.

What Is It? How Does It Work?

Anatomy is the study of the body's structures. **Physiology** is the study of how these structures interact and function. The basic component of all living things is the **cell**. Cells combine to form different kinds of tissues. Tissues combine to form **organs,** which are groups of tissues that perform specific tasks or functions in the body. Organs work together in organ systems that provide for the body's essential needs.

Medical terminology for organ systems

We'll begin with the organization of the body on a large scale and work down to the smallest level of organization. **Organ systems** are groups of organs that work together to carry out the body's essential functions. Table 2-1 shows the locations and functions of these systems.

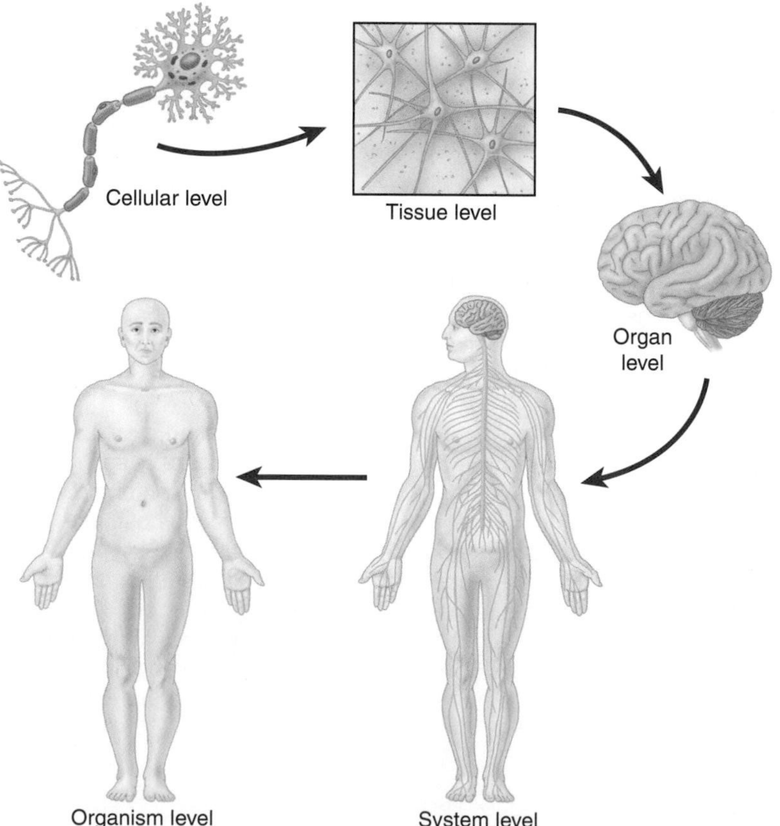

Figure 2.1: Levels of organization of the body

TABLE 2-1: Organ Systems and Their Functions

Organ (Body) System	Functions
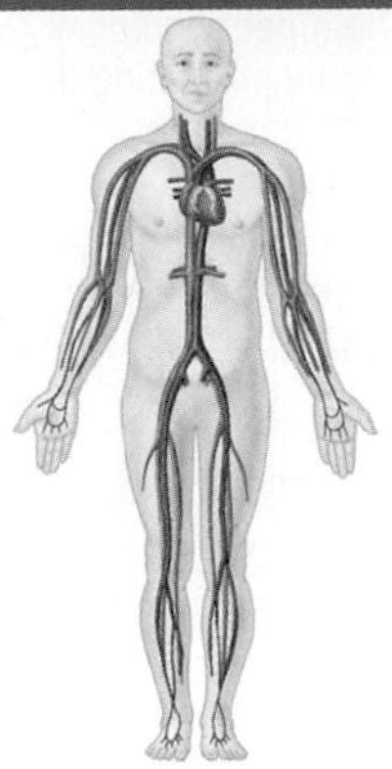 Cardiovascular or circulatory system	Transports oxygen and other nutrients to the tissues of the body; removes metabolic waste products such as carbon dioxide
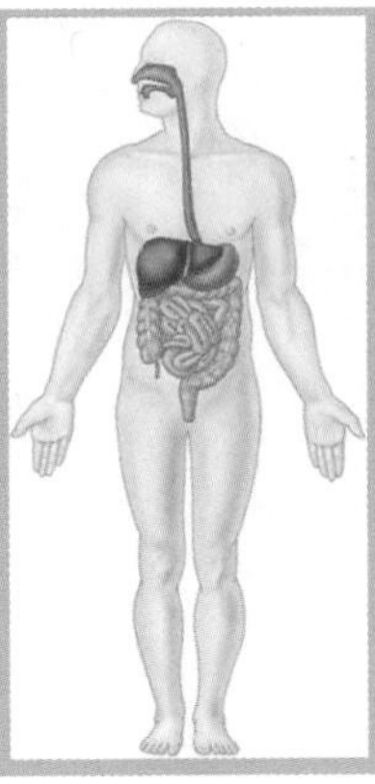 Digestive or gastro-intestinal system	Metabolizes (breaks down) food into nutrients that can be absorbed by the body; excretes waste products such as undigested matter and secretes waste from the body
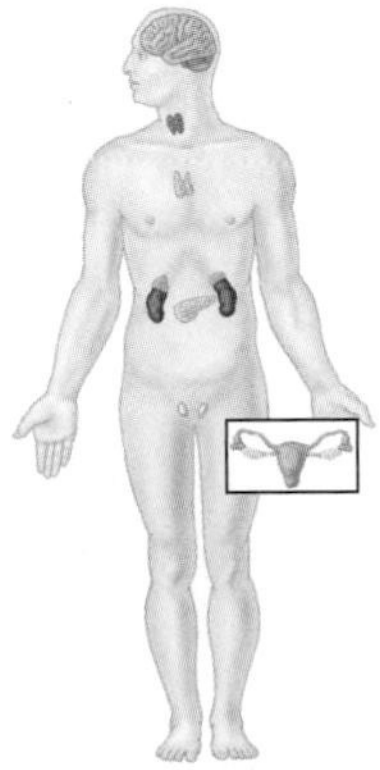 Endocrine system	Secretes hormones that regulate growth, metabolism (various internal processes of the body), and sexual development and function
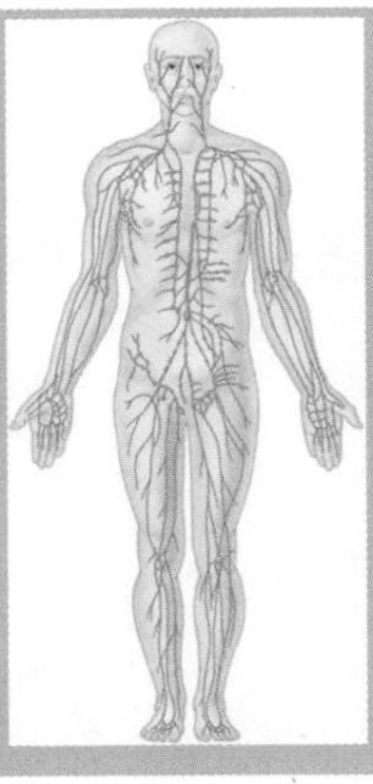 Immune system (including the lymphatic system)	Protects against harmful microorganisms such as viruses and bacteria

Continued

TABLE 2-1: Organ Systems and Their Functions—cont'd

	Organ (Body) System	Functions
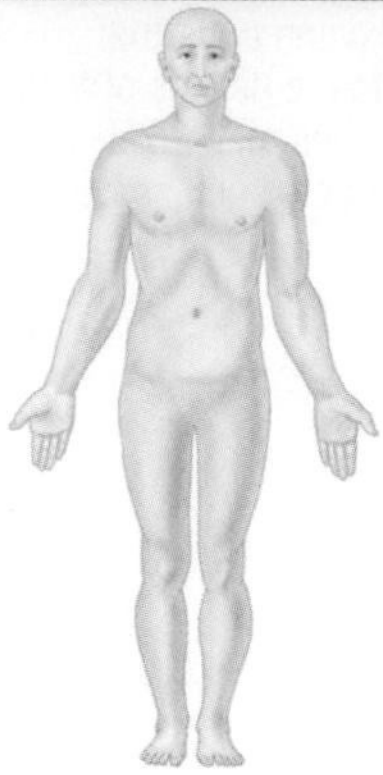	Integumentary system	Maintains the inner conditions of the body by protecting it; cotributes to homeostasis (internal equilibrium), temperature regulation, sensory reception, and absorption; synthesizes vitamin D, melanin, and carotene (pigment)
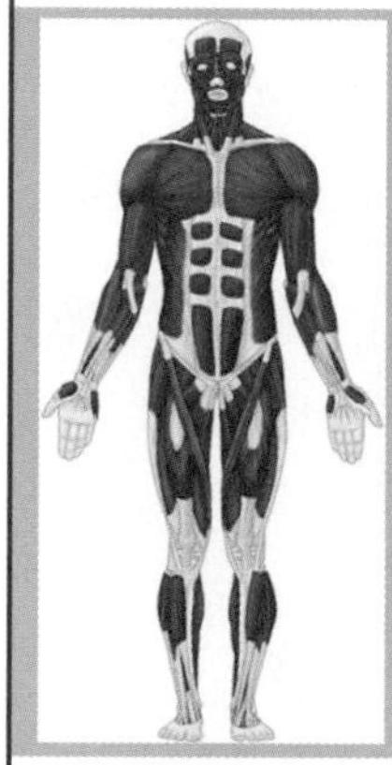	Muscular system	Provides movement of the body through the skeletal muscles, as well as organ function, through necessary contraction and expansion
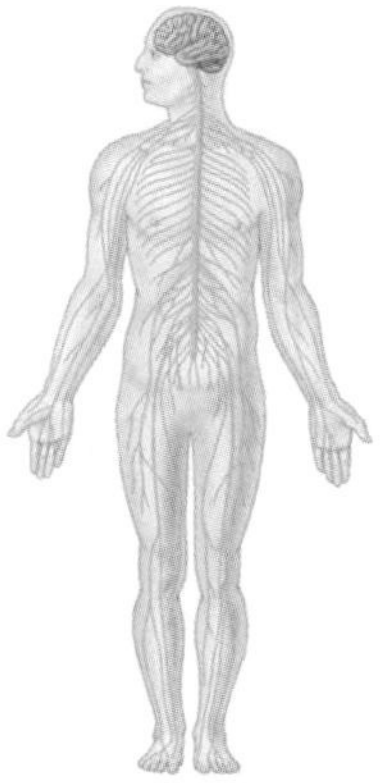	Neurological system	Processes nerve impulses; enables the communication of all sensations and sensory responses to stimuli; controls and coordinates movement, emotional responses, and thinking
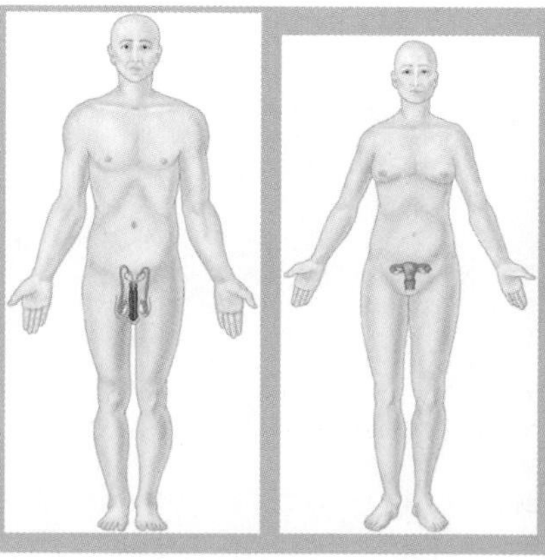	Reproductive system	Controls functions related to reproduction and birth

TABLE 2-1: Organ Systems and Their Functions—cont'd

	Organ (Body) System	Functions
	Respiratory system	Supplies oxygen to the body; eliminates nonessential gases; assists with the maintenance of pH balance
	Skeletal system	Supports the body in shape and posture; protects the brain and other internal organs; helps the bones act as levers at the point of the joints
	Urinary system	Removes fluid wastes; regulates electrolyte balance (acid-base balance); maintains blood volume, blood pressure, and tissue volume

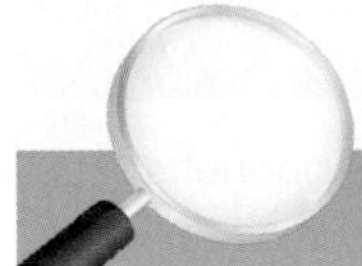

FOCUS POINT: Organ Systems

Sometimes the term *excretory system* is used, but the excretory organs are actually part of the digestive system. Often the muscular and skeletal systems are considered together as one system: the *musculoskeletal system.*

The term *organ system* is often used interchangeably with *body system*.

TABLE 2-2: Medical Roots Used to Name Organ Systems

Organ System	Root or Combining Form
Cardiovascular or circulatory system	cardi(o), meaning *heart* vascu, meaning *small vessels* circ, meaning *to go around as in a circuit*
Digestive or gastrointestinal system	digest(i/o), meaning *to break down or chemically alter* gastri(o), meaning *stomach* intesti, meaning *pertaining to the intestine*
Endocrine system	crin/krin-, meaning *to secrete*
Immune system (including the lymphatic system)	immune(o/e), meaning *safe* lymph(o,a), meaning *lymph (a type of tissue fluid)*
Integumentary system	integ, meaning *to make whole or cover*
Muscular system	muscul(o), meaning *muscle*
Neurological system	neuro, meaning *nerves*
Reproductive system	product(i/o), meaning *to produce*
Respiratory system	respir, meaning *to breathe; breathing*
Skeletal system	skeleto, meaning *a dried or dry body; bones*
Urinary system	ur(o), meaning *urinary*

Refer to Table 2-2 to learn the meanings of the roots used to create terminology that concerns the organ systems.

Build a Word

Use the following hints to correctly name the organ system that is being described.

1. bones + the suffix *-al* ____________________
2. lungs and breathing + the suffix *-tory* ____________________
3. pregnancy ____________________
4. eating + digesting + eliminating ____________________
5. skin + the suffix *-ary* ____________________

Mix and Match

Match each function with the body system that carries it out.

1. eliminating fluid waste	muscular system
2. removal of nonessential gases	respiratory system
3. concerned with contraction and expansion	neurological system
4. responds to pain	immune system
5. protects against infection	urinary system

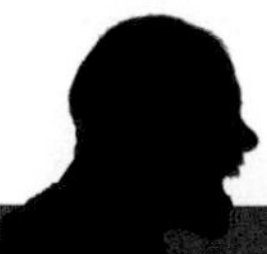

PRONUNCIATION PRACTICE

Say these words aloud to a friend or classmate, if you can. Here you are given the phonetic pronunciation. Your instructor can help you with pronunciation, or you can visit

http://www.MedicalLanguageLab.com. 

integumentary	ĭn-tĕg-ū-**mĕn**´tă-rē
neurological	nū-rō-**lŏj**´ĭk-ăl
cardiovascular	kăr″dē-ō-**văs**´kū-lăr

circulatory	**sĭr**″kū-lă-tōr′ē
respiratory	rĕs-**pīr**′ă-tō-rē or **rĕs**′pĭ-ră-tō″rē
endocrine	**ĕn**′dō-krīn or **ĕn**′dō-krĭn or **ĕn**′dō-krēn
lymphatic	lĭm-**făt**′ĭk
gastrointestinal	găs″trō-ĭn-**tĕs**′tĭn-ăl
reproductive	rē″prō-**dŭk**′tīv
urinary	**ū**′rĭ-nār″ē

Anatomical terms for organs

One of the easiest ways to learn and remember terminology related to the organs of the body is to learn the organs by the system to which they belong. For example, bones, cartilage, tendons, and ligaments belong to the skeletal system. Study Table 2-3 to learn the important organs in each organ system.

Figure 2-2 identifies some of the body's major organs by showing where they are found within the body. Study these now. Later in the chapter, you will be asked to name their location or position using medical terminology.

Figure 2-3 identifies the vital organs of the body. The word **vital** is derived from a Latin root meaning *life*. The functions performed by the vital organs are essential, necessary to maintain the life of the body.

TABLE 2-3: Organ Systems and Constituent Organs

Body System	Constituent Organs (organs that constitute or make up part of the system)
Cardiovascular or circulatory system	Heart and blood vessels
Digestive or gastrointestinal system	Mouth, tongue, pharynx, pancreas, esophagus, stomach, gallbladder, liver, small and large intestines, rectum, and anus
Endocrine system	Glands such as the hypothalamus; the pancreas; testes and ovaries; and the pituitary, thyroid, and adrenal glands
Immune system (including the lymphatic system)	Lymph vessels, lymph nodes, thymus, spleen, adenoids, appendix, blood vessels, bone marrow, and tonsils
Integumentary system	Skin (the largest organ in the body)
Muscular system	In addition to the voluntary muscles that enable the body to move, this system also includes organs that have muscle tissue that allows them to contract and expand, such as the heart, bladder, and lungs
Neurological system	Brain and spinal cord
Reproductive system	Female: ovaries, uterus, vagina, and fallopian tubes Male: penis, testes, and seminal vesicles; the prostate gland is sometimes included here as an organ
Respiratory system	Nose, trachea, and lungs
Skeletal system	Bones, cartilage, tendons, ligaments, and joints
Urinary system	Kidneys, bladder, ureters, and urethra

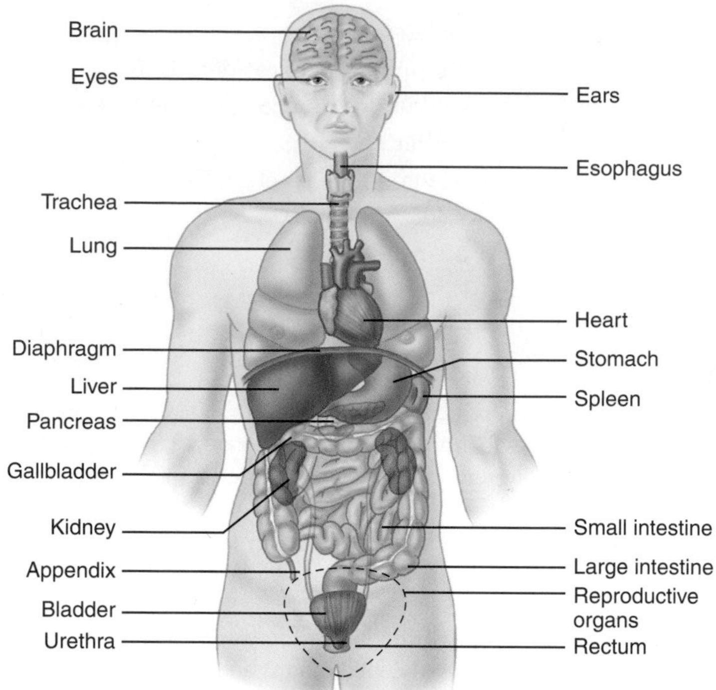

Figure 2.2: Organs of the body

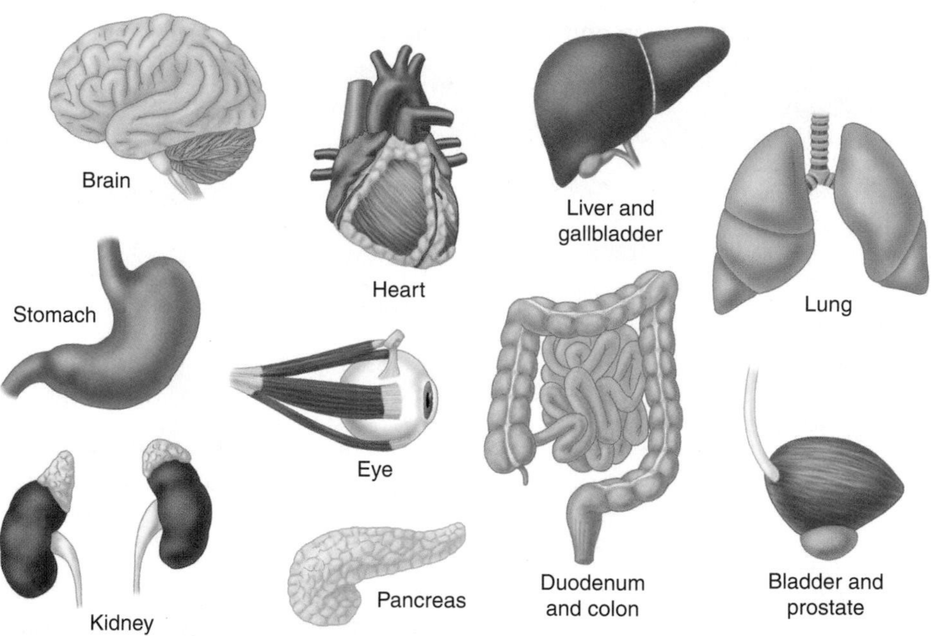

Figure 2.3: Vital organs

Let's Practice

Next to each body part, write the name of the system or systems to which it belongs.

1. heart ______________________________
2. kidney ______________________________
3. stomach ______________________________

4. brain ______
5. skin ______
6. ovaries ______
7. lungs ______
8. biceps ______
9. esophagus ______
10. trachea ______
11. artery ______
12. testes ______
13. lymph nodes ______
14. thyroid ______
15. bladder ______
16. large intestine ______

Critical Thinking

This exercise challenges you to think critically about the origins of the medical term *vital.* Consider whether modern science and technology have changed the essence of what is vital and what is not, even though terminology that is centuries old rarely changes. Draw from your own knowledge and life experiences as you answer these questions from a 21st-century perspective.

1. Is an eye really essential? Can you live without this organ?

   ______

2. Can a person live without a stomach? Is it essential to life? Is it vital?

   ______

3. Is it vital to have a large intestine (colon)? Can you live without it?

   ______

4. Is it vital to have both kidneys?

   ______

Right Word or Wrong Word: *Colon or Large Intestine?*

You have seen the word *colon* used in a question about the large intestine. Are these two terms interchangeable? Consider these examples:

The patient has been diagnosed with a disease of the *colon.*
The patient has been diagnosed with a disease of the *large intestine.*
Check your answer in the Answer Key.

Cells and tissues: the basics of physiology

Organs are made up of different types of **tissues**, which are groups of cells that are similar in structure and function. These cells carry out the basic processes of the body. To understand the body's physiology, you need to understand the structure and processes of the cells and the tissues that they form.

Medical terminology for cells

Cells are the smallest units of life. Each cell contains a nucleus, cytoplasm, and a cell membrane. The **nucleus** contains the genetic information of the cell, including its **deoxyribonucleic acid (DNA)** and **ribonucleic acid (RNA)**. Working together, DNA and RNA communicate with the rest of the cell to synthesize proteins. **Cytoplasm** is the gel-like substance in the cell, and it contains **organelles** that are responsible for the cell's reproduction and survival. A **cell membrane** protects the cell while allowing for the transportation of nutrients into it and the secretion of waste products outward.

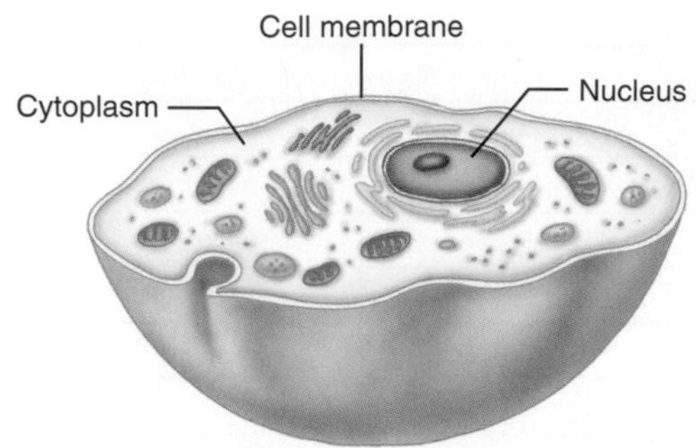

Figure 2.4: Basic parts of a human cell

TABLE 2-4: Medical Roots That Describe Cells

Root or Combining Form	Meaning
cyt/o	cell
nucle/o	pertaining to the nucleus

Medical terminology for tissue

Tissue is an aggregate (collection) of cells that are similar in structure and function. There are a number of types of tissue in the human body, with the most common being epithelial, connective, nerve, and muscle tissue.

Epithelial tissues are divided into two main types. *Covering and lining epithelia* cover and protect internal organs, cavities, and the external surface of the body. *Glandular epithelia* form glands, which are structures that secrete chemicals that promote important processes in the body.

Connective tissues consist of a variety of different cell types. They connect organs and other tissues; thus, the name *connective* is descriptive of their function. Types of connective tissue include bone marrow, cartilage, tendons, ligaments, blood vessels, nerves, and organs.

Nerve tissues, which are also referred to as *nervous tissues,* are aggregates of three types of neurons: motor neurons, sensory neurons, and interneurons. Each transmits and receives nerve impulses for a specific purpose.

Muscle tissues are designed to flex, contract, or move. There are three categories of muscle tissue: visceral, cardiac, and striated.

Medical terminology for membranes

Membranes are thin layers of tissue that surround organs and cells. By doing this, they protect the viability (life) of these body structures. Three significant types are the pleural, pericardial, and peritoneal membranes.

- **Pleural membranes** surround the lungs by lining the pleural cavity.
- **Pericardial membranes** surround the heart and the roots of the great blood vessels that originate within the heart.
- **Peritoneal membranes** surround and line the abdominal cavity.

Membranes have inner and outer layers. The layer that faces inward (toward the inside of a cell, organ, or structure) is called the **visceral** layer. Visceral membranes line organs found within the body cavities. Those layers that line the outside of a cell, organ, or structure are called the **parietal** layers. Parietal membranes line the walls of the body cavities.

Refer to Table 2-6 to learn the meaning of roots used to name and describe the three significant types of membranes noted previously.

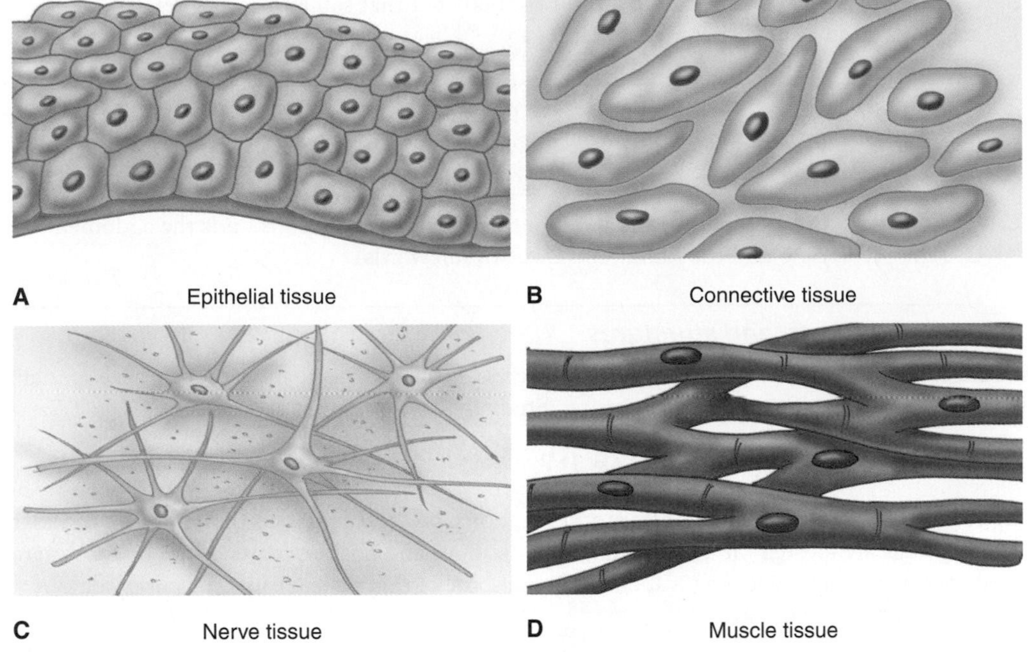

Figure 2.5: **a** Epithelial tissues, **b** Connective tissues, **c** Nerve tissues, **d** Muscle tissues

TABLE 2-5: Medical Roots That Describe Tissues

Root or Combining Form	Meaning
hist/o/io	tissue
epitheli/o	tissue that forms skin or a protective surface
viscer/o	internal organ
glan/s	gland
myo/mylo	muscles
neur/o	nerve
stria	striped or furrowed

TABLE 2-6: Medical Roots That Describe Membranes

Root or Combining Form	Meaning
pleur(o,a)	the ribs; the region of the ribs
cardi(o,a)	the heart
periton	the peritoneum or the lining of the abdominal cavity

Build a Word

Work with the roots in Table 2-6 to complete this exercise. Add a suffix or prefix to build a new word that is also a medical term. Use the clues that have been provided.

1. Use the prefix *peri-* (meaning *surrounding*), and add it to the root for *heart.* Then, add a suffix that means *relating to.*

   ____

2. Use the root that describes the lining of the abdomen, and add a suffix that means *relating to.*

   ____

3. Use the root that refers to the rib area of the body but that sometimes also refers to the lung area. Add a suffix that means *relating to.*

____

4. Create a term to describe the outer layer of the membrane that surrounds the heart. Use the prefix *peri-* and the suffix *-um.* Use two full words.

____

5. Create a term to describe the inner layer of the membrane that surrounds the abdomen. Use the prefix *peri-* and the suffix *-um.* Use two full words.

____

Elements, aspects, and structures

In the context of anatomy and physiology, the terms **element**, **aspect**, and **structure** have specialized meanings that can sometimes be confusing. Study the examples that are given in Table 2-7.

Where Is It? How Can I See It?

In addition to naming body structures and functions, medical professionals also need to describe where things are located on the body and how to move and position parts of the body. Whatever medical career you pursue, you will probably use some of this basic terminology every day.

Anatomical terms for body cavities

In health care, the term **cavity** refers to a hollow space within the body. Anatomical terms for the body cavities are used to locate and describe. There are two major cavities: the dorsal cavity and the ventral cavity. **Dorsal** is a medical and anatomical term that is derived from the root *dorso,* meaning *the back or posterior.* The dorsal cavity is divided into two parts: the **cranial** cavity and the **vertebral** canal, which is also referred to as the **spinal** cavity.

The term **ventral** is derived from the Latin *ventro,* meaning *the belly.* The ventral cavity is located on the front or anterior portion of the body. It, too, is divided into two regions: the thoracic region and the abdominopelvic region.

As you can see, these terms have roots, prefixes, and suffixes that originate in Latin and early Greek. Figure 2-7 identifies the cavities of the body.

TABLE 2-7: Elements, Aspects, and Structures

Term	Meanings	Examples
element	a. basic or fundamental part b. part of a process	a. Oxygen is an essential *element* of the body. b. *Elements* of wound healing include the body's ability to produce epidermal tissue, to synthesize products of arginine and glutamine, and to produce collagen.
aspect	a. part or area b. facet c. viewpoint	a. The x-ray shows the lateral *aspect* of the femur head. b. There are multiple *aspects* that contribute to the illness. c. From the surgical team's *aspect,* the tumor was inoperable.
structure	a. composition or makeup b. organization or arrangement	a. The nucleus is a vital part of the cell's *structure.* b. The *structure* of a cell determines its function.

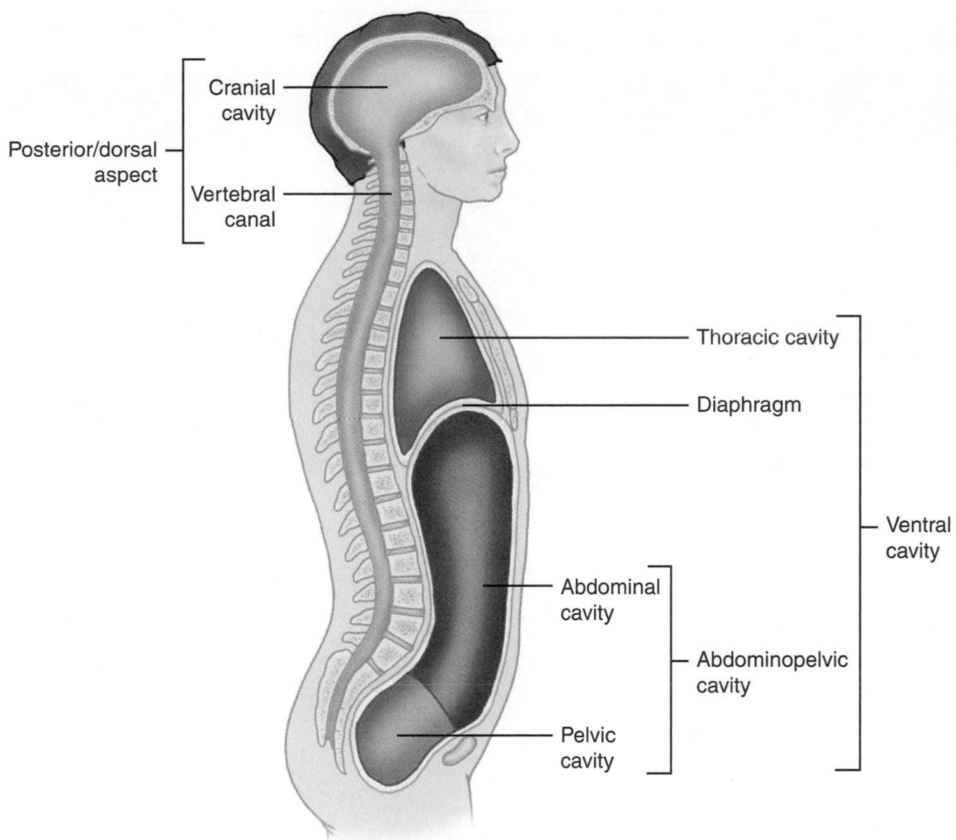

Figure 2.6: Body cavities

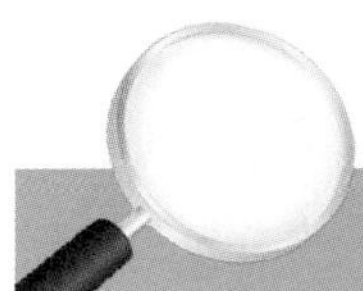

FOCUS POINT: The Spinal Canal

Although some anatomy textbooks identify a spinal *cavity,* others refer to this area as a *canal,* instead. In this textbook, the spinal canal is not considered a cavity.

Fill In the Blanks

Work with new words. Refer to the diagram of the body cavities to complete this exercise.

1. The brain is located in the ____________cavity.
2. The ____________ cavity contains the large intestines and the bladder.
3. The lungs, heart, esophagus, and lymph glands are located in the ____________ cavity.
4. The liver, gallbladder, stomach, and kidneys are found in the ____________ cavity.
5. The ____________ cavity houses the reproductive organs.

Locations and directions

Cavities, organs, and other body parts can also be identified by where they are situated (located)on or within the body. Medical terms for location are essential for accurate descriptions and reports. Study Table 2-8 and Figures 2-7 and 2-8 to learn these important terms.

TABLE 2-8: Medical Terms for Locations and Directions

Term	Combining Form	Meaning	Example
distal	dist(o)	farther from the center or point of attachment	The wrist is *distal* to the elbow.
proximal	proxim(o)	nearer the center or point of attachment	The elbow is *proximal* to the wrist.
superior	super(o)	upper; above other structures or parts	The nose is *superior* to the lips.
inferior or caudal	infer(o) caud(o)	lower; below other structures or parts; pertaining to the tail or the tail end	The lips are *inferior* to the nose.
anterior or ventral	anter(o) ventr(o)	front	The ribs are bones on the *anterior* side of the body.
posterior or dorsal	poster(o) dors(o)	back	The spinal column is on the *posterior* side of the body.
lateral	later(o)	toward the side	The hips are *lateral* to the abdomen.
medial	medi(o)	toward the center	The abdomen is *medial* to the hips.
superficial	superfic(i)	near the surface	A scar is a *superficial* injury.
deep	(none)	below the surface	The heart lies *deep* within the body.

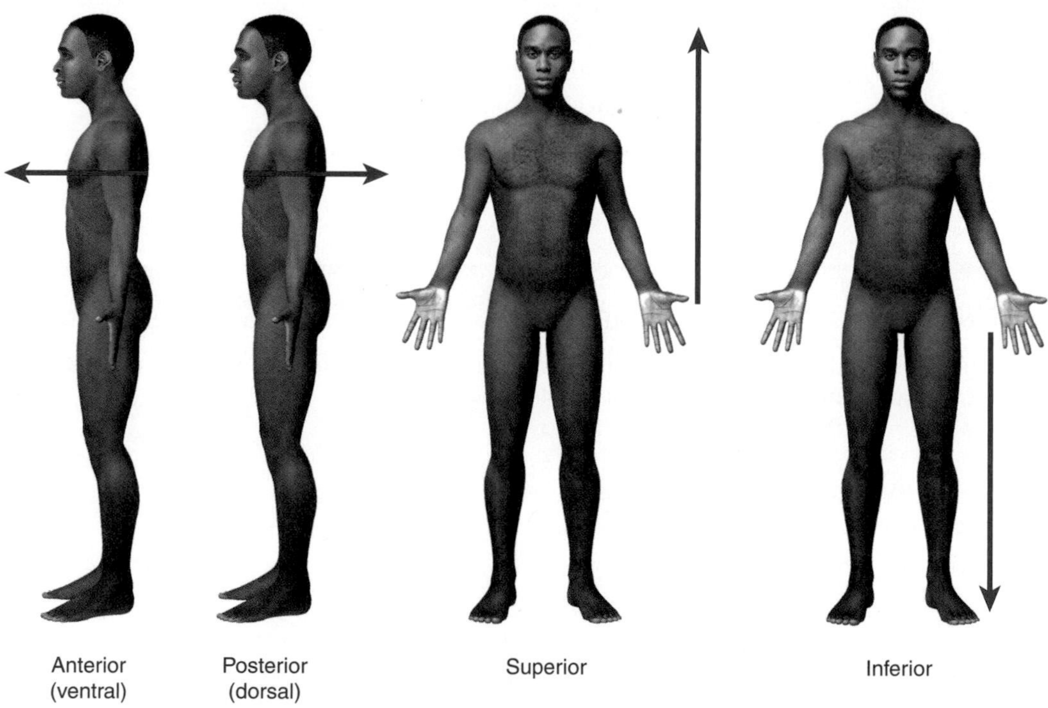

Figure 2.7: Body locations

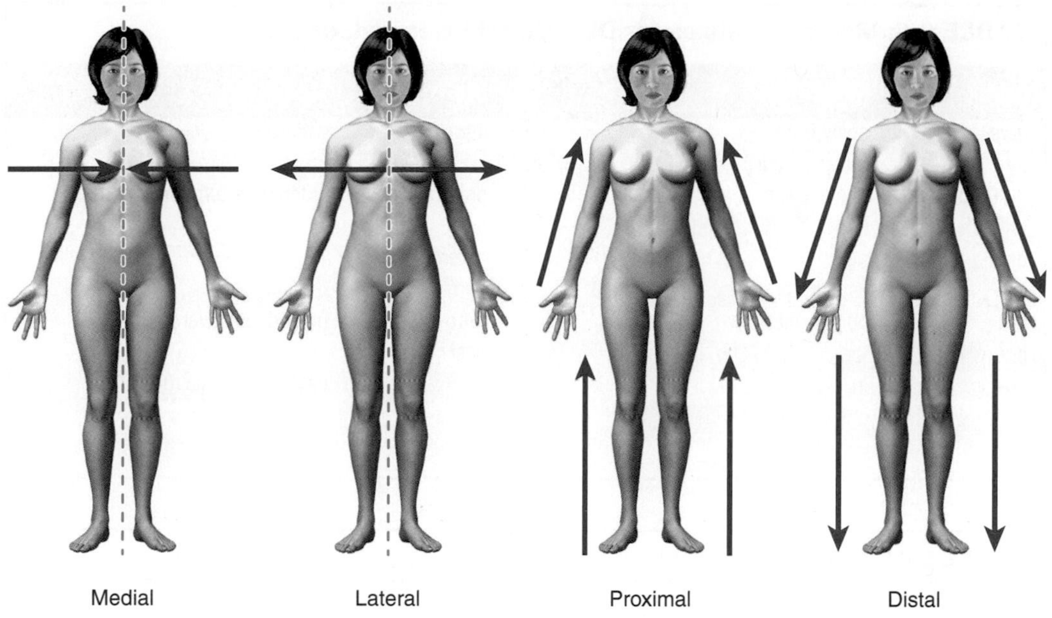

Figure 2.8: Body directions

Fill in the Blanks

Use terms to locate these body parts. The term **torso** refers to the trunk or main part of the body.

1. The thoracic cavity is located on the _______________ side of the body.
2. The head is _______________ to the torso.
3. The wrist is _______________ to the hand and _______________ to the shoulder.
4. The peritoneal cavity is _______________ to the thoracic cavity.
5. The navel is _______________ to the abdomen.
6. The arms are _______________ to the body.
7. The knees are _______________ to the torso.
8. The lungs are _______________ within the body.
9. A mole is _______________ to the body.
10. The cranial cavity is _______________ to the face.

Mix and Match

Find the antonym. Draw a line between the two terms that have opposite meanings.

1. superficial	ventral
2. anterior	posterior
3. dorsal	distal
4. inferior	deep
5. lateral	medial
6. proximal	superior

Prefixes that indicate direction, movement, and place

Medical prefixes combine with roots to give a more exact description of where an organ, body part, or structure is located or in which direction it can move. Table 2-9 highlights some of these prefixes.

Table 2-10 gives examples of how these prefixes are used to form terms that describe body movements. These are sometimes referred to as terms for range of motion, but they can be used to describe body movements in general.

TABLE 2-9: Medical Prefixes for Direction, Movement, or Place

Prefix	Meaning	Prefix	Meaning
ab/s-	away from	intra-	within
ad-	toward, near	ir-	against, toward, into, or not
cycl/e/o-	circle, cycle	pre-	anterior, before, or in front of
de-	down, away, or from	pro-	
dext-	right	anter/o-	
dia-	across, through	per/i-	through, around, or by means of
e-	out of, out from	retro-	behind, backward, after
es-	into	post-	
en-	in, on	ana-	upward, backward
ex-	out, off, without, or outside of	supra-	over, above
in-	not or in		

TABLE 2-10: Body Movements

abduction	a movement away from the base or core
adduction	a movement back in toward the base or core
extension	an opening or straightening of a limb or muscle
flexion	a bending or contraction of a limb or muscle
eversion	a turning movement away from the base or core; away from the center

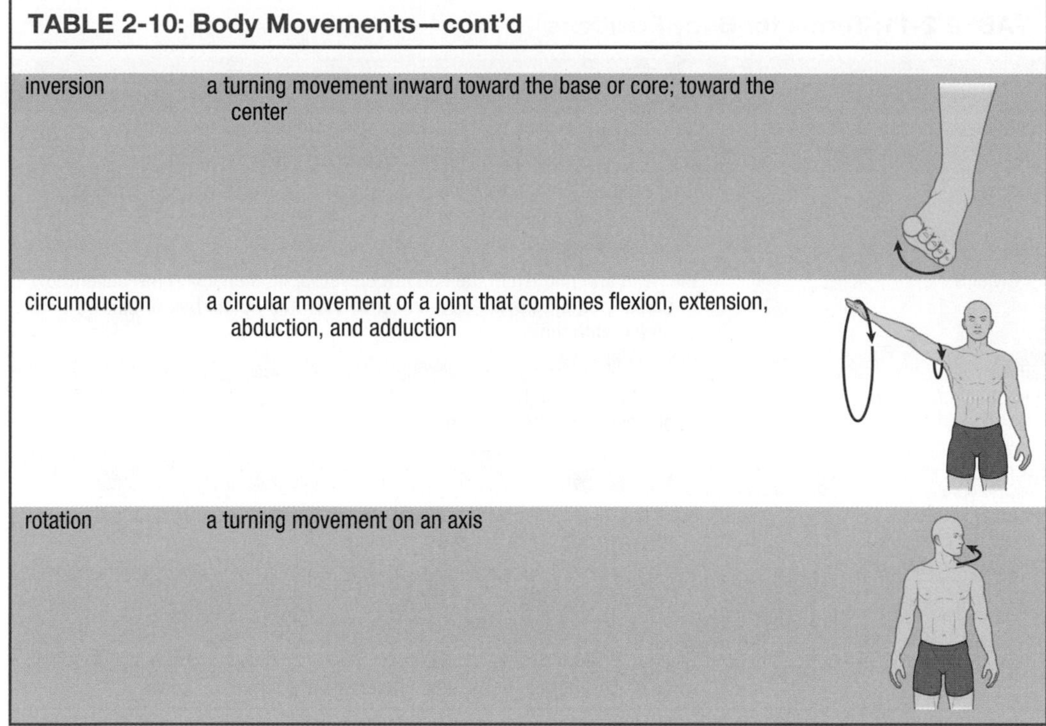

TABLE 2-10: Body Movements—cont'd

inversion	a turning movement inward toward the base or core; toward the center
circumduction	a circular movement of a joint that combines flexion, extension, abduction, and adduction
rotation	a turning movement on an axis

Let's Practice

The characters in the scenario that opened this chapter used many of the movements described in Table 2-9. Write the correct terms for the movements described.

1. When EMT Wallis turned to look at her colleague, Manuel, she had to perform which movement with her head?

    ____

2. EMT Manuel wanted his patient to step up into the rescue unit for further examination. What movements and body parts will the elderly gentleman have to use to accomplish this task?

    ____

3. EMT Manuel's patient had his hands clasped together. What movements are necessary to hold your hands in this position?

    ____

4. EMT Wallis reached out to touch her patient, Stevie-Rose Davis, and to guide Ms. Davis to the rescue vehicle. What movements and limbs did this EMT use?

    ____

5. Mr. Davis is sitting. What body movements are necessary to accomplish this position?

    ____

Medical terminology for positions

Positional terms are particularly useful when examining patients and recording findings. For example, placing a patient in a very specific position is often necessary to obtain clear, accurate, and precise x-rays or other radiographic images of an injury or disease. When victims are found at the scene of an accident or trauma, their position is noted before they are moved and treated. This information helps the health-care provider to understand what has happened and what organs or body parts may be involved.

During surgery, stays in the hospital, and treatment for medical conditions at home, proper positioning is crucial for the optimal functioning of the human body. Refer to Table 2-11 for a list of related terms and their meanings. Figures 2-9A through 2-9F provide visual representations to

TABLE 2-11: Terms for Body Positions

Term	Meaning
supine or horizontal recumbent	lying flat on the back with the arms at the sides or above the head
dorsal recumbent	lying on the back with the knees bent and the feet flat on the bed
prone	lying on the stomach with the head turned to one side and the arms at the sides or alongside the body
erect	vertical or straight
Fowler's	the head and mid leg of the bed are elevated, thus enabling the patient to partially sit up; the knees are slightly elevated by the bed or pillows underneath them
semi-Fowler's	only the head of the bed is elevated
knee–chest	on the knees with the chest and elbows on the bed; the head is turned to one side, and the legs are separated
Sim's	lying on the left side with right knee drawn up (flexed); the left arm is behind the body but the right arm is positioned as comfortably as possible
dorsal lithotomy	lying flat on the back with the knees bent, the legs separated, and the heels in stirrups at the end of the bed
lateral recumbent or recovery	rolled to one side with the superior knee moderately flexed and the superior elbow placed alongside the front of body; the mouth faces slightly downward, but the chin is positioned slightly upward
sitting	seated; in situ meaning *to be seated or settled in one position or place;* the torso is upright, and the hips and knees are flexed

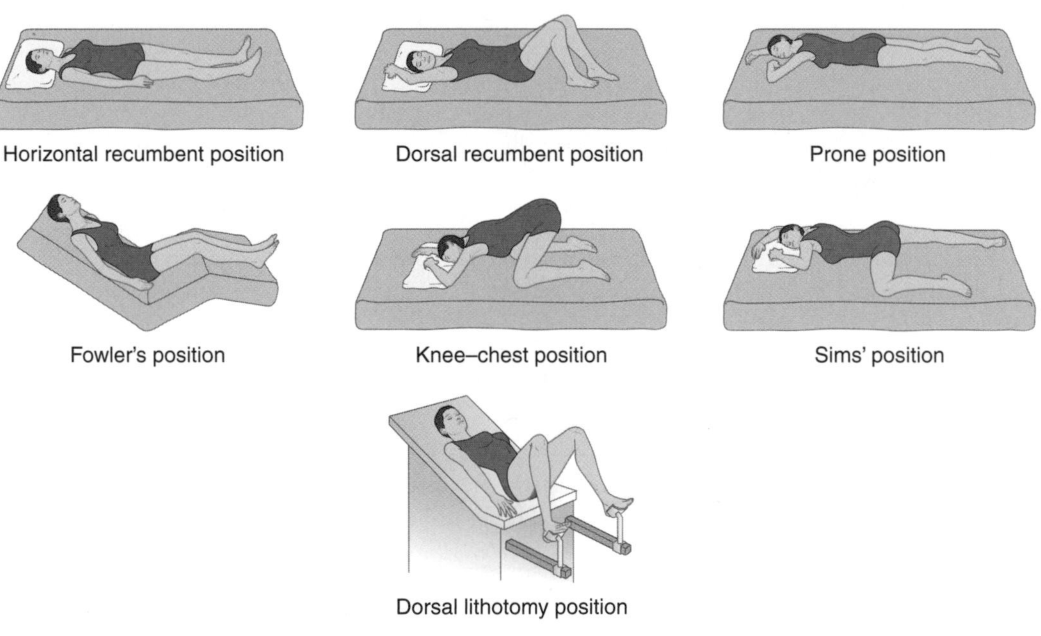

Figure 2.9: Body positions

support your understanding of each position. In later chapters, you will be given many examples of when and why different body positions are important.

Anatomical terms for planes of the body

Examinations are often performed by viewing the body from different planes or angles. There are three main planes: the coronal, transverse, and the sagittal. These planes separate the body into regions; see Figure 2-10.

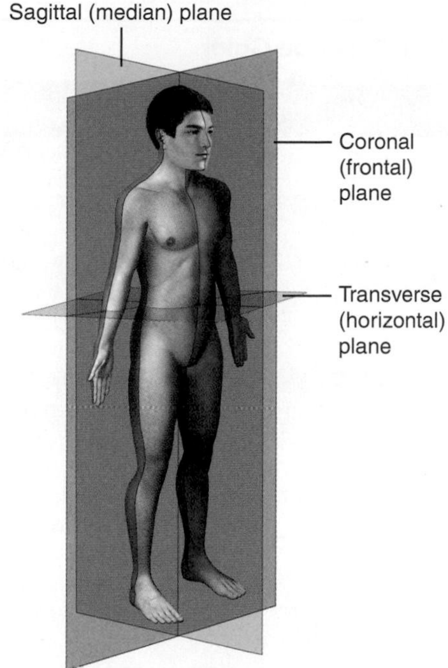

Figure 2.10: Anatomical planes

The **coronal plane** is also called the *frontal plane.* It divides the body into front and back (anterior and posterior).

The **transverse plane** is also called the *horizontal plane.* It divides the body crosswise into upper and lower (superior and inferior) halves horizontally at an invisible line at the middle of the body.

The **sagittal plane** is also called the *median plane.* It runs lengthwise, and it divides the body into two parts: the left and right lateral planes.

Let's Practice

For each body plane below, write an alternative term that has the same meaning.

1. transverse ______________________________
2. coronal ______________________________
3. sagittal ______________________________

Descriptors

In the health-care professions, the term **descriptor** is used to identify descriptive words that can be adjectives, adverbs, or phrases. Illnesses have descriptors; so do situations, events, and people in this context. The following sentences from the chapter-opening scenario contain descriptors:

As she did so, Wallis noted a fine tremor in the woman's arm and hand, and she also noticed some disfigurement of the woman's fingers.

EMT Wallis is using descriptive language as she assesses her patient's health status by observing the patient's outward and overt signs and symptoms.

Prefixes that describe

Many descriptors include medical prefixes that identify color, shape, size, quantity, and other important details. Prefixes that describe color are frequently used in medicine. As you study Table 2-12, notice that prefixes that originate in both the Greek and Latin languages are used to indicate colors.

Other prefixes can be used to describe quantity or size. Table 2-13 highlights some of these.

TABLE 2-12: Prefixes That Describe Color

Color	Prefix from Greek	Prefix from Latin	Medical Examples
black	melan/o- mal/o-		melanoma = a darkly pigmented tumor
blue	cyano-	liv-	cyanosis = a bluing of the lips and tissues as a result of lack of oxygen lividity = bluish skin discoloration from a bruise
gray; ash colored	polio-		polioclastic = destructive to the gray matter of the brain
green	chlor/chloro-		chloropia = a condition in which viewed objects appear green
orange-yellow; reddish yellow	cirrho-	icter-	cirrhosis = a disease of the liver that leads to a yellowish color of the skin and of the sclera of the eyes icterus = jaundice (the yellowing of the skin and sclera)
red	erythr/o-	rub/e/o- rubr- sang/ui	erythrocyte = a mature red blood cell rubella = a type of measles that produces a reddish rash sanguineous = bloody
pale, sallow, ashen		pall-	pallid = pale or lacking color
purple	porphyry-	purpr/purpureo-	porphyrias = disorders of porphyrin metabolism that can cause purplish rashes and lesions on the skin purpura = a type of rash caused by leakage from blood cells into the skin or mucous membranes that results in a purplish, bruise-like color
white	leuco/leuko-	albu-	leukocyte = white blood cell leukemia = a disease that depletes the red blood cells and leads to an abnormal increase in white blood cells albino = a person who is affected by the disease albinism, which involves an absence of any pigment or color
yellow	xantho-	flav-	xanthosis = a yellowing of the skin as a result of the excessive intake of yellow or orange vegetables or other foods such as carrots, squash, or egg yolks flavivirus: a family of viruses that includes yellow fever, which can lead to jaundice

TABLE 2-13: Prefixes That Describe Size and Quantity

Size	Prefix	Example
breadth or width	ampl-	ample = more than enough amplitude = abundance, fullness, breadth, or width
short, small, or brief	brach- brevis-	brachydactylia = an abnormal shortness of the fingers and toes brevicollis = a short neck
large, long, or inclusive	macr/o-	macrobrachia = an abnormally large or long arm
large	meg/a/alo-	megacolon = a condition in which the colon is greatly enlarged or dilated
small or very small	micr/o-	microcyte = a very small erythrocyte
small or lesser	min-	minimal = the smallest size or amount possible

TABLE 2-13: Prefixes That Describe Size and Quantity—cont'd

Quantity or Amount	Prefix	
all	pan-	panacea = a cure for all illnesses or troubles
many	multi- poly-	multiparity = referring to a woman who has been pregnant more than once (whether or not she gave birth) polypharmacy = the prescribing or use of multiple pharmacological agents (medications)
one or single	uni-	unibasal = only one base
only, sole, or singular	mon/a/er/o-	monocular = affecting only one eye
two, twice, or double	bi- di-	bilateral = encompassing or involving both sides dioxide = containing two oxygen molecules
ten	deca-	decagram = 10 grams
one tenth	deci-	decigram = 1/10 of a gram
hundred	hect/o-	hectogram = 100 grams
one hundredth	cent/i	centigram = 1/100 of a gram
one thousand	kilo-	kilogram = 1000 grams
one thousandth	mill/e/i/o-	milligram = 1/1000 of a gram
one half	hemi- semi-	hemisphere = half of a sphere semicircular = half of a circle
equal or same	equi-	equilibrium = a state of balance in which contending forces are equal
whole, complete, holistic, or entire	hol-	holotonia = a muscle spasm of the entire body
few, scant, or not many	oligo-	oliguria = a condition that describes a very low output of urine per day

Fill in the Blanks

In this exercise, use prefixes to describe medical situations. Fill in the blanks by adding the appropriate prefix to the word or word part provided.

1. Lack of oxygen gave the patient a _________*tic* look.
2. Red blood cells are more properly called _________*cytes.*
3. The study of tiny organisms such as bacteria is called _________*biology.*
4. _________*brachia* is the term for an arm of abnormal size or length.
5. The sagittal plane divides the body into _________*spheres.*
6. To assess circulation, pulses and blood pressure are often taken _________*laterally.*

Putting it all together

Like any language, medical language is a system for conveying messages. It includes specialized terminology, abbreviations, and jargon for naming and describing body parts, body locations, medical conditions, and health-care procedures. (The term **jargon** refers to slang words that are used by a specific group of professionals.)

However, learning a language involves more than just learning its vocabulary. Like other languages, medical language also has its own grammar and syntax, which are the rules for how words are ordered and arranged into phrases and sentences. Table 2-14 compares sentences that are written in everyday English grammar and syntax with how the same information would be communicated in medical language in a patient's record.

In the patient scenarios that you've read and listened to so far, you've heard dialogues that show how health-care professionals put medical language to use in on-the-job situations. You'll be reading and listening to many more dialogues as you progress in your knowledge of medical language. The more experience that you have with how the language is used in "real life," the easier it will be for you to remember it.

TABLE 2-14: Comparison: Everyday English Grammar and Syntax versus Medical Language Grammar and Syntax

Everyday English Grammar and Syntax	Medical Language Grammar and Syntax
He's had the measles for at least a week now.	Measles. Onset × 1wk.
She miscarried her first child, but she has had three children since then.	Para 3, Gravida 1 or Para 3, Grava 4, Abortus 1 (miscarriage) or GPA: G4, P3, A1
The patient knows what time it is, where she is, and who she is.	Oriented × 3.

CHAPTER SUMMARY

Chapter 2 has introduced the medical terminology used to name and describe body structures and their functions. There have been opportunities to work with medical terminology through word-building exercises that reinforce the recognition of word parts as an aid to understanding full terms. Anatomy and physiology have been introduced, in addition to the language that involves anatomical locations, movements, and the planes of the human body.

See How Much You've Learned

For audio exercises, visit **http://www.MedicalLanguageLab.com.** 

FOCUS POINT: Patient or Client?

The term *patient* is often used interchangeably with the term *client.*

Chapter 2 has introduced you to some medical abbreviations. These abbreviations have been organized into a study table here for quick reference. You will recognize some of these terms immediately, and some will reappear throughout the following chapters with more explanation and application.

TABLE 2-15: Medical Abbreviations: Review

Medical Abbreviation	Full Term	Medical Abbreviation	Full Term
DNA	deoxyribonucleic acid	RNA	ribonucleic acid

Key Terms

anatomy
aspect
cavity
cell membrane
cell
connective tissues
coronal plane
cranial
cytoplasm
deoxyribonucleic acid (DNA)
descriptor
dorsal
element
epithelial tissues
jargon
membranes
muscle tissues
nerve tissues
nucleus
organ systems
organelles
organs
parietal
pericardial membranes
peritoneal membranes
physiology
pleural membranes
ribonucleic acid (RNA)
sagittal plane
spinal
structure
tissues
torso
transverse plane
ventral
vertebral
visceral
vital

CHAPTER REVIEW

Critical Thinking

Answer the following questions. Use medical terminology. Share your answers with a peer, if possible, before looking at the Answer Key.

1. Study the body positions shown in Figure 2-10. Which one do you think is the best choice for a patient who has difficulty breathing?

____

2. What is the term for the plane that separates the body into upper and lower (superior and inferior) planes?

____

3. Which medical term refers to something that is away from the core or the main point of attachment?

____

4. Both Mr. and Mrs. Davis need to get into the rescue unit vehicle for further assessment and transport to the hospital. To step up onto something, it is necessary to bend at the joint. What is the term for this movement?

____

Break It Down

Break these words down into their component parts of prefix-root-suffix, as applicable. Name each element.

1. irradiate _______________
2. disfigurement _______________
3. reproductive _______________

Translate the Terminology

Use your new skills to decipher medical language. On the line provided, explain what is being said to the best of your ability. Try to do so without the use of a medical dictionary.

1. She proceeded to *palpate the cranium* and *cervical spine* of her patient.

____

2. Since Mrs. Davis was *ambulant,* Wallis touched her elbow and gently began to direct her toward a grassy spot on the median of Shawnee Boulevard.

____

3. She gently examined the bones of the face proceeding from the *proximal* point of the nose at the brow line and working outward from there for *bilateral* assessment.

____

Label the Body Cavities

Write the name of each body cavity on the appropriate line. Begin at the top left of the figure, working down, then around to the right.

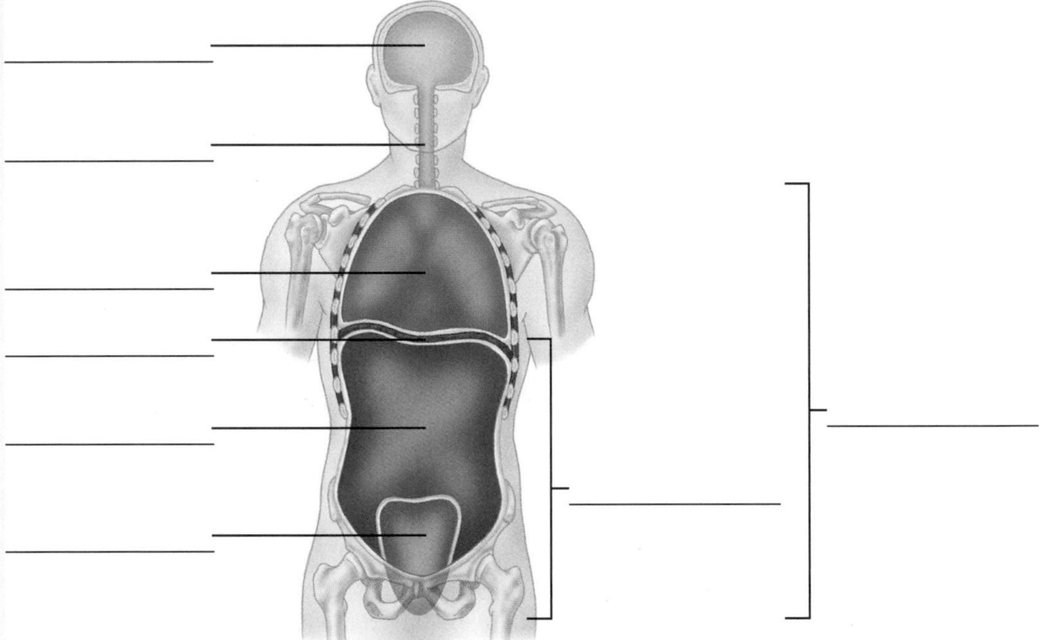

Name the Root

Read the definition, and then write the appropriate root.

1. This system is responsible for the continuous movement of blood throughout the body. The root of this word means *to go around.* The root is ______________________.
2. This system secretes hormones within the body. The root is ______________________.
3. The root of this word means *to cover.* We usually refer to it as "the skin." The root is ______________________.
4. The root of this word means *the lining of a cavity in the lower abdominal region.* The root is ______________________.

Name the Prefix

Read the definition, and then write one or more prefixes that add this meaning to a root.

1. red ______________________________
2. outside of, outer ______________________________
3. not ______________________________
4. many ______________________________
5. one, only ______________________________

Mix and Match

Match the term for a type of movement or range of motion in the left column with its opposite in the right column. Draw a line to connect the terms.

1. abduct	median/medial
2. flexion	posterior
3. proximal	dorsal
4. lateral	adduct
5. ventral	distal
6. anterior	extension

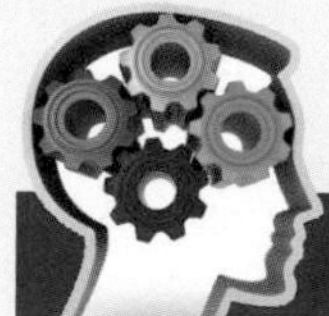

MEMORY MAGIC

Remembering body locations, planes, and positions requires using your visual memory. When the eye is exposed frequently to images, it "takes pictures" of the images (and the words associated with them) and files them into the memory. This requires frequent exposure to the target images. In this case, you have two targets: body organs and planes.

Complete this activity by yourself, and do it freehand. You will need two index cards or pieces of paper that are approximately 3 inches by 5 inches in size.

Draw a diagram of the human body. It can be as simple as you like.
Now, sketch the major organs of the body where they belong and label them.
Check your answers using the diagrams in this chapter.
Keep this card in your pocket or taped to your refrigerator or mirror, where you will see it frequently for at least 7 days.
Draw another diagram of the human body. It can be the same as the first, but place it on a new card.
Now draw lines that divide the body by planes, and label each plane.
Check your answers using the diagrams in this chapter.
Keep this card in your pocket or taped to your refrigerator or mirror, where you will see it frequently for at least 7 days. However, do not put it in the same place as your other card.

Glory Loeppky is a 32-year-old married woman. Her husband is Gil Loeppky. Mrs. Loeppky is currently 7½ months pregnant. This is the couple's first baby, and they are very happy about it. Mrs. Loeppky works as a receptionist at a local business. Today, she's been in a motor vehicle accident.

Mrs. Loeppky cannot remember all of the details of the accident. However, she recalls vaguely that the door to the truck fell open. She got out, and she called for Gil. She saw that he was unconscious and bleeding, still behind the wheel. She hurried to her husband's side of the cab, having to go around a power pole embedded in the front of the vehicle. She reached his door and tried to open it. She desperately wanted to pull Gil to safety, but she couldn't do it. She remembers suddenly crying out in pain. The next thing she knew, she was sitting on the grass near the truck. Someone was sitting at her side and had wrapped a blanket over her shoulders. A man in a uniform was talking to her, and eventually she was put on a stretcher and taken away from the scene in an ambulance.

The paramedic of Ambulance NM421 deemed Mrs. Loeppky to be a Level 2 priority for care. Through Emergency Dispatch, the nearest appropriate facility was found and Mrs. Loeppky was transported to Fayette General Hospital for urgent care. On arrival, she would receive further medical assessment and treatment. Her priorities of care were determined as a deep left leg laceration and a possible fracture to her left hand. In addition, the status of her fetus would be monitored and the potential for labor and delivery assessed.

Patient Update

"Ma'am, how are you doing?" asked a physician as Mrs. Loeppky was wheeled into the emergency room. Mrs. Loeppky was sitting up in a semi-Fowler's position, and she could see the busy department. Beside her, an emergency medical technician and his partner were pushing the stretcher.

"Um, I don't know. Am I okay? Is my baby okay? Where's Gil?" Mrs. Loeppky looked around. She saw that a nurse had joined them and noticed that the nurse's nametag read "Teresa, LPN." Mrs. Loeppky asked, "Nurse, where is my husband? Do you know? Is Gil okay?"

"Gil's her husband," interjected a paramedic. "He's gone to Okla Trauma Center. This is Glory Loeppky. She's 7½ months pregnant. Incontinent at the scene. No evidence of labor. Fetus's vitals seem okay. Deep laceration to upper left thigh. Tourniquet in place. BP is high, and so is pulse: thready and tachycardic at 108. Resps are quick but not abnormally so for the situation. Pain and localized swelling to left thumb. Might be a fracture. Appears to have fainted at the scene. Out × 3 or 4 minutes according to a bystander who stopped to help her. No evidence of head trauma. Oriented × 3. We've started her on oxygen, 2 liters per minute."

"Mrs. Loeppky, your husband is at another hospital right now. You're here at Fayette General," the licensed practical nurse, Teresa said reassuringly.

"Okay, fellas, thanks. We'll take it from here," said the physician to the ambulance team as they transferred Mrs. Loeppky onto a hospital stretcher in an ER bay. They placed Mrs. Loeppky in a supine position for her initial assessment. A number of other hospital staff appeared. Someone put two pillows under Mrs. Loeppky's head to prop her up just slightly and to take the weight of her pregnancy off her lower back. She groaned loudly throughout the move.

"Here's her purse. ID is in it, and an insurance card with an HMO," said another paramedic, as he and his partner took leave of the situation and moved off to Admissions to file their reports.

"Oh, my baby. Check my baby. Is my baby okay?" Mrs. Loeppky asked in a soft but anxious voice. As she spoke, she ran her hands over her swollen belly.

"I'm Dr. Abrams," said the emergency physician. "I just need to feel for your baby, ma'am. How far along are you?" He began to gently palpate Mrs. Loeppky's belly and then to listen with his stethoscope.

"7½ months," Mrs. Loeppky responded. "Is my baby okay?" As she waited for the answer, the treatment team began to take off her sandals and slacks, and someone helped her out of her blouse. A nurse on her right side wrapped the blood pressure cuff around her arm and clipped something to the middle finger of her right hand. These devices were both attached to a large monitor at the bedside. Digital numbers appeared on a monitor. Mrs. Loeppky looked around her; she was confused by the bustling of the treatment team.

"Hi," said the nurse at her side, noticing her perplexed look. "I'm Marnie, and I'm an RN here at Fayette General. We're going to take good care of you and your baby. This machine reads your vital signs."

"Babe looks okay," stated the doctor to both the team and the patient. "Mrs. Loeppky, are you having any labor pains? Has your water broken?" he asked, continuing his examination below her belly now and noticing that the skin of her inner thigh and pelvic area was damp. A nurse quietly showed him the litmus test she'd just taken. It was negative. He nodded.

"No, no labor, no, I don't think so. I'm just worried that maybe my baby is hurt or frightened. Did my baby get hurt in the accident?" The doctor continued his examination with the assistance of the nurses.

"Ma'am, your baby looks fine right now, and it doesn't look like you're in labor. We're going to do a few more tests just to be sure. Nurse, get hold of Obstetrics. Let's get a fetal monitor and order an ultrasound," he said. "But now, let's have a look at that leg wound," he said. He began unwrapping the dressing and tourniquet put in place by the emergency responders. Immediately blood began to flow at the site, and Mrs. Loeppky groaned loudly in pain. Nurses rushed to staunch the blood flow with gauze.

"Tell me where you feel the pain," said the nurse beside Mrs. Loeppky.

"Oh, my leg! What's happening to my leg?" Mrs. Loeppky said to the doctor. He explained how the sudden pain was related to the release of the tourniquet and the return of blood flow to this deep laceration.

"I'll want a complete blood count, hematocrit, and HGB," the doctor ordered. "Missed the artery, but it's deep. We're going to want to start some antibiotics, but let's just hold off for a bit till the lab work's in."

"The call's in. The Lab will be here in a minute, Doctor," replied one of the nurses. The patient grimaced while the team worked on the wound. As this was being done, Marnie, the RN, examined Mrs. Loeppky's hands. She noticed that the left hand was particularly red and swollen at the base of the thumb and that a bluish discoloration was extending up the patient's forearm. Marnie touched the area gently, and the patient startled and cried out.

"Looks like this thumb might be dislocated, if not fractured, Dr. Abrams," reported Marnie.

"Right. I'll get to it in a minute," he replied in a calm, businesslike voice. "Raza, is there a problem with the IV? We need it now," he said to one of the other nurses. The nurse replied that he didn't want to put a line into the injured hand or arm, and he didn't think using the arm with the automatic blood pressure cuff on it was wise, either. He wanted direction from the doctor.

"Okay, try the dorsum of the foot for now," advised Dr. Abrams, and the nurse moved to the patient's feet to insert the IV catheter. "We'll need to suture this wound right now," he said, and the team went to work.

Reflective Questions

Reflect on the story that you've just read.

1. Where has Mrs. Loeppky been transported?

   ____

2. In the emergency department, the treatment team is attending to three priorities during the assessment of this patient. What are they?

   ____

3. Are Mr. and Mrs. Loeppky being treated in the same facility?

   ____

4. What type of examinations or tests has the doctor ordered?

   ____

5. At the end of the scenario, the team has gone to work on something. What is that?

   ____

For audio exercises, visit **http://www.MedicalLanguageLab.com.** 

Learning Objectives

After reading Chapter 3, you will be able to do the following:

- Recognize and use medical language for physical assessment.
- Appreciate the education and training of nurses.
- Recognize and use medical terms for the muscular system.
- Recognize medical terminology related to the injury of the muscular system.
- Recognize and use medical terminology related to blood.
- Have a beginning knowledge of pregnancy and maternal health assessment.
- Understand the basic concepts and terms for sonography/ultrasound.
- Appreciate the education and training of sonographers.

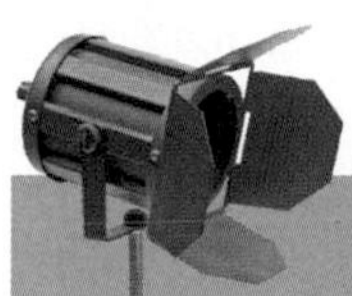

CAREER SPOTLIGHT: Nurses

Nurses play a key role in initial and ongoing patient assessment in all health-care situations. Of all of the health professions, nurses statistically spend the most time performing direct patient contact. Nursing education prepares nurses to assess, treat, and care for patients in the hospital, the community, and at home.

Nurses function within a scope of practice. This means that certain activities and practices are clearly outlined and defined as being within the skill set of nurses. An example of this scope of practice is that a registered nurse can assist with surgery but cannot actually perform surgery; surgery is within the scope of the physician.

Nurses also abide by the standards set by their regulatory bodies. Standards are clear descriptions of the focus of nursing activities. They identify who the recipients of the activities can and will be, and they set the criteria for professional accountability and responsibility.

The scope of practice and the standards are regulated by a specific regulatory organization, legislation such as a Nurse Practice Act, or both.

Finally, nurses are required to abide by a Code of Ethics that is set by their specific regulatory bodies and that is related to professional conduct and patient care.

There are three types of nurses in the United States.*

Registered Nurse (RN): RNs require knowledge and skills of the science and art of caring, including clinical judgment, critical thinking, and problem solving. At the entry level, they complete a 2-year associate degree, a 3-year diploma, or a 4-year baccalaureate degree in nursing. They also successfully complete a national licensing examination. RNs are regulated with regard to their scope, standards, and ethics of practice by national and state nursing boards. RNs may choose to expand their knowledge and skills by studying in master's degree programs or attaining their doctoral degrees (PhD, EdD, DNS, or DNP). At each level of education, the RN maintains the "R" in the title *RN;* it is a permanent part of the RN's professional identity.

Registered Nurse Practitioner (RN, APN): The nurse practitioner is an advanced practice nurse (APN) with a good deal of autonomy (independence) in the areas of diagnosing, clinical decision making, treatment, and care. Many nurse practitioners are able to prescribe medications. In addition to achieving a minimum of a master's degree in nursing, this type of nurse must successfully pass the American Academy of Nurse Practitioners Advanced Nursing examination to be certified.

Licensed Practical Nurse (LPN): LPNs focus on the direct care of patients, specifically at the bedside, within their own scope of practice; this is generally similar to but more limited

Continued

than the scope of practice of an RN. A diploma or certificate program of at least 1 year or 1100 hours of classroom and clinical experience are the common standards of education for this type of nurse. LPNs must also pass a licensing examination for admission into the profession. LPNs are sometimes referred to as licensed vocational nurses (LVNs).

In Canada and a number of other countries around the world, Registered Psychiatric Nurses also exist. These nurses specialize in the care of patients with mental health concerns, mental illness, addictions, and psychological and emotional disorders and challenges across the life span. These individuals complete 4-year baccalaureate degree programs to attain designation as a BPN or a BScPN. Psychiatric nurses in the United States are generally qualified at a master's degree level.

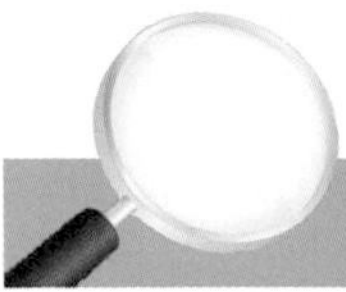

FOCUS POINT: Certified Nursing Assistant

A certified nursing assistant (CNA) is not a nurse. A CNA is a care aide who provides direct care to patients, such as assisting with activities of daily living (i.e., bathing, toileting, feeding, bed making, spending time with clients, and so on). CNAs are invaluable members of many care teams, and they come to know their clients very well. To become a CNA, most States require training from an approved school, at which the teachers are most often RNs. In many states, CNAs must successfully pass an examination to become certified. CNAs might also be called *long-term care aides, residential care aides, home health aides,* or *personal care attendants.*

Emergency Assessment

We begin the chapter with an introduction to the language of assessment that is used in the emergency department. When patients arrive, they are assessed to determine treatment priorities; this process is called **triage.** A quick overall assessment is done, and this focuses on airway, breathing,

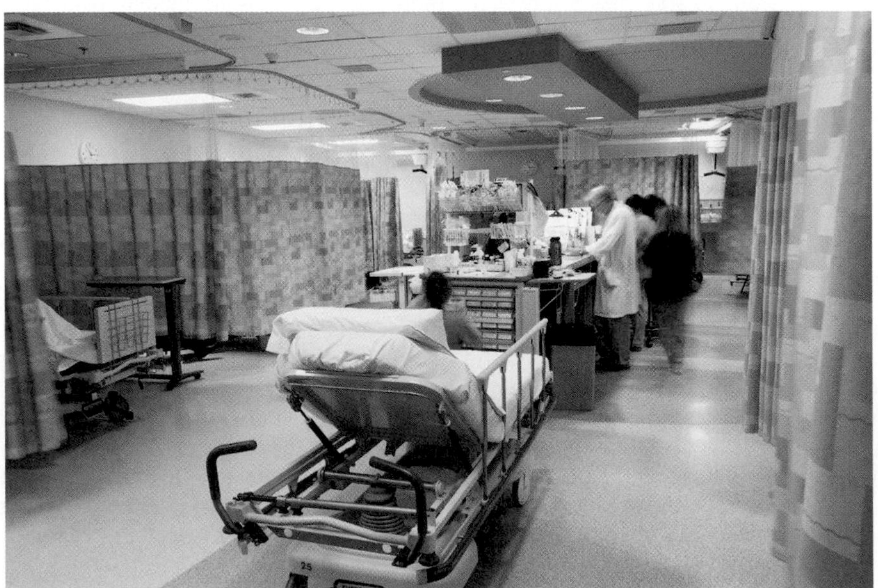

Figure 3.1: Hospital emergency department (© Thinkstock/Getty Images/Jupiterimages)

and circulation (i.e., the **ABCs**). This assessment is completed by the emergency responders on the scene of an accident or medical emergency. However, the ABCs become a priority once again on the patient's admission to a hospital. If the patient's ABCs are sufficiently stable to proceed, then the next step in assessment is to attend to the presenting complaint or health issue. Mrs. Loeppky has been triaged by the emergency medical technicians and the emergency department physician.

A: Airway: The patient was able to talk, so the airway was not blocked.

B: Breathing: The emergency medical technician reported that Mrs. Loeppky's respiration rate was a bit high. To assist her with breathing, she was given oxygen.

C: Circulation: Attention was turned to this priority of care: the open wound on the patient's thigh that had a tourniquet in place to prevent further bleeding. This meant that circulation was temporarily impeded in that extremity. The emergency team's goal would be to restore circulation to the limb.

Mrs. Loeppky's unborn child was also triaged, but in a general way. The status of the fetus's health was quickly assessed and found to not be urgent or emergent, so the treatment team was able to move on with the mother's assessment.

A **patient complaint** is the patient's subjective, personal report of why he or she is seeking medical attention. It can also be referred to as the *presenting complaint,* the *current complaint,* the *chief complaint,* or the **presenting condition.** After this condition is identified, the physician and treatment team perform a focused examination to determine the severity of the situation. This assessment entails acquiring laboratory test results, x-rays, and other tests as warranted by the nature of the medical condition. Treatment then ensues.

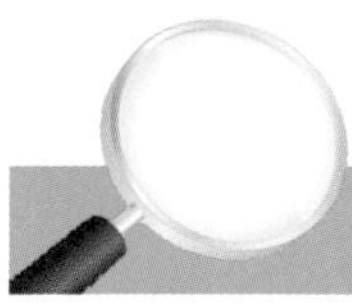

FOCUS POINT: *Emergent* vs. *Urgent*

There are three levels of acuity in hospital emergency departments.

Level 1: Emergent. This patient requires assessment, treatment, and reassessment immediately to save his or her life. Examples of health conditions that require emergency care are head injury with which there is a coma or a prolonged state of unconsciousness, respiratory or cardiac arrest, massive bleeding, severe burns, and so on.

Level 2: Urgent. This patient requires quick assessment, treatment, and reassessment within a period of approximately 20 minutes to 2 hours. Examples of urgent medical cases include chest pain, shortness of breath, and maternity and delivery issues.

Level 3: Non-urgent. This patient has an injury or condition that does not require immediate or quick attention; however, they do require treatment in an emergency room setting. Examples of these conditions include bone fractures and sprains.

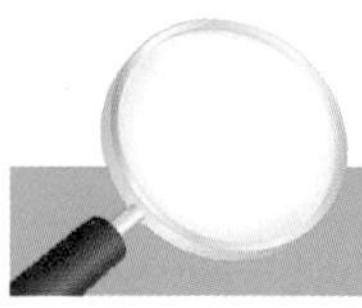

FOCUS POINT: *Fetus* or *Baby*?

A number of terms can be used to refer to an unborn child. The choice of a term is often dependent on the situation. Medically speaking, the term *embryo* is used during the earliest days and weeks of pregnancy. The embryo stage of development begins four days after conception and continues until week 8. After that and for the rest of the pregnancy, the medical term for the unborn child is *fetus*. Technically, the fetus is not referred to as a baby until birth. For some people, however, the terms *embryo* and *fetus* seem too coldly clinical. They prefer to refer to the unborn child as a *baby* or *babe*, even before it is born. In your professional contact with pregnant patients, it is best practice to follow the lead of the patient and to refer to the unborn child in the same terms used by the parent.

The language of emergency assessment

The care team in an emergency department functions like a well-oiled machine or a well-choreographed dance troupe. Health and allied-health professionals work together to provide assessment and treatment for patients who are in urgent or emergent health situations. On arrival, the ambulance attendants or emergency medical personnel who are transporting the patient provide a verbal report of the patient's medical status. The doctors and nurses then take over, completing the primary physical assessment of the patient. They attend to wounds and other presenting complaints, take vital signs, collect a medical history, and initiate treatment. They also speak to each other using abbreviations and jargon that are common to health care, including *STAT* (immediately), *PRN* (as needed), and *IV* (intravenous).

To understand this language, it is important to learn frequently used key terms, concepts, and word parts. Let's begin with the word parts used in the terms *urgent, emergent,* and *present.*

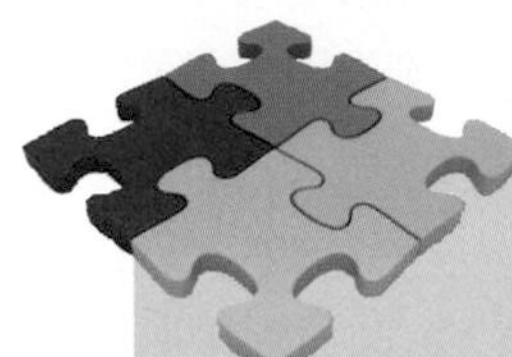

WORD BUILDING: Formula for Creating Words with the Combining Forms *Emerg, Urg(e),* and *Present*

1. emerg: a combining form originating in Latin meaning *unforeseen or suddenly arising, appearing, or making itself known.* NOTE: The term *Emerg* (capitalized) is the short form that is used in health care to identify the emergency room or the emergency department. This abbreviated form is never used to indicate an emergency situation.

emerg + e = *emerge*

Definition: to awaken, rise, or appear. *verb*

Example: When the patient *emerges* from his medically induced coma, he will not have any cognitive impairment.

emerg + ence = *emergence*

Definition: appearance or arrival. (The suffix *-ence* means *the act, state, or condition of.*) *noun*

Example: The *emergence* of the norovirus in multiple countries attests to the fact that viruses can be global.

emerg + ency = *emergency*

Definition: an unexpected serious event that requires immediate assessment and medical intervention. (The suffix *-ency* means *the state or condition of.*) *noun* or *adjective*

Example: Glory Loeppky was in a car accident today and required *emergency* assessment and treatment for her injuries at the scene.

emerg + ent = *emergent*

Definition: sudden and unforeseen or growing out from. (The suffix *-ent* means *having the characteristics of.*) *adjective*

Example: If Mrs. Loeppky suddenly goes into labor, her medical status will change from urgent to *emergent.*

2. urg(e): a combining form of the Latin word *urgere* meaning *to push, to press, or a strong need to act.*

urg + ency = *urgency*

Definition: a condition in which quick or immediate attention is important or necessary. (The suffix *-ency* means *the state or condition of.*) *noun*

Example: Bladder control issues during pregnancy and later in life can lead to a sense of *urgency* to void.

urg + ent = *urgent*

Definition: requiring quick or immediate attention or action. (The suffix *-ent* means *having the characteristics of.*) *adjective*

Example: En route to the hospital, a woman in labor may be in *urgent* need of attention. However, if she begins to deliver the baby in the car, this is an *emergent* situation: it is an emergency.

urg + ent + ly = *urgently*

Definition: acting without delay. (The suffix *-ly* means *how something is done* or *in a certain way.*) *adverb*

Example: The urge to vomit causes a person to *urgently* seek a toilet.

3. present: a root word originating in Latin meaning *to give, pose (i.e., a question), show, appear, introduce,* or *be in attendance with others.*

present + ation = *presentation*

Definition: appearance. (The suffix *-ation* means *the act or process of.*) *noun*

Example: In obstetrics (i.e., maternity and childbirth), the term *presentation* refers to the position of the fetus when it is examined through the vagina.

present + ed = *presented*

Definition: appeared. (The suffix *-ed* turns this verb into a past-tense form.) *verb*

Example: The patient *presented* to the emergency department with a complaint of abdominal pain.

present + ing = *presenting*

Definition: introducing, giving, or attending. (The suffix *-ing* makes this a present participle of the verb *to present.*) *adjective*

Example: The *presenting* evidence leads the doctor to determine that the patient's life is not at risk.

Let's Practice

Begin to use new terminology by choosing terms to complete the following sentences. By doing so, you will become more familiar with terms in their proper context.

1. The assessment of a ________________ in the emergency room begins with the ABCs.
2. The ________________ process identifies priorities of care, which are the injuries or conditions that should be dealt with first.
3. Another way to say that a patient arrives at the emergency department with a health concern is to say that the patient ________________ to the emergency department with one.
4. The letter *C* in the ABCs stands for ________________.
5. A ________________ nurse has a larger scope of practice than an LPN.

Fill in the Blanks

Fill in each blank by writing a word that begins with *emerg, urg(e),* or *present* to create a logical sentence. Work on your own or with a partner, if you can.

1. Marnie is a registered nurse who works in the ________________ department at Fayette General Hospital.
2. Mrs. Loeppky ________________ wants to know if her unborn child is okay.
3. The ambulance crew describes Mrs. Loeppky's ________________ condition to the emergency department doctor.
4. Mrs. Loeppky's health status is not critical; her life is not a risk, so she did not go to a trauma center, as her husband did. Mrs. Loeppky's level of medical acuity is ________________, not ________________.

5. Mrs. Loeppky _______________ to the emergency department with a deep laceration in her leg and a possibly fractured thumb.

Key terms: emergency room

Working together to care for a patient in an urgent or emergent situation requires clear and concise communication by the members of the treatment team. Recall this scene from the opening scenario of the chapter, when the EMT gave a report of his patient to the ER physician. Key terms and concepts are highlighted below.

> "...7 ½ months pregnant. *Incontinent* at the scene. No evidence of labor. Fetus's *vitals* seem okay. *Deep laceration* to upper left thigh. *Tourniquet* in place. *BP* is high, and so is pulse: *thready* and *tachycardic* at 108. *Resps* are quick but not abnormally so for the situation. Pain and *localized* swelling *to left thumb,* might be a *fracture.* Appears to have fainted at the scene. Out × 3 or 4 minutes according to a bystander who stopped to help her. No evidence of head trauma. *Oriented × 3.* We've started her on oxygen, 2 liters per minute."

How many of these terms and abbreviations did you already know or figure out on your own? Check your understanding as you read the meanings of these key terms:

incontinent: involuntarily emptying the bladder

vitals: vital signs: temperature, pulse, respirations, and blood pressure (TPR and BP)

deep laceration: a cut or incision that goes beyond the skin and into the musculature or organs

tourniquet: a device or tool such as a long strip of elastic or cloth that is used to staunch or stop bleeding

BP: blood pressure

thready: describes a pulse that is fine or barely perceptible

tachycardic: referring to a faster-than-usual pulse rate or heart rate, which is measured in beats per minute; a normal pulse rate for a person who has been sitting for a period of time (i.e., riding in an ambulance) should be between 88 and 100 beats per minute (bpm)

resps: respirations (breaths) per minute

localized: appearing in only one specific area or location

to left thumb: the word *to* is frequently used in medicine in place of the word *of*

fracture: a break or a broken bone *out × 3 or 4 minutes:* unconscious for 3 or 4 minutes; just as it is in math, the symbol × is used as an abbreviated way of saying "times"; in this context, "times" refers to duration or how long the patient was out

oriented × 3: the three spheres of orientation are normal: the patient is aware of person, place, and time and she is not confused; in this example, Glory Loeppky has been evaluated and is aware of who she is, she knows that she is in the company of ambulance and hospital staff, and we are left to understand that she also knows the approximate time of day or the day of the week

Right Word or Wrong Word: *Oriented* or *Orientated*?

These two words are often used interchangeably. Is this correct? Do these words actually mean the same thing?

The language of blood and bleeding

Mrs. Loeppky's most urgent problem in the ER was bleeding from a deep laceration in her leg. No matter where you work in health care, blood and bleeding are major topics of concern. This section will help you develop a vocabulary related to blood.

Read the following update about Mrs. Loeppky's condition.

Patient Update

To examine Mrs. Loeppky's leg wound, Dr. Abrams inspected it first with the tourniquet in place. The nurse removed the soiled dressing and swabbed the wound bed with gauze to dry it. Dr. Abrams explored for damage to tissues, muscles, and blood vessels. He determined that the major artery of the leg, the femoral artery, had not been severed, although other minor vessels had.

The doctor then removed the tourniquet. It had been in place for almost 30 minutes, and circulation to the left leg and foot had been impeded. It was critical that circulation be returned. However, the removal of the tourniquet would cause blood to flow into the site from the damaged blood vessels. The staff arrested the bleeding and prepared to suture the vessels, muscles, and tissues. Dr. Abrams asked the patient about the cause of her injury.

Mrs. Loeppky was unsure how it had occurred, but she wondered if she had caught her leg on the side of the truck door or the grill as she exited the vehicle and went around it to help her husband. She remembered that the door was stuck and that she had to force it open; the window was shattered. She said that she did not know she was bleeding until she looked down and saw a great amount of blood. That was the last thing she remembered until someone was patting her face gently and asking her to wake up.

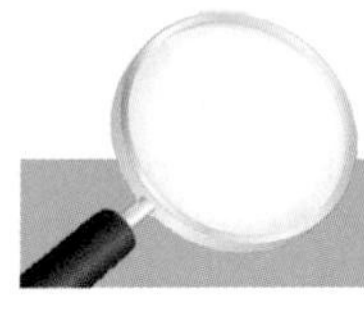

FOCUS POINT: *Impaired* vs. *Impeded*

These are two very different descriptors that are frequently used in health care. Notice the difference in the degree of severity that each word implies. One word refers to partial restriction, and the other refers to full restriction. Notice also use of the prefix *im-*, meaning *not.*

The word *impaired* means *damaged or harmed; not fully functioning.*

The word *impeded* means *obstructed, blocked, or held back; not functioning; incapable of movement.*

Learn roots related to blood

Many medical terms relating to blood and bleeding include the Latin roots *hema/o/ato* and *sangui.*

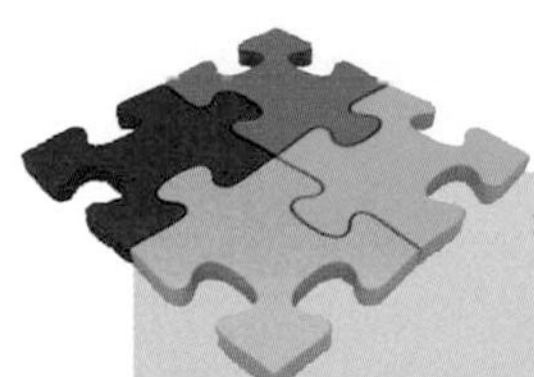

WORD BUILDING: Formula for Creating Words with the Combining Forms *Hem-, Hema-, Hemo-,* and *Hemato-*

Hem-, hema-, hemo-, and hemat- are combining forms of the Greek root meaning *blood.*

hem + angio + oma = *hemangioma*

Definition: a benign (non life threatening; harmless) tumor of a dilated blood vessel. (*Angio-* is a combining form of a root meaning *vessel.* The suffix *-oma* means *tumor.*) *noun*

Example: Babies can be born with a strawberry *hemangioma,* which is a temporary birthmark on the skin that disappears after 2 to 3 months.

hema + chrosis = *hemachrosis*

Definition: an abnormal redness of the blood. (*Chrosis* means *color* or *coloring.*) *noun*

Example: *Hemachrosis* is sometimes seen in patients who are suffering from carbon monoxide poisoning.

Continued

hemat + ocrit = *hematocrit*
Definition: the percentage of blood that consists of red blood cells. *noun*

Example: A decreased *hematocrit* test result can occur during pregnancy as a result of increased fluid in the bloodstream.

hemat + o + cyt + o + penia = *hematocytopenia*
Definition: a condition in which the patient has too few blood cells. (The root *cyt* means *cell,* and the suffix *-penia* means *too few or an abnormal decrease in amount.*) *noun*.

Example: *Hematocytopenia* is a symptom that is found in patients with leukemia, anemia, and lupus.

hemat + o + cyt + ur + ia = *hematocyturia*
Definition: a condition in which red blood cells are found in the urine. (The root *ur* means *urine.* The suffix *-ia* means *a condition or abnormal state.*) *noun* (NOTE: An alternate term for this condition is *hematuria.*)

Example: *Hematocyturia* can be the result of a serious genitourinary, lower abdominal, or pelvic injury.

hemo + dia + lysis = *hemodialysis*
Definition: a process of clearing urea, nitrogen, and other toxic wastes from the bloodstream when the kidneys are unable to do so. (*Dia-* means *through.* The suffix *-lysis* means *the process of dissolving, breaking down, or breaking up.*) *noun*

hemo + globin = *hemoglobin*
Definition: pigments in the blood that contain iron, which gives blood its red color. Hemoglobin is commonly referred to as the *red blood cells* or *RBCs.*

Example: Because the patient's blood was low in *hemoglobin,* it was not as red as it should have been.

hemo + rrhage = *hemorrhage*
Definition: loss of blood, usually in excess. (*Rrhage* stems from the Latin word *rhegny,* meaning *to burst forth or flow.*) *noun* or *verb*

Example: When an artery is cut, *hemorrhage* is to be expected; without treatment, the patient can exsanguinate (bleed to death).

hemo + philia = *hemophilia*
Definition: a hereditary bleeding disorder in which there are insufficient amounts of the proteins that are needed for the clotting of the blood. (The suffix *-philia* means *a tendency toward.*) *noun*

Example: Children with *hemophilia* cannot risk a bump or bruise for fear of internal hemorrhage.

hemo + stat = *hemostat*
Definition: a piece of equipment that is used to stop the flow of blood by compressing a blood vessel. (The root *stat* means *to stand still.*) *noun*

Example: The doctor used a stainless steel *hemostat* to clamp the blood vessel that was bleeding profusely into the wound.

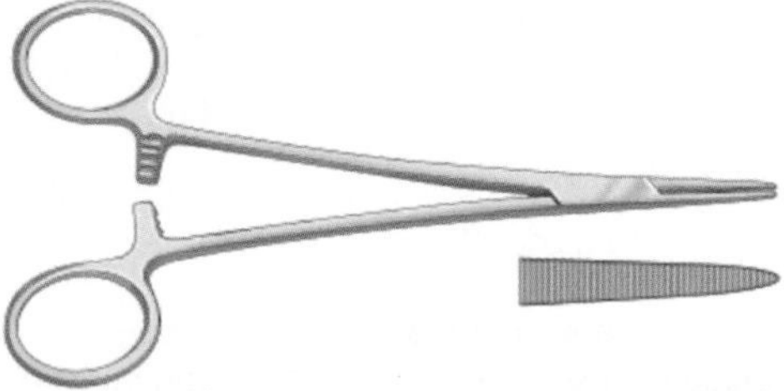

Figure 3.2: Hemostat (From Eagle S, Brassington C, Dailey C, Goretti C: *The Professional Medical Assistant: An Integrative, Teamwork-Based Approach.* Philadelphia: FA Davis, 2009, p. 385. With permission.)

Free Writing

Use the clue words given to write sentences that include medical terms with the roots *hem-*, *hema-*, *hemo-*, and *hemat-*. You will need to add some of your own words to make these sentences logical. Work with a partner or in a small group.

Example: urine, bloody, diagnosed

Sentence: The patient with bloody urine was diagnosed as having hematocyturia.

1. bleeds easily, lacks, clot

____

2. artery, cut, bleed heavily

____

3. skin, infant, tumor, temporary

____

4. pigment, red, blood, patient

____

5. compress, doctor, stop, bleeding, tool

____

Right Word or Wrong Word: *Hematocyturia* or *Hematuria*?

Study the word parts in these two words. Try to decide if these words mean the same thing. Do they, or do they have different meanings?

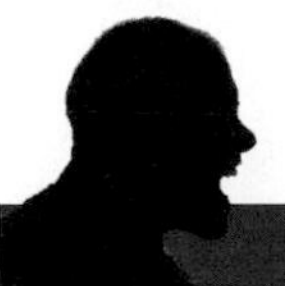

PRONUNCIATION PRACTICE

Say these words aloud to a friend or classmate if you can. You are given the phonetic pronunciation. Your instructor can help you with pronunciation,

or visit **http://www.MedicalLanguageLab.com.** 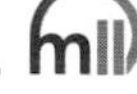

incontinent	ĭn-**kŏnt**´ĭn-ĕnt
tachycardic	tăk″ē-**kăr**´dĭk
hemangioma	hē-măn″jē-**ō**´mă
hemachrosis	hĕm″ă-**krō**´sĭs
hematocrit	hē-**măt**´ō-krĭt
hematocyturia	hĕm″ă-tō-sī-**tū**´rē-ă
hematuria	hē″mă **tū**´rē-ă or hĕm″ă-tū´**rē**-ă
hemodialysis	hē″mō dī-**ăl**´ĭ-sĭs or hĕm″ō-dī-**ăl**´ĭ-sĭs
hemoglobin	hē″mō **glō**´bĭn or hĕm″ō-**glō**´bĭn
hemorrhage	**hĕm**´ē-rĭj
hemophilia	hē″mō **fĭl**´ē-ă or hĕm″ō-**fĭl**´ē-ă
hemostat	**hē**´mō-stăt

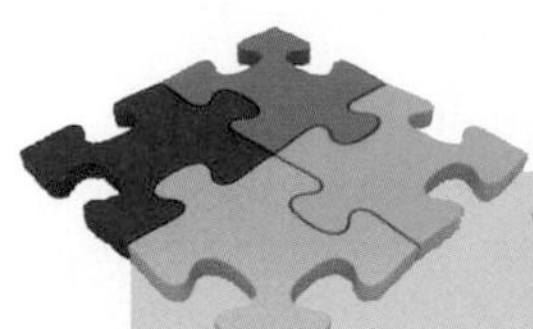

WORD BUILDING: Formula for Creating Words with the Combining Form *Sangui-*

Sangui is the combining form for a Latin root meaning *blood.*

sangui + ne = *sanguine*

Definition: bloody or consisting of blood. *adjective*

Example: The lack of color in Mrs. Loeppky's left foot, particularly in the toes, alerted Dr. Abrams that her extremity was no longer fully *sanguine.* The tourniquet needed to be removed.

sangui + n + eous = *sanguineous*

Definition: consisting of or full of blood. (The suffix *-eous,* in this case, means *full of.*) *adjective*

Example: When Dr. Abrams removed the tourniquet from the patient's upper left thigh, the wound bed was immediately *sanguineous,* making visibility and treatment difficult.

sero + sangui+ neous = *serosanguineous*

Definition: having the appearance of or actually containing both serum and blood. (The combining form *sero* refers to serum, which is the watery portion of the blood that contains antibodies.) *adjective*

Example: When the nurse removed the dressing, it appeared *serosanguineous;* it was wet and slightly pink in color. He knew that this meant there was a slight amount of blood mixed with the serum that is normal to wound healing.

sangui + ferous = *sanguiferous*

Definition: describing an organ or vessel that carries blood. (*Fer* is the combining form of the root *ferre,* which means *to carry.* The suffix *-ous* means *containing or full of.*) *adjective*

Example: The heart and liver are *sanguiferous* organs.

sangui + no + purulent = *sanguinopurulent*

Definition: describing a condition in which pus and blood coexist. In other words, the blood is infected. (*Purulent* is a root word meaning *full of pus.* Pus is the result of infectious bacteria.) *adjective*

Example: If Mrs. Loeppky's leg wound becomes infected, it is very possible it will be *sanguinopurulent.*

ex + sangui + nate = *exsanguinate*

Definition: to bleed out. (The prefix *ex-* means *out, away from, or outside.* The suffix *-ate* means *the end result of a process.*) *verb*

Example: When an artery is severed, it is possible for a person to *exsanguinate* in a very short time.

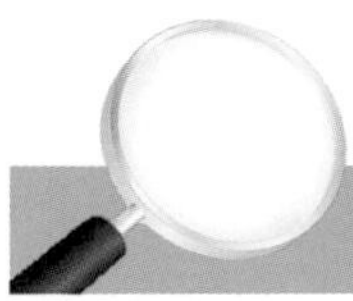

FOCUS POINT: *Sanguineous* and *Plethoric*

These two terms are synonymous: both of them mean *bloody or having an excess of blood.* The root of *plethoric* is *plethora,* meaning *an abundance.*

Let's Practice

Write the term with the combining form of *sangui-* that fits each description or definition below.

1. This adjective describes blood vessels. ______
2. This adjective describes a dressing that is slightly pink because not all of the fluid on it is blood. ______
3. The liver is this type of organ. ______
4. This verb tells what can happen if an artery is severed and treatment is not available immediately. ______

PRONUNCIATION PRACTICE

Say these words aloud to a friend or classmate if you can. You are given the phonetic pronunciation. Your instructor can help you with pronunciation,

or visit **http://www.MedicalLanguageLab.com.** 

sanguine	**săng**´gwĭn
sanguineous	săng-**gwĭn**´ē-ŭs
serosanguineous	sē˝ rō-**săn**-gwĭn´ē-ŭs
sanguiferous	săng-**gwĭf**´ĕr-ŭs
sanguinopurulent	săng˝ gwĭ-nō-**pū**´rū-lĕnt
exsanguinate	ĕks-**săn**´gwĭn-āt
plethora	**plĕth**´ō-ră
plethoric	plĕ **thor**´ ĭk

Key terms: the physiology of blood

There are three major types of blood cells: erythrocytes, leukocytes, and platelets.

Erythrocytes are red blood cells. They function to provide oxygen to the cells and to partially remove carbon dioxide.

Leukocytes are white blood cells. They function as part of the body's autoimmune system, defending against invaders in the form of bacteria, infection, allergy, and disease.

Platelets are actually thrombocytes rather than hemocytes. Unless they are diseased or otherwise compromised, platelets are clear or colorless. They function to clot the blood.

Together, platelets and white blood cells make up 45% of the blood by volume. The term **hematic cells** or **hemocytes** refers to erythrocytes and leukocytes only.

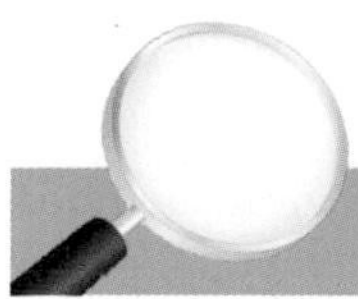

FOCUS POINT: Histamine and Antihistamine

Histamine is a natural substance that is released by the immune system in the body to create an allergic response, thereby putting the body on alert. An *antihistamine* is a chemical that can counteract the allergic response that is caused by histamine. Antihistamines are also known as *histamine-blocking agents* or *histamine-blocking drugs.* They do not occur naturally in the body.

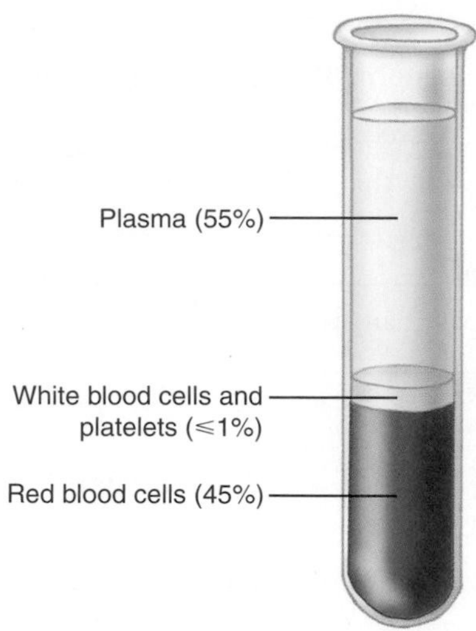

Figure 3.3: The composition of blood

TABLE 3-1: Blood Cells: Root and Prefixes

BEGIN with a Prefix	ADD a Root	COMBINE to Create a New Medical Term	Meaning
erythr(o)- (red)	cyte (cell)	erythrocyte	red blood cell
leuk/o- or leuc- (white)	cyte (cell)	leukocyte	white blood cell

TABLE 3-2: Types of Leukocytes (White Blood Cells)

Type	Function	When They Multiply
Basophils	To release histamine and other chemicals in response to an allergic reaction or a generalized, non-specific inflammation	They increase in response to radiation therapy, some food sensitivities, or chronic inflammation.
Eosinophils	To destroy parasites and counter allergic reactions by releasing histamine	They increase when there is a parasitic infection, an allergic response, or an inflammation of the skin.
Lymphocytes	To provide immune protection	They increase in cases of viral infections, including human immunodeficiency virus, as well as in response to some cancers and radiation therapy.
Monocytes	To provide defense against inflammation	They increase in response to a myriad of infections and inflammatory disorders.

Learn the language of blood tests

Although we are not suspecting that our patient, Glory Loeppky, has any pathalogical condition (disease or disease process) that can be detected in her blood, Dr. Abrams has ordered blood tests from the laboratory just to be sure. Blood tests can tell us many things. Understanding the terminology of blood tests is important when interpreting lab results and data on a patient chart.

Study Table 3-3 to learn about some important blood tests, their purposes, and the abbreviations that are used to refer to them.

The following tests are included in a **complete blood count (CBC)**, which is sometimes referred to as a **hemogram**:

- White blood cell count
- White blood cell differential
- Red blood cell count
- Hemoglobin level
- Hematocrit level
- Platelet count
- Mean corpuscular volume (MCV)
- Mean corpuscular hemoglobin concentration (MCHC)
- Red cell distribution width (RDW)

For more information about blood and the circulatory system, see Chapter 5.

Mix and Match

Use the new terminology that you have learned for talking about blood cells. Connect the medical term with its definition. Draw a line from the term on the left to its description on the right.

1. erythrocytes	red blood cells
2. basophils	counter allergic reactions by releasing histamine
3. lymphocytes	white blood cells
4. eosinophils	respond to allergies or inflammation by releasing histamine
5. leukocytes	provide an immune defense

TABLE 3-3: Blood Tests: What They Measure and Screen for (All of these tests are included in a complete blood count.)

Name of Test	Abbreviation	Measures	Screens for
Red blood cell count	RBC	Actual number of red blood cells in a given volume of blood	Decrease may indicate anemia; increase may indicate fluid loss (i.e., dehydration, diarrhea)
Hemoglobin	HGB	Amount of oxygen-carrying protein in the blood	Anemia (i.e., a reduction in the mass of red blood cells)
Hematocrit	HCT	Percentage of blood cells in a certain volume of blood	Ongoing bleeding, anemia, and dehydration
Platelet count (also known as *thrombocyte count*)	PLT	Number of platelets in a given volume	Decrease may indicate excessive bleeding or clotting, leukemia, pernicious anemia, or other disorders
Red cell distribution width	RDW	Variation in size of red blood cells	Pernicious anemia (i.e., a potentially fatal form of anemia)
White blood cell count	WBC	Actual number of white blood cells in a given volume of blood	Increase can indicate infection; decrease or extremely high count may be related to severe bleeding and clotting or may indicate leukemia
White blood cell differential (also known as *leukocyte differential* or *peripheral differential*)	WBC diff or Diff	Proportion of each type of white blood cell present; each is given as a percentage of the total number of white blood cells	Parasitic and viral infections, leukemia, severity of allergic or drug reactions

Critical Thinking

Identify the blood tests that would help during the assessment of the following cases. Use terminology related to blood and blood tests only, and then discuss your answers with another student, a colleague, or in class.

1. Jaycee is a 35-year-old woman who feels tired "all the time." You notice that she is also pale and lethargic. She has no other signs or symptoms of illness or allergy.
   a. What is the term for her condition (based on her appearance)? ____________________
   b. What two blood tests might the physician order? ____________________
2. Fred was hiking in the woods, and he forgot to take a water bottle with him. His thirst increased as the day wore on. He found a small, dirty-looking pond. He knew that he shouldn't drink out of it, but he was very thirsty. He also knew that it would be equally dangerous or even more dangerous to become dehydrated while out in the forest. So he took a drink. Within a few hours, he developed a minor fever and a slight rash over his body, and he noticed that he was wheezing a bit. Luckily, he made it back to town, where a friend was waiting for him. They then went to the nearest clinic.
   a. What blood tests might the physician order?
   ____

Assessment and the Muscular System

Patient Update

Mrs. Loeppky's wound has been stabilized, and her condition is stable (not urgent or emergent). She has had an x-ray taken of her painful, swollen left thumb and hand. The bones are not broken, but she has an ulnar collateral ligament injury. The nurse questioned Mrs. Loeppky about the probable cause of the injury.

Listen to the language: muscular system

Read the following dialogue between Mrs. Loeppky and her nurse. They are discussing the injury to the patient's thumb. The nurse has the responsibility to explain treatments and care to all patients. Notice that she does not use a lot of medical terminology but instead makes word choices that best suit the patient and that enhance her ability to establish rapport (i.e., the nurse-patient relationship) with Mrs. Loeppky.

Notice, too, that Mrs. Loeppky now identifies that she prefers to be called by her first name, and she invites the nurse to do this. This is proper protocol. Staff may call patients by their first names only if they ask the patients first or if the patients invite them to do so.

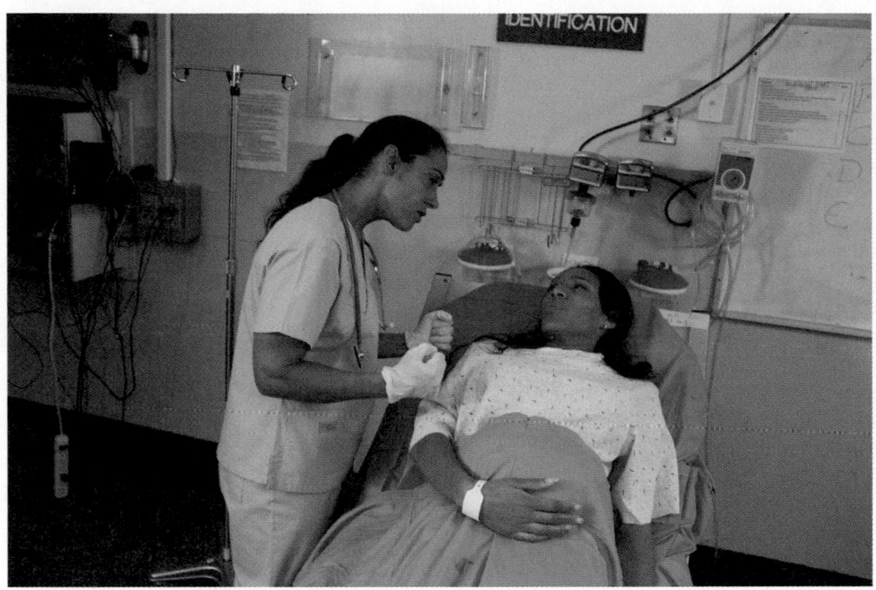

"Mrs. Loeppky, as the doctor told you, your thumb is not broken, but it is injured. It's going to require a splint to immobilize it," said Nurse Marnie. "Do you know what happened to it? How you injured it?"

"Please, call me Glory. I'd like it if you just called me Glory," came the reply. "All I can remember for sure is that we were driving along and I was uncomfortable with the seat belt on. But I wanted to keep it buckled. I know it's important to wear a seat belt. So, it was bothering me on the left side of my belly. I hooked my thumb inside the seat belt to keep the edge of it away from my skin a bit so it wouldn't feel like it was cutting into me. That's the last I remember about my hand."

"I see," said Marnie. "Well, there are a couple of things that might have happened. In the force of the accident, that thumb might have remained hooked in the belt. It would have been pushed and pulled with a great deal of force when you were hit and then again as you came to a stop. That's usually how these types of injuries occur. You've damaged what are called the ulnar collateral ligaments. Is there any possibility that you might have torn the ligaments by reaching out to brace the dashboard?"

"No, I don't think so. I don't remember doing that, because we got hit on my side of the truck. I remember a loud bang and being pushed toward Gil."

"I see. Well, as Dr. Abrams pointed out, the good news is that the ligament did not tear completely, and you won't need surgery for it. Luckily, you didn't dislocate the joint, either. Dr. Abrams will be back in a little bit to apply a thumb spica cast: that's really just a type of splint. In the meantime, I'm just going to wrap that thumb securely against your hand. Immobilizing it like that will protect it from any further injury and help you to avoid any extra pain and discomfort," the nurse explained as she worked.

"It's really turning black and blue now, isn't it?" commented Mrs. Loeppky. "Is that normal?"

"Yes, discoloration is quite normal, Glory. And it will be very sensitive to touch right around the middle joint. That's why we'll splint it. The splint will also prevent you from trying to use it to grasp things until the ligament heals and the thumb is strong enough to do so. That's going to take 3 to 6 weeks. It's susceptible to reinjury when it's healing. The thumb won't be strong enough to hold any weight."

TABLE 3-4: Medical Terminology Related to the Patient's Status

Medical Term	Prefix	Root	Suffix
stabilized (unchanged or unchanging)		stable (fixed in one place; not likely to suddenly change in any significant way)	-iz(e) (to make) -ed (creates the past tense of a verb)
ulnar (related to the ulna, which is a bone in the arm)		ulna (the larger bone of the forearm)	-r (related to)
collateral (accompanying or side by side)	co(n)- (together)	latero- (side or to the side) (	-al (related to)
ligament (band of tissue that supports muscles and other body parts)		ligamentum (band or binding)	
dislocate (to displace or force something out of its normal place)	dis- (not, not with, or apart)	loc(a)- (place)	-ate (to perform an act or undergo a process)
joint (the junction or place where two bones meet)		junct(io)- (place where two things come together)	
immobilizing (preventing movement)	im- (not)	mobili- (movable)	-ize (to make) -ing (indicates ongoing action)
susceptible (at risk for being affected by something)		susceptibil(i) (having the capability of being affected by or receiving something)	

Learn the terminology: muscular system

Our patient, Glory, actually has two muscular injuries. One is a torn ligament of the left thumb next to the middle joint and the web space of the thumb. The elements involved in this injury are the *metacarpal phalangeal* joint (MCP) and the *ulnar collateral* ligament (UCL). The other injury is the result of a deep cut on her left thigh along the *vastus lateralis* muscle.

To fully understand what is happening with this patient, it is necessary to develop a vocabulary related to the muscular system. We begin with the muscular system in general and then proceed more specifically to the muscles, tendons, and ligaments. We will use Glory Loeppky's injuries as specific examples of how medical terminology is used for this system. Figure 3-4 introduces some of the major muscles of this system.

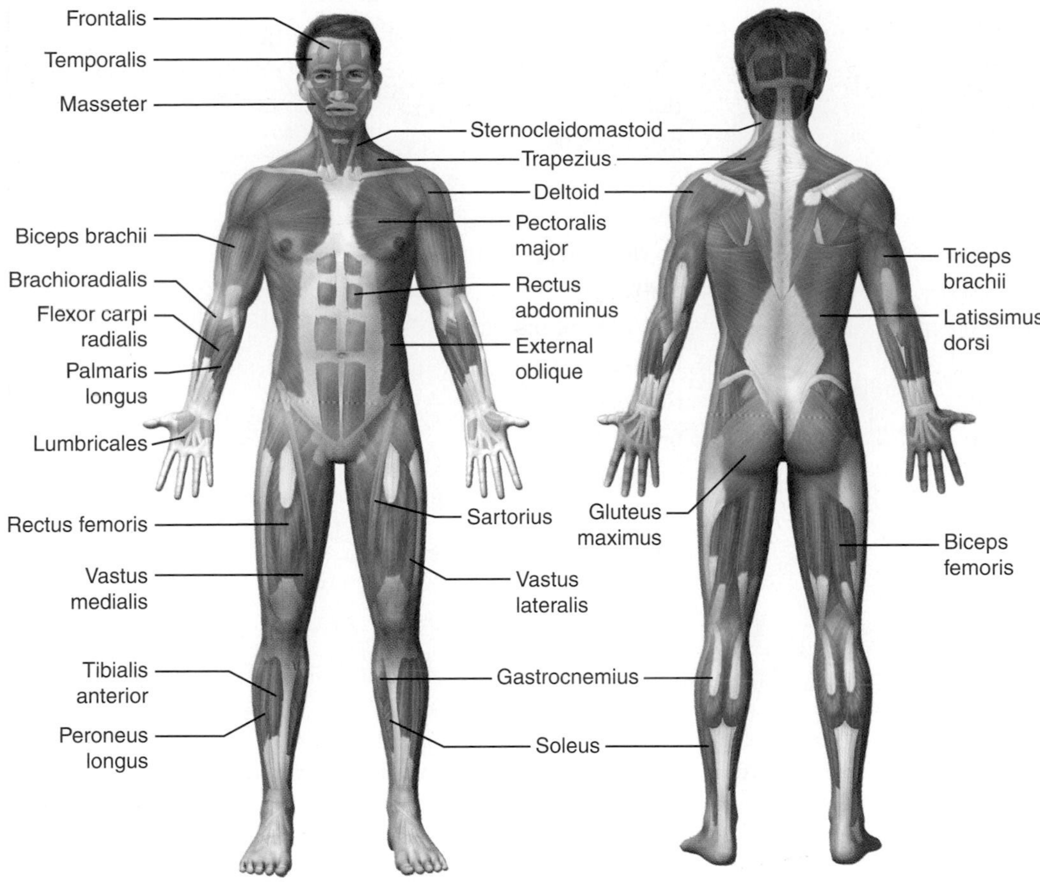

Figure 3.4: The muscular system

Let's Practice

Write the name of the muscle that fits each description.

1. located on the anterior portion of the lower leg ____________________
2. located on the outer side of the thigh ____________________
3. located posterior to the collarbone and into the upper back ____________________
4. located on the inner thigh ____________________
5. located medially on the forearm ____________________

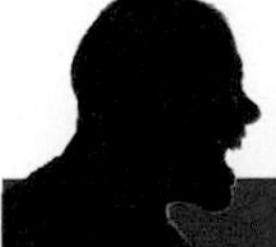

PRONUNCIATION PRACTICE

Say these words aloud to a friend or classmate if you can. You are given the phonetic pronunciation. Your instructor can help you with pronunciation,

or visit **http://www.MedicalLanguageLab.com.**

metacarpal	mĕt″ă-**kăr**′păl
phalangeal	fă-**lăn**′jē-ăl
ulnar	**ŭl**′năr

Continued

spica	**spī**´kă
trapezius	tră-**pē**´zē-ŭs
deltoid	**del**´toyd
pectoralis	pĕk˝tō-**rā**´lĭs
oblique	ō-**blēk**´
rectus	**rĕk**´tŭs
abdominus	ăb-**dŏm**´ĭ-nŭs
sartorius	săr-**tō**´rē-ŭs
gastrocnemius	găs˝trŏk-**nē**´mē-ŭs
tibialis	tĭb˝ē-**ā**´lĭs
femoris	**fĕm**´or-ĭs
brachio	**brā**´kē-ō-
brachi	**brā**´kē
radialis	rā˝dē-**ā**´lĭs
flexor	**flĕks**´or
carpi	**kăr**´pē
biceps	**bī**´sĕps

The muscular system is the site of many common injuries, including strains, sprains, spasms, bruising, and tearing. Disorders can include symptoms of weakness, stiffness, and pain, and these can possibly even lead to paralysis. Diseases such as muscular dystrophy specifically attack this system. Many of these conditions have been given the names of the people who discovered them or experienced them. Study Eponyms: Muscle Disorders and Diseases.

Eponyms: Muscle Disorders and Diseases

Becker's muscular dystrophy is an inherited disease in which the muscles dystrophy (weaken) slowly over time, and it is mostly seen in men. The disease was identified by the physicians Peter E. Becker and Franz Keiner in Germany in 1955. It is also known as *benign pseudohypertrophic muscular dystrophy.*

Bell's palsy or Bell's paralysis is a weakness of the muscles of only one side of the face that may progress to full paralysis. The cause is still unknown. Pregnant women are more than three times more likely to acquire this condition than the general population. People with diabetes are even more at risk. Bell's palsy is named after Sir Charles Bell, a Scottish anatomist and surgeon who was one of the first to describe this condition during the 19th century.

Duchenne muscular dystrophy is a rapidly worsening form of muscular dystrophy. Symptoms usually occur before the age of 6 years and lead to dependency on a wheelchair for mobility. This disease is named for Guillaume B. A. Duchenne, the French neurologist who first discovered it circa 1861.

Isaac-Mertens syndrome involves intermittent and persistent rippling muscle movement that is brought on by a peripheral nerve disease that leads to a stiffening and exhaustion of the muscles themselves. It occurs during late childhood and early adulthood. The condition is named for Hyam Isaacs, a 20th-century South-African neurophysiologist, and Hans-George Mertens, a German neurologist.

Lou Gehrig's disease is a progressive motor neuron disease that involves nerves and nerve conduction in the muscles and that negatively affects the voluntary control of the muscles. Eventually, all muscle control is lost, and death results. Lou Gehrig was a professional baseball player who was afflicted by the disease in the mid 20th century. His struggle was well publicized, and it increased public awareness of the disease, as well as interest in finding a cure.

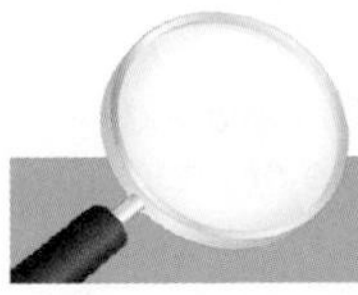

FOCUS POINT: Joints and Bones

Joints and bones are not part of muscular system; they belong to the skeletal system. This will be explored in detail as you follow Glory Loeppky's husband, Gil, through his assessment, treatment, and rehabilitation. Joints are also discussed when you encounter the patient Stevie-Rose Davis.

Roots related to muscles

The root *mys* originates in Greek and means *muscle.* The combining form is *my* or *myo-*. The root *musculus* originates in Latin and also means *muscle.* The combining form is *musculo-*.

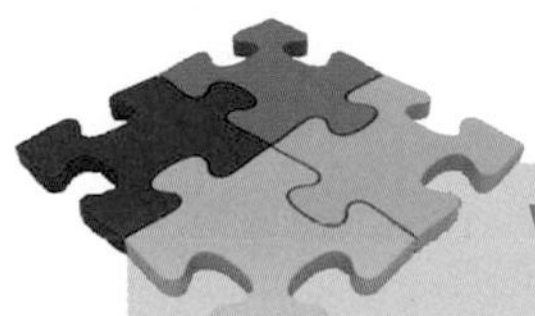

WORD BUILDING: Formula for Creating Words with the Combining Forms *Myo-* and *Muscul/o/a*

1. myo- = muscle

my + algia = *myalgia*

Definition: muscle pain. (The word is made up of two roots. The combining form *algia* means *pain.*) *noun*

Example: The patient has been diagnosed with *myalgia,* but the true cause of the pain is not yet known.

my + asthenia = *myasthenia*

Definition: muscle weakness that is usually accompanied by abnormal muscle fatigue. (The second root, *asthenia,* is derived from Greek and means *weakness.*) *noun*

Example: *Myasthenia* gravis is a disease in which there is increasing difficulty with using and voluntarily directing muscles. Motor activity (movement) becomes disordered.

myo + card + itis = *myocarditis*

Definition: inflammation of the heart muscle. (The second root, *cardi/o,* meaning *heart,* is found in its combining form. The word ends with the prefix *-itis,* meaning *inflammation.*) *noun*

Example: The doctor discovered that the patient had a viral infection called sarcoidosis, which has led to his treatment for *myocarditis.*

electro = myo = graph + y = *electromyography*

Definition: preparation or study of the graphic records of the activity of certain muscles when they are electronically stimulated. The record "observes" the muscles at rest and in action. (The root *electro* means *electricity.* The root *graph* means *record or writing.* The suffix *-y* means *the act of. noun*

Example: The patient is scheduled for *electromyography* to ascertain if the specific muscles are weak as a result of nerve conduction problems related to the muscle or because of a disease process in the muscle itself.

Continued

myo + kym + ia = *myokymia*
Definition: persistent twitching or rippling of a muscle or a portion of a muscle. (The second root in this word is *kym,* a Greek word meaning *wave.* The suffix *-ia* means *the state of.*) *noun*

Example: Isaac-Mertens syndrome is a form of *myokymia.*

myo + path + y = *myopathy*
Definition: muscle disease. (The second root in this word derives from *path/o,* meaning *disease.* The suffix *-y* means *the state of.*) *noun*

Example: Rheumatologists, physiotherapists, and registered massage therapists all have expertise in treating clients with varying types of *myopathy.*

myo + sarc + oma = *myosarcoma*
Definition: a malignant cancer of the muscle tissue. (The second root, *sarc,* means *flesh.* The suffix *-oma* means *tumor.*) *noun*

Example: *Myosarcoma* can occur in the large and small intestines, the prostate, or the bladder.

myo+ vascul + ar = *myovascular*
Definition: referring to the blood supply to the muscles. (The second root is *vascul/o,* meaning *blood vessel.* The suffix *-ar* means *referring to.*) *adjective*

Example: When a person has *myovascular* insufficiency (not enough blood flow to the muscles), he or she can experience symptoms of pain and aching. In the heart muscle, this is referred to as *angina.*

poly + my + algia = *polymyalgia*
Definition: muscle pain in many muscles. (The prefix *poli/y* means *many.* The second root is *algia,* meaning *pain.*) *noun*

Example: *Polymyalgia* rheumatica is a disease that begins with moderate to severe aching in the muscles of the neck and the extremities that is accompanied by fatigue and weight loss.

2. muscul/o/a- = muscle

muscul + ar = *muscular*
Definition: pertaining to the muscles or well-developed muscles. The suffix *-ar* means *pertaining to.*) *adjective*

Example: The Olympic athletes are very *muscular.*

muscul + o + skelet + al = *musculoskeletal*
Definition: referring to the muscular and skeletal body systems, combined as one. (The combining form of the root *skeleto-* is added, followed by the suffix *-al* meaning *referring to or about.*) *adjective*

Example: The *musculoskeletal* system provides the shape, posture, and movement of the body.

muscula + t + ure = *musculature*
Definition: the arrangement of muscles. (The suffix *-ure* changes this word into a noun.) *noun*

Example: The *musculature* of the leg includes the quadriceps muscles and others.

muscul + aris = *muscularis*
Definition: any layer of smooth muscle. (The suffix *-aris* is derived from *arius,* meaning *pertaining to.*) *noun*

Example: The *muscularis* of the heart is complex.

Free Writing

Use one of the terms that begins with *myo-* or *musculo/a-* to write a logical sentence. Use the clue words that are given, and work with a partner or in a small group. Note: You will have to add some of your own words to make the sentence complete.

1. weakening of, muscles tire easily, diagnosis

 ____

2. muscles, insufficiency of blood, condition

 ____

3. bones, muscles, erect, ability, stand, system, us

 ____

4. name, diseases, muscles

 ____

5. twitching, eye, persistent, condition, could be

 ____

Name the Term and Break it Down

Write the term that fits each definition or description. Next, break down the term into its separate word parts, and write the meaning of each part.

1. pain in a muscle
 term: ____________ parts: ____________
2. a test of impulse conduction on a muscle to see it work
 term: ____________ parts: ____________
3. an uncontrollable twitching
 term: ____________ parts: ____________
4. describing well-developed muscles
 term: ____________ parts: ____________
5. pain in multiple muscles
 term: ____________ parts: ____________

Anatomy and physiology: muscular system

Key terms: muscle tissue

Muscles are made up of contractile connective tissues. The primary function of muscles is to produce movement and maintain posture. There are three specific types of muscle tissue: visceral, cardiac, and striated. With the exception of visceral muscle, most connective tissue in the muscular system is **fibrous**, which means that it is composed of thin, threadlike structures or fibers.

Visceral muscles are also known as smooth muscles. They are found in hollow organs such as the lungs, the gastrointestinal tract, and the blood vessels. Visceral muscles are **involuntary**; we do not have conscious control over them.

Cardiac muscle, which is found in the heart, is a very specific type of muscle. It functions like other smooth muscles, but it has the appearance and strength of striated muscles. This muscle is also involuntary.

Striated or **skeletal muscles** are those that permit movement and that support the skeleton. Our bodies are made up of more than 600 skeletal muscles, all of which are under voluntary control.

Fascia is a fibrous membrane that covers, supports, and separates the muscles internally. Fascia also exists just below the surface of the skin, where it connects the skin with the muscles.

Fascicules are long muscle fibers that form bundles and that are joined by connective tissue. They help to give shape to muscles and to protect them.

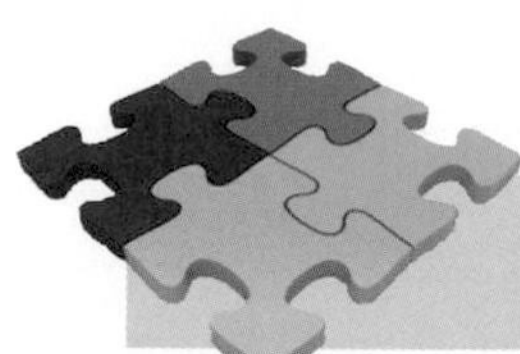

WORD BUILDING: Formula for Creating Words with the Combining Form *Viscer/a/o*

Viscer/a/o is the combining form of the word *viscera,* meaning *internal organs.*

viscer + al = *visceral*

Definition: referring to internal organs. (The suffix *-al* means *pertaining to.*) *adjective*

Example: Glory Loeppky and her husband were at risk for *visceral* injury when their seat belts dug into their bellies and sides during the motor vehicle accident.

viscero + gen + ic = *viscerogenic*

Definition: originating in the viscera. (The second root, *gen,* means *to produce or generate.* The suffix *-ic* means *pertaining to.*) *adjective*

Example: X-rays and thermographic scans can be used to help assess the causes of *viscerogenic* pain.

viscero + trop/e + ic = *viscerotropic*

Definition: affecting the viscera. (The second combining form, *trop/e,* means *turning.* The suffix *-ic* means *pertaining to.*) *adjective*

Example: The yellow fever virus causes *viscerotropic* diseases, which means that the virus primarily affects the internal organs.

e + viscer + ate = *eviscerate*

Definition: to move or remove organs from the inside to the outside of the body. (The prefix *e-* means *outside,* and the suffix *-ate* means *an act or process.*) *verb*

Example: The patient tried to lift his suitcase onto his bed much too soon after the abdominal surgery. This tore open the sutures, and his intestines began to *eviscerate* or protrude from the wound site.

TABLE 3-5: Terms Including the Roots *Stria, Fibr/o,* and *Fasci/o*

Term	Meaning
stria (plural: striae)	a line, strip, or furrow that sits just below or above the tissue that surrounds it
striate	striped
striae atrophica	stretch marks on the skin that may have resulted from obesity, a tumor, or other circumstances
striae gravidarum	stretch marks on the skin as the result of a pregnancy
fiber	any thin, threadlike structure
fibrous or fibroid	made up of or resembling fibers
fibromyalgia	a condition of chronic pain in the muscles and soft tissues that surround the joints
fibromyoma	a fibroid tissue muscle tumor in the uterus that is made up of more fiber than muscle; this is a common condition in women
fascia	a fibrous membrane
fasciculus	a small bundle; used to refer to small bundles or nerve or muscle fibers
fasciitis	inflammation or swelling of the fascia

Fill in the Blanks

Use the new language and terms that you have learned in a meaningful way. Complete these sentences by filling in the blanks

1. ________________________ is the proper term for the stretch marks that a woman may develop as her belly swells during pregnancy.
2. If the belly is opened, it is possible that the organs will ________________________.
3. The combining form of the root word that means *internal organs* is ________________.

Tendons

Tendons are a type of fibrous tissue that forms into strong cords. Tendons connect muscles to bones. The term tendon is synonymous with *sinew.*

One of the best-known tendons is the *Achilles tendon* at the back of the heel. It connects the calf muscles to the ankle. The *abdominal aponeurosis* is also known, particularly to women. This is the tendon of the abdomen that stretches during pregnancy.

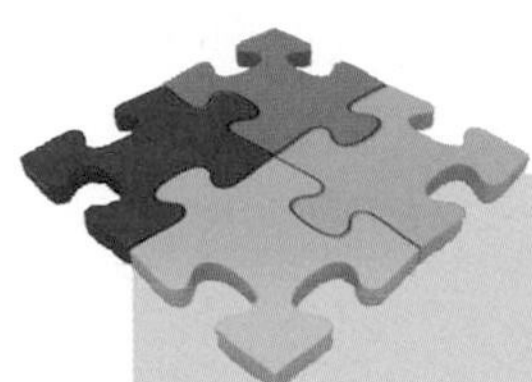

WORD BUILDING: Formula for Creating Words with the Combining Forms *Teno-*, *Tendo-*, and *Tendin/o*

Teno, tendo- or tendin/o are the combining forms of the root *tendo,* meaning *tendon.*

tendon + itis = *tendinitis*

Definition: inflammation of a tendon. (The suffix *-itis* means *inflammation.*) *noun*

NOTE: This word can also be spelled *tendonitis.*

Example: Did you know that wearing high heels frequently can lead to a shortening of the Achilles tendon and the calf muscle? After a long time, it can lead to *tendinitis.* It will be painful and difficult to put your heel flat on the ground when you are standing in bare feet.

tendin + *osis*

Definition: degeneration of a tendon. (The suffix *-osis* means *condition.*) *noun*

Example: Wear and tear through repetitive strain on a tendon can eventually cause the degenerative condition of *tendinosis.*

tendo + plasty = *tendoplasty*

Definition: surgery to repair a tendon. (The suffix *-plasty* means *to mold.*) *noun*

Example: If a tendon is ruptured (comes apart) and detaches from the bone, *tendoplasty* will likely be necessary to reconnect it.

teno + desis = *tenodesis*

Definition: surgical fixation (binding) of a tendon. *noun*

Example: Recurring inflammation, pain, and damage to a tendon can require *tenodesis* to fix, attach, or bind the tendon back to the bone and to restabilize the joint.

teno + odyn + ia = *tenodynia*

Definition: pain in a tendon. (The second root, *odyne,* means *pain.* The suffix *-ia* means *state of.*) *noun*

Example: After his full leg cast was removed, the patient found it very painful to step down on his heel. At first, he thought that the pain was in his heel itself, but he quickly came to realize that the pain was in the Achilles tendon. He was suffering from *tenodynia.*

teno + suture = *tenosuture*

Definition: suturing of a tendon. The root word *suture* derives from *sutura,* meaning *seam.* This is also known as *tendinosuture* or *tenorrhaphe* (*rhaphe* meaning *seam or ridge.*) *noun*

Example: Dr. Abrams used a *tenosuture* to repair the patellar tendon of Glory Loeppky's quadriceps muscle injury.

tenon + ectomy = *tenonectomy*

Definition: excision of a portion of a tendon. (The combining form *-ectomy* means *excision, cutting out, or removal.*) *noun*

Example: *Tenonectomy* is sometimes part of the surgical treatment of the eye for patients with glaucoma.

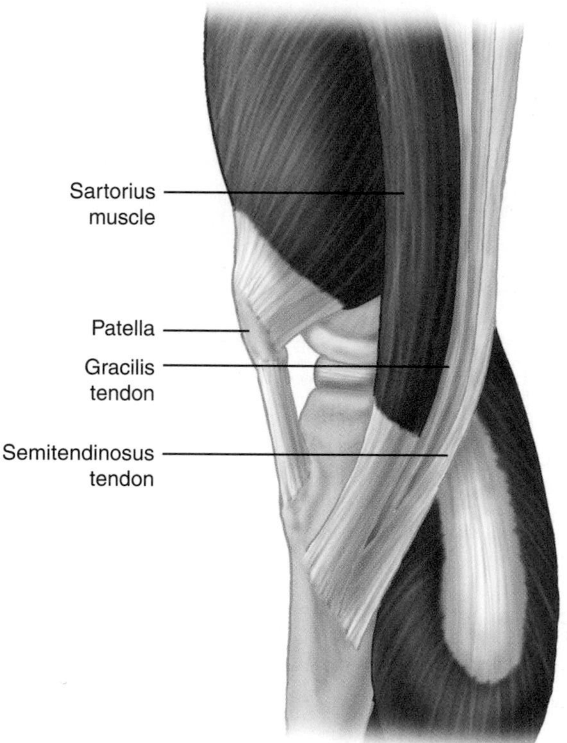

Figure 3.5: Muscles and tendons of the knee (medial view)

Ligaments

Ligaments are a type of fibrous connective tissue that connect the articulating ends of bones (i.e., the joints) and bind them together. Ligaments can also consist of aggregates or bands of ligamentous tissue that connect bones, cartilage, and other structures. These support or attach to muscle or to the fascia of muscles.

For example, a number of different ligaments support the shoulder. They attach to the scapula (shoulder blade), the clavicle (collar), and the humerus (upper arm) bones and the surrounding muscles to support them all or to keep them in place. There are ligaments like this that work throughout the muscular system.

The term *ligament* is rarely broken down or combined with other medical terms, except in the case of the adjective *ligamentous.*

As you know, Glory Loeppky has an injury to her hand. More specifically, it is to her thumb and the ulnar collateral ligament at the middle joint of the thumb. The function of this ligament is

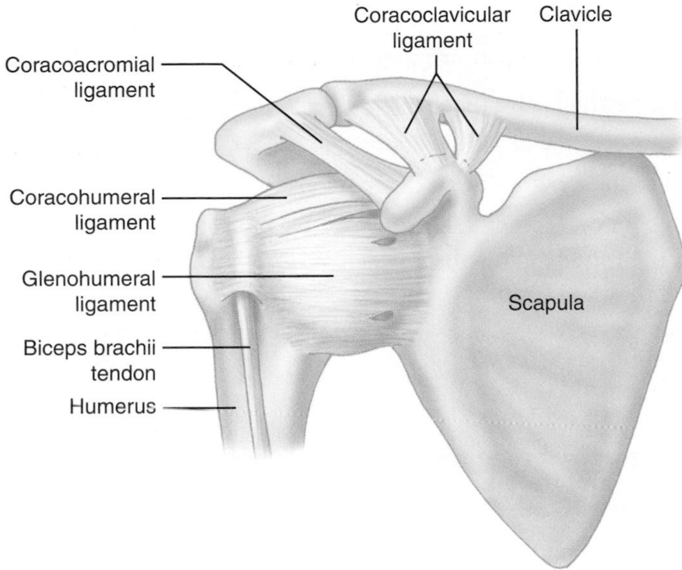

Figure 3.6: Ligaments of the shoulder (anterior view)

to stabilize the thumb; it holds the thumb in place alongside the hand and allows for some flexion and extension. Any hard force on the thumb that wrenches it away from the hand can cause the ligament to tear away. A complete tear is called a *rupture.* Dr. Abrams does not suspect that the ligament is ruptured, and he has ruled out the need for surgery. Figure 3-7 shows how this damage may occur.

Name the Term and Break it Down

Write the term that fits each definition or description. Next, break down the term into its separate word parts, and write the meaning of each part.

1. surgery to repair a tendon

term: ______________________ parts: ______ ______ ____

2. chronic pain in the soft tissues around the muscles and in the muscles themselves

term: ______________________ parts: ______________________

3. inflammation of the fibrous membranes around the muscles

term: ______________________ parts: ______________________

4. connects bone to bone

term: ______________________ parts: ______________________

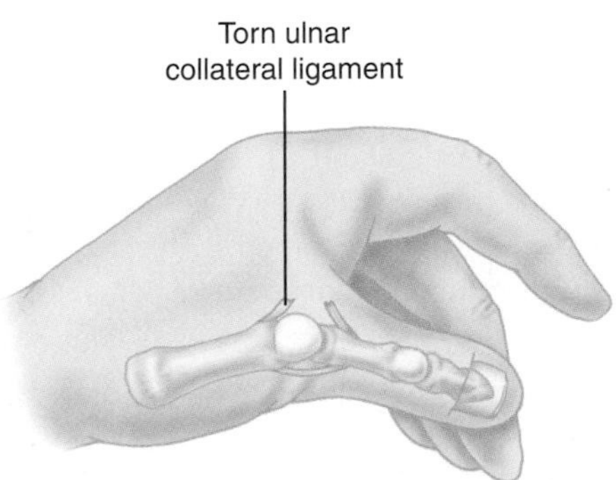

Figure 3.7: How an ulnar collateral injury occurs

Let's Practice

Write the term that identifies each part or system described.

1. made up of contractile connective tissues ______________________________
2. provides support and movement for the body ______________________________
3. contributes to the formation of muscles ______________________________
4. connects muscle to bone ______________________________
5. envelops muscles to protect and support them ______________________________

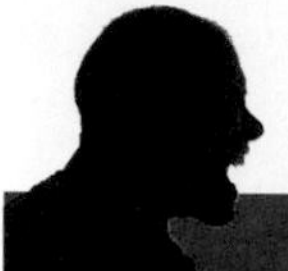

PRONUNCIATION PRACTICE

Say these words aloud to a friend or classmate if you can. You are given the phonetic pronunciation. Your instructor can help you with pronunciation, or visit **http://www.MedicalLanguageLab.com.**

electromyography ē-lĕk″ trō-mī-**ŏg**′ră-fē
eviscerate ē-**vĭs**″ĕr-ā′t
fibromyalgia fī″ brō-mī-**ăl**′jē-ă
fibromyoma fī″ brō-mī-**ō**′mă
fasciitis făs″ē-**ī**′tĭs
musculoskeletal mŭs″kū-lō-**skĕl**′ē-tăl
myasthenia mī-ăs-**thē**′nē-ă
myokymia mī-ō-**kĭm**′ē-ă
myopathy mī-**ŏp**′ă-thē
polymyalgia pŏl″ē-mī-**ăl**′jē-ă
stria **strī**′ă
sternocleidomastoid stĕr″nō-klī″dō-**măs**′toyd
scalene **skā**-lēn′
tendinitis tĕn″dĭn-**ī**′tĭs
tenodesis tĕn-**ŏd**′ē-sĭs
tenonectomy tĕn″ō-**nĕk**′tō-mē
viscerogenic vĭs″ĕr-ō-**jĕn**′ĭk
viscerotropic vĭs″ĕr-ō-**trŏp**′ĭk

Muscle origin and insertion

Muscles attach to bones at a point of origin and a point of insertion. Muscles work in pairs: when one muscle contracts, the opposing muscle relaxes. When muscles contract, they cause movement. The type of movement is dependent on the type of muscle. Extension occurs when muscles straighten. Some muscles are under our voluntary control, whereas others, such as cardiac muscle, are not.

Key terms: origin, insertion, and basic function of muscles

point of origin: A muscle *begins* at a stationary bone, which is a bone that does not move. An example of a stationary bone is the tibia in the lower leg (the shin bone). The gastrocnemius muscle (calf) has its point of origin at the proximal end of the tibia.

point of insertion: A muscle *ends* at a moveable bone. For example, the biceps and triceps brachii muscles of the humerus (upper bone of the arm), at their distal head, connect with the proximal end of the ulna bone of the lower arm. This connection occurs at the elbow joint.

contraction: shortening or bending; also referred to as *flexion*

extension: opening, lengthening, straightening, or expanding

opposes/opposing: works or stands against; also referred to as *agonists* and *antagonists*

relax/relaxes: at ease; resting in a straighter or more open position; sometimes also referred to as *extension,* although a relaxed muscle is not always fully or rigidly straight

voluntary control: under conscious control and moving as a person chooses to move it

involuntary control: impossible to control by will or thought

Fill in the Blanks

Use the new language and terms that you have learned in a meaningful way. Complete these sentences by filling in the blanks

1. When I clench my fist, I am ______________________ my hand muscles.
2. People can smile whenever they choose because most of the facial muscles are under ______________________.
3. When you open your hand and raise it to wave goodbye, you are ______________________ the muscles of your hand and arm.
4. If you turn your thumb into your palm and leave it there, this position is called ______________________.

Right Word or Wrong Word: *Ligament* or *Tendon*?

If a ligament is a tough band of connecting tissue that connects muscle to bone, what is a tendon? Are they the same thing?

Names of common muscles

It would be impossible to learn the terms for all of the body's muscles in one chapter of a book. Learning the meaning of the word parts of the names of body structures is more important than learning the terms for every structure.

Look back at Figure 3-4 as you work through the following medical and anatomical terms that relate to the muscular system. Only a portion of the many muscles of the body are listed. These examples will help you to see how medical terms are combined, formed, and used to name and describe aspects of the muscular system. For ease of learning, the following examples have been categorized by their location in the body.

TABLE 3-6: Some Muscles of the Head, Neck, and Arms

Muscles of the Head and Neck	Muscles of the Arms
Sternocleidomastoid Located on the anterior side of the trunk and laterally to the neck Originates at the sternum, crosses the clavicle, and extends up the side of the neck to insert at the base of the skull Supports and rotates the head and the neck	**Deltoid** Located in the upper arm Originates at the scapula Inserts at the humerus Abducts arm and provides for some arm movement
Scalene • located in the neck • originate in the first, second, or third rib and insert into the cervical (neck) spine • elevate the ribs and rotate the neck; flex the neck	Biceps bracchi • located in the upper arm • originates and inserts at different points on the scapula • flexes the forearm and supinates it from a neutral position
Masseter (cheek) • located at the back of the jaw • originates at the zygomatic arch (cheek bone) and inserts laterally on the mandible (jaw) • opens the jaw and extends and protracts it	Brachioradialis • located in the forearm along the radial bone • originates at the side of the humerus and inserts distally at the radius, near the thumb • flexes the forearm at the elbow joint
Frontalis (forehead) • located above the eyes • originates along the anterior scalp line and inserts into the skin around the nose and eyebrows • allows for wrinkling of the forehead and movement of the eyebrows	Triceps brachii • located in the upper arm • originates in the scapula and inserts at the proximal head of the ulna • extends the elbow and supports the action of pushing
Temporalis • located at the temples • originates along the temporal bones of the skull and inserts just above the jaw (mandible) • allows the jaw to be closed and kept closed	Extensor carpi • a number of muscles all originating within the forearm and extending down into the hands and fingers • the extensor carpi radialis brevis and extensor carpi radialis longus extend and abduct the hand

TABLE 3-7: Some Muscles of the Trunk and Legs

Muscles of the Trunk	Muscles of the Legs
Trapezius • located along the upper back and shoulders • originates at the base of the skull (occipital bone) and inserts at the lateral clavicle, scapula, and spine • elevates and rotates the scapula (shoulder) and extends the neck	Gastrocnemius (calf) • located in the lower leg • originates at the medial and lateral side of the lower femur and inserts at the calcaneus (heel) • flexes the ankle; stabilizes the knee and ankle when standing
Intercostals (serratus anterior) • located between the ribs, internally and externally • originate at the ribs and insert at the distal end of the scapulae • allow for the elevation, expansion, and contraction of the rib cage for breathing, as well as the movement and stability of the shoulders	Biceps femoris • located in the upper leg • originates at the coccyx bone (tailbone) and inserts at the head of the fibula and the side of the tibia • extends the thigh, flexes the knee, and can rotate the leg

TABLE 3-7: Some Muscles of the Trunk and Legs—cont'd

Muscles of the Trunk	Muscles of the Legs
Pectoralis major and pectoralis minor • located in the chest • attached to the clavicle, the sternum, and the humerus • originate in the clavicle and sternum and insert into the humerus • allow for shoulder rotation and flexion as, well as adduction of the humerus	Sartorius • located in the upper leg • originates at the iliac spine (lower backbone and pelvis) and inserts at the proximal tibia • flexes the knees and hips
Internal and external obliques • located diagonally in the trunk • originate at the ileum and insert at the ribs • allow for movement at an angle or sideways and for the rotation of the trunk	Gluteus maximus • located posterior, on the dorsal side of the body • originates at the coccyx, the ileum, and the sacral bones and inserts at the femur • extends the hip and abducts and rotates the thigh laterally
Rectus abdominus • located medially along the anterior of the trunk • originates along the pubic bone and inserts at the ribs and the sternum • Allows for trunk motion and flexes the spine • sometimes referred to as the *abs* or *six pack*	Adductor longus • located inside the upper leg from the groin to below the knee • originates at the pubic bone and inserts medially and distally on the femur • adducts and flexes the thigh at the hip
Transverse abdominis • located laterally around the abdomen • originates at the ileum and inserts at the sternum and the pubic bones • provides stability for the trunk	Tibialis anterior • located along the front of the lower leg (shin) • originates laterally on the tibia and inserts into the foot at the base of the toes (metatarsals) • allows for the inversion of the foot and dorsal flexion (i.e., pointing the toes upward)
Latissimus dorsi • located along the back laterally • originates in the lower spine and ileum and inserts at the humerus • extension: allows for weight bearing and for lifting with the hands and arms	Fibularis longus (peroneus longus) • located in the calf • originates laterally on the fibula and inserts laterally at the foot • allows for eversion of the foot and plantar flexion (i.e., pointing the toes)
Erector spinae • located in the back • originate along the sacrum and the ileum and insert at the lower ribs • keep posture erect; allow for movement of the spine and stabilize spine	Soleus • located at the back of the leg in the calf area • originates on the posterior proximal half of the tibia and fibula and inserts at the calcaneus • allows for plantar flexion and the ability to stand on the toes

TABLE 3-8: Muscles That Comprise the Quadriceps

Quadriceps Muscles
Rectus femoris • located deep within the upper leg • originates on the pelvis and crosses the hip joint • extends the knee and flexes the hip
Vastus intermedius • located along the front and side of the thigh bone • originates at the anterior and lateral surface of the femur and inserts at the base of the patella and the top of the tibia • extends the leg at the knee
Vastus lateralis • located along the outside of the upper part of the leg (thigh) • originates at the head of the femur (thigh bone) and inserts at the patella (knee) and the proximal end of the tibia • extends the leg at the knee
Vastus medialis • located at the top of the femur, along the inside • originates at the medial edge of the trochanter (head) of the femur and inserts into the base of the patella and the proximal end of the tibia • extends the leg at the knee

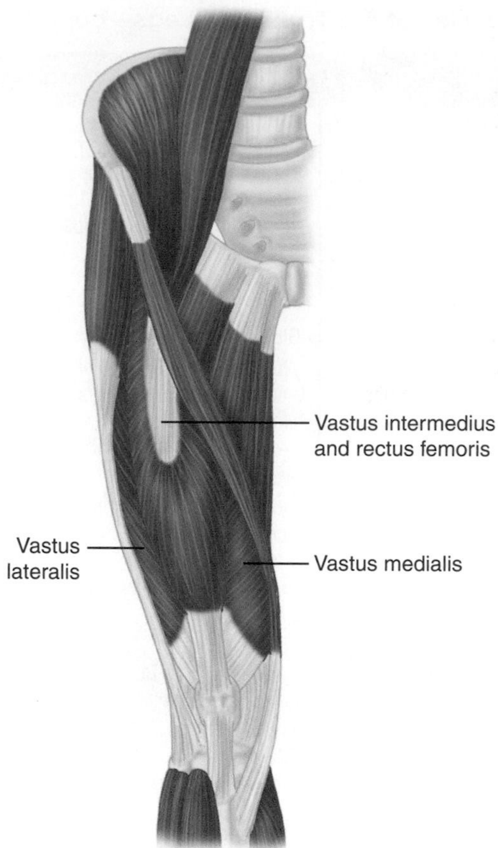

Figure 3.8: Quadriceps muscles of the leg (anterior view)

The **quadriceps** are four specific muscles that sit on the anterior aspect of the thigh. They include the *rectus femoris,* the *vastus intermedius,* the *vastus lateralis,* and the *vastus medialis.* The quadriceps work cooperatively to extend to straighten the leg and to contract to bend the knee.

Glory Loeppky has a deep laceration wound to her left thigh. This means that her quadriceps have been injured; specifically, they have been lacerated or cut. When the physician sutured her wound, he first applied sutures internal to the wound by suturing the vastus lateralis muscle, the accompanying tendons, and the damaged blood vessels. He then sutured the wound closed at the level of the skin.

Fill in the Blanks

Use the new language and terms that you have learned in a meaningful way. Complete these sentences by filling in the blanks.

1. The ______________________________ muscles allow you to keep your mouth closed when it is not in use.
2. ______________________________ is another name for the calf muscle.
3. The ______________________________ is sometimes known as "the abs."
4. The ______________________________ keeps the body erect and stabilizes the spine.
5. All of the ______________________________ help to extend the knee and flex the hip.
6. The ______________________________ muscles allow a person to raise his or her eyebrow when feeling skeptical.
7. The ______________________________ wraps around the trunk and provides stability for it.
8. A large muscle on the buttocks is the ______________________________.

9. The two muscles that are commonly known simply as the chest muscles or “the pecs” are the ______________________ and the ______________________.

10. The ______________________ holds up or supports the shoulder and the surrounding area.

It's All Greek to Me

Stop now and reflect on what you've just been reading about the muscular system. Notice how many of the terms you've been asked to write. This is a clear example of the learning challenges that medical terminology brings to learners. Many of the terms for muscles look like a foreign language, don't they? Well, indeed they are. They originate not only in Greek but in Latin as well. This is why simply memorizing words like these is not the best approach to learning them. Recognizing word parts and understanding their meanings are the keys to success when learning medical terminology and language.

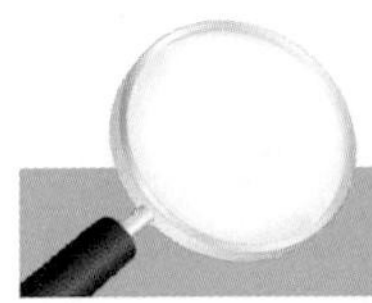

FOCUS POINT: Latin or Greek?

Please note that is *not* important to know which words originated in Latin and which are from the Greek. It is sufficient for your career needs simply to appreciate that these words have been with us for a long time and to see that the way these words were constructed helped readers and speakers to glean their meanings. Now you, too, are learning those skills.

Learn the word parts of muscle names

Study the following table. It will help you to understand the word parts that are often used to name muscles.

For more information about the muscular system, see Chapter 10

TABLE 3-9: Word Parts Used to Name Muscles

Medical Term Derived From Latin or Greek	Word Parts	Meaning
abdominus	abdomin/o + us	abdominal
brachii	brachi/o or bracchi-	arm
brachioradialis	brachi/o + radialis	a muscle on the lateral side of the forearm
frontalis	front/o + alis	forehead or anterior
temporalis	tempor/a + alis	temporal: located at the temples
pectoralis	pector or pectoris + alis	pectoral: located at the chest
femoris	femor + is	femur: pertaining to the femur bone of the leg
spinae	spina/e	the spine or referring to the spine
sternocleidomastoid	sterno + cleid/al + masto/id	sternum: breastbone cleidal: clavicle mastoid: breast (In combination, these terms form the descriptive name of a muscle found in proximity to these areas.)

Mix and Match

Use your new language skills to create terms from the parts below. Draw a line from the word part on the left to the appropriate part on the right to create a proper medical term related to the muscular system.

1. femor	maximus
2. abdomin	spinae
3. gluteus	viscerate
4. erector	lateralis
5. vastus	is
6. e	myopathy
7. cardio	us

TABLE 3-10: Descriptive Terms Used in Body Systems

Medical Term	Meaning	Medical Term	Meaning
rectus	straight	vastus	huge
trapezius	shaped like a triangle		

Right Word or Wrong Word: ***Brachi/o*** **or** ***Bracchi/o*** **vs.** ***Brachy-*?**

Do both of these combining forms stem from the root *brachys*?

Let's Practice

Provide the Latin or Greek term that fits each description. Think carefully. Not all of these terms were in the table that you just reviewed, but they do appear in this chapter.

1. the temples on the side of your head ____________________
2. a modern word for backbone that looks much like (but not exactly like) the original word for it ____________________
3. abdomen ____________________
4. a muscle with a name that is very similar to an English word that describes a high-flying circus act in which a person is suspended by something (much as your shoulder is suspended by muscles) ____________________
5. a term meaning *erect* ____________________

Pregnancy Assessment: An Introduction

Patient Update

Mrs. Loeppky's wound has been stabilized, and her condition is not urgent or emergent. She has had an x-ray of her painful and swollen left thumb and hand. The bones are not broken, but she does have an ulnar collateral ligament injury. The deep laceration to her thigh has been sutured, and she was given a local anesthetic to relieve the pain of that procedure. At first she was reluctant to receive the anesthetic out of fear of harming her unborn child, but both the doctor and the nurse were able to allay her fears.

"A local anesthetic is one that is given directly to the site that we are working on. It won't cause any harm to your baby. I'll just inject it here and here, around your leg wound, so that I can put the sutures in," advised Dr. Abrams.

"Are you sure, doctor? Are you sure about my baby? I thought I wasn't supposed to take any medications," Glory said.

"Ah, yes. Well, that is correct. Medications can have harmful effects on a fetus. This varies throughout the pregnancy, when the babe is more or less vulnerable to the effects of certain drugs. You are in the third trimester of your pregnancy, and I'm giving you a local anesthetic to numb the pain. There is plenty of scientific evidence that local anesthetics don't harm the growth and development of the unborn child. You and your baby will be quite safe." Glory nodded.

Dr. Abrams completed the procedure, and Nurse Marnie dressed the wound with gauze and tape. The nearby LPN put the head of the bed back up into a semi-Fowler's position to improve the patient's comfort. Glory smiled at the LPN in thanks. Glory had been very uncomfortable on her back, even though the team had propped pillows under her left side. She heard someone say that a side-lying position put less stress on the abdominal muscles and the placenta than laying supine. She didn't know if that was true, but it certainly felt much better to her when she could sit up a bit and take the weight of her baby off of her lower back.

"I've ordered some acetaminophen with codeine for your pain if you need it, Glory. It's quite safe to take this as well," Dr. Abrams said as he pulled off his gloves. "If you are comfortable now, let's get you over for a sonogram. I'd like to get a couple of pictures of your abdomen, your placenta, and your baby, okay?" Dr. Abrams touched her gently on the shoulder and then left the ER bay.

"Nurse, do you believe what he said about my baby and the medications?" asked Glory.

"Absolutely, Glory. It's quite safe for you and the baby to have that local anesthetic and to have a couple of pain medications when you need them right now. You've been through a lot today already, and I'm not sure you realize how sore you just might be after you start to settle down from the accident." The nurse smiled and spoke directly to Glory, showing her patient confidence and caring. "What do you think? Would you like a pain pill now?" Glory nodded. The nurse left for a moment and returned with a medication cup, a small white pill, and a glass of water. Glory took the medication.

"Hey, Marnie, how's it going?" someone called.

The nurse nodded and smiled. "Hi, Willy."

"I'm looking for Glory Loeppky," said Willy. "Is this Ms. Loeppky?" The nurse nodded and introduced the patient to Willy, the porter. "How are you, Mrs. Loeppky?" Willy greeted the patient. "I'm here to wheel you down to get some pictures taken. You ready for that?" The nurse and Glory nodded simultaneously.

Within moments, Glory and Willy approached the Diagnostic Imaging Department. Willy entered and turned left. Another sign said Sonography, and Glory noticed the corridor next to it said Radiology. Willy entered Sonography and was met by a middle-aged man in a white lab coat.

"Hi, Ranjeet. This is Mrs. Glory Loeppky. She likes to be called by her first name, Glory." He looked at the patient. "Glory, this is Ranjeet. He's probably the best sonographer we've got. You're in good hands." He patted Glory on the shoulder and left. "Just give me a call when Glory wants a ride back to the ER," Willy called on his way back down the corridor.

"Hello, Glory," said Ranjeet as he wheeled Glory into a quiet, dark room. "I'm going take a few pictures of your abdomen and of your baby. Have you had a sonogram before?" Glory nodded yes. "All right then, you know what the procedure is. This machine is an ultrasound machine. It allows me to take a look at what's going on inside of you. First, I'm just going to put some of this gel on your belly. I know it might feel a bit cold, but that only lasts a minute or two. There, we're ready." Ranjeet pulled a computer monitor attached to the ultrasound machine nearer to Glory's bedside and began the scan. He worked gently, moving the transducer probe gently up and down; he occasionally stopped

and then worked in a close concentric circle before moving back to larger sweeps of her belly. Sometimes he stopped and entered data or clicked directions on the central processing unit (CPU), the ultrasound machine's computer. "I'm just taking a sonogram," he advised. "Did you know that still pictures taken with this machine are called sonograms or sonographs? It's the technology itself—the machine—that's called an ultrasound." Glory nodded and mentioned that she had not known the difference before.

"How far along are you, Glory?" Ranjeet asked calmly, as he kept his eyes on the scanner. She told him. "Yes, yes," he responded, "7½ months, yes. That's a 7-month-old fetus, all right." He smiled.

"Is my baby okay, Ranjeet? Is there anything wrong?"

"Well, ma'am, I am not at liberty to say. As you probably know from your last sonogram, only the radiologist or your doctor can actually make those kinds of determinations. It's protocol. A sonographer is not qualified to diagnose." All the while, Glory watched for any changes in Ranjeet's facial expression and to see if his eyes seemed to brighten as if he'd seen something unusual. She saw none, and when he spoke to her, he remained calm and professional. She felt reassured by that, although she wished he could say more. But he was right; these were the rules, and she knew it. She'd have to wait till she was back in the ER with Dr. Abrams.

Reflective Questions

1. Why has Glory been sent to sonography?
____

2. Is the sonographer able to tell Glory anything about her medical status or the status of her fetus? Why or why not?
____

3. Is it safe to have a local anesthetic when treating an injury if you are pregnant? Why or why not?
____

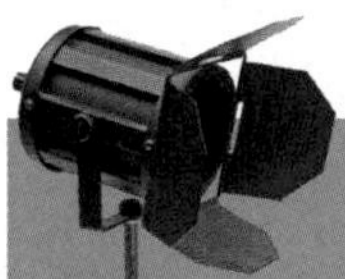

CAREER SPOTLIGHT: Sonographer

A sonographer is a professional who is not a physician. Sonographers work specifically with ultrasound technology, although they may assist with other procedures and tasks in the diagnostic imaging department. Their education can range from 1 to 4 years.

In the United States, sonographers are accredited and licensed (registered) by the American Registry of Diagnostic Medical Sonographers.

There are many subspecialties in sonography; the following list identifies some of them. Notice that the names for some of these specialties do not include the term *sonograph,* although most have derivative forms of the two roots *sono* (meaning *sound*) and *graph* (meaning *record*). Those word parts are highlighted.

Subspecialties of sonography include the following:

- Obstetrics and gynecology *sonograph*er: examines and assesses the female reproductive system
- Breast *sonograph*er: examines and assesses the breast
- Echocardio*graph*er: examines and assesses the heart and the blood flow
- Neuro*sono*logist: examines and assesses the brain and spinal cord
- Ophthalmology *sonograph*er: examines and assesses the eye, orbital structures, and related muscles
- Vascular technologist: examines and assesses the circulation of the peripheral vascular system and the abdominal vessels
- Abdominal *sonograph*er: examines and assesses all organs, blood vessels, and tissues of the abdomen

Right Word or Wrong Word: ***Sonogram*** **or** ***Ultrasound*****?**

The terms *ultrasound* and *sonogram* are often used interchangeably. Is this proper?

Learn the terminology: ultrasound assessment

Ultrasound technology is quite commonly used for the assessment of a patient's health status. For diagnostic purposes, an ultrasound provides a view of the internal organs. It does so by emitting a high-pitched sound through the transducer wand and into the body. These sound waves echo off of dense or solid masses. Depending on the purpose of the examination, the ultrasound technician or sonographer will stop from time to time to take a picture; this is also done through the transducer wand. The image or **sonogram** appears on the attached computer monitor, where it is captured as part of the examination record, which is called **sonograph**. Because ultrasound technology uses sound waves rather than x-rays, there is no risk of harm to the patient's health. In addition, this is a noninvasive procedure: nothing enters or invades the patient's body.

Ultrasound technology is frequently used for the ongoing assessment of pregnant women and the child in utero. This may be done on a routine basis throughout the pregnancy. Recall that our patient Glory Loeppky is 7½ months pregnant. For this reason, the ER doctor will automatically have ordered sonography of her abdomen and pelvic area to assess the status of both the fetus and the mother. Ultrasound or sonography is preferred as a diagnostic tool over x-ray methods when pregnancy is involved.

Critical Thinking

Work with a partner or small group to answer the following questions.

1. For what reason is an ultrasound examination (rather than an x-ray) preferred when a woman is pregnant?

   ____

2. What is meant by the term *noninvasive procedure*?

   ____

3. In the case of Glory Loeppky, Ranjeet may be a generalist in ultrasound technology, or he may have a specific specialty in that field. What might his specialty be?

   ____

4. What is the professional title of a person who uses the ultrasound machine?

   ____

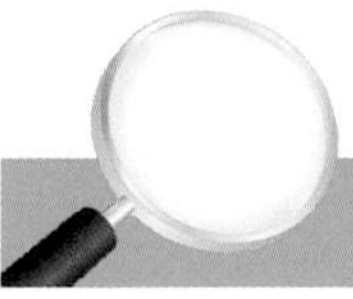

FOCUS POINT: *Noninvasive* vs. *Invasive*

In medicine, when a procedure is deemed to be *noninvasive,* it means that nothing will enter the body through the skin or a body orifice. Alternatively, if a procedure is *invasive,* then the body will somehow be entered. This could be through an orifice or through the skin (i.e., via an injection or a surgical incision).

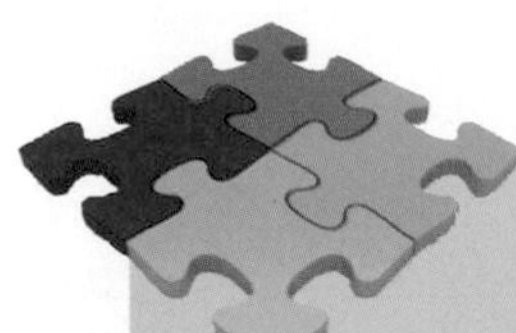

WORD BUILDING: Formula for Creating Words with the Combining Form *Son/o*

Whether you choose a career in sonography or not, you will likely encounter these terms in your role as a health-care provider. Sonograms and ultrasound images are very common tools for assessment.

son/o = combining form of a root that means *sound*

son + ic = *sonic*

Definition: referring to sound and its ability to be heard or its speed of transmission. (The suffix *-ic* means *pertaining to.*) *adjective*

Example: Some jets fly at supersonic speeds. A few moments after they pass overhead, you can hear a *sonic* boom; this is the noise wave that they make.

son + i + cate = *sonicate*

Definition: to expose someone or something to sound waves. *verb*

Example: Bacteria can be interrupted or destroyed by exposing them to high-frequency sounds. In other words, it can be beneficial to *sonicate* bacteria.

son + o + meter = *sonometer*

Definition: a special device used by dentists to cause sound for the production of anesthesia. *noun*

Example: Patients who do not tolerate some forms of anesthesia may find themselves exposed to a *sonometer* to help numb pain receptors and to alleviate pain.

sono + graph = *sonograph*

Definition: a record of the procedure in which computerized pictures of internal organs and body structures are taken by sound waves. *noun*

Example: Some parents like to keep a *sonograph* of their baby in utero, before he or she is born, to look at and show to family and friends.

sono + rous = *sonorous*

Definition: an adjective that describes a loud and resonant sound or loud, deep tones. This term may be used in medicine, diagnostic imaging, or when describing someone's voice. *adjective*

Example: A cello is a *sonorous* musical instrument. The continuous loud hum of hospital equipment can also be *sonorous,* and staff may wear hearing protectors.

Free Writing

Use each of the words below and add a term that begins with *son/o-* to create a sentence. You will need to add a few of your own words to make a complete, logical sentence. Work with a partner or in a small group, if you like.

1. pictures, record, sound waves

   ____

2. professional, examines, ultrasound

   ____

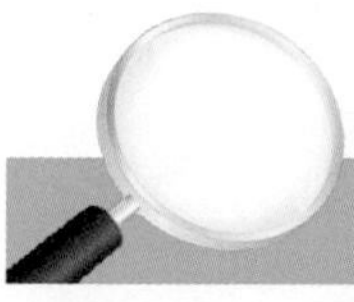

FOCUS POINT: *Sonometer* vs. *Centimeter*

Be very careful with these two words. They are homonyms of a sort: they sound alike when they are pronounced quickly, and people frequently make mistakes when interpreting their meaning.

A *sonometer* is a device that is used to produce anesthesia through sound waves.

A *centimeter* is a measurement in the metric system. For example, there are 2.54 centimeters in 1 inch. In medicine and health care, you may very well hear terms for the metric system used with regard to measurements and scientific or laboratory reports.

Learn the language: obstetrics

When Glory Loeppky arrived in the ER, her maternal health status was quickly assessed. In most emergency situations like this one, hospitals follow something called an OB/GYN protocol. The abbreviation *OB* stands for **obstetrics.** This is the medical field that specializes in pregnancy and childbirth. The abbreviation *GYN* stands for **gynecology**. This field of medicine treats women only, and it is particularly focused on reproductive health.

In the opening scene of this chapter, the ER physician, Dr. Abrams, orders someone on the team to contact OB/GYN so that someone from that department will come to assess the patient as well. Protocol demands that the ABCs of a pregnant patient in the ER are the primary and priority responsibilities of the attending ER physician, but that ER physician must also triage the status of the pregnancy. When the ER physician determines that there is no trauma to the fetus or to the pregnancy, OB/GYN may simply be contacted to provide a second opinion and to stand by in case of any sudden changes. The ER physician remains in charge of the patient's assessment, care, and treatment. Should the attending ER physician determine that the pregnancy or the life of the mother or fetus is at risk, an obstetrician or obstetrical surgeon will step in to provide emergency care. Table 3-10 provides insight into terms that refer to these medical specialties.

TABLE 3-11: Roots: Obstetrics and Gynecology

Root or Combining Form	Add Another Root, a Prefix, or a Suffix	Create a Medical Term
obstetrics (root) obstetr/o (combining form) Meaning: midwife		obstetrics: the branch of medicine focused on all aspects of pregnancy and childbirth
obstetr/i (combining form of obstetrics)	-ician	obstetrician: a physician who specializes in pregnancy and childbirth
gyne (root) Meaning: woman, female	-cic	gynecic: pertaining to women
gynec/o gyno- gyn- (combining forms of *gyne*)	-ology	gynecology: the field of study of conditions and diseases specific to the female reproductive system
gynec/o gyno- gyn- (combining forms of *gyne*)	-ologist	gynecologist: a physician who specializes in medicine that addresses female reproductive health and illness

Fill in the Blanks

Use the new language that you have learned in a meaningful way. Complete these sentences by filling in the blanks.

1. The term for a set of rules that guide practice (action), such as the one that Dr. Abrams followed, is _______________.
2. When a patient's health status during an emergency is assessed, the procedure is called _______________.
3. The _________________ specializes in maternal health and childbirth.
4. _______________ is a field of medicine that focuses on the female reproductive system.
5. If there is no assessment of trauma to the unborn child or to the mother's abdomen, then the _______________ continues to hold full responsibility for treating a pregnant patient who has been in an accident.

The language of pregnancy: an introduction

Pregnancy is a 9-month process. It begins with conception, and it ends with birth. The time in between these two events is pregnancy. Pregnancy is divided into **trimesters**. The term *trimester* means *a 3-month period of time*. That means that the 9 months of pregnancy are divided into three equal time periods:

- Trimester one: The period from conception to week 12 is marked by significant hormonal changes in the mother's body. Symptoms can include swelling of the breasts, nausea, and vomiting (i.e., morning sickness).
- Trimester two: During weeks 13 through 28, evidence of the growth of the fetus is noticeable. The pregnant woman can perceive the movement of the fetus.
- Trimester three: From week 29 until birth at week 40, the fetus completes its growth and development. Other people may be able to observe fetal movement or outlines of parts of the fetus's anatomy on the mother's enlarged belly. Our patient, Glory Loeppky, is in the third trimester of her pregnancy.

Critical Thinking

Use proper medical terminology as you answer the following questions.

1. What is a trimester? ____
2. How many trimesters are there in a pregnancy? ______________________________
3. At what point during pregnancy are the hormonal changes in the pregnant woman most significant? ____

Physical assessment: pregnancy

During the physical examination of a pregnant woman, the following types of assessment are used by the nurse or doctor:

Subjective Report

The woman will be asked a number of questions about the pregnancy, her history with childbirth, the prenatal care that she has received, and her general health (both currently and historically).

Observation

- Of the breasts for symmetry, size, color, texture, status of milk production, and any observable abnormalities
- Of the abdomen for size (appropriate to the number of months of pregnancy) and evidence of movement of the fetus
- Of the vaginal area for any signs of bleeding (In a healthy low- or no-risk pregnancy, there should be no bleeding.)

Palpation (touch)

- Of the breasts for texture, elasticity, tenderness, temperature, and masses (lumps)
- Of the abdomen for any pain or discomfort (After the fourth or fifth month of pregnancy, this examination can also locate the fetus, identify the fetal position, and detect any fetal movement.)

Objective Investigation

Assessments of the woman and her fetus can be followed up and confirmed by a sonogram and blood tests. Fetal heart monitors or listening with a stethoscope can also assist with locating and assessing the fetus.

Blood tests and pregnancy

Glory Loeppky is 7½ months pregnant. It is likely that when she first suspected that she was going to have a child, she was given a blood test called a **quantitative blood serum** test or **beta hCG** to confirm it. This test measures the presence of the hormone human chorionic gonadotropin (hCG). Before her admission to the hospital and during the early months of her pregnancy, Mrs. Loeppky would have had several routine blood tests. Learn the names of the terms listed in Routine Blood Tests during Pregnancy.

Today, at Fayette General Hospital, the doctor has ordered blood work (lab tests using blood) for Glory Loeppky, for a number of reasons. He is not only interested in the potential for infection from her leg wound, but he is also assessing her overall maternal health. In addition to a complete blood count, Dr. Abrams has also ordered a glucose screening. During pregnancy, women run the risk of acquiring **gestational diabetes**, which is a type of diabetes that only occurs during pregnancy. Under stress (such as a motor vehicle accident), blood glucose (sugar) levels may be adversely affected, thereby clouding the patient's judgment and leading to symptoms such as confusion and fainting. If left untreated, gestational diabetes can cause some harm to the fetus as well.

For more information about pregnancy and the female reproductive system, see Chapters 8 and 17

Let's Practice

Write the term that identifies what is being talked about in each sentence.

1. The source of a ____________________ report about a patient's condition is the patient himself or herself.
2. The abbreviation *hCG* stands for ____________________.
3. The abdominal palpation of a woman who is 7½ months pregnant can identify ____________________, ____________________, and ____________________.
4. ____________________ bleeding is not usually observed during a healthy pregnancy.

TABLE 3-12: Routine Blood Tests during Pregnancy

Test	Purpose
Blood group	This test simply identifies the blood type: A, B, AB, or O. Blood group O is the most common. This knowledge is important before giving birth (or before any surgery that a person might have) so that the medical team can have a blood transfusion on hand in case of emergency.
Rhesus factor (Rh factor)	This test identifies the presence of a certain protein in the blood. Ideally, the biological parents of the child should have the same Rh factor. If one is negative and the other is positive, then the fetus's ability to survive may be at risk.
Hemoglobin level	Anemia is sometimes seen during pregnancy, and an anemic pregnant woman experiences a great deal of fatigue and a low energy level. Knowledge of the iron (ferrous) level of the blood allows the care team (i.e., the family doctor, obstetricians, midwife, or nurse practitioner) to intervene with suggestions for dietary supplements.
Hepatitis B (and perhaps C)	This blood test screens for the presence or absence of hepatitis B, a liver disease that may be undetected without the test. Hepatitis B can be passed on to a baby before or at birth, and this potentially leads to liver damage in the child.
Human immunodeficiency virus/acquired immunodeficiency syndrome (may be optional)	Screening for these diseases with a blood test can prevent transmission to the child during childbirth.

CHAPTER SUMMARY

In this chapter, we have followed our patient, Glory Loeppky, from her arrival at Fayette General Hospital through her assessment and treatment in the ER. Key terms to use during a physical assessment in an emergency situation and with a pregnant patient have been explored. The language of blood was also introduced. Anatomical and medical terms for the muscular system were presented; this included opportunities to break words into their component parts and to create words by combining prefixes, roots, and suffixes. Career Spotlights focused on nurses and sonographers, and there was an introduction to the language of ultrasound technology and sonography.

See How Much You've Learned

For audio exercises, visit **http://www.MedicalLanguageLab.com.** 

Chapter 3 has introduced you to some medical abbreviations. These have been organized into a study table here for quick reference. Some of them you will recognize immediately, and some will reappear throughout the following chapters with more explanation and application.

TABLE 3-13: Medical Abbreviations: Review

Medical Abbreviation	Full Term	Medical Abbreviation	Full Term
ABC	airway, breathing, and circulation	LPN	licensed practical nurse
BP	blood pressure	LVN	licensed vocational nurse
BMD	Becker's muscular dystrophy	MCV	mean corpuscular volume
BPMD	benign pseudohypertrophic muscular dystrophy	MCHC	mean corpuscular hemoglobin concentration
CBC	complete blood count	MCP	metacarpal phalangeal
CPU	central processing unit	OB	obstetrics
CNA	certified nursing assistant	PLT	platelet count
EMT	emergency medical technician	PRN	as needed
ER	emergency room (synonymous with *emergency department*)	resps	respirations
GYN	gynecology	RN	registered nurse
hCG	human chorionic gonadotropin	RCDW	red cell distribution width
HMO	health maintenance organization	Rh	Rhesus factor in blood
HGB	hemoglobin	RBC	red blood cell
HCT	hematocrit	STAT	short for *statim,* meaning *immediately or right now*
HIV	human immunodeficiency virus	UCL	ulnar collateral ligament
ID	identification	WBC	white blood cell
IV	intravenous	WBC diff	white blood cell differential

Key Terms

ABCs
beta hCG
BP
cardiac muscle
complete blood count (CBC)
contraction
deep laceration
erythrocytes
extension
fascia
fascicules
fibrous
fracture
gestational diabetes
gynecology (GYN)
hematic cells
hemocytes
hemogram
incontinent
involuntary
involuntary control
leukocytes
ligaments
localized
obstetrics (OB)
opposes/opposing
palpation
patient complaint
platelets
point of insertion
point of origin
pregnancy
presenting condition
quadriceps
quantitative blood serum
relax/relaxes
resps
skeletal muscles
sonogram
sonograph
striated
tachycardic
tendons
thready
tourniquet
triage
trimesters
ultrasound
visceral muscles
vitals
voluntary control

CHAPTER REVIEW

Critical Thinking

Use your new knowledge of medical terms to answer these questions.

1. What is palpation?

____

2. Who is able to diagnose what is found on a sonogram?

____

3. In health care, who makes a subjective report?

____

4. Which trimester is Glory in? How do you know?

____

Name the Term

Read the description given and identify the correct muscle.

1. a muscle on the lateral side of the forearm ______________
2. a major muscle in the chest that body builders pay close attention to ______________
3. a muscle that works with the longest bone in the leg ______________
4. a muscle along the upper back that supports the clavicle and the scapula ______________

Break It Down

Break these words into their component parts of prefix-root-suffix, as applicable. Name each element.

1. hematology ______________
2. sonograph ______________
3. fibromyalgia ______________

Translate the Terminology

Use your new skills to decipher medical language. Try to do so without the use of a medical dictionary. You may, of course, look back through this chapter for help.

1. Dr. Abrams informed Glory Loeppky that a local anesthetic could be safely administered during the third trimester of her pregnancy.

   ____

2. When she presented at the ER, Glory was reported to be *oriented × 3.*

   ____

3. Dr. Abrams applied a hemostat to prevent the hemorrhaging of the laceration in Glory's leg.

   ____

4. The sonographer used the transducer wand to view Glory's fetus.

   ____

Fill in the Blanks

Fill in the blanks with the missing part of each term.

1. ____________ology is the field of medicine that specializes in women's health, particularly as it is related to their reproductive and sexual health.
2. The term ____________*rrhage* refers to excessive blood loss.
3. The ____________ceps are a specific group of muscles in the upper leg.
4. The term ____________*myalgia* means *pain in many muscles.*

Name the Suffix

Read each definition and then write a suffix with that meaning.

1. ____________ an act or process; the end result of an action
2. ____________ to form or shape
3. ____________ inflammation or swelling
4. ____________ the immediate, current state of something
5. ____________ containing or full of

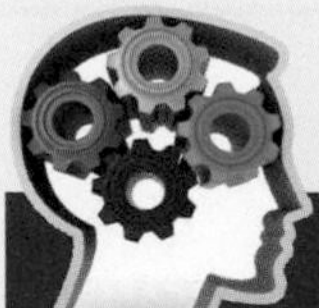

MEMORY MAGIC: The SAMPLE Mnemonic

First responders and emergency health providers often use this simple mnemonic (memory technique) to help them remember the steps to take to perform a health assessment. You might find it helpful, too. Write this mnemonic out on a card, and keep it in your pocket for future reference. After a while, you'll have memorized the whole process!

S = Signs and symptoms

A = Allergies, if any, as well as types of reactions

M = Medications being used, including prescription and non-prescription drugs, herbal preparations, and vitamins, as well as the time of the last dose

P = Past medical and surgical history, including pregnancy, if applicable

L = Last meal and fluids taken

E = Events leading up to this injury, illness, or situation

Even if you don't envision yourself doing assessments, this mnemonic is still helpful. It demonstrates the logical process that care providers go through. If you work in medical records or transcription, you will see this flow in your written work and dictations. If you create medical forms, these pieces may very well fit into the first section of that form.

CHAPTER FOUR

Diagnostic Imaging

Focus: Neurological System and Skeletal System

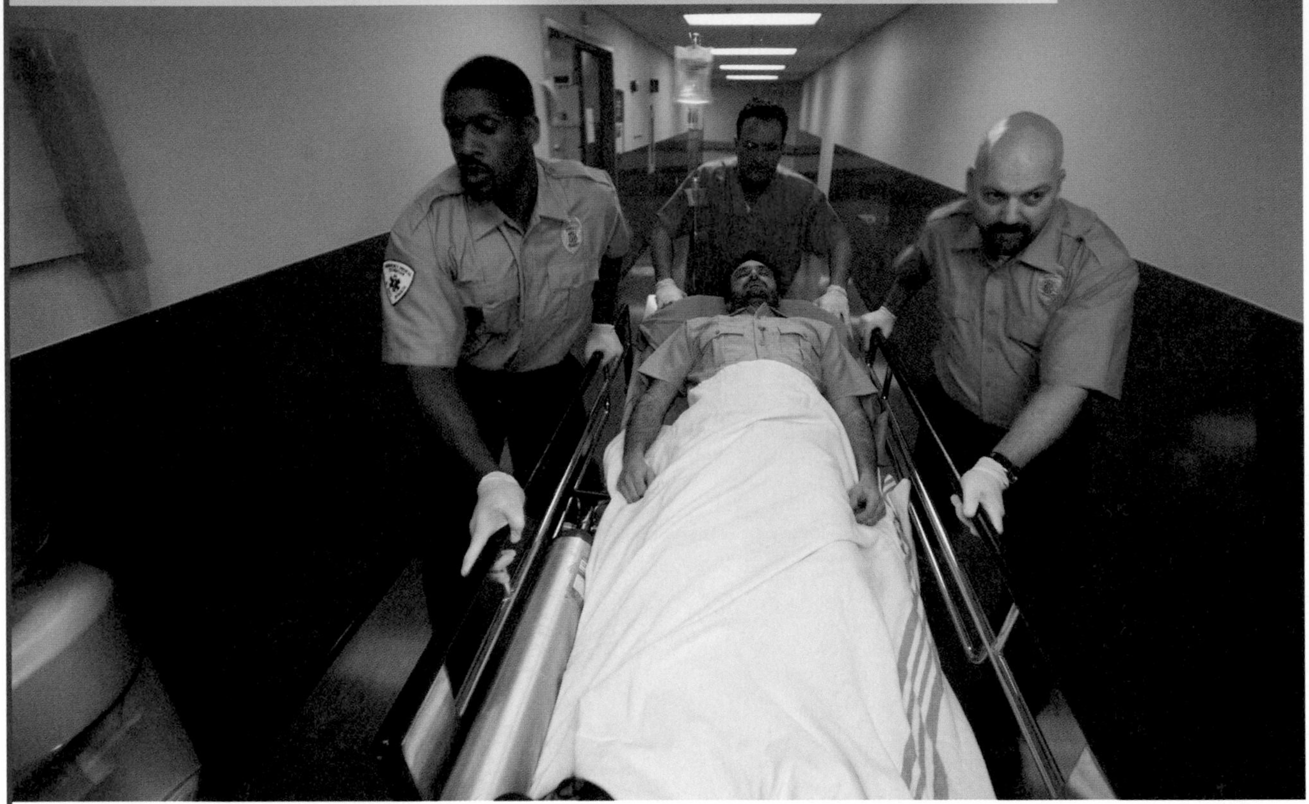

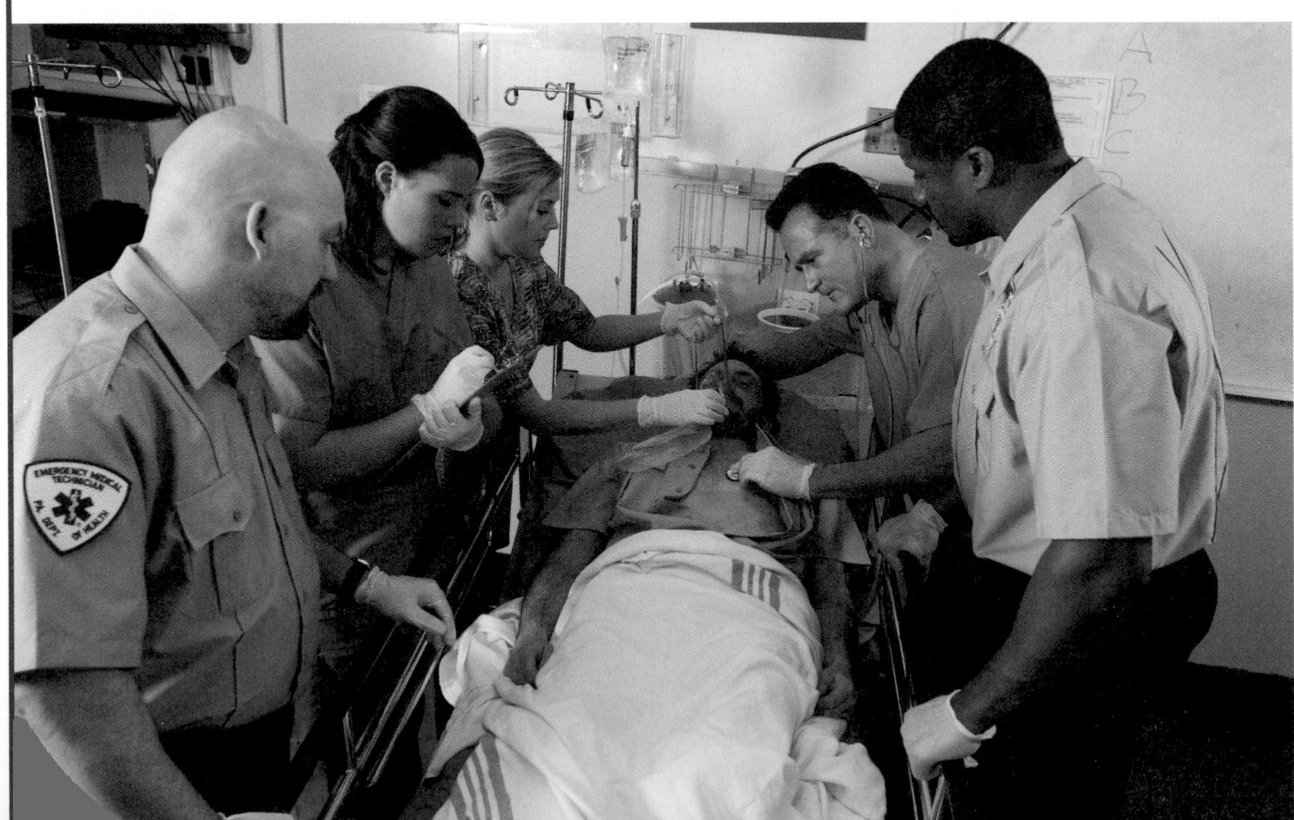

Gilbert Loeppky is a 36-year-old married man. He drives a delivery truck in a busy city. He often works long days, sometimes putting in more than 16 hours a day. He works hard, and he is well liked and respected by colleagues, friends, and family. He occasionally wears glasses to read.

Today, Mr. Loeppky—or Gil, as he likes to be called—was in a motor vehicle accident on a main street in a commercial district. Two vehicles (his truck and a car) collided at an intersection around noon. The impact sent his truck swerving across the road and up onto the sidewalk. The truck came to a stop when it slammed into a power pole. The left front side of the vehicle was severely damaged.

According to police on the scene, Gil was not wearing his seat belt at the time of the accident. The force of the crash pushed the hood of the truck inward. Gil's head came into contact with the windshield and molding. His feet and legs appeared to be trapped, but the EMT had no difficulty extracting him.

Gil was found in an unconscious state by emergency personnel. He was suffering from facial lacerations, head trauma, and a fractured leg. As a result of the seriousness of his injuries, Gil was immediately transported to the Emergency Room of Okla Trauma Center by Rescue Unit 112 of the Fire Department.

Patient Update

"What have we got?" called out the emergency physician as the Emergency Room doors swung wide on their electric hinges.

"Adult male. Name's Gil Loeppky. Head trauma; loss of consciousness. Reactive to pain, so may not be a spinal injury. We put the collar on him. Vitals stable but high. BP 140/80, pulse thready at 100 and holding. ECG okay. No apparent internal injuries. Looks like a fracture of the right femoral. Superficial bleeding from lacerations to the face. Hematoma, left and right orbital. No apparent fracture there," reported EMT Stanley as he and EMT Raybuck unloaded Gil Loeppky from their rig and rushed him in through the hospital doors. "We started an IV. O_2 by nasal prongs."

"Sir, sir... can you hear me?" queried the physician, with his face close to the patient and his voice loud, while running alongside the gurney. "Sir, can you hear me?" As they approached the trauma bay, nurses and technicians swarmed into it. As a team, they carefully lifted the patient up and onto the hospital stretcher. Gil groaned loudly when this occurred. "Mr. Loeppky, this is Dr. Raymond. You've been in an accident. You're at Okla Trauma Center." Dr. Raymond began the emergency assessment: He checked Gil's airway, breathing, and circulation, and he then assessed for Gil's level of consciousness. Once again, Gil responded to the pain assessment, but he did not awaken.

"Let's get him up for x-rays, guys. I'll want a head CT while we're at it," ordered Dr. Raymond. "Keep that backboard and head block on him until we know what we're dealing with." The ER staff prepared to move Gil.

"Get x-rays of the femur, and do the chest and abdomen," added Dr. Raymond.

The team moved with precision clockwork to hang the IV, to connect a portable O_2 tank to the nasal prongs in situ, and to cleanse Gil's head wound. Other staff cut off Gil's clothes while being careful not to jostle his spine, neck, or head. They then covered him with a blanket. The emergency team moved quickly, and, by the time Dr. Raymond completed his assessment and orders, they were already wheeling Gil Loeppky to Diagnostic Imaging.

Reflective Questions

Reflect on the story you've just read as you answer these questions.

1. EMT Stanley is giving a running report to someone who works in the Emergency Room at Okla Trauma Center. Whom is he talking to?

   ____

2. The patient's name is Gilbert Loeppky. He likes to be called Gil, but why does the physician refer to him as "Mr. Loeppky"?

   ____

3. EMT Stanley reports that the patient is unconscious, but he does not use those words. Instead, he uses a short descriptive phrase to convey that message. What is that phrase?

   ____

4. Break down the medical terminology to decipher its meaning. In plain English, what does "hematoma, left orbital" mean?

   ____

For audio exercises, visit **http://www.MedicalLanguageLab.com.** 

Learning Objectives

After reading Chapter 3, you will be able to do the following:

- Recognize and define the vocabulary used to diagnose and discuss assessment of the neurological system and the brain.
- Recognize and define the vocabulary used to diagnose and discuss assessment of the skeletal system.
- Identify and use anatomical terms related to the skeletal system, specifically the spine, cranium, femur, hip, and pelvic girdle.
- Identify diagnostic imaging (DI) personnel.
- Name two key diagnostic imaging (DI) tests.
- Interpret the abbreviations that are associated with medical professionals, procedures, and anatomical systems.
- Improve your word recognition skills for word parts and derivatives.
- Expand your vocabulary as it pertains to injury and trauma.
- Successfully use new medical terms and language in writing and conversation.

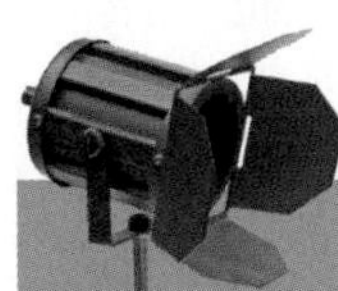

CAREER SPOTLIGHT: Physicians and Surgeons

Physicians are highly trained medical professionals. Their main responsibilities are diagnosis and treatment, and they are also able to prescribe medications. In addition, physicians can carry out a variety of procedures and medical investigations, such as biopsies. According to the American Medical Association, physicians require undergraduate degrees followed by four years of medical school. Residency (internship) begins after medical school and can last from 3 to 5 years in the United States.

During their residency, physicians may choose to specialize. Although all physicians will have a clinical rotation experience in surgery, they are not all certified as *surgeons.* Criteria for this advanced certificate or licensure may be set by a state or regulatory body for physicians and surgeons. Surgeons receive specialized training and experience during their residency, and they can go on to a fellowship in their field. Trauma surgeons have advanced training in emergency medical situations, including a minimum of 2 years of residency in surgery.

Physicians and surgeons are both legally qualified to practice medicine.

Assessment Through Diagnostic Imaging

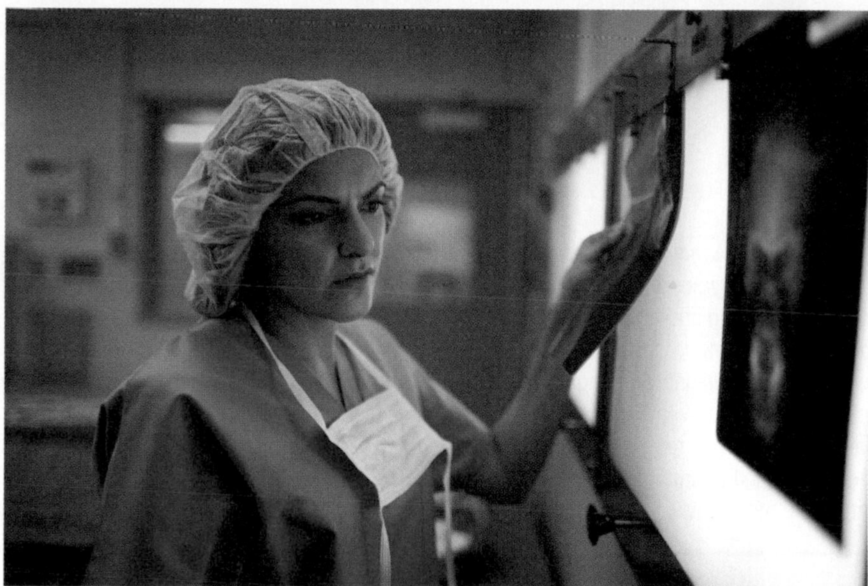

Figure 4.1: Diagnostic imaging department

We begin this chapter with an introduction to the language of the diagnostic imaging department. Here, a full range of radiology services is provided for assessment, diagnostic imaging, and image-guided treatments. In the latter case, treatments usually fall under the heading of medical imaging. Some hospitals and clinics will have different names for these departments, but Radiology, Diagnostic Imaging, and Medical Imaging are the most common.

Read the following information about our patient, Gil Loeppky. You are not expected at this point to know all of the terms and procedures that are mentioned. The purpose of this story and the following exercises is not to understand everything being said but rather to practice your skills of "getting the big picture" of the situation by analyzing context and word structure.

Patient Update

Mr. Loeppky has now arrived in the diagnostic imaging (DI) department for emergency radiology. (*Emergency radiology* is a medical term that is commonly used to signify the urgent need for these examinations to be performed.) Although the patient's vital signs are stable, his health status remains at great risk as a result of the injuries that he received during the motor vehicle accident. The priority of care is to keep him alive. Although Gil is not presently showing signs of hemorrhaging, it is critical to assess this possibility through imaging. Second, the treatment team needs to assess the patient's brain. Finally, Gil's fracture or fractures will be identified.

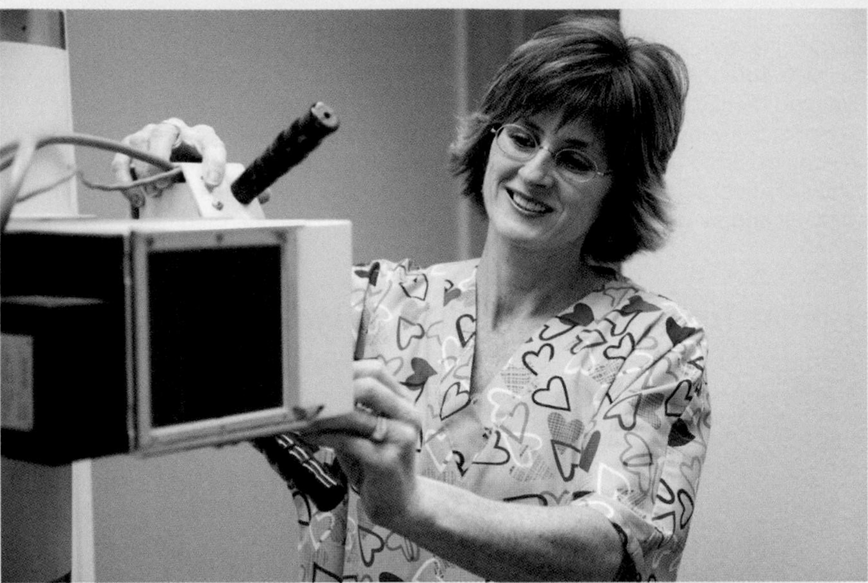

A radiologist and a radiological technician quickly read the accompanying chart and organize the imaging. They see that Dr. Raymond in the ER wants images of the patient's head, torso, and abdomen to rule out internal hemorrhaging and brain injury, as well as to assess for other injuries.

The radiological nurse, Maggie, will also attend the patient while his images are being taken. She will stay with him while diagnostic imaging procedures are completed. It will be essential that she monitor the patient's vital and neurovital signs and that she be on hand should his condition worsen.

Plain radiography (x-ray) will be the first procedure in Mr. Loeppky's assessment. This is a quick and informative method for internal assessment of the head and the abdomen. Images will be obtained, and the patient will be moved directly afterward to have a CT scan of the head, neck, and spine performed.

The language of radiology and assessment

Radiology plays a key role in patient assessment. To understand what happens in a diagnostic imaging department, you will need to learn how medical terms are formed from the combining forms *rad, radi,* and *radio,* as well as about the symbols and abbreviations that are used to refer to these terms.

Many terms used in diagnostic imaging derive from the Latin root *radix,* meaning *root.* The combining form for this root is *rad.* Notice that *rad* and *radical* have multiple meanings.

rad:

1. combining form meaning *root or cause*
2. the approved medical abbreviation signifying a radiation-absorbed dose
3. In America, RAD (capitalized) is a medical abbreviation that refers to the diagnostic term *reactive adjustment disorder,* which is found in children.

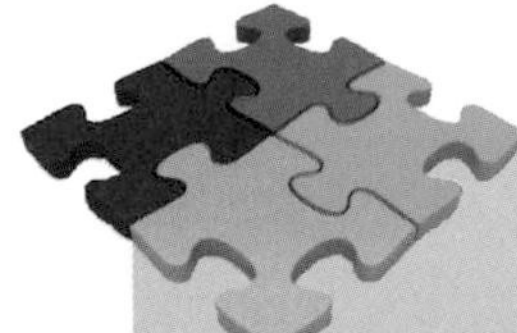

WORD BUILDING: Formula for Creating Words with the Combining Forms *Rad, Radi-,* and *Radio*

radi- = combining form meaning *beam or spoke.*

rad + ical = *radical*

Definitions: 1) signifying a group of atoms that, when formed together, produce a component of a particular compound. *noun* 2) a medical term used to describe an unusual or extreme measure taken to eradicate disease or interrupt a disease process. *noun* or *adjective*

Example: A *radical* mastectomy or the complete removal of a breast may be called for as part of cancer treatment.

radi + um = *radium*
Definition: a metallic element that is radioactive and fluorescent. *noun*

Example: *Radium* is no longer used for cancer treatment, because it settles in the bone and can itself cause leukemia.

radi + ate = *radiate*
Definition: to spread out from a common center or core; to be emitted in rays. *verb*

Example: A transducer wand *radiates* ultrasound frequencies into the body.

radi + ation = *radiation*
Definition: energy in the form of emitted ionizing rays, which are used for diagnosis or therapy. *noun*

Example: The use of *radiation* to kill cancer cells is called *radiation therapy.*

radio + active = *radioactive*
Definition: having the ability to emit radiation as a result of exposure to radium. *adjective*

Example: *Radioactive* isotopes are often used for diagnostic and assessment purposes.

radio + logy = *radiology*
Definition: the study of radiation and radioactive substances; the field of medicine that uses these substances. *noun*

Example: *Radiology* is an important diagnostic tool.

radio + ologist = *radiologist*
Definition: a medical specialist doctor who obtains and interprets x-rays or radiographic images. *noun*

Example: *Radiologists* have been quick to embrace the new technologies of MRI, CT, and PT scans.

radio + graph = *radiograph*
Definition: an x-ray image produced on film that shows the internal structure of an object that has been exposed to radiation. *noun*

Example: While the patient underwent a series of operations to repair a shattered leg bone, *radiographs* of the leg were examined before each stage of treatment.

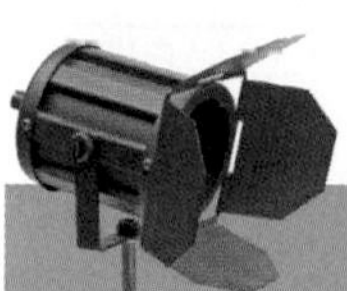

CAREER SPOTLIGHT: Careers in Diagnostic Imaging

A *radiologist* is a physician who is an expert at obtaining and interpreting medical images. A radiologist is a qualified and certified physician with a specialty in radiology. This doctor's training will have included a minimum of 4 years of residency (graduate medical education) in radiology.

A *medical imaging technologist* is a health-care professional with specific training and education in the use of diagnostic imaging equipment. Training can range from a 1-year certificate to a full baccalaureate degree. Some medical imaging technologists may go on to earn a master's degree in their field.

A *radiologic technologist (RT)* is a health-care professional who carries out medical imaging using x-rays or other radiation-based diagnostic tools. These can include computed tomography scans (CTs) and magnetic resonance imaging (MRIs). The RT assists the radiologist. The work includes explaining procedures to patients, reassuring them, and obtaining their cooperation for positioning. The RT also moves the imaging equipment into position and controls it to obtain

Continued

exposures of the inside of the patient's body. This professional may also operate mobile x-ray equipment that can be taken to the emergency department, the operating room, or the patient's bedside. This technologist is often referred to as "the RT," "the radio-tech," or simply "the technician."

The *x-ray technician* is a radiologic technologist whose focus is radiography with the use of x-ray films.

The *radiologist assistant (RA)* is a health-care professional with a more advanced level of education and training than the RT. The RA person works under the close supervision of a radiologist, and he or she performs and assists with imaging tasks that require an advanced level of skill. The RA is also involved in patient management and evaluation in the diagnostic imaging department. These professionals can also make judgments about image quality and patient status related to those images, which they forward to the radiologist.

The *radiological nurse (R-RN)* is a nurse who develops and manages care plans to facilitate an understanding of diagnostic imaging procedures for patients and their families. The R-RN follows the patient through imaging procedures and monitors the patient's recuperation from these procedures. He or she provides physical, mental, and emotional care to patients who are undergoing diagnostic imaging procedures, records procedures on the patient's chart, and confers with the radiologist and the patient's assigned physician.

Fill in the Blanks

Fill in each blank by writing a word that begins with *radi* or *radio* to create a logical sentence. Work with a partner or in a small group.

1. The most common form of diagnostic imaging is the x-ray or ____________________.
2. A person who is exposed to the element ____________________ can become ____________________.
3. The x-ray technician wears a lead apron to protect himself or herself from ______________ when taking images.
4. A doctor who makes assessments on the basis of diagnostic images is a specialist in ____________________. He or she is referred to as a ____________________.

Let's Practice

Complete the following exercise related to our patient, Mr. Loeppky, and the diagnostic imaging (DI) department. Use the new medical terms and titles that you have learned.

1. What are the professional titles of the DI staff who will be working with Mr. Loeppky?
   ____
2. Who has made the decision to send the patient to the DI department?
   ____
3. Who has made x-rays the top priority in the patient's care?
   ____

TABLE 4-1: Radiology Symbols and Abbreviations

Abbreviation or Symbol	Notice	Meaning
Ra	There is no hyphen at the end.	the chemical symbol for *radium,* which is a chemical element
Ra-	There is a hyphen at the end of the prefix.	a prefix used to form terms that relate to the element radium
RAI	This abbreviation is in all capital letters, with no periods.	the medical abbreviation for *radioactive iodine*
RAIU	This abbreviation is in all capital letters, with no periods.	the medical abbreviation for *radioactive iodine uptake*

Right Word or Wrong Word: *Ra* or *RA*?

The symbol *Ra* should not be confused with the abbreviation *RA*. Why not?

Fill in the Blanks

Begin to use new terminology by choosing terms to complete the following sentences. By doing so, you will become more familiar with medical terms in their proper context.

1. A __________ is a physician who works specifically in the diagnostic imaging department.
2. The quickest method of viewing and assessing the internal body is with __________.
3. In large medical or trauma centers, you may find a __________ working in the DI department, but it is not common to see him or her in smaller or more general health facilities.
4. From your knowledge of the health care system, you know that a __________ is likely to complete a full assessment and to report on a patient who has been assessed with the use of diagnostic imaging.
5. To work in the field of __________ __________ requires education and training that can include one-year technology certificates or degrees.

Listen to the language of radiology and assessment

Read aloud or listen to the following dialogue between the radiologist, Dr. Krenshaw, the radiological nurse, R-RN Maggie, and the radiologic technologist, RT Juanita.

Patient Update

Dr. Krenshaw: Okay, what do we have here?

R-RN Maggie: Head injury from an MVA in a 36-year-old male. Unconscious. Vital signs are normal at the moment, but we're worried about the potential for brain hemorrhaging. He's breathing on his own, so the airway isn't impeded, and the spinal cord seems intact because he moans when we touch his broken leg. Dr. Raymond has ruled out quadriplegia and paraplegia.

Dr. Krenshaw: All right, and you're saying no evidence of esthesioneurosis or sensory impairment, as far as you can tell. I'm assuming that you've been doing some pain response tests?

R-RN Maggie: Yes. I've been doing a coma scale on him every 15 minutes. No epileptic activity. Looks like a right hip and maybe an ankle fracture, too, probably from trying to brake to prevent the crash.

Dr. Krenshaw: Right. His color isn't good, but that's understandable due to the traumas. Certainly has raccoon eyes. *Backboard* and *cervical collar*? Yes, good. We'll take a look at his spine to be safe and get a *thoracic* shot while we're at it. Okay, let's get him to *x-ray* STAT. Where's the RT... Juanita...

Oh, there you are. Good. Let's start with some cranial pictures, then the cervical spine and the chest. When you're done, get those films to me STAT, will you? I want those pictures first and then get him to CT for a head scan. You can do the hips and lower extremities after I see what's going on.

RT Juanita: Yes, of course.

The RT and the R-RN wheel the patient into the x-ray examination room.

R-RN Maggie: Let me help you position him. You'll need another hand.

RT Juanita: Thanks. I can see he has been in an accident of some sort. What happened?

R-RN Maggie: MVA. Hit a pole and the motor came right in on him. Looks like he hit the frame of the windshield or something. As you can see, both of his eyes are now turning black and blue, and the left one's swollen shut.

RT Juanita: Okay, so we're looking for head injuries and brain trauma. Here, let's get a frontal view first, since he's wearing a collar. We can leave him supine, in this position. Then you can help me as we get lateral views, left and right. But I won't actually do that until we get an *exposure* of the cervical spine. I'll do that immediately, run the film to the radiologist, and then we'll get those lateral pictures.

R-RN Maggie: Okay, good.

RT Juanita: He seems to be breathing okay on his own, although his breaths are shallow, so I am assuming you don't suspect fractured ribs, lung impairment, or spinal cord injury?

R-RN Maggie: Correct. But we'll take that chest x-ray, just in case. And the doctor wants a picture of his full spine. He didn't have his seat belt on, you know.

RT Juanita: Oh, that's why the Doc wants pictures of his knees and hip, too, huh?

R-RN Maggie: Yes, we're suspecting a right hip fracture from braking hard when he saw he was going head-on into a pole.

RT Juanita: Wow. I guess his left knee probably hit the dashboard then? And the force of the crash pushed his right leg up into his *pelvis*. Maybe the pelvis is fractured, too. Or maybe just his hip is fractured. I guess we'll know in a moment.

R-RN Maggie: Yes. The doctor thinks his right ankle is broken, too, but that's not a priority for us right now.

RT Juanita: Okay, I'll check with the radiologist before taking those hip, knee, and ankle shots. They are important but of lower priority than these others. So, just to summarize so we are both clear on what's going to happen now, I'm going to take images of the head, neck, and spine first. That will give us some indication of the status of his neurological system in general. After I run those by the radiologist, we'll get some x-rays of his femur and pelvic area to assess for fractures. Okay, let's begin.

Key terms: radiology and assessment

A number of key medical terms appeared in the dialogue. Learn these words, which are often used during radiological assessment.

x-ray: a form of electromagnetic radiation that involves the use of photons. Another term that is sometimes used for this is *ionizing radiation.* The term *x-ray* also refers to a type of image that is produced on radiographic film by exposing the body to x-rays.

exposure: the general meaning is *the process of revealing something*. However, in the context of imaging, the term derives from the field of photography. An image is exposed in its negative form onto film to create an image. When an x-ray image is being taken, the technician leaves the room for a moment and tells the patient not to move. At that time, a sound is heard as the technician exposes the patient to radio waves or rays, which imprint an image onto the radiographic film that is on or very near the patient.

STAT: a standard medical abbreviation derived from the Latin word, *statim,* which means *immediately.* The full word is rarely used.

thoracic: adjective describing the thorax, the chest, or the upper part of the torso, both internally and externally

cervical collar: a protective and supportive device that encircles the neck to prevent the movement of the head and neck and that also helps to support the weight of the head. This device is most often used at the scene of an accident when there is a potential risk of spinal injury.

backboard: a protective and supportive device that is placed under a patient or an accident victim to prevent the movement of the spine

pelvis: part of the skeleton in the lower abdominal area that gives shape, protection, and support to the organs and structures located within

TABLE 4-2: Medical Terminology Related to a Patient's Status

Medical Term	Prefix	Root	Suffix
unconscious	un- (not)	consc (combining form of the Latin root *conscius*, meaning *aware*)	-ous (having the characteristics of)
hemorrhaging		hemo (blood)	rrhag (combining form of *rhexis,* used as suffix, meaning *burst, rupture, or discharge*) + -ing (happening now)

TABLE 4-3: Forming Adjectives with the Suffixes *-al* and *-ic*

Noun or Root	Add Suffix	Adjective
spine	-al	spinal (relating to the spine)
cranium	-al	cranial (relating to the cranium or skull)
front	-al	frontal (relating to the front of the body)
later-	-al	lateral (relating to the side of the body)
cervic-	-al	cervical (relating to the neck)
pelvis	-ic	pelvic (relating to the pelvis)
thorax	-ic	thoracic (relating to the chest area)

Learn the word parts of radiology and assessment

Read the dialogue again. This time, notice how often Maggie and Juanita use terms with the suffixes *-al* and *-ic*. In addition, study Table 4-3.

Fill in the Blanks

Write the correct adjective to complete each sentence.

1. RT Juanita does not want to take images of the patient from the side first. She wants ______________ images.
2. Mr. Loeppky may have fractured his skull. Drs. Raymond and Krenshaw believe that ______________ x-rays are important to assess this.
3. The patient remains on a backboard until the treatment team discerns whether or not he has a ______________ injury.
4. The patient was not wearing a seatbelt during the accident and may have fractured his ribs on the steering wheel. As a result, it will be important to obtain ______________ x-rays.
5. The patient's neck has been stabilized with the use of a head block. A radiograph of the ______________ spine will be necessary before these blocks are removed.
6. RT Juanita will take x-rays of Mr. Loeppky's ______________ area to make sure that he has not fractured his hip.

Right Word or Wrong Word: *Radiology* or *Medical Imaging*?

Is there a difference between the terms *radiology* and *medical imaging*? Discuss your answer with a partner or your peers, and share your conclusion with the class. Check with your instructor or consult the Answer Key to confirm your answer.

Assessment: The Language of the Neurological System

Before we can proceed with our updates regarding Gil Loeppky's medical condition, it is necessary to develop a vocabulary related to the neurological system. Refer to Figure 4-2 as you read the following information about this system.

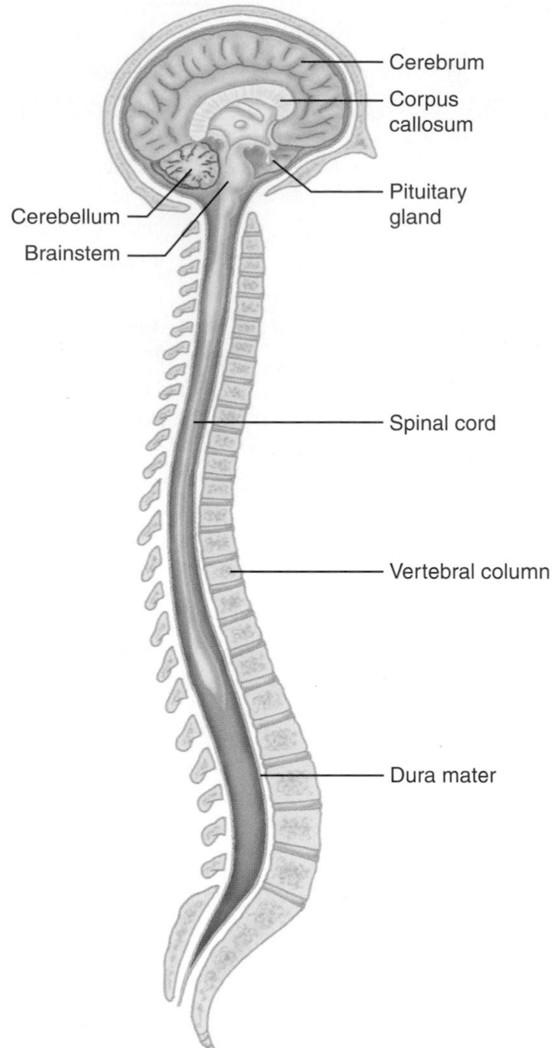

Figure 4.2: Neurological system

The neurological system

The neurological system begins with the brain, which is housed in the cranium or the skull. The brain is also known as the *cerebrum.* The cerebrum is connected to the cerebellum and then to the spine. Working together, these parts of the neurological system coordinate all of the body's activities through a system of neurons, sensory receptors, neurotransmitters, and neuropathways. The neurological system is also known as the *nervous system.*

Remember that Mr. Loeppky is unconscious. The trauma team has already ruled out any kind of paralysis, and R-RN Maggie has not observed any signs of epileptic activity. Although the entire neurological system cannot be assessed through diagnostic imaging at this time, Mr. Loeppky does require head x-rays STAT (immediately), followed by a CT scan to help provide a diagnostic assessment for his head injury. These tests will focus in on the brain and skull, and they will look for any evidence of fracture, bleeding, or other trauma. (In Unit 3, you will encounter Mr. Loeppky again. At that time, you will learn even more about the medical terminology and language related to the neurological system.)

Study the following terms and word parts related to the neurological system.

Key terms: neurological system

cranium: skull

cerebrum: anterior portion and largest part of the brain; commonly referred to simply as "the brain." The cerebrum is responsible for higher-level functions such as judgment, reasoning, problem solving, learning, memory, and sensations. It is divided into two hemispheres or halves: the left hemisphere and the right hemisphere.

cerebellum: posterior portion of the brain. The cerebellum is located at the superior end of the spinal cord, and it is responsible for coordination of voluntary movements such as walking. Injury here could lead to the paralysis of the arms and legs.

dendrite: an extension of a nerve cell. The dendrite is the first part to receive electrical or chemical stimuli during the process of nerve conduction. It is also referred to as a *sensory receptor.*

neurons: nerve cells. They receive stimuli or impulses in an action–reaction response.

neurotransmitters: chemical substances emitted by the neurons, which are then sent into the body in response to a stimuli. Examples of neurotransmitters include dopamine, serotonin, acetylcholine, and epinephrine (adrenalin). Brain injury or chemical imbalances in the brain can affect mood and behavior by adversely affecting neurotransmission.

neuropathways: routes throughout the body that lead to and from the neurons. Neuropathways carry impulses and neurotransmitters. Any damage to or disease of the neuropathways can cause impairment of sensation, emotion, behavior, or voluntary movement.

Let's Practice

Write the term that identifies each symptom or part of the neurological system described.

1. Mr. Loeppky's neck has been stabilized so that he cannot move it. The treatment team is worried about potential injury to which part of the neurological system?

   ____

2. A first priority of care is to get an x-ray and CT scan of which bony part of Mr. Loeppky's body?

   ____

3. The ER physician, Dr. Raymond, is worried about injury or bleeding in which part of Mr. Loeppky's neurological system?

   ____

4. The treatment team worries that, if Mr. Loeppky's neck is broken, the spinal cord may be severed, thereby causing a full loss of movement from that point downward. What is this condition called?

   ____

5. Brain injury can lead to seizures. What is this condition called?

   ____

Right Word or Wrong Word: *Contusion* or *Concussion*?

Is there a difference between a *contusion* and a *concussion*? This is a very important question! Discuss your answer with a small group of peers. If you have any reference books or a laptop with you, feel free to look this up, and then check the answer in the Answer Key.

TABLE 4-4: Suffixes and Combining Forms: Neurological System

Suffix or Combining Form	Meaning	Example
-algesia (suffix)	pain or sensitivity	analgesia (absence of pain or sensation)
-esthesia (suffix) esthesi/o (combining form)	feeling or sensation	paresthesia (a stinging, burning, or prickling sensation or a feeling of numbness as a result of nerve injury) esthesioneurosis (impairment of nerve conduction)
-kinesia (suffix) kinesi/o (combining form)	movement	dyskinesia (difficulty moving or impaired movement) kinesiology (the science or study of movement)
-lepsy -leptic (suffixes)	seize	epilepsy (a neurological disorder involving recurrent seizures that results from abnormal electrical discharges within the brain) catalepsy (a condition that results from parietal lobe cerebrovascular accidents or a psychotic or trance-like state in which the body remains in a rigid position)
-paresis (suffix)	weakness	hemiparesis (a condition in which one side of the body suffers from weakness)
-plegia (suffix)	paralysis; loss of movement	quadriplegia (full paralysis of the body from the neck [cervical spine] downward)

The combining form neuro

The neurological system plays a key role in all patient assessment, whether the patient has a head injury or not. This is because the status of the nervous system determines the patient's ability to sense, to think, and to act and react in response to stimuli. The combining form **neuro** is used frequently in medicine, and it refers to any aspect or condition of the neurological system. Whichever medical career you pursue, you will often use words that are built from the combining form *neuro.*

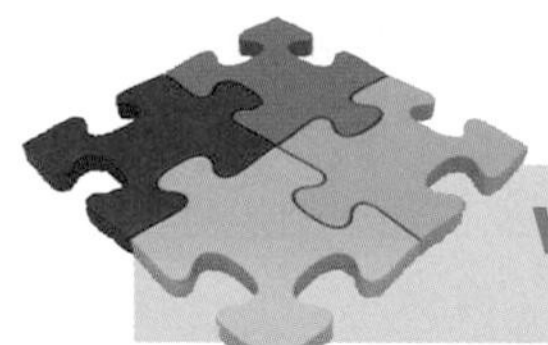

WORD BUILDING: Formula for Creating Words with the Combining Form Neur/o

neuro = combining form meaning *nerve*

neur + algia = *neuralgia*

Definition: nerve pain. *noun*

Example: Shingles is a virus-based skin rash that causes acute *neuralgia.*

neuro + anatomy = *neuroanatomy*

Definition: the structure of the nervous system. *noun*

Example: Nerve cells are important structures of human *neuroanatomy.*

neuro+ n = *neuron*

Definition: a nerve cell. A neuron consists of an axon, dendrites, and a cell body. It is the basic element of the neurological system. *noun*

Example: *Neurons* transmit nerve impulses.

neuro + nal = *neuronal*

Definition: relating to nerve cells. *adjective*

Example: Strokes, Parkinson's disease, and Alzheimer's disease are all potential causes of *neuronal* death.

neuro + logy = *neurology*

Definition: the study or science of the neurological system. *noun*

Example: A brain surgeon has advanced knowledge of *neurology.*

neuro + logical = *neurological*

Definition: relating to the nervous system (i.e., neurological examination, neurological disease). *adjective*

Example: Epilepsy and brain tumors are examples of *neurological* impairments.

neuro + logist = *neurologist*

Definition: a doctor who specializes in disorders and diseases of the neurological system. *noun*

Example: The *neurologist* identified the patient's hand tremors as a symptom of Parkinson's disease.

neuro + pathy = *neuropathy*

Definition: a pathology of or in the nervous system. *noun*

Example: Carpal tunnel syndrome is a type of *neuropathy* that causes pain and numbness of the hand and wrist.

neuro + sis = *neurosis*

Definition: a type of mental disorder that is mild in nature and very common. *noun*

Example: Anxiety is a common symptom of *neurosis.*

neuro + surgery = *neurosurgery*

Definition: surgery to any part of the neurological system; the term is often used to refer specifically to brain surgery. *noun*

Example: A patient with a skull fracture may require *neurosurgery.*

neuro + surgeon = *neurosurgeon*

Definition: a surgeon who specializes in operations on the neurological system. *noun*

Example: A *neurosurgeon* was consulted when the patient with a severe head injury was rushed to the emergency department.

neuro + transmitter = *neurotransmitter*

Definition: a chemical that transmits nerve impulses or stimuli between nerves. *noun*

Example: Some examples of *neurotransmitters* are dopamine and serotonin.

neuro + science = *neuroscience*

Definition: the scientific study of the neurological system. *noun*

Example: Recent advances in *neuroscience* are helping us to understand how human beings perceive and respond to the world around them.

Continued

neuro + vitals = *neurovitals*

Definition: a specific group of vital signs that measure neurological response, as well as basic physical signs. It is an abbreviated form of the term *neurovital signs. noun, slang*

Example: Nurses kept a close watch on the accident victim's *neurovitals.*

Break It Down

If you look closely at the words created with the root *neuro,* you will see that you can break them down into even smaller parts. For example:

neurovitals = *neuro* (root) + *vit* (root meaning *life*) + *al* (suffix meaning *relating to*) + **s** (suffix signifying plural)

Break down the following words into their roots and suffixes. Label and define each part. Feel free to refer to Chapter 1 if you need help.

1. neurotransmitter

   ____

2. neuropathy

   ____

3. neurological

   ____

4. neuronal

   ____

5. neuralgia

   ____

The combining form cereb

The brain (or the cerebrum) is not only the center of thought and emotion; it also controls and regulates the nervous system. In fact, it is a massive container of nervous tissue and neuroglia. Neuroglial cells support neurons by binding them together within the brain. In fact, the term **glia** originated in the early Greek and means *glue.* Learn the following terms, which are formed from the combining form *cereb.*

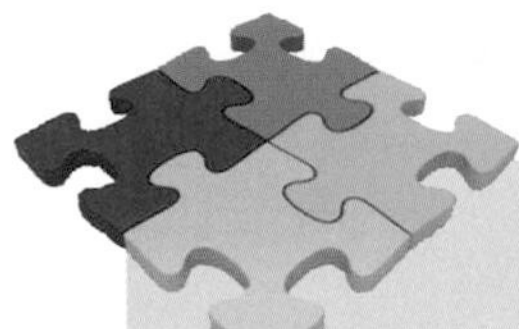

WORD BUILDING: Formula for Creating Words with the Combining Form *Cereb-*

cereb- or cerebro- = the brain

cerebr + al = *cerebral*

Definition: 1) referring to intellect or the higher functions of the brain, such as thinking and reasoning. *adjective* 2) referring to the front area of the brain. *adjective*

Example: *Cerebral* palsy is caused by injuries to a fetus's developing brain during pregnancy.

cerebro + spinal = *cerebrospinal*

Definition: a descriptive term that refers to anything related to the connection between the brain and the spinal cord, such as cerebrospinal fluid. *adjective*

Example: *Cerebrospinal* fluid conducts nerve impulses from the brain through the spinal cord and out to the rest of the body.

cerebro + physi + ology = *cerebrophysiology*

Definition: the study or science of the physiology of the brain. *noun*

Example: The study of blood circulation through the brain is one aspect of *cerebrophysiology.*

Break It Down

If you look closely at the words created with the root *cereb,* you'll see that you can break them down into even smaller parts. For example:

cerebrospinal = *cerebro* (root meaning *brain*) + *spin* (root meaning *spine or backbone*) + *al* (suffix meaning *relating to*)

Break down the following words into their roots and suffixes. Label and define each part. Feel free to refer to Chapter 1 if you need help.

1. cerebrophysiology (phys = root word originating in Greek and meaning *nature*)

____

2. cerebrovascular

____

3. cerebration (meaning *thinking or mental activity*)

____

4. cerebrotomy (meaning *dissection of the brain*)

____

PRONUNCIATION PRACTICE

Say these words aloud to a friend or classmate if you can. You are given the phonetic pronunciation. Your instructor can help you with pronunciation, or visit

http://www.MedicalLanguageLab.com. mll

cerebrum	**sĕr**´ĕ-brŭm or sĕr-ē´brŭm
cerebellum	sĕr-ĕ-**bĕl**ŭm
cerebral	**s**ĕ**r**´ă-brĭl or să-**r**ē´brĭl
cranial	**krā**´nē-ăl
neuron	**n**ŭ´rŏn

Let's Practice

Write the term that begins with *neuro* or *cereb* that fits each definition or description.

1. an adjective that means *intellectual* or that describes the front part of the brain

____

2. a highly specialized physician who works with the brain and nervous system

____

3. the part of the neurological system responsible for the coordination of walking and movement

____

4. a sensory receptor cell

____

5. a chemical produced by a neuron

____

6. a surgeon who specializes in operations on the nervous system

____

7. something that is more commonly (although not completely accurately) referred to as "the brain"

____

8. someone who worries a lot or who is preoccupied with his or her thoughts may be diagnosed with this condition

____

9. the study of the physiology of the brain

____

10. the nervous system

____

Anatomy and physiology of the brain

Continue to learn more about the language of the brain through the exploration of its anatomy and physiology.

Structures of the brain

The brain is divided into two main parts or hemispheres, which are located in the largest part of the brain, the cerebrum. However, the brain is actually much more than just the cerebrum. It includes the cerebellum, located at the base of the brain, and the nearby pons and medulla. Together, the pons and medulla are referred to as the **brainstem**. The **pons** connects the cerebrum and cerebellum with the other parts of the brain. The **medulla** (more properly called the **medulla oblongata**) connects the spinal cord to the brain. The function of the brainstem is vital to sustain life because it regulates the constriction and dilation of blood vessels and automatically regulates heart rate and breathing. The **midbrain** is more formally called the **mesencephalon**. This structure, which is part of the brainstem, is responsible for embryonic brain development. Later, it is responsible for the creation and maintenance of motor (movement) pathways in the developed brain.

The **pituitary** is also housed in the brain. It is a gland that is responsible for the growth of bone. The pituitary also contributes to metabolism and activates sexual growth and development through the release of hormones. It exerts control over the most of the endocrine system (see Chapter 7 for more information about the endocrine system). The **thalamus** relays sensations of pain, pleasure, and so on. The **hypothalamus** is so named because it is smaller (hypo) than the thalamus and located within it. The function of the hypothalamus is to control the pituitary gland and to regulate sleep, appetite, and emotions.

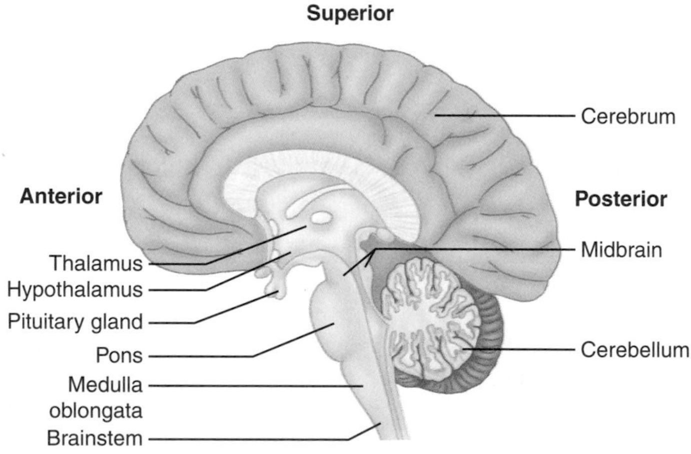

Figure 4.3: Structures of the brain

Critical Thinking

Define, describe, or explain the following terms in your own words. Work in small groups, if possible.

1. On the basis of its word parts, what does *hemisphere* mean?

____

2. Look at the diagram of the brain. Why is the term *hemisphere* applied to parts of the brain?

3. In which part of the brain are the hemispheres located?

4. What is the purpose of the hypothalamus?

5. Which part of the brain is responsible for regulating the heart and breathing rates?

6. Which parts of the brain are sometimes referred to as the *brainstem*?

Let's Practice

Name the part of the brain that fits each description.

1. Which gland is responsible for the growth of bone and the regulation of growth hormones?

2. Which structure is highly influential with regard to the brain development of an embryo during early pregnancy?

3. What is an important structure that connects the brain to the spinal cord?

4. Where are sensations of pain and pleasure recognized?

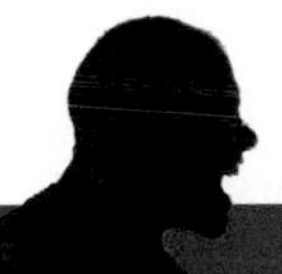

PRONUNCIATION PRACTICE

Say these words aloud to a friend or classmate if you can. You are given the phonetic pronunciation. Your instructor can help you with pronunciation, or visit http://www.MedicalLanguageLab.com.

medulla	mĕ-**dŭl**′lă
oblongata	ŏb″lōng-**gă**′tă
pons	pŏnz
pituitary	pĭ-**tū**′ĭ-tār″ē
thalamus	**thăl**′ă-mŭs

Lobes of the brain

The cerebral hemispheres are divided into four **lobes** or sections, each with its own special functions. The **frontal lobe** is involved with reasoning, judgment, emotions, planning, and strategizing, as well as some memory and speech functions. The **parietal lobe** has the ability to distinguish the five senses and controls some language functions. The **temporal lobe** is actually divided into two parts, one on each side of the brain. These parts are responsible for speech, making meaning from sensory input, and hearing. The **occipital lobe** is responsible for vision and the ability to recognize objects.

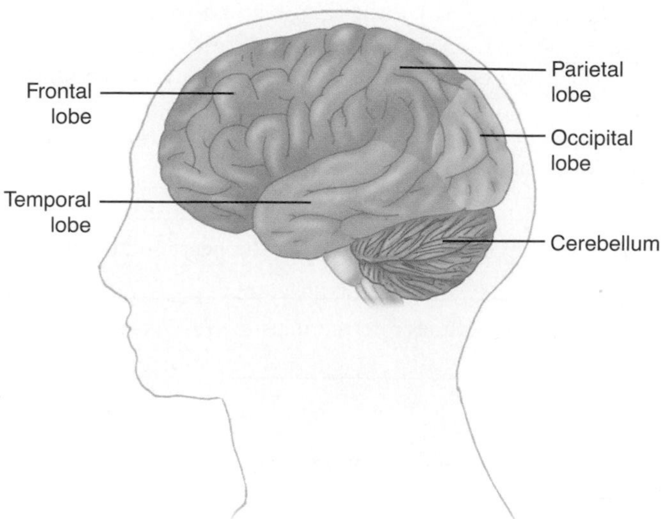

Figure 4.4: Lobes of the brain

Let's Practice

Write the name of the brain lobe that controls each function described.

1. Which lobe is responsible for reasoning and judgment?

   ____

2. Name the lobe responsible for vision.

   ____

3. Identify the lobe responsible for speech, language, and communication.

   ____

Fill in the Blanks

In Chapter 2, you learned medical terminology for sites and locations in the body. Apply that knowledge here. Refer to Figure 4-4 to help you locate the position of each lobe of the brain. Use the following word choices. You may use each word more than once.

anterior　　superior　　caudal　　posterior

1. The temporal lobes are located __________ to the occipital lobe.
2. The occipital lobe is located in the __________ portion of the cerebral cortex.
3. The parietal lobe is located __________ to the occipital lobe and __________ to the frontal lobe.
4. The frontal lobe is located in the __________ portion of the cerebral cortex.

Assessment: neurological and vital signs

You have now seen that the brain and spinal cord work together to sustain life. Mr. Loeppky is undergoing diagnostic imaging testing while he is unconscious. It is imperative that Maggie, the R-RN, monitor this patient's neurological and vital signs; his *neurovital signs.* The R-RN will use a number of assessment tools and techniques to accomplish this monitoring.

Levels of consciousness (LOC)

Neurological assessment is critical in all cases of head injury or suspected head injury, whether the patient is conscious or not. Because the brain is responsible for sustaining breathing and heart rates, it is equally critical to assess vital signs at the same time. A change in either the neurological status or vital signs can be life threatening.

A person is **conscious** when he or she is fully alert and aware of his or her surroundings. This person can interpret what is happening and is oriented to persons, places, and things (i.e., the person can name what he or she is seeing). **Unconsciousness** is a sign of neurological dysfunction. It has a number of stages. These are referred to as *states* or **levels of consciousness (LOC).**

When alertness is reduced and the patient acts confused when aroused, a **semiconscious** state of arousal is determined. This drowsy state is also called **obtundation**.

Hypersomnia is the next state of consciousness. This is like a very deep sleep. The only way to awaken someone from hypersomnia is by shaking or other strong stimuli, such as pain. Even so, these patients may not completely awaken. If they do, they will be confused and only partially alert before drifting back into hypersomnia.

Stupor is a state of deep unconsciousness from which the person cannot be awakened or aroused without a stimulus such as a very loud noise or strong pain. Even then, he or she may only awaken briefly before slipping back into this level of unconsciousness. Gil Loeppky is in this state.

Finally, a patient who cannot be roused by any stimuli whatsoever is said to be in a **coma**. The neurological assessment will pay particular attention to the patient's ability to breathe on his or her own and will determine whether the patient's circulation is impaired. The patient's eyes will be checked for reactiveness and movement. CT and MRI scanning are the best diagnostic assessment tools to use with comatose patients.

Mr. Loeppky is diagnosed as being in an unconscious state. The nurse uses an assessment tool called the **Glasgow Coma Scale** (GCS) to routinely test his level of consciousness. The GCS is an internationally recognized scale that assesses neurological functions such as reflexes and responses to sound and touch, including shaking, pinching, and attempts to elicit a pain response. It outlines a standardized procedure that will be explored further regarding its terminology and meaning in Unit 3.

TABLE 4-5: Glasgow Coma Scale

Eye Opening Response	Score	Verbal Response	Score	Motor Response	Score
Spontaneous; open with blinking at baseline	4	Oriented	5	Obeys commands for movement	6
To verbal stimuli, command, or speech	3	Confused conversation but able to answer questions	4	Purposeful movement to painful stimulus	5
To pain only (not applied to face)	2	Inappropriate words	3	Withdraws in response to pain	4
No response	1	Incomprehensible speech	2	Flexion in response to pain (decorticate posturing)	3
		No response	1	Extension response in response to pain (decerebrate posturing)	2
				No response	1

References
Centers for Disease Control and Prevention: *Glasgow Coma Scale*. Retrieved from http://www.bt.cdc.gov/masscasualties/gscale.asp. Accessed July 25, 2012.
Teasdale G, Jennett B: Assessment of coma and impaired consciousness, *Lancet* 1974;2(7872):81-84.
Teasdale G, Jennett B: Assessment and prognosis of coma after head injury, *Acta Neurochir (Wien)* 1976;34(1-4):45-55.

Critical Thinking

Apply your understanding of terms related to different levels of consciousness by answering the following questions.

1. On the basis of what you know so far, what is Mr. Loeppky's level of consciousness?
   ____
2. What does the abbreviation *GCS* stand for? ______________________________
3. When neurological status and vital signs are assessed together, what term is used?
   ____
4. On the basis of your reading so far in this chapter, whom do you think is responsible for obtaining the neurovital signs? ______________________________
5. In which state of consciousness can the person not, under any circumstances or with the use of any stimuli, be aroused? ______________________________

6. What medical term is used to indicate a body part or system that is not functioning well?

____

7. Someone in which state of consciousness may have experienced an excessive intake of alcohol during their very recent past? _______________________

Patient Update

Mr. Loeppky has suffered a head trauma and possibly a brain trauma. Although he remains unconscious during testing, he has begun to rouse from his stupor and to become more alert sometimes. His eyes flutter open briefly, and he moans a bit. He will suddenly blink his closed eyes in response to being exposed abruptly to a bright light overhead. To assist with assessment and decision making regarding his status, the treatment team will use a clinical pathway to guide them. Clinical pathways are tools that are commonly used in the health-care field. Refer to Figure 4-5 for an example of a clinical pathway. Notice that the language choices in the example are simple, clear, and concise for easy interpretation. They are also specific to the diagnosis.

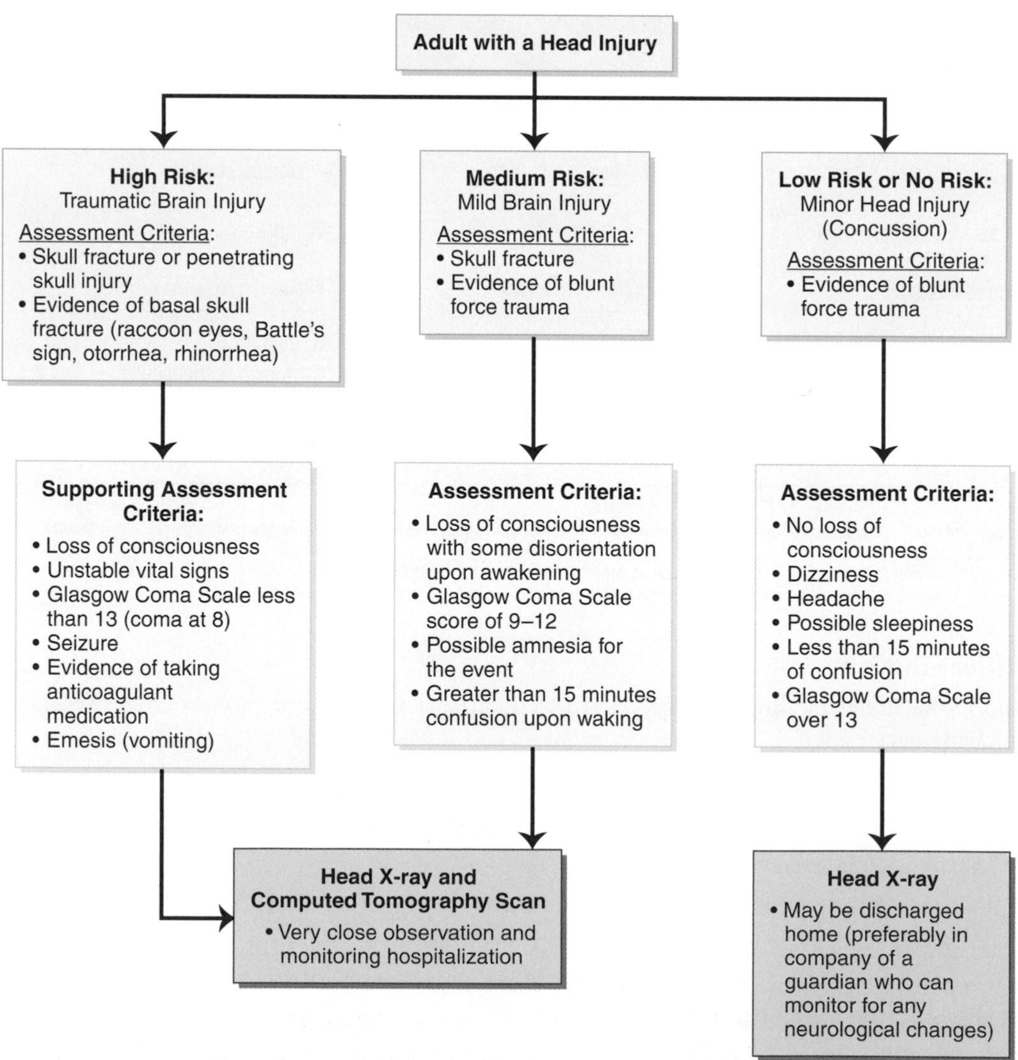

Figure 4.5: Clinical pathway: adult/blunt head injury

Critical Thinking

This exercise will help you see how words are used in the context of care. Study Figure 4-5, and locate Mr. Loeppky on the scale. Then explain how you know this is (provide your rationale). When you are ready, check the Answer Key to see if you are correct.

____

____

Head injury: signs and symptoms

By applying the Clinical Pathway for an Adult with a Blunt Head Injury, it is possible to see how and why diagnostic imaging assessment will proceed. Study the following signs and symptoms of head injury:

- localized tenderness and possible swelling at the site of the injury or fracture
- headache
- confusion
- changes in pupil size, either unilaterally or bilaterally
- drowsiness
- nausea and vomiting
- partial amnesia (memory loss)
- shock
- anxiety
- pupils not appropriately reactive to light
- temporary loss of consciousness

Skull fracture: signs and symptoms

Review the following signs and symptoms of skull fracture:

- loss of consciousness
- convulsions or seizures
- cerebrospinal fluid leaking from the nose (**rhinorrhea**) or ears (**otorrhea**)
- retrograde amnesia (memory loss)
- restlessness or irritability
- symptoms of dysarthria, including slurred speech and the inability to articulate words
- difficulties with balance and coordination
- visual disturbances, such as double vision
- neck stiffness
- swelling or bruising around the eyes (**periorbital hematoma** or raccoon eyes) or behind the ears (**mastoid hematoma** or Battle's sign)
- bleeding from a head wound, the ears, or the nose (Blood may collect behind the eardrum. If the eardrum is ruptured, blood may drain from the ear. It can also pool in the sinuses and drain from there if the nose is also fractured.)
- paralysis

Fill in the Blanks

Use the language and medical terms that you have just studied in the context of a head injury. Fill in the blanks.

1. ____________________ may drain from the sinuses as a result of a head injury.
2. Blood may drain from the ear in the same circumstances, but this drainage might also contain ____________________ fluid.
3. One pupil may be discovered to be unequal in size to the other after a blunt head injury. When both pupils are tested, the test is referred to as a ____________________ assessment.
4. ____________________ is the medical term for loss of fluid through the nose.
5. ____________________ is the medical term for loss of fluid through the ear.
6. Mr. Loeppky has the visual signs of an injury that are often referred to as *raccoon eyes.* The medical term for this injury is ____________________.

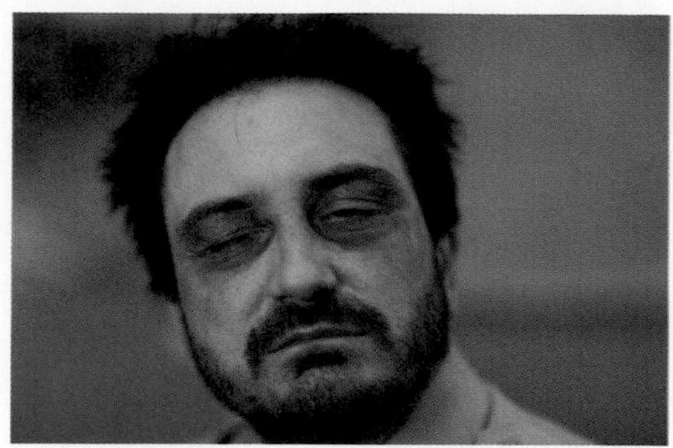

Figure 4.6: Patient with "raccoon eyes"

Medical terminology: the prefix peri-

The prefix *peri-* appears in many medical terms. It simply means *around or about.* For example, the term *periorbital,* meaning *around the eyes,* has been used a number of times in Mr. Loeppky's case. This prefix can also be added to other roots and combining forms to create medical terms.

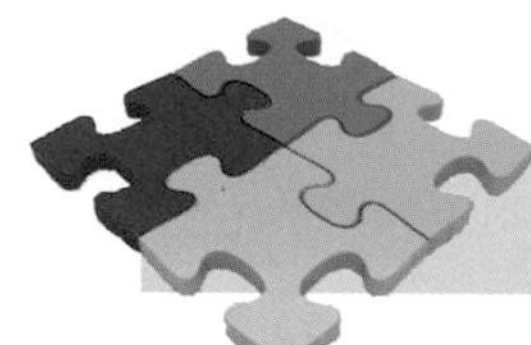

WORD BUILDING: Formula for Adding the Prefix *Peri-*

peri + orbital = *periorbital*

Definition: related to or occurring in the area and tissue around the eye socket. The word *orbital* derives from the root *orb,* meaning *circle. adjective*

Example: Puffiness under the eyes is a form of *periorbital* edema (gathering of fluid).

peri + meter = *perimeter*

Definition: the outer edge of something or the measure of this outer edge. The word *meter* is derived from the Greek root *metron,* meaning *measure. noun*

Example: The *perimeter* of the liver can be identified by the palpation of the outer right upper quadrant of the abdomen.

peri + cardium = *pericardium*

Definition: a sac-like structure that surrounds the heart. *noun*

Example: The function of the *pericardium* is to protect and support the heart within the chest cavity.

peri + o + dontal = *periodontal*

Definition: relating to or occurring within the structures that surround the teeth. The gums are an example of a periodontal structure. *adjective*

Example: *Periodontal* diseases involve the inflammation of the tissue that surrounds the teeth.

peri + osteum = *periosteum*

Definition: a naturally occurring cover for the bones that protects their surface. The periosteum contains bloods vessels that nourish the bones. In addition, it attaches ligaments and tendons to the bone. *noun*

Example: The *periosteum* facilitates the healing of damaged or diseased bone.

Break It Down

Break down the following words and identify any prefixes, roots, and suffixes that they contain. Next, write the meaning of each word part. For example:

otorrhea = *oto* (root meaning *ear*) + *rrhea* (root meaning *flow, discharge, or burst*)

1. rhinorrhea

   ____

2. periorbital

   ____

3. bilaterally

   ____

4. unilaterally

   ____

5. dysarthria

   ____

Let's Practice

Identify the prefix in each term, and then write the meaning of the prefix.

1. unilateral ____________ ______________________
2. unequal ____________ ______________________
3. dysarthria ____________ ______________________
4. periorbital ____________ ______________________
5. dysfunction ____________ ______________________
6. hypersomnia ____________ ______________________
7. hemisphere ____________ ______________________
8. hypothalamus ____________ ______________________

Right Word or Wrong Word: *Trauma* or *Injury*?

Gil Loeppky is being treated at a trauma center as a result of the injuries that he sustained during a motor vehicle accident. Mrs. Davis is at a general hospital for her injuries. What is the difference between a *trauma* and an *injury*?

Computed tomography (CT)

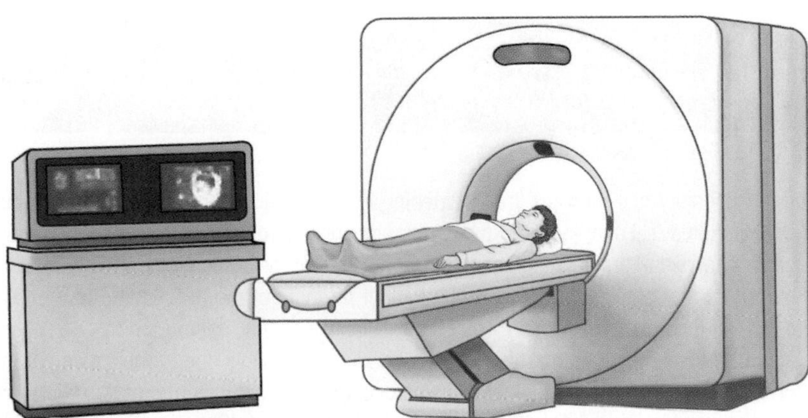

Figure 4.7: Computed tomography scanner (From Eagle S, Brassington C, Dailey CS, Goretti C: *The Professional Medical Assistant: An Integrative, Teamwork-Based Approach.* Philadelphia: FA Davis, 2009, p. 457. With permission.)

The next step in the diagnostic imaging assessment for Mr. Loeppky is to have a **computed tomography (CT or CAT)** scan of his head and spinal cord, core components of the neurological system. Although the patient shows no overt or visible signs of brain injury, skull fracture, or paralysis, this test will clearly determine whether he has in fact suffered any of these traumatic injuries. CT scans provide highly detailed image scans of the body's internal organs and structures.

Patient Update

Mr. Loeppky has now been assessed with a complete round of neurological x-rays and CT scans. The radiologist has seen the films and conferred with the attending physician in the emergency department. They both agree that the patient has had an accelerated-impact, blunt-force injury to his head and lower extremities. The mechanism of injury was an average-speed motor vehicle accident.

The patient does not have a skull fracture or any internal bleeding of the brain or abdomen. His ribs and spinal cord are intact. However, he did suffer a serious concussion that has rendered him unconscious. His badly bruised eyes are the result of his collision with the frame of the windshield in his vehicle. Initially, the trauma team suspected that his black eyes were the result of a basilar skull fracture. However, the diagnostic images do not support this diagnosis. The attending physician and the radiologist conclude that the patient's black eyes are a result of the blunt force trauma to his brow and upper nose as a result of a facial injury. The radiographs show that the ethmoid bones (the bones that support the nasal cavity and form part of the orbits of the eyes) are not actually fractured.

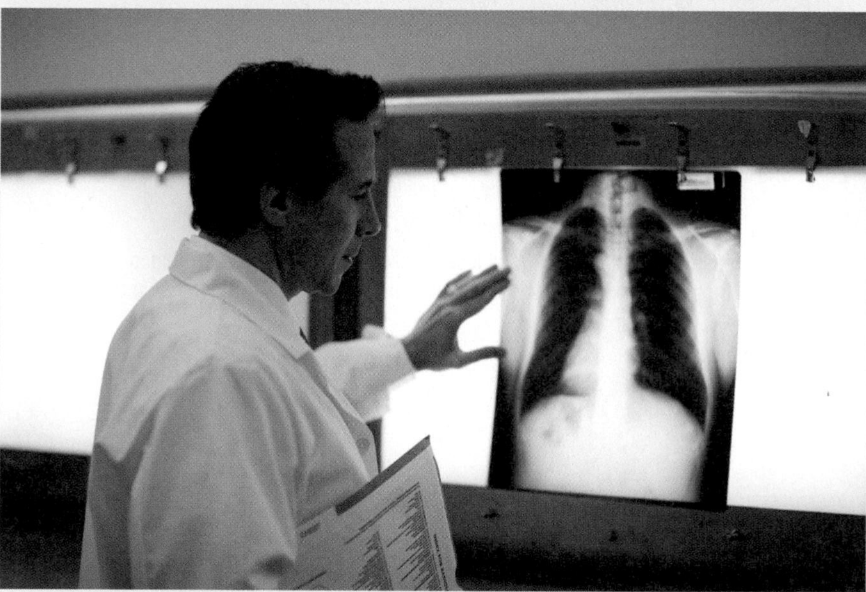

Because Mr. Loeppky has no overt life-threatening injuries and remains stable although unconscious, the doctor decides that Mr. Loeppky can remain in the diagnostic imaging department to complete the rest of the assessment tests that are needed. The doctor is aware that the patient is now in and out of consciousness, and he orders that the nurse stay with the patient throughout the procedures to monitor neurovital signs and to care for the patient as needed. The ER physician wants the patient monitored frequently because the risk of an intracranial bleed (hemorrhage) is still a possibility. This is due to the jostling of the head that occurred during the MVA. An intracranial bleed could occur if the meninges (the membranes that cover the brain) are torn or if any blood vessels rupture as a result of the trauma. (Chapter 10 enhances and advances terminology related to the brain and neurological system.)

It is now possible for the DI staff to take x-rays of the patient's pelvis, knee, femur, and ankle. The staff have noticed that the patient moans both when his right hip is moved and also when his right ankle is jostled. R-RN Maggie notes that the pain must be quite severe to cause him to rouse from time to time. She and RT Juanita move the patient back into the x-ray area of the department. They will proceed with a top-down, head-to-toe approach to taking films now. This type of approach is standard protocol for all aspects of health assessment. As they begin, Juanita explains to Maggie which bones in particular she will be targeting with her assessment.

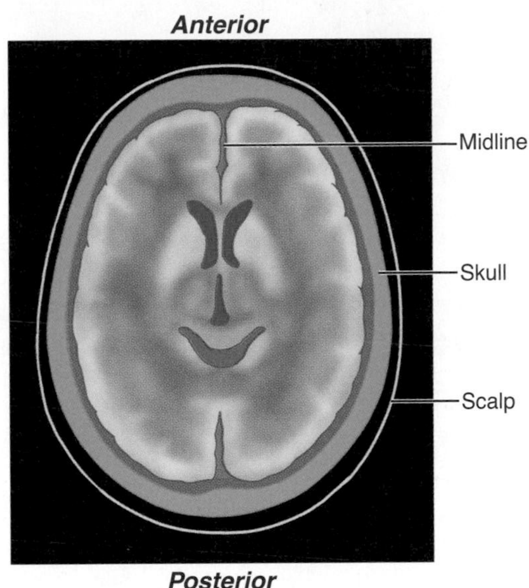

Figure 4.8: Normal computed tomography scan of the head

The Language of the Skeletal System

Bones, cartilage, and joints

Before we can proceed any further, you will need to develop vocabulary related to the skeletal system (the *skeleton).* This includes the language of bones, cartilage, and joints.

Refer to Figure 4-9. Read the names of all of the bones silently to yourself. Work from top to bottom to get used to working with a head-to-toe approach to assessment and care. Next, read all of the names of the bones aloud to yourself for practice with pronunciation.

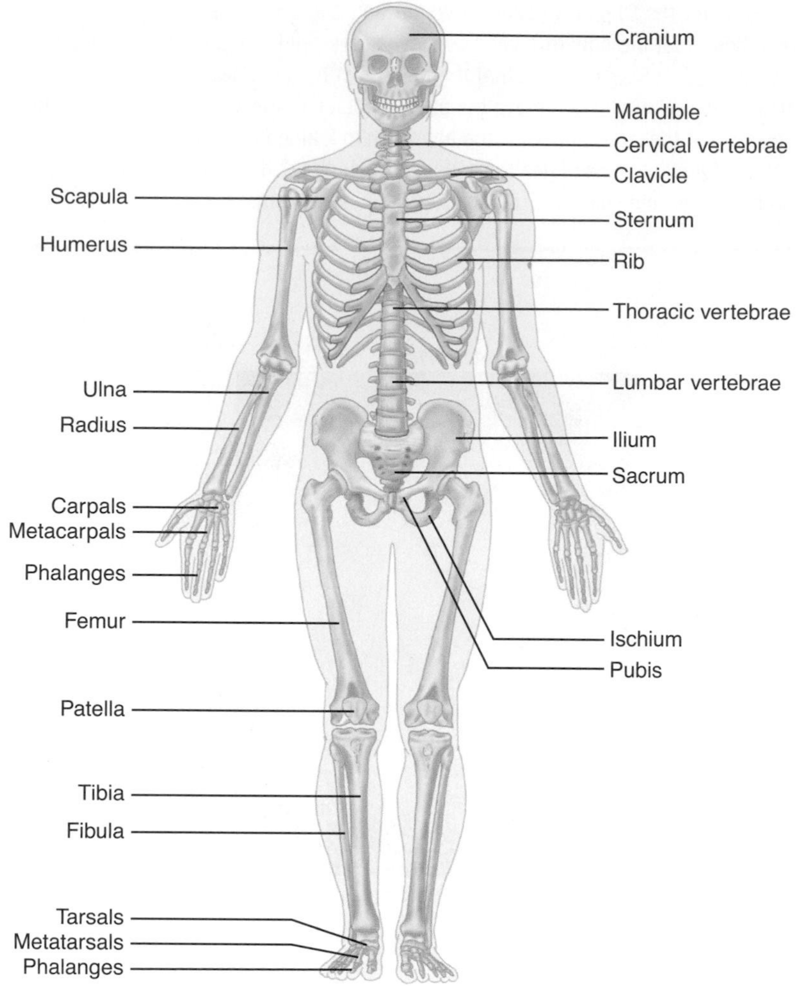

Figure 4.9: Skeletal system

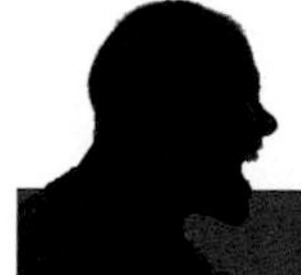

PRONUNCIATION PRACTICE

Say these words aloud to a friend or classmate if you can. You are given the phonetic pronunciation. Your instructor can help you with pronunciation, or visit **http://www.MedicalLanguageLab.com.** mll

cranium	**krā´**nē-ŭm	pubis	**pū´**bĭs
mandible	**măn´**dĭ-bl	carpal	**kăr´**păl
clavicle	**klăv´**ĭ-k'l	metacarpal	mĕt″ă-**kăr´**păl
sternum	**stĕr´**nŭm	ischium	**ĭs´**kē-ŭm
humerus	**h**ŭ´mĕr-ŭs	femur	**fē´**mŭr
rib	rĭb	patella	pă-**tĕl´**ă
lumbar	**lŭm´**băr	fibula	**fĭb´**ū-lă
vertebra	**vĕr´**tĕ-bră	tibia	**tĭb´**ē-ă
ulna	**ŭl´**nă	metatarsal	mĕt″ă-**tăr´**săl
radius	**rā´**dē-ŭs	phalanges	fă-**lăn´**jēz

ilium	**ĭl**´-ē-ŭm	coccyx	**kŏk**´sĭks
pelvis	**pĕl**´vĭs	tarsal	**tăr**´săl
sacrum	**sā**´krŭm		

Let's Practice

Here is a list of common, everyday terms that identify the bones of the body. Change these to professional anatomical term. Work alone, and then check your work with a partner.

1. jaw ____________
2. backbone ____________
3. bones of the hand ____________
4. fingers and toes ____________
5. bones of the feet ____________
6. small bone in the lower arm ____________
7. tailbone ____________
8. thighbone ____________
9. kneecap ____________
10. collarbone ____________

TABLE 4-6: Common Medical Roots: Skeletal System

Medical Root	Basic Meaning or Pertaining to	Medical Root	Basic Meaning or Pertaining to
carp(o)	wrist	clavicul(o)	collarbone
crani(o)	skull	femor(o)	thighbone
mandibul(o)	jaw	oste(o)	bones
scapula	shoulder	tars(o)	ankle

Let's Practice

Identify the bones from their description. Use proper terminology.

1. provides support for the entire skeleton ____________
2. longest bone in the leg ____________
3. affects whether or not you can chew or bite ____________
4. these make up the foot ____________
5. it is very, very common to take a pulse near this bone ____________
6. large, flat bones that are located dorsally ____________
7. protects the lower abdomen ____________
8. situated in your lower back ____________
9. located at the distal end of the spine ____________
10. protects the organs of the thorax ____________

Classifying bones

There are 126 bones in the human body, and each bone has its own name. Bones can also be categorized or sorted into groups according to their length and shape.

The **long bones** are important to the main skeleton because they provide the core support for the body. They also link with one another to allow for movement. These bones are longer than they are wide. The long bones include the radius, ulna, metacarpals, clavicle, humerus, femur, tibia, fibula, and metatarsals.

Short bones provide for movement and flexibility of the body. They also provide shock absorption and elasticity. They are less dense than the long bones. Their internal consistency is more spongy than that of most other bones, and, as a protective measure, they are covered with a thin layer of compact bone. Short bones include the carpal and tarsal bones.

Sesamoid bones are another type of short bones that function to modify the angle of bone where it is inserted into a muscle. Sesamoid bones are embedded within tendons or joint capsules. The patella (kneecap) is an example of a sesamoid bone.

Flat bones provide protection for the body. They also function as attachment sites for muscles. The sternum, scapula, and ribs are flat bones.

Medical terminology: the root oste(o)

The anatomical term for a bone is **ossa**. Its combining forms *oss, oste,* and *osteo* are used to create a variety of words related to the skeletal system.

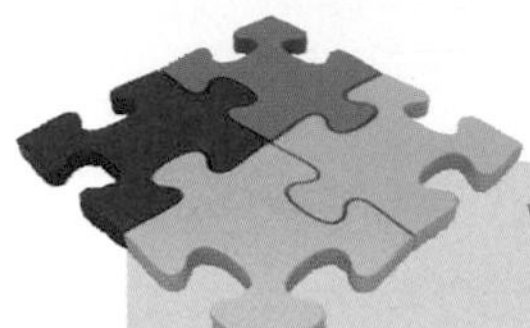

WORD BUILDING: Formula for Creating Words with the Combining Forms *Oss* and *Oste/o*

oss = bone (derives from Latin)
osteo = bone (derives from Greek)

oss + ific + ation = *ossification*

Definition: the process of bone formation. The word part *ific* derives from the Greek word *facere,* meaning *to produce or to become. noun*

Example: *Ossification* begins at 8 weeks' gestation in the human fetus.

oss + eous = *osseous*

Definition: a type of tissue found in bones. This term is also used as an adjective to refer to anything that is like bone. *adjective*

Example: The *osseous* system is the technical term for the skeletal system.

oste + itis = *osteitis*

Definition: inflammation of the bone. *noun*

Example: Symptoms of *osteitis* include bone pain, enlargement of the bone, and tenderness.

osteo + arthr + it is = *osteoarthritis*

Definition: a condition in which there is an inflammation and deterioration of the cartilage of joints and vertebrae. *Arthr(o)* is a combining form of the root *arthr,* meaning *joint. noun*

Example: As people age, their chances of developing *osteoarthritis* increase.

osteo + porosis = *osteoporosis*

Definition: a condition in which there is a depletion of calcium in the bone, which results in thin and brittle bones. The suffix *-porosis* means *porous. noun*

Example: Women in their 50s and 60s often develop *osteoporosis.*

osteo + blast

Definition: a bone cell that contributes to bone tissue formation . The suffix *-blast* identifies a very young embryonic cell. *noun*

Example: In patients with osteoporosis, *osteoblasts* no longer exist to replace damaged or diseased bone.

osteo + clast = *osteoclast*

Definition: a type of bone cell that absorbs and then removes unwanted bone tissue. The suffix *-clast* means *to break. noun*

Example: *Osteoclasts* reabsorb old bone, whereas osteoblasts create new bone.

Free Writing

Use a term that begins with *oss, oste,* or *osteo* to create a logical sentence that includes the words that are given as clues. Work with a partner or in a small group.

EXAMPLE: calcium, supplements, older women, prevent

Sentence: Many older women take calcium supplements to prevent osteoporosis.

1. fingers, joints, swelling, suspect, elderly

   ____

2. child, process, slowly, soft bones

   ____

3. covering, bones, inflamed

   ____

Listen to the language of the skeletal system

Read or listen to the following dialogue between the radiologist, the radiologic technologist, and the radiology nurse as they discuss Mr. Loeppky's x-rays.

Patient Update

RT Juanita: Here are Mr. Loeppky's films of his femur and pelvic area, Doctor.

Radiologist, Dr. Krenshaw: Thank you. Okay, let's see what we have. Right hip. Okay, here ... and here. There is a complex spiral fracture at the distal end of the femur, where it impacted with the acetabulum. The femoral neck and the trochanter both seem to be involved. Well, the acetabulum looks okay, but we're going to have to operate on that femur. The condyle is definitely involved. No evidence of fracture to any part of the pelvic girdle. Good. Let me see the ankle now.

RT Juanita: Here are the x-rays. It's the right ankle. It doesn't look good.

Dr. Krenshaw: Hmmm ... no, it's not good. This looks like an impacted fracture. Look here, where a small portion of the talus has been forcefully pushed into the base of the tibia, causing a fracture there, too. This one's going to require surgery, too. All right, let's take a look at the knee.

RT Juanita: OK. Here's the left, and here's the right.

Dr. Krenshaw: OK, no visible fracture of either patella, but the left is certainly inflamed. I'd say acute patellar injury: contusion to the patella. Must have hit the dashboard somehow. He's lucky the right one's okay. I suspect the surgeons will want to attend to the fractures first during surgery and worry about any articular cartilage or tendon damage to the knee after that. First things first, right?

R-RN Maggie: Yes. Shall I take the patient back to the ER now? He's starting to waken.

Dr. Krenshaw: Yes, why don't you do that. I'll call the Attending right now and let him know what I've been able to assess, and then I'll write it up. What's his name again?

R-RN Maggie: The Attending? Dr. Raymond. He's a trauma surgeon. He'll want to see the films. Can I take them along?

Dr. Krenshaw: Yes, please do so.

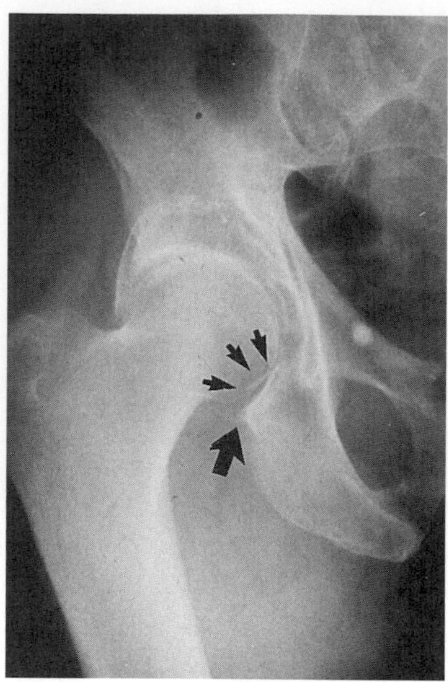

Figure 4.10: X-ray: broken hip (From McKinnis LN: *Fundamentals of Musculoskeletal Imaging,* 3rd ed. Philadelphia: FA Davis, 2010, p. 345. With permission.)

Critical Thinking

Answer the following questions by yourself or with a peer. You may or may not know the answer, but try to work it out on the basis of what you have learned so far in this book and from your own life experiences.

1. Which of Mr. Loeppky's bones are fractured? Answer using proper anatomical terms.

 ____

2. Why won't any special treatment or intervention be given to the patient's knee right now?

 ____

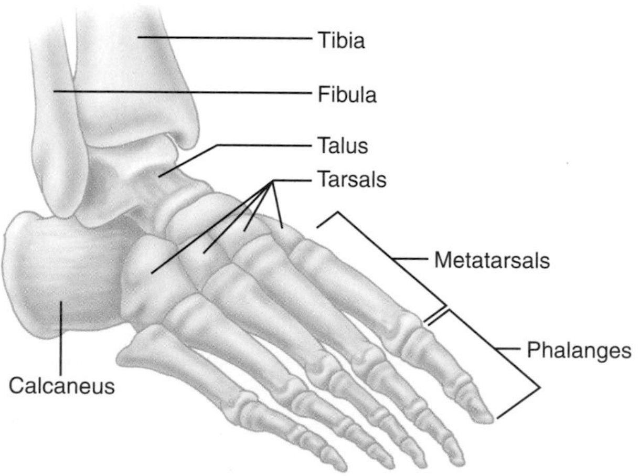

Figure 4.11: Bones of the foot and ankle

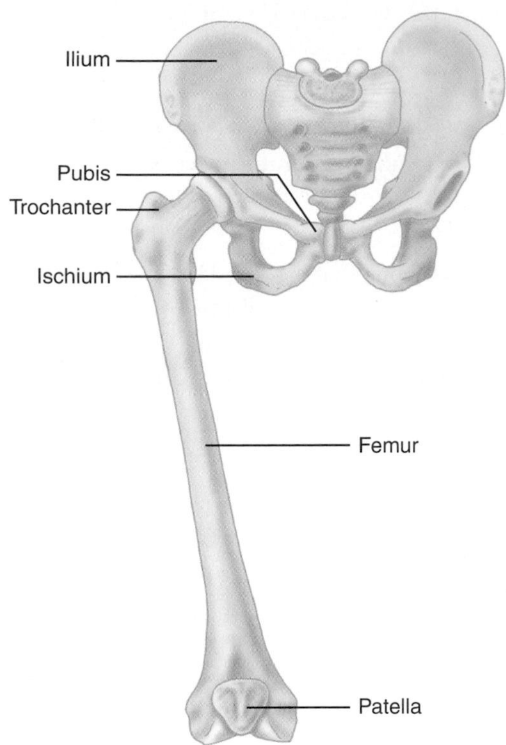

Figure 4.12: Pelvic girdle

Key terms: skeletal system

A number of key medical terms appeared in the dialogue. Learn these words related to the skeletal system.

Bones of the leg:

femur: the longest and strongest bone in the body, located in the upper leg. The top or proximal head of the femur forms part of the ball-and-socket joint, which is commonly referred to as the *hip*. The femur itself is most commonly referred to as the *thighbone*. The distal or lower end of the femur articulates with the patella.

tibia: the largest bone of the lower leg, it is situated between the knee and the ankle, anterior to the fibula. The tibia actually articulates with the femur (above it) through the process of the knee joint as well as with the talus in the ankle. The tibia is commonly referred to as the *shinbone*.

fibula: the smaller bone of the lower leg. It lies posterior to the tibia. The fibula is one of the thinnest and longest bones in the human body, and it articulates with the tibia and the talus.

Bones of the knee:

patella: a sesamoid bone situated in the tendon that is located at the front (anterior aspect) of the knee. It is commonly referred to as the *kneecap*.

Bones of the ankle:

tarsus: the combination of all seven small bones that make up the ankle: the talus, the calcaneus, the navicular, the cuboid (outer bone of the instep), and three cuneiform bones (small internal, external, and middle). Together, these seven bones are generally referred to as the *ankle*.

talus: the ankle bone that articulates with the tibia and fibula, as well as with other bones of the ankle

Bones of the pelvis:

innominate bones: the ilium, the ischium, and the pubis, form the pelvis

pelvic girdle: the structure of bones that attach the upper parts of the skeleton (i.e., the head and the trunk) to the lower parts. It is commonly referred to as the *pelvis.*

Bones of the hip:

acetabulum: the part of the pelvic bone that is shaped like a saucer and that provides a socket for the head of the femur

condyle: a rounded, knuckle-like process (i.e., not a true, separate bone) at the end of any bone that becomes part of a moving ball-and-socket joint. Condyles are found in the hip and the shoulder.

Build a Word

Practice expanding words to create derivatives. Use the following roots:

- The root word *femur.* As this root expands, the *u* is replaced with an *o* to create the combining form *femor/o-*.
- The root *tibia.* As this root expands, the *a* is replaced with an *o* to create the combining form *tibi/o-*.
- The root *patella.* The combining form of this root word is varied: *patella/e/i/o-*.

1. Combine *femor/o-* with the name for the inner, larger bone in the lower leg.

   ____

2. Change a noun to an adjective: add a suffix to change *femur* to an adjective that describes a quality or characteristic of the femur.

   ____

3. Think carefully here. Can you turn *femur* into it plural form? (You might want to refer back to Chapter 1 for a hint.)

   ____

4. Add a suffix to *tibia* to create an adjective that means *concerning the tibia.*

   ____

5. Combine *tibia* with *femur* to create an adjective that describes the interaction between these two bones.

   ____

6. Combine *tibia* with *fibula* to create an adjective that describes an interaction between these two bones.

   ____

7. Combine *tibia* with *tarsus* to create an adjective that describes an interaction between the tibia and the ankle.

   ____

8. Add a short suffix to *patella* to create an adjective that means *concerning the patella.*

   ____

9. Create a surgical word that refers to the removal of the patella.

   ____

10. Combine *patella* with the name of the longest bone in the body to create an adjective that describes the interaction between these two bones.

    ____

Break It Down

Identify the combining forms and suffixes in the following terms that relate to bones.

1. Referring to the chest: *thoracic* ______________________________
2. Referring to the collarbone: *clavicular* ______________________________
3. Referring to the neck: *cervical* ______________________________
4. Referring to the bone in the upper arm: *humeral* ______________________________
5. Referring to the jaw: *mandibular* ______________________________

Key terms: joints

Joints are formed when two or more bones meet. The joint is the point of **articulation,** the place where movement occurs. There are three main types of joints:

Synovial joints

Synovial joints consist of the following:

synovial fluid: a viscous (thick and sticky) fluid found in joints that helps them to move smoothly

synovial membrane: a layer of connective tissue that lines the cavities of joints

bursa: a sac-like membrane that contains and secretes fluid to facilitate joint movement

Examples: hip, shoulder

Cartilaginous joints

Cartilage is not bone; however, it is an essential component of the skeletal system. **Cartilage** is a highly specialized type of tissue that surrounds bones. It is found in the joints between vertebrae and between any bones that articulate. The ends of bones in a synovial joint are covered with cartilage to provide smooth movement.

Example: the spine

Fibrous joints

Fibrous joints are formed from connective tissue that may eventually harden. Movement is possible in this type of joint, but it is not freely occurring.

Example: the symphysis pubis, which can expand for childbirth

Joints are also classified by their movement. Refer to Figure 4-13 to learn about these classifications.

Mix and Match

Match the type of joint with its example.

1. ball-and-socket	neck
2. ellipsoidal	elbow, knee
3. hinge	shoulder, hip
4. pivot	wrist

TABLE 4-7: Common Medical Roots for Joints

Medical Root	Basic Meaning or Pertaining to	Medical Root	Basic Meaning or Pertaining to
arthr(o)	joint	articul(o)	join
burs(o)	sac	chondr(o)	cartilage

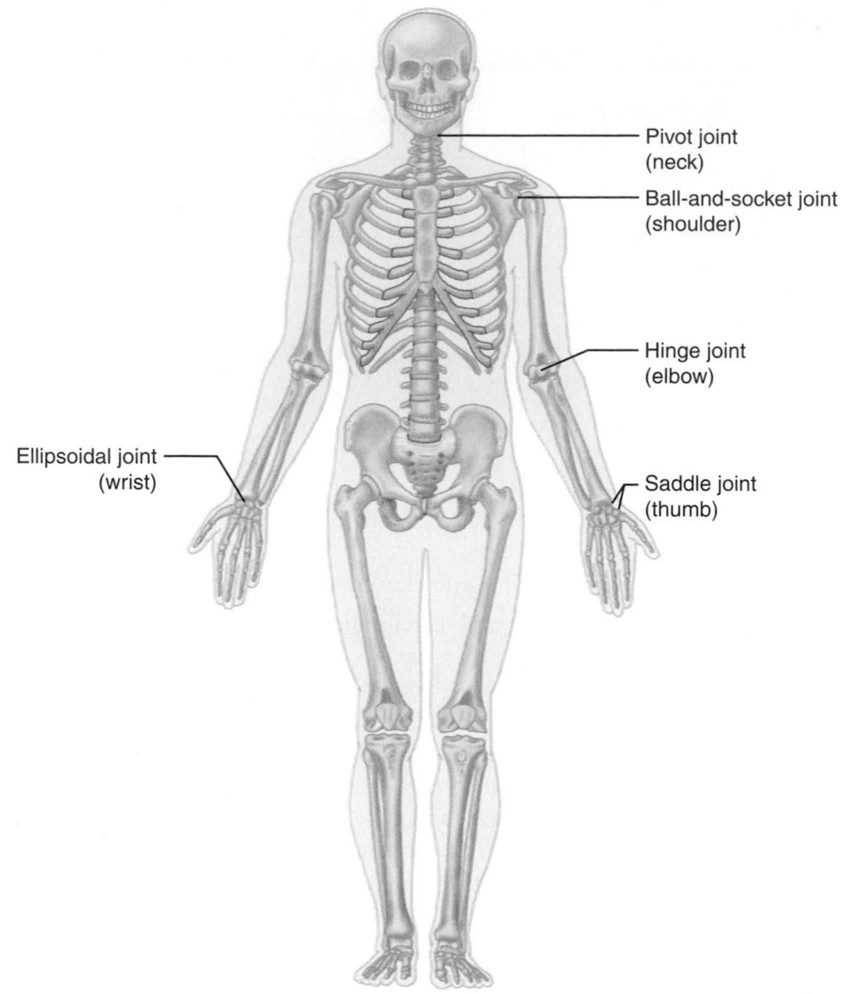

Figure 4.13: Joints identified by types of movement

Build a Word

Use medical roots that apply to the skeletal system to build words that fit the following descriptions:

1. Elderly people often suffer from this disease (To build the word, use the root that means *joint,* and add a suffix meaning *inflammation.*).

   ____

2. To bend, two bones must work together to produce the movement. What verb describes this action of working together (Use the root that means *join,* and add the suffix *-ate.*)?

   ____

3. Sometimes referred to as "tennis elbow," this term begins with a root that means *sac* and ends with a suffix that means *inflammation.*

   ____

Key terms: anatomy of the spine

Throughout this chapter, we have been concerned about our patient's brain and spine. The spinal cord is part of the neurological system. The spine itself, however, is part of the skeletal system. Composition of the spine

spinal cord: a column of nerve fibers and neuropathways that extends from the brain to the end of the first lumbar vertebra of the spine through a hole in the center of each vertebra

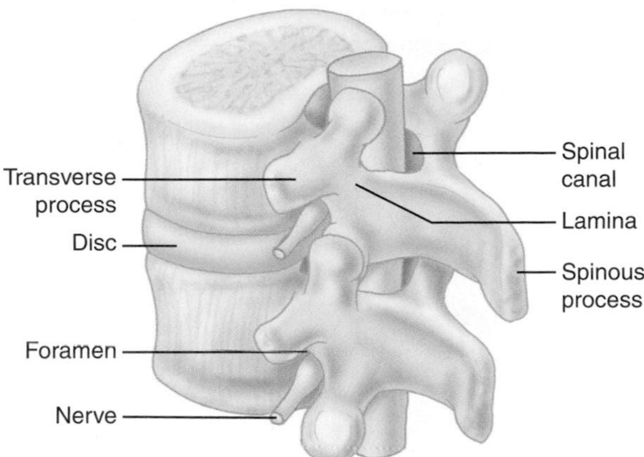

Figure 4.14: Anatomy of the spine

vertebrae: the 24 small bones that form the spine. These bones protect and support the spinal cord as it extends through the spinal canal, the hollow center of the vertebra. These hard bones are somewhat visible through the skin. Together, vertebrae form the **spinal column**. Vertebrae are stacked one on top of the other, and they are held together by ligaments. Between each vertebra and the next is a soft, spongy matter known as a *disc.*

discs: soft pads of tissue that prevent the vertebrae from exerting pressure on each other. This tissue can be injured, inflamed, pinched by imposing vertebrae, or displaced, thereby causing pain and limited movement of the spine.

facet joints: synovial joints that link vertebrae and provide flexibility in the spine

Regions of the spine

cervical spine (neck): consists of seven vertebrae. This region begins at the base of the skull and extends to the thoracic spine. Unlike other vertebrae, these contain a small opening through which blood vessels bring blood to the brain. The atlas and axis vertebrae of the cervical spine are designed specifically to accommodate the rotation of the head.

thoracic spine (mid back): consists of 12 vertebrae that connect to the ribs and form the back

lumbar spine (lower back): consists of five vertebrae that eventually connect the spine to the pelvis. This region of the spine bears most of our weight. It is the site of a great deal of body movement, such as bending and turning.

sacrum: consists of five conjoined vertebrae. This triangular-shaped structure is found at the base of the spine.

coccyx (tailbone): a small bone at the very end (base) of the spinal column.

Mix and Match

Read each description and match it with the correct part or region of the spine.

1. bears most of our weight	vertebrae
2. sometimes called the *tailbone*	synovial fluid
3. a soft pad	lumbar spine
4. an example is the spine	cartilaginous joint
5. bones that stack into a column shape	disc
6. found in a sac and makes movement easier	coccyx

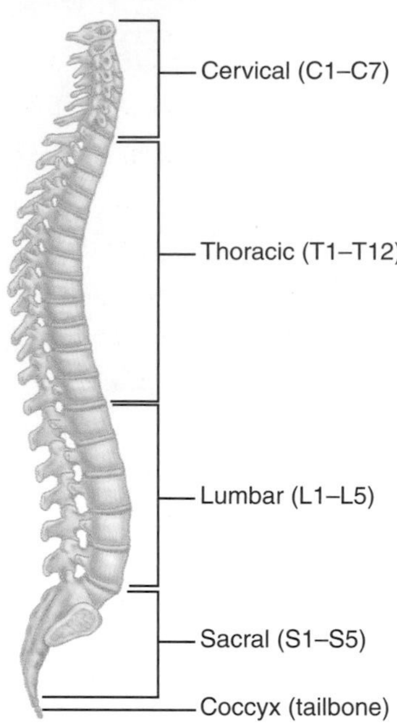

Figure 4.15: Regions of the spine

CHAPTER SUMMARY

Chapter 4 has introduced medical language and terminology related to the neurological and skeletal systems in the context of diagnostic imaging. It provided key terms and explanations that will serve as a strong foundation for future chapters. Opportunities were available to practice word building, breaking words into their component parts, and using new words in contextual sentences.

In Chapter 4, Gil Loeppky was followed through an assessment of his neurological and skeletal systems. This patient will appear again in Chapters 10 and 15.

Chapter 4 also introduced the qualifications and responsibilities of a physician, a radiologist, a radiology technician, and a radiological registered nurse. Dialogues offered insight into how these medical professionals communicate with one another.

See How Much You've Learned

For audio exercises, visit **http://www.MedicalLanguageLab.com.** 

Chapter 4 has introduced you to some medical abbreviations. These have been organized into a study table here for quick reference. Some of them you will recognize immediately, and some will reappear throughout the following chapters with more explanation and application.

TABLE 4-8: Abbreviations: Review

Medical Abbreviation	Full Term	Medical Abbreviation	Full Term
EEG	electroencephalogram	RA	radiologist assistant
O_2	oxygen	RT	radiologic technologist or radiological technician
CT or CAT	computed axial tomography	GCS	Glasgow Coma Scale
DI	diagnostic imaging		
Ra	chemical symbol for *radium*		

Key Terms

acetabulum
articulation
backboard
brainstem
bursa
cartilage
cerebellum
cerebrum
cervical collar
cervical spine (neck)
coccyx (tailbone)
coma
computed tomography (CT or CAT)
condyle
conscious
cranium
dendrite
discs
exposure
facet joints
femur
fibrous joints
fibula
flat bones
frontal lobe
Glasgow Coma Scale (GCS)
glia
hypersomnia
hypothalamus
innominate bones
joints
levels of consciousness (LOC)
lobes
long bones
lumbar spine (lower back)
mastoid hematoma
medulla
medulla oblongata
mesencephalon
midbrain
neuro
neurons
neuropathways
neurotransmitters
obtundation
occipital lobe
ossa
otorrhea
parietal lobe
patella
pelvic girdle
pelvis
periorbital hematoma
pituitary
pons
rhinorrhea
sacrum
semiconscious
sesamoid bones
shot bones
spinal column
spinal cord
STAT
stupor
synovial fluid
synovial membrane
talus
tarsus
temporal lobe
thalamus
thoracic
thoracic spine (mid back)
tibia
unconsciousness
vertebrae
x-ray

CHAPTER REVIEW

Critical Thinking

Answer the following questions about the patient, Gil Loeppky. Use medical terminology whenever this is possible. Share your answers with a peer, if possible, before looking in the Answer Key.

1. Why does Mr. Loeppky have black eyes?

____

2. Why is the radiological nurse required to stay with Mr. Loeppky while he undergoes additional diagnostic imaging procedures?

____

3. What specific types of diagnostic imaging does the patient undergo?

____

4. Mr. Loeppky's blackened eyes are not the result of a head injury. What type of injury are they the result of?

____

5. What type of systematic approach are the health professionals in the scenario using as they begin to take x-rays?

____

6. What do you think is meant by a *head-to-toe assessment*?

____

Break It Down

Break these words into their component parts of prefix-root-suffix, as applicable. Name each element.

1. radiograph ____
2. vertebral ____
3. cranial ____

Translate the Terminology

Use your new skills to decipher medical language. On the line provided, explain what is being said to the best of your ability. Try to do so without the use of a medical dictionary. You may, of course, look back through this chapter for help.

1. Mrs. Davis suffers from arthritis.

   Meaning: ____

2. Evan experiences some numbness and tingling in his feet and hands from time to time. He may have an undiagnosed neuropathy.

   Meaning: ____

Fill in the Blanks

Write the root that completes each definition.

1. ________ *ology* is the field of medicine that uses x-rays, radiation, and radiological substances to view the inside of the body.
2. ________ *pathy* is the term for a disease or disorder of the nervous system.

Name the Root

Read the definition, and then write the appropriate root.

1. There are 126 bones in our body. The anatomical term for *bone* is ______________________.
2. A disease of the joints that is commonly found in the elderly uses which or what root?

   ____

3. Medical references to the system that contains the brain, the spinal cord, and the nerves use which or what root? ____

Name the Suffix

Read the definition, and then write one or more suffixes that add this meaning to a root.

1. having a characteristic or property of ____
2. identifying a process or act ____
3. pain ____
4. inflammation ____
5. creates the name of a health care professional ____

MEMORY MAGIC

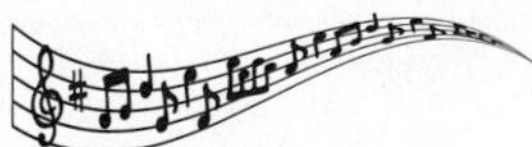

Wondering how to remember the bones of the body?

Try singing about them.

You could make up your own song or rap, or you could sing a childhood song about bones. You can start with the common names for bones and then switch to the anatomically correct terms.

For example, do you remember...

- Childhood favorite "Head, Shoulders, Knees, and Toes"
- "Dem Dry Bones" by J.W. Johnson
- "Everybody Knows the Bones," an adaptation of "Doin' the Bone Dance," written by Miley and Billy Ray Cyrus

CHAPTER FIVE

Laboratory Diagnostics

Focus: Cardiovascular System and Urinary System

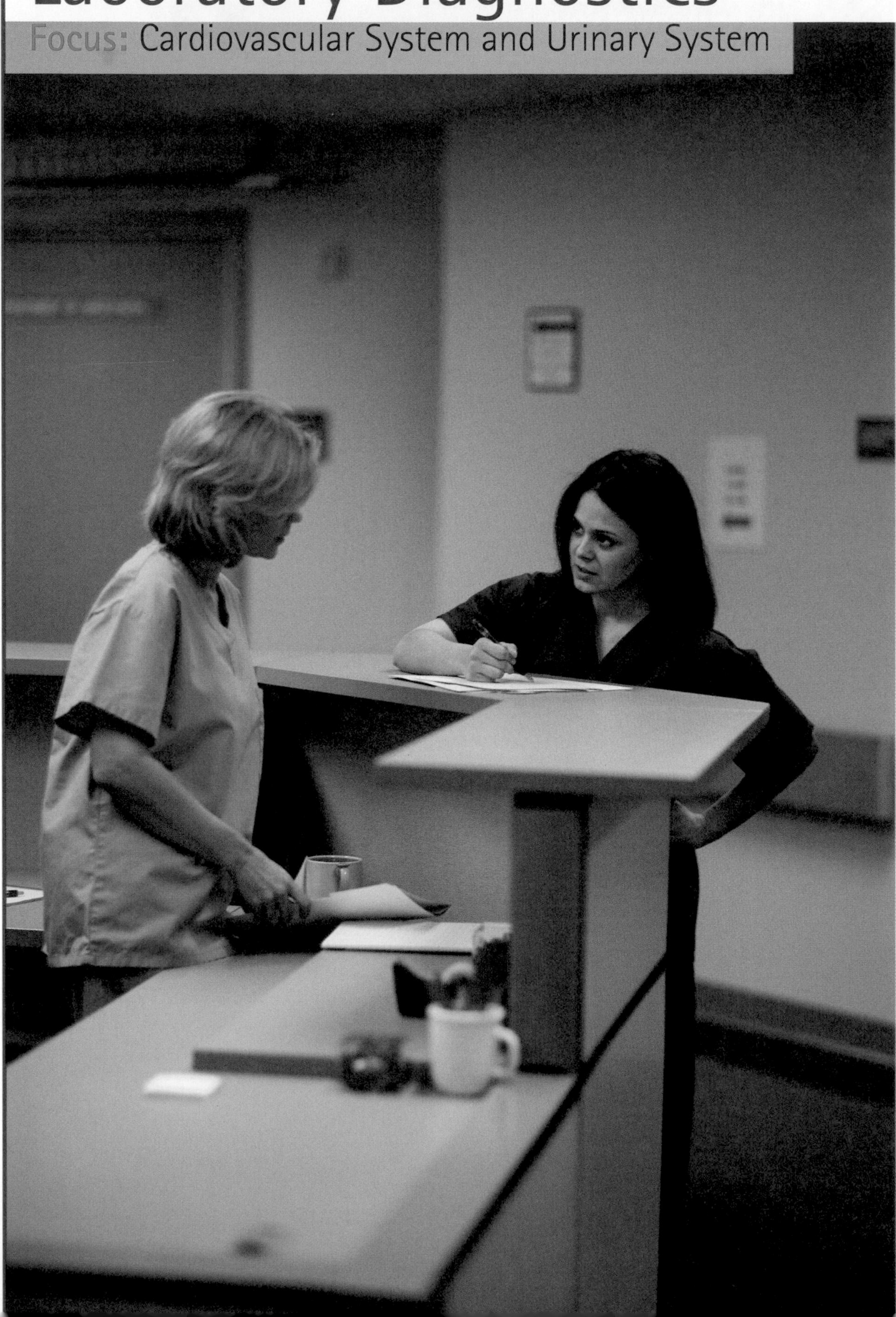

You first met Mr. Zane Davis in the audio dialogue at the beginning of Chapter 2. A victim of a motor vehicle accident, Mr. Davis was attended to by an emergency medical technician (EMT) at the scene. At that time, Mr. Davis was ambulant, but he was also somewhat confused. Even so, Mr. Davis was able to tell EMT Manuel Orantes that he has a history of a "bad heart." His actual diagnosis was never made clear.

Mr. Davis is a 74-year-old married man. He, his wife Stevie-Rose Davis, and their grandson Clay Davis were all in the Davis's vehicle at the time of the accident. Mrs. Davis has been transported to Fayette General Hospital for assessment. Clay Davis, who is 7 years old, is expected to arrive at Okla Trauma Center shortly. Neither Mr. Davis nor the staff knows any of this yet.

Patient Update

En route to the hospital, Mr. Davis began to slur his words. He became increasingly confused, and he was unable to understand what was going on around him or what was being said to him. EMT Orantes immediately assessed the patient's neurological signs. During one test, Mr. Davis' ability to grip the EMT's hand on command was slow and uncoordinated. When he did take the EMT's hand, the strength of his grip was weak. Also during this time, Mr. Davis was incontinent of urine. Due to his age and the potential for elderly patients' health to deteriorate rapidly, he was brought to the Okla Trauma Center rather than to a general hospital as the EMT had originally planned.

Upon arrival at the trauma center, EMT Orantes advised the attending physician in the ER of the possibility of a transient ischemic attack and recounted the patient's symptoms to her. A CT scan and blood work were immediately ordered. The patient was attached to a 12-lead *electrocardiogram* and given oxygen by mask. The team proceeded with the immediate medical and neurological assessment of Mr. Davis's condition in preparation for his transport to Diagnostic Imaging for the CT. The laboratory had been notified of an incoming case, and a laboratory technician would soon arrive to take initial blood tests. The attending physician, Dr. Crowchild, also ordered a urinalysis to be done as soon as possible to rule out a possible urinary tract infection.

At the ER nursing station, a young woman in a white lab coat introduced herself and inquired about a patient. "Hi, I'm Tracey from the lab. I'm looking for a Mr. Zane Davis. Can you tell me where he is?"

Graciella, the medical assistant, looked up from the desk. "Sure," she replied. "Bed 3, over there. You might have to wait a minute, though. The treatment team is still working with him. I'm not sure if they want you first or a CT scan. Protocol says CT first. Just wait. I'll go ask."

"Okay," Tracey responded. Moments later, the medical assistant returned. "Tracey, the doctor wants you to stand by for just a minute. Then she wants you to take the blood specimens STAT so they can transport the patient over to CT. CT is standing by. You'll have to hurry when they call you, or you might even have to follow the patient to CT and take the blood there," explained Graciella.

"Okay," said Tracey. "Since I have a minute then, can you tell me what's going on with this patient?"

"He's an elderly gentleman brought in by emergency medical services from an MVA. It happened around noon today. I haven't heard a peep from the patient, and I didn't see a lot of blood or anything when they wheeled him by on the stretcher, so I'm not really sure what the story is. I've got a few orders here for lab work and for a CT scan STAT. I saw them wheel in the *defibrillator*, but they haven't used it. I know they have an ECG started, because I can see the *readout* here at the desk. No one's called a *Code*. I'm wondering if they are suspecting an *MI* or a *CVA* or something. I guess we'll know soon enough. I suppose if he did have some sort of heart attack or stroke it might explain the car accident."

"Was the patient the driver?" Tracey asked. "Did he hit someone?"

"Honestly, I don't know. I was just speculating. Please don't take anything I say about the accident as the gospel truth. We'll have to wait 'til the chart comes back to the desk to find out what's really going on. Or the nurse or the doctor will tell me."

"Okay. My lab req. asks for a CBC, platelets, INR, PT, and PTT. So you might be right. They very well might be trying to rule out a cardiovascular event. Oh, I see they're ready for me. Gotta go," said Tracey. She turned from Graciella and proceeded to ER Bay 3.

Reflective Questions

Reflect on the dialogue that you've just read as you answer these questions.

1. What is the patient's name?

2. Name the doctor and the emergency medical technician who are involved in this case.

3. Can you tell what the priority of care for this patient is right now? If so, identify it.

4. On the basis of this scenario and what you've learned in previous chapters, what is a CBC?

5. There are two reasons why Mr. Davis was brought to Okla Trauma Center instead of to Fayette General Hospital. What are they?

6. What types of tests are ordered and being performed to assess the patient?

For audio exercises, visit **http://www.MedicalLanguageLab.com.** 

Learning Objectives

After reading Chapter 5, you will be able to do the following:

- Recognize and use language that is used in laboratory diagnostics.
- Appreciate the education and training of laboratory technicians.
- Appreciate the education and training of electrocardiographic technicians.
- Understand the basic concepts and terms for laboratory work, its processes, its core supplies, and its equipment.
- Understand the clinical pathway for triage of a patient suspected of having a circulatory impairment to the brain.
- Recognize and use anatomical and medical terms for the cardiovascular system.
- Recognize medical terminology related to and pathology of the cardiovascular system.
- Recognize and use anatomical and medical terms for the urinary system.
- Recognize medical terminology related to diagnostics of the urinary system.

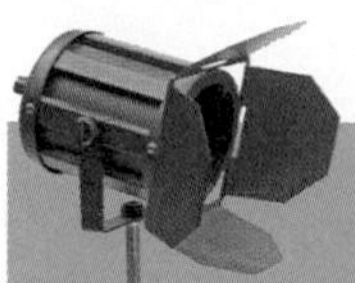

CAREER SPOTLIGHT: Medical Laboratory Technician/ Medical Technologist

Medical laboratory technicians, medical technologists, and *clinical laboratory technicians* are all known by the familiar abbreviated term *lab techs.* Lab techs working in hospitals, clinics, and outpatient laboratories are essential members of the health-care team. They not only collect specimens of blood, urine, feces, and cells, but they also complete rigorous scientific testing of these specimens in the laboratory (lab). They may analyze specimens for their constituents, identify abnormalities in blood and body fluids, and detect harmful bacteria, parasites, and other microorganisms. Lab techs can also analyze drug levels in the blood, urine, and hair to detect abnormalities and to determine whether a patient is responding positively to a treatment. In some laboratory settings, lab techs analyze blood and tissue for DNA, genes, and fertility.

In other settings, medical laboratory technicians may set up and perform electrocardiograms and other diagnostic tests of the heart. Laboratory technicians may also screen for blood types and crossmatch blood for transfusion purposes. The data collected through laboratory diagnostics help to inform physicians of a patient's health status, contribute to forming a diagnosis, and lead to clinical decisions about treatment and health-promoting interventions.

To become a laboratory technician, it is necessary to study in a state-approved program that leads to a certificate, diploma, or degree. Some of the specialties available are in microbiology, hematology, immunology, virology, and chemistry. Graduates can then take one of several national certification tests, which are administered by one of the following bodies: the Board of Registry of the American Society of Clinical Pathologists, the American Medical Technologists organization, or the National Certification Agency for Medical Laboratory Personnel. Successful completion of these tests leads to the credential of Certified Medical Laboratory Technician (MLT).

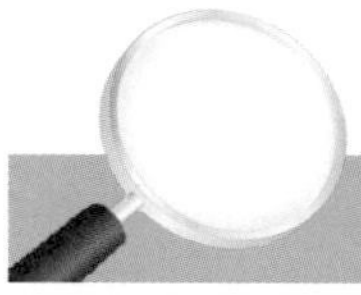

FOCUS POINT: Technicians and Technologists

Technicians work under the supervision of a *technologist,* who has more education than a technician. This generally means that the technologist has a bachelor's degree or a higher level of education and more experience in the field. In addition, because of their advanced training and experience, the medical laboratory technologist may have a specialty and can perform more complex laboratory tests and procedures as compared with a technician.

The Language of Laboratory Diagnostics

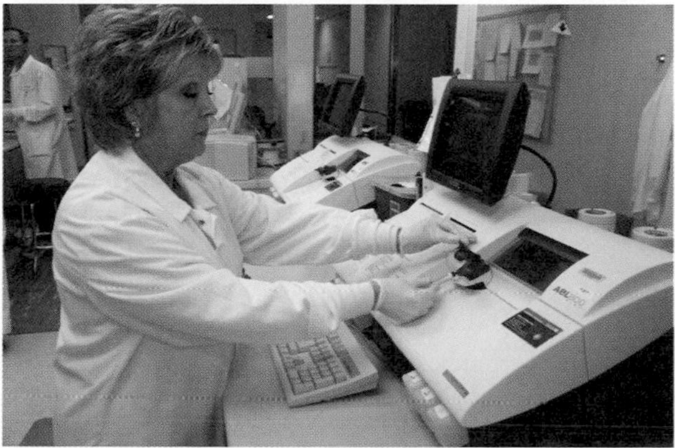

Figure 5.1: Hospital diagnostics lab (From Strasinger S, Di Lorenzo M: *The Phlebotomy Textbook,* ed 3. Philadelphia: FA Davis, 2011, p. 349. With permission.)

Key terms: assessment

We begin the chapter with an introduction to the language of assessment that is used by laboratory technicians (lab techs) and other medical professionals. In the dialogue between Graciella and Tracey in the chapter opener, you may have noticed that Graciella used a number of terms and phrases that Tracey seemed to understand immediately. Their conversation shows how staff members use medical language to communicate across disciplines or health-care career fields. Let's look at some passages from the dialogue. Key terms, phrases, and abbreviations are italicized in the example and highlighted below with the explanation.

> "He's an elderly gentleman brought in by emergency medical services from an MVA. It happened around noon today."
>
> "I've got a few *orders* here for *lab work* and for a CT scan STAT."

orders: the short form of the term *doctor's orders,* meaning requisitions, treatments, or medications ordered specifically by a doctor

lab work: medical jargon. This term is used very broadly to refer to diagnostic tests and testing. Physicians or nurse practitioners order lab work, lab technicians collect and analyze specimens or data from other diagnostic procedures within their field, and nurses and physicians read the results. An example of a question a nurse or doctor might ask is, "Is the lab work back yet?" or "What does the lab work say?" A more formal way to frame these questions would be, "Are the results from the laboratory tests back yet?" or "What are the results from the laboratory tests?"

> "I saw them wheel in the *defibrillator,* but they haven't used it."

defibrillator: a device that is used to send an electrical impulse into the heart to either restart it or to change a life-threatening arrhythmia (abnormal rhythm). The medical term *fibrillation* means *a quivering or contraction of muscle fibers.*

wheel in the defibrillator: defibrillator machines are portable and can be moved from bedside to bedside or patient to patient, as needed Many sit on carts with wheels.

> "I know they have an *ECG* started, because I can see the *readout* here at the desk."

Electrocardiogram (ECG): This is a device that monitors and records the electrical activity of the heart. You will learn more about ECGs later in this chapter. An ECG can be started by physicians, nurses, and certain medical laboratory technicians.

readout: the written record of the data acquired by a computer or a computer-assisted device. A readout (or trace) can appear on a computer monitor screen, or it may be a piece of paper that is continuously printed out by the device. In health care, these readouts become part of the patient's medical record.

> "No one's *called a Code.*"

Code: medical jargon that refers to a protocol and policy for responding to an emergency. All codes are emergency alerts. In hospitals, it is common to hear the terms *Code, Code Blue, Code Red,* and *Code White* called out on a public address (PA) system. Health professionals may also receive these alerts on their pagers. The meaning of each color of code is dependent on the facility. For example, a Code Red might be for fire, and a Code White might be for an incident involving violence and aggression. The most common code, a Code Blue, generally refers to a cardiopulmonary emergency.

called a Code: medical jargon meaning that an alert has gone out. In this scenario, Graciella is referring to a cardiopulmonary emergency code because she believes that the patient is being assessed for his cardiovascular status.

> "I'm wondering if they are suspecting an *MI* or a *CVA* or something."

MI: myocardial infarction: a heart attack

CVA: cerebrovascular accident; a stroke

(explained in detail later in the chapter)

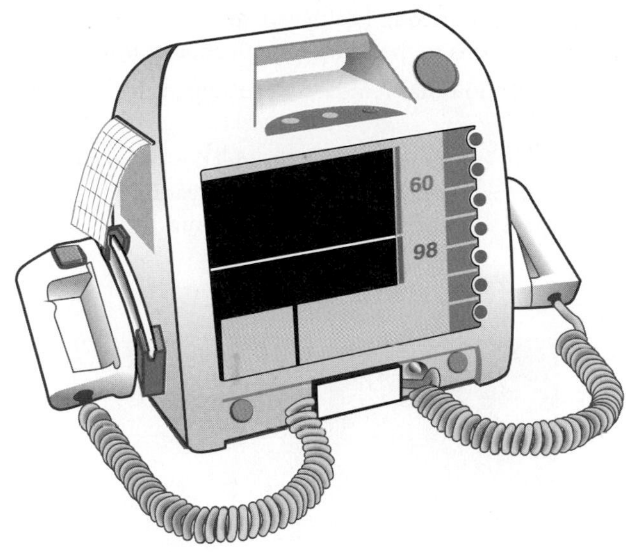

Figure 5.2: Defibrillator

Right Word or Wrong Word: *STAT* or *A.S.A.P.*?

Do *STAT* and *A.S.A.P.* have the same meaning? Can they be used interchangeably?

Infection control in laboratory diagnostics

All health-care personnel follow protocols to minimize the risk of infection for patients, staff, and everyone else in the facility. Infection control is particularly important to laboratory technicians, who work with specimens of body fluids, feces, viruses, bacteria, parasites, and other microorganisms.

Key terms: infection

Infection is the result of the transmission of infectious agents or microorganisms. Infection spreads in the body (i.e., the host) because these agents are able to reproduce.

Infectious agents are organisms that cause communicable (contagious) diseases. These agents include bacteria, viruses, fungi, and protozoa.

The **inflammatory response** is the automatic defense process that begins when tissue is damaged. The goal of this response is to protect the body. The inflammatory response can be set in motion by infectious agents or injuries that can lead to serious illness and possibly death. Laboratory diagnostic tests for leukocytes (white blood cells [WBCs]) can determine when the inflammation process is at work.

Sepsis is a medical term meaning *decay, putrefaction, or the decomposition of animal matter.* Sepsis is a serious medical condition that can occur as a result of uncontrolled infection, and it can lead to blood clots, organ failure, and gangrene. Another name for sepsis is **systemic inflammatory response syndrome (SIRS)**.

Key terms: infection control

Infection control refers to a policy and protocol adhered to by all health professionals and facilities. The goal is to prevent the spread of infection by limiting the potential for contamination and containing the spread of infection should one occur. Infection control procedures include frequent hand washing (hand hygiene), gloving, gowning, and the sterilization of equipment.

Asepsis means *preventing or being free from disease, infection, or putrefaction.* This is achieved through rigorous cleanliness and good hygiene practices.

Medical asepsis is a technique that is used in health care to remain free of infectious agents and to prevent their spread. Asepsis is supported by an infection control protocol.

Surgical asepsis refers to sterilization that removes all pathogens from surgical areas and equipment.

Isolation precautions are used in health care when an infectious agent or a communicable disease is present and there is a risk of the infection spreading to others. This protocol requires full gowning, as well as the use of gloves, face masks, booties, and perhaps even surgical caps.

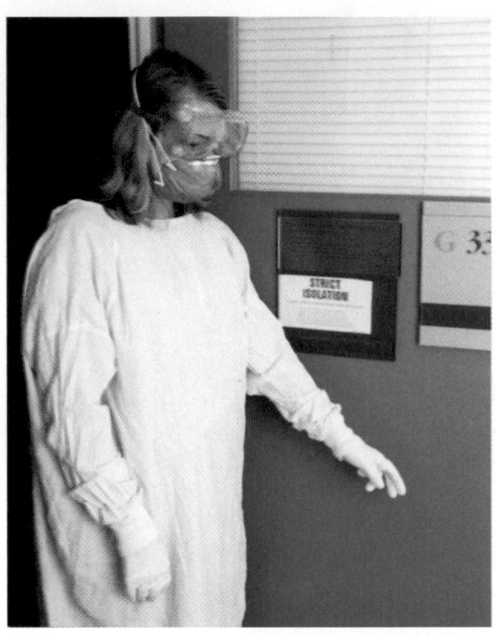

Figure 5.3: Isolation precautions (From Williams LS, Hopper PD: *Understanding Medical Surgical Nursing,* ed 4. Philadelphia: FA Davis, 2011, p. 114. With permission.)

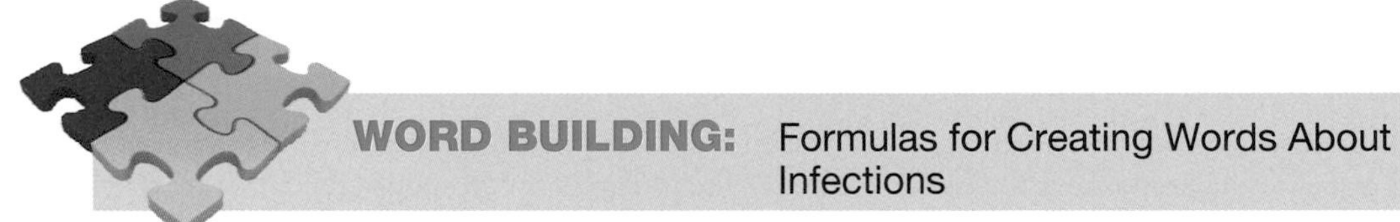

WORD BUILDING: Formulas for Creating Words About Infections

patho + gen = *pathogen*

Definition: a microorganism that can cause disease. (*Path/o* is the combining form of the Greek root meaning *disease; gen* is a root meaning *to produce.*) *noun*

Example: Viruses are *pathogens* because they cause disease.

patho + logy = *pathology*

Definition: disease or the study of disease. (The root *logy* means *reason.*) *noun*

Example: Scientists who study *pathology* may find new cures for fatal diseases.

patho + log + ist = *pathologist*

Definition: a medical professional who studies tissues, cells, and body fluids for evidence of disease (The suffix *-ist* means *a person who does a certain job.*) *noun*

Example: The *pathologist* examined the cancer cells under a microscope.

bacteria

Definition: plural form of *bacterium,* a broad class of microorganisms that live in soil, water, plants and animals; some are beneficial to people, and others are pathogens. *noun*

Example: Some *bacteria* are essential to good health, whereas others cause disease.

dia + rrhea = *diarrhea*

Definition: a condition in which a person experiences frequent watery bowel movements. (*Dia* is a root meaning *through or moving through; rrhea* is a suffix meaning *to flow.*) *noun*

Example: *Diarrhea* can be caused by the bacteria *Clostridium difficile.*

col + itis = *colitis*

Definition: inflammation of the colon. (*Col/o* is a combining form of the word *colon,* meaning *large intestine; -itis* is a suffix meaning *inflammation.*) *noun*

Example: The symptoms of *colitis* include pain, chills, fever, diarrhea in waves, and sometimes blood in the stool (feces).

gastro + entero + itis = *gastroenteritis*

Definition: inflammation that includes both the stomach and the intestinal tract. (*Gastro* is a root meaning *stomach; enter/o* is a combining form of the root *enteron,* meaning *intestines*; *-itis* is a suffix meaning *inflammation.*) *noun*

Example: One of the causes of *gastroenteritis* is the bacteria *Escherichia coli.* This condition is commonly referred to as the stomach flu, although the intestines are also involved. Symptoms can include pain, cramping, and diarrhea.

tubercul + osis = *tuberculosis*

Definition: a contagious respiratory disease that is commonly known as "TB." (*Tubercul* is a combining form of *tuberculum,* meaning *a little swelling; -osis* is a suffix meaning *a condition or disease.*) *noun*

Example: Symptoms of *tuberculosis* include the coughing up of sputum from the lungs, chest pain, shortness of breath, fever, weight loss, and fatigue.

gono + rrhea = *gonorrhea*

Definition: an infectious sexually transmitted disease caused by bacteria. (*Gono* is a combining form of *gonos,* meaning *genitals; -rrhea* is a suffix meaning *to flow.*) *noun*

Example: Symptoms of *gonorrhea* include inflammation of the urethra and genitalia, which causes a burning sensation and urethral discharge.

hepat + itis = *hepatitis*

Definition: a disease of the liver that includes inflammation of this organ. (*Hepat* is a combining form of the root meaning *liver; -itis* is a suffix meaning *inflammation.*) *noun*

Example: There are several forms of *hepatitis.* Some of the symptoms of hepatitis A include nausea, vomiting, low-grade fever, fatigue, jaundice (yellowing of the skin and sclera of the eyes), and dark-colored urine.

TABLE 5-1: Common Pathogens

Pathogen	Type	Causes or Contributes to These Major Infections
Candida albicans	Yeast	Candidiasis (infections of moist areas such as the mouth, the vagina, and the skin)
Staphylococcus aureus	Bacteria	Wound infection Food poisoning Pneumonia
Staphylococcus epidermidis	Bacteria	Wound infection Bacteremia (infection of the blood)
Streptococcus A	Bacteria	Strep throat Rheumatic fever Scarlet fever Wound infection
Streptococcus B	Bacteria	Urinary tract infection Wound infection Postpartum infection or sepsis
Herpes simplex virus type I (HSV-1)	Virus	Cold sores or lesions of the mouth
Herpes simplex virus type II (HSV-2)	Virus	Genital herpes (may include lesions of the mouth)
Human immunodeficiency virus (HIV)	Virus	Acquired immunodeficiency syndrome (AIDS)
Trichophyton	Fungus	Tinea pedis (athlete's foot)

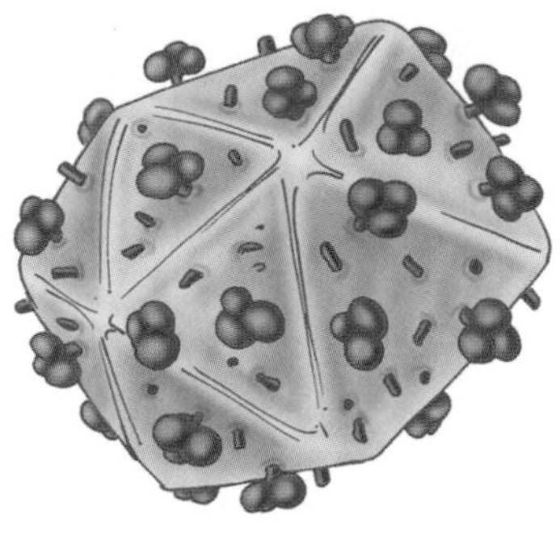

Virus

Figure 5.4: Microscopic view of the human immunodeficiency virus (HIV)

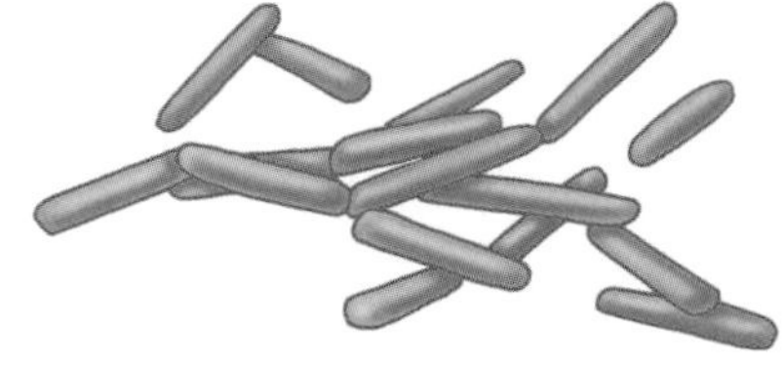

Bacteria

Figure 5.5: Microscopic view of *Escherichia coli* bacteria

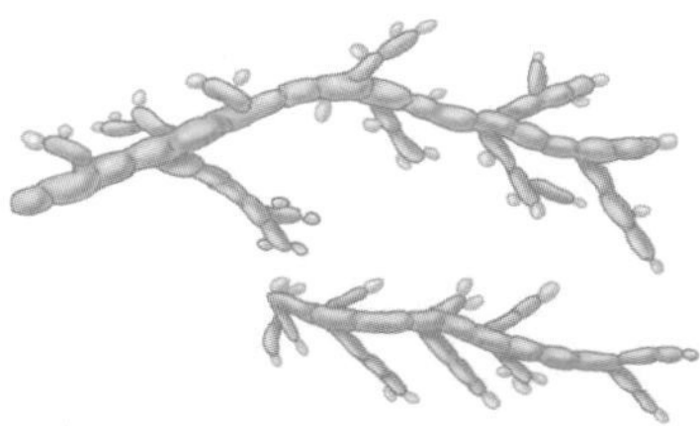

Fungus

Figure 5.6: Microscopic view of tinea fungus

Critical Thinking

Why are infection control techniques particularly important for lab techs? Consider how a medical laboratory technician who did not follow infection control protocols could infect others. Write your ideas here, and share them with another student, a colleague, or an instructor to explore their perspectives.

____

____

____

____

Build a Word

This exercise will reinforce the skill of understanding medical terms from their component parts. The following word parts are scrambled. Arrange each set of parts in a logical order to create a medical term, and then write a definition for the word that you have created.

	TERM	DEFINITION
1. -ic, path/o, gen		
2. -ology, physi, patho/o		
3. toxic, bacteri/o		
4. osis, bacteri/o		
5. colon/o, scopy		
6. -emia, bacter/i/o		
7. rrhea, gono, -al		

Let's Practice

Write the term or terms that best identify what is being described.

1. yeast infections ______________ ______________
2. cold sores ______________ ______________
3. tinea pedis ______________ ______________
4. food poisoning ______________ ______________
5. coughing up of sputum from the lungs, weight loss, fatig ______________
6. frequent watery bowel movements ______________ ______________
7. *Escherichia coli,* stomach ______________
8. inflammation of the large intestine ______________

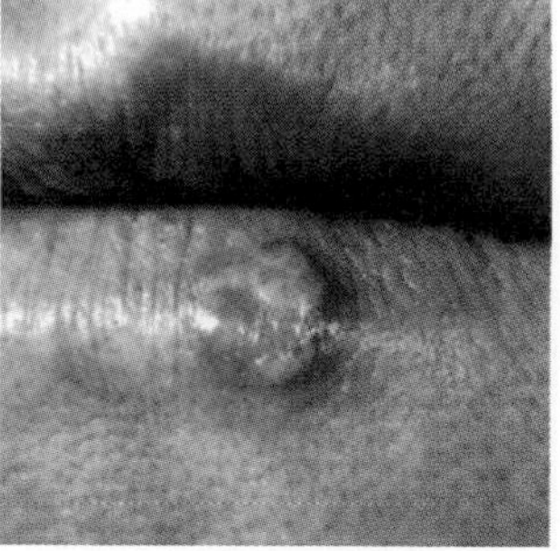

Figure 5.7: Herpes simplex I: cold sore (Courtesy of the Centers for Disease Control and Prevention and Dr. Hermann.)

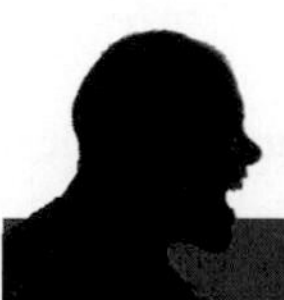

PRONUNCIATION PRACTICE

Say these words aloud to a friend or classmate if you can. You are given the phonetic pronunciation. Your instructor can help you with pronunciation,

or visit **http://www.MedicalLanguageLab.com.**

asepsis	ā-**sĕp**´sĭs
albicans	**ăl**´bĕ-kănz″
bacteriotoxic	băk-tē″rē-ō-**tŏk**´sĭk
candida	kăn´**dĭ**-dă
candidiasis	kăn″dĭ-**dī**´ă-sĭs
colitis	kō-**lī**´tĭs
gastroenteritis	găs″trō-ĕn-tĕr-ī´tĭs
staphylococcus	stăf″ĭl-ō-**kŏk**´ŭs
streptococcus	strĕp″tō-**kŏk**´ŭs
tricophyton	trĭ-**kŏf**´ĭ-tĭn

Read aloud

Return to Table 5-1. Read aloud the name and information about one pathogen three times in succession, and then repeat this process for each pathogen. This exercise will help you to build confidence with the use of new words that may seem difficult or unusual to pronounce.

The Language of Blood Work

Key terms: drawing blood

In the opening scenario, the laboratory technician has arrived in the ER to draw blood from Mr. Davis for analysis. She will be using the technique of venipuncture. To do this work, she must have a certificate in phlebotomy and be licensed in the state in which she practices. Here are some key terms used in the process of drawing blood.

venipuncture: the process of drawing blood from a vein.

capillary puncture: the process of drawing blood from a capillary.

phlebotomy: the process of puncturing or cutting into a vein. This might be done with the use of a surgical instrument, such as a needle or a small blade called a *lancet.*

phlebotomist: a technician with specialized training and certification that permits him or her to take blood from a vein or capillary for the purpose of blood donation or diagnostic testing.

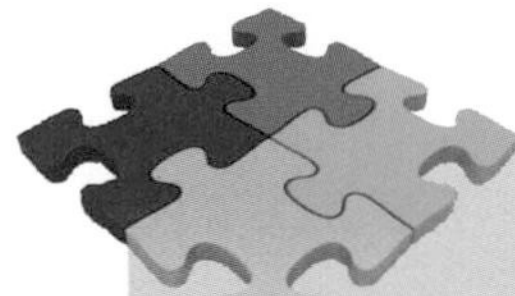

WORD BUILDING: Formula for Creating Words with the Combining Form *Ven/o/a* and *Phleb/o*

1. vena = vein the combining form is *ven/o/a*, which refers to *veins* or the *blood*.

ven + ous

Definition: referring to blood passing through the veins or to the veins themselves.

Example: It is not yet known whether or not Mr. Davis is suffering from impaired *venous* circulation.

veni + puncture = *venipuncture*

Definition: puncture of a vein. An exception to the rule, *ven/a/o* uses the letter *i* to create its combining form. (*Puncture* derives from the combining form *punctur/a,* meaning *point, prick, or pierce.*) *noun*

Example: Medical laboratory technicians often use *venipuncture* to collect blood specimens.

veno + graph + y = *venography*

Definition: a procedure in which a dye (contrast medium) is inserted into the veins to visualize them with the use of radiography (x-ray).

Example: *Venography* can help to determine the presence of narrowing and clotting in the veins.

2. phleb/o = combining form referring to veins or blood vessels in general

phlebo + tom + y = *phlebotomy*

Definition: bloodletting by incision into a vein. (The second root *tome* is found in its combining form, *tom/e/i/a,* meaning *incision or cutting.*) *noun*

Example: To practice *phlebotomy,* you need to be a licensed health professional.

phleb + itis = *phlebitis*

Definition: inflammation of a vein. *noun*

Example: *Phlebitis* can occur as a result of injury, pregnancy, smoking, obesity, or sitting in one position for too long.

phlebo + mano + meter = *phlebomanometer*

Definition: a medical device that is used to measure venous pressure (pressure in the veins). (*Mano* derives from Greek and means *thin; meter* is a root word meaning *measure.*) *noun*

Example: A *phlebomanometer* can be used to study venous hypertension and intravascular status (the status of the blood vessels).

Fill in the Blanks

Begin to use new terminology by choosing terms to complete the following sentences. By doing so, you will become more familiar with terms in their proper context.

1. The quickest method of assessing the blood is to take a specimen by ________________.
2. Penetrating a vein is referred to as the process of ________________________
3. A certificate in ________________ allows a health professional to draw blood.
4. Many medical words that refer to veins begin with the combining form *ven/a/o.* What is the exception to this rule? ________________________
5. During long periods of sitting or lying, when the veins of the lower extremities struggle to return blood flow upward to the heart, what might occur? ________________
6. If the physician suspects that a patient's veins are beginning to narrow or that they may be inflamed, what radiographic test might he or she order? ________________________

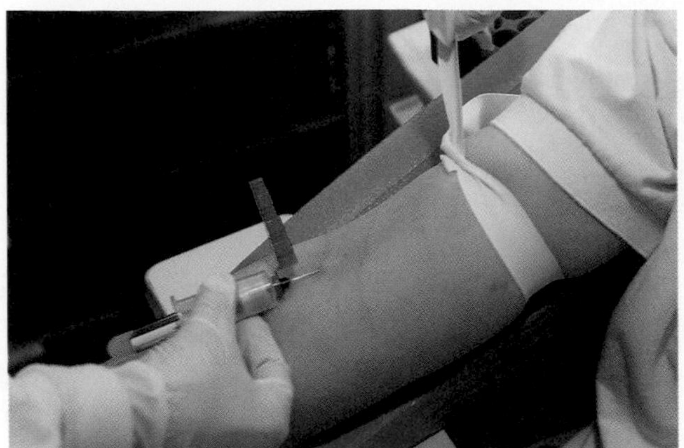

Figure 5.8: Venipuncture
(From Strasinger S, Di Lorenzo M: *The Phlebotomy Textbook,* ed 3. Philadelphia: FA Davis, 2011, p. 207. With permission.)

Key terms: blood tests

In Chapter 3, you began learning about blood and blood tests. Now you have the opportunity to learn more about blood tests. Dr. Crowchild has ordered laboratory work for diagnostic purposes. Mr. Davis is having these tests because if he has had or is about to have a cerebrovascular accident or a stroke, then bleeding may occur in the brain. The body's normal response to bleeding is to send clotting agents into the circulatory system to stem the flow of blood.

Recall the statement by Tracey, the laboratory technician, about the blood tests that had been ordered for Mr. Davis. In the following excerpt, key abbreviations are highlighted and explained. To learn more about abbreviations that are commonly used in laboratory testing and other medical fields, see Table 5-2.

> "My lab *req.* asks for a CBC, *platelets, INR, PT,* and *PTT.*"

req.: an abbreviated form of requisition, meaning *request*

platelets: particles in the blood that are involved in the clotting process

INR: international normalized ratio: An INR test measures the level of coagulation in the blood. In our case, Dr. Crowchild knows that the patient, Mr. Davis, has a "bad heart," but she does not know if he is taking any medication for it. Mr. Davis may be taking an anticoagulant, and she needs to find out this information immediately. An **anticoagulant** is a medication that prevents blood from clotting and is often referred to as a *blood thinner.* An INR test will reveal if Mr. Davis is undergoing anticoagulant therapy. An INR is often used to replace the need for a PT test.

PT: prothrombin time: the time that it takes for the blood to thicken and clot. This test is given to identify the cause of unexplained bleeding, the status of the liver, and the effectiveness of anticoagulant medication such as warfarin (Coumadin) or heparin.

PTT: partial thromboplastin time. This test is ordered in cases of unexplained bleeding (a thrombotic episode), bruising (thromboembolism), or recurrent miscarriage. It also evaluates the function of all coagulation (clotting) factors.

Thrombus is an important medical term for the assessment of our patient, Mr. Davis. The word refers to a blood clot that adheres to the wall of a blood vessel. The following are derivatives of this root word.

Thrombin is an enzyme that is the basis of a blood clot.

Thromboplastin is a substance in the blood and tissues that increases clotting time.

Thromboemboli are blood clots. **Emboli** (the plural form of *embolus*) is the term for large masses of material (i.e., a blood clot) that block blood vessels.

Thrombosis is the presence of a blood clot in the circulatory system. This occurs when a thrombus has come loose from the walls of a vessel and is moving through the system. It is a life-threatening condition.

In addition to the blood tests mentioned by the lab tech, Dr. Crowchild will also have ordered O_2SATs to be monitored and arterial blood gases (ABGs) to be tested.

O_2SATs is medical jargon. It is an abbreviated form of the term **oxygen saturation**. This is a diagnostic measure of the amount of oxygen that is bound to hemoglobin in the blood (oxyhemoglobin). Normal saturation is recorded as 95% to 100%. O_2SATs can be measured by using a pulse oximeter device or by collecting a blood specimen of arterial blood gases.

To assess O_2SATs, a device called a **pulse oximeter** is commonly used. This device measures any changes in blood volume in the skin, and it also measures the patient's pulse. A pulse oximeter can be used continuously and left clipped to a patient's finger. Most health professionals are permitted to apply and read a pulse oximeter.

Arterial blood gases (ABGs) are determined with the use of an invasive test that also measures O_2SATs. Blood is drawn from an artery, usually at the inner aspect of the wrist. The test measures the levels of oxygen and carbon dioxide in the blood and the blood's acidity (determined by pH or the level of hydrogen ions). The pH of blood is normally between 7.35 and 7.45. An ABG test is used diagnostically to help determine heart or kidney failure, diabetes, lung disorders, and other diseases. The laboratory will need to know if the patient is receiving oxygen therapy before or during the test because oxygen therapy can significantly affect the results of the test. Only certified and approved health professionals are permitted to perform this procedure because it punctures an artery and thus involves the potential for blood loss and infection.

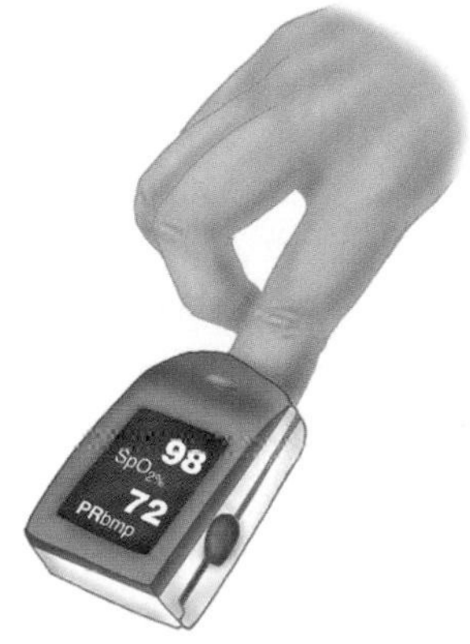

Figure 5.9: Pulse oximeter

TABLE 5-2: Common Medical Abbreviations Used in Lab Tests

Abbreviation	Full Term	Abbreviation	Full Term
BUN	blood urea nitrogen	O_2	oxygen
Na	sodium	O_2SATs	oxygen saturation; oxyhemoglobin
K	potassium	CBC	complete blood count
Cl	chloride	FBS	fasting blood sugar
CO_2	carbon dioxide	TBIL	total bilirubin test
Ca	calcium	Li	lithium
INR	international normalized ratio		
PT and PTT	prothrombin time and partial prothrombin time		

Key terms: laboratory instruments and equipment

capillary tube: a device that is usually used for the accurate measurement of small amounts of liquid. A capillary tube looks like a very small drinking straw that is made of glass. When the tube touches liquid, the liquid moves up inside the tube because of the attraction between water molecules and the glass (i.e., adhesion). The liquid will move up until the force of adhesion is matched by the force of gravity. Different sizes of capillary tubes will hold different amounts of liquid. (Note that pipettes are now used more often than capillary tubes for measuring small amounts of liquid in laboratories.)

pipette or pipettor: a device that is used to measure liquid. The word *pipette* is more often used to describe a device that is operated by hand. The word *pipettor,* however, is more often used to describe a device that operates with the assistance of electricity or that is automated. Both devices use vacuum suction to draw up a measured amount of fluid. Both devices use changeable or disposable plastic tips or barrels.

blood gas analyzer: a device for measuring the pH of blood and the amount of oxygen and carbon dioxide in the blood. A blood gas analyzer usually measures the gases in arterial blood (ABGs), but sometimes venous blood is used. Chemicals, pressure, or both may be used to separate the gases from the liquid blood. After these substances are separated, they may be attracted to a special electrode with a sensor that can measure them.

centrifuge: a device that is used to separate components of a substance such as blood. The process used is centrifugal force, which is the result of a rapid spinning motion.

coagulation analyzer: a device that measures the time that it takes for a sample of blood to clot. Automated coagulometers operate by different methods. Some measure the decrease in the amount of light that can pass through a sample as it changes from liquid blood to a solid clot; others measure how clotting affects movement in the blood sample.

chemistry analyzer: a device that measures sugars, salts, and other small molecules and ions in body fluids. Chemistry analyzers measure components such as glucose, blood urea nitrogen (BUN), creatinine, Na, K, CI, CO_2, Ca, and total protein.

hematology analyzer: an instrument that is used to count the different kinds of cells found in blood. A hematology analyzer is used to give the values for the complete blood count (CBC). Many newer hematology analyzers also count cells in other body fluids, as well as in blood.

immunology analyzer: a device that identifies and measures molecules such as antibodies, hormones, and drugs. Each antibody will bind (attach) to only one specific thing. Immunological analyzers use known antibodies to identify different molecules in samples such as blood, urine, or other body fluids and tissues.

urine analyzer: a device that identifies and measures molecules in urine. An automated urine analyzer identifies factors such as pH, protein, sugar, bilirubin, ketones, nitrites, and blood cells in urine. Most of these are measured with the use of chemicals that change color or that react when they contact the molecule that they are measuring. Some automated urine analyzers will also measure urine density and cloudiness (turbidity).

electrolyte analyzer: a device for measuring and comparing the amounts of ions such as Na, K, Cl, Ca, Li, and phosphate in the serum, plasma, and urine. Many electrolyte analyzers have functions that overlap with chemistry analyzers.

Critical Thinking

Consider what you've been learning about the types of laboratory tests that can help the physician diagnose Mr. Davis's condition.

1. Dr. Crowchild has ordered an INR, a PT, and a PTT STAT. What might she be looking for with regard to Mr. Davis's immediate health?

   ____

2. It is very likely that Dr. Crowchild will order urine testing (urinalysis) later as well. Keeping in mind what you know about laboratory tests so far, which urine test do you think she might order? Why? ______________________________

3. Mr. Davis is being given oxygen by the treatment team. Which test involving a machine might this oxygen negatively affect (i.e., cause interference with the results)?

____

4. On the basis of the blood tests that have been ordered for Mr. Davis, identify three machines or devices that will be used in the laboratory to analyze his blood samples.

____

Mix and Match

Match each abbreviated term on the left with the full term on the right by drawing a line to connect them.

1. K	complete blood count
2. Ca	blood urea nitrogen
3. PPT	fasting blood sugar
4. BUN	partial prothrombin time
5. CBC	potassium
6. FBS	calcium
7. Na	sodium

TABLE 5-3: Key Prefixes: Laboratory Analysis

Prefix	Meaning	Prefix	Meaning
a-	absent, absence of; not	ab-	away from
an-	absent, absence of; not	anti-	opposite, against

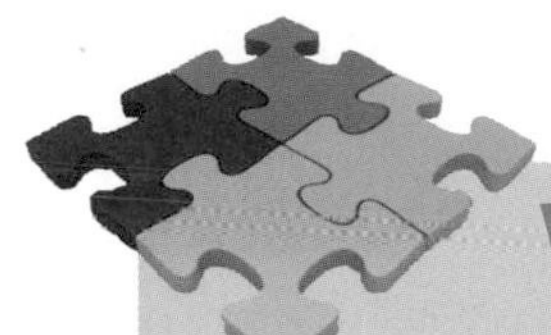

WORD BUILDING: Formula for Creating Words with the Prefixes *A-/Ab-/An-/Anti-*

ab + norm + al = *abnormal*

Definition: not as expected or not standard. (The prefix *ab-* means *not*; the root *norm* means *standard.*) *adjective*

Example: *Abnormal* results in a lab test can be cause for concern.

a + typic + al = *atypical*

Definition: unusual or uncharacteristic. (The prefix *a-* means *not;* the combining form *typic* means *in the original form.*) *adjective*

Example: *Atypical* results of a diagnostic assessment are those that are not typically expected.

an + ox + ia = *anoxia*

Definition: lack of oxygen in the blood. (The prefix *an-* means *without or lacking; ox* is a combining form of *oxygen.*) *noun*

Example: *Anoxia* can cause brain damage and threaten life.

anti + body = *antibody*

Definition: a naturally occurring substance in the body that is present as part of the reaction to the presence of a foreign cells. (The root word *body* originates in Old English and refers to a *collection.* In this word, *body* refers to a collection of foreign cells.) *noun*

Example: *Antibodies* are elements of the immune system that are sometimes referred to as *antitoxins.*

Continued

anti + gen = *antigen*

Definition: a specialized type of cell that can distinguish between the body's own cells and foreign cells; when it recognizes foreign cells, it triggers an immune response. (The prefix *anti-* means *not or opposite;* the root *gen* means *producing.*) *noun*

Example: Each type of antibody can attach to a particular kind of foreign *antigen.*

anti + coagul + ant = *anticoagulant*

Definition: 1) a substance that hinders the clotting of blood; 2) describing the properties of such a substance. (The prefix *anti-* means *not or opposite. Coagul* derives from the root *coagulans,* meaning *congealing or solidifying.*) *noun or adjective*

Example: Individuals who have had a heart attack are often prescribed an *anticoagulant* medication to prevent the clotting of blood.

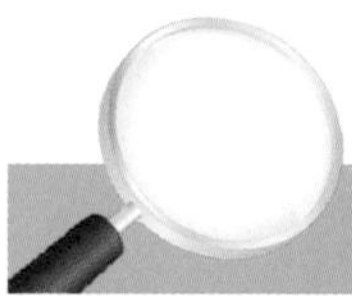

FOCUS POINT: Anomaly

The term *anomaly* is a root word meaning *an irregularity or an unusual finding; a deviation from normal.* In medical laboratories, it is common to hear this term used to refer to the results of laboratory diagnostics. The plural form is *anomalies.*

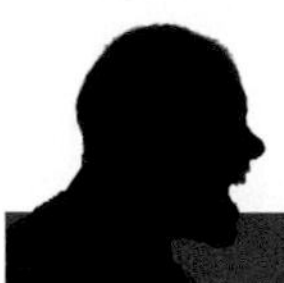

PRONUNCIATION PRACTICE

Say these words aloud to a friend or classmate if you can. You are given the phonetic pronunciation. Your instructor can help you with pronunciation,

or visit **http://www.MedicalLanguageLab.com.** 

anomaly	ă-**nŏm**´ă-lē
antibody	**ăn**´tĭ-bŏd″ē
antigen	**ăn**´tĭ-jĕn
atypical	ā-**tĭp**´ĭ-kăl
capillary	**kăp**´ĭ-lăr″ē
coagulant	kō-**ăg**´ū-lănt
manometer	măn-**ŏm**´ĕt-ĕr
phlebomanometer	flĕb″ō-mă-**nŏm**´ĕ-tĕr
phlebotomy	flĕ-**bŏt**´ō-mē
pipette	pī-**pĕt**´
thrombus	**thrŏm**´bŭs
thromboemboli	thrŏm″bō-**ĕm**´bō-lī
urea	ū-**rū**´ă
venipuncture	**vĕn**´ĭ-pŭnk″chūr

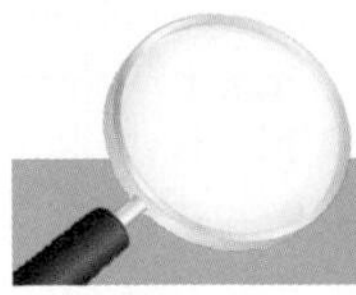

FOCUS POINT: Subjective Data vs. Objective Data

There are two very important sources of data in health care: the patient's own *subjective* report of his or her symptoms and personal history and the *objective* data obtained through science. Objective data derive from scientifically verified and approved testing, and it may or may not include laboratory diagnostics. For example, the Glasgow Coma Scale, which is based on professional observation and the patient's vital signs, is an accepted standard for measuring neurological function and levels of consciousness. Objective tests are conducted with the use of the scientific method, and they provide results that can be compared with standardized empirical results.

The Language of the Cardiovascular System

Mr. Davis is going through the triage process in the emergency department of the trauma center. Before Mr. Davis's arrival, the EMT had advised the care team that Mr. Davis might present with an urgent condition involving his cardiovascular (circulatory) system.

Emergency assessment: cardiovascular system

You may recall that the EMT reported the patient's history of a "bad heart" and then described signs and symptoms of neurological impairment. This information led the care team to immediately assess Mr. Davis for a cerebrovascular accident (CVA) and a transient ischemic attack (TIA). Each of these conditions involves the cardiovascular system and the brain. Protocol requires the team to follow a clinical pathway for care in this type of case (see "Triage Protocol: Signs and Symptoms of CVA").

Note that Mr. Davis is not being assessed specifically at this time for a myocardial infarction (MI; a heart attack). Although the physician and her team have been made aware of the patient's "bad heart," their first priority of care involves the patient's blood circulation because of the potential for brain damage that could result from a blood clot or hemorrhage impeding circulation to the brain and as the heart. Mr. Davis has not exhibited symptoms of an MI. Even so, the monitoring and diagnostic tests that will be performed on this patient will also provide the care team with important data about Mr. Davis's heart.

Key terms: cerebrovascular emergencies

A **cerebrovascular accident (CVA)** is the same thing as a stroke. A **stroke** is a sudden loss of brain function caused by interruption of blood flow or excessive blood flow to the brain. Contributing factors to a CVA are a history of heart disease and prior incidents of transient ischemic attacks (TIAs). A stroke may also be the result of a brain injury. Some of the symptoms include the sudden onset of slurred speech, confusion, visual impairment, confusion, and an inability to understand what is going on.

An **ischemic stroke**, which is also called a *cerebrovascular accident* (CVA), is the result of a blood clot (thrombus) impeding circulation and cutting off blood supply to the brain. This condition can be caused by the disease atherosclerosis, which involves the hardening of the arteries. *Ischemia* means *lack of blood.*

A **hemorrhagic stroke** is the result of bleeding into the brain via an intracerebral or subarachnoid hemorrhage. This condition is the result of a broken blood vessel caused by an aneurysm, a break in the thin, brittle arteries as a result of atherosclerosis. In some cases, hemorrhagic stroke can be caused by uncontrolled high blood pressure. Damage or injury to the head and neck can also cause bleeding within the brain and mimic the signs and symptoms of a hemorrhagic stroke.

A **transient ischemic attack (TIA)** is a temporary interruption in the blood flow to the brain. The symptoms are the same as those of a CVA, but they pass in minutes or hours. Contributing factors can include a history of heart disease, cardiac arrhythmias, and high blood pressure. TIAs require medical attention and are considered potential precursors to full CVAs. They are often referred to as *mini-strokes*.

An **aneurysm** is a balloon-like widening or bulge in an artery. Aneurysms can occur in the chest, the brain, and other parts of the body. They usually occur in the aorta of the heart. Dr. Crowchild will be interested in finding out if Mr. Davis has a cerebral aneurysm that may be causing his stroke-like symptoms. When an aneurysm bursts, it can cause excessive bleeding and lead to death.

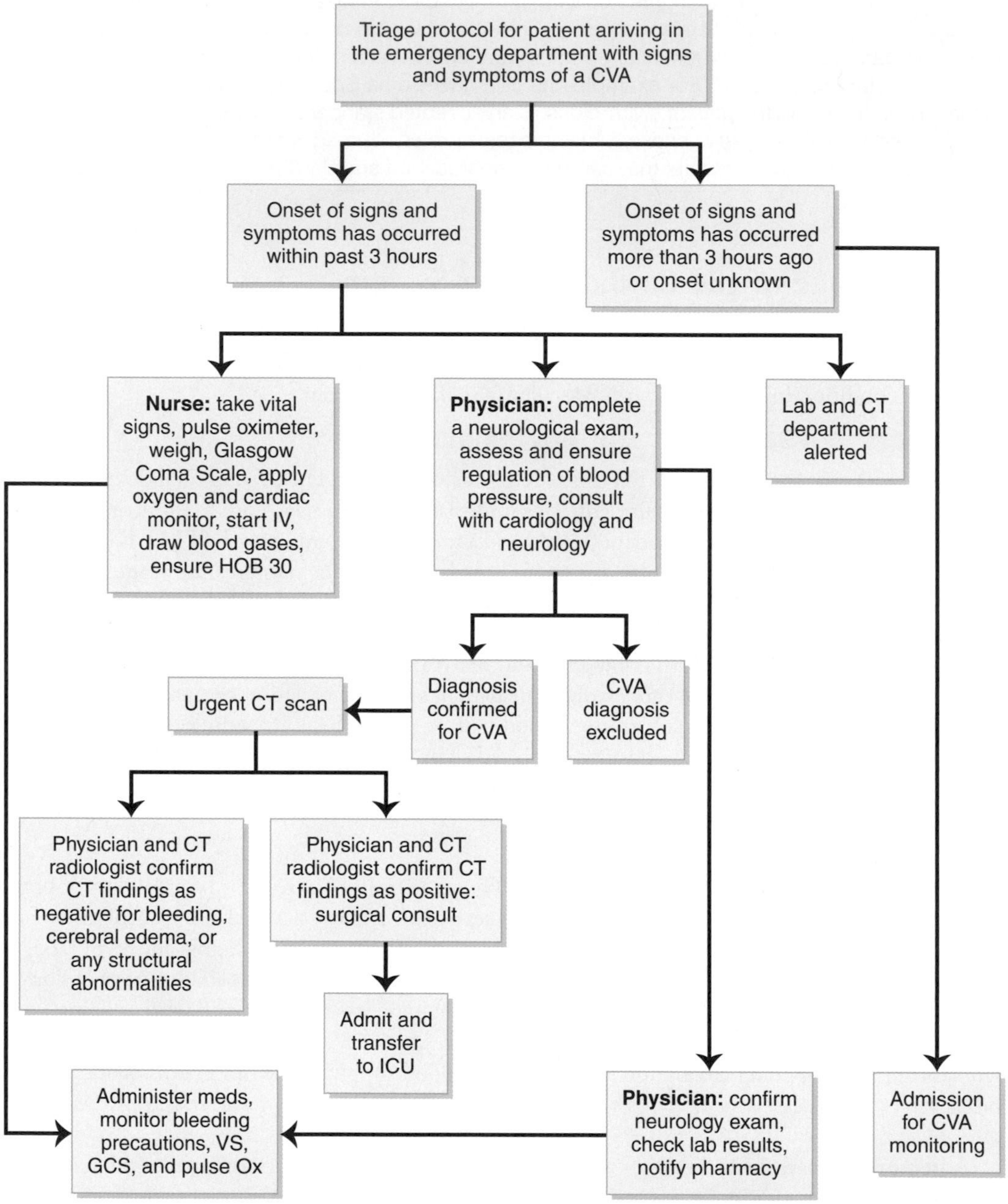

Triage protocol for patient arriving in the emergency department with signs and symptoms of a CVA

Onset of signs and symptoms has occurred within past 3 hours

Onset of signs and symptoms has occurred more than 3 hours ago or onset unknown

Nurse: take vital signs, pulse oximeter, weigh, Glasgow Coma Scale, apply oxygen and cardiac monitor, start IV, draw blood gases, ensure HOB 30

Physician: complete a neurological exam, assess and ensure regulation of blood pressure, consult with cardiology and neurology

Lab and CT department alerted

Diagnosis confirmed for CVA

CVA diagnosis excluded

Urgent CT scan

Physician and CT radiologist confirm CT findings as negative for bleeding, cerebral edema, or any structural abnormalities

Physician and CT radiologist confirm CT findings as positive: surgical consult

Admit and transfer to ICU

Administer meds, monitor bleeding precautions, VS, GCS, and pulse Ox

Physician: confirm neurology exam, check lab results, notify pharmacy

Admission for CVA monitoring

Figure 5.10: Clinical pathway: triage protocol for a cerebrovascular accident

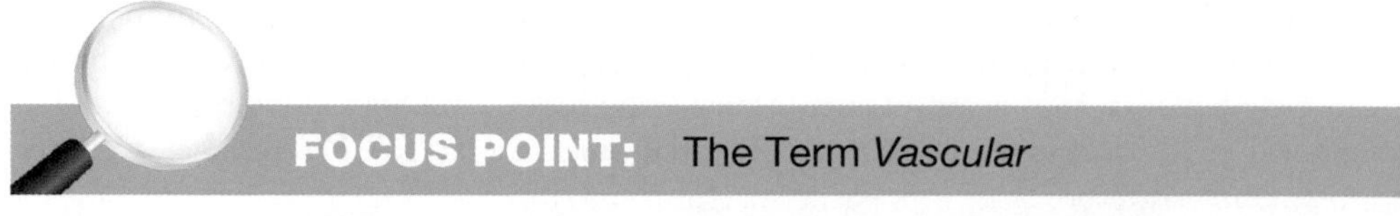

Vascular is a medical term that refers to the blood vessels, the blood, or the components or composition of blood.

Critical Thinking

Dr. Crowchild suspects that Mr. Davis is having a cerebrovascular accident. She wishes to determine the severity of it and as the potential for another incident. Answer the following questions with that in mind.

1. Break down the term *cerebrovascular,* and explain how the two parts of the body that this term refers to are normally and naturally related.

 ____

 ____

2. Use your critical thinking skills to suggest what impairment or dysfunction might have caused Mr. Davis's symptoms.

 ____

 ____

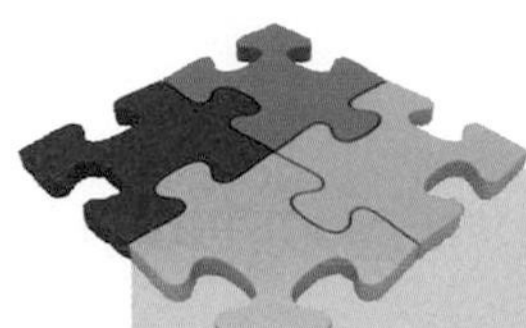

WORD BUILDING: Formula for Creating Words with the Combining Form *Ather/o*

ather/o = combining form of the Greek root *athere,* meaning fatty plaque or patch

ather + oma = *atheroma*

Definition: fatty degeneration or thickening of the walls of the larger arteries as a result of plaque buildup. (The suffix *-oma* means *tumor.*) *noun*

Example: Aging and high blood pressure (hypertension) are risk factors for the development of *atheroma.*

ather + oma + tous = *atheromatous*

Definition: describing an obstruction within an artery that is the result of an atheroma. *adjective*

Example: The CT scan detected an *atheromatous* plaque in the femoral artery.

athero + scler + osis = *atherosclerosis*

Definition: a condition in which deposits of fatty material build up in the lining of an artery, possibly restricting blood flow. *noun*

Example: *Atherosclerosis* is also called *coronary artery disease* (CAD).

athero + genesis = *atherogenesis*

Definition: the formation of plaque on arterial walls. (*Genesis* is a root word meaning *birth or production.*) *noun*

Example: The likelihood of *atherogenesis* in a middle-aged person who smokes cigarettes and who is obese is greater than that for someone the same age who does not smoke and who maintains a healthier weight.

Anatomy and physiology: blood vessels and circulation

Before we can proceed any further with updates on Mr. Davis's medical condition, it is necessary to develop a vocabulary related to the structures and functions of the cardiovascular system. First, we will look at the vessels that carry blood to and from the heart. Figure 5-11 provides an overview of these blood vessels. Note that, in medical diagrams, arteries are always red in color, whereas *veins* are always blue. The reason for this is that arteries contain oxygen, which brightens the blood. Alternatively, veins have a blue appearance, and many can be seen through the skin. Their color is a result of a diminished level of oxygen in the blood.

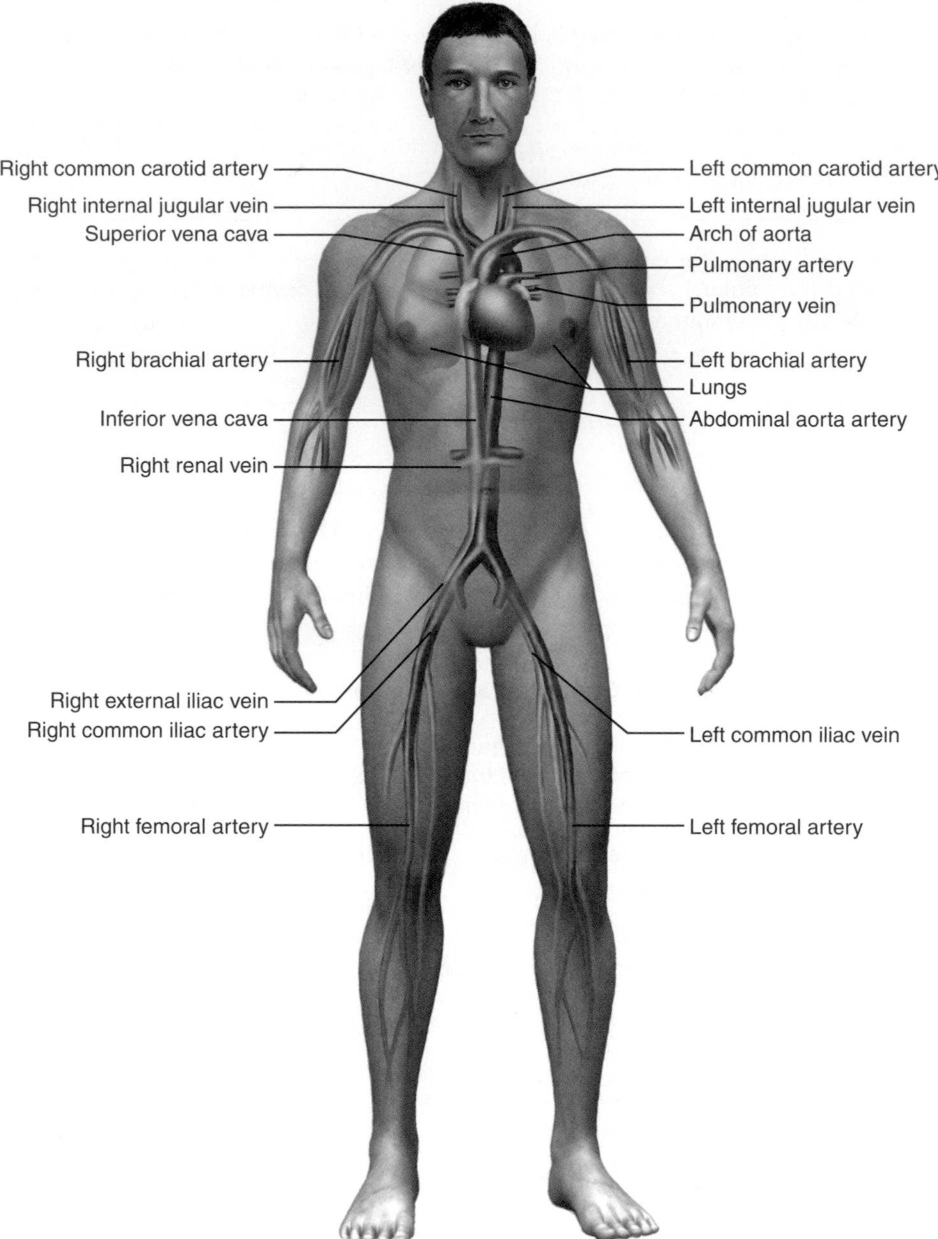

Figure 5.11: Blood vessels and circulation

Cardiovascular functions

The cardiovascular system is concerned with the circulation of blood through the body. The major components of the system are the heart, the arteries, and the veins. (We will study the heart in more detail in the next section.) Arteries and veins are the blood vessels through which blood flows. Blood carries important nutrients, hormones, electrolytes, and oxygen to the body. Arteries are the supply vessels for the body, whereas veins help to remove waste products from the body.

The second purpose of the cardiovascular system is to defend against disease. It does this through the production and distribution of white blood cells and lymph. **Lymph** is the clear, watery component of blood plasma. It contains oxygen, glucose, proteins, and white blood cells.

The third purpose of the system is to transport heat and assist with the maintenance of body temperature. This process is called **thermoregulation**. Thermoregulation is accomplished through the distribution of heat generated by the liver and the transportation of secretions from the hypothalamus (see Chapter 7) in response to perceived temperature changes.

The cardiovascular system can also be discussed by dividing it into two subsystems: systemic circulation and pulmonary circulation. **Systemic circulation** refers to the circulation of oxygenated blood. **Pulmonary circulation** is concerned with the oxygenation of blood in the lungs.

Key terms: blood vessels

Arteries are blood vessels that circulate blood *away* from the heart. The compression of the heart as it beats pumps blood into the arteries with a regular and rhythmic fluctuation of increasing pressure followed by decreasing pressure. Arterial muscles then provide enough pressure to keep the blood circulating through the body. The major arteries eventually subdivide into arterioles and capillaries.

Arterioles are smaller arteries. Arteries become narrower the further from the heart that they go. When they reach a certain size, they become arterioles, which play a major role in the regulation of blood pressure. Arterioles branch into capillaries.

Capillaries are very thin, tiny, tubular extensions that branch off of arterioles. They are best seen under a microscope. Each capillary has a permeable membrane that is made up of microscopic openings. These serve to diffuse (deliver) essential nutrients and other matter into the cells of the body. In return, capillaries are able to collect nonessential microscopic matter from body cells and to then transport it to the veins, which will in turn assist in the removal of this matter from the body.

Veins are blood vessels that carry blood *to* the heart. Veins empty into the right atrium of the heart. From there, the blood proceeds through the right ventricle and into the pulmonary artery, which empties into the lungs. Four pulmonary veins (two per lung) then transport the newly oxygenated blood into the left atrium of the heart, and circulation begins again. Note that the distinction between veins and arteries is about the direction of the flow of blood: either to or away from the heart. It is not about whether the blood within the vessel carries oxygen, because the pulmonary veins, like arteries, also carry oxygenated blood. You will learn more details of this process when you study the anatomy of the heart.

Venules are very small veins. They connect to the capillaries.

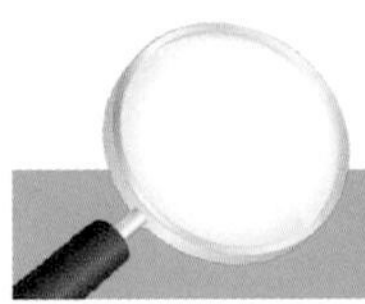

FOCUS POINT: Pulmonary Arteries

There are two pulmonary arteries. They are an exception to the definition that arteries oxygenate and nourish the body through the circulatory system. These arteries do not take oxygenated blood into the body. Instead, they take blood only to the lungs. The right pulmonary artery enters the right lung, and the left pulmonary artery enters the left lung.

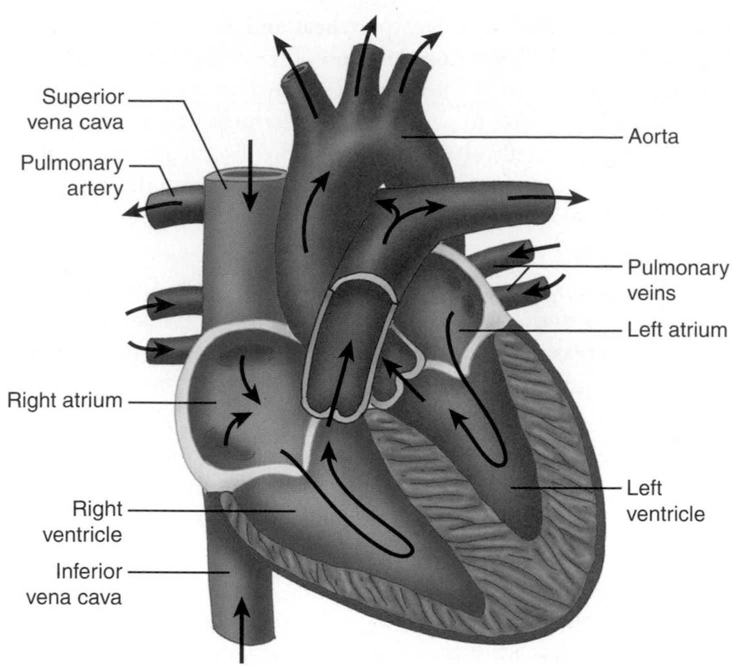

Figure 5.12: Blood circulation through the heart, simplified (see Figure 5-17 for a more detailed view)

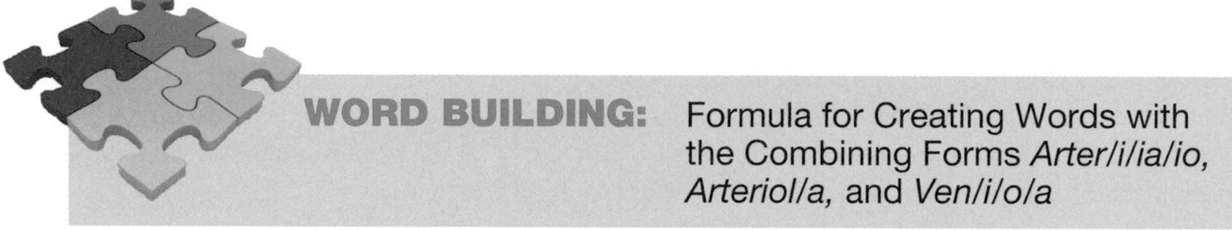

WORD BUILDING: Formula for Creating Words with the Combining Forms *Arter/i/ia/io, Arteriol/a,* and *Ven/i/o/a*

1. arteria = artery. The combining forms are *arteri/ia/io.*

arter + ectomy = *arterectomy*

Definition: incision into an artery; the surgical removal of part of an artery. (The suffix *-ectomy* means *removal or cutting out.*) *noun*

Example: It may be necessary for the surgeon perform an *arterectomy* to remove a thrombus before it loosens from the wall of the artery.

arterio + gram = *arteriogram*

Definition: a radiograph of an artery in which a contrast medium that cannot be penetrated by radiation is injected to illuminate the artery on the x-ray or scan. *noun*

Example: Coronary *arteriograms* are part of a diagnostic workup to explore the condition of the heart, as well as symptoms of angina and myocardial infarction.

arterio + rrhexis = *arteriorrhexis*

Definition: rupture of an artery. (The root *rrhexis* means *rupture. Rrhexis* and *rhexis* are both accepted spellings for this root.) *noun*

Example: *Arteriorrhexis* can lead to sudden death.

arterio + rrhaph + y = *arteriorrhaphy*

Definition: suture of an artery. (The root *rhahe* or *rrhaphe* means *seam or ridge.*) *noun*

Example: The surgeon was called to do an immediate *arteriorrhaphy* of a patient whose femoral artery was cut in an accident.

2. arteriola = an arteriole; a small artery. The combining forms are *arteriol/o.*

arteriolo + necr + osis = *arteriolonecrosis*
Definition: the death or destruction of an arteriole. (The root *necro* or *nekros* means *corpse or death.* The suffix *-osis* means *condition.*) *noun*

Example: *Arteriolonecrosis* is also referred to as *necrotizing arteriolitis.* It is seen in cases of ongoing severe hypertension.

arteriolo + sclera + osis = *arteriolosclerosis*
Definition: the thickening of the walls of arterioles, thereby causing them to lose elasticity and contractibility. (The root *scler* means *hard,* and the suffix *-osis* means *disease or abnormal increase.*) *noun*

Example: *Arteriolosclerosis* is seen in cases of chronic hypertension (high blood pressure).

3. vena = vein or blood vessel. The combining forms are *ven/a/i /o/e.*

ven + ectas + ia = *venectasia*
Definition: the condition or situation of dilation (widening, expanding) of a vein. (*Ectas* is derived from the Greek root *ektasis,* meaning *dilation.*) *noun*

Example: *Venectasia* may be used to rectify or clear varicose veins.

ven + ule = *venule*
Definition: a little vein. (The suffix *-ule* means *little.*) *noun*

Example: *Venules* are tiny veins that function with capillaries to receive waste materials from the blood.

veni + suture = *venisuture*
Definition: suturing of a vein. *noun*

Example: *Venisuture* may be used in varicose vein surgery.

veno + stasis = *venostasis*
Definition: the trapping or pooling of blood in an extremity (limb) via the compression of a vein. (The root *stasis* means *standing still.*) *noun*

Example: *Venostasis* can occur as a result of immobility, or it can be done intentionally to reduce the amount of blood returning to the heart for a particular medical reason.

Right Word or Wrong Word: *Arteritis* or *Arthritis*?
Are these two words the same? Is one of them misspelled, or are they two different words with two different meanings?

TABLE 5-4: Key Suffixes: Blood Vessels

Suffix	Meaning	Suffix	Meaning
-ole	small	-osis	disease; condition; process or action
-ule	small	-ectomy	removal of; taking out
-ous	having the qualities of; full of		

Mix and Match

Match the term in the left column with its synonym in the right column. Draw a line to connect them. The goal of this exercise is to test your ability to recognize word parts and to understand their meaning.

1. arterectomy	phlebectasia
2. venipuncture	coronary artery disease
3. abnormal	phleborrhaphy
4. venisuture	atypical
5. venosclerosis	phlebosclerosis
6. arteriogram	angiogram
7. venectomy	arteriectomy
8. atherosclerosis	phlebectomy
9. vectasia	venipuncture

Build a Word

Use the combining forms *ather/o, arter/i/ia/io, arteriol/o,* and *ven/a/i.*

Combine each set of word parts to create a medical term. Some you will know, and others will be new to you. However, you will be able to understand them by analyzing the meaning of each part.

1. athero osis sclera ____________________

2. arterio rrhexis ____________________

3. osis arteriolo necr ____________________

4. ven peri ous ____________________

5. sectio vene n ____________________

6. periton e ostomy veno ____________________

7. necr athero osis ____________________

8. otomy arterio ____________________

9. ven arterio ous ____________________

10. itis arteriol ____________________

Fill in the Blanks

Use medical language and terminology in context to complete the following sentences.

1. The cardiovascular system ______________ heat and assists with the temperature regulation of the body.

2. Blood flows through ______________ in the cardiovascular system.

3. The tiniest form of blood vessel is the ______________.

4. Circulation serves ______________ main functions.

5. ______________ take blood away from the heart and lungs and into the body.

6. ______________ lack oxygen and may appear blue or bluish in color through the skin.

7. ______________ is a root word meaning *vessel.*

8. With the medical condition cyanosis, a person's lips and nailbeds may appear bluish. This is a sign of ______________ in the blood.

Naming blood vessels: modern vs. traditional terms

Turn your attention now to Figure 5-13. In this diagram, the blood vessels are labeled with their traditional Greek and Latin names. Compare the terms on this diagram with those used in Figure 5-11. From time to time, both forms of the terms may be encountered in the health field, so it is important to be familiar with both forms. Many of the traditional terms are still recognized and used internationally.

Table 5-5 lists both the modern and traditional names for each major blood vessel, and it includes a description of each vessel's location and function. Study this table in preparation for the exercises that follow.

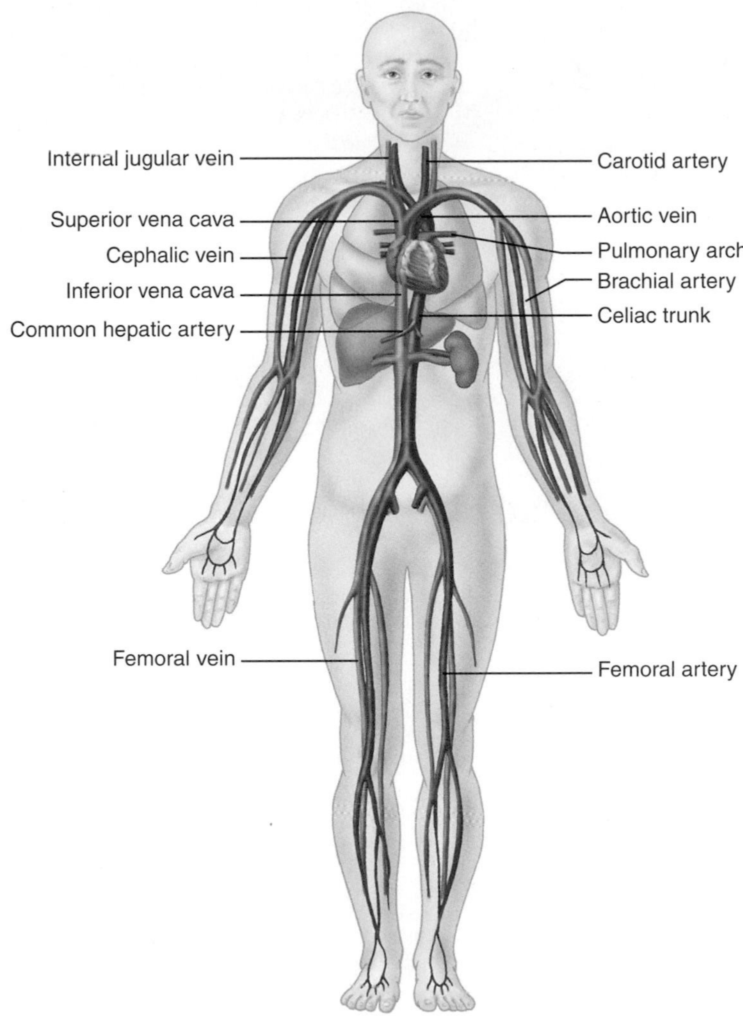

Figure 5.13: Blood vessels: traditional names

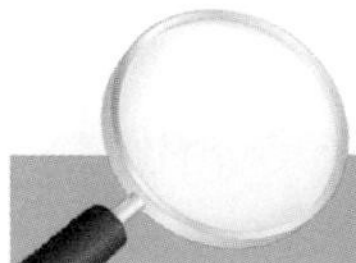

FOCUS POINT: Etymology of the Term *Carotid*

The word *carotid* is derived from the early Greek root *karotis,* meaning *deep sleep or to plunge into a deep sleep.* The word is used in reference to the carotid artery because, if enough pressure is exerted on this artery, a person may lose consciousness. In fact, too much pressure applied to the carotid artery can affect blood supply to the brain and actually cause brain damage.

TABLE 5-5: Blood Vessels: Modern and Traditional Names

Modern Term	Traditional Term	Word Deconstruction	Meaning
carotid artery, common carotid artery	arteria carotis communis	arteria: artery carotis: deep sleep communis: common	a large palpable artery in the neck that supplies blood to the head
aortic arches, arches of aorta	arcus aortae	arcus: arch or bow shape aortae: plural form of aorta, the main trunk of the arteries in the body	the uppermost part of the aorta (The aorta is the main artery that transports blood away from the heart.)
brachial artery	arteria brachialis	brachi: arm	the main artery of the arm, which is found toward the inner aspect of the upper arm and that then divides into the radial and ulnar arteries in the forearm
common hepatic artery	arteria hepatica communis	hepat/o/a: liver	a short artery that supplies the liver, the pancreas, part of the small intestine, and part of the stomach
femoral artery	arteria femoralis	femor/o: thigh	the large artery that originates in the lower abdomen and that extends into the thigh
femoral vein	vena femoralis	vena: vein or blood vessel	the largest vein in the groin, which carries blood from the lower extremities back to the heart
celiac trunk	truncus coeliacus	celiac/coeliacus: belly truncus: trunk or stem	the main stem that arises from the aorta and that supplies blood to the major organs of the abdomen
inferior vena cava	vena cava inferior	cava: trunk or stem	the main stems that return venous blood to the heart from the lower portion of the body
cephalic vein	vena cephalica	cephalica/cephalic: above or superior to	the large vein in the arm; the brachial vein
superior vena cava	vena cava superior		the main stems that return venous blood to the heart from the upper portion of the body
internal jugular vein	vena jugularis interna	jugularis: pertaining to the throat	the vein that returns blood to the heart from the head and neck; it sits deep within the throat and is only slightly visible to the eye

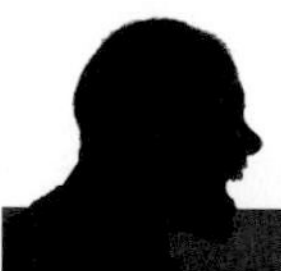

PRONUNCIATION PRACTICE

Say these words aloud to a friend or classmate if you can. You are given the phonetic pronunciation. Your instructor can help you with pronunciation,

or visit **http://www.MedicalLanguageLab.com.** mll

anoxia	ăn-**ŏk´**sē-ă
atheroma	ăth-ĕr-**ō´**mă

atherosclerosis	ăth″ĕr-ō″ sklĕ-**rō**′sĭs
arterectomy	ăr-tĕ-**rĕk**′tō-mē
arteriogram	ăr-tē″ rē-ō-grăm
arteriorrhexis	ăr-tē″ rē-ō-**rĕk**′sĭs
arteriorrhaphy	ăr-tē″ rē-**or**′ă-fē
cardiovascular	kăr″ dē-ō-**văs**′kū-lăr
carotid	kă-**rŏt**′ĭd
cerebrovascular	sĕr″ĕ-brō-**văs**′kū-lăr
celiac	**sē**′lē-ăk
jugular	**jŭg**′ū-lăr
vena cava	vē′nă **kā**′vă
venectasia	vē″ nĕk-**tā**′zē-ă

Anatomy and physiology: the heart

The heart is the core of the cardiovascular system and of life itself. Understanding the language of the anatomy, physiology, and function of the heart is crucial in health care.

Key terms: anatomy of the heart

Anatomically, the heart is divided into four chambers: two *atria* and two *ventricles.* It has two *atrioventricular (AV) valves* and two *semilunar valves.* The AV valves are called the *tricuspid* and *mitral* valves. The semilunar valves are the *aortic* and *pulmonary* valves. Study Figures 5-14 and 5-15 to locate these important structures of the heart, and then refer to Table 5-6 to explore how these terms are constructed and what they mean.

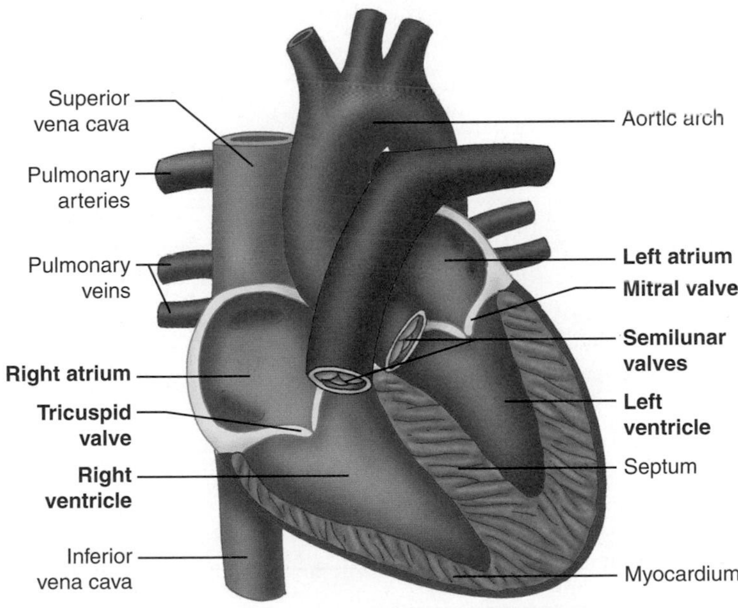

Figure 5.14: Anatomy of the heart

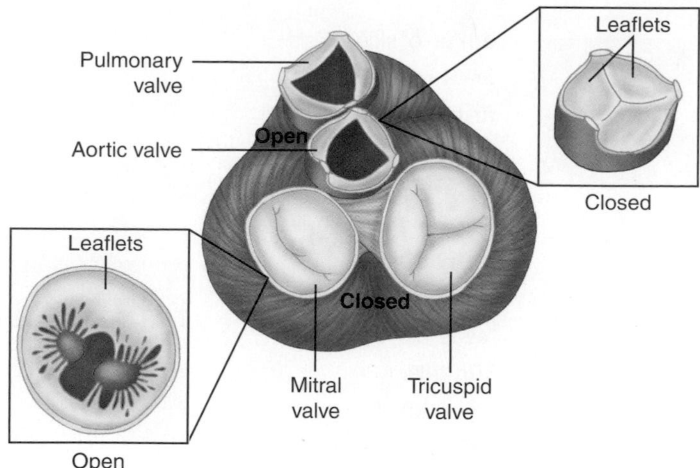

Figure 5.15: Valves of the heart

TABLE 5-6: Medical and Anatomical Terms for the Heart

Medical or Anatomical Term	Word Deconstruction	Meaning
pulmonary	pulmon + ary pulmo = lungs	concerning or involving the lungs
atrium	atri + um atri = entrance or entrance room	a cavity of the body; more specifically, an upper chamber of the heart
tricuspid	tri + cuspid tri = three cuspid = point	three points
valve	(This is a root word.)	a membranous structure that opens and closes; valves that are located in a hollow organ or vessel permit fluid to pass through in one direction when they are open
ventricle	ventr + icle ventr = small chamber	a hollow chamber of the heart
septum	Latin root meaning *partition*	a partition or a wall between two cavities or chambers
mitral	miter = a bishop's hat	resembling or shaped like a bishop's hat
semilunar	semi + lun + ar semi = partly or half lun = moon	shaped like a crescent moon

Let's Practice

Use new terminology to identify what is being described.

1. a flap-like structure that opens and closes ______________
2. contains three points ______________
3. opens and closes the aorta ______________
4. refers to the lungs ______________
5. has an inferior and superior stem ______________
6. location of the mitral valve ______________
7. sit proximal yet inferior to the pulmonary arteries ______________
8. pulmonary arteries exit from this chamber ______________

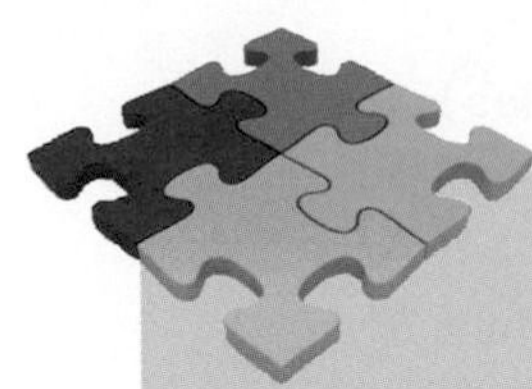

WORD BUILDING: Formula for Creating Words with the Combining Forms *Aort/o, Cardio, Valvul/o,* and *Ventricul/o*

1. aorta = the main trunk of the arteries of the body. The combining forms are *aort/o.*

aort + algia = *aortalgia*

Definition: pain in the aorta or in the area near the aorta. (The suffix *-algia* means *pain.*) *noun*

Example: *Aortalgia* may be a symptom of an aneurysm.

aort + clasia = *aortoclasia*

Definition: rupture of the aorta. (The suffix *-clasia* means *break, breaking, or crushing.*) *noun*

Example: *Aortclasia* is most often caused by trauma and produces a high risk of bleeding to death.

aorto + plasty = *aortoplasty*

Definition: surgical repair of the aorta. (The suffix *-plasty* means *remolding or reshaping surgically.*) *noun*

Example: *Aortoplasty* is called for STAT in the case of aortclasia.

2. cardia = heart. The combining forms are *cardi/a/o.*

cardio + myo + pathy = *cardiomyopathy*

Definition: disease of the heart muscle. *noun*

Example: *Cardiomyopathy* can be caused by a number of pathological conditions, but its most common cause is ischemia.

cardi + asthma = *cardiasthma*

Definition: dyspnea (shortness of breath; difficulty breathing) as a result of heart disease. (The root word *asthma* means *panting.*) *noun*

Example: People with congestive heart failure suffer the symptoms of *cardiasthma.* This condition is usually referred to simply as *cardiac asthma.*

cardio + inhibit = ory = *cardioinhibitory*

Definition: inhibiting the action of the heart. (The word *inhibit* means *to restrain or hold back.*) *adjective*

Example: Medications designed to regulate cardiac arrhythmias (unusual irregular rhythms) can be *cardioinhibitory.*

3. valve = *The original root means folding door or leaf. In English, a valve is a device that is used to control the flow of liquid, and it works much the same as a door in that it opens and closes. The combining forms are valv/ul/o.*

valvo + tom + y = *valvotomy*

Definition: incision of a valve; also called *valvuloplasty. noun*

Example: If a valve is malfunctioning, a surgeon may perform a *valvotomy* by inserting an expanding balloon into the valvular opening.

valvul + a = *valvula*

Definition: a small valve. *noun*

Example: The tricuspid valve is really a *valvula.*

Continued

4. ventricle = a small cavity; a chamber; a belly or womb. There are ventricles in the heart and the brain. The combining forms are *ventricul/o.*

ventriculo + atrio + stoma + y = *ventriculoatriostomy*

Definition: a procedure performed by a plastic surgeon to drain a ventricle of the brain by creating a stoma (mouth; opening) with a one-way valve that allows excessive fluid to drain. *noun*

Example: A *ventriculatriostomy* is performed in the case of hydrocephalus (an excess of cerebrospinal fluid in the brain) to allow a cerebral ventricle to connect to the right atrium of the heart to assist with drainage.

ventricul + ar = *ventricular*

Definition: pertaining to a ventricle. *adjective*

Example: The patient's heart showed *ventricular* abnormalities.

ventricul + itis = *ventriculitis*

Definition: inflammation of a ventricle. *noun*

Example: *Ventriculitis* is treated with antibiotics.

Build a Word

Use your word-building skills to create medical terms from the following word parts, and then define the term in your own words.

1. rrhaphy aorto ____________ Meaning: ____________
2. scler aorto osis ____________ Meaning: ____________
3. tomy aorto ____________ Meaning: ____________
4. ic gen cardio ____________ Meaning: ____________
5. logist cardio ____________ Meaning: ____________
6. y cardio graph ____________ Meaning: ____________
7. ar ventricul ____________ Meaning: ____________
8. tom ventriculo y ____________ Meaning: ____________
9. plasty valvulo ____________ Meaning: ____________
10. ectomy valv ____________ Meaning: ____________

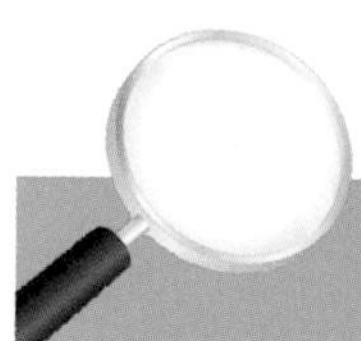

FOCUS POINT: The Word *Corona* and the Combining Form *Coron/o*

The term *corona* identifies any structure that resembles a circular crown. The related word *coronary* is used to refer to the heart because the vessels that supply blood to the heart encircle it like a crown.

Right Word or Wrong Word: *Cardia* or *Cardio*?

Are these two terms the same? Do they share the same combining forms?

TABLE 5-7: Cardiology: Prefixes and the Suffix *-itis*

BEGIN with a Prefix	ADD the Root or Combining Form of *cardia*	ADD a Suffix	CREATE a New Term
endo (within)	card	itis	endocarditis (inflammation or infection of the lining of the heart or the heart valves)
	myo (muscle) card	itis	myocarditis (inflammation of the heart muscle)
peri (around or about)	card	itis	pericarditis (inflammation of the pericardium [a saclike structure that encases the heart and its large vessels])

Key terms: physiology of the heart

The heart is a muscle, and it contracts and expands by a process of electrical conduction that occurs within it. This process is referred to as the **cardiac conduction system.** The physiology of this conduction process includes five main parts that work together as a unit:

1. The **sinoatrial (SA) node** is a mass of cardiac muscle cells in the right atrium that serves as the natural pacemaker of the heart by releasing electrical stimuli at regular intervals (beats). It causes a wave of contraction to occur in both atria of the heart.
2. The **atrioventricular (AV) node** picks up stimuli from the SA node as the atria begin to refill after contraction. It conducts the stimuli onward to the bundle branches and the Purkinje fibers.
3. The **bundle of His** also picks up the electrical stimuli as the atria begin to refill. It too sends the impulse forward into the bundle branches and the Purkinje fibers.
4. The **bundle branches** are very fine branches off of the bundle of His. They ensure that the heart actually pumps and that the contraction and relaxation of cardiac muscle occur.
5. **Purkinje fibers** are specialized conductive fibers. They lie within the ventricular walls, and they conduct electrical impulses throughout the cells of the ventricles, thus causing them to contract and empty.

Eponyms: His and Purkinje

Wilhelm His, Jr. (1863-1934) was a Swiss biochemist, internist, and cardiologist. He discovered the fibers that are now known as the *bundle of His* in the cardiac conduction system. He also coined the term *heart block.*

Johannes (Jan) Evangelista von Purkinje (1787–1869) was a Bohemian physiologist with an interest in microscopic anatomy and physiology. In 1838, he discovered the nerve fibers on the surface of the heart that now bear his name.

The sequence of steps in the cardiac conduction system creates the **cardiac cycle.** This cycle consists of a continuous rhythm of alternating contraction and relaxation of the heart muscle or **myocardium,** which is coordinated by the actions of the five parts of the heart that were described previously. Note that the two atria always contract at the same time. When the atria relax, the two ventricles contract. The contraction phase is called **systole,** and the relaxation phase is called **diastole.** These are two terms with which you will become more familiar when you learn the language of blood pressure. A normal heart rate beat lasts for approximately 1 second, which is why we are able to count heartbeats and measure pulse rates.

TABLE 5-8: More Anatomical and Medical Terms for the Cardiovascular System

Anatomical or Medical Term	Meaning
systemic	affecting the body as a whole or pertaining to one system
conduction	transmission of electrical energy
node	a small bundle or knot of tissue
bundle of His	a bundle of fibers that conducts electrical impulses in the heart; also known as the *atrioventricular bundle*
Purkinje fibers	a network of fibers found in the ventricles
pacemaker	a group of cells or a device that can regulate activities and rhythms
sino, sinus	a cavity with a narrow opening; in the case of the heart, the term refers to the dilation of a passageway for venous blood flow

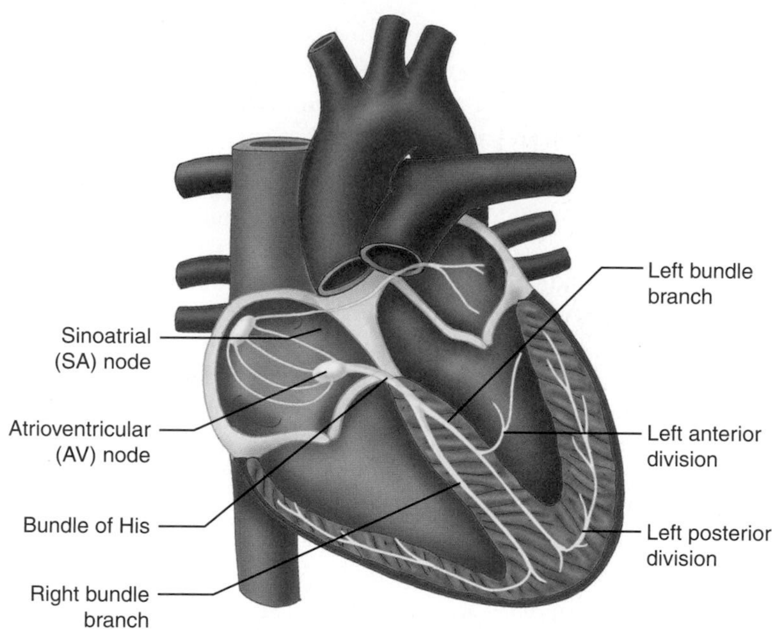

Figure 5.16: The cardiac conduction system

Fill in the Blanks

Use the new terminology that you have learned to complete the following sentences.

1. The function of the AV node is to ______________________________.
2. The ______________________ serve to stimulate the ventricles to contract or relax.
3. The ______________________ is responsible for initiating contraction and expansion (relaxation) of the heart.
4. The ______________________ branches into smaller bundles.
5. The ______________________ is the natural pacemaker of the heart.

The process of conduction: from cardio to vascular

You have now learned the details of how the heart and blood vessels supply the body with blood. Figure 5-17 summarizes the process by which cardiac contractions conduct blood into the vascular or circulatory system, which carries the blood to the rest of the body.

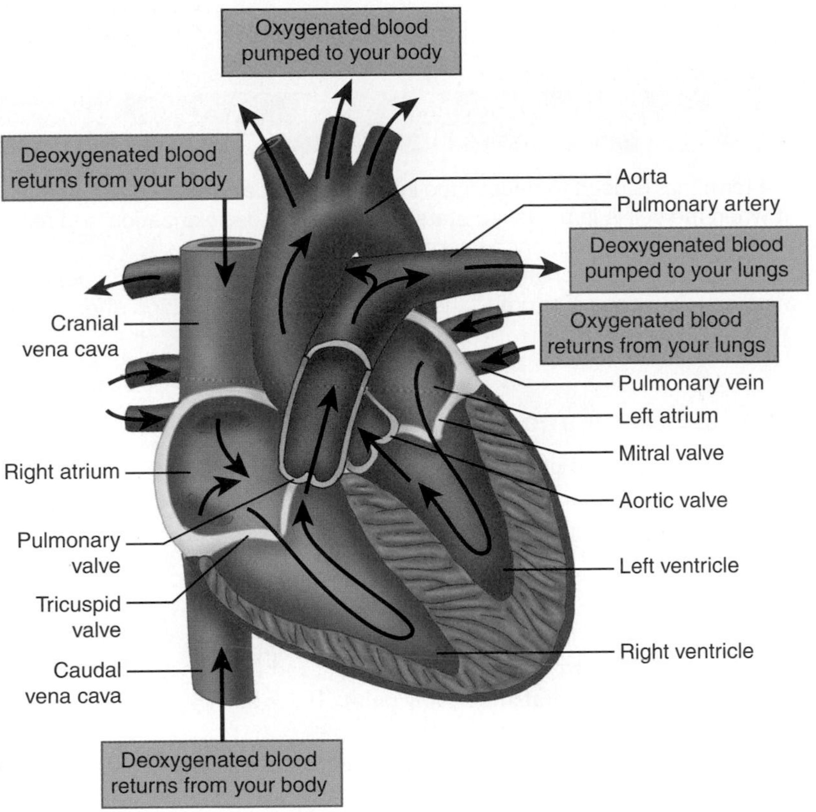

Figure 5.17: Blood circulation through the heart, detailed

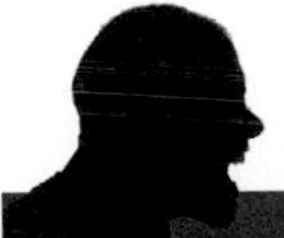

PRONUNCIATION PRACTICE

Say these words aloud to a friend or classmate if you can. You are given the phonetic pronunciation. Your instructor can help you with pronunciation,

or visit **http://www.MedicalLanguageLab.com.**

aorta	ā-**or**´tă
aortalgia	ā″or-**tăl**´jē-ă
aortoclasia	ā″or-tō-**klā**´zē-ă
aortoplasty	ā-or″tō-**plăs**´tē
aortosclerosis	ā-or″tō-sklĕr-**ō**´sĭs
cardiomyopathy	kăr″dē-ō-mī-ŏ**p**´ă-thē
membranous	**mĕm**´bră-nŭs
mitral	**mī**″trăl
myocarditis	mī″ō-kăr-**dī**´tĭs
pulmonary	**pŭl**´mō-nĕ-rē
semilunar	sĕm″ē-**lū**´năr
sinoatrial	sīn″ō-**ā**´trē-ăl
tricuspid	trī-**kŭs**´pĭd
ventriculatriostomy	vĕn-**trĭk**″ū-lō-ā″trē-**ŏs**´tō-mē

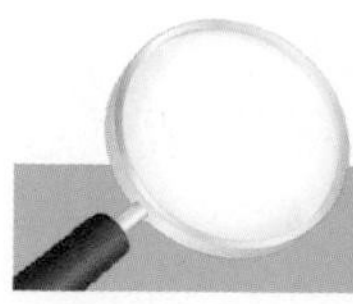

FOCUS POINT: Polarization of the Heart

Polarization is a term that is used to refer to the internal electrical state of a cell in relation to the cells around it when the cell is in a relaxed state. A process of depolarization and repolarization of the cells of the heart occurs with each heartbeat.

Depolarization is a reversal or change in the internal electrical state (or charge) of a cell.

Repolarization simply means a return to the normal state of polarization after depolarization.

The language of assessment: cardiovascular system

The assessment and measurement of the level of functioning of the cardiovascular system includes the language of waves, beats, pulses, and blood pressure. Equipment and procedures that are used to measure cardiovascular functioning include electrocardiograms, echocardiograms, stethoscopes, sphygmomanometers, and blood pressure cuffs.

Key terms: cardiovascular assessment

Cardiac waves

A **wave** is any rhythmic motion with a defined amplitude and frequency. The *amplitude* of a wave is the difference between its high point and its low point. The *frequency* is how many times a pattern repeats during a given time period.

The healthy heart has a normal rhythm; **cardiac waves** run in a steady sequence. Abnormal heart rhythms, which are called **arrhythmias,** can be detected by taking the patient's pulse, listening to the patient's heartbeat, and observing the patient's cardiac wave pattern with the use of an *electrocardiogram (ECG)* or an *echocardiogram.* A cardiac wave begins when the heart contracts: this is the heartbeat. **Interval** is the term used to identify the time lapse between waves. Waves are referred to as *pulse waves* and *heart pressure waves.*

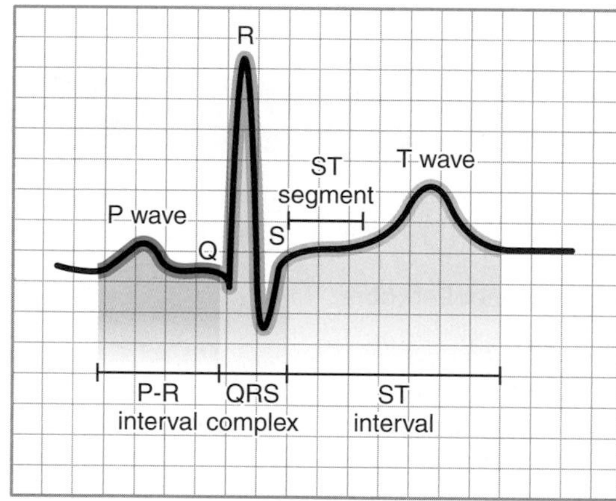

Figure 5.18: Waves in the cardiac cycle

TABLE 5-9: Waves in a Cardiac Cycle

Wave or Interval	Description
P	the result of electrical activity in the atrium; the period of atrial depolarization, when the atria rest between contractions
QRS	the period of ventricular depolarization, which occurs as the atria repolarize; this occurs as the impulse arrives in the ventricles and triggers their contraction; the Q interval measures the beginning of this wave
T	the period of ventricular repolarization
ST segment	the interval between ventricular depolarization and the beginning of ventricular repolarization

Electrocardiogram

An electrocardiogram (ECG) monitors the electrical activity of the heart by recording the depolarization and repolarization of the cardiac muscle. There are three types of cardiac waves that can be monitored by ECG: P waves, QRS waves, and T waves. Refer to Table 5-9 to learn more about these.

To take an ECG, a system of 12 leads is attached to the patient's chest in the precordial area, which is the skin over the heart and the lower thorax. A **lead** is an electrocardiographic conductor or electrode. Nurses, laboratory technicians, and other health professionals are qualified to do this procedure. (Note that there are also three-lead and five-lead ECGs available.)

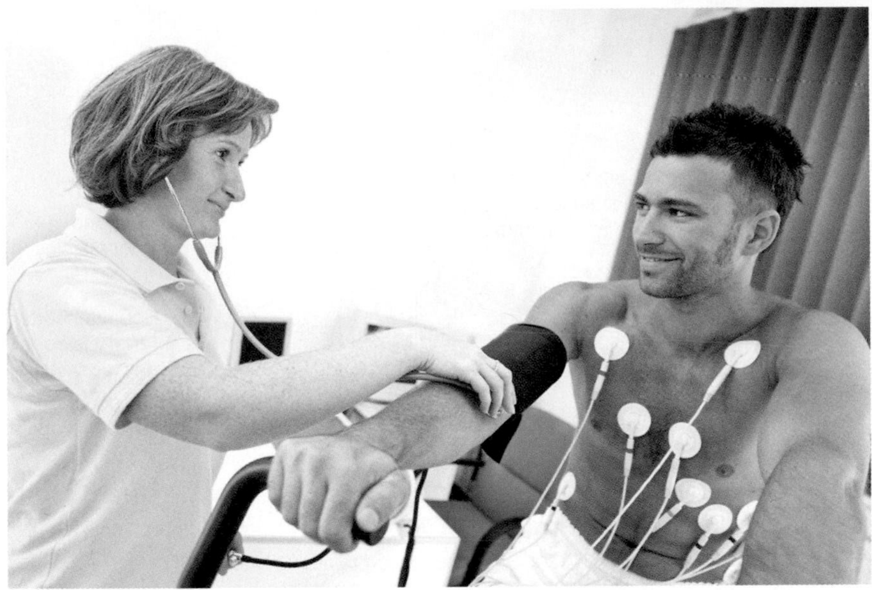

Figure 5.19: Patient receiving an electrocardiogram (© Thinkstock/IT Stock)

Right Word or Wrong Word: *Electrocardiogram* or *Echocardiogram*?

Are these two words interchangeable? Are they synonyms? Are they antonyms? Are they related to each other in any way?

Blood pressure

As the blood is forced under pressure out into the circulatory system, **blood pressure (BP)** is created. This is the amount of force that the blood is actually exerting on the vessels as it passes through them. BP can be measured by listening to an artery with a stethoscope, a blood pressure cuff, and a sphygmomanometer. A patient's blood pressure is reported as two numbers, such as 120/80 mm Hg. The first number is the systolic pressure; the second number is the diastolic pressure:

Systolic pressure is the highest number measured on the sphygmomanometer. It is the sound of the heart beating as it exerts pressure on the blood vessels.

Diastolic pressure is the sound that is heard when the heart is at rest, thus relieving the pressure on the vessels.

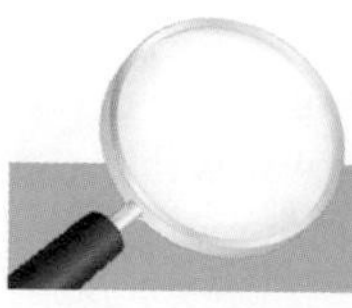

FOCUS POINT: Sphygmomanometer

A *sphygmomanometer* is a device that is used to identify blood pressure levels in the body. It is a type of pressure gauge, and it must be used in conjunction with an inflatable blood pressure cuff. Systolic and diastolic blood pressures are read on the gauge; they are also heard through a stethoscope after the cuff has been inflated and slowly released. A typical blood pressure reading for an adult is 120/80 mm Hg. A systolic reading of more than 140 suggests hypertension (high blood pressure). A systolic measure of less than 110 can be indicative of hypotension (low blood pressure).

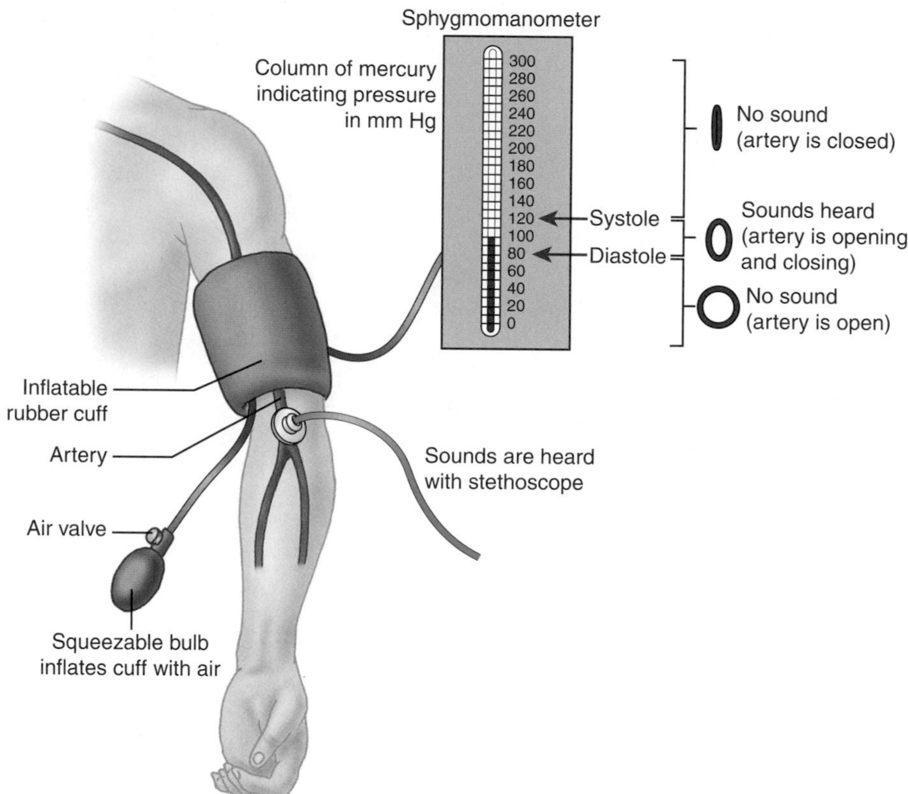

Figure 5.20: Equipment for measuring blood pressure

Pulse rate

Each time the heart contracts (beats), it causes pressure in the arteries, which can be felt through the skin. A person's **pulse rate** is the number of times that the heart beats per minute. A pulse can be read at any point on the body where an artery lies close to the surface of the skin. Refer to Figure 5-20 to learn the names and locations of pulse sites on the body.

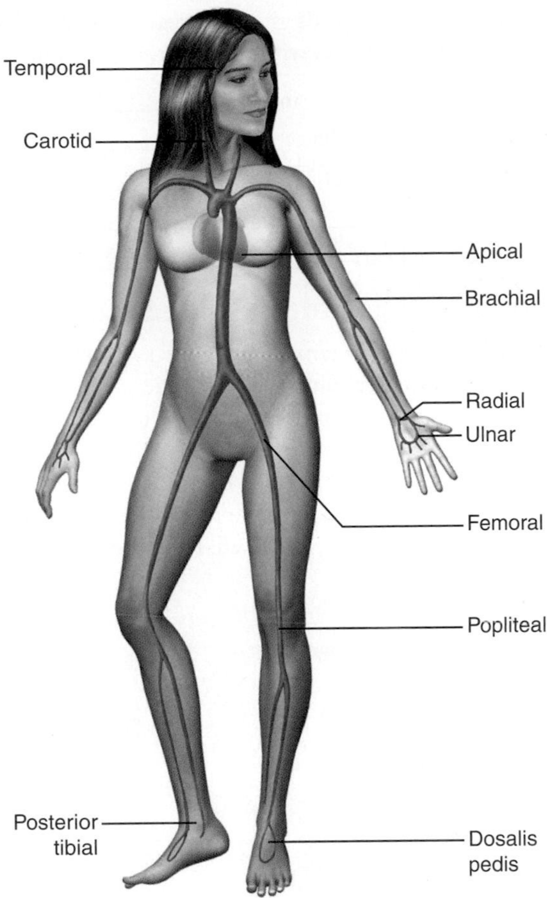

Figure 5.21: Pulse sites

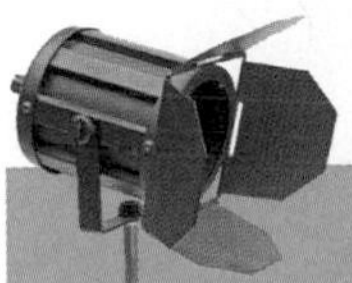

CAREER SPOTLIGHT: Electrocardiographic Technician

Although nurses, physician assistants, and medical laboratory technicians may all become qualified in ECG technology, there are also *electrocardiographic technicians* whose sole responsibility is to perform ECGs. With advanced training, an electrocardiographic technician can also perform Holter monitoring and exercise ECG testing. A *Holter monitor* is a device that is worn continuously over a period of one or more days and that records the activity of the heart over time. Exercise ECG testing involves monitoring the patient's heart while having him or her perform increasingly stressful physical exercise.

Free Writing

Use each of the medical terms and other words given to create a logical sentence. You may need to add verbs, articles, and so forth. Work alone, with a partner, or in a small group.

1. velocity echocardiogram heart within determines ______________________
2. worn continuously activity monitor cardiac ______________________
3. conduction refers to cardiac activity electrical heart ______________________
4. pulse pressure arteries beat heart ______________________
5. Purkinje ventricles fibers surface heart ______________________

Listen to the language of laboratory assessment

Mr. Davis remains in the ER of Okla Trauma Center for assessment and care. He has had his blood drawn by the medical laboratory technician, and an emergency CT scan has been performed. Mr. Davis is in no grave danger at the moment, but Dr. Crowchild, the consulting radiologist, the cardiologist, and the neurologist all agree that Mr. Davis is at risk for a cerebrovascular or cardiovascular accident. As a team, they have decided to transfer him to the Intensive Care Unit for observation and monitoring of his condition. He will remain there for at least the next 48 hours. In he interim, he will have more diagnostic tests completed. Read the following aloud as Dr. Crowchild consults with the ER staff.

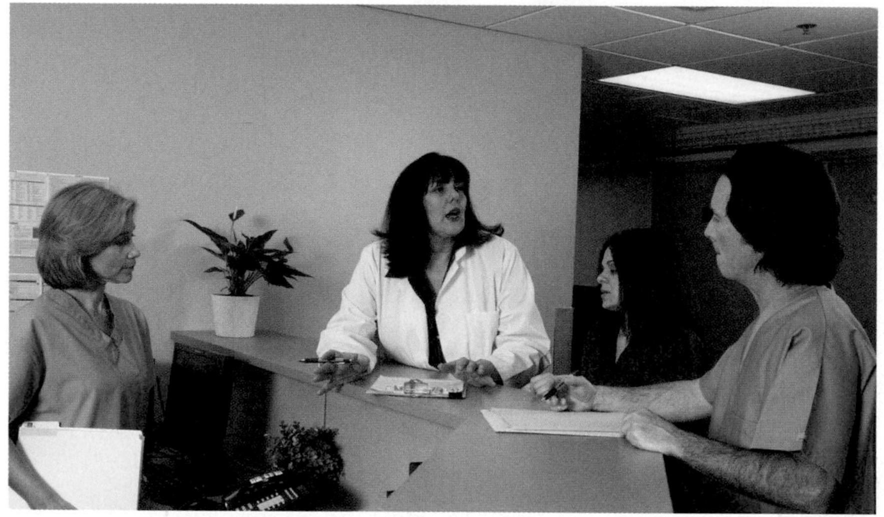

Patient Update

"Thank you all for coming so promptly. Doctors Krenshaw, Fillmore, Hamidi, and I have reviewed the tests for Mr. Davis, our 74-year-old MVA patient. As you may know, he arrived with a report of having, in his words, a "bad heart." We have yet to determine what that diagnosis is. The ECG provides some evidence of cardiac arrhythmia. The CT confirms CAD, but there is no evidence of a rupture. We are interested in a couple of potential sites, and emboli are still a concern. So, it appears that Mr. Davis might have had a TIA. All of the signs were there: he was slightly confused, his speech was slurred, and so on when he arrived, but that has resolved. He has some lingering retrograde amnesia for the event, but we expect that to clear. At the moment, we've got a working diagnosis of probable TIA at the scene of the accident, as well as while en route here, but we'll have to look at all of this patient's test results before we know for sure. We're moving him to ICU STAT. I've given the orders, and the porters are transporting him as we speak. Roxie, you'll need to get your notes to ICU as quick as you can. I want that file completed and on their desk A.S.A.P."

"Yes, doctor," replied the nurse.

"Graciella, make sure that the lab reqs. have been sent upstairs STAT as well. Are they on the computer?"

"Yes, ma'am, I entered them immediately. I just need to change the room number for the patient, and the lab will take it from there."

"When we catheterized the patient, I obtained the first urine specimen for the lab. Unfortunately, it was small, since he'd been incontinent," commented Roxie.

"Right. I don't want those orders for follow-up *U/A* to get lost. We still don't know if infection or diabetic reaction played any role in this accident. U/A and the other blood tests will tell us. And I've just ordered an *echo*," added Dr. Crowchild.

"I did get a glucometer reading at the bedside, Dr. Crowchild. His blood sugars were good at the time, relevant to his circumstances."

"Yes, Roxie, thanks. That's why it's important for the lab reqs. to follow him upstairs. We'll need an FBS, too."

LPN Kamila joined in, "Did anybody contact the family?"

"I went through his wallet and found his ID," Graciella responded. "He has a wife at the same address, but there was no answer when I phoned. I think the EMT said she was also in the accident. Mr. Davis doesn't have any other contact numbers with him. Do you want me to call the other hospitals or Emergency Dispatch to try to find her?"

"Yes, do that. Thanks. Find out where she is. Let her know he's here, that he's stable, and that we're keeping him for a bit," said the physician.

"He'll probably want to know where she is, too, once he starts thinking more clearly," added Roxie.

"Okay, team, our patient didn't have any other major injuries, so we'll hand this case over to ICU. That's it. Good work." Dr. Crowchild ended the patient update just as a code bell went off.

"Code Blue, third floor; Code Blue, third floor," came the message over the public address system. The doctor's pager buzzed at the very same moment. She looked down, read the message, and looked up again.

"We've got incoming, ladies and gentleman: a small child; ETA 5 minutes. Multiple injuries. Let's move it!" Dr. Crowchild directed. Under her breath, she muttered, "It's turning out to be quite the day around here!"

Critical Thinking

How well did you understand the dialogue that took place among the hospital staff? On the basis of the patient update, answer the following questions.

1. Judging from the interaction between Dr. Crowchild and the nurse named Roxie, what do you think the term *U/A* stands for? ______________________
2. What does the expression *we've got incoming* mean?
   ____
3. How did Dr. Crowchild know that a patient was "incoming"?
   ____
4. What does the term *en route* mean? ______________________
5. Roxie performed a certain diagnostic test at the bedside with the patient. The doctor wants this followed up with an FBS. What do you think these initials stand for?
   ____

The Language of the Urinary System

To diagnose the cause of Mr. Davis's incontinence, as well as his confusion, Dr. Crowchild has ordered a **urinalysis (UA or U/A)**, which is a biochemical analysis of the patient's urine. In the elderly population, symptoms of urinary incontinence and urinary infection are common. They need to be assessed for their etiology (cause) before treatment can be determined.

Anatomy and physiology: urinary system

To understand Mr. Davis's incontinence, it is important to learn the language of the urinary system. We begin with its anatomy and physiology of this system. Figure 5-21 and Table 5-10 will help you better understand the urinary system.

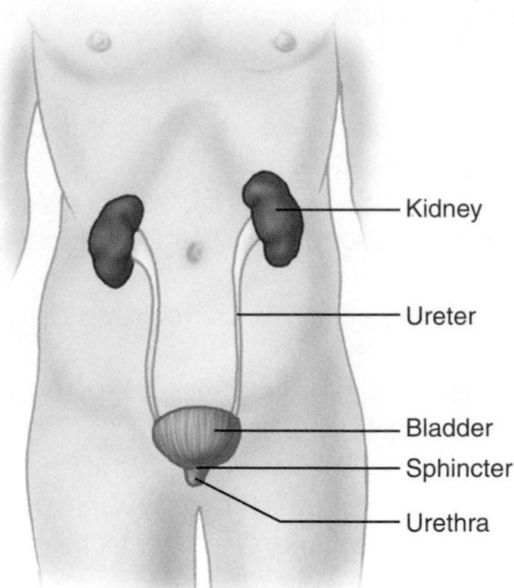

Figure 5.22: The urinary system

Key terms: anatomy of the urinary system

The major organs and structures of the urinary system are *the kidneys, bladder, ureters*, and *urethra*. Notice that there are two kidneys and two ureters and that they sit bilaterally in the abdomen. The renal pelvis is the name given the proximal end of the ureters. The urinary meatus is the opening at the distal end of the urethra that is controlled by a *sphincter muscle*.

TABLE 5-10: Combining Forms: Urinary System

Combining Form	Structure It Refers To
cyst/o/i	bladder
vesic/o	bladder
glomerul/o	glomerulus; glomeruli
nephr/o	kidneys or nephrons of the kidneys
ren/o	kidneys
ur/o/e	urine
ureter/o	ureters: the urinary tubes that transport urine away from the kidneys and into the bladder
urethra/o	urethra: the tube through which urine passes from the bladder to the outside of the body
meatu/o	referring to the meatus, which is the opening at the distal end of the urethra

Build a Word

You have become acquainted with the roots and combining forms of key terms for the anatomy of the urinary system. Using your knowledge of how medical terminology is constructed, complete the following exercise by creating new terms from the word parts given, and then write a definition of each term.

1. gram cyst/o ____________ Meaning: ____________
2. itis nephr/o ____________ Meaning: ____________
3. ureter/o scope cyst/o ____________ Meaning: ____________
4. algia nephr/o ____________ Meaning: ____________
5. genesis ur/o/e ____________ Meaning: ____________
6. cyst/o urethra/o itis ____________ Meaning: ____________
7. vascul ren/o ar ____________ Meaning: ____________

8. path glomerul/o y ______________ Meaning: ______________
9. cyst itis ______________ Meaning: ______________
10. nephr/o ectom ureter/o y ______________ Meaning: ______________

Right Word or Wrong Word: ***Vesico, Viscer/o,*** **or** ***Vasculo*?**
Are these combining forms synonyms?

Key terms: physiology of the urinary system

The function of the urinary system is to filter and excrete liquid waste and excess water from the body. By doing so, the system maintains the body's chemical balance. The kidneys are the major organs of this system.

The **kidneys** sit just below the ribs and closer to the back in the human abdomen. They contain the *renal artery, renal vein, nephrons,* and *glomeruli*. The kidneys filter almost 42 gallons of blood per day as they remove liquid and soluble waste from the circulating blood.

The function of the kidneys is to remove *urea* and other nonessential or harmful soluble or liquid waste from the blood. The kidneys do this with the use of fine filters called **nephrons.** Each nephron includes **glomeruli**, which are small balls or bundles of capillaries. The kidneys also filter blood through the renal tubes. Kidneys produce urine, and, by doing so, they allow the body to maintain homeostasis and an electrolyte balance.

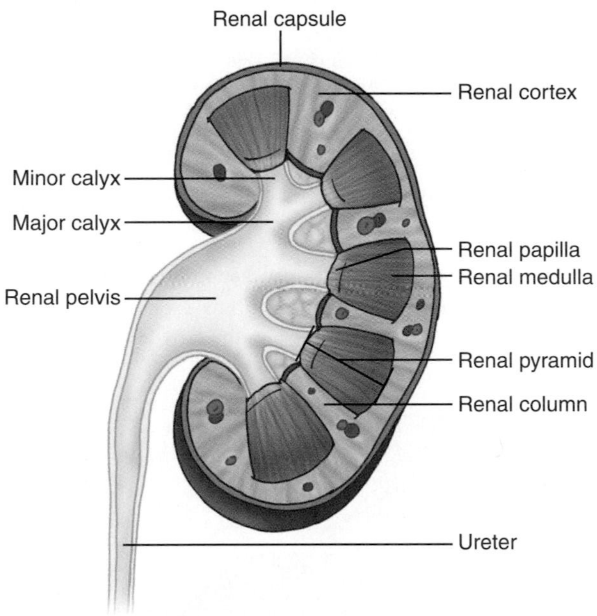

Figure 5.23: The kidney (cross-sectional view)

Urine is composed of urea and other soluble substances that have been filtered through the kidneys.

Urea is not created in the kidneys. It is produced when foods that contain protein are metabolized in the body. When this metabolism occurs, urea is transported via the bloodstream into the kidneys, where it is filtered out. Urea is also called *carbamide.*

Homeostasis means *equilibrium.* The maintenance of a constant balanced internal environment is necessary for the body to function normally. This state is achieved through structural, functional, and behavioral activities that are both voluntary and involuntary. Some examples are thirst (i.e., the need for fluids in the body) and urination (i.e., the need to expel waste fluid). The inability of the body to fulfill these needs can lead to serious imbalances, which can result in pathology and even death. The kidneys are just one part of the many systems that make homeostasis possible.

Electrolytes are essential to life. They are ions (i.e., atoms or groups of atoms). When immersed in fluids, these ions gain the ability to conduct electrical impulses. The most common electrolytes are sodium, potassium, chloride, and bicarbonate. The kidneys monitor the amounts of electrolytes in the blood and intervene as needed to increase output or reserve concentration levels. (You will learn more about electrolytes in Unit 3.) Kidney disease is just one condition that can lead to life-threatening electrolyte imbalances.

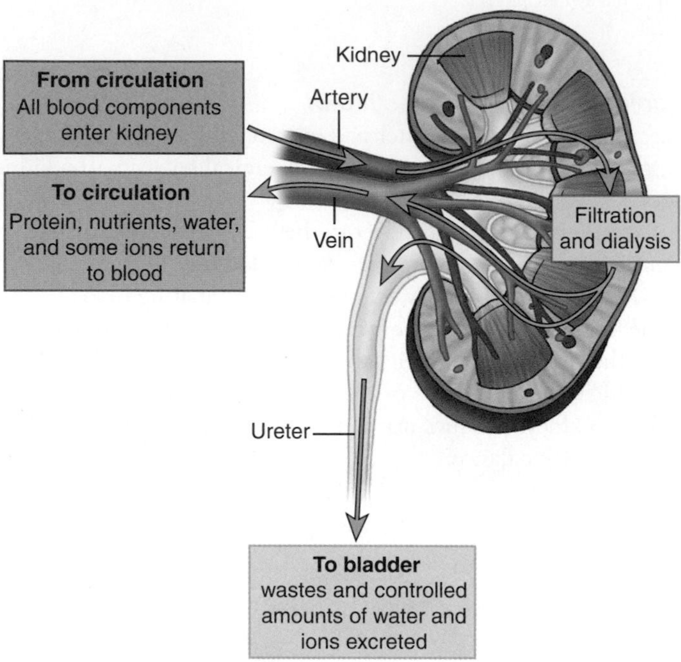

Figure 5.24: Directional flow through the kidney

The function of the *bladder* is to collect, store, and release urine produced by the kidneys. An average healthy adult bladder has the capacity to store up to 2½ cups (600 cc) of urine, but the urge to void usually occurs when the bladder contains about 1 to 1⅓ cups (200 to 300 cc) of urine.

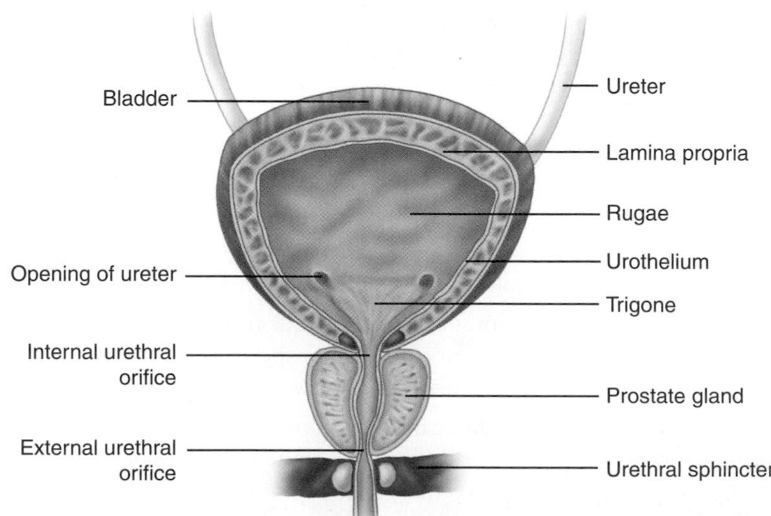

Figure 5.25: The bladder

The language of urinary incontinence

When the bladder is nearly full, the brain sends nerve impulses that cause the bladder muscles to tighten. This process is called the **innervation** of the bladder. After they have been stimulated, the bladder muscles contract and force urine out of the bladder through the *sphincter muscles*. These relax and open to allow urine to exit the bladder through the *urethra*. When all the signals occur in the correct order, normal urination occurs.

Humans are able to exert self-control over the need to urinate or *void* by the time that they are 2 to 3 years old. In the situation of **urinary incontinence,** the ability to exert self-control over this emptying is diminished. This loss of control may be due to changes in the musculature of the bladder, which may cause elasticity to be lost. In that circumstance, the bladder will fill and overflow. Incontinence can also be the result of disease or dysfunction in nerve transmission into the bladder (i.e., innervation), wherein the bladder does not respond to cues that it is full. Instead, it empties on overflow or without any warning. Incontinence can also occur as the result of urinary tract infection, disease, injury, or normal aging processes later in life.

Mix and Match

Match each term with its definition or description.

1. innervate	a circular band-shaped muscle at an orifice
2. sphincter	loss of self-control over urination
3. void	the act of supplying or stimulating a body part
4. incontinence	urinate; to pass urine

Right Word or Wrong Word: *Innervate* or *Enervate*?

Are these synonyms, or are they examples of Greek or Latin words being modernized into English?

Laboratory diagnostics: urinary system

Urinalysis simply means *analysis of urine.* It is an assessment tool used to diagnose a urinary tract infection or kidney disease and to detect the presence of certain drugs, hormones, or alcohol in the system. To do this, a specimen must be taken. When patients are unable to collect their own urine for the purpose of analysis, a specimen might be taken via the temporary introduction of a urinary catheter.

Composition of urine

Normal urine is sterile. It is composed of 95% water and 5% waste products called **solutes**. These solutes include naturally occurring ions, as well as solutes that originated outside of the body but that are now being excreted in the urine. Medications, alcohol, and illicit drugs are examples of such solutes. Organic molecules are also excreted in the urine and thus become part of its composition. These organic molecules include creatinine, uric acid, hormones, enzymes, and carbohydrates, to name a few. Healthy urine does not contain bacteria.

Urine is always collected in a clean container and stored in a cool place until it is tested. It should not be allowed to sit for long periods. Urine is a bodily fluid, and, although urine is sterile, it is necessary to wear gloves when collecting or working with urine specimens, because each and every one has the potential to contain viruses, harmful bacteria, infections, and other microorganisms that can be harmful to a person who comes into contact with it. Procedures for the analysis of urine include visual inspection, chemical analysis, and microscopic analysis.

Sensory characteristics of urine

The assessment of urine begins with a visual inspection. Its color, odor, and transparency all have meaning.

Normal color: Healthy urine is amber yellow, although this color can be diluted by drinking large amounts of water. It is sometimes described as being “straw” colored.

Normal odor: Fresh urine has a moderate smell, whereas urine that has been sitting for some time begins to smell more like ammonia.

Transparency: The clarity or cloudiness of urine can indicate health or illness, as can the presence of blood or fine mucous threads in it. Sometimes this visual examination is called assessing the *turbidity* (cloudiness) of the urine.

A full urinalysis is a composite of many tests. Table 5-11 identifies and describes some of the more common U/A tests. Prefixes related to those tests and their results are provided in a Table 5-12.

TABLE 5-11: Common Tests in Urinalysis

Test	Description and Purpose
Specific gravity	This test measures urine density by testing the weight of a volume of urine as compared with an equal weight of distilled water. For normal urine, the measure should be almost comparable. Urine that contains more soluble matter will be heavier.
Hydrogen ion concentration (pH)	The normal pH balance is 4.8 to 7.5
Protein	Protein is normally found in the urine. However, increased levels can indicate nephrotic syndrome (proteinuria).
Glucose	Only a trace of glucose is normally present in the urine. Higher amounts may indicate diabetes or other pathology. Glycosuria means that there is an excessive amount of sugar in the urine.
Ketones	Ketones are not normally found in the urine. Their presence could indicate starvation or diabetes.
Hemoglobin	Blood and hemoglobin are not normally found in the urine. Their presence can indicate lower urinary tract bleeding or renal disease.
Bilirubin (a bile pigment involved in the breakdown of hemoglobin in the liver)	Trace amounts of bilirubin may appear in healthy urine. Increased amounts can indicate liver or hemolytic disease.
Leukocytes (WBC)	WBCs are only present in the urine if an infection is present.
Nitrates	The presence of nitrates means that bacteria such as *Escherichia coli* are present in the urine.

TABLE 5-12: Prefixes: Urine diagnostics

Prefix	Full Term	Prefix	Full Term
azo/t- (nitrogenous waste or compounds)	azote (an archaic Greek term for nitrogen)	glyco- (sugar and/or glycerin)	glycose
glycos/o- gluco- glucoso- (sugar, sweetness)	glucose	ket/o- (acids and acetone)	ketones
		nitr- (salt)	nitrates

Reflective Questions

Review and reflect upon what you have been learning about urine and urinalysis as you answer these reflective questions.

1. Name two reasons for collecting a urine specimen.

____

2. Which three procedures are included in urinalysis?

____

3. Name four elements that are not normally found in healthy urine.

____

Let's Practice

Write the medical term that fits each description.

1. This term refers to the appearance of urine. ______________________________
2. This term tells us what electrolytes are. ______________________________
3. These two combining forms are used in words that refer to the kidneys. ______________
4. This term applies to situations in which children wet their pants. __________________
5. This term refers to a bundle or knot of capillaries in the kidneys. __________________

Listen to the language of the urinary system

Read the following dialogue between ER Nurse Roxie and her patient, Mr. Davis, as she prepares to collect a urine specimen.

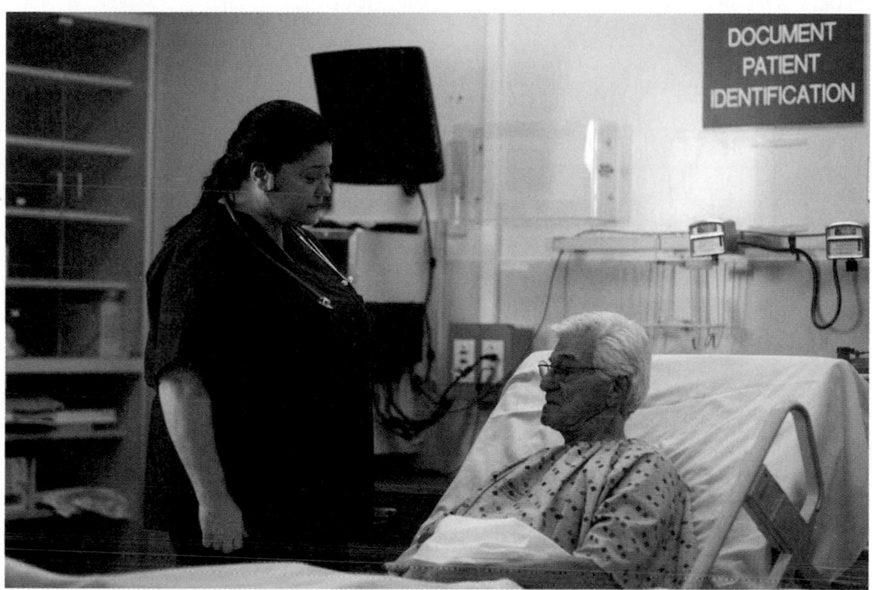

Patient Update

"Hello, Mr. Davis, I'm Roxie, one of the nurses here. Please don't pull on that tube. We've inserted a catheter, sir, to help you void. I know it might be a bit uncomfortable just now, but it's important that you leave it in place."

"Huh? What? What's going on?" replied Mr. Davis as Roxie gently moved his hands away from the catheter tube.

"Sir, you are in the ER of Okla Trauma Center. You've been in a motor vehicle accident, and we're taking care of you. You were incontinent of urine on your way here, so we've put in a catheter to help you with that for the time being."

"Catheter? What do you mean?" Mr. Davis asked as he began to fumble with the oxygen mask covering his mouth and nose. The nurse gently moved his hands away from it, too, and held them for a few seconds.

"Mr. Davis, that's your oxygen mask. You need to keep it on right now. Just relax and take a deep breath. You're in the hospital, and we're here to help you," Roxie said soothingly.

"I have to pee. Let me go now. I have to go to the bathroom," Mr. Davis mumbled. "I have to go. Please help me." He tried to sit up, and he moved his legs. Two other nurses helped Roxie to gently restrain Mr. Davis using their own hands.

"No, sir, you've got to lie still a bit longer. You've been in a car accident, and we're doing some assessments to see if you're okay," explained Roxie. "You have a urinary catheter in place. It's a small tube that we've inserted up through your penis, through your urethra, and into your bladder. It will drain your bladder for you. You don't have to worry about going to the bathroom. Just relax when you feel that need to void, and the catheter will take care of emptying your bladder for you. It's hooked up to a bag here; there's a catheter bag hung just at the side of your bed, below you."

"Yeah ... yes, okay. Oh, I know, I know what you mean now. I know. I've had one before, I think," Mr. Davis responded as he lay back on the bed.

"Sir, I'm just going to take a quick urine specimen from this bag before they wheel you down to have a CT scan." Roxie bent down then and opened the port on the catheter bag. She drained some urine into a specimen cup labeled with the patient's name, date, location, and attending physician.

Reflective Questions

Consider what you've just read or heard as you answer the following questions.

1. How did the nurse collect a urine specimen from Mr. Davis?

____

2. What did Mr. Davis remember while the nurse was explaining the catheter to him?

____

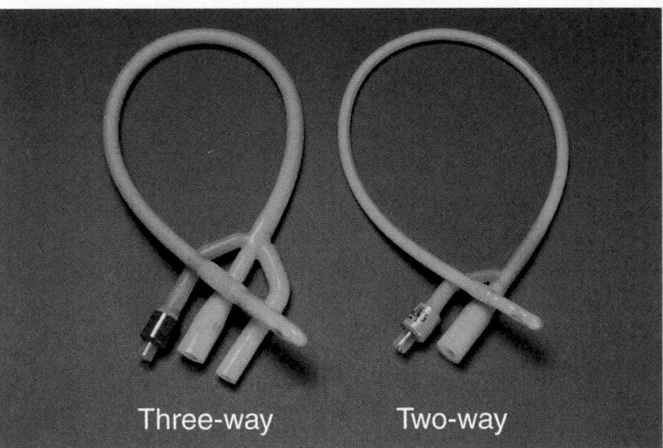

Figure 5.26: Three-way and two-way urinary catheters (From Rutherford CJ: *Differentiating Surgical Equipment and Supplies.* Philadelphia: FA Davis, 2010, p. 101. With permission.)

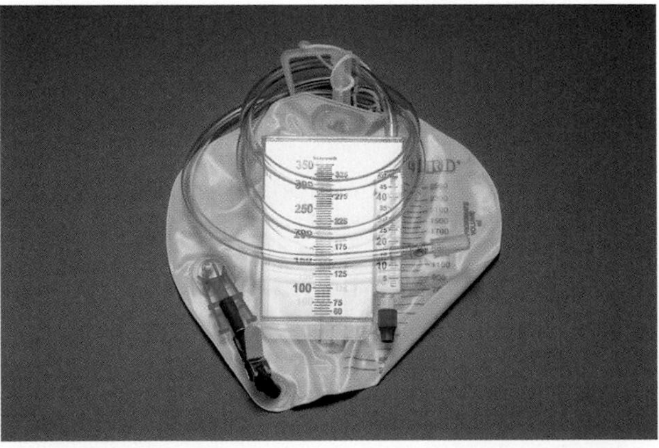

Figure 5.27: Urinary drainage bag with a urometer attached (From Rutherford CJ: *Differentiating Surgical Equipment and Supplies.* Philadelphia: FA Davis, 2010, p. 102. With permission.)

PRONUNCIATION PRACTICE

Say these words aloud to a friend or classmate if you can. You are given the phonetic pronunciation. Your instructor can help you with pronunciation,

or visit **http://www.MedicalLanguageLab.com.**

bilirubin	**bĭl**-ĭ-roo´bĭn
calyx	**kā**´lĭx
catheter	**kăth**´ĕ-tĕr
homeostasis	hō″mē-ō-**stā**´sĭs
incontinence	ĭn-**kŏnt**´ĭn-ĕns
ketones	**kē**´tōnz
meatus	mē-**ā**´tŭs
medulla	mĕ-**dŭl**´lă
renal	**rē**´năl
sphincter	**sfĭngk**´tĕr
turbidity	tŭr-**bĭd**´ĭ-tē
urinary	**ū**´rĭ-năr″ē
urea	ū-**rē**´ă
ureter	**ū**´rĕ-ter
urethra	ū-**rē**´thră

CHAPTER SUMMARY

Chapter 5 has followed Mr. Davis's assessment and care since his arrival at Okla Trauma Center's emergency department. Much of his assessment involved laboratory diagnostics. Key terms that are used to refer to laboratory procedures, analyses, and equipment have been studied. Both anatomical and medical terms for the cardiovascular and urinary systems have been presented, with opportunities made available to construct and deconstruct new terminology, to apply critical and reflective thinking to new learning, and to observe how medical language is used within the context of these body systems, as well as within the context of patient care and assessment. Career spotlights featured laboratory, medical laboratory, and electrocardiograph technicians.

Chapter 5 has introduced you to some medical abbreviations. These have been organized into a study table here for quick reference. Some of them you will recognize immediately, and some will reappear throughout the following chapters with more explanation and application.

TABLE 5-13: Abbreviations: Review

Medical Abbreviation	Full Term	Medical Abbreviation	Full Term
ABGs	arterial blood gases	CBC	complete blood count
AIDS	acquired immunodeficiency syndrome	CT	computed axial tomography
A.S.A.P.	as soon as possible	CV	cardiovascular
AV	atrioventricular	CVA	cerebrovascular accident
BUN	blood urea nitrogen		
CAD	coronary artery disease	Cl	chloride

Continued

TABLE 5-13: Abbreviations: Review—cont'd

Medical Abbreviation	Full Term	Medical Abbreviation	Full Term
CO_2	carbon dioxide	PQRST	heart waves (see the table entitled "Waves in a Cardiac Cycle")
Ca	calcium	PT	prothrombin time
ECG	electrocardiogram	PTT	partial thromboplastin time
E. coli	*Escherichia coli*	reqs.	requisitions
HSV-1	herpes simplex virus type I	STAT	statim; immediately
HSV-2	herpes simplex virus type II	SIRS	systemic inflammatory response syndrome
INR	international normalized ratio	SA	sinoatrial
ICU	intensive care unit	TIA	transient ischemic attack
K	potassium	TB	tuberculosis
Li	lithium	UA or U/A	urinalysis
MI	myocardial infarction		
Na	sodium		
O_2SATs	oxygen saturation		
pH	parts hydrogen; hydrogen ion concentration		

Key Terms

aneurysm
anticoagulant
arrhythmias
arterial blood gases (ABGs)
arteries
arterioles
asepsis
atrioventricular (AV) node
blood gas analyzer
blood pressure (BP)
bundle branches
bundle of His
capillaries
capillary puncture
capillary tube
cardiac conduction system
cardiac cycle
cardiac waves
centrifuge
cerebrovascular accident (CVA)
chemistry analyzer
coagulation analyzer
code
defibrillator
diastole
electocardiogram (ECG)
electrolyte analyzer
electrolytes
emboli
glomeruli
hematology analyzer
hemorrhagic stroke
homeostasis
immunology analyzer
infection
infection control
infectious agents
inflammatory response
innervation
international normalized ratio (INR)
interval
ischemic stroke
kidneys
lead
lymph
myocardial infarction (MI)
myocardium
nephrons
oxygen saturation (O_2SATs)
partial thromboblastin time (PTT)
phlebotomist
phlebotomy
pipette or pipettor
platelets
prothrombin (PT)
pulmonary circulation
pulse oximeter
pulse rate
purkinje fibers
readout (trace)
sepsis
sinoatrial (SA) node
solutes
stroke
systemic circulation
systemic inflammatory response syndrome (SIRS)
systole
thermoregulation
thrombin
thromboemboli
thromboplastin
thrombosis
thrombus
transient ischemic attack (TIA)
urea
urinalysis (UA or U/A)
urinary incontinence
urine
urine analyzer
veins
venipuncture
venules
wave

CHAPTER REVIEW

Critical Thinking

Use your new knowledge of medical terms and medical language to answer these questions.

1. What is a Code Blue? ____________________
2. If healthy urine is sterile, why is it necessary to wear gloves when you come into contact with it?

   ____
3. Why might a urinalysis be ordered for a person who is exhibiting confusion?

   ____

Name the Term

Write the term that fits each definition or description.

1. Filters blood and removes waste ____________________
2. A urinary passageway to the outside of the body ____________________
3. A blood clot ____________________
4. A blood clot that has come loose from the wall of an artery and that is moving with the flow of blood through the vessels ____________________
5. Requires a credential or certification that permits the taking of blood by venipuncture

   ____

Break it Down

Break these words into their component parts of prefix-root-suffix, as applicable.

1. cardiovascular ____________________
2. phlebotomy ____________________
3. nephritis ____________________

Right Word or Wrong Word: *Ureters* or *Uterus*?

Do these two terms mean the same thing, despite their slightly different spelling?

Translate the Terminology

Use your new skills to decipher medical language. On the line provided, rewrite each statement in your own words.

1. "Ask the lab to get us the ketone levels A.S.A.P."

   ____
2. "I'll have to get it from the bag, then. He has a catheter."

   ____
3. "Let's get an ECG started and run it continuously for now."

   ____
4. "Take those pulses bilaterally at the radius and dorsalis pedis."

   ____

Fill in the Blanks

Fill in the blanks with the missing part of each term.

1. ________ ology is the field of medicine that specializes in the urinary system.
2. A ________ ologist is a specialist in kidney health and disease.
3. ________ ology refers to the science of the heart.

Name the Prefix

Read the definition and then write the prefix that it describes.

1. glycerin or sugar ________________________________
2. acids or acetones ________________________________
3. sweet or sugar ________________________________

STUDY TIP

Depending on where your career aspirations are going to take you, you may or may not have to remember all of the laboratory tests discussed in this book. You might instead just want to become familiar with some of the most common lab tests so that you can recognize them and place them in context when you see them, as we have done here for tests involving the urinary and cardiovascular systems. However, if you want to study laboratory tests further or even memorize the key points of some of them, you may wish to purchase the wonderful book entitled *Davis's Comprehensive Handbook of Laboratory and Diagnostic Tests with Nursing Implications,* which was written by A.M. Van Leeuwen, D.J. Poelhuis-Leth, and M.L. Bladh and published by the F.A. Davis Company.

CHAPTER SIX

Dental and Burn Assessment

Focus: Craniofacial Structures and the Integumentary System

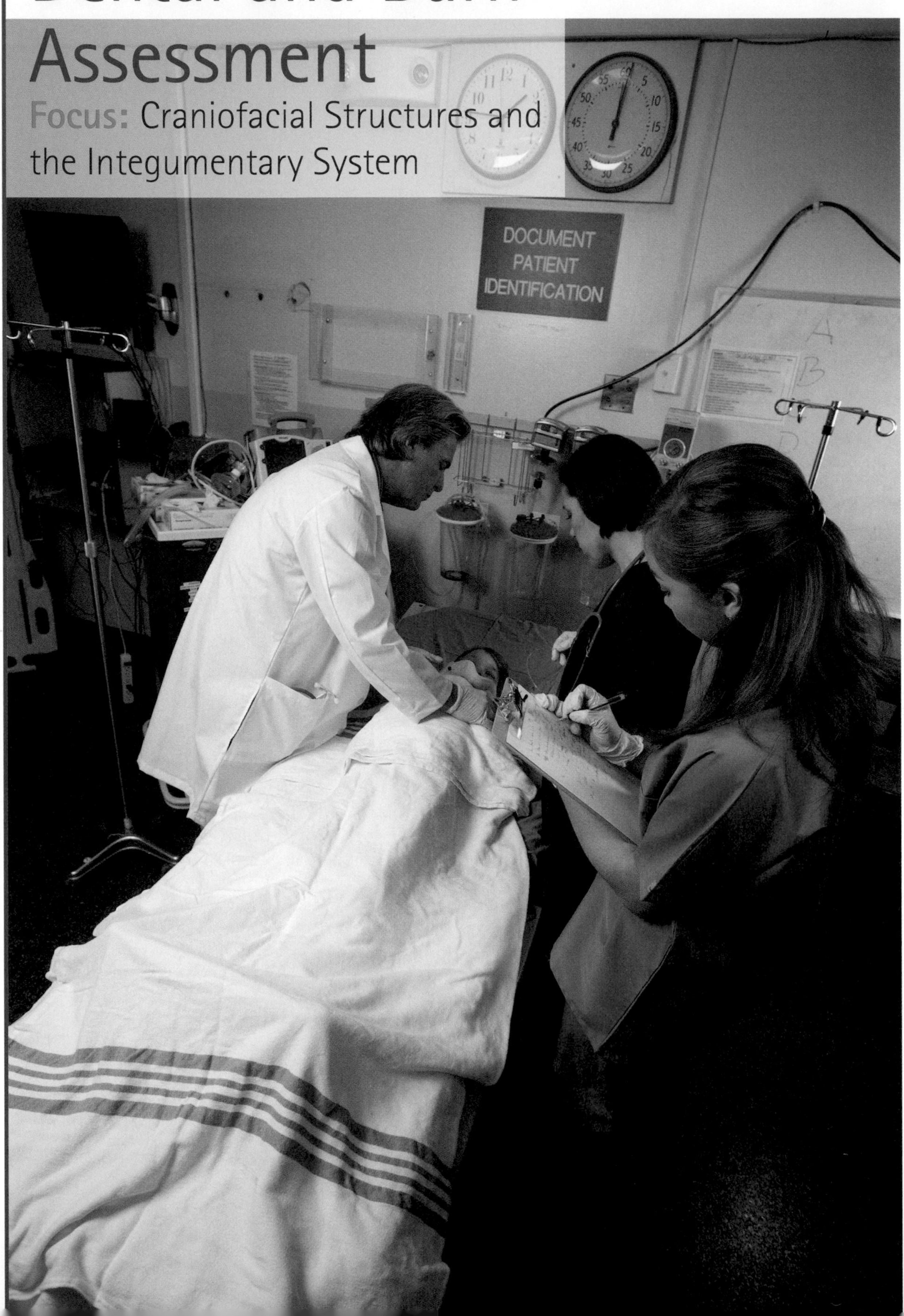

Clay Davis is a 7-year-old child who is being treated at Okla Trauma Center for severe injuries received in a motor vehicle accident this afternoon. Clay was apparently sitting in the backseat of the car when the accident occurred. The EMT reports that the child did not have a seatbelt on and that Clay appears to have hit the back upper edge of the front seat with his jaw. ABCs were done on the scene and in the ambulance on the way to Okla Trauma.

At the time of the incident, Clay was in the company of his grandparents, Zane and Stevie-Rose Davis. He had no identification on him, and, although his grandfather is also being treated at this facility, the staff has not yet made the connection. The paramedic who brought the child in gave the staff the patient's name; he told the staff that he got the information from another EMT on the scene, who was attending to the child's grandmother.

Patient Update

"I'm Dr. Lincoln from Peds. What have we got here?" asked the physician as he entered the ER bay. He noted that the team was busily involved with patient care, and he watched for a moment as a nurse gently removed the child's oxygen mask while being careful not to jostle the child's head or neck. The patient's mouth was bloody and swollen. Nasal prongs were quickly placed. The child's head was still in the spinal fixation collar from Emergency Services.

"Suction standing by," interjected one of the nurses as the staff continued their work. The child moaned loudly, tried to move, and tried to push away the helping hands.

The ER physician, Dr. Raymond, was talking to the boy. "It's all right, son. I know you're in a lot of pain. You've been in an accident, and we're going to help you now. I'm Dr. Raymond. I have to get a look at your face." He paused a moment then to turn to the newly arrived pediatrician, Dr. Lincoln. "Good to have you here, Steve," Dr. Raymond said. "We've got a 7-year-old male, blunt force trauma to the face. I've just started the assessment, but feel free to take over if you like. Kids are your specialty."

"Thanks. I got your page and came as quick as I could," replied Dr. Lincoln. "Let's see what we can do together. You'll stay?" Dr. Raymond nodded in agreement.

"Right, well, first things first. I see he's breathing on his own, but with that trauma to his mouth and a burn across his upper torso ... well, this could soon be compromised. What are his O_2SATS, nurse?" Dr. Lincoln asked.

"95%, doctor."

"Okay. This facial trauma comes first, before what appears to be a partial-thickness scald burn on his torso. I'm worried about the lower jaw. Have you taken a look at his spine, Dr. Raymond?"

"No, not yet," said Dr. Raymond. "He just arrived seconds before you did. As you can see, we've left the head block on until we can get some x-rays. He's conscious, alert, and moving, so I don't suspect spinal or cerebral involvement at this time, but we can't rule that out just yet."

Dr. Lincoln moved in closer to the patient's side and began to examine the child's face for wounds and fractures. He quickly noted what appeared to be a split lip. Although the mouth was bloody, the child was clearly not aspirating any blood or teeth. Dr. Lincoln observed the swelling, bruising, and asymmetry of the lower jaw. He began the craniofacial examination in accordance with standard protocol. He palpated bimanually, beginning at the cranial vault and then proceeding to the forehead and the orbital rims. "No bruising or evidence of fracture here," he said. "What do we know about the burn?" Dr. Lincoln asked as he continued the examination of the boy's face and neck.

"According to the paramedic, they found the child on the floor of the backseat. He wasn't wearing a shirt, and there was a wet towel nearby. EMT and the police were not sure what happened, but they think that the grandparents could have been taking the boy to the hospital for the burn when the accident occurred. Maybe the wet towel was covering the burn," offered Daniel, the RN at hand.

"And the mouth? The jaw? What was the mechanism of injury?"

"He wasn't wearing a seatbelt," Daniel replied.

"Uh-huh. Hit the back of the front seat? That would explain the split lip and the bruising around the mouth. His lips were probably crushed against his teeth. Makes me worry about the jaw, though." Dr. Lincoln turned to the patient. "Well, the good thing is, you're here with us in the hospital, and you're breathing on your own despite the blood in and around your mouth." Dr. Lincoln smiled at the child, and he noticed that the boy was crying silently.

Dr. Lincoln returned to the assessment. "He's in a good deal of pain," Dr. Lincoln said to the team, "and I'd like to help him with that a.s.a.p." Dr. Lincoln's hands returned to the examination of the facial bones. "Zygomatic arches intact. Let's check the nose now. Young man, I'm just going to touch your nose, gently." Clay looked up at him with tears in his eyes. In a kind, warm voice, the doctor acknowledged him. "I know, I know you're hurting. We've just got a few more things to do here. Hang on for bit, will ya trooper?" Dr. Lincoln smiled reassuringly at the child. He moved his fingertips gently over the boy's nose, listening for crepitus and observing for tenderness. He noticed no evidence of a displacement or a fracture, but he ordered an x-ray to be sure. "Now," he said to the treatment team, "Let's take a look at the mouth and the jaw. Did someone call Dental?"

"Yes, sir, they've been paged. Emergency Dispatch let us know that the patient had a possible jaw fracture while they were in transport. Dr. Sandor is in surgery at the moment, finishing up. She'll be here momentarily," replied an LPN. "She asked me to be sure that the panorex was made ready, and it is. They're standing by in D.I."

"Good, we're going to need her." Dr. Lincoln turned his direct attention back to the boy. "Clay ... is that your name?" The child nodded ever so slightly, blocked by the head restraint. "Clay, I've got to touch your jaw and your mouth now. Especially your mouth. I've got to have a look in there to see what's going on." The child moaned loudly in protest, and his eyes suddenly grew very wide. He tried to raise a hand up to prevent his mouth from being touched. Dr. Raymond gently took the boy's hand and lowered it back onto the bed so that Dr. Lincoln could proceed with the intraoral examination.

"Let's get Social Services down here," Dr. Raymond instructed. "We can't treat this child until we get parental consent."

One of the nurses toward the foot of the bed responded, "They were here when he arrived and are tracking his parents down now, Doctor."

Suddenly, a side drape was pulled back, and a woman said, "I'm Dr. Sandor. I got here as fast as I could."

Reflective Questions

Reflect on the story that you've just read.

1. How many physicians are working on Clay Davis right now? Give their names and titles.

____

2. Who is expected to appear in the ER shortly to assist? What is his or her title?

____

3. This child has two observable traumatic injuries. What are they?

____

4. The doctors are talking to each other about priority emergency assessment data. What are they referring to? (A nurse answers one of the relevant questions.)

____

5. List at least two reasons that the medical staff are concerned about this patient's breathing.

____

6. Why does one of the nurses make a point of saying that suction equipment is standing by?

____

7. What does the term *mechanism of injury* mean?

____

For audio exercises, visit **http://www.MedicalLanguageLab.com.** 

Learning Objectives

After reading Chapter 6, you will be able to do the following:

- Understand the basic concepts and terms related to emergency dental assessment and equipment.
- Understand the clinical pathway for triage of a patient with suspected dental trauma.
- Recognize and use language that pertains to emergency dental diagnostics.
- Understand basic concepts and terms related to dentistry.
- Appreciate the education and training of dentists and dental surgeons.
- Recognize and use anatomical and medical terms for the face and the facial skeleton.
- Recognize medical terminology as it relates to diagnostics and trauma of the structures of the craniofacial complex, including the cranial nerves.
- Recognize and use key anatomical and medical terms for the integumentary system.
- Recognize and use standardized terminology that pertains to burns.

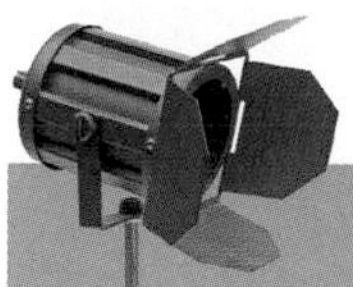

CAREER SPOTLIGHT: Dentists and Dental Surgeons

Dentistry is the field of medicine that is concerned with the teeth and the structures of the oral cavity (mouth). Dentistry is concerned with preventing, diagnosing, and treating diseases, malformations, and injuries of the teeth, jaw, and mouth. *Dentists* practice dentistry. They are medically trained, but they are not physicians. They earn a credential of doctor of dental surgery (DDS) or doctor of dental medicine (DDM).

A *dental surgeon* is highly specialized in dentistry as either an oral or maxillofacial surgeon. Extensive education and training beyond a baccalaureate in dentistry are required for these professionals. Just like dentists, dental surgeons must be licensed by a professional regulatory body. Dental surgeons are able to diagnose and treat diseases, injuries, and deformities of the hard and soft tissues of the oral and maxillary regions of the face. They may do this through surgery and other treatments. Their focus of practice may be functional, aesthetic, or both. A specialty in dentistry must be formally recognized by the American Dental Association.

The Language of Facial and Dental Trauma

Facial and dental traumas are among the most frequently seen injuries in emergency treatment centers and dental clinics. They are the result of blunt force trauma to the face, particularly to the area of the mouth. Although many of these facial injuries are related to broken teeth and dental work, they also include split lips and subluxation (displacement) of the teeth. Mandibular fractures (fractured lower jaws) are the second most frequent facial bone fractures seen among the pediatric population. (Broken noses are the most frequent.)

Triage assessment: dental trauma

Our patient, Clay Davis, requires immediate attention by the dental surgeon at Okla Trauma Center, Dr. Reka Sandor. Whenever facial injuries are traumatic and involve the jaw or the mouth, assessment by a dentist or a dental surgeon is required. Clay has multiple traumas, so a dental surgeon will be attending him. The pediatrician, Dr. Lincoln, completed the triage assessment for facial and dental trauma in anticipation of the dental surgeon's arrival. He followed a protocol or a clinical pathway for assessing these injuries.

Study the clinical pathway for the triage assessment of a dental trauma. Next, reread the opening scenario, and then compare what the doctors said and did with the steps listed on the pathway. Notice that, because the child could not speak and was not accompanied by a family member, it was impossible for the treatment team to learn much about the patient's medical or dental history. Even so, the treatment team members were able to make some clinical decisions on the basis of the data that they received from the EMT and on the observations that they made themselves.

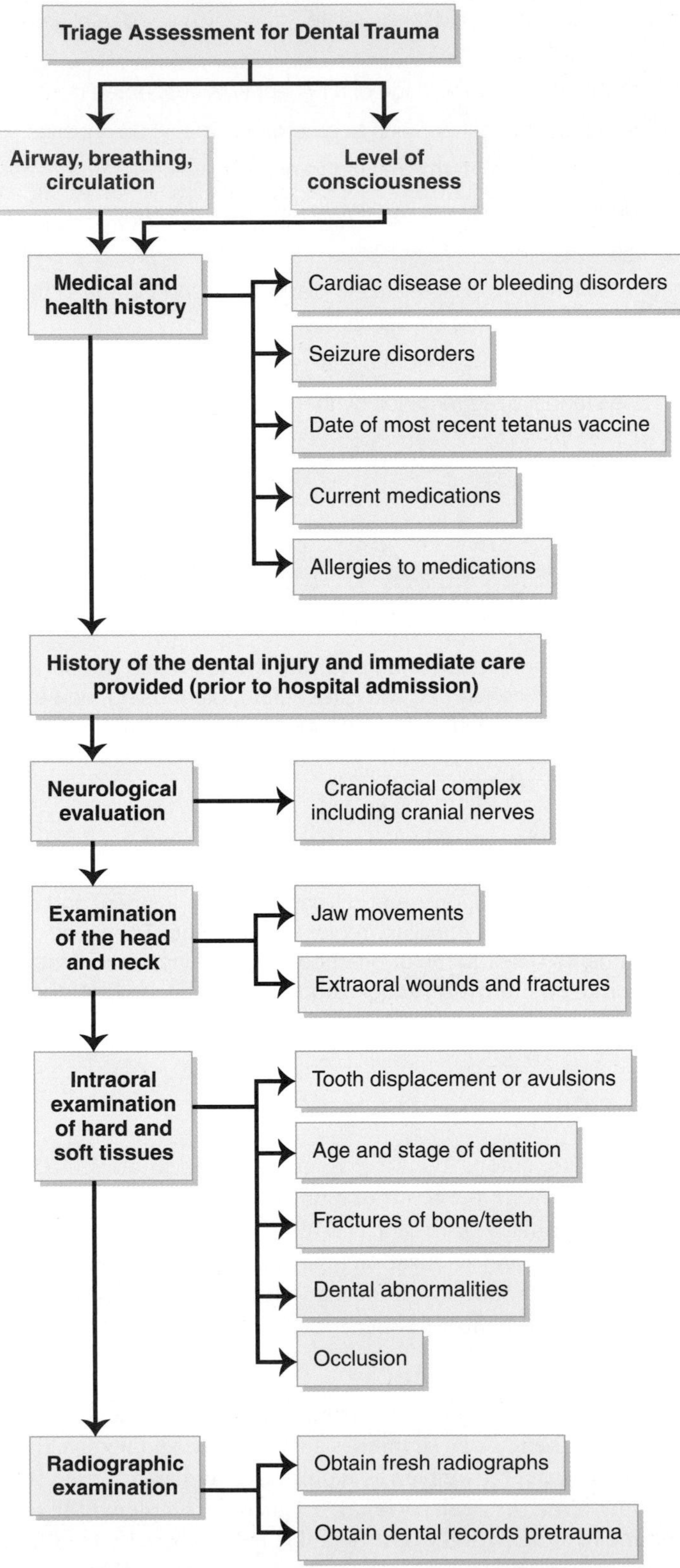

Figure 6.1: Triage assessment: dental trauma

Key terms: triage assessment of dental trauma

The chapter opener included a number of key medical terms and phrases that were used to describe how Dr. Lincoln assessed the patient's dental trauma. Let's look at some passages from the opening scenario. The key terms and phrases are italicized in the example and highlighted below with the explanation.

> "He quickly noted what appeared to be a *split lip*. Although the mouth was bloody, the child was clearly not *aspirating* any blood or teeth."

A **split lip** is a trauma to the lip in which the skin is broken. It occurs when the soft tissues of the lips are crushed against the teeth by a forceful blow. A tooth or teeth cut the lip, thereby splitting it open. Because of the high level of vascularity of the mouth, any injury to this area can bleed heavily.

In this context, **aspirating** means *inhaling an object*. The fear is that, with trauma to the lip and mouth, teeth may be knocked out of their sockets and inhaled. In addition, when there is blood in the mouth, there is risk of aspirating that blood. This is the reason that the child has not been laid flat on a stretcher.

> "Dr. Lincoln observed the swelling, bruising, and *asymmetry* of the lower jaw."

Asymmetry of the lower jaw means that the jawline is not evenly shaped bilaterally.

> "He began the *craniofacial examination* ..."

A **craniofacial examination** is an examination of the head and face. This is discussed in more detail later in the chapter.

> "He *palpated bimanually* ..."

The term **palpated bimanually** means that the doctor used both hands to touch and assess both sides of the patient at the same time.

> "... beginning at the *cranial vault* and then proceeding to the forehead and the *orbital rims*."

The **cranial vault** is the portion of the skull that houses and protects the brain.

The **orbital rims** are the eye sockets.

> "'*Zygomatic arches intact.*'"

The **zygomatic arches** are the cheekbones.

Intact means *undamaged and unharmed.*

> "... listening for *crepitus* ..."

Crepitus is the medical term for a crackling or rattling sound.

Let's Practice

Write the term or terms that best identify what is being described.

1. broken lower jaw bone ____________________
2. trauma that opens the tissue of the oral labia ____________________
3. cheekbones ____________________
4. used both hands ____________________
5. sucking something other than air into the trachea or windpipe ____________________
6. refers to time before the injury ____________________
7. lack of balance, proportion, or regular shape ____________________
8. sound of crackling ____________________

Critical Thinking

Review the clinical pathway again to respond to the following questions.

1. Identify which steps of the triage assessment pathway Dr. Lincoln was able to assess.

____

____

2. Identify which steps of the triage assessment pathway Dr. Sandor will address.

____

____

3. Identify which elements or parts of the triage assessment pathway cannot be completed until the patient's parents, next of kin, or guardian can be consulted.

____

____

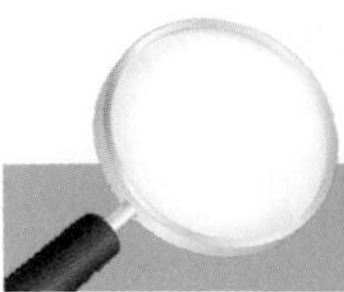

FOCUS POINT: Age of Consent

The term *age of consent* refers to the client or patient's age and capacity or legal right to consent to medical treatment. In the United States, the age of consent is 18 years. However, there may be deviations in this age on a state-by-state basis. As a health-care professional, you will want to inform yourself regarding the age of consent (also known as the *age of majority*) in your jurisdiction specifically as it relates to medical treatment. There are many legal, ethical, and moral implications for not following this statute.

Anatomy and physiology: face and facial skeleton

Medically speaking, the face is the anterior portion of the head, and it extends from the forehead to the chin. Laterally, it extends only to the ears, but it does not include them. The face consists of many muscles that are responsible for facial movement and expressions. It also contains the oral and nasal cavities.

Structures of the face

Anatomical references to the face often include the term *surface anatomy of the face.* The face consists of skin, muscles, and vascular structures. Exterior to the facial skeleton are the **oral labia** (lips), the nose, the eyes, and the eyebrows.

Facial ossa (bones) give shape to the face. There are fourteen stationary (fixed) bones in the facial skeleton, as well as one that is mobile. The mobile bone is the mandible (lower jaw), which is able to move by way of the temporomandibular joint (TMJ). Many facial bones come in pairs. Interestingly, the frontal bone (forehead) is considered a cranial bone or a bone of the skull rather than a bone of the face.

Bones of the face

lacrimal (2): These are the smallest bones in the face. They are situated at the inner corners of the eyes, and they form part of the orbits.

maxillae (2): These are the largest bones of the face. They form part of the orbits (eye sockets), the hard palate (roof of the mouth), the base of the nose, and the tooth sockets.

mandible (1): This is the lower jaw bone; it is the strongest bone of the face, and it also forms the chin (mental tuberosity) and the sides of the face. This bone has a horseshoe shape.

nasal (2): These oblong-shaped bones form the bridge of the nose.

palatines (2): These bones are situated behind the maxillae. They also form part of the hard palate at the back and base of the nose.

turbinator or inferior nasal conchae (2): These thin bones form the sides of the nasal cavity.

vomer (1): This bone forms part of the floor of the nasal cavity and part of the nasal septum. The vomer has the shape of a plow.

zygomatic bones or malar bones (2): This pair of bones forms the cheekbones and part of the orbits.

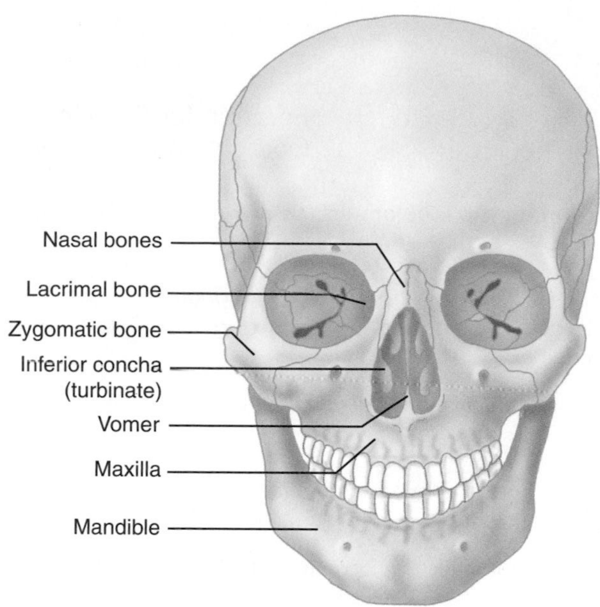

Figure 6.2: Facial bones

TABLE 6-1: The Prefix *sub-* in Terms That Relate to the Face

BEGIN with a Prefix	ADD a Root or Combining Form	ADD a Suffix	CREATE a New Term
sub-	zygomat-	-ic	subzygomatic (beneath the zygomatic [cheek] bone)
sub-	naso-	-al	subnasal (below [underneath] the nose)
sub-	orbit	-al	suborbital (beneath the orbit)
sub-	mandibul-	-ar	submandibular (beneath the mandibular ossa)
sub-	mental (from the Latin root *mentum,* meaning *chin*)		submental (under the chin)

Fill in the Blanks

Refer to Figure 6-2 and use your own knowledge of anatomy and physiology for this exercise. Practice using medical terminology related to location. You are given the names of two bones or structures of the face. On the blank between them, write *interior, exterior, superior, inferior, anterior,* or *posterior.*

1. The vomer is ______________ to the nasal bones.
2. The zygomatic bone is ______________ to the maxilla.
3. The turbinators are ________________ to the nose.
4. The teeth are ____________________ to the maxilla and mandible.
5. The nasal bones are ____________ and ____________ to the turbinate bones.
6. The skull is ______________ to the face.
7. The zygomatic bones are ____________________ to the temporal bones.
8. The frontal bone is ____________________ to the zygomatic and nasal bones.

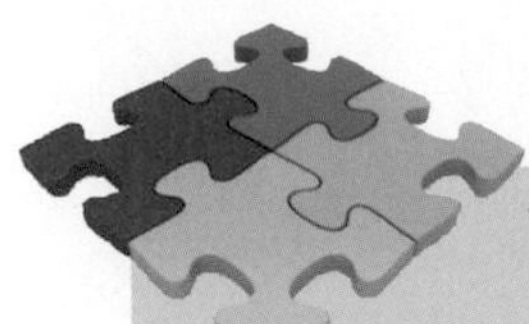

WORD BUILDING: Formula for Creating Words with the Combining Form of *Facies*

facies = the medical term for the face or surface of something. The combining form is *faci/o.*

facio + lingu + al = *faciolingual*

Definition: pertaining to both the face and the tongue together. (The second root is *lingua,* meaning *tongue.*) *adjective*

Example: Orthodontists may deal with *faciolingual* abnormalities and the arrangement or positioning of the teeth.

facio + plasty = *facioplasty*

Definition: plastic or cosmetic surgery of the face. (The suffix *-plasty* means *to form.*) *adjective*

Example: In recent years, requests for *facioplasty* have become more common among both men and women.

Build a Word

Use your word-building skills to create medical terms from the following word parts, and then define each term in your own words.

1. dent maxilla al ____________________ Meaning: ____________________
2. face al maxilla ____________________ Meaning: ____________________
3. cervix face al ____________________ Meaning: ____________________

Fill in the Blanks

Use medical language and terminology in context to complete the following sentences.

1. Rebecca is 85 years old and suffers from arthritis and other chronic conditions. Recently, she has been experiencing pain and stiffness when she tries to yawn or open her mouth wide. This is likely due to pathology of the ____________________.
2. Brett plays hockey. He had recent ____________________ surgery because of an injury in which a hockey puck hit him in the mouth and knocked out two of his front upper teeth.
3. Speaking and pronunciation require contact of the tongue with the teeth and lips. When the teeth are not arranged as they should be, a ____________________ assessment is needed.

Critical Thinking

Answer the following question with the your new knowledge of the vocabulary of the face and the facial skeleton.

1. Proximal to the lacrimal bone is the lacrimal duct. What do you think this duct produces?

   ____

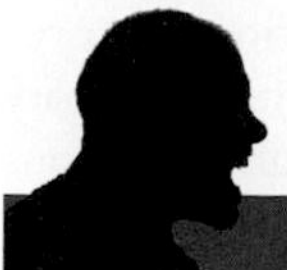

PRONUNCIATION PRACTICE

Say these words aloud to a friend or classmate if you can. You are given the phonetic pronunciation. Your instructor can help you with pronunciation,

or visit http://www.MedicalLanguageLab.com.

conchae	**kŏng**´kā
dentofacial	dĕn˝tō-**fā**´shăl
faciolingual	fā˝shē-ō-**lĭn**´gwăl
faciocervical	fā˝shē-ō-**sĕr**´vĭ-kăl
lacrimal	**lăk**´rĭm-ăl
mandible	**măn**´dĭ-bl
maxillae	măk-**sĭl**´ā
maxillodental	măk-sĭl˝ō-**dĕn**´tăl
palatines	**păl**´ă-tīns
turbinate	**tūr**´bĭ-nāt
temporomandibular	tĕm˝pō-rō-măn-**dĭb**´ū-lăr
vomer	**vō**´mĕr
zygomata	zī˝gō-**măt**´ă

Structures of the nose and the nasal cavity

The **nose** or **proboscis** is the organ of inspiration, expiration, and smell. The bridge of the nose is formed by the union of the *nasal bones*. The nose sits externally and medially on the face. The tip of the nose is called its *apex*. The fleshy part of the nose is called the **nasal septum.** The medical term for the nostrils is **nares.** The fleshy external structures that flare open for breathing and that close to protect the nasal cavity are called the **alae nasi.**

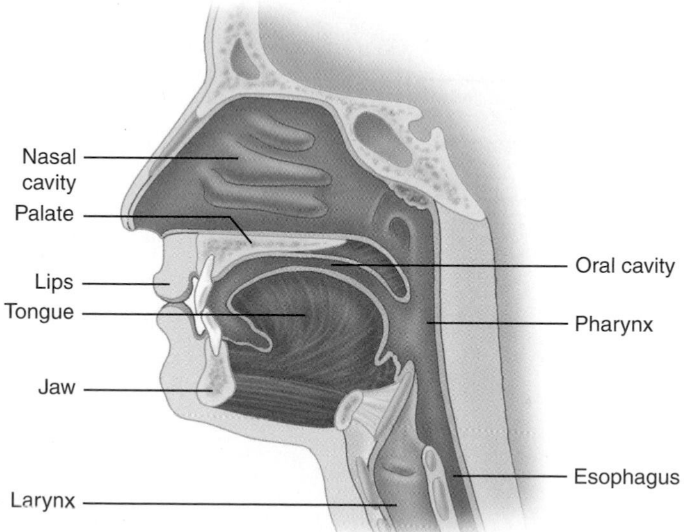

Figure 6.3: Anatomy of the nose and the nasal cavity

The *nasal cavity or nasal fossa* is the uppermost part of the respiratory tract. Its function is to prepare air that has been breathed in through the nose or mouth to be received into the respiratory tract. **Cilia** (small hairs) and mucous line the naval cavity to protect it. The nasal cavity also functions as an olfactory organ (organ of smell).

Sinuses are small air pockets within the craniofacial complex that are connected to the nasal cavity by small tubes. These tubes permit airflow into the nasal passages and allow for the drainage of mucous. There are four pairs of sinuses. Two are located bilaterally to the nose; this position is referred to as **paranasal**. Another pair of sinuses sits at the superior aspect of the nose and across the medial portion of the forehead, as well as behind the eyes. Sinuses are lined with mucous, which moistens the air that is breathed before that air is transported into the rest of the respiratory tract. This mucous also traps unwanted particles and expels them from the body.

Assessment of the nose

Assessment includes the inspection of the nose from the inside and the outside. If the nose has been injured, this can be painful, because the physician will use instruments to view the interior aspects and use fingertip palpation to examine the exterior.

The external assessment of the nose involves examination for placement, alignment, symmetry, discharge, the patency of the nares, tenderness, and masses. The term **patency of the nares** refers to whether or not the nasal airways are open and whether air is able to travel in and out of the nares. The examiner purposefully occludes one naris at a time to determine whether there is any difficulty with breathing or any blockage. If the nares are clear, they are patent.

The internal assessment of the nose includes hyperextending the neck backward and pushing hard against the tip of the nose upward. A small penlight is then used to examine the inside of the nares. This examination will provide information about the status of the mucosal lining of the nose, the condition of the septum (or its deviation), and the health of the sinuses.

Dr. Lincoln has performed a cursory assessment of Clay's nasal cavity and nose because any blunt force trauma to the face has great potential for involving the nose (i.e., slamming into the back edge of the front seat in a vehicle). The doctor found no overt signs or symptoms of injury, but x-rays will confirm this.

Medical terminology for the nose involves the use of two roots: nasus and rhinos. Each of these has its own combining forms.

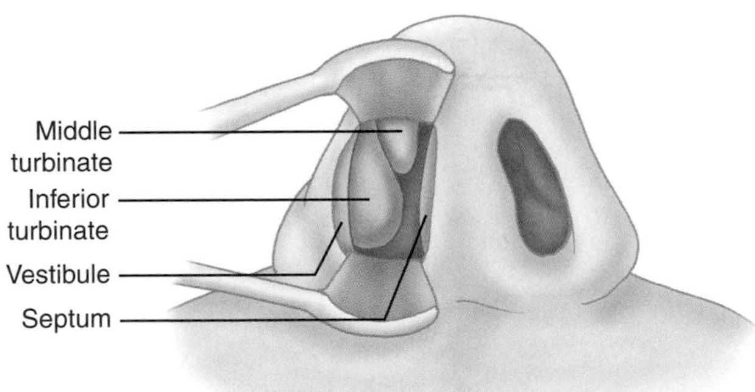

Figure 6.4: Internal examination of the nose

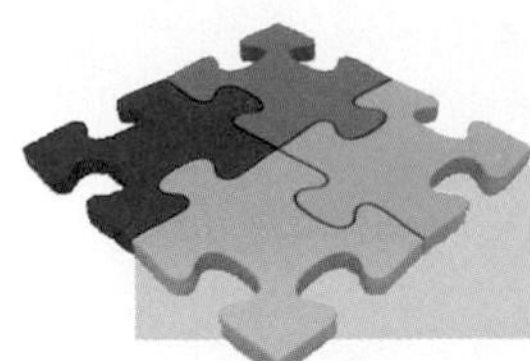

WORD BUILDING: Formula for Creating Words with the Combining Forms *Nas/o* and *Rhin/o*

1. nasus = Latin root meaning *nose.* The combining form is *nas/o.*

nas + al = *nasal*

Definition: pertaining to the nose. *adjective*

Example: You may have *nasal* congestion when you cannot breathe properly through your nose.

nas + endo + scope = *nasendocscope*

Definition: an instrument inserted into the nostril to view the interior of the nasal cavity. *noun*

Example: After suffering from chronic sinus pain, the patient finally has an appointment for an examination by *nasendoscope.*

naso + gastr + ic = *nasogastric*

Definition: pertaining to both the nose and the stomach. (The second root, *gaster,* is used in its combining form *gast-.* It means *stomach.*) *adjective*

Example: Clay Davis may require a *nasogastric* tube for feeding if his jaw needs to be surgically wired shut.

2. rhinos = Greek root meaning *nose.* The combining form is *rhin/o.*

rhin + itis

Definition: inflammation of the mucosa of the nose. *noun*

Example: Allergic *rhinitis* is commonly known as *hay fever.*

rhino + antr + itis = *rhinoantritis*

Definition: inflammation of the nasal cavity and one or both of the maxillary sinuses. (The word part *antr* is the combining form of the root *antron,* meaning *cavity.*) *noun*

Example: Sinusitis may accompany *rhinoantritis;* both of these conditions are inflammations that are caused by infection or allergens.

rhino + plasty = *rhinoplasty*

Definition: plastic surgery of the nose. *noun*

Example: Today, many people choose *rhinoplasty* to enhance their looks.

TABLE 6-2: More Medical and Anatomical Terms for the Nose

Medical or Anatomical Term	Word Deconstruction	Meaning
mucosa	muc/o/i + sa combining form of the root *mucus;* the letters *sa* simply complete the term	a moist tissue layer or mucous membrane that lines the body's cavities and hollow organs
turbinate (synonym for *conchae*)	turb/o/i + nate *turbo* is a Latin root meaning *a child's top (toy)*	lateral scroll-shaped bones in the nasal cavity
conchae (synonym for *turbinate*)	concha + e plural form meaning *shell or shell-shaped (i.e., conch shell)*	lateral scroll-shaped bones in the nasal cavity

Right Word or Wrong Word: *Turbinates* or *Conchae*?

Consider what you've just learned. Are these two words synonyms? Do they have the same meaning?

Build a Word

This exercise will reinforce the skill of understanding the meaning of words on the basis of their component parts. In this exercise, the word parts are scrambled. Put them into logical order to create a medical term, and then write a definition of the word that you have created. (You may need to change the spelling of some of the word parts to complete the exercise.)

1. labi/a naso -al ______
2. gram sino- ______
3. naso para- -al ______
4. muc/o/i -eous sanguine ______
5. -al sept ______
6. laryng/o rhin/o itis ______
7. -al front nas/o ______
8. -ologist rhin/o ______
9. -it is muco- ______
10. -tomy septo ______

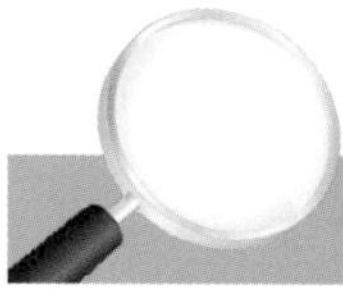

FOCUS POINT: A Bleeding Nose

The medical term for a bleeding nose is *epistaxis.* It is also called *rhinorrhagia.* You may hear, read, and use both terms.

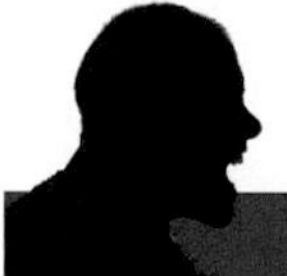

PRONUNCIATION PRACTICE

Say these words aloud to a friend or classmate if you can. You are given the phonetic pronunciation. Your instructor can help you with pronunciation,

or visit **http://www.MedicalLanguageLab.com.** 

mucosanguineous	mū″kō-săn-**gwĭn**′ē-ŭs	nasogastric	nā″zō-**găs**′trĭk
mucus	**mū**′kŭs	patency	**pā**′tĕn-sē
mucositis	mū″kō-**sī**′tĭs	rhinolaryngitis	rī″nō-lăr″ĭn-**jī**′tĭs
nasendoscope	nāz″**ĕn**′dŏ-skōp″		

Structures of the oral cavity

The term **oral cavity** refers to the inside of the mouth. The oral cavity includes the hard and soft palates, pharynx (throat), tonsils, the associated muscles, salivary glands, teeth, gums, uvula, and the tongue. The lips, teeth, and jaw make it possible for the mouth to open and close. The cheeks form the interior walls of the mouth. Except for the teeth, the oral cavity is covered by **oral mucosa,** which is a mucous barrier against temperature, irritants, and trauma.

As you learn the language of the mouth, jaw, and teeth, notice references to digestion, and then consider how our young patient, Clay Davis, is going to be able to eat or drink if the diagnosis of a broken jaw is confirmed. (The links will become even more clear as you explore the language of the digestive system in Chapter 11.)

Key terms: the oral cavity

palates: structures that separate the nasal cavity from the mouth.

The *hard palate* forms the anterior portion of the roof of the mouth.

The *soft palate* lies posterior to the hard palate.

larynx: the voice box; an organ of muscle and cartilage at the upper end of the trachea (windpipe) that is involved in the production of sound (the voice) and that protects the entrance to the main respiratory tract.

pharynx: the throat. The pharynx sits posterior to the oral and nasal cavities and is connected to both.

tongue: a large mass of muscular tissue situated on the floor of the mouth and that extends into the upper pharynx. The purpose of the tongue is to assist with speech and to move food and fluids backward through the mouth to the esophagus for digestion. The tongue is also the primary organ of taste; the taste buds are located on the tongue.

uvula: the fleshy appendage (attachment) of tissue that appears at the posterior of the mouth, above the tongue. The uvula closes the nasal fossa (cavity) during swallowing.

saliva: the substance that is produced by the salivary glands near the oral cavity. The purposes of saliva are to keep the oral cavity moist and to assist with the transport of food by moistening it. Saliva carries digestive enzymes and actually initiates digestion. Saliva is commonly referred to as *spit*.

tonsils: small masses of lymphoid tissue found at the base of the tongue. The tonsils are located in the mucous membranes of the pharynx. (Older adults may no longer have their tonsils if the tonsils were surgically removed when these individuals were young.)

Our patient, Clay Davis, will be assessed for the position and status of the structures of the oral cavity, including the following:

- ips (at least one of which was split open);
- teeth (to determine if they are in situ [in their correct position] or if have been damaged);
- tongue (which he may have bitten down on); and
- jaw (which may be dislocated or fractured).

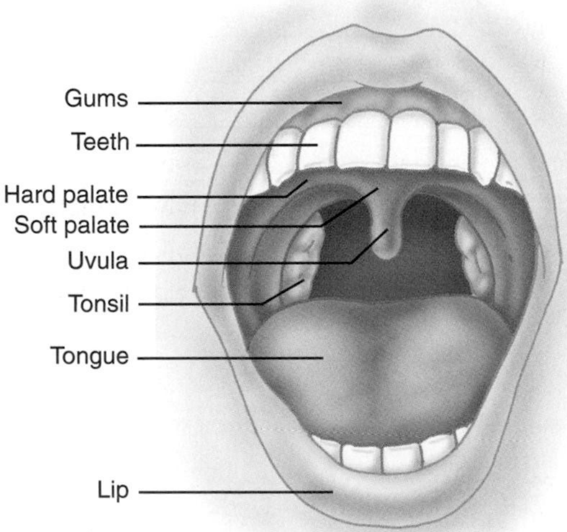

Figure 6.5: The oral cavity

TABLE 6-3: Medical and Anatomical Terms for the Oral Cavity

Medical or Anatomical Term	Word Deconstruction	Meaning
buccal	bucc/o + al combining form of *bucca,* meaning *cheek*	relating to the cheek or mouth
gingivae	gingiv/o + ae combining form of the root *gingival,* meaning *gum;* the *-ae* ending makes the word plural	the gums; the tissue surrounding the sockets of the teeth
glossology	gloss/o + ology combining form of *glossa,* meaning *tongue*	the study of the tongue and its diseases; also known as *glottology*
linguoversion	lingu/o + version combining form of the root *lingua,* meaning *tongue; version* is a noun that is formed from the root *versio,* meaning *to turn or turning*	the turning of or displacement of a tooth toward the tongue
laryngopathy	laryngo/o + pathy combining form of *larynx,* meaning *upper windpipe; -pathy* means *disease*	disease of the larynx
oral labia	*oro-* means *pertaining to the mouth;* *labia* is the plural form of *labium,* meaning *lips or a fleshy border*	lips of the mouth; oral lips
pharyngeal	pharyng/o- + eal combining form of *pharynx,* meaning *throat*	concerning the throat
tonsillectomy	tonsil/a + ectomy combining form of *tonsilla,* meaning *tonsil*	surgical removal of the tonsils

Build a Word

You have become acquainted with the roots and combining forms of key terms for the anatomy of the oral cavity. Using your knowledge of how medical terminology is constructed, complete the following exercise by creating new terms from the word parts given. You may not yet be familiar with all of these terms. Take your time, and use your new knowledge and word-recognition skills to help you decipher them. Remember, you may need to change the spelling of some of the word parts that you have been given. When you are ready, check your answers in the Answer Key.

1. gingiv/a -al bucc/o ____________ Meaning: ____________
2. plasty pharyng/o ____________ Meaning: ____________
3. laryng/o -eal pharyng/o ____________ Meaning: ____________
4. gingiv/o itis gloss/o ____________ Meaning: ____________
5. -ectomy laryng/o pharyng/o ____________ Meaning: ____________
6. gingiv -al linguo ____________ Meaning: ____________
7. graph gloss/o ____________ Meaning: ____________
8. gloss/a -al pharyng/o ____________ Meaning: ____________
9. itis tonsil/a ____________ Meaning: ____________
10. -ar tonsil/a ____________ Meaning: ____________

Right Word or Wrong Word: *Palate* or *Pallet*?

These two words sound the same, but do they have the same meaning?

Key terms: the teeth

Each tooth has two main parts: the crown and the root. The *crown* is made up of enamel, dentin, and pulp. *Enamel* covers the tooth and hardens it. *Dentin* is the main substance of the tooth. *Pulp* is made up of the nerves and blood vessels that supply the tooth.

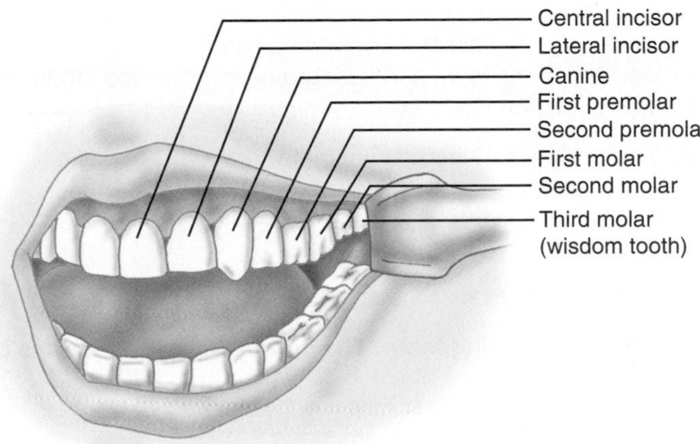

Figure 6.6: The teeth

Names of Teeth

Adults have 32 permanent teeth, which are identified by their location and function. Figure 6-6 shows the names of different kinds of teeth.

Surfaces of Teeth

Dentists also need to identify which side or surface of a tooth they are assessing or treating.

A *facial surface* is a tooth surface that faces the outside of the mouth. There are two kinds of facial surfaces. Teeth with a *labial surface* face the lips; these include the incisors and the canines. Teeth with a *buccal surface* face the cheeks; these include the molars and premolars.

A tooth surface that faces the inside of the mouth is called *lingual* or *palatal*. The back of a bottom tooth has a *lingual surface*, which faces the tongue. The back of a top tooth has a *palatal surface*, which faces the palate.

Molars and premolars also have an *occlusal surface*, which is the part of the upper and lower molars that comes in contact when a person bites down or clenches the teeth.

To learn more words related to teeth, study the combining forms of *dent/o/i* and *odont/o* that follow.

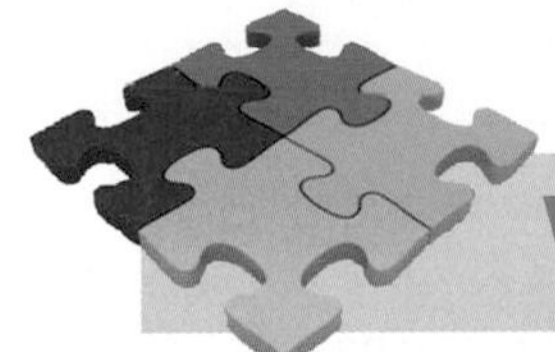

WORD BUILDING: Formula for Creating Words with the Combining Forms *Dent/o/i* and *Odont/o*

1. dens = Latin root meaning *teeth.* The combining form is *dent/o/i.*

dento + faci + al = *dentofacial*

Definition: concerning the teeth and the face. (The combining form of the root *facies* is *faci,* meaning *face.*) *adjective*

Example: *Dentofacial* abnormalities, such as a smile with excessive presentation of the gums, are not uncommon.

denti+ labi + al = *dentilabial*

Definition: pertaining to both the teeth and the lips. The combining form of the root *labia* means *lips. adjective*

Example: A *dentilabial* analysis studies the relationship between the teeth and the lips, such as an assessment of a smile.

Continued

denti + tion = *dentition*

Definition: the development of the teeth and their arrangement in the mouth; referring to all of the natural teeth in the mouth. *noun*

Example: Adult *dentition* includes 32 permanent teeth.

dent + algia = *dentalgia*

Definition: tooth pain. *noun*

Example: *Dentalgia* is another word for *toothache.*

2. odous = early Greek root meaning *teeth.* The combining forms form is *odont/o.*

odonto + genesis = *odontogenesis*

Definition: the origin and formation of new teeth. *noun*

Example: *Odontogenesis* begins in the embryo and proceeds to the eruption of teeth after birth.

odonto + rrhagia = *odontorrhagia*

Definition: hemorrhage from the socket when a tooth is extracted or knocked out. *noun*

Example: Clients suffer *odontorrhagia* when their front teeth are knocked out during sports injuries.

odont + erism = *odonterism*

Definition: chattering teeth. (The second word part derives from the Greek word *erismos,* meaning *quarrel.*) *noun*

Example: When the body gets cold, muscles contract to produce heat-generating shivering and *odonterism.*

peri + odont + al = *periodontal*

Definition: referring to bacterial infection around the teeth and gums. (The prefix *peri-* means *around or surrounding.*) *adjective*

Example: Gingivitis (gum disease) is a mild form of *periodontal* disease.

Let's Practice

Write the term or terms that best identify what is being described.

1. gum disease ______________________
2. bleeding, tooth missing ______________________
3. pain or swelling along the jaw and tooth ______________________
4. pertaining to cosmetic dentistry and smiles ______________________
5. concerned with the assessment, diagnosis, and treatment of the teeth and the structures of the mouth ______________________

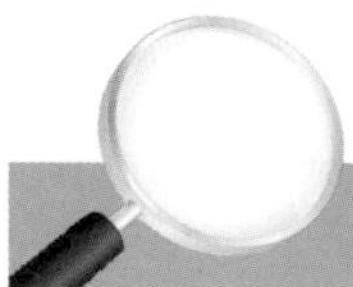

FOCUS POINT: Endodontists and Orthodontists

Endodontists and orthodontists are dental specialists. *Endodontists* are experts in diagnosing and relieving mouth pain, and they are concerned with dental pathology. *Orthodontists* specialize in the assessment, prevention, treatment, and care of irregularities in the arrangement of teeth.

Key terms: the jaw

The jaw is made up of three large bones: the mandible and two maxillae. All of these bones contain and anchor the teeth.

maxillae: bones that sit anterior on the skull inferior to the cranium and that connect at the zygomatic bone. The maxillae are fused together and give the appearance of one solid bone that is slightly arched and horizontal across the face. The maxillae form the upper jaw. They function to shape and protect the oral and nasal cavities and the floor of the orbits. The maxillae are fixed (immovable).

mandible: bone that sits inferior to the maxillae. The mandible is a large horseshoe- or u-shaped bone that stretches between the ears and includes the chin. The mandible forms the lower jaw. It is a movable bone by way of its bilateral joints. Its ability to move permits both biting and chewing.

temporomandibular joints (TMJs): bilateral joints that connect the mandible to the upper facial skeleton near the ears. The temporomandibular joints are hinge joints.

condyle: the rounded end of the mandible that fits into the joints. There is one condyle on each side or end of the bone.

coronoid process: triangular area of the distal end of the mandible that connects a muscle of mastication (chewing) with the bone. There are coronoid processes on the mandible.

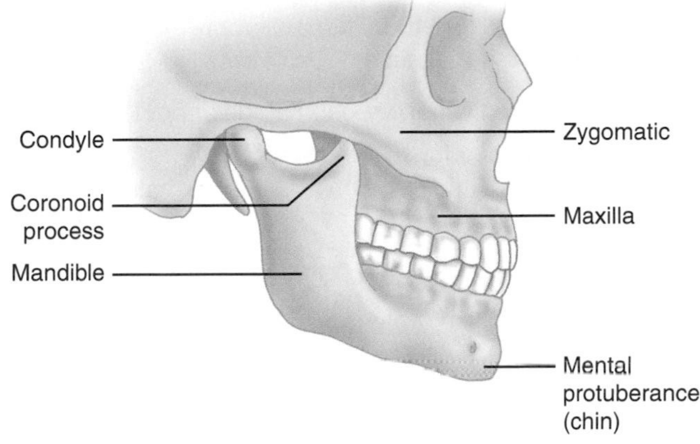

Figure 6.7: The jaw

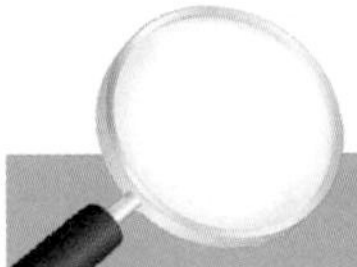

FOCUS POINT: The Chin

The anatomical term for the chin is the *mentum* or the *mental protuberance.* It is part of the mandible.

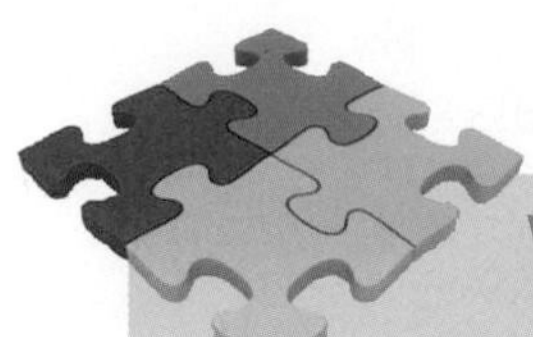

WORD BUILDING: Formula for Creating Words with the Combining Forms of *Maxilla*

maxilla = the upper jawbone. The combining form is *maxillo-*.

maxilla + ary = *maxillary*

Definition: pertaining to the upper jaw. *adjective*

Example: Acute *maxillary* sinusitis is a bacterial infection.

maxillo + jugal = *maxillojugal*

Definition: pertaining to the maxilla and the zygomatic bones. The second root *jugal* means *connected* and refers to the zygomatic bones. *adjective*

Example: The point where the maxilla and the zygomatic bones come together is called the *maxillojugal suture.*

maxillo + mandibul + ar = *maxillomandibular*

Definition: pertaining to both the maxilla and mandibular bones; the full jaw. *adjective*

Example: *Maxillomandibular* fixation is commonly referred to as "wiring the jaws."

maxillo + tomy = *maxillotomy*

Definition: surgical incision of the maxilla. *noun*

Example: A *maxillotomy* is performed when a section of the upper jaw is malformed, injured, or requires reshaping.

Let's Practice

Write the term or terms that best identify what is being described

1. joint that connects the upper and lower jaws ____________________
2. movable bone in the face ____________________
3. pyramid-shaped region of bone that connects to jaw muscles ____________________
4. anatomical term for the chin ____________________
5. wiring the jaws shut ____________________

Free Writing

Use each of the words and word parts given to create a logical sentence. You may need to add verbs, articles, and so on. Work alone, with a partner, or in a small group.

Example: voice lost -itis
Sentence: She is suffering from laryngitis and has lost her voice.

1. tonsils when -ectomy 10 years old ____________________
2. dentist -itis gingival inflammation gums ____________________
3. joints dislocate possible temporomandibular jaw ____________________
4. term bucca cheek ____________________

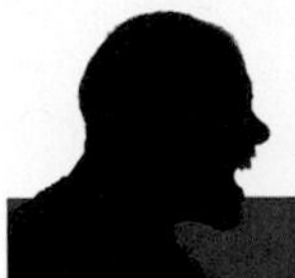

PRONUNCIATION PRACTICE

Say these words aloud to a friend or classmate if you can. You are given the phonetic pronunciation. Your instructor can help you with pronunciation,

or visit **http://www.MedicalLanguageLab.com.**

buccal	**bŭk´**ăl
buccogingival	bŭk″kō-**jĭn´**jĭ-văl
condyle	**kŏn´**dīl
coronoid	**kor´**ō-noyd
gingivae	jĭn-**jī´**vā
gingivoglossitis	jĭn″jī-vō-glŏs-**sī´**tĭs
glossology	glŏ-**sŏl´**ō-jē
labia	**lā´**bē-ă
larynx	**lăr´**ĭnks
laryngopathy	lăr″ĭn-**gŏp´**ă-thē
laryngopharyngectomy	lăr″ĭn″gō-făr-ĭn-**jĕk´**tō-mē
maxillojugal	măk-sĭl″ō-**jū´**găl
occlusal	ŏ-**kloo´**zăl
pharynx	**făr´**ĭnks
pharyngeal	făr-**ĭn´**jē-ăl
pharyngolaryngeal	fă-rĭng″gō-lă-**rĭn´**jē-ăl
saliva	să-**lī´**vă
uvula	**ū´**vū-lă

The language of craniofacial assessment

The face can be divided into three anatomical regions. The upper third includes the area above the *superior orbital margin*. The second third includes the area between the superior orbital margin and the *occlusal plane* below it. The lower third of the face is the mandible. Notice that Dr. Lincoln assessed the patient, Clay Davis, by describing each of these regions. All diagnostic imaging methods (radiographs, computed tomography scans, and so on) refer to these three regions as well. However, it would be unlikely that x-rays would be ordered for routine facial assessment unless there was some evidence of trauma. Assessment under normal circumstances is performed via visual inspection and palpation. In the case of facial trauma, inspection, palpation, and radiography are employed.

The middle third of the face is also delineated by invisible lines called *Le Fort lines* (see Figure 6-8). It is equally as common to hear health professionals refer to these lines.

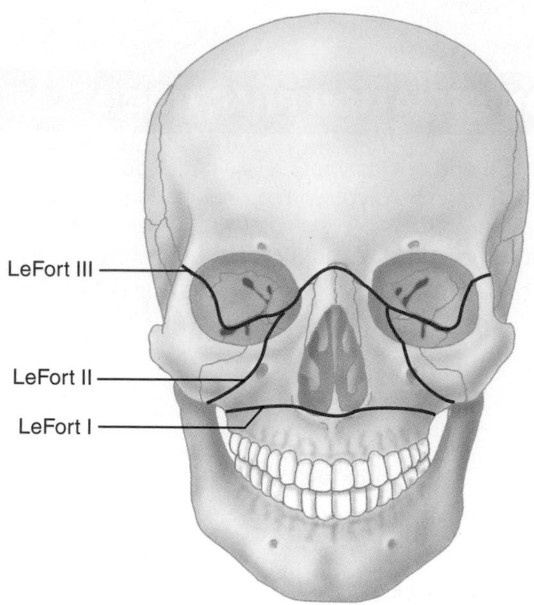

Figure 6.8: Facial skeleton: Le Fort lines

The craniofacial complex

The **craniofacial complex** includes the dental, oral, and craniofacial tissues that house the sense organs. Sight, sound, smell, and taste result from signals that come from the cranial nerves. Craniofacial assessment includes not only the overt exterior structures of the face but also the fine microscopic workings of the cranial nerves.

Our patient, Clay Davis, will eventually have a cranial nerve assessment because of the trauma to his face. As you can see from Table 6-4 and Figure 6-9, a number of cranial nerves are located in this area of trauma.

Cranial nerves

Craniofacial tissues and other tissues are innervated or stimulated by the cranial nerves. There are 12 of these nerves, and they come in pairs. They are always referred to in writing by Roman numerals: for example, cranial nerve IX. Cranial nerves transmit both sensory or motor messages. There are two main types:

Afferent nerves: These are sensory nerves that carry messages from the sense organs toward the spinal cord and the brain.

Efferent nerves: These are motor nerves that carry messages from the brain to the spinal cord and into the body.

TABLE 6-4: Numbers, Names, and Functions of the Cranial Nerves

Cranial Nerve Number	Name	Function
I	olfactory	sensory: smell • transmits smell from the nasal mucous membranes to the brain
II	optic	sensory: vision • transmits visual impulses from the eyes to the brain
III	oculomotor	motor: movement of the eyelids and the eyeballs • contracts the eye muscles, constricts the pupils, elevates the eyelids, and controls eye movements (interior, lateral, medial, and superior)
IV	trochlear	motor: turns the eye downward and laterally • contracts a single eye muscle that is responsible for eye movement centrally and below the orbit
V	trigeminal	sensory and motor: face and mouth sensation, chewing, and biting • transmits sensory impulses of pain, touch, and temperature from the face to the brain • influences chewing and biting through clenching and lateral jaw movements
VI	abducens	motor: moves and turns the eye to the side • controls lateral eye movement
VII	facial	Sensory and motor: facial expressions, taste, saliva, and tears • senses taste on the anterior two thirds of the tongue • stimulates secretions from the salivary glands that are located at submaxillary and sublingual sites • stimulates secretions from the lacrimal glands (tear ducts) • innervates facial muscles and facilitates expressions
VIII	acoustic or vestibulocochlear	sensory: balance and hearing • consists of the sensory fibers that affect hearing and equilibrium
IX	glossopharyngeal	sensory and motor: senses the carotid blood pressure; also affects taste and swallowing • senses taste on the posterior third of the tongue • stimulates the gag reflex of the pharynx • stimulates the parotid salivary glands • promotes swallowing movements
X	vagus	sensory and motor: senses the aortic blood pressure, affects the heart rate, stimulates digestion, and senses taste • transmits sensations from the pharynx, larynx, heart, lungs, bronchi, gastrointestinal tract, and abdominal organs • stimulates the slowing of the heart rate • promotes swallowing and talking • promotes digestion
XI	spinal accessory	motor: controls the neck muscles and facilitates swallowing • innervates the trapezius and sternocleidomastoid muscles, thus promoting the movement of the shoulders and head rotation • promotes some movement of the larynx (voice box)
XII	hypoglossal	motor: influences tongue movement • innervates the tongue muscle, thus promoting the movement of food and talking

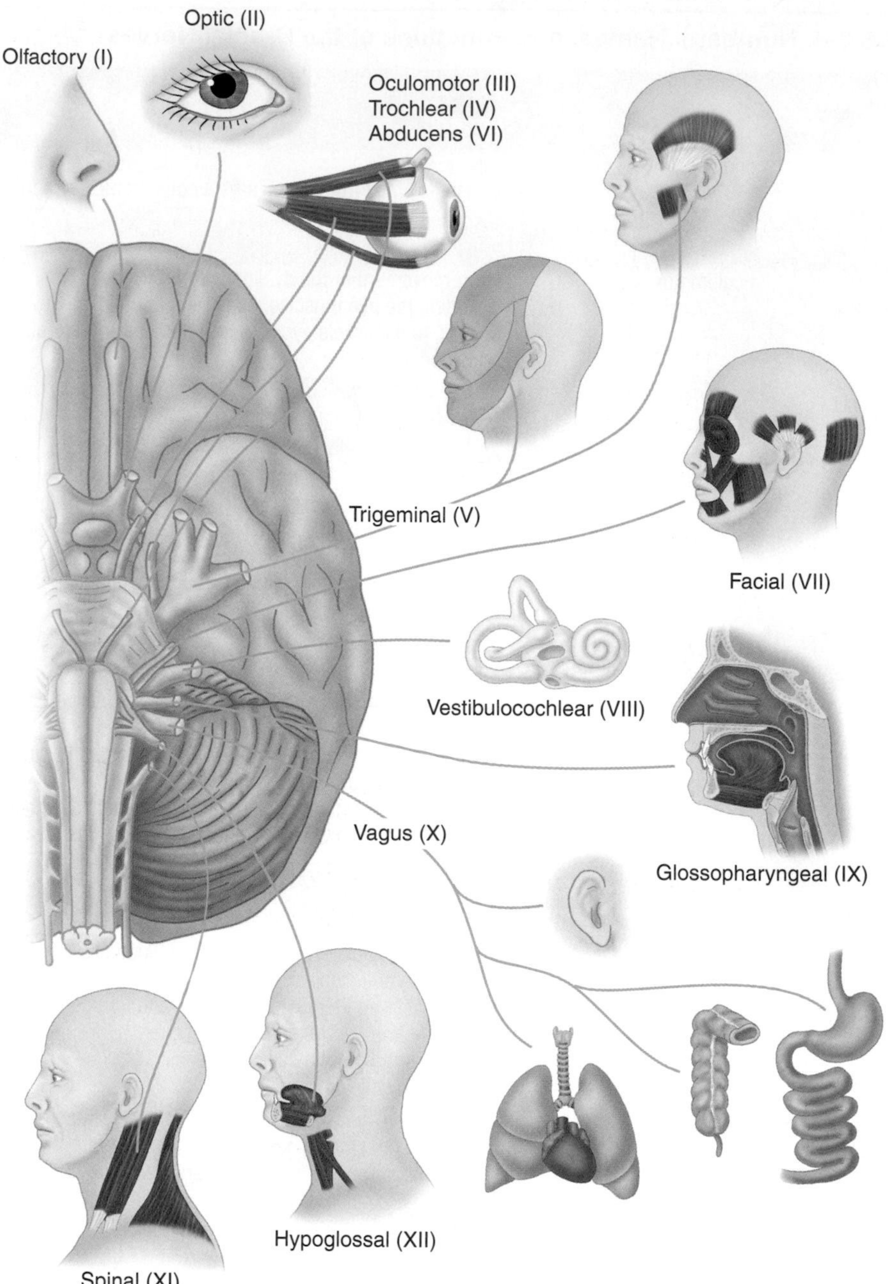

Figure 6.9: Cranial nerves

Critical Thinking

Use your new knowledge and language skills to answer the following questions.

1. Four of the cranial nerves transmit both motor and sensory impulses. Identify them.

 ____

 ____

2. What is an afferent nerve? ______________________

3. Which cranial nerve is responsible for hearing and equilibrium? ______________

4. In general, what is the function of cranial nerves? ______________________

5. Clay Davis is a candidate for a cranial nerve assessment, and so is the patient Gil Loeppky, whom you read about in Chapter 4. Explain why Mr. Loeppky might require this type of assessment.

____

Mix and Match

Match the function on the left with the cranial nerve on the right by drawing a line to connect them. This exercise requires that you apply your new terminology and critical thinking skills.

1. dizziness	I. olfactory
2. kiss	II. optic
3. wink	III. oculomotor
4. sight	VIII. vestibulocochlear
5. gag	IX. glossopharyngeal
6. tears	VII. facial
7. smell	VII. facial

PRONUNCIATION PRACTICE

Say these words aloud to a friend or classmate if you can. You are given the phonetic pronunciation. Your instructor can help you with pronunciation,

or visit **http://www.MedicalLanguageLab.com.**

abducens	ăb-**dū**´sĕnz
glossopharyngeal	glŏs″ō-fă-**rĭn**´jē-ăl
olfactory	ŏl-**făk**´tō-rē
oculomotor	ŏk″ū-lō-**mō**´tor
trigeminal	trī-**jĕm**´ĭn-ăl
trochlear	**trŏk**´lē-ăr
vagus	**vā**´gus

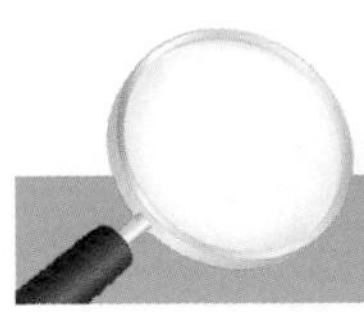

FOCUS POINT: Otolaryngologist

An otolaryngologist is a physician with a specialty in illnesses of the ears, nose, and throat. This specialist is also referred to as "an ENT." The foci of otolaryngology include the ears, nose, throat, sinuses, face, and neck.

The language of dental diagnostics

Patient Update

A hospital social worker has been able to locate Clay Davis's parents. They are in transit now, and they are expected at the trauma center momentarily. Mr. and Mrs. Davis have given verbal permission for their son to have further assessment tests. Dr. Sandor, the dental surgeon, suspects that Clay has a mandibular fracture. The patient is now quickly being transported to the diagnostic imaging department, where he will undergo a panorex radiograph, a series of x-rays, and a computed tomography (CT) scan. The diagnostic images will focus particularly on the bones and structures of the face, with attention paid to the nose and jaw as well, and they will include radiographs of the skull per the orders of the pediatrician, Dr. Raymond.

Clay is conscious, and he remains in the spinal fixation collar. He is being transported by stretcher in a semi-Fowler's position to promote ease of oral and nasal drainage, thereby limiting the risk of aspiration or choking. A urinary catheter is in situ to facilitate his need to remain immobile for now, and his burn has been covered with a sterile burn sheet. He has been started on intravenous (IV) fluids to ensure that he remains hydrated. A low pediatric dose of the analgesic morphine was administered through the IV because Clay is unable to take any medication by mouth. The medication has helped to relieve some of the acute pain from his jaw and burn. Clay's face has been cleansed by one of the ER nursing staff. He is in a hospital gown, and he understands that his mom and dad will be arriving shortly.

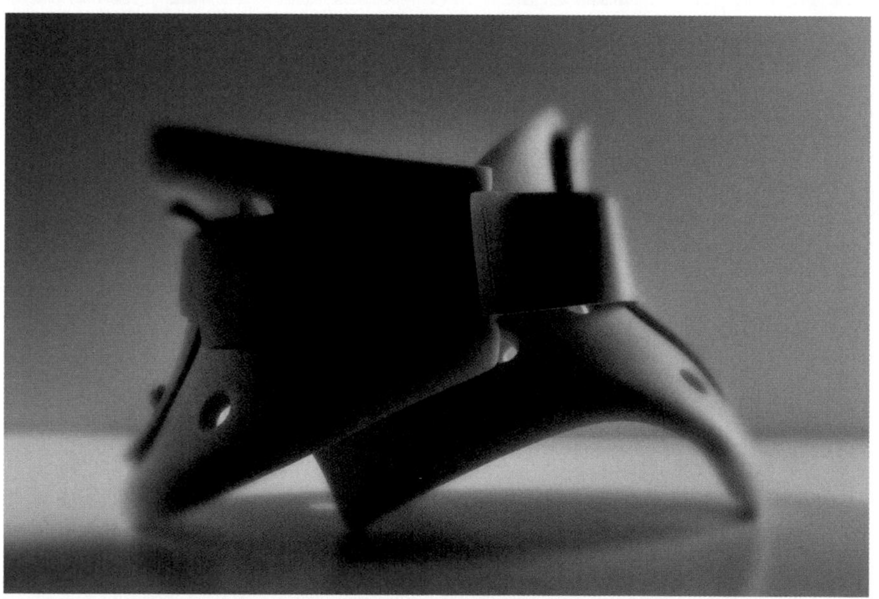

Critical Thinking

Answer the following questions on the basis of the patient update.

1. Dr. Sandor suspects that Clay has experienced which serious injury?

   ____

2. In which position is the patient being transported? ____________________
3. For what is the patient still at risk? ____________________

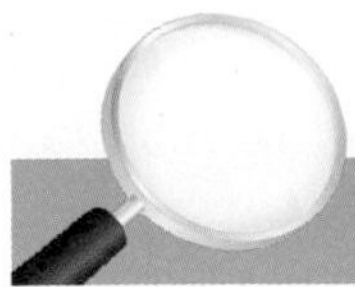

FOCUS POINT: Sterile Burn Sheet

Sterile cotton burn sheets are designed to prevent infection and further trauma to a burn site. The emergency medical technician or the hospital treatment team will make a clinical decision regarding whether the burn sheet should be used wet or dry. These sheets are used dry for third-degree burns, and they may be either wet or dry for first- and second-degree burns. (You will learn more about burns later in this chapter.)

TABLE 6-5: Diagnostic Terms: Dental Emergencies

Diagnostic Terms: Dental Emergencies	Meaning
avulsion(s)	separation of a tooth from the gums, usually as a result of trauma; during the process, the tooth may cut into or split the lip; synonymous with *evulsion*
extraoral wounds	facial injuries around the oral cavity
intraoral examination	examination inside of the mouth or oral cavity
intraoral wounds	injuries inside the oral cavity
parasymphyseal fracture	a fracture of the bones in the areas bilateral to the midline (symphysis) of the jaw but excluding the midline
subluxation	a partial or incomplete dislocation of the jaw, a tooth, or teeth
symphyseal fracture	a fracture at the midline of the mandible, usually caused by direct blunt force trauma or violence

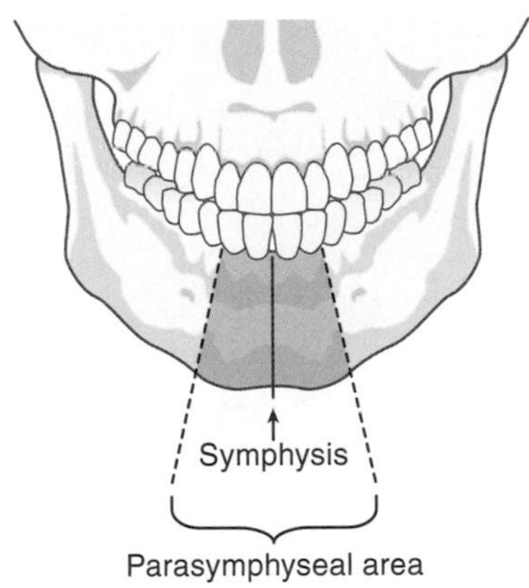

Figure 6.10: Mandible: symphyseal and parasymphyseal areas

Let's Practice

Write the term or terms that best identify what is being described.

1. tooth has cut into the lip ____________________
2. involving half of the face ____________________
3. laceration above the upper lip ____________________
4. tooth remains in socket after injury but is facing the wrong direction ____________________
5. the ability to bite or close the teeth together is affected ____________________

TABLE 6-6: Prefixes Used in Dental Assessment and Diagnosis

Prefix	Meaning	Prefix	Meaning
extra-	in addition to; outside	mal-	bad; not good; poor or abnormal
hemi-	half	sub-	below or beneath; underneath
intra-	within		

Right Word or Wrong Word: *Intra-* or *Inter-*?

Do these two prefixes mean the same thing?

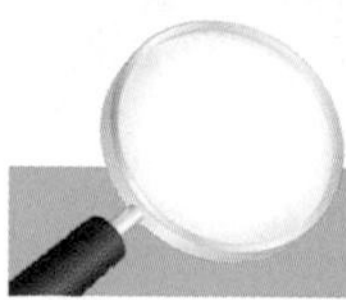

FOCUS POINT: Subluxation

The term *subluxation* is not used solely in dentistry; it is used for the assessment and treatment of the skeletal system as well. For example, you can expect to see, hear, and use the word *subluxation* in the fields of orthopedics, orthotics, and chiropractic physical therapy.

Mix and Match

Match the prefix with the proper term.

1. sub-	lingual
2. intra-	facial
3. hemi-	maxillary
4. extra-	ocular
5. inter-	cranial

Maxillofacial radiographs

As you will recall from the opening scene of this chapter, Clay Davis was about to be treated by Dr. Sandor, a maxillofacial dental surgeon. She has ordered a series of routine and maxillofacial radiographs of the patient's face.

Maxillofacial radiographs are a series of x-rays that begin at the upper portion of the face, which is called the **nasoethmoid**, and that then proceed downward to the mandible. These x-rays provide pertinent images for the diagnostic process by revealing fractures, deformities, occlusion, and malocclusion. **Occlusion** refers to the relationship between the upper and lower teeth when the jaw is closed.

Dr. Sandor is particularly interested in obtaining a *mandibular series* of *diagnostic images (mandibular radiographs)*. This series includes images taken from a posteroanterior (PA) view, a Towne view (also known as an anteroposterior [AP] axial view), and bilateral oblique views. Table 6-7 describes the differences among these types of images.

A computed tomography scan has also been ordered for the patient. Along with panorex imaging (see Table 6-7 and Figure 6-11), this type of imaging is considered the best diagnostic tool for assessing the bones, facial structures, and tissues. However, a CT scan that focuses on a possible mandibular fracture may be difficult to attain. The patient would have to hyperextend his neck, but this is impossible because he is in a spinal fixation collar.

Other types of facial radiographs include the following:

Occlusal radiographs are taken with the film placed between the teeth. These images can confirm a symphysis fracture, which is one that occurs midline on the mandible.

Lateral radiographs assess all parts of the face. They are particularly used to view the mandible and the ramus, which is the vertical portion of the mandible. These radiographs can be done at the bedside or in a dental chair; the patient can be in a supine position.

Occipitomental radiographs view the maxilla, the zygomatic area, and the orbital floor.

TABLE 6-7: Mandibular Series of Radiographic Views

Type of Radiographic View	Focus
posteroanterior (PA)	assesses the mandible; can identify a parasymphyseal fracture; shows the orbital rims, the nasal septum, the nasal fossa, and the sinuses
Towne view (anteroposterior [AP] axial)	assesses the mandibular condyles, the mandibular symphysis, and the occipital bone
bilateral oblique	assesses the mandible as a whole
panoramic topographic (panorex)	views the entire mandible, particularly the condyles (Note: A panorex machine may not always be available in smaller facilities, so general x-rays will suffice.)

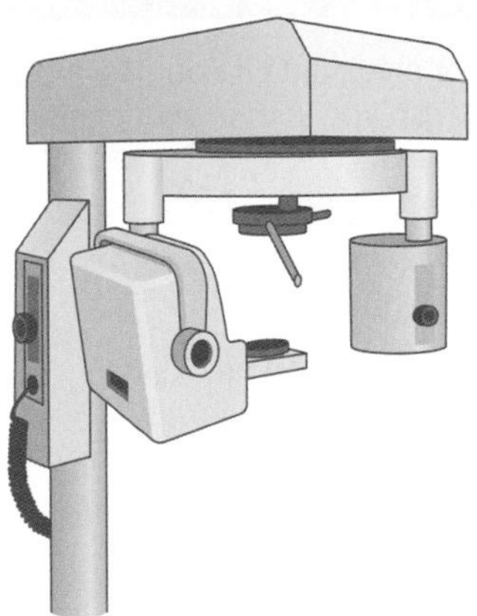

Figure 6.11: Panorex machine

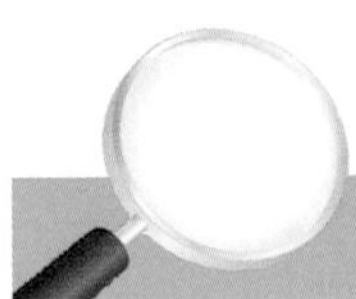

FOCUS POINT: Orthopantomogram

An orthopantomogram is a newer piece of radiographic technology that allows the entire dentition and the surrounding bone to be captured on one continuous image. This machine is not yet available in all facilities. The image that it creates is called an *orthopantomograph.*

Eponyms: René Le Fort

René Le Fort was a prominent French surgeon of the late 19th and early 20th centuries, and his specialty was facial fractures. Le Fort I, II, and III fractures occur along one of the Le Fort lines of the face; the term for each type of fracture includes the number of the corresponding Le Fort line.

Le Fort I fracture: a transverse maxillary fracture in which the nose is not compromised.

Le Fort II fracture: a fracture that spans the frontal process of the maxilla and involves the orbital floor but that does not involve the midface.

Le Fort III fracture: a fracture that includes a complete craniofacial separation and that involves the nasofrontal suture line and the frontozygomatic sutures.

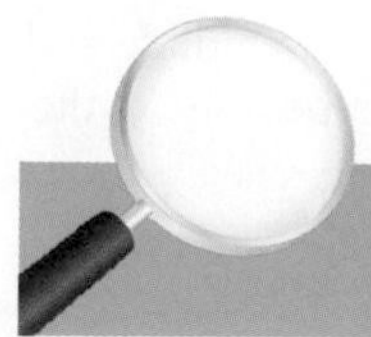

FOCUS POINT: A Le Fort Fracture vs. a Le Fort I, II, or III Fracture

Be very careful. In medical terminology, it is critical that you use terms correctly and specifically.

When referring to a Le Fort fracture of the facial skeleton, you MUST NAME it by including the number. Without a number following it, the term *Le Fort facture* refers to a longitudinal break in the distal fibula of the leg. Although Le Fort I, II, and III facial fractures are named after the French physician René Le Fort, the Le Fort leg fracture is named after Léon Clément Le Fort, who was another French surgeon.

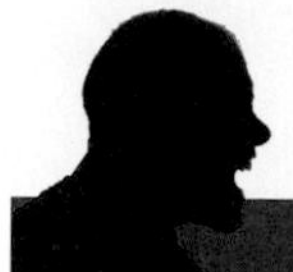

PRONUNCIATION PRACTICE

Say these words aloud to a friend or classmate if you can. You are given the phonetic pronunciation. Your instructor can help you with pronunciation,

or visit **http://www.MedicalLanguageLab.com.**

avulsion	ă-**vŭl**´shŭn
maxillofacial	măks-ĭl″ō-**fā**´shăl
occipitomental	ŏk-sĭp″ĭ-tō-**mĕn**´tăl
orthopantograph	or″thō-**păn**´tō-grăf
subluxation	sŭb″lŭks-**ā**´shŭn
symphyseal	sĭm-**fĭz**´ē-ăl

The Language of the Integumentary System

In addition to his facial and dental trauma, Clay Davis has a secondary injury: a partial-thickness burn (dermal burn) to his upper torso. To understand burn injuries, you need to learn the language of the skin and integumentary system.

Anatomy and physiology: the integumentary system

The integumentary system consists of the skin and the accessory organs of the nails, hair, sebum, and sweat. The skin is an organ that is made up of three layers:

- The **epidermis** is the top or outer layer of the skin.
- The **derma or dermis** is the layer of skin just under the epidermis. It is known as the "true skin." Synonyms for this word are *corium* and *cutis vera* (which means *true skin*).
- The *subcutaneous layer* is a thin layer of tissue under the dermis. This tissue contains nerve cells and tiny blood vessels. It is sometimes referred to as the **hypodermis.**

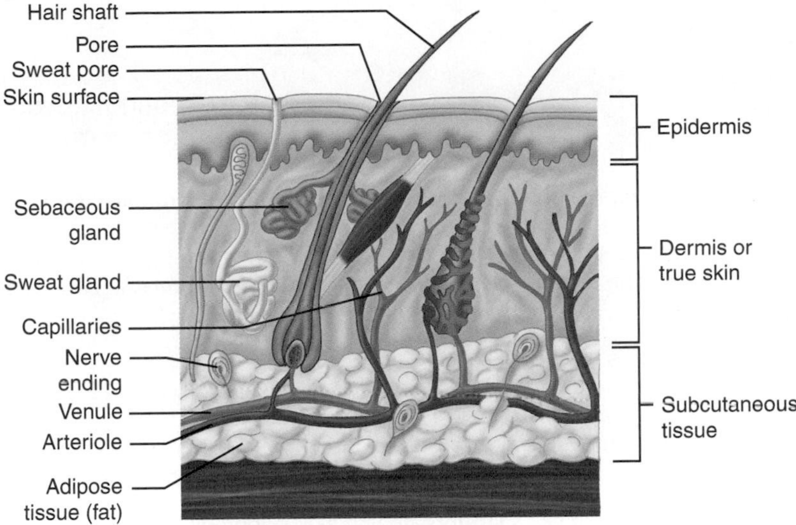

Figure 6.12: Cross section of the skin

The integumentary system also includes a variety of membranes (see Chapter 11). The function of the integumentary system is to protect the inner body from external threats such as temperature, injury, bites, stings, and contact allergens. The skin is the body's first line of defense.

Key terms: integumentary system

integument: a root word meaning covering. The integumentary system provides external coverage for the entire body.

sebum: a fatty, grease-like secretion that originates in the sebaceous glands of the skin.

sweat or perspiration: an emission of clear, odorous moisture through the pores of the skin. Sweat originates in the sudoriferous (sweat) glands within the skin and subcutaneous tissues. The purpose of sweat is to cool the skin and the body as it evaporates off the surface of the skin.

unguis: the nail of the finger or toe.

TABLE 6-8: Medical Terms: Integumentary System

Medical or Anatomical Term	Word Deconstruction	Meaning
dermatitis	Word Deconstruction derm or derma roots meaning *skin* -itis	inflammation of the skin caused by disease or allergens
cutaneous	suffix meaning *inflammation* cutaneo- combining form of the root *cutis,* meaning *both the epidermis and dermis layers of the skin tissue* -ous	pertaining to the skin
sebaceous	suffix meaning *having a certain quality* sebo- combining form of *sebum,* meaning *grease* -eous prefix meaning *having a certain quality*	describing a grease-like or oily substance, particularly on the body or in the hair
polyunguia	unguia combining form of *unguis,* meaning nail	an excessive number of nails; also known as *polyonychia,* which is a rare congenital condition

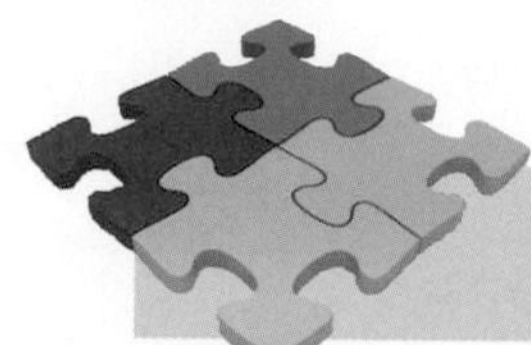

WORD BUILDING: Formula for Creating Words with the Combining Forms *Derm/at/ato-*

derma or dermis = Greek root meaning *skin.* The combining forms are *derm/at/at-*.

dermato + cyst = *dermatocyst*

Definition: a skin cyst. The second root, *cyst,* means *a sac or bladder-like structure filled with fluid. noun*

Example: A *dermatocyst* is filled with fluid.

dermato + fibr + oma = *dermatofibroma*

Definition: a benign, firm, movable skin nodule found under the skin; also known as a *histiocytoma.* (The combining form *fibra* means *fiber.* The suffix *-oma* means *tumor.*) *noun*

Example: A *dermatofibroma* is not a life-threatening skin condition.

derma + tome = *dermatome*

Definition: an instrument used for cutting fine slices of skin, such as those used for skin transplantation. (The suffix *-tome* means *incision.*) *noun*

Example: *Dermatomes* are instruments that are used in skin grafting and plastic surgery.

dermato + path + y = *dermatopathy*

Definition: skin disease, including bacterial and fungal infections; also known as *dermopathy. noun*

Example: A dermatologist assesses and treats many different kinds of *dermatopathy.*

dermato + phyte = *dermatophyte*

Definition: a fungal infection of the skin. (The suffix *-phyte* means *plant* and is used in medical terms to refer to fungi and fungal parasites. *noun*

Example: A well known *dermatophyte* is the tinea, which causes athlete's foot (also known as *dermatophytosis*).

dermato + rrhexis = *dermatorrhexis*

Definition: a rupture of the skin and its capillaries. *noun*

Example: *Dermatorrhexis* is a skin laceration in which the cut is superficial and there is minimal (if any) bleeding.

TABLE 6-9: Prefixes and Suffixes: Integumentary System

BEGIN with a Prefix	ADD a Root or Combining Form	ADD a Suffix	CREATE a New Term
epi- (over, upon, or in addition to)	dermis		epidermis (the outermost or surface layer of the skin) Example: The sun can burn the *epidermis.*
hypo-	dermis		hypodermis (below the skin) Example: The subcutaneous layer of skin is also known as the *hypodermis.*
sub-	cutaneo	-eous	subcutaneous (under the skin) Example: The patient received a *subcutaneous* injection.

Build a Word

Combine each set of word parts to create a medical term, and then define each term in your own words. Some terms you will already know, whereas others will be new to you. However, you will be able to figure out the definitions of these words by analyzing the meaning of each word part.

1. cranium epi ____________ Meaning: ____________
2. mucosa sub ____________ Meaning: ____________
3. epi itis derm ____________ Meaning: ____________
4. vascul derma -ar ____________ Meaning: ____________

PRONUNCIATION PRACTICE

Say these words aloud to a friend or classmate if you can. You are given the phonetic pronunciation. Your instructor can help you with pronunciation,

or visit **http://www.MedicalLanguageLab.com.** mll

cutaneous	kŭ-**tā**´nē-ŭs
derma	**dĕr**´mă
epidermitis	ĕp″ĭ-dĕr-**mī**´tĭs
integument	ĭn-**tĕg**″ū-mĕnt
polyunguia	pŏl″ē-**ŭng**´gwē-ă
sebum	**sē**´bŭm
sebaceous	sē-**bā**´shŭs
sudoriferous	sū-dor-**ĭf**´ĕr-ŭs
unguis	**ŭng**´gwĭs

The language of burns

A **burn** is a type of tissue injury that can be caused by chemicals, electricity, radioactive agents, or exposure to temperatures of more than 120°F. When a burn is severe, blood flow to the site is impaired. As a result, the body may be unable to heal, and cell death can occur. Burns can also send the body into shock. The body is at risk for dehydration and organ system failure when responding to extreme heat.

Types of burns

Identification of the type of burn is critical to the provision of care.

Thermal burns are caused by fire, steam, hot liquids, or hot objects. They are identified by the percentage of the body involved and the depth of the burn into the skin.

Chemical burns are caused by contact with acids and other chemicals that destroy living tissue.

Electrical burns are the result of contact with an electrical current or lightning.

Light burns are caused by exposure to intense light sources, including ultraviolet light (i.e., the sun).

Radiation burns can also be caused by ultraviolet light as well as by nuclear radiation.

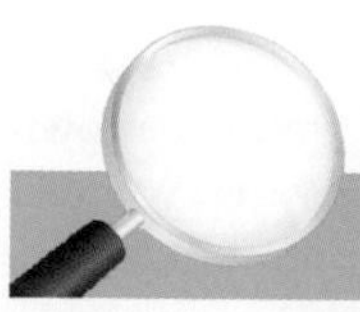

FOCUS POINT: Shock

Shock is a medical term that identifies a crisis of the body or mind. A traumatic event puts the complete human organism into a state of alert to cope. The natural "fight-or-flight" response kicks in to preserve life: adrenaline is released to provide strength for the core organs so that they might tolerate and cope with the situation, and the heart and respiration rates increase as well. Various steroids are released to provide muscle strength, and the pupils dilate. The abilities to look and listen become highly focused on the perceived threat at hand and nothing else.

Physical trauma can be life threatening in its own right, but the addition of the systemic natural shock process, also called *shock syndrome,* can complicate treatment and recovery. Assessment for shock and the prevention of the adverse physical effects of shock are key elements of emergency care.

Scalds

It appears that our patient, Clay Davis, may have a scald burn. Scalds are the most commonly seen type of burn in young children. They are usually the result of contact with hot liquids, foods, or cooking utensils. Although scalds are dangerous and can be physically and emotionally scarring, they are rarely life threatening. This depends, of course, on the length of time of contact with the scalding agent and the depth of the burn.

Burn assessment: The Rule of Nines

One standard method for assessing burns is the Rule of Nines. The **Rule of Nines for Burns** identifies the total *body surface area (BSA)* affected by the burn (see Figure 6-13). It is a universally accepted tool used to assess the extent of burns and also to calculate safe and appropriate medication dosages and amounts of IV fluids to be administered. For example, the anterior surface of the torso makes up 18% of a person's total body surface area. Clay Davis has a burn to the anterior upper torso, so between 9% and 18% of his total body surface has been burned. In addition, Dr. Lincoln identified Clay's injury as a partial-thickness, second-degree burn.

Burn assessment: by degree

First-degree burns are limited to the epidermis. They heal themselves within days, and they do not leave a scar. There is mild pain and discomfort associated with this burn. An example of a first-degree burn is common sunburn. Medical treatment is not required. First-degree burns are also called **superficial burns**.

Second-degree burns extend into the dermis but do not injure or destroy all of the dermis. The skin appears swollen and red, and blisters form. There is a good deal of pain involved during the acute phase of this type of burn, and medical treatment may be required. These are also known as **partial-thickness burns**.

Third-degree burns involve the destruction of the dermis. Subcutaneous tissue is left exposed. There is no pain involved because the nerve endings have been destroyed. Visually, these burns look leathery and dry, and they may be white in color. Medical treatment is absolutely required. These are also known as **full-thickness burns**.

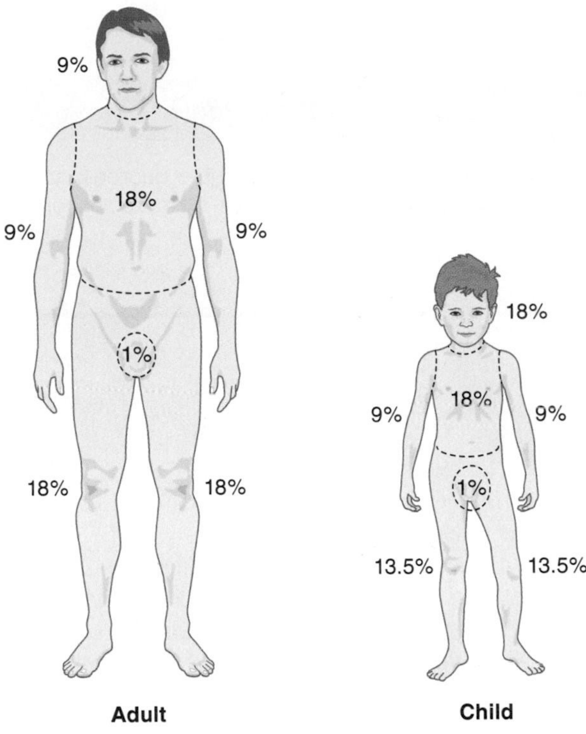

Figure 6.13: Burn assessment: the rule of nines

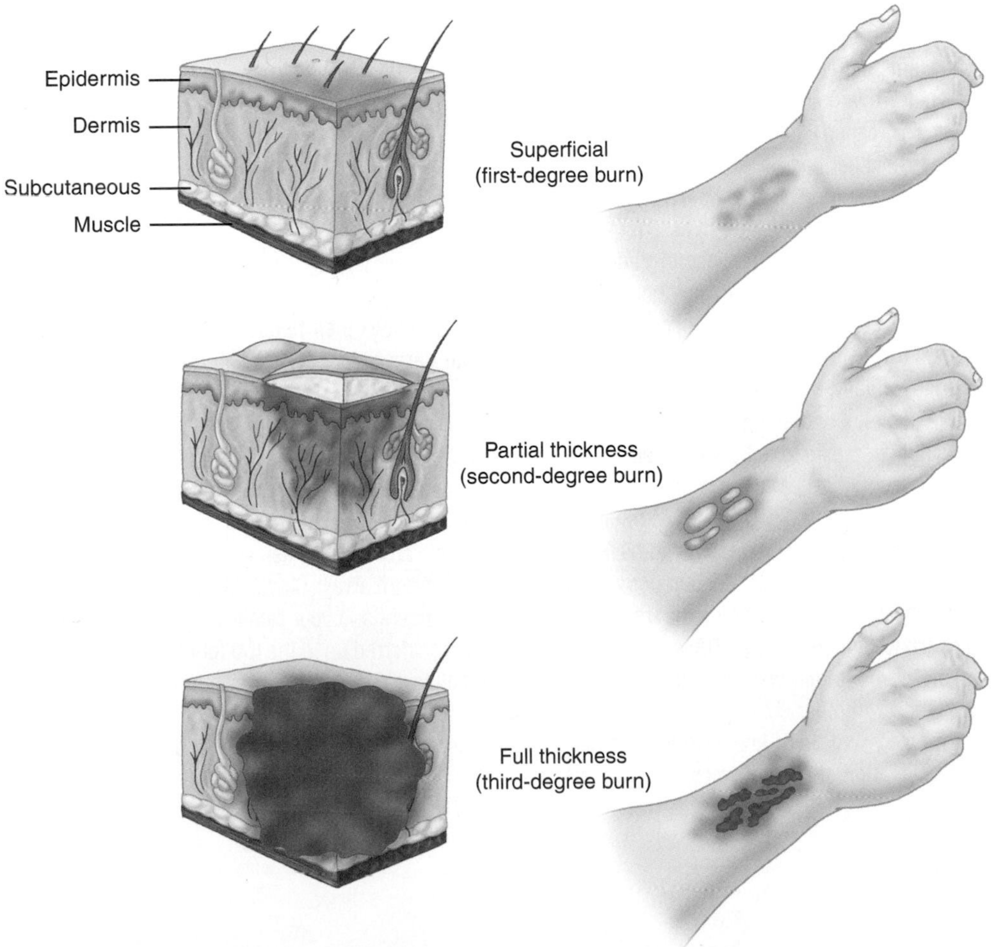

Figure 6.14: Assessing the severity of burns

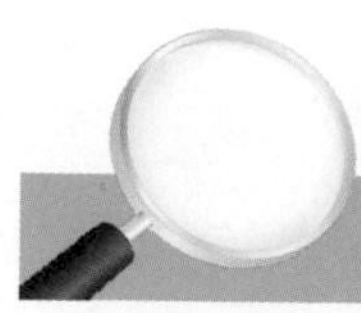

FOCUS POINT: Fourth-Degree Burns

Fourth-degree burns are rarer than those of the other three degrees, and they are often lethal. Fourth-degree burns extend through all tissues and into the muscles, organs, and bones. They are also called *transmural burns.*

Patient Update

Clay Davis has returned from Diagnostic Imaging just as his parents arrived in the ER. They are with Doctors Sandor and Lincoln right now. Listen to their conversation.

"Mr. and Mrs. Davis?" A couple seated in the waiting room nod. "I'm Dr. Sandor, a dental surgeon here at Okla Trauma. This is my colleague, Dr. Lincoln, a pediatric surgeon. Please sit down."

"No, no, I can't," hastily interjected Mrs. Davis. "I can't. I need to see Clay. Is he all right? Where is he? They said there was an accident when they called. What happened? Where is my son? And where are his grandparents?" Mr. Davis took Mrs. Davis's arm to calm her. Dr. Sandor explained that Clay was just returning from having his x-rays and that they would be able to see him momentarily. Mrs. Davis sat down. Her husband joined her.

"Your son has two substantial injuries that we are attending to right now. I'm just waiting for the results of the x-rays, but it looks like he has a mandibular fracture," said Dr. Sandor. Both parents looked at him blankly for a second. "A fracture of the lower jaw," she added quickly. "We're going to need to stabilize that quickly, and, depending on the results of his tests, he may need surgery to repair the fracture."

"What are you saying?" asked Mr. Davis. "You're going to have to wire his jaw shut? Is it that bad?" Mrs. Davis groaned in the background and began to cry softly. "My poor baby," she muttered quietly to herself. Mr. Davis held her hand.

"Yes, sir, we may have to do that. We'll know very shortly," replied Dr. Sandor. "Dr. Lincoln will tell you now about the second priority of care for your son."

"Yes, Clay arrived with a second-degree burn across his upper chest," said Dr. Lincoln. "It looks like a scald burn. Do you know anything about that?"

"What?" came the startled response of both parents. They shook their heads in unison. "A scald burn," repeated Mr. Davis. "How did he get a scald burn?" Both parents looked at each other and then at the surgeons for answers.

"We don't know that, and he's in no condition to tell us at this moment. His grandfather is also here, but he has not been able to tell us much either," commented Dr. Lincoln.

"His grandfather!" Mr. Davis cried out and jumped to his feet. "Where is he? That's my dad. Where is he? Is he okay? Why didn't someone tell me he was here, too? What's going on in this place? Why didn't someone tell us this? Where's my mother?" he demanded, his anxiety increasing.

"We didn't make the connection between the two patients right away. Clay arrived sometime after your father, who was being seen by a different treatment team. I understand your father was confused on arrival and may have suffered from a TIA: a mini-stroke. He's been transferred up to the ICU for observation. I believe someone in your family was contacted," Dr. Sandor informed them. Mr. and Mrs. Davis gasped, both standing now. "And my mother?"

"I'm sorry, we don't know. She's not here at Okla. She may have gone to Fayette General," replied Dr. Lincoln. "Come. I'll take you to see your son now."

Reflective Questions

Think about how the doctors and the parents communicated in this scene. Discuss the dialogue with a friend, another student, or a colleague, if you like, and then answer these questions. There are no right or wrong answers here.

1. Place yourself in the role of one of the parents. In this situation, would you have responded to the doctors in the same way that Mr. and Mrs. Davis did? Why or why not? Discuss your answers, and provide your rationale.

2. Place yourself in the role of one of the doctors. In this situation, would you have communicated with the parents in the same way that Doctors Sandor and Lincoln did? Why or why not? Discuss your answers, and provide your rationale.

CHAPTER SUMMARY

Chapter 6 has followed a child, Clay Davis, through triage and diagnostic assessment for his primary injury of dental trauma. It also introduced the subject of his second priority of care, which is a partial-thickness burn to his upper torso. The field of dentistry related to dental trauma has been introduced through the perspective of a dental surgeon's assessment of the patient. The anatomy, physiology, and language of craniofacial assessment have been presented, and the medical terms related to the integumentary system and burn assessment have also been introduced. Word-recognition skills have been used to construct and deconstruct new terminology and to apply critical-thinking skills within the context of new learning. The language of diagnostics has included the naming of procedures and equipment, and the career spotlight was placed on dentists and dental surgeons.

See How Much You've Learned

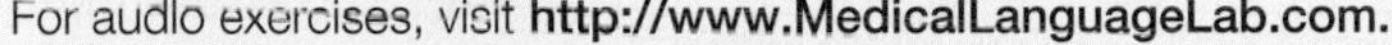
For audio exercises, visit **http://www.MedicalLanguageLab.com.** 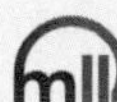

Chapter 6 has introduced you to some medical abbreviations. These have been organized into a study table here for quick reference. Some of them you will recognize immediately, and some will reappear throughout the following chapters with more explanation and application.

TABLE 6-10: Chapter 6 Abbreviations

Medical Abbreviation	Full Term	Medical Abbreviation	Full Term
Peds	pediatrics	PA	posteroanterior view
O_2SATs	oxygen saturation	AP	anteroposterior view; Towne's view
panorex	panoramic topographic		
DI	diagnostic imaging	BSA	body surface area
DDS	doctor of dental surgery	NG	nasogastric
DDM	doctor of dental medicine		

Key Terms

alae nasi
aspirating
Asymmetry
burn
cilia
condyle
coronoid process
cranial vault
craniofacial complex
craniofacial examination
crepitus
derma or dermis
epidermis
first-degree burns (superficial burns)
hypodermis
intact
integument
lacrimal
larynx
mandible
maxillae
nares
nasal
nasal septum
nasoethmoid
nose (proboscis)
occlusion
oral cavity
oral labia
oral mucosa
orbital rims
palates
palatines
palpated bimanually
paranasal
patency of the nares
pharynx
Rule of Nines for Burns
saliva
sebum
second-degree burns (partial thickness burns)
sinuses
split lip
sweat (perspiration)
temporo-mandibular joint (TMJ)
third-degree burns (full-thickness burns)
tongue
tonsils
turbinator (inferior nasal conchae)
unguis
uvula
vomer
zygomatic arches
zygomatic bones (malar bones)

CHAPTER REVIEW

Critical Thinking

1. What is the body's first line of defense? ______
2. How does the term *mental protuberance* relate to craniofacial anatomy?
______
3. What is a proboscis? ______
4. If Clay Davis does indeed have a broken jaw, will he be able to eat and drink normally for the next week or so?
______
5. What is the Rule of Nines? ______

True or False?

1. A *protuberance* is the same as a proboscis. ______
2. The prefixes *inter-* and *intra-* mean the same thing. ______
3. The maxillary bone is really two bones fused together. ______
4. Clay Davis is able to sign his own consent forms for treatment. ______
5. *Afferent* and *efferent* have different meanings. ______

Fill in the Blanks

1. Sebum originates in the ______ glands.
2. Two combining forms for words that mean *tongue* are ______ and ______.
3. The ______ form the roof of the mouth.
4. Clay Davis may have a broken mandible but not a broken ______.
5. The medical term for the lips of the mouth is ______.
6. Cranial nerves originate in the ______.

Mix and Match

Match each description to its medical term.

1. inflammation of the voice box and some or full loss of voice	Le Fort I, II, and III
2. medical field for diseases of the nose and larynx	split lip
3. blisters may appear on the surface	avulsion
4. crushing may force the tissue to separate	laryngorhinology
5. invisible lines across the facial skeleton	pharyngitis
6. forcefully removed from a socket	second-degree burn

Identify the Abbreviations

Throughout the chapter, you have encountered a number of abbreviations. Did you notice them? Recall them here, and write out the words expressed by each abbreviation.

1. TMJ ______________________________
2. BSA ______________________________
3. PA ______________________________
4. ENT ______________________________
5. NG ______________________________
6. IV ______________________________

Right Word or Wrong Word: *Sublingual* or *Subungual*?

Are these two words the same? Do they sound the same? Do they have the same meaning?

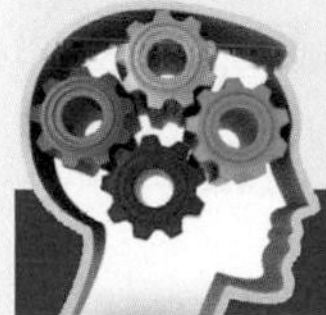

MEMORY MAGIC

If you want to or need to remember the names of the cranial nerves, try this simple mnemonic (memory device) to help you do so. Take the first letter of each word in this silly sentence, and match each of the cranial nerves in numerical order:

"**O**n **O**ld **O**lympus' **T**owering **T**op, **A** **F**inn **A**nd **G**erman **V**iewed **S**ome **H**ops."

CHAPTER SEVEN

Mental Health, Drug Use, and Endocrine Assessment

Focus: Psychoneuroendocrinology

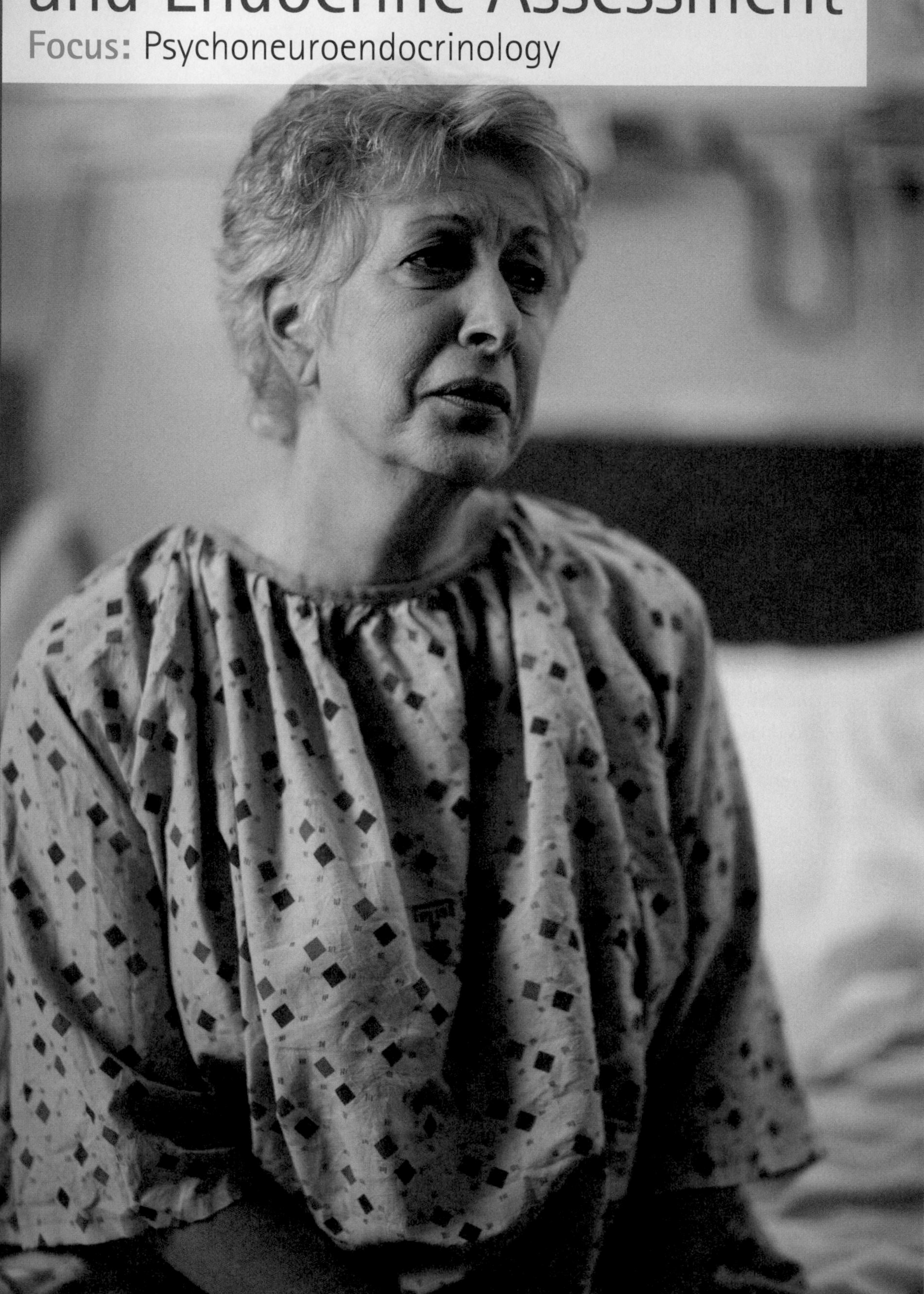

Mrs. Stevie-Rose Davis has been in a motor vehicle accident today. Although she had no apparent injuries, she was a bit unsteady on her feet, nervously wringing her hands and pacing. She was also confused and unable to give a recount of the accident to the emergency medical technician who tended to her at the scene. Because of her age, her confusion, and the difficulty that EMT Wallis had assessing her, Mrs. Davis was transported to the hospital for further assessment. (To review Mrs. Davis's condition at the scene of the accident, you can listen to the Chapter 2 opening scenario on DavisPlus Audio.)

Patient Update

Mrs. Davis arrived at Fayette General Hospital 2 hours ago, and all of her initial assessments have been performed. A few diagnostic tests remain to be completed. She has a small bump on her forehead, high above her right eyebrow. She has a light-colored bruise forming over her left kneecap that was not visible at the scene of the accident. At present, she remains in the ER, and she appears to be sleeping. It's approximately 3 pm now, and the nurses and care aides are changing shifts. Listen as RN Marnie hands over the care of Mrs. Davis in her report to Caroline, the RN on the afternoon shift.

"Hi, Caroline. Good to see you," said Marnie, smiling warmly.

"It looks busy here this afternoon," said Caroline.

"Yes," Marnie replied. "It's busy, but not really too hectic. Not like a Saturday night can be," she laughed. The two nurses take their seats in the Report Room of the nursing station. "Let me tell you a bit about our new patient, Mrs. Davis, before everyone else arrives for Report, okay? You'll be taking over her care now." Caroline nodded.

"The patient, 72-year-old Mrs. Stevie-Rose Davis, was brought in around 1330 hours by EMS. She'd been in an MVA. The EMT found her walking around at the scene, confused. Dr. Jensen attended her and did the initial workup. No major injuries. Her right knee is bruised, and she has a minor concussion where she struck her head on something. She was moderately confused on arrival. Admission vitals were T 98°, P 100, R 18, BP 130/88. Neurologically, she is alert, she responds to voice and pain stimuli, and her pupils are normal and reactive.

"Because her vitals were slightly elevated but her neurological signs were stable and she seemed to be telling us she was a diabetic, the doctor ordered a glucometer test STAT. Her sugars were low at 55 mg/dL. We immediately gave her some orange juice. Her confusion began to lift within the half hour, but it hasn't completely resolved. We got a second blood sugar value on her and it was up to 75, which is within normal range. The patient was able to tell us about herself and was oriented to place and person. However, she is confused about time and some other things. For example, she thinks that it's 1971 and that she's 28 years old. Like I said, she's really 72. Mrs. Davis is still experiencing some recent memory loss for the accident as well. Dr. Jensen wants to keep her overnight because of these findings, at least until all of the test results are in. He's also ordered a mental health assessment. Meagan's on duty in the ER this evening, so I thought you might like to ask her to do the preliminary psych assessment to see whether we need to call in a psychiatrist. As you know, she's working toward her MHNP, and she would likely jump at the opportunity."

"Great idea. I'll ask her," replied Caroline. Then she clarified, "You're saying the patient appears to be physically fine, but there may be something cognitively or emotionally happening with her?"

"Yes. We're not ruling out physical causality for her symptoms yet," said Marnie. We need to continue to take her neurovitals every hour as a precaution. We also need to do glucose testing tonight at 1900 and 2300 and then again tomorrow morning at 0600 hours. If the glucose levels are stable, we can discontinue those tests then. Dr. Jensen will call in this evening to check on the patient. He says he'll likely discontinue neurological and vital signs testing at that time, if nothing untoward has occurred."

"All right. I'll spend some time with her, too, to assess her levels of orientation and memory," added Caroline. Marnie nodded in agreement.

Marnie continued: "She's been asking about her husband and her grandson. Apparently they were with her in the vehicle at the time of the accident. They haven't come here, so Social Work was trying to track them down. It turns out that they are both at Okla Trauma Center. I don't know the details, but their injuries must be significant because they were directed there by EMS. She was made aware."

The nurse continued her patient report by providing Caroline with a health history that she had gathered through an interview with Mrs. Davis just a short time ago. She explained that Mrs. Davis had previously been diagnosed with type 2 diabetes and that it is diet controlled. She has arthritis in her hands and fingers, which is quite noticeable. The patient takes glucosamine (an unknown amount) and ibuprofen (250 mg tid) to relieve pain and inflammation in her joints. She is also taking levothyroxine (150 mcg daily) for hypothyroidism. This led the doctor to order thyroid tests to rule out thyroid involvement in the patient's behaviors.

"The doctor's left some orders that still need to be completed," said Marnie. She noted that Dr. Jensen wanted an FBS in the morning for further assessment of the patient's diabetic status and a TSH for thyroid function. She relayed that the physician was very concerned about the amount and types of medication that Mrs. Davis was taking and that he wanted a complete rundown of these for assessment. A drug screen and a toxicology report were ordered, but specimens still needed to be collected. Both nurses nodded at this, knowing that these tests will determine the amount of medication that the patient has in her system.

"Yes, good idea," added Caroline. "Because polypharmacy is not unusual in the elderly, it could account for some of her confusion, beyond the initial low glucose level." Marnie nodded.

"Sure, you bet," said Marnie. Medication plus low blood sugar, the body's response to the trauma of a car accident, and even thyroid levels could all complicate the picture. So could dementia. I've been wondering about that. The patient does think that it's 1971, as I've said. Other than that, I haven't seen any other evidence that might hint at dementia, but we'll see what the mental health assessment determines."

"Anything else?" asked Caroline, as a few other staff members began to file into the room for shift change. She was told that Mrs. Davis was currently resting quietly in Bed 6 and that, when she was seen moments ago, she had appeared to be falling asleep. "The stress of today has probably worn her out," observed Caroline. "Did you order a diabetic diet for her?" Marnie stated that she had.

"Oh, and has anyone in her family been contacted?" asked Caroline.

"Glad you asked," replied Marnie. "Yes, we've contacted one of her sons. It took some time. We had his home phone number from her, but there was no answer. As she became more clear headed, she remembered that his cell phone number was in her purse, and we helped her to find it. It was just a slip of paper with no name on it, just a phone number. When we reached him, he was on his way to Okla Trauma to see his father. He gave us the numbers of his other brother and a sister, and we're still attempting to reach them. The social worker said that she'd left messages asking them to contact Fayette General and to ask for the ER."

"Okay, thank you for the good information," said Caroline. "I see that they're not quite ready for handover yet, so I'm going to take a quick peek at Mrs. Davis myself. Have a nice evening." She smiled and rose to leave the room. Marnie waited for the others to arrive to share in the handover of patient care from the day shift to the afternoon shift.

Reflective Questions

Reflect on the story that you've just read.

1. Is Mrs. Davis fully oriented? Explain.

   ____

2. Who took on the responsibility for finding the patient's next of kin?

   ____

3. What conditions might be contributing to Mrs. Davis's abilities to concentrate and to remember?

   ____

4. What do the initials *EMS* stand for?

   ____

5. What is the priority of care for Mrs. Davis at this point?

   ____

6. How old is Mrs. Davis?

   ____

For audio exercises, visit **http://www.MedicalLanguageLab.com.** 

Learning Objectives

After reading Chapter 7, you will be able to do the following:

- Recognize and use the language and terminology found in a mental health assessment.
- Appreciate the education and training of a psychiatric nurse.
- Understand the basic concepts and terms involved with mental health assessment.
- Appreciate the links between neurological assessment and mental health assessment.
- Appreciate the interplay of diabetes and thyroid dysfunction with regard to mental health.
- Recognize and use anatomical and medical terms for the endocrine system.
- Recognize medical terminology related to diagnostics of the endocrine and exocrine systems specifically as it relates to the thyroid and the pancreas.
- Recognize medical terminology related to the diagnostics and pathology of the thyroid and the pancreas.
- Appreciate the education and training of a biomedical technologist, especially as it relates to drug screening and other diagnostics.
- Recognize the basic principles and language of pharmacology and pharmacokinetics.

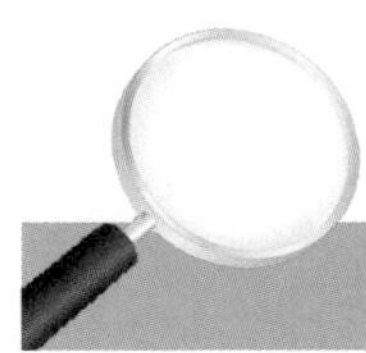

FOCUS POINT: TPR

The abbreviation *TPR* refers to *temperature, pulse, and respirations.* The normal or typical TPR values for an adult are as follows: temperature, 97.8° to 99.1°F; pulse, 60 to 100 beats per minute; and respirations, 16 to 20 breaths per minute. All health-care providers understand the term *TPR* when it is written or spoken aloud.

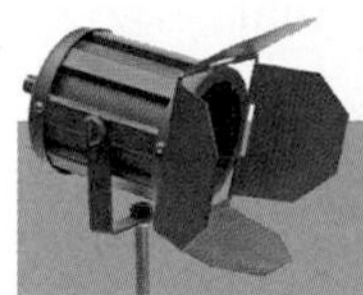

CAREER SPOTLIGHT: Psychiatric/Mental Health Nurse

In the United States, a registered nurse with a generalist education in nursing may assess and treat clients with mental health concerns. However, with additional education and clinical training, many will choose to become psychiatric or mental health nurses. To earn the title of an RN-PMH (registered nurse, psychiatric mental health) or an MHNP (mental health nurse practitioner), a minimum of a master's degree in this specialty must be completed. This will include a minimum of 600 hours of clinical practice. MHNPs are advanced practice nurses who are recognized by the American Nurses Association and the American Psychiatric Nurses Association. They are clinical nurse specialists, and, as such, they provide direct patient care and expert consultation. They may also have medication-prescribing privileges. Individual states set out specific requirements to qualify MHNPs for the right to prescribe medication.

Continued

Psychiatric and mental health nurses work with clients across a broad spectrum of mental health challenges and across many different age groups. Grief, loss, trauma, suicide, drug and alcohol addiction, eating disorders, behavioral disorders, cognitive and intellectual disabilities, bipolar disorders, schizophrenia, and depression are just a few of the areas that may be included in their practices. They are concerned with the physical and psychosocial states of their patients. The MHNP is permitted to make psychiatric diagnoses and to determine medical disorders that involve psychiatric symptoms. He or she is able to manage the total care of the patient.

Assessment: Ruling In and Ruling Out

In the dialogue between the nurses named Marnie and Caroline in the chapter opener, you may have noticed that they used a number of terms, phrases, and abbreviations that both of them understood and were quite comfortable with. Their language included a mixture of medical terminology, medical jargon, and everyday language. This is quite normal among colleagues.

Marnie and Caroline discussed the ongoing assessment of Mrs. Davis' condition. They understand that Dr. Jensen is attempting to rule in or rule out various possible causes of the patient's mental confusion. Potential contributing factors include a thyroid condition, diabetes, a possible mental disorder or disease, and minor head injury. The doctor also wonders if Mrs. Davis's current prescribed medications are interfering with her cognition and memory. He is exploring these possibilities through a variety of diagnostic tests.

The following passages from the opening scenario show some of the processes that are used to rule in or rule out potential causes of a condition to make a diagnosis. Key terms, phrases, and abbreviations are italicized in the example and highlighted below with the explanation.

IS THE CONDITION CAUSED BY DIABETES?

> "... and she seemed to be telling us she was a diabetic, the doctor ordered a *glucometer* test STAT."

glucometer: a glucose-monitoring device that uses a droplet of blood from the fingertip. A glucometer runs on batteries and is portable.

> "Her *sugars were low at* 55 mg/dL."

sugars were low at 55: a shorthand reference to glucose levels in the patient's blood; a blood glucose level of 55 is less than normal.

> "... *glucose* testing at *1900 and 2300* tonight and then again tomorrow morning at *0600 hours.*"

glucose: the medical term for sugar; glucose is a type of sugar that is used by the body for energy.

1900, 2300, and 0600 hours: times on the 24-hour clock, meaning 7 pm, 11 pm, and 6 am. Almost all of health care uses this form of time keeping (see Figure 7-1).

> "The patient takes *glucosamine* (an unknown amount) and *ibuprofen* (250 mg tid) to relieve pain and inflammation in her joints."

glucosamine: an over-the counter substance that is used to treat the pain of arthritis; a health-food supplement.

ibuprofen: an anti-inflammatory analgesic (pain-relieving) medication.

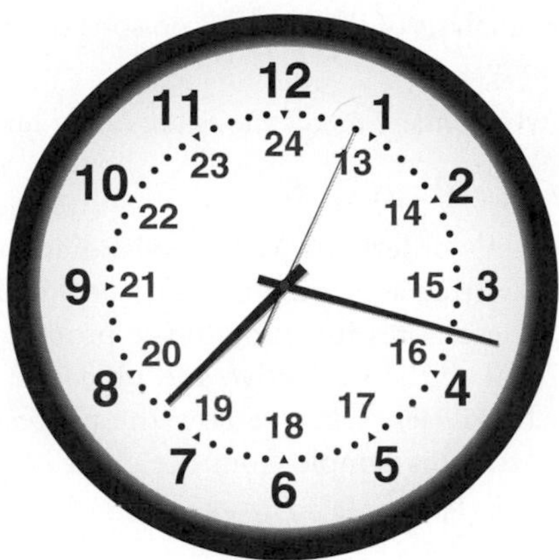

Figure 7.1: 24-hour clock

IS THE CONDITION CAUSED BY A MENTAL DISEASE OR DISORDER?

"... ask her to do the preliminary *psych assessment* to see whether we need to call in a psychiatrist."

psych assessment: medical jargon referring to a mental health assessment. *Psych* can refer to psychiatry or psychology.

"... but there may be something *cognitively* or *emotionally* happening with her?"

cognitively: involving the mental processes of thinking, judging, imagining, reasoning, and so on.

emotionally: pertaining to feelings and the ability to express or respond with emotion.

"... I haven't seen any other evidence that might hint at *dementia.* ..."

dementia: a type of mental or organic brain dysfunction.

IS THE CONDITION CAUSED BY A HEAD INJURY?

"We need to continue to take her neurovitals every hour as a *precaution.*"

as a precaution: in the context of this sentence and this case, the nurse is saying that monitoring both neurological and vital signs periodically and on a schedule is required to ensure that the patient's minor concussion has not caused any internal injury to the brain.

IS THE CONDITION CAUSED BY A THYROID DYSFUNCTION OR DISEASE?

"She is also taking *levothyroxine* (150 µg daily) for *hypothyroidism.* This led the doctor to order thyroid tests to rule out thyroid involvement in the patient's behaviors."

hypothyroidism: a condition of low levels of thyroid hormones in the body.

levothyroxine: a thyroid preparation given to supplement low thyroid levels.

150 µg: the amount of levothyroxine that the patient is taking. The unit of measurement is µg, µq, or mcg. **Mcg** is a medical abbreviation used to identify micrograms. This is read aloud as "150 micrograms."

DOES THE CONDITION REFLECT THE TOXIC EFFECTS OF MIXING MEDICATIONS?

"A *drug screen* and a *toxicology report* were ordered ..."
"Since *polypharmacy* is not unusual in the elderly ..."

drug screen: a laboratory analysis of the types of drugs in the body.

toxicology report: a laboratory analysis of the levels of poisons or of substances deemed noxious or harmful in the body.

polypharmacy: a situation in which many medications are being taken at the same time.

The written language of ruling out

Dr. Jensen has written physician's orders for Mrs. Davis' diagnostic tests, medications, and directions for care. He has also written admitting notes describing his findings and impressions about the case to this point. These notes incorporate the process of ruling out. By using this diagnostic process, eventually all of the subjective and objective data collected will lead the doctor to a firm diagnosis or diagnoses. Observe how the process of ruling out is written by Dr. Jensen in Mrs. Davis's chart. This sample from the chart is found within a larger section called "Physician's Notes."

Date/time	Physician's Notes
June 23, *1500 hrs*	*r/o hypoglycemic reaction* *r/o dementia* *r/o thyroid disease* *r/o minor concussion, gr. 2* *? medications/polypharm*

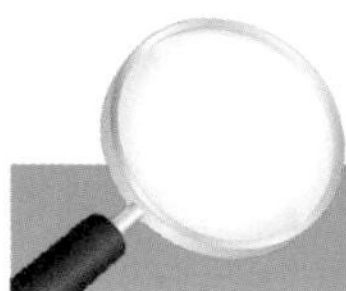

FOCUS POINT: Query

Notice in the physician's notes that Dr. Jensen is querying the effects of medications or the possibility of polypharmacy on the patient's mental status. A query such as this can be written in shorthand form with the question mark in front of the terms. Read aloud, it means the following: "Query medications and polypharmacy." This means that the team needs to find out whether medications or polypharmacy are contributing to the patient's condition.

Priority of Care

As the treatment team continues to assess and care for Mrs. Davis, they are working by priority. Judging from the information gathered about and from this patient during the initial assessment by Dr. Jensen, she does not appear to be in physical distress or danger at this time. The doctor has diagnosed a mild **concussion**, also referred to as a mild concussion or **mild traumatic brain injury** or **MTBI**, which involves a temporary impairment of mental functioning. He is aware of Mrs. Davis's history of type 2 diabetes and thyroid disease (type not yet determined). Therefore, the priorities of care for the next 6 to 12 hours will be the following:

1. Ongoing neurological assessment and monitoring related to mild concussion, confusion, and memory impairment
2. Mental health assessment and monitoring related to confusion and memory impairment
3. Ongoing diabetic assessment, monitoring, and treatment related to hypoglycemia and confusion at time of admission
4. Thyroid function assessment and treatment (if needed) related to confusion
5. Medication assessment related to confusion and memory impairment

Assessing a concussion

Mrs. Davis has exhibited symptoms that are indicative of a mild concussion. The symptoms of a mild concussion (MTBI) include the following:

- Vomiting
- Confusion
- Amnesia: The amnesia may be **retrograde**, which means that it involves memory loss of events that occurred just before the injury. It may also be **anterograde**, which involves memory loss of events that occurred after the accident. Anterograde amnesia is more common; it is also called post-traumatic amnesia (PTA).
- Visual disturbances
- Unconsciousness: If unconsciousness occurs, it will be of less than 30 minutes' duration.

Concussions are *graded by* their level of severity. On the chart, Dr. Jensen placed Mrs. Davis' concussion at Grade 2. There are five grades of a concussion, and these identify the signs, symptoms, and gravity of the injury. Beginning at Grade 2, if the symptoms last for more than 15 minutes, the risk of developing permanent brain damage increases. For this reason, our patient's neurological signs continue to be monitored

- Grade 1 concussion: this is the mildest level, with only the symptom of confusion
- Grade 2 concussion: includes confusion and anterograde amnesia that last for more than 5 minutes
- Grade 3 concussion: includes confusion, anterograde amnesia, loss of consciousness for less than 5 minutes, and retrograde amnesia
- Grade 4 concussion: includes all of the above symptoms, plus unconsciousness for more than 5 minutes
- Grade 5 concussion: this level is same as Grade 4 but with a much longer period of unconsciousness

The Language of Mental Health

According to the National Institute of Mental Health,[1] approximately 26% of Americans are diagnosed with a mental disorder each year; that is just over one quarter of the population. Therefore, in the health-care field, the language of mental health is important when working with people from all walks of life and all different circumstances.

Mental health concerns the mind, and the mind involves more than just the brain. Assessing a patient's mental health requires examining a variety of factors in the patient's life. This section introduces the medical language and terminology that relate to mental health. It differentiates between mental health and mental illness, and it explores the language of mental health assessment.

Mental health factors

In simple terms, the term **mental health** describes a disease-free level of cognitive and emotional well-being. However, mental health or mental well-being is much more than that. It is the result of striking a balance in all domains (dimensions) of our lives: biological, psychological, socioeconomic, spiritual, and environmental. When these are in balance, we are able to mentally function at a higher level; this leaves us free to be trusting, loving, creative, and altruistic, and our self-esteem is intact. Mental health also includes the ability to enjoy life. Flexibility, resiliency, and self-actualization are important assets for the development and maintenance of mental health.

In summary, mental health is a subjective and objective state of wellness that is related to how we think about and interact with our internal and external worlds.

A state of mental health is hard to achieve and maintain in our complicated lives. It is very possible that, over a lifetime, we will slip away from optimal mental health and then

---

[1]National Institute of Mental Health, US Department of Health and Human Services. http://www.nimh.nih.gov. Last reviewed July 23, 2010.

retain it several times. Crises, illnesses, and other difficult situations can affect our state of mental health. Mental health and mental illness are anchors at opposite ends of a continuum (see Figure 7-2).

Mental health assessment usually—but not always—falls in the realm of psychiatry. **Psychiatry** is the field of medicine concerned with the diagnosis, treatment, and prevention of mental illness. (In written notes, the symbol Ψ is often used to denote psychiatry). Diagnoses of various mental illnesses can only be made by psychiatrists, psychologists, certain other physicians, and mental health nurse practitioners (MHNPs).

Key terms: mental health factors

biological health: referring to physical or physiological health.

psychological health: referring to the mind and the processes of the mind, including thinking, remembering, and the capacity for emotion. Emotional health includes the ability to feel and express emotions. Collectively, the expression of emotions, emotional response, and mood are referred to as the **affect**.

socioeconomic health: referring to the social world and membership in families, groups, communities, and societies. This term also refers to a financial state that provides adequate food, clothing, and shelter (without which an individual is under a great deal of stress and anxiety).

spiritual health: referring to an inner sense of meaning, direction, and purpose in one's life; this can be religious or philosophical. Some elements of spiritual health include morals, ethics, values, hope, compassion, caring, and sharing.

environmental health: referring to the world in which we live at the micro and macro levels (i.e., the home, office, community, country, and world).

cognition: thought processes that include thinking, knowing, reasoning, learning, applying what is learned, deciding, judging, remembering, language, awareness, imagination, problem solving, and more. Cognition includes perception—the ability to recognize, interpret, and understand (make meaning of) stimuli and information.

altruistic: referring to altruism, an unselfish concern for the health and welfare of others.

wellness: the absence of disease and a subjective sense of mental and physical well-being.

resiliency: the ability to bounce back from adversity and to cope and do well again afterward.

flexibility: a positive response to change and to the unpredictability of life.

self-actualization: the process of becoming the person we always truly wanted to be. The achievement of self-actualization usually takes a lifetime.

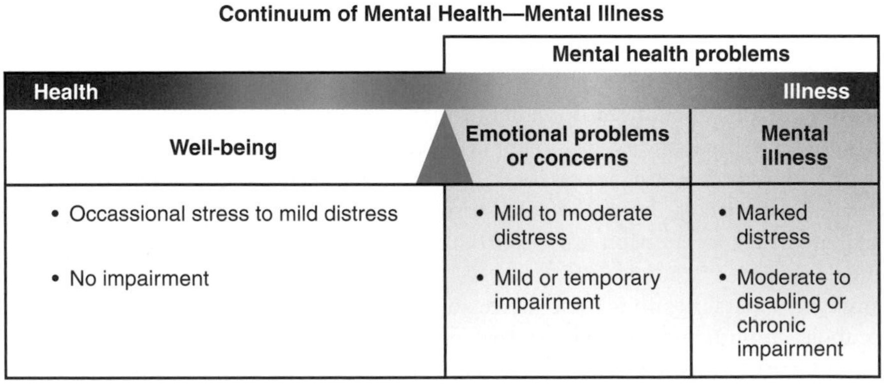

Continuum of Mental Health—Mental Illness

	Mental health problems	
Health		Illness
Well-being	Emotional problems or concerns	Mental illness
• Occassional stress to mild distress • No impairment	• Mild to moderate distress • Mild or temporary impairment	• Marked distress • Moderate to disabling or chronic impairment

Figure 7.2: Mental health and mental illness continuum

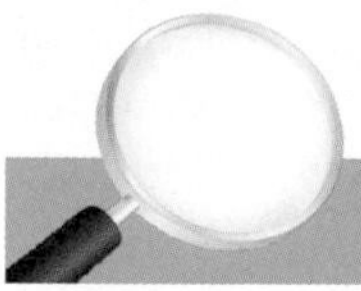

FOCUS POINT: Mind and State of Mind

The term *mind* refers to the mental functioning of consciousness, which includes awareness and perception. There are many philosophical, religious, and scientific explanations for the mind. These include the consideration of the activity of the brain as it affects the mind and psychological functioning (referred to as the *mind-body connection*) and the consideration of the interaction of the brain and the human spirit. The term *state of mind* refers to one's ability to think clearly, as well as to a person's emotional state or mood.

Critical Thinking

Answer the following questions about mental health. Whenever possible use new terminology that you have learned.

1. What are the five dimensions of mental health?

 ____

 ____

2. Identify a term that describes one's ability to bounce back from hardship, trauma, and illness.

 ____

3. In addition to adaptability, what is another element of healthy coping?

 ____

4. Complete this statement: Optimal mental health is ____________ to ______________ over a lifetime, but not impossible.
5. What is *affect*?

 ____

What is mental illness?

In America, close to one in five people will experience some form of mental illness during their lives. For this reason, learning the terminology for mental illness is important for those who work in the health field. **Mental illness** involves a broad range of psychiatric and emotional disorders. These are not all chronic or lifelong, and they do not all require treatment in a hospital, mental institution, or psychiatric facility. Some examples of mental illnesses include depression, post-traumatic stress disorder, schizophrenia, bipolar disorder, and addictions. (These and other mental illnesses are defined and explained in Tables 7-2 and 7-3.) The severity and duration of mental illnesses vary from individual to individual.

In the United States and Canada, psychiatric illnesses are identified by following the criteria for assessment, diagnosis, and treatment found in the latest edition of *Diagnostic and Statistical Manual of Mental Disorders* (DSM), published by the American Psychological Association. This manual provides descriptions and statistics, identifies the effects of treatment, and offers common treatment approaches for clinicians and psychiatrists. Assessment criteria are divided into five axes (dimensions), and references to each axis are made by numbers written as Roman numerals. These number references are frequently used in health care, and you should at least be familiar with them. (However, unless you work specifically in mental health or addiction services, it will not be necessary to recall these specifically or in detail.)

- Axis I: clinical syndromes: symptoms that cause impairment of functioning
- Axis II: developmental and personality disorders
- Axis III: medical conditions and physical disorders
- Axis IV: psychosocial and environmental problems
- Axis V: global assessment of functioning: a summary or conclusion of the impact of other findings (per Axes I through IV) on the client's life for children and teens who are younger than 18 years old

Mental illnesses are also referred to as *mental disorders, mental diseases,* or *psychiatric illnesses.* Terminology specific to the field of mental health and mental illness includes the root words *mentis, psyche,* and *phren,* all of which mean *the mind.* Study the examples of how to create words with the combining forms of these roots to explore and learn new terminology.

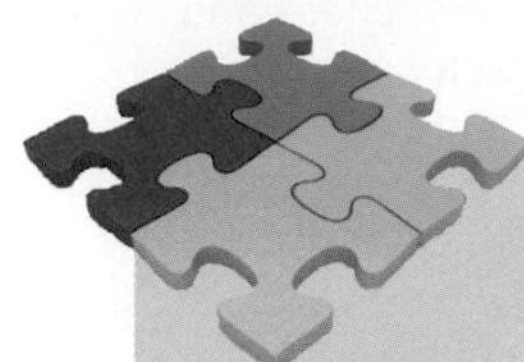

WORD BUILDING: Formula for Creating Words with the Combining Forms *Ment/o, Psycho/o,* and *Phren/o*

1. mentis = the mind. The combining form is *ment/o.*

ment + al + ity

Definition: mental activity or mental power. *noun*

Example: When a group of people all decide to do the same thing, we say that they are exhibiting a herd *mentality.*

ment + ation = *mentation*

Definition: mental activity. (The suffix *-ation* means *the state or condition of.*) *noun*

Example: Psychometric testing can assess *mentation.*

2. psyche = the mind or the soul. The combining form is psych/o.

psych + osis = *psychosis*

Definition: a mental condition that involves a severe loss of contact with reality and the presence of hallucinations, disorganized speech, bizarre behavior, and delusions. (The suffix *-osis* means *condition.*) *noun*

Example: *Psychosis* can occur as a result of substance abuse and withdrawal, as an effect of medications, and as a feature of acute schizophrenia or bipolar disorder.

psycho + bio + logy = *psychobiology*

Definition: the study of the relationship between biology and the psyche (mind) and of the relationship between a person and the environment. (The second root is *bios,* meaning *life.* The suffix is *-logy,* meaning *the study or science of.*) *noun*

Example: *Psychobiology* studies the mind-body connection and seeks to find biological reasons for psychological behaviors and beliefs.

psycho + logic + al = *psychological*

Definition: pertaining to the mind and its mental processes, including its effects on behavior. *adjective*

Example: The loss of a loved one can have a profound *psychological* effect on a person.

psycho + motor = *psychomotor*

Definition: regarding or causing physical activity associated with the mind, such as thinking, will, and so on. (The second root, *motor,* means *move.*) *adjective*

Example: The learning of a *psychomotor* skill (i.e., taking a blood pressure) requires concentration and the ability to plan and follow through steps to turn ideas into actions.

psycho + metr + ic = *psychometric*

Definition: describing types of tests that measure psychological variables, such as intelligence levels, emotional reactions, interests, and aptitudes. (The root *metron,* used here in its combining form, means *measure.*) *adjective*

Example: An IQ test is one type of *psychometric* test.

3. phren = the mind. The combining form is phren/o.

phren + etic = *phrenetic*

Definition: frenzied, agitated, manic, and excitable. This term is more commonly spelled *frenetic* today. (The suffix *-etic* is used to form an adjective.) *adjective*

Example: A person with a bipolar disorder may exhibit *phrenetic* behavior.

phren + ology = *phrenology*

Definition: the study of the shape of the skull, which was once believed to reveal personality characteristics and mental abilities. *noun*

Example: *Phrenology* is always included in courses and readings that discuss the history of mental illness and treatment.

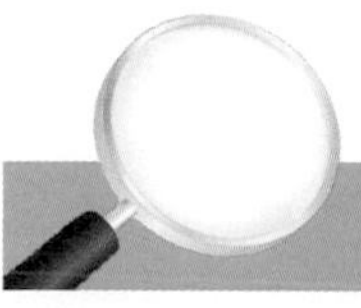

FOCUS POINT: Caution Regarding *Phren/o*

Be very careful with words that use the combining forms *phren* or *phreno.* They can refer to one of two things: the mind or the diaphragm (part of the respiratory system). Indeed, most medical terms that begin with *phren/o* are related to the diaphragm rather than the mind.

Who are mental health professionals?

Assessment of the brain and the mind may involve specialists in the medical fields of neurology and psychiatry, as well as professionals in the non-medical field of psychology. Study the differences among these professions in Table 7-1.

TABLE 7-1: Neurology, Psychiatry, and Psychology

Focus of Neurology	Focus of Psychiatry	Focus of Psychology
• a medical science that is focused on diseases and disorders of the brain and the nervous system • includes research and assessment of the function of the brain and the nervous system • biological focus	• a medical science that is focused on the prevention, diagnosis, and treatment of disorders and diseases of the mind • includes research and assessment of the brain, as well as the mind • biopsychosocial focus (the integration of biological and psychosocial aspects of mental health) • treatment with medication and psychotherapies for behaviors, thought processes, and emotions	• the cognitive science of the mind • includes research and assessment of behaviors, thoughts, and feelings • humanistic focus • treatment with psychotherapies for behaviors, thought processes, and emotions

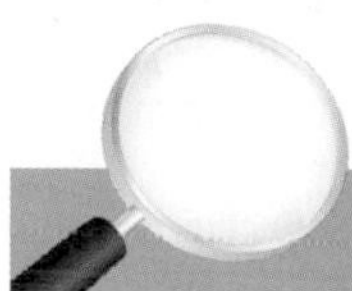

FOCUS POINT: Psychiatrist vs. Psychologist

A *psychiatrist* is a medical doctor with an advanced specialty in psychiatry and mental illness. A clinical *psychologist* holds a PhD or PsyD doctoral degree in psychology.

Critical Thinking

Use your new knowledge of the language of mental health and mental illness to answer these questions.

1. What is the difference between mental health and mental illness?
   ____
2. What is the medical term that explains our ability to cope with and bounce back from crisis?
   ____
3. What do the initials *DSM* stand for? ______________________________
4. Can a psychologist prescribe medications? ______________________________
5. What is the name of the medical specialty that deals specifically with mental illness?
   ____

Build a Word

Use your word-building skills to create medical terms from the following word parts, and then define each term in your own words.

1. ic phren ______________________ Meaning: ______________________
2. -ology path psych/o ______________________ Meaning: ______________________
3. gen psych/o -ic ______________________ Meaning: ______________________

Psychopathology: mental disorders and diseases

Although there is no suggestion so far that our patient, Mrs. Davis, has a mental illness, she will be examined shortly to rule this out. A mental health assessment is not required for every patient nor for every elderly patient. Mrs. Davis is only being assessed because of her state of confusion and memory loss, which has not fully resolved.

Psychopathology is mental illness; this is a medical condition in which there is a pattern of psychological and behavioral disruption that involves alterations in mood, cognition, and behavior. Some conditions are marked by **flat affect**, or a lack of emotional response, whereas others are characterized by extreme *lability* (i.e., mood swings).

This section provides an introduction to the pathology of mental disorders and diseases. Although these two terms are often used interchangeably, there may be some fine distinctions. *Diseases* are physiological and biological in origin, whereas *disorders* generally are not. However, both are pathological, both can be defined by set criteria, and both describe a disruption or impairment in normal functioning.

Remember that the purpose of this book is to expose you to medical terminology that you may come across during your health-care career; it is not to teach you all the fine details of every illness. With that in mind and for ease of studying, mental illnesses that are commonly identified as disorders are listed in Table 7-2, and those that are commonly thought of as diseases appear in Table 7-3.

TABLE 7-2: Mental Illnesses Classified as Disorders

Mental Disorder	Medical Abbreviation	Definition	Primary Signs and Symptoms
anxiety disorders	—	a group of disorders related to abnormal or pathological levels of anxiety or fear	panic, phobic reactions, inability to think clearly, heightened fear, palpitations, shortness of breath
attention deficit disorder	ADD	a pattern of the inability to pay attention, focus, or concentrate for more than a very short period of time	restlessness, distractibility, inability to concentrate, low frustration tolerance, irritability

TABLE 7-2: Mental Illnesses Classified as Disorders—cont'd

Mental Disorder	Medical Abbreviation	Definition	Primary Signs and Symptoms
attention deficit-hyperactivity disorder	ADHD	a behavioral disorder that usually occurs before the age of 7 years	overactivity, chronic inattention, difficulty dealing with multiple stimuli, irritability, little or no frustration tolerance, potential for acting out impulsively and aggressively
amnestic disorders	—	cognitive disorders of memory	short- and long-term memory deficits, inability to recall previous information, inability to learn new information
anorexia nervosa	—	a disorder that involves a preoccupation with food and eating, the suppression of the desire to eat, an uncontrollable need to be thin, and body dysmorphia (the inability to see the true size and shape of one's body)	extreme weight loss, social withdrawal, low blood pressure, anemia, cardiac arrhythmias, loss of bone density (more fractures), fatigue
bipolar disorder	BPD	a mood disorder that includes one or more manic episodes and usually one or more depressive episodes	in mania: grandiosity, hyperactivity, mood lability (mood swings), inability to concentrate for long periods, insomnia, very poor judgment
bulimia nervosa	—	An eating disorder that involves cycles of binge eating followed by purging	episodes of excessive and uncontrollable intake of large amounts of foods that alternate with activities to compensate for this, such as vomiting, taking laxatives, and taking diuretics; self-starvation
dissociative disorders	—	a group of disorders in which there is a disturbance in the normal integration of perception, consciousness, memory, and the identification of the self	feelings of detachment from the environment or the outer world, amnesia (missing memories and missing time), sometimes a fugue state (going somewhere and doing something without conscious awareness)
generalized anxiety disorder	GAD	uncontrollable and often irrational worry every day; excessive worry that is constant	nervousness, sleep disturbances, labile mood, fatigue, difficulty concentrating
multiple personality disorder or dissociative identity disorder	MPD or DID	a severe dissociative* disorder in which one or more distinct subpersonalities exist within an individual and which surface on a recurring basis	sporadic changes in speech patterns and behavior, interests, mannerisms and so on; memory impairments
panic disorder	—	a sudden and overwhelming anxiety of extreme intensity	disorganization, loss of rational thought, inability to communicate
post-traumatic stress disorder	PTSD	a type of anxiety disorder that is the result of exposure to a terrifying trauma or event	persistent frightening thoughts and memories about the traumatic event, sleep disturbances (including nightmares), labile mood, easily startled, flashbacks to the event or trauma, detachment and increasing social isolation

Continued

TABLE 7-2: Mental Illnesses Classified as Disorders—cont'd

Mental Disorder	Medical Abbreviation	Definition	Primary Signs and Symptoms
psychotic disorders or psychoses	—	severe mental disorders; extreme responses to psychological or physical stressors that lead to the pronounced distortion or disorganization of cognition, affect, behavior, and motor functioning; mostly transient (temporary)	hallucinations (false perceptions), delusions (fixed false beliefs), paranoia
seasonal affective disorder	SAD	a mood disorder that most often occurs during the winter or "darker" months and that is affected by seasonal changes in climate and exposure to light	during the winter months: hypersomnia (excessive sleep), fatigue, weight gain, irritability, avoidance of social activities

*Dissociation is an unconscious defense mechanism in which overwhelming anxiety is blocked from awareness.

TABLE 7-3: Mental Illnesses Classified as Diseases

Mental Illness	Medical Abbreviation	Definition	Primary Signs and Symptoms
Alzheimer's disease or dementia of the Alzheimer's type	AD or DAT	primary cognitive impairment	progressive deterioration of the following: memory, problem solving, judgment, ability to complete familiar tasks, orientation and awareness, spatial and visual awareness, speech and word choice, social skills and social interests; personality changes and labile and unpredictable mood
addiction or drug dependence	—	physiological dependence on drugs despite adverse (harmful) effects in all dimensions of life	preoccupation with attaining and using the drug, manipulation of others, antisocial behaviors, symptoms of withdrawal when drug not available
alcoholism	ETOH abuse	physiological dependence on alcohol that is beyond the individual's control	repeatedly neglecting responsibilities, legal difficulties related to drinking, socially inappropriate drinking and behaviors, symptoms of withdrawal when alcohol not available
depression	—	a mood disorder that is characterized by a depressed (low) mood and an inability to enjoy life	lack of interest and enjoyment in usual activities, changes in sleep patterns, changes in eating patterns, low self-esteem, self-doubt, difficulty concentrating
dementia (also known as *senile dementia* or *chronic organic brain syndrome*)	—	a collection of symptoms that progressively adversely affect the brain and that impair cognition	gradual memory loss, increasing tendency to repeat oneself, increasing episodes of confusion, increasing mood lability
schizophrenia	schiz	a group of illnesses characterized by severe psychological disturbances	disorganized and disordered thinking, hallucinations (auditory, visual, tactile, olfactory), delusions, preoccupations, flat affect, decreased socialization or isolation

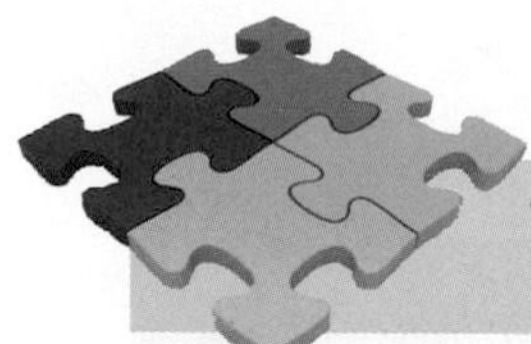

WORD BUILDING: Formula for Creating Words with the Combining Form *Schiz/o*

skhizein = to split. The combining form is *schiz/o/a,* which means *division or divided.*

schizo + phren + ia = *schizophrenia*
Definition: a mental illness of marked thought disorder, hallucinations, disorganization of speech and behavior, delusions, and more. (The second root, *phren,* means *mind.*) *noun*

Example: *Schizophrenia* can be a debilitating disease, particularly when it is left untreated.

schiz + oid = *schizoid*
Definition: severely introverted, socially isolated, and unable to become less so. (The second root is *eidos,* meaning *to form or shape.*) *adjective*

Example: A person diagnosed with a *schizoid* personality has a serious mental disorder, unlike a person who is merely shy and introverted.

schizo + aphasia = *schizophasia*
Definition: speech that is hard to follow. It is marked by a looseness of associations and a flight of ideas; flow, content, and logic could be said to be divided. (The second root is *phasis,* meaning *speech.*) *noun*

Example: *Schizophasia* may be present in patients with schizophrenia, patients with psychosis, and possibly in patients with dementia and delirium.

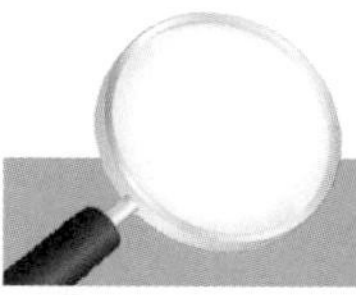

FOCUS POINT: Hallucinations

Hallucinations are false perceptions that have no relationship to reality. They cannot be explained by an external stimulus. Hallucinations are not the sole purview of schizophrenia or psychosis: Anyone can experience a hallucination under the right circumstances. Causes might include medications and anesthetics, drug withdrawal, the use of illicit substances that are hallucinogenic in nature, and some types of mental illness. Many people have experienced *hypnagogic* hallucinations as they are falling asleep. In this situation, a person experiences a sense of falling or sinking or has difficulty determining if he or she is asleep, awake, or in a dreamlike state. Types of hallucinations include visual, olfactory (smell), gustatory (taste), auditory (sound; hearing voices), and tactile (touch). Tactile hallucinations are not uncommon during alcohol withdrawal.

Right Word or Wrong Word: *Schizophrenia* or *Multiple Personality Disorder*?

Sometimes we hear that the word *schizophrenia* means *split personality.* If that is true, is schizophrenia synonymous with multiple personality disorder? Look back at the information presented in this chapter to find the answer before checking the Answer Key.

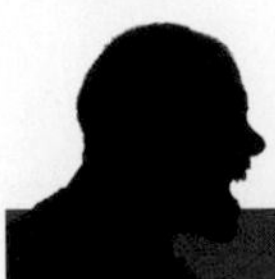

PRONUNCIATION PRACTICE

Say these words aloud to a friend or classmate if you can. You are given the phonetic pronunciation. Your instructor can help you with pronunciation, or visit **http://www.MedicalLanguageLab.com.** mll

anorexia	ăn-ō-**rĕk**´sē-ă	olfactory	ŏl-**făk**´tō-rē
Alzheimer's	**ălts**´hī-mĕrz	psychiatry	sī-**kī**´ă-trē
amnestic	ăm-nĕ**s**´tĭk	psychosis	sī-**kō**´sĭs
bulimia	bū-**lĭm**´ē-ă	psychometric	sī˝kō-**mĕ**´trĭk
dementia	dĭ-**mĕn**´shă	schizoid	**skĭz**´oyd
gustatory	**gŭs**´tă-tō-rē	schizophasia	skĭz˝ō-**fā**´zē-ă
hypnagogic	hĭp-nă-**gŏj**´ĭk	schizophrenia	skĭz˝ō-**frĕn**´ē-ă
mentation	mĕn-**tā**´shŭn		

Right Word or Wrong Word: *Psychotic* or *Schizophrenic*?

Are the words *psychotic* and *schizophrenic* interchangeable? Why or why not?

The language of amnestic disorders

Amnesia means loss of memory. Occasionally, we all may forget people, things, events, and information. This type of memory loss is not indicative of a disorder unless it is severe and persistent, thus impairing a person's ability to function in day-to-day life.

Amnestic disorders are actually quite uncommon. Their causes include head trauma, hypoxia (lack of oxygen to the brain), thiamine (vitamin B complex) deficiency, brain swelling (i.e., encephalitis), and substance abuse. These disorders may include severe and persistent memory loss, as well as the inability to learn new information or recall old information. Both short- and long-term memory may be affected. The person with an amnestic disorder may also exhibit a bland or flat affect and apathy about life, and he or she may also **confabulate** (make up stories to fill in gaps in memory).

There are three types of amnestic disorders: those caused by traumatic brain injury, those caused by substance abuse, and those with an unknown cause, which are referred to as *amnestic disorders not otherwise specified* (NOS). Our patient, Mrs. Davis, will be assessed for these amnestic disorders to rule them out as the cause of her own current memory problems.

The language of dementia and Alzheimer's disease

Dementia is a mental disorder; this means that it is a collection of symptoms that affect the brain rather than a disease. It involves progressive decline in both occupational and social functioning abilities. It primarily affects cognition, which in turn manifests itself (appears) in behavioral and psychological symptoms. Dementia results in the death of neurons (nerve cells) in the brain and impairs communication between them as well.

There are many types and causes of dementias, but the most common type and cause is *Alzheimer's dementia (AD),* also known as dementia of the Alzheimer's type (DAT). The risk of developing a dementia increases with age, particularly after 60 years. As a very large segment of the American population grows older (i.e., the baby boomer phenomenon), you can expect to hear, see, and read the language of dementia across all health and allied health careers.

Cardinal (primary) symptoms of dementia include the following:

- Cognitive impairment in abstract thinking, judgment, insight, language, tasks, and recognition, as well as personality change
- Memory impairment
- Spatial disorientation (the inability to determine one's own physical position or location in relationship to the environment)
- Altered affect
- Decline in intellectual function (including the first sign of difficulty with numbers and arithmetic)
- Altered judgment and decision-making ability

Eponyms: Alzheimer's disease

Alzheimer's disease is named after Alois Alzheimer, the German neuropathologist and psychiatrist who first described the condition in 1906.

Let's Practice

Write the medical term or word part that fits each description and that accurately answers the question.

1. This abbreviation refers to a developmental pathology related to concentrating, problem solving, deciding, and behaving in youngsters. ______________________
2. ______________________ describes a condition in which a person's mood is significantly altered only at certain times of the year.
3. What is the medical term for a mental disorder that occurs as the result of a trauma? ______________________
4. Identify the combining form found in the name of an illness that includes hallucinations, thought disorders, and speech difficulties as part of its makeup. ______________________
5. ______________________ is the term for a loss of appetite.
6. Identify a mental illness that uses the root *polus* in its combining form. ______________________
7. This word means *mood swings.* ______________________
8. What is the general term for a progressive decline in cognitive, occupational, and social functioning? ______________________
9. What is another medical term meaning *addiction?* ______________________
10. This term describes a condition of impatience, lacking patience, or the inability to be patient. ______________________

Mix and Match

Match the medical term or abbreviation on the left to the definition on the right by drawing a line to connect them.

1. hypoxia	denies self food
2. B_{12} complex	expression of emotion
3. NOS	condition of the mind with a loss of contact with reality
4. cardinal	false perceptions of reality
5. affect	thiamine
6. psychosis	not otherwise specified
7. manic	primary
8. AD	lack of oxygen
9. self-starvation	Alzheimer's dementia
10. hallucinations	phrenetic or excited

Critical Thinking

To answer this question, you will need to think critically about how signs and symptoms can sometimes lead to a variety of different diagnoses. Think about the symptom of anorexia or loss of appetite. Did you ever experience a loss of appetite? At that time, did you think you were physically ill, mentally ill, or neither of these? Explain your answer to a friend, another student, or a teacher. Explain how you ruled in or ruled out a diagnosis of physical illness or mental illness.

____

____

____

Right Word or Wrong Word: *Psychiatrist* or *Psychologist*?

Read the following sentences, and then fill in each blank with the correct word:

A ______________ sees clients in counseling and can also treat them in the hospital.

A ________________ sees clients in counseling but cannot treat them in the hospital.

Classifications of Mental Illnesses

Mental illnesses are also classified by type. You may encounter these categories in your career, whether you are working in mental health or not. Here are a few examples:

- Schizophrenia and other psychotic disorders
- Mood disorders
- Anxiety disorders
- Substance-related disorders
- Cognitive disorders
- Eating disorders
- Sleep disorders
- Somatoform disorders (*soma* means *body*)
- Dissociative disorders
- Delirium, dementia, and amnesia

Prefixes and the language of mental illness

Prefixes play an important role in diagnosing, describing, and discussing mental illnesses. A simple addition of a prefix can change the meaning of a term to indicate the absence of an element of health or a degree of psychopathology. Refer to Table 7-4 to explore some common prefixes that are used in the mental health field.

TABLE 7-4: Word Building: Prefixes and Psychopathology

BEGIN with a Prefix	ADD a Medical Root Word	COMBINE to Create a Diagnostic Term
an- (not)	orexis (appetite	anorexia (no appetite or loss of appetite)
ab- (away from)	usus (to use)	abuse (improper use or maltreatment)
bi- (two, twice, or double)	polus (pole)	bipolar (consisting of two poles on the ends of a continuum: depression ←→ mania)
eu- (well, healthy, or normal)	phoros (carrying or bearing)	euphoria (an exaggerated sense of well-being)
hypo- (below or less than)	mania (madness or insanity)	hypomania (a mild stage of mania and excitement that includes only a few changes from normal behavior)

TABLE 7-4: Word Building: Prefixes and Psychopathology—cont'd

BEGIN with a Prefix	ADD a Medical Root Word	COMBINE to Create a Diagnostic Term
hyper- (above, more than, or excessive)	active (in motion; liveliness or briskness)	hyperactivity (increased or excessive levels of activity)
im- (causing)	pejor (worse; to make worse)	impair (to cause a worsening or diminished capacity of ability, strength, or value)
im- (not)	balance (equilibrium or equality and harmony among parts)	imbalance (lack of or absence of harmony among parts)
mis- (wrongly)	use (to put something into action)	misuse (to use incorrectly or improperly)
post- (after)	trauma (wound)	post-traumatic (occurring after a wound [which may be physical or emotional])

Build a Word

Combine each set of word parts to create a medical term. Some you will know, whereas others will be new to you. However, you will be able to understand them by analyzing the meaning of each part. Remember that you may need to change the spelling of some of the word parts to fit them together appropriately and accurately.

1. al norm ab __________ Meaning: __________
2. diagnose mis -ed __________ Meaning: __________
3. -ed impair un- __________ Meaning: __________
4. percept -ion mis- __________ Meaning: __________
5. an- -genic oerixis __________ Meaning: __________
6. phor/i -ant eu- __________ Meaning: __________
7. function hypo- __________ Meaning: __________
8. mnesis hypo- __________ Meaning: __________
9. sensus hyper- -ivity __________ Meaning: __________
10. exposure post- __________ Meaning: __________

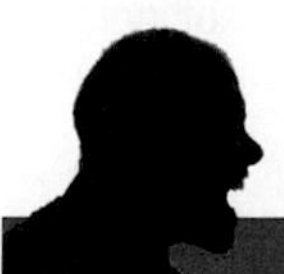

PRONUNCIATION PRACTICE

Say these words aloud to a friend or classmate if you can. You are given the phonetic pronunciation. Your instructor can help you with pronunciation,

or visit **http://www.MedicalLanguageLab.com.** mll

anorexigenic	ăn″ō-rĕk′sĭ-**jĕn**′ĭk
somatoform	sō-**măt**′ă-fŏrm″
neuropathology	nū″rō-pă-**thŏl**′ō-jē

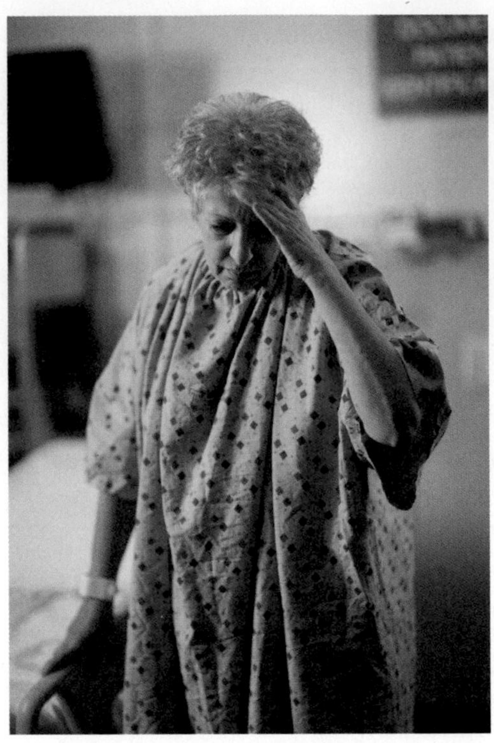

Patient Update

Mrs. Davis has risen from a short nap and is disoriented and unsure about where she is and why she is there. She recognizes that this is a hospital and draws some conclusions. She gets up and steps into the open area near her bed, and she reaches out toward a nursing assistant who is coming her way.

"Oh, you there! Nurse! There you are," Mrs. Davis begins. "Why did you let me sleep? I thought I heard helicopters. Why didn't you wake me? Where's Dr. Morgan?" She runs a hand through her hair in an attempt to straighten it. The nursing assistant stops and looks at her for a moment; she is confused by what Mrs. Davis is saying.

"Can I help you, ma'am?" she asks.

"Well, yes, of course you can help me! Help me find my shoes and get the rest of the nurses up. They'll be in their tents. Tell them to get a move on, we've got in-coming," Mrs. Davis directed in an authoritarian tone, her voice rising somewhat. A passerby glanced over at her. "Nurse, what is that civilian doing here?" Mrs. Davis demanded as she began to walk toward the nursing station.

"Ma'am, my name is Sandra. You are in Fayette General Hospital. You've been in an accident, and you're confused. Let me help you." The nursing assistant reached out and gently touched Mrs. Davis on the forearm. Mrs. Davis stopped momentarily, confused by this touch and the words.

"What ... what are you saying?" Mrs. Davis asked, and then she paused to think. Caroline the RN approached them. "Hello, Mrs. Davis, how are you feeling?" Caroline inquired.

"Lieutenant Davis," came a quick retort. Caroline and Sandra glanced at each other. Sandra explained the circumstances and Mrs. Davis's behaviors. The RN nodded and reoriented the patient, just as the nursing assistant had. Mrs. Davis paused again to consider what they were telling her.

"I'm in the hospital. Here in the States," she said, as if thinking aloud. Sandra and Caroline both nodded in agreement. Mrs. Davis looked around again, as if searching for something familiar to reassure her of this. Again, she ran a hand through her hair.

"Mrs. Davis, do you know where you are right now?" asked the nurse. The patient nodded.

"Yes, I'm on leave in Hawaii. I must have been dreaming. I thought I heard helicopters, and I thought I was back with my Unit."

"Ma'am, do you know what year it is?" continued the nurse. Mrs. Davis nodded and said, "1971."

"Mrs. Davis, you are in Fayette General Hospital. It's 2015. You've been in a car accident, and we're taking care of you now. I'm your nurse, Caroline." The RN gently reoriented her patient. "Come with me, Mrs. Davis. Let's get you back in bed for a bit. You seem a bit confused, and I want to help you with that." Caroline touched Mrs. Davis's elbow and was able to escort her back to her bed. "Sandra, can you tell Meagan that Mrs. Davis is awake now if she'd like to talk to her?" Mrs. Davis sat down on the side of her bed, looked around, and said, "Oh, this is a hospital. I'm not in Hawaii. I don't know why I thought that. It must have been a dream."

Critical Thinking

Answer the following questions based on the patient update that you have just read.

1. Is Mrs. Davis oriented × 3? How do you know? ______________________
2. Both the nursing assistant and the nurse attempt to do something to alleviate Mrs. Davis' confusion. What do they do? ______________________
3. From the context of what Mrs. Davis is saying, what do you think her previous occupation was?
____
4. Mrs. Davis woke up because she thought she heard the sound of helicopters. Now she thinks this might have been a dream. Based on what you've learned in this chapter, what else might it be? ______________________

Putting it all together: mental health assessment

Mrs. Davis's behaviors indicate an ongoing state of disorientation and confusion. She has misidentified the time, the place, and the people to whom she was talking.

A **mental status examination** is an examination of an individual's mental state. It includes a number of target areas from which diagnostic criteria can be identified. This type of examination can include assessments for the following:

- Presenting complaint: the current symptoms that may appear to be psychological or psychiatric in nature
- Present and past medical history
- General behavior, appearance, and attitude
- Emotional state
- Thought content and processes
- Characteristics of speech
- Orientation
- Memory: remote and recent, as well as retention and recall; a general grasp of what is happening or what has just occurred
- Insight and judgment
- History of mental illness (including family history and any hospitalizations for this)
- History of addictions or substance abuse (including family history and any hospitalization or rehabilitation for this): the use of alcohol, drugs, caffeine, or tobacco
- Occupation or occupational history
- Level of education
- Marital and family status, including significant others: intimate (close or private) interpersonal relationships
- Religious, spiritual, or cultural practices

Critical Thinking

Consider Mrs. Davis's circumstances and her current mental state as you think about the following questions.

1. Identify some reasons why a mental health assessment is warranted in the case of Mrs. Davis. ______________________
2. What might the reason be for including questions about a person's level of education during a mental health assessment? ______________________

Listen to the language: mental status examination

Patient Update

Go to DavisPlus Audio to listen to the dialogue between Meagan the RN and Mrs. Davis as they complete a mental status examination. The nurse asks the patient questions to gain subjective data, but she also collects a good deal of data by observing the patient's appearance, behavior, affect, and mood. The RN listens closely not only to evaluate the content of the answers but also to identify any thought and perceptual disturbances; she also observes for the patient's rate of speech, other speech disturbances, and overall cognition. Listen carefully to see if Meagan addresses what she observes regarding Mrs. Davis's appearance and behavior from time to time.

For audio exercises, visit **http://www.MedicalLanguageLab.com.** 

The Language of the Endocrine System

A person's mental state may reflect disturbances in the function of certain glands that regulate the body's functioning. These connections between mind and body are studied in the fields of *psychoneuroendocrinology* and *psychoendocrinology*. Dr. Jensen and the treatment team are doing a broad assessment workup on Mrs. Davis to determine if her state of confusion has any physical causes. Remember that our patient has a medical history of diabetes (pathology of the pancreas) and, on the basis of all appearances upon admission to the ER, hypothyroidism, for which she is taking a thyroid supplement. To ascertain the status of these chronic conditions and to assess whether or not they are involved in the patient's current situation, an understanding of the endocrine system and its medical terminology is necessary. A brief overview of this system follows, with special attention given to the thyroid and pancreas because they are relevant concerns for this patient.

Anatomy and physiology: endocrine system

The **endocrine** system is composed of a number of glands and organs that have the purpose of maintaining a stable internal environment in the body. This system does so through the secretion of hormones. **Hormones** are chemically regulatory substances; this means that they regulate the internal body, much as a thermostat might regulate the internal environment of a house. Make no mistake, however: hormones are responsible for much more than temperature regulation.

Observe how this medical term breaks down into its component parts.

endo	+	crine	=	endocrine
↓		↓		
prefix meaning *inside/within*	+	suffix meaning *to secrete*		

Definition: secretions that are directed within the body

Break It Down

Divide each word into its meaningful parts. Write the meaning of each part, and then define the word.

1. psychoneuroendocrinology
   - **a.** Word parts: ____________________
   - **b.** Meaning of each part: ____________________
   - **c.** Definition of term: ____________________
2. psychoendocrinology
   - **a.** Word parts: ____________________
   - **b.** Meaning of each part: ____________________
   - **c.** Definition term: ____________________

Organs of the endocrine system

The endocrine organs include the ovaries, pancreas, testes, and a number of glands. There are pairs of adrenal and parathyroid glands and one each of the pineal, pituitary, thymus, and thyroid glands. You will learn more about the ovaries and testes in Chapters 9 and 17, when you learn the language of the reproductive systems of males and females. The word part that identifies a gland is the suffix *-crine.*

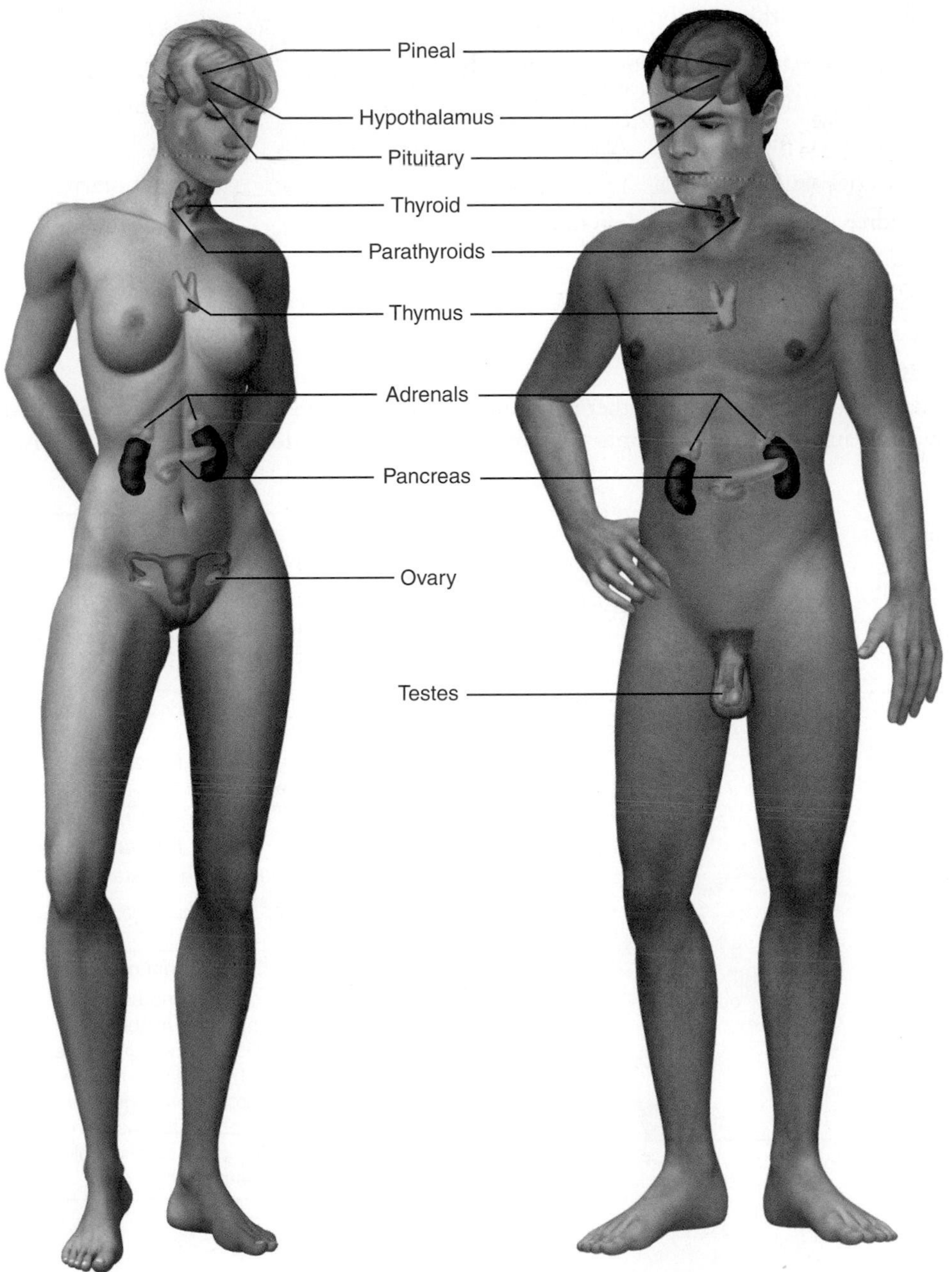

Figure 7.3: Endocrine system: female and male

Let's Practice

For this exercise, refer only to the diagram of the endocrine system. Use medical terminology to locate the organs of the endocrine system. Use the terms *external, superior, posterior, bilateral, medial, distal,* and *anterior* in their appropriate forms. (To review these terms that indicate body position, see Chapter 2.)

Example:

Q: Where are the ovaries located?

A: Bilaterally within the abdomen and superior to the womb

1. Where are the testes located on or in the body? ______________________
2. The pineal gland is ______________ and ______________ to the hypothalamus
3. The thyroid gland sits ______________ in neck on the ______________ side.
4. The ovaries are located ______________________ to the pituitary gland.
5. The adrenal glands are located on the ______________________ of the kidneys.

Functions of the endocrine system

The endocrine system takes on many roles and responsibilities in the body. Refer to Figure 7-4 to explore these.

Glands

Glands are tissues that work together to synthesize (produce) substances to be secreted within the body. The glands secrete directly into the bloodstream or by diffusion (spread) into the cells. Some

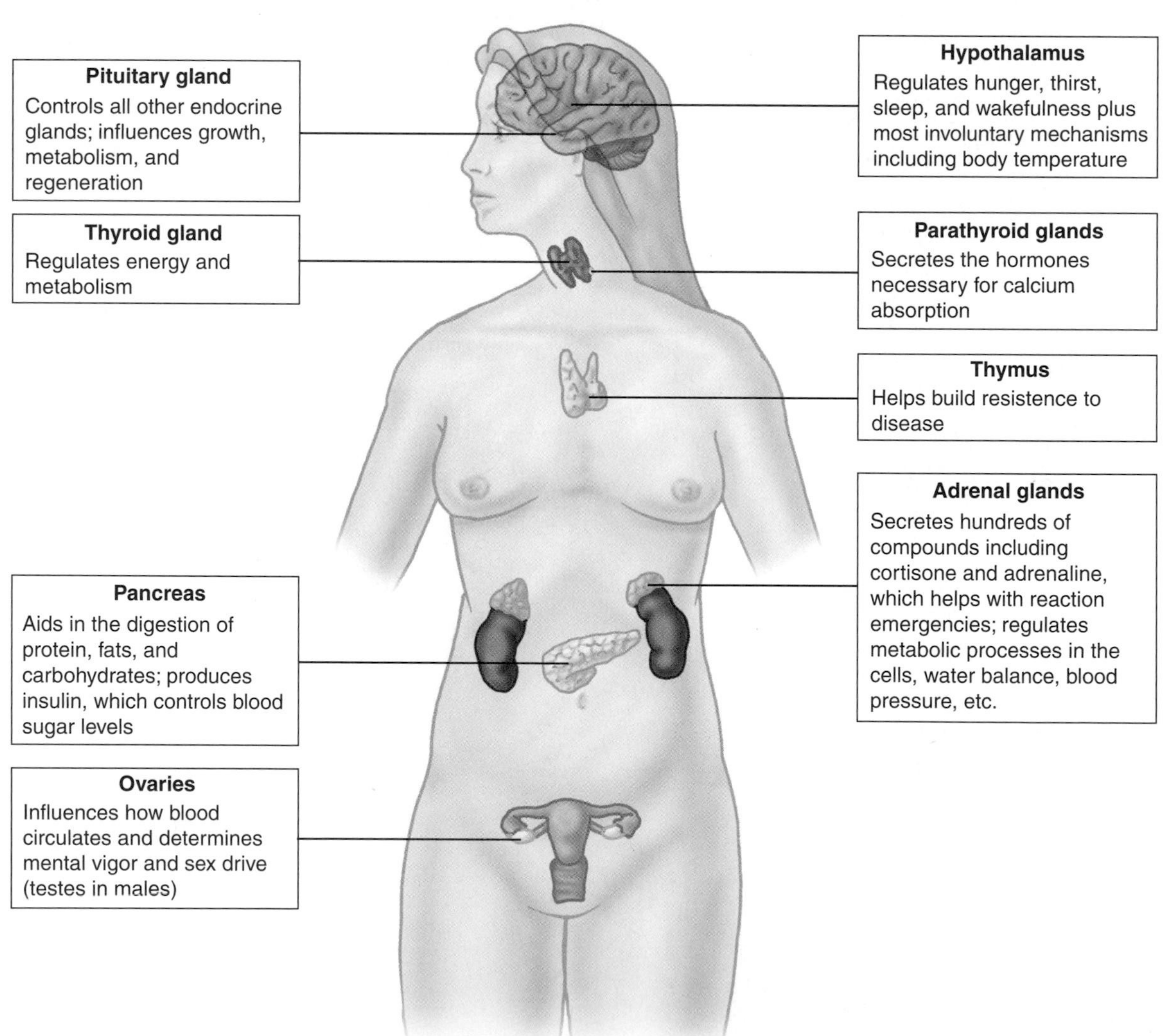

Figure 7.4: Endocrine system: functions

glands have **ducts** or special openings through which chemicals are secreted (see "The Language of the Exocrine System" later in this chapter). Endocrine glands do not have ducts.

Explore the medical and anatomical terms for the endocrine glands, and become familiar with their combining forms in Table 7-5.

TABLE 7-5: Endocrine Glands: Roots and Combining Forms

Gland	Roots/Combining Forms	Gland	Roots/Combining Forms
adrenal glands	aden/o adren/o adrenal/o	pineal gland or epiphysis	pineal/o
		pituitary gland or hypophysis	pituitar/o
		thymus gland	thym/o
parathyroid glands	parathyroid/o		

Mix and Match

Match the function with its gland. Draw a line between the two to connect them. (The word *pancreas* intentionally appears twice here.)

1. facilitate urgent or emergency needs for energy	pancreas
2. important for metabolism	hypothalamus
3. controls levels of blood sugar	pancreas
4. integral to male sexual development	adrenal glands
5. important for digestion	testes
6. involved in female reproduction	thyroid
7. regulates core biological functions such as sleep, hunger, and thirst	ovaries

Pituitary gland

The **pituitary** gland is more technically known as the **hypophysis**. It controls most of the other glands within the endocrine system, and it participates in the maintenance of homeostasis in the

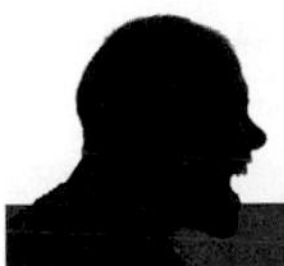

PRONUNCIATION PRACTICE

Say these words aloud to a friend or classmate if you can. You are given the phonetic pronunciation. Your instructor can help you with pronunciation, or visit **http://www.MedicalLanguageLab.com.**

adrenal	ăd-**rē**´năl
adenohypophysis	ăd″ĕ-nō-hī-**pŏf**´ĭ-sĭs
adrenocorticotropic	ăd-rē″nō-kor″tĭ-kō-**trŏp**´ĭk
calcitonin	kăl″sĭ-**tō**´nĭn
epiphysis	ĕ-**pĭf**´ĭ-sĭs
endocrine	**ĕn**´dō-krīn or krĭn or krēn
hypophysis	hī-**pŏf**´ĭ-sĭs
hypothalamus	hī″pō-**thăl**´ă-mŭs
neurohypophysis	nū″rō-hī-**pŏf**´ĭs-ĭs
melanocyte	mĕl´**ăn**-ō-sīt
oxytocin	**ŏk**″sē-tō´sĭn
pineal	pĭn´ē-ăl

Continued

pituitary	pĭ-**tū**´ĭ-tăr″ē
parathyroid	păr-ă-**thī**´royd
psychoneuroendocrinology	sī″kō-nū″rō-ĕn″dō-krĭn-**ŏl**´ō-jē
somatotropin	sō″măt-ō-**trō**´pĭn
thymus	**thī**´mŭs
tri-iodothyronine	trī″ī-ō″dō-**thī**´rō-nēn

body. It is very tiny yet very significant. The pituitary gland is divided into three lobes: the *adenohypophysis* (anterior), the *neurohypophysis* (posterior), and the *intermediate lobe*, each of which serves different functions (see Figure 7-5). The pituitary gland is attached to the hypothalamus, which is located at the base of the brain.

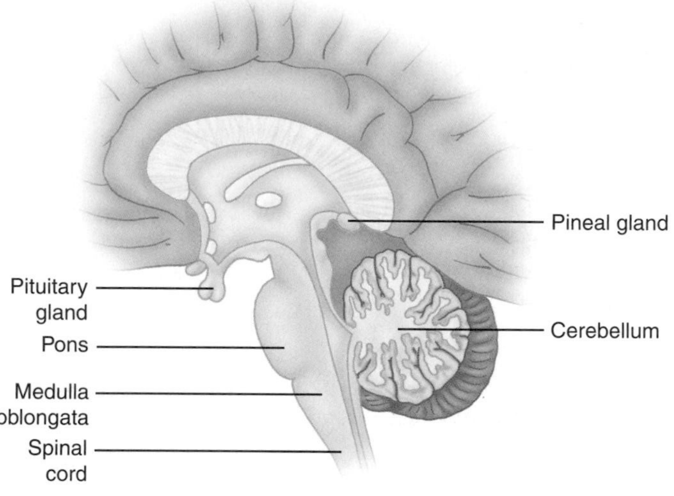

Figure 7.5: Anatomy of the pituitary gland

TABLE 7-6: The Pituitary Gland: Hormones and Lobes

Hormone	Role or Purpose	Location by Lobe
adrenocorticotropic hormone (ACTH)	regulates the activity of the adrenal cortex; stimulates the adrenal gland	adenohypophysis (anterior)
antidiuretic hormone (ADH)	increases water absorption from the kidneys into the blood; decreases urine formation and output	neurohypophysis (posterior)
follicle-stimulating hormone (FSH)	stimulates the growth and reproductive activities of the ovaries and testes	adenohypophysis
human growth hormone (HGH)	controls the process of growth	adenohypophysis
luteinizing hormone (LH) (also known as *luteotropic hormone* [LTH] or *prolactin hormone* [PRL])	stimulates the growth and reproductive activities of the ovaries and testes	adenohypophysis
melanocyte-stimulating hormone	controls skin pigmentation	intermediate
oxytocin	contracts the uterus during childbirth and stimulates milk production	neurohypophysis
thyroid-stimulating hormone (TSH) (also known as *somatotropin*)	stimulates the thyroid gland	adenohypophysis

Explore the word parts of the hormones that are released by the pituitary gland. These will help you to recognize new terms related to the pituitary.

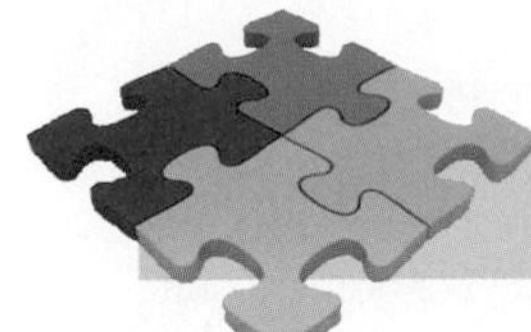

WORD BUILDING: Word Building for Pituitary Hormones

adrenocorticotropic = *ad* + *ren/o* + *cortic/o* + *tropic*

ad = toward (prefix)
ren/o = kidneys (combining form)
cortico = cortex; outer surface of an organ or structure (combining form)
tropic = a hormone secreted by the pituitary gland that stimulates the release of other hormones

prolactin = *pro* + *lactin*

pro = ahead of, in front of, or before (prefix)
lactin = milk (derived from the root *lac*)

melanocyte = *melano* + *cyte*

melano = black; pigment (combining form)
cyte = cell

antidiuretic = *anti* + *diuretic*

anti = against or opposite (prefix)
diuretic = increasing production of urine (derivative of *diuresis*, meaning to *urinate*)

adenohypophysis = *adeno* + *hypo* + *physis*

adeno = gland (combining form)
hypo = below or under (prefix)
physis = growth

neurohypophysis = *neuro* + *hypo* + *physis*

neuro = nerve (root)
hypo = below or under (prefix)
physis = growth

somatotropin = *somat/o* + *tropin*

somat/o = body (combining form)
tropin = effect of a substance (a combining form used as a suffix)

Free Writing

Use the clue words given to write sentences that include medical terms made up of word parts that refer to the endocrine system.

EXAMPLE: result of, height, childhood, spurts, release, hormone
Sentence: During childhood, spurts in height are the result of the release of human growth hormone.

1. skin color, natural, cells ______________________________
2. formation stimulates hormone urine ______________________________
3. TSH gland stimulates to ______________________________

Mix and Match

Match the term on the left with the description on the right. Draw a line to connect them.

1. antidiuretic	growth
2. oxytocin	increases urine output
3. physis	decreases urine output
4. diuretic	stimulates the uterus to contract during labor

Thyroid gland

The **thyroid** is a gland that is located internally just below the larynx and on the anterior surface of the throat. This gland has two lobes: one on each side of the esophagus. Following a chain of events, the hypothalamus stimulates the pituitary gland, which then stimulates the thyroid gland to produce and secrete thyroid hormone. The thyroid requires iodine to produce its hormones. **Iodine** is a non-metallic chemical element; it is a natural element in digestion, and it occurs in low doses in the human body.

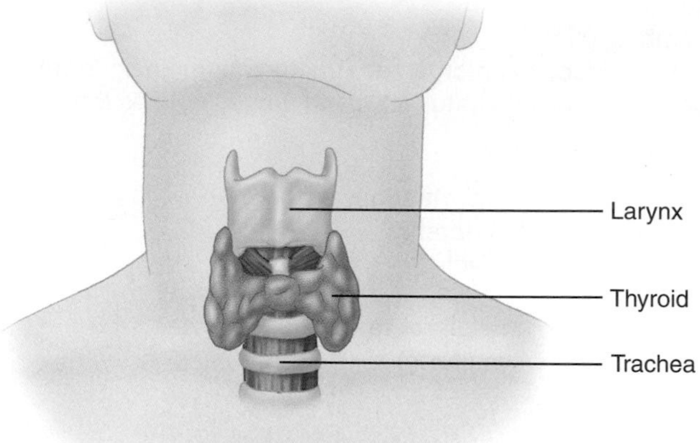

Figure 7.6: Thyroid gland

The thyroid gland is composed of two cell types:

- *Follicular cells* of the thyroid gland secrete the hormones thyroxine (T4) and tri-iodothyronine (T3).
- *Parafollicular cells* secrete the hormone calcitonin.

The function of the thyroid gland is to regulate the body's metabolism and its calcium balance. **Metabolism** refers to the chemical activity within the cells during which energy is released from nutrients or energy is used to create other substances (i.e., proteins).

Thyroxine and tri-iodothyronine stimulate the production of protein and regulate the rate of metabolism.

Calcitonin works in conjunction with the *parathyroid glands* to regulate calcium levels in the blood and the bones. There are four tiny parathyroid glands that sit adjacent to and behind the thyroid gland.

The combining forms of the root *thyroid* are *thyr/o* and *thyroid/o.*

Function of the Thyroid

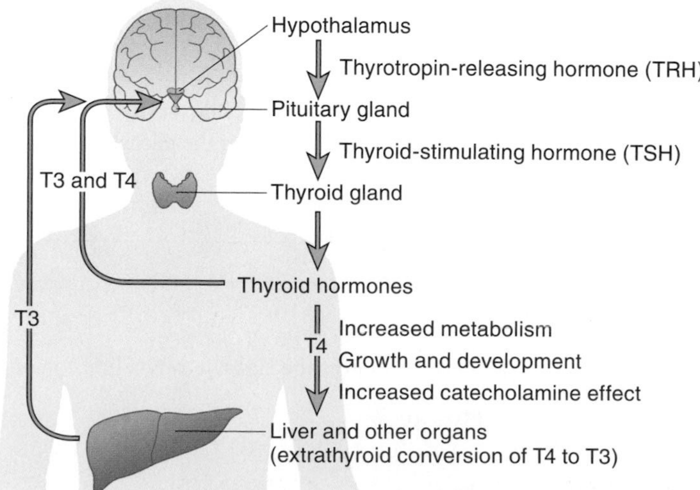

Figure 7.7: Functions of the thyroid gland

TABLE 7-7: Hormones Secreted by the Thyroid Gland

Hormone	Role or Purpose
thyroxine (T4)	increases the use of food for the production of energy; increases the rate of protein synthesis (the formation of chemical compounds or combinations of compounds)
tri-iodothyronine (T3)	helps to control metabolism and body temperature; helps to regulate growth and development
calcitonin	responsible for the maintenance of bone density and strength, as well as blood calcium levels

Pathology of the thyroid gland

Numerous references have been made to the relationship between our patient, Mrs. Stevie-Rose Davis, and an unknown thyroid disorder or disease that she seems to have. One of the nurses suggested that Mrs. Davis suffered from hypothyroidism. She drew this conclusion from the fact that the patient had a prescription with her for 150 μg of levothyroxine. Levothyroxine is a thyroid hormone replacement or supplement that is used when the thyroid is not producing its hormones adequately or at all. It has also been suggested that Mrs. Davis's thyroid condition or her usage of a thyroid supplement may be contributing to her current mental state. It may even be possible that Mrs. Davis's mental state contributed to the motor vehicle accident in some way. Study Table 7-7 to learn more about thyroid pathology, and then think critically about why the treatment team at Fayette General Hospital has included thyroid function testing for Mrs. Davis.

TABLE 7-8: Signs and Symptoms of Thyroid Pathologies

Hyperthyroidism	Hypothyroidism	Thyroiditis	Thyroid Cancer
• difficulty with concentration (particularly among elderly patients) • muscle weakness • agitation • nervousness • difficulty swallowing • perspiration • irritability • racing heart • weight loss • difficulty sleeping • brittle hair • frequent bowel movements • Graves' disease	• lethargy • depression • dry skin and hair • muscle cramps • development of a goiter (enlargement of the thyroid gland) • weight gain • sensitivity to cold	• inflammation of the thyroid • decreased thyroid levels in the blood or a sudden rapid increase • may mimic either hyperthyroidism or hypothyroidism • can be acute, chronic, or transient (temporary) • examples: Hashimoto's thyroiditis, postpartum thyroiditis	• a lump (nodule) is present and may be the only sign or symptom • the most common of the endocrine cancers; it can be effectively treated

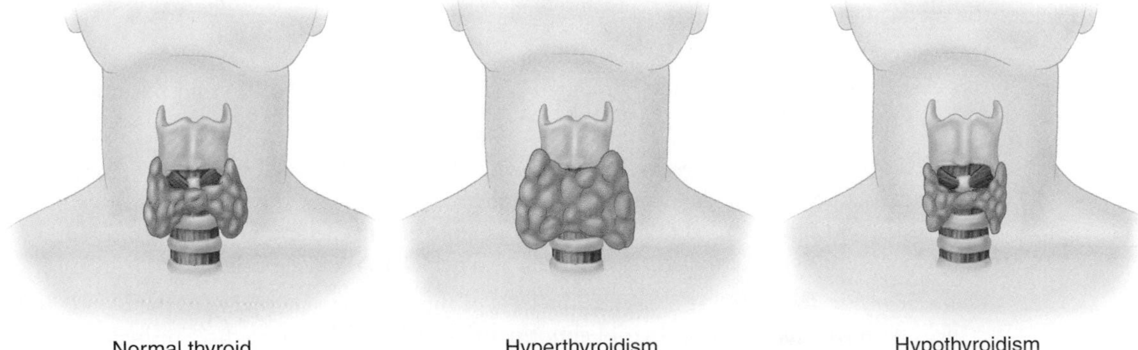

Figure 7.8: Levels of thyroid functioning

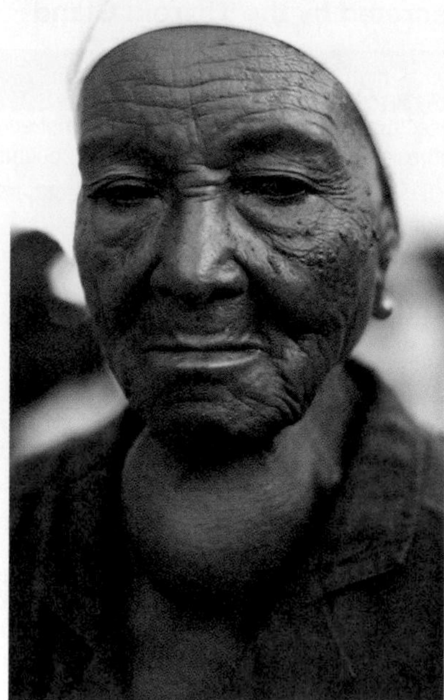

Figure 7.9: Patient with a goiter (Courtesy James Gray, MissionFoto, Gosport, Indiana)

Critical Thinking

Refer to Table 7-7 to help you answer these questions.

1. Has Mrs. Davis exhibited any signs and symptoms of a thyroid disease since she was brought into the emergency department? If so, name them.

____

____

2. Notice that Mrs. Davis has symptoms of hyperthyroidism yet she is receiving medication for hypothyroidism. Think deeply about this. What else might be happening in relation to the thyroid gland that leads to confusion about which diagnosis is correct? (This is a difficult question. The answer will become even more clear as this chapter continues. Try not to look at the Answer Key just yet.)

____

The language of diagnostics: thyroid function tests

Diagnostic testing for thyroid function includes blood tests, screening by diagnostic imaging, and the medical procedure of taking a biopsy.

Blood tests

Blood samples are collected and compared against normal ranges of thyroid hormones and calcitonin in the bloodstream.

TSH: This blood test measures the level of *thyroid-stimulating hormone* or *thyrotropin* in the blood. It is used as a first step in the detection of any thyroid dysfunction. It detects hypothyroidism or hyperthyroidism, it is used to monitor thyroid replacement therapy, and it may be used to screen newborns for hypothyroidism. A TSH can also help with the diagnosis of female infertility.

Total T4 or free T4: This test measures the level of the hormone thyroxine in the blood, and it can help with the detection of thyroid abnormalities such as hypothyroidism or hyperthyroidism. It is often used conjointly with TSH testing to provide the most accurate assessment of thyroid function.

Total T3 or free T3: This test measures levels of the hormone tri-iodothyronine in the blood. It is used to detect hyperthyroidism.

Thyroid antibodies: This test detects and identifies different types of thyroiditis.

Calcitonin: This test detects the presence and production of calcitonin in the blood.

Screening

Thyroid ultrasound allows for the measurement of the thyroid gland. It is able to show whether a nodule (lump) on the thyroid is solid or fluid.

Thyroid scans involve the use of putting radioactive iodine in the body and then subsequently scanning for where it accumulates to evaluate the functioning of the thyroid gland and any related abnormalities.

Thyroid biopsies are medical procedures in which a small amount of tissue is removed from the thyroid or a nodule by a small needle and then sent to the laboratory for examination.

Treatment

At the beginning of this chapter, you learned that Mrs. Davis is taking a thyroid replacement drug; she had a prescription for this drug among her belongings. As you become more familiar with her symptoms and assessment, you may very well be able to diagnose her condition before you learn the results of her blood tests, which are given in Chapter 12. Challenge yourself.

Thyroid replacement therapy is indicated when diagnostic data confirm that the thyroid is not functioning as it should. Hypothyroidism is the most common reason for thyroid replacement therapy.

Anti-thyroid therapy is indicated for conditions of hyperthyroidism. In this instance, anti-thyroid medication is prescribed to inhibit or arrest the production of the thyroid hormones.

Radioactive iodine treatment is an effective and permanent treatment for hyperthyroidism. Radioactive iodine is taken once by mouth, and, within a month or two, the thyroid cells are killed. Although this is highly effective and quite a common solution for hyperthyroidism, it often leaves the patient in a state of hypothyroidism; thyroid replacement therapy may be necessary after this treatment.

Diagnostics and biomedical technology

The assessment of Mrs. Davis's thyroid condition required the collecting of blood and urine specimens, which will be analyzed in the laboratory. **Biotechnology** is the analysis of specimens from the human body, such as blood, body fluids, and tissue. *Chemical pathology* is a subfield of biotechnology in which normal and abnormal blood chemistry is examined; this includes hormone and blood glucose levels. *Cellular pathology* is another subfield that examines abnormal changes in cells and tissues, including cancer. Mrs. Davis's blood and urine specimens may well be examined by a biomedical technician in the hospital laboratory, particularly if this is a teaching or research facility.

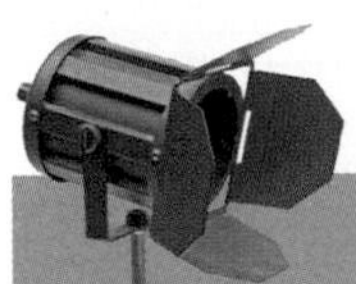

CAREER SPOTLIGHT: Biomedical Technician

There is some confusion regarding the practice and training of a biomedical technician. In the United States, there seem to be two diverse groups and two separate streams of education.

1. One type of biomedical technician works in a laboratory analyzing human samples. He or she rarely if ever has any contact with the specimen donors, unlike the laboratory technicians that you learned about in Chapter 3. Tests and analyses are performed with the use of modern technology (see Chapter 3 for some examples). This is a field of basic and applied medical research. The education of these technicians includes courses in laboratory sciences. These biomedical technicians will work in microbiology, chemical pathology, cellular pathology, and hematology. They are also referred to as *clinical laboratory technologists* and *medical laboratory technologists.*

Continued

2. Another type of biomedical technician repairs medical equipment and devices. Examples of such devices include heart monitors, complicated life-saving electronic equipment, oxygen machines, electric wheelchairs, and mechanical lifts. This type of biomedical technician may go on to pursue studies and obtain credentials in biomedical engineering technology.

Critical Thinking

On the basis of what you have just learned, answer the following questions.

1. What is the difference between a TSH test and a total T4 test? ______________________
2. Which thyroid treatment might very likely lead to hypothyroidism? ______________________
3. What is the medical term for a lump? ______________________
4. What does the abbreviation *TSH* stand for? ______________________
5. The thyroid gland produces another hormone in addition to the thyroid hormones. What is it? ______________________

Build a Word

Use your skills at combining word parts to create words related to the thyroid that you have not yet learned, and then use your understanding of each part's meaning to write a definition.

1. toxin thyroid/o ______________________ Meaning: ______________________
2. -ectomy thyroid/o ______________________ Meaning: ______________________
3. tome thyr/o ______________________ Meaning: ______________________
4. uria calci ______________________ Meaning: ______________________

Let's Practice

Spelling is an important skill in health care, particularly if you are required to write by hand and do not have the benefit of a spellchecker on a computer. For this exercise, unscramble the words, and then spell them correctly. These terms refer to the pituitary and thyroid glands.

1. i d t y h o r ______________________
2. l u l r a r a p f a o l c i ______________________
3. t a f r o n o i m ______________________
4. t t p o n r i a o o a m ______________________
5. d i a t e r i i c n t u ______________________
6. p s i h y s p y h o ______________________
7. l u e z i g n i t i n ______________________
8. d n i o i e ______________________

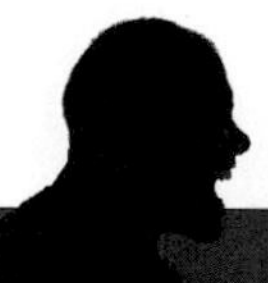

PRONUNCIATION PRACTICE

Say these words aloud to a friend or classmate if you can. You are given the phonetic pronunciation. Your instructor can help you with pronunciation,

or visit **http://www.MedicalLanguageLab.com.** 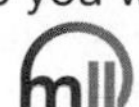

calciuria	kăl″sē-ū′rē-ă	thyroidectomy	thī″royd-**ĕk**′tō-mē
iodine	ī′ă-dīn″	thyrotome	**thī**′rō-tōm
thyroidotoxin	thī″royd-ō-**tŏk**′sĭn	thyroxine	thī-**rŏks**′ĭn

The Language of the Exocrine System

Mrs. Davis has a medical history of diabetes, which arises in the endocrine and **exocrine** systems. The exocrine system is normally discussed under the broader category of the endocrine system, and although it is connected to that system, it is different. An introduction to the exocrine system follows, with a focus on the pancreas and its role in diabetes.

Anatomy and physiology: exocrine system

Exocrine glands secrete into ducts that reach the surface of the skin. These include the sweat, sebaceous, and mammary glands, as well as the glands that secrete digestive enzymes (i.e., the salivary glands in the mouth).

exo + crine = exocrine

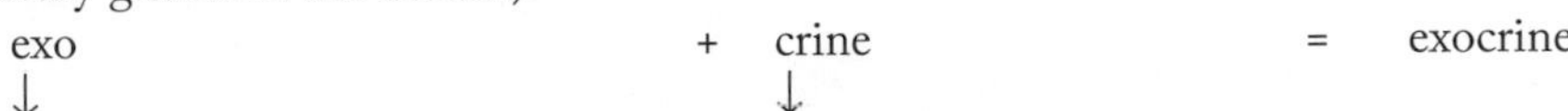

↓ ↓

prefix meaning outside/external + suffix meaning to secrete

Definition: secretions that are directed externally or toward the outside of the body.

Organs of the exocrine system

The exocrine system includes the pancreas, the liver, and numerous glands, each of which has a duct or opening through which the exocrine glands secrete chemicals to the internal and external surfaces of the body. Internally, glands may secrete into organs and body cavities. For example, the liver secretes bile; the pancreas secretes insulin and pancreatic fluid.

Functions of the exocrine system

The function of the exocrine glands is to maintain homeostasis, which is a state of internal equilibrium. This state is achieved via such activities as sweating, digestion, and lubrication.

Key terms: exocrine glands

holocrine (sebaceous) glands: glands located in the skin and hair. These glands secrete a fatty substance called sebum into the pores of the skin. Each pore contains a hair follicle, and the sebum travels up the follicle to the external surface of the body.

merocrine (eccrine) glands: sweat glands found throughout the skin. These glands secrete water and sodium (NaCl). The sweat glands play a major part in the thermoregulation (temperature regulation) of both the skin and the internal body.

apocrine glands: sweat glands around the hair follicles of the armpits, the perineum, and the nipples. They secrete water, sodium, and bacteria, which can lead to an odor.

mammary glands: specialized glands in females that secrete milk for newborns.

salivary glands: glands in the oral cavity that secrete a number of substances that come together as saliva. These secretions contain enzymes and begin the process of digestion.

The language of the pancreas

The **pancreas** is both an endocrine and exocrine gland. It is located deep within the abdomen, between the stomach and the spine, and adjacent to the duodenum (small intestine).

Function of the pancreas

The pancreas is integral to the maintenance of appropriate blood glucose or sugar levels in the body, and it is also an integral part of the digestive system (see Chapter 16). Under stress (i.e., a motor vehicle accident), blood glucose levels may be adversely affected, thereby clouding the patient's judgment and leading to symptoms such as confusion and fainting.

Physiology of the pancreas

The pancreas consists of a number of endocrine cells and exocrine ducts. The main duct is the *pancreatic duct*, which runs the length of this small organ and which drains pancreatic fluid into the *bile duct*. Endocrine cells secrete directly into the tissue and blood.

The **islets of Langerhans** are endocrine cells that produce the pancreatic hormones insulin and glucagon. These hormones help with the maintenance of normal glucose levels in the blood. Glucose provides energy for the body.

Insulin promotes the removal of glucose from the blood and stores it in the liver as glycogen, fats, and protein.

Glucagon has the opposite effect of insulin. It raises the level of blood glucose by changing stored glycogen back to glucose. Glucagon is usually secreted between meals to maintain a normal blood glucose level.

Acinar cells are exocrine cells that secrete enzymes. **Enzymes** are catalysts; they allow cells to carry out chemical reactions. Pancreatic fluid, which contains enzymes, is produced by the acinar cells to assist with digestion and then to transport the waste products of digestion out of the body. Together with the secretions of the bile duct, the pancreatic duct secretions empty into the duodenum.

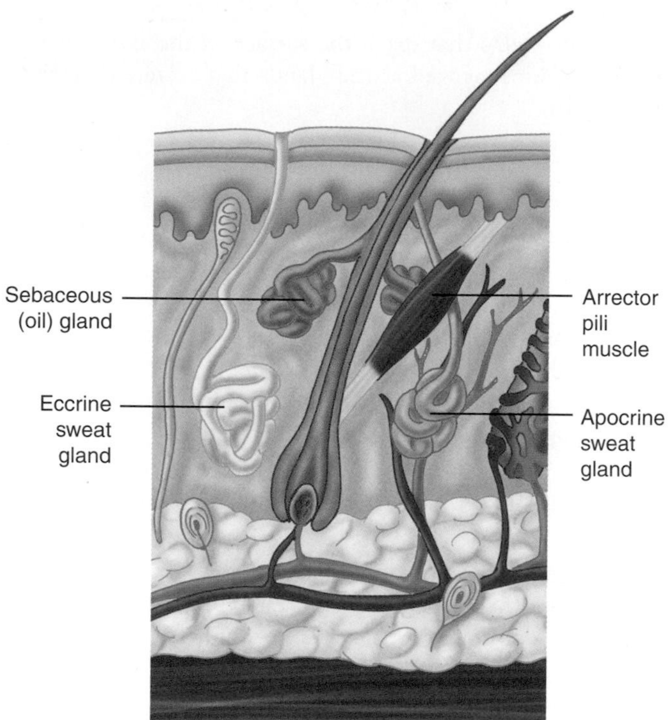

Figure 7.10: Apocrine and eccrine glands

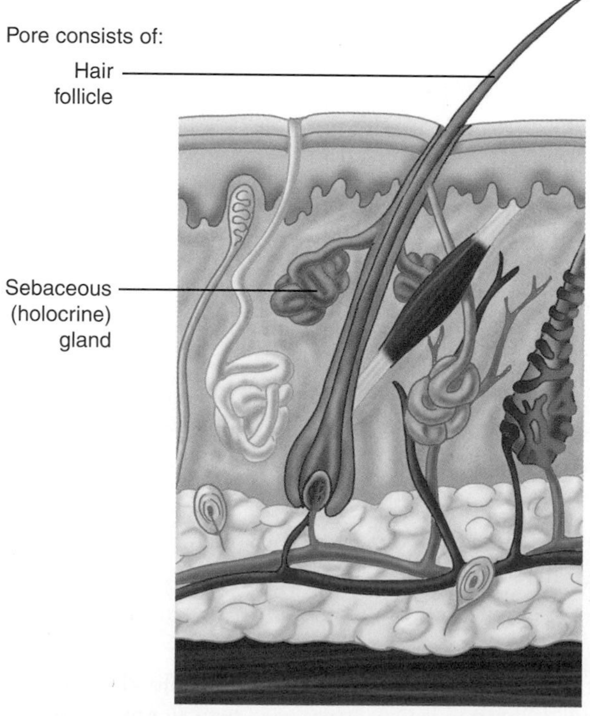

Figure 7.11: Holocrine or sebaceous glands

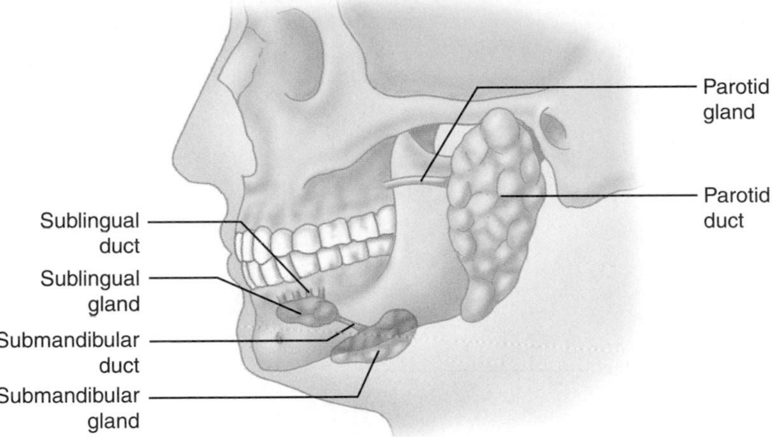

Figure 7.12: Salivary glands

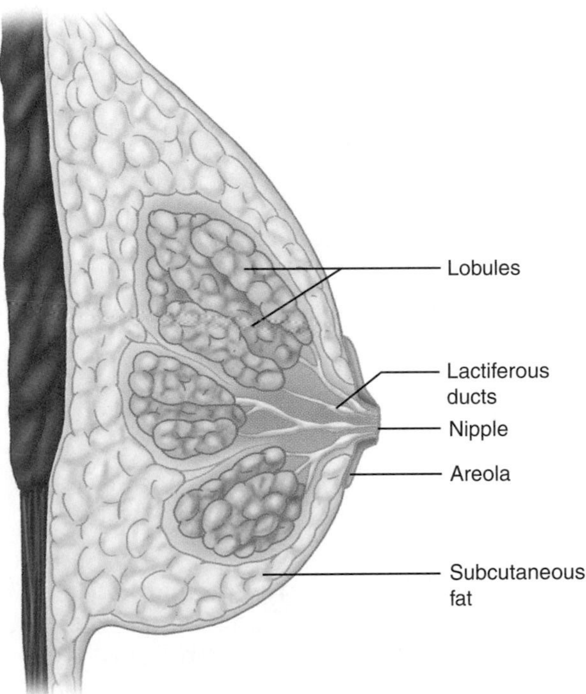

Figure 7.13: Mammary glands

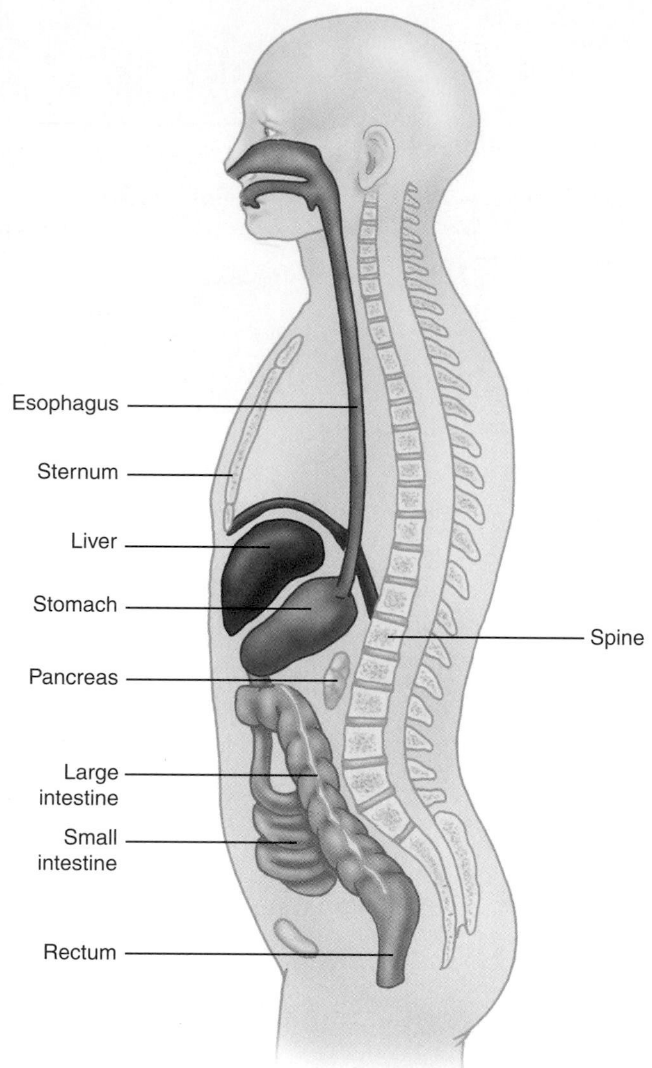

Figure 7.14: Location of the pancreas

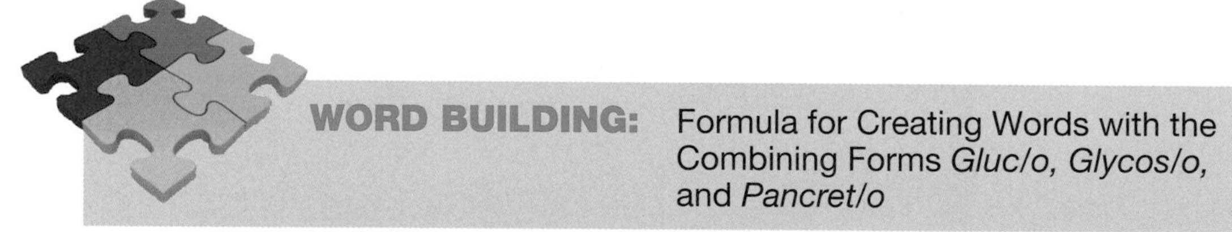

WORD BUILDING: Formula for Creating Words with the Combining Forms *Gluc/o, Glycos/o,* and *Pancret/o*

1. gluekos = Greek root meaning *sweet.* The combining forms *gluc/o* and *glucoso* mean *sugar or having a relationship to sweetness.*

gluco + meter = *glucometer*

Definition: a device for measuring blood glucose levels from a few drops of blood from the finger. (The second root is *meter,* meaning *measure.*) *noun*

Example: Mrs. Davis had a STAT *glucometer* test in the ER.

gluco + penia = *glucopenia*

Definition: low blood sugar. (The suffix *-penia* means *lack.*) *noun*

Example: *Glucopenia* is another name for hypoglycemia.

glucos + uria = *glucosuria*
Definition: the presence of glucose in the urine. (The second root is a combining form of the word *urine.*) *noun*

Example: *Glucosuria* is a symptom that can be identified with a urinalysis test.

2. glykys = Greek root meaning *sweet or sweetness in specific reference to sugars or the presence of glycerol* (present in fats). The combining form are *glyc-* and *glycos/o.*

glyc + emia = *glycemia*
Definition: the level of glucose in the blood. (The suffix *-emia* stems from the root word *haima,* meaning blood.) *noun*

Example: Endocrinologists and laboratory diagnosticians are interested in the maintenance of *glycemia* levels.

glyco + clastic = *glycoclastic*
Definition: pertaining to the digestion and hydrolysis (decomposition by water) of sugars. (The second word part derives from *klastos,* meaning *broken or divided into pieces.*) *adjective*

Example: Studies of the *glycoclastic* processes in the human body are part of the focus of diabetic research.

3. pancreas = an organ that secretes enzymes and insulin. (The word part *pan* means *all.* The original root *kreas* means *flesh.* The combining form is *pancret/o.)*

pancreato + graphy = *pancreatography*
Definition: endoscopic and radiographic examination of the pancreas. *noun*

Example: A radiographic medium (substance) is injected into the pancreas before beginning *pancreatography.*

pancreato + lytic = *pancreatolytic*
Definition: describing something that can cause the destruction of the pancreas. (The suffix *-lytic* is derived from *lysis,* meaning *dissolution.*) *adjective*

Example: Pancreatitis can lead to a *pancreatolytic* condition if it is left untreated.

eu + pancreat + ism = *eupancreatism*
Definition: the normal condition of the pancreas; a healthy state of the pancreas. (The suffix *-ismos* means *condition.*) *noun*

Example: Most people can be said to be in a state of *eupancreatism.*

Build a Word

Combine these word parts to create terms that you have not yet learned. Using your knowledge of each part's meaning, discuss the definition of each term with a partner.

1. genesis glyco ____________________
2. poly glyc/o uria ____________________
3. -ism glyc/o metabol ____________________
4. genesis gluc/o ____________________
5. pathy pancreat/o ____________________

Diabetes

Diabetes is the term that is used for a group of medical conditions in which both the pancreas and the adrenal glands are implicated. Diabetes and metabolism are closely tied. A cardinal symptom of diabetes is excessive urination (**polyuria**).

The *pancreas* of a diabetic does not produce enough insulin to meet the body's needs; alternatively, the cells of the body do not respond appropriately to insulin when it is received.

The *adrenal glands* secrete three types of hormones. One type that is important in the pathology of diabetes is the **glucocorticoid** hormones. Glucocorticoids affect the metabolism, and they facilitate an increase in the level of blood glucose. These hormones have the potential to create insulin resistance. They can also induce **hyperglycemia**; this is an excess level of glucose in the blood, which is the prime symptom of diabetes. Diet, exercise, and blood glucose monitoring can effectively treat glucocorticoid-induced hyperglycemia.

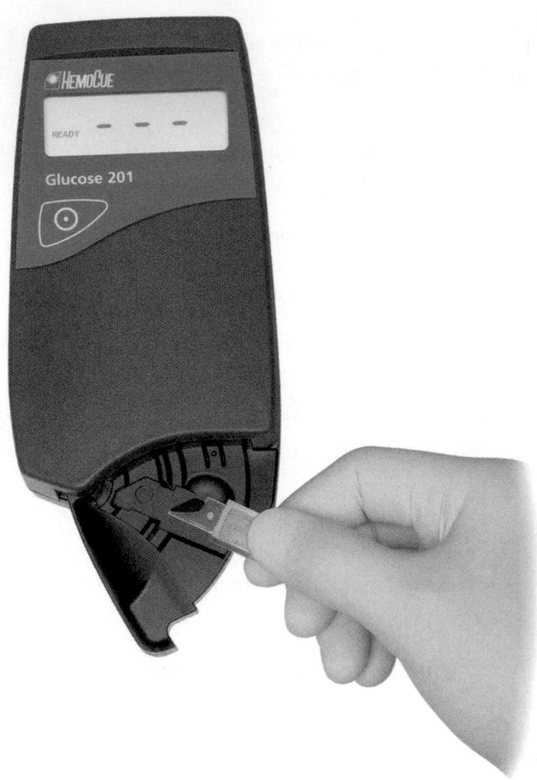

Figure 7.15: Types of glucometers (From Strasinger S, Di Lorenzo M: *The Phlebotomy Textbook,* ed 3. Philadelphia: FA Davis, 2011, p. 380. With permission.)

Types of diabetes

There are three main types of diabetes. They are referred to either by number or by their formal medical names.

Type 1 Diabetes (Diabetes Mellitus)

This illness begins before the age of 40 years. In the United States, the peak age of onset is around 14 years. The cause (etiology) is an insulin deficiency. The body does not have enough insulin to maintain normal blood glucose levels, which leads to symptoms of hyperglycemia. Type 1 diabetes is a pancreatolytic autoimmune disorder. Treatment involves subcutaneous insulin injections or the use of an insulin pump, which is a medical device attached to the body that allows for the easier delivery of multiple doses of insulin. Dietary restrictions are critical. Type 1 diabetes was formerly known as *juvenile diabetes.*

Type 2 Diabetes (Adult Onset)

Type 2 diabetes generally occurs after middle age. It is caused by insulin resistance, which is the inability of the body to accept and use insulin. As a result, glucose cannot be removed from the blood. Without intervention, an eventual buildup of excessive blood glucose can be toxic to the pancreas, thereby causing less insulin production. Contributing factors for type 2 diabetes are obesity, a high caloric intake, and a genetic predisposition (i.e., others in the family may have it, too). Treatment may include oral medications and dietary restrictions.

Gestational Diabetes

Gestational diabetes is a temporary condition that occurs during pregnancy for some women. After the birth of the child, it usually clears. However, women who experience this type of diabetes during pregnancy have an increased risk of developing type 2 diabetes later in life.

Critical Thinking

Refer to the signs and symptoms of diabetes for this exercise.

1. Are there any signs and symptoms of diabetes that Mrs. Davis may have been experiencing at the time of the motor vehicle accident or while in the hospital? If so, name them. (To review her symptoms at the scene of the accident, refer to the opening scenario of Chapter 2.)

   ____

   Identify a synonym for *hypoglycemia.* ______________________

Free Writing

Use the clue words given to write sentences that use medical terms associated with the pancreas and diabetes.

1. insulin blood organ produces ______________________
2. pregnancy temporary diabetes form ______________________
3. metabolism glucocorticoids glucose ______________________
4. subcutaneous type insulin ______________________
5. pancreas adrenal diabetes implicated ______________________

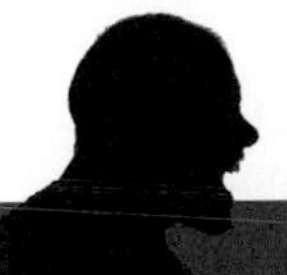

PRONUNCIATION PRACTICE

Say these words aloud to a friend or classmate if you can. You are given the phonetic pronunciation. Your instructor can help you with pronunciation,

or visit **http://www.MedicalLanguageLab.com.** 

apocrine	**ăp**´ō-krĕn	glycometabolism	glī″kō-mĕ-**tăb**´ō-lĭzm
acinar	**ăs**´ĭ-năr	glucogenesis	gloo″kō-**jĕn**´ĕ-sĭs
exocrine	**ĕks**´ō-krĭn	holocrine	**hŏl**´ō-krīn
eccrine	**ĕk**´rĭn	merocrine	**mĕr**´ō-krīn
eupancreatism	ū-**păn**´krē-ă-tĭzm	islets	ī´lĕts
glucagon	**gloo**´kă-gŏn	Langerhans	**lăng**´gĕr-hănz
glycemia	glī-**sē**´mē-ă	mammary	**măm**´ă-rē
glycoclastic	glī″kō-**klăs**´tĭk	pancreatography	păn″krē-ă-**tŏg**´ră-fē
glucosuria	glĭ″kō-**s**ū´rē-ă	pancreatolytic	păn″krē-ăt-ō-**lĭt**´ĭk
glucopenia	gloo″kō-**pē**´nē-ă	polydipsia	pŏl″ē-**dĭp**´sē-ă
glucometer	gloo-**kŏm**´ĭ-tĕr	polyphagia	pŏl″ē-**fā**´jē-ă
glucocorticoid	gloo″kō-**kort**´ĭ-koyd	pancreatopathy	păn″krē-ă-**tŏp**´ă-thē
glycogenesis	glī″kō-**jĕn**´ĕ-sĭs	salivary	**săl**´ĭ-vĕr-ē
glycopolyuria	glī″kō-pŏl″ē-**ū**´rē-ă	sebaceous	sē-**bā**´shŭs

Eponyms: The Endocrine and Exocrine

Graves' disease is an autoimmune disease in which antibodies mistakenly attack the thyroid. This causes inflammation of the thyroid gland and the excessive production of thyroid hormone. This hyperthyroid disease is named after 19th-century physician and educator Robert James Graves of Ireland, who was one of the first doctors to describe it. It was also described by one of Graves' contemporaries, Karl Adolph von Basedow. The condition is known as *Graves' disease* in English-speaking countries and as *von Basedow's disease* in Europe.

Hashimoto's thyroiditis is a chronic autoimmune disease of the thyroid gland that causes inflammation and the decreased production of thyroid hormone. This hypothyroid disease is named after Hakaru Hashimoto, the Japanese surgeon who first described it in 1912.

The islets of Langerhans were named after the German pathologist and anatomist Paul Langerhans, who first described this pancreatic tissue in 1869. In 1893, which was 6 years after Langerhans' death, these anatomical features were named after him.

Pharmacology and Pharmacokinetics: An Introduction

During the last assessment of Mrs. Davis's presenting condition in the ER, the nurses were concerned about the medications that the patient was taking. The treatment team as a whole worries about the potential adverse effects that may result when patients take one or more drugs together, particularly if the drugs are not taken as prescribed or if they are combined with over-the-counter medications. To explore these concerns, knowledge of the terminology of pharmacology and pharmacokinetics is helpful. (You will learn more about pharmacology and the language of medication administration in Unit 3.)

Pharmacology is the study of the science of drugs, including how they work and interact with the body, as well as with other drugs.

Pharmacokinetics is a field that focuses specifically on the metabolism of drugs, how they are absorbed and distributed, how the body excretes them, how long it takes for them to achieve a therapeutic effect, and the duration of the desired effect.

Drugs are metabolized, which means that they are chemically altered by the body. For most drugs, this process occurs in the liver. *Metabolization* produces *metabolites*, which are chemicals that are responsible for producing the desired therapeutic effects. As a person ages, the ability of the liver to maintain a desired level of functioning decreases. This means that the elderly, like infants and children, require much smaller doses of medications. Many older adults do not understand this fact about their changing metabolisms. It is common to find older individuals taking the same adult-strength doses of a drug that they did when they were younger, not realizing that the drug will now remain in their bodies longer and have the potential to create adverse or even toxic effects. This is why the treatment team at Fayette General Hospital ER has ordered a drug screening for Mrs. Davis. The combination of drugs that she has been taking recently may be at least partly responsible for her current state of mental confusion.

The language of drug assessment

Drug tests and drug screens

A **drug screen** is a technical analysis of the urine, hair, blood, sweat, and tissue to determine if there are drugs in the body now or if they were present there recently. This technology can also be used to screen for certain types of drugs, specifically amphetamines, barbiturates, and opioids. However, there are many categories of drugs, and there is no one test that can screen for all of them. Some examples of drug categories are antihistamines, antibiotics, anxiolytics, cardiovascular medications, cholesterol drugs, analgesics, antipsychotics, antidepressants, sleep aids, cough and cold remedies, insulin, digestive agents, thyroid hormones, and so on. To test for these, the physician orders them by name. For example, he or she may order a screen for acetaminophen levels.

Key terms: drug screens

Amphetamines are stimulants, which are medications that promote wakefulness.

Barbiturates are medications called **hypnotics**, which produce sleep. They are designed to calm and to promote a sense of tranquility.

Opioids are medications that are designed to alleviate pain, and they are highly addictive. Examples include codeine, meperidine (Demerol), and oxycodone (OxyContin).

Toxicology screens

The term **toxic** means *lethal, noxious,* or *poisonous.* **Toxicology screens** are also technical analyses of urine, hair, blood, sweat, and tissue, but they often serve different purposes than drug tests and drug screens. Notice the different purposes served by the types of toxicology screens listed below.

Therapeutic drug management: the monitoring of blood to assess for the desired therapeutic range of a known prescribed medication. For Mrs. Davis, this would include her thyroid replacement drug, levothyroxine.

Emergency toxicology: the screening of the blood for drugs and poisons that are posing an urgent threat to a person's life. There is a rapid response time involved because of the emergency, and hundreds of chemicals and compounds can be tested with this method.

Metals and biological monitoring: these tests analyze for exposure to and the presence of heavy metals in the body, most often as a result of occupational exposure.

Forensic toxicology: testing that is done under specific legal protocols of evidence collection and analysis. Forensic toxicology can also often identify the cause of death.

Oftentimes, patients do not recall offhand the *over-the-counter (OTC) medications* that they are taking, and they may omit these from the history taken by their health-care provider. Sometimes patients are taking a medication or drug that they do not wish their health-care team to know about. Drug screens can help to provide a clear picture of what is really going on.

The concept of polypharmacy

Mrs. Davis is taking a number of prescribed medications, but we do not know if she takes any OTC medications (other than the supplement glucosamine) in addition to these. The term **polypharmacy** is used to describe the use of more than one medication at a time. Pharmacists, physicians, and nurse practitioners are required to know how drugs interact with one another before prescribing them. To prescribe drugs safely, these individuals require a clear, specific, and honest list of all other medications, health supplements, and herbal remedies that a patient is already taking. Nurses are also responsible for this knowledge because they are the ones to administer the medications and to teach the patients to self-administer.

Medications and other preparations (as noted previously) all have a desired or intended effects, but they also have a likelihood of producing side effects, including adverse effects. Mrs. Davis's lab work will help the treatment team to assess whether the mixture of medications and herbal supplements that she is taking is affecting her mental and physical functioning. Table 7-9 provides some examples of common medications and their desired effects, as well as their possible side effects, including their potential adverse effects.

The term **side effects** is used to describe any effects other than the intended ones that a drug may cause. Side effects may be temporary or permanent and mild or severe. For example, the medication lithium carbonate, which is used to treat bipolar disorder, has a negative side effect of hand tremors, which can develop to such a degree that the person has difficulty writing, eating, and so on. When the lithium is discontinued, the tremors disappear. However, some side effects can be positive. An example of a medication that may have positive side effects is prednisone, which is a drug that is prescribed for its anti-inflammatory effects. Many patients who take prednisone experience positive side effects, such as the lessening of everyday aches and pains and an improvement in mood or state of mind.

The term **adverse effects** is used to describe side effects that are actually harmful, even when a drug is taken in its normal, appropriate dose. Adverse effects are particularly important to be aware of when someone is pregnant and when these effects could harm the embryo or fetus. An example of such a drug is lorazepam, which is an antianxiety medication. It is not recommended during pregnancy or breastfeeding.

Drug interactions

Many drugs should not be used concurrently, even at their recommended dosages. Drugs and other medicinal preparations interact chemically within the body as they are metabolized, and some drug interactions can have dangerous results. An example of an adverse drug interaction is the mixing of alcohol with a sedative or a sedative-hypnotic medication that is used for sleep. This combination can decrease respiration and cardiac rates significantly, possibly leading to coma or death.

TABLE 7-9: Effects of Common Medications

Medication	Desired Effects	Side Effects	Adverse Effects
acetylsalicylic acid (aspirin)	• analgesia (pain relief) • anti-inflammatory • anti-pyretic (anti-fever) • anti-coagulant (decreases blood clotting)	• stomach irritation • bruising • ringing in the ears	• stomach ulcer • excessive bleeding
diphenhydramine Trade names: Benadryl, Dramamine	• relief from allergy symptoms • sleep aid • cough suppressant	• drowsiness • dry mouth • confusion • blurred vision • impaired coordination • slowed reaction time • agitation	• overdose can lead to coma, cardiorespiratory collapse, or death when mother takes it, risk to infant of stimulation and seizures from receiving drug through breast milk
acetaminophen Trade name: Tylenol paracetamol	• analgesic • antipyretic	• rare	• overuse can cause liver damage; recent studies (2010) suggest that use by adolescents leads to an increased incidence of asthma in that age group
ibuprofen or ibuprophen Trade names: Advil, Motrin	• analgesic • anti-inflammatory	• rash and itching • constipation or diarrhea • ringing in the ears	• serious damage to the small intestine • severe bleeding in the stomach • increased risk of heart attack or stroke

The language of addiction and substance abuse

The realm of mental illness includes addiction and substance abuse. Mrs. Davis is taking a number of medications for her chronic illnesses. Her symptoms in the emergency department might be caused by the combination of these drugs in her body. Mrs. Davis might also be misusing her prescription medications; she may not understand the repercussions of that misuse on her mental health, including her ability to remember, think clearly, and function normally. In addition, it is also possible that Mrs. Davis has become dependent on one or more of her medications, particularly those she uses for pain. If this is true, she is addicted to them. Each of these scenarios poses a number of health and mental health issues for Mrs. Davis, so the treatment team is exploring whether any of these situations exist. The answer could have huge consequences for Mrs. Davis if she was the driver of the car in the accident. The team will find their answers, both subjectively by interviewing Mrs. Davis and her next of kin and objectively through the results of her blood work and urinalysis (see Chapter 12).

Key terms: addictions and substance abuse

An **addiction** is an ongoing and compulsive dependence on a substance or behavior; it can be a psychological addiction or a physical addition. One type of addiction is **chemical dependency**, which is the persistent use of a certain drug or drugs. A few powerful drugs, such as crack cocaine and heroin, can cause immediate or almost immediate states of dependence or addiction. The longer a person uses the drug, the more they build a **tolerance** to it. This means that the user needs ever-increasing doses of the substance to achieve the same effects that smaller doses initially provided. When used in a medical context, the term *tolerance* means the threshold level or point at which a substance, pain, or exertion is able to affect the body or mind without causing undue adverse effects.

The term **substance abuse** refers to a use pattern of drugs, alcohol, or other substances (i.e., glue) that are harmful to the body or mind and that have the potential to adversely affect all dimensions of health. Some substances, when abused, can lead to severe brain damage; some can lead to addiction, whereas others do not. Substance abusers participate in this potentially harmful behavior to achieve what they perceive to be desirable effects.

The term *substance abuse* does not apply only to illicit or illegal substances. Indeed, abuse is common with prescribed and over-the-counter medications. As tolerance levels build with the use of these medications or when the client discovers a desired effect of them, self-medication may become a health issue. No longer are the prescribed or recommended doses taken. Instead, clients decide their own dosages, which are often above the prescribed doses. Substance abuse also includes the sniffing of aerosol sprays, glues, paints, gasoline, and so on.

Because substance abuse is widespread and because it affects people of all ages and socioeconomic classes, health-care workers need to be familiar with its terminology. Refer to Table 7-10 for a list of commonly abused substances, their medical terms, their types, and their desired and potentially adverse effects.

TABLE 7-10: Commonly Abused Substances

Substance	Medical Term	Type of Substance	Desired Effect by Abuser	Potential Adverse Effects
alcohol	ethanol, ethyl alcohol	depressant	relaxation, enhanced mood, intoxication	increased risk for brain damage, increased risk for liver damage and disease
cocaine	cocaine hydrochloride	stimulant	heightened alertness, euphoria, increased energy	heart attack, respiratory failure, seizures
codeine	codeine	opioid, opioid derivative, analgesic	pain relief, euphoria, drowsiness	respiratory depression and arrest, addiction, unconsciousness
ecstasy or MDMA	methylene-dioxymethamphetamine	synthetic stimulant with psychoactive properties	mental stimulation, emotional warmth, enhanced energy, mild hallucinations, increased sense of touch	nausea, sweating or chills, clenched teeth, muscle cramps, blurred vision; hyperthermia: the inability to regulate temperature, which can lead to death
LSD or acid	lysergic acid diethylamide	hallucinogen	hallucinations, euphoria	increased body temperature, increased blood pressure and heart rate, anorexia
marijuana and hashish	cannabis	cannabinoid	sense of euphoria or tranquility (mellow mood), increased sense of humor, silliness	memory impairment, difficulty thinking and problem solving; chronic use leads to apathy and some withdrawal symptoms
OxyContin	oxycodone hydrochloride	narcotic, analgesic	pain relief, euphoria, drowsiness	respiratory depression and arrest, addiction, unconsciousness
Vicodin	hydrocodone bitartrate, acetaminophen	opioid, opioid derivative, analgesic	pain relief, euphoria, drowsiness	respiratory depression and arrest, addiction, unconsciousness

Right Word or Wrong Word: *Abuse* or *Misuse*?

Is there a difference between these two terms? They are often used interchangeably, but should they be?

Self-medicating behaviors

The term **self-medicating** means that an individual takes medications or drugs in a manner that he or she thinks is appropriate to achieve a desired effect. This is misuse.

If our patient, Mrs. Davis, is taking levothyroxine and ibuprofen at the prescribed or recommended dosages, she will not likely suffer any adverse effects. However, if she self-medicates, she runs the risk of setting in motion adverse effects or adverse drug interactions. Self-medication will be an important factor in her diagnoses, especially if she tells the team later that she also takes a number of other over-the-counter medications as well.

Ibuprofen is an analgesic, anti-inflammatory, antipyretic, anti-coagulant medication. Mrs. Davis uses it to manage her arthritis. Symptoms associated with the misuse of ibuprofen (which generally means excessive use) include the risk of bleeding and orthostatic hypotension (i.e., weakness, dizziness, and a drop in blood pressure upon standing).

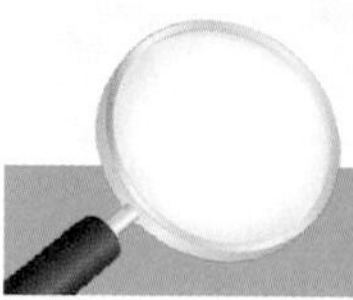

FOCUS POINT: Over-the-Counter Medications

The term *over-the-counter medication* refers to any medication or pharmaceutical product that can be purchased in a store without a prescription. The abbreviation *OTC* is very common in health care.

Fill in the Blanks

Use medical language and terminology in context to complete the following sentences about mental illness, substance abuse, and addictions.

1. Codeine is a ____________ prescribed for pain.
2. ______________ is a mood disorder that refers to and includes two poles or extremes of emotions.
3. OTC medications do not require a ______________________________.
4. It is not necessarily true that all illicit drug use results in ________________________.
5. _____________________ is a psychological or physical response to persistent substance abuse.
6. Unfortunately, prescription drugs can also be ______________________.
7. Another way to say adverse effects is ________________ *effects.*
8. ____________________ is a term that describes taking your medication or other substances at dosages that you determine rather than at the dosages prescribed by a physician or nurse practitioner.
9. Ecstasy, cocaine, marijuana, and even heroin all have the ability to create a chemical state of well-being or ________________ for the user.
10. A desired effect of cocaine for users is ________________________.

Putting It All Together

Before concluding Chapter 7, let's review the facts as they appear related to the multiple possible diagnoses for Mrs. Davis. Recall that Dr. Jensen is trying to rule each one in or out to determine exactly what is happening for this patient today so that targeted treatment interventions may begin.

Ruling Out: Complete the Table

Complete this table by writing each of Mrs. Davis' symptoms under the appropriate heading.

TABLE 7-11: Your Turn: List Mrs. Davis' Symptoms by Potential Diagnosis

Minor Concussion	Mental Health or Illness	Hypoglycemia	Thyroid Disease	Polypharmacy

CHAPTER SUMMARY

In Chapter 7, you have learned about mental health and illness, the endocrine system, the exocrine organs and glands, and the various pathologies of these. At many junctures, you were asked to consider how what you have been learning pertained to our patient at Fayette General Hospital, Mrs. Stevie-Rose Davis. You have continued to learn terminology related to health assessment and diagnostic procedures. A very brief introduction to the language of pharmacology, pharmacokinetics, and drug testing was provided.

Chapter 7 also introduced a number of new abbreviations. Many of them appear again here in a concise table to promote their study.

TABLE 7-12: Abbreviations

Abbreviation	Meaning	Abbreviation	Meaning
AD	Alzheimer's disease	MHNP	mental health nurse practitioner
ADD	attention deficit disorder	OTC	over-the-counter (when referring to medications)
ADHD	attention deficit-hyperactivity disorder	ψ	psychiatry or psychology
ATA	anterograde amnesia (post-traumatic amnesia)	t.i.d.	three times per day
ADR	adverse drug reaction	TSH	thyroid-stimulating hormone
ACTH	adrenocorticotropic hormone	T3	tri-iodothyronine
FSH	follicle- stimulating hormone	T4	thyroxine
HGH	human growth hormone	µug	micrograms
IQ	intelligence quotient		
MTBI	mild traumatic brain injury; (mild concussion)		

Key Terms

acinar cells
addiction
adverse effects
affect
amnesia
amphetamines
anterograde
barbiturates
biotechnology
chemical dependency
cognition
cognitively
concussion
confabulate
dementia
diabetes
drug screen
ducts
emotionally
endocrine
enzymes
exocrine
flat affect
gestational diabetes
glands
glucocorticoid
glucometer
glucosamine
glucose
hormones
hyperglycemia
hypnotics
hypothyroidism
ibuprofen
iodine
islets of Langerhans
levothyroxine
mental health
mental illness
mental status examination
metabolism
micrograms (mcg, ug)
mild-traumatic brain injury (MTBI)
opioids
pancreas
pharmaco-kinetics
pharmacology
pituitary (hypophysis)
polypharmacy
polyuria
psych assessment
psychiatry
psycho-pathology
resiliency
retrograde
self-medicating
side effects
substance abuse
thyroid
tolerance
toxic
toxicology report
toxicology screens
wellness

See How Much You've Learned

For audio exercises, visit **http://www.MedicalLanguageLab.com.** 

CHAPTER REVIEW

Critical Thinking

1. What is the difference between the endocrine glands and the exocrine glands? ______________________________

2. Identify the word part that means *to secrete.* ______________________________

3. Are substance abuse and addiction the same thing? Explain. ______________________________

4. Many medications are named by using a certain prefix to say what they are not. What is this prefix? ______________________________

5. What is the difference between an adverse effect of a drug and a side effect of a drug? ______________________________

Right Word or Wrong Word: ***Disorder*** **or** ***Disease*?**

Can these two words be used interchangeably? Why or why not?

Right Word or Wrong Word: ***Schizoid Personality*** **or** ***Multiple Personality*?**

Are these two words synonymous? Explain.

Right Word or Wrong Word: ***Oxytocin*** **or** ***OxyContin*?**

Do these two words refer to the same thing? Are they just spelled slightly differently? What do they mean?

Identify the Abbreviations

Throughout this chapter, you have encountered a number of abbreviations. Do you remember what they mean? Spell out the words that are expressed here in an abbreviated form.

1. ADD ______________________________
2. LTH ______________________________
3. GAD ______________________________
4. BPD ______________________________

Fill in the Blanks

Fill in the blanks with the missing part of each term

1. ____________ ology is the non-medical specialty concerned with the mind and behavior.
2. ____________ ology is the specialized field of medicine concerned with hormones.
3. ____________ ology refers to the study of the effects of the endocrine system on the functioning of the mind.

Name the Prefix

Read each definition, and then write the prefix that it describes.

1. normal, well ______________________
2. after ______________________

Break It Down

Break these words into their component parts of prefix-root-suffix, as applicable.

1. parafollicular ______________________
2. antibodies ______________________
3. thyroiditis ______________________
4. melanocyte ______________________
5. glycemia ______________________

Label the Organs of the Endocrine System

1. ______________________
2. ______________________
3. ______________________
4. ______________________
5. ______________________
6. ______________________
7. ______________________
8. ______________________
9. ______________________

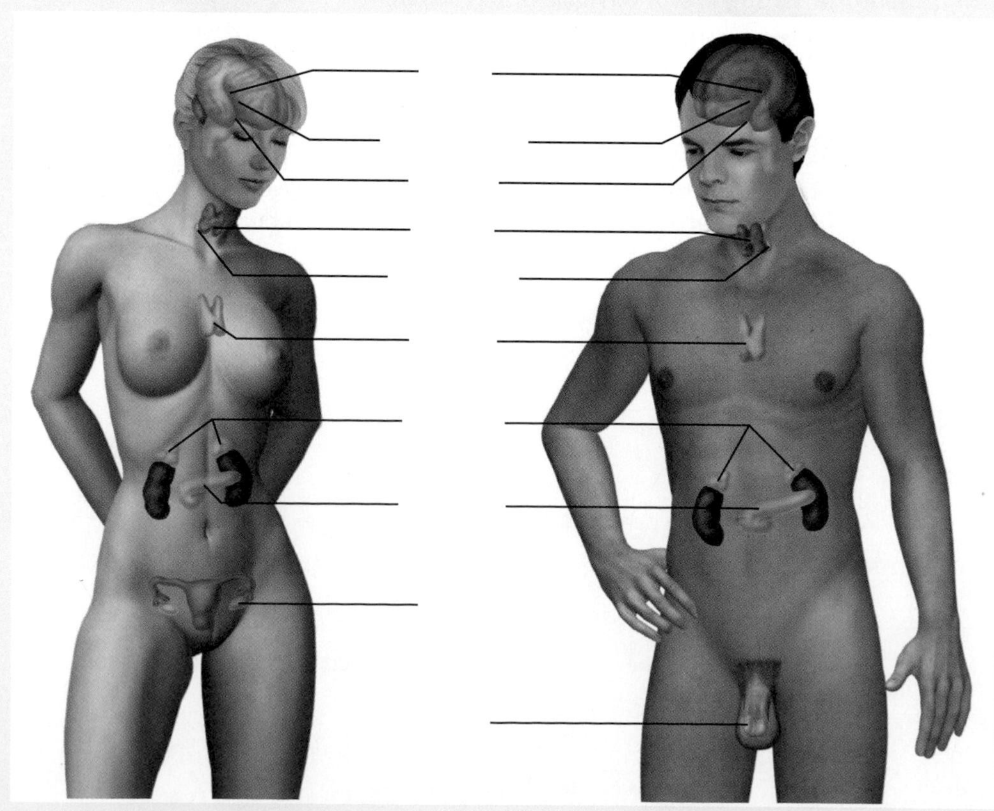

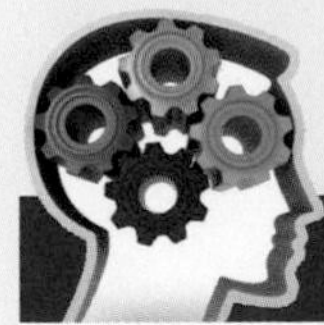

MEMORY MAGIC

Here is a helpful mnemonic for remembering the symptoms of hypothyroidism. Use the acronym *SLUGGISH.*

S = sleepiness or fatigue

L = loss of memory

U = unusually coarse, dry skin

G = goiter

G = gradual personality and mood changes (depression)

I = increase in weight, bloating, or edema (swelling)

S = sensitivity to cold

H = hair loss or increasing sparseness of hair

Here is one more Memory Magic strategy. This one is to help you remember how thyroid disease relates to TSH levels. TSH levels and thyroid function are inversely related; this means that means that an increase in TSH levels reveals a decrease in thyroid function and that a decrease in TSH levels reveals an increase in thyroid function.

↑ TSH means ↓ thyroid

↓ TSH means ↑ thyroid

In other words:
High TSH means hypothyroidism.
Low TSH means hyperthyroidism.

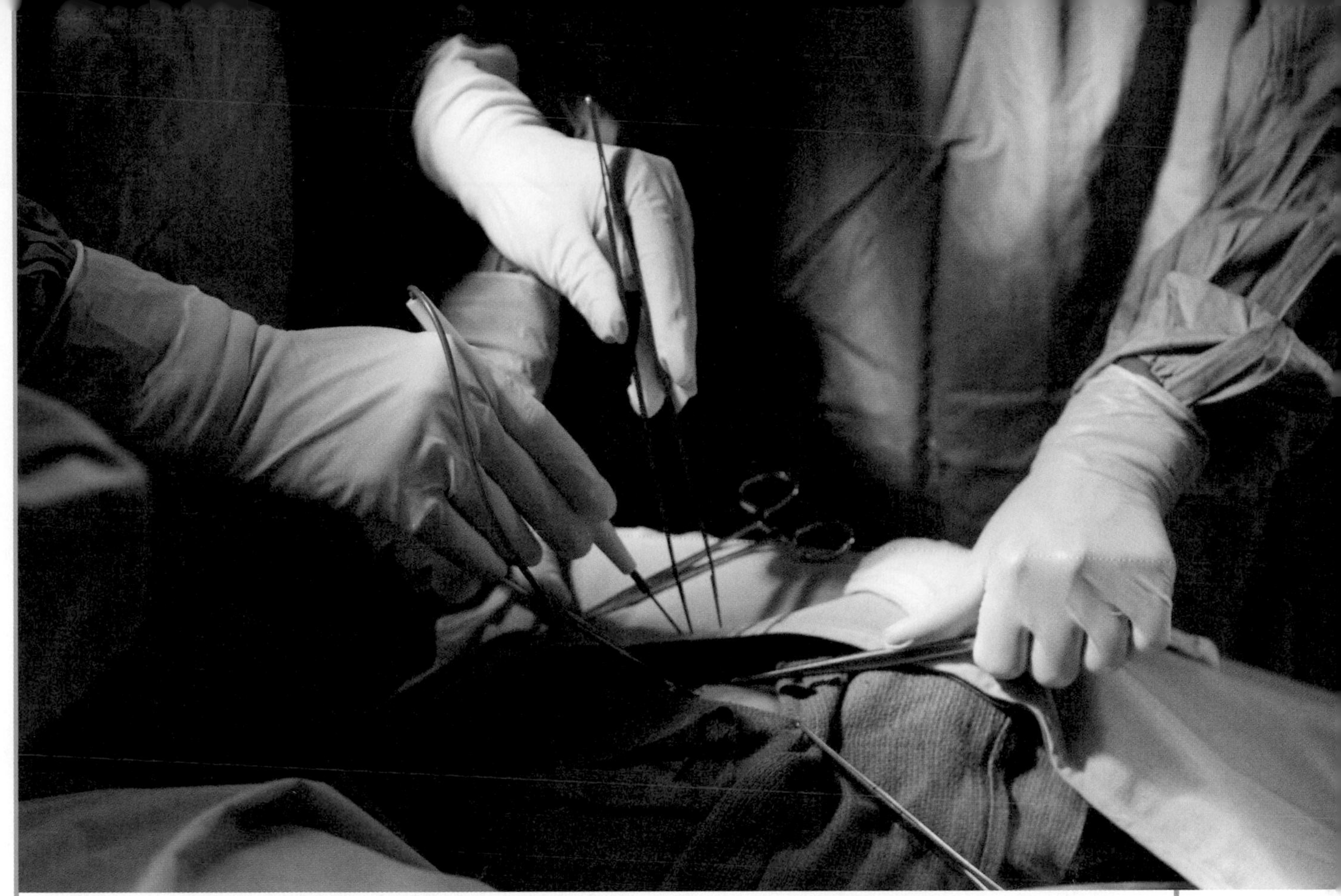

UNIT THREE

The Language of Treatment

CHAPTER EIGHT

Obstetrics, Labor, and Delivery

Focus: Female Reproduction

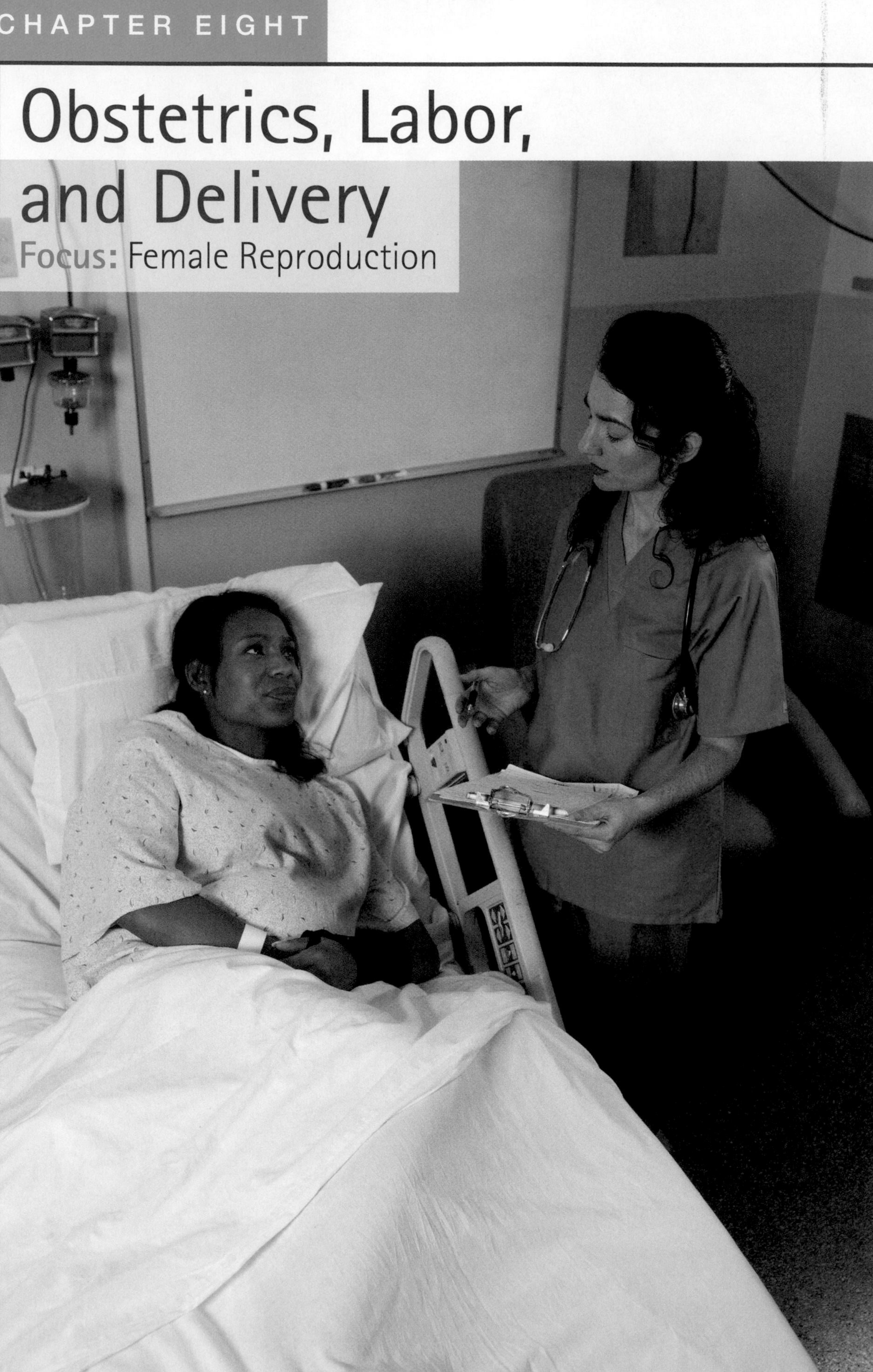

Mrs. Glory Loeppky has been assessed in the emergency department of Fayette General Hospital. She has been treated for a deep laceration to her left thigh, and she received a number of sutures to close the wound. She also has a spica cast on her left thumb and hand as treatment for an ulnar collateral injury to the thumb. The attending physician, Dr. Abrams, has contacted an obstetrician, Dr. Bedard, because Glory is 7½ months pregnant and she and the baby are under stress as the result of a motor vehicle accident (see Chapter 3). The two physicians decided that because of her pregnancy, Glory should be admitted to the antepartum unit for observation and ongoing fetal assessment for the next 24 hours. Glory has just been admitted to that unit and is speaking with the nurse.

Patient Update

"Hello, Mrs. Loeppky. I'm Laura, your nurse here. How are you feeling right now?" She inquired, gently touching the patient's hand.

"Oh, please call me Glory. Do you know where my husband is? I need to see my husband. The nurse in the ER said he's at another hospital. Why is that? Is he badly injured? Can you help me find out? Please, I need to know about Gil," replied Glory, her eyes filling with tears.

"Glory, everything's all right now. Please take a deep breath with me," said Laura. "That's it, deep breath in and out. Good," she said. "Yes, I understand from your chart that your husband was with you today and that you were both in a car accident. And yes, he's at another facility. He's at Okla Trauma Center, but I don't have any information about him. Our medical social worker is trying to find out more for you, and we'll let you know as soon as we can." The nurse went on to explain to Glory the importance of focusing on the here and now: on her own health and that of her baby.

"Yes, I am worried about my baby," said Glory. "But the doctors said I wasn't in labor and that the baby was okay. Isn't that true? I'm really not sure why I'm here in this unit. Isn't this where you go to have your baby?"

Laura explained why Glory had been admitted to the antepartum unit and the importance of monitoring both her and her unborn child's health status. Laura said, "I know you're worried about a lot of things right now, but I'm going to try to help you keep as calm as possible so we can get some good assessments from our monitors." Glory nodded. "You're in very good hands here," said Laura. "You've been assigned to Dr. Bedard, and she's an excellent obstetrician. She'll be in to see you in awhile. Rest assured, as soon as we find out anything about your husband, we'll let you know. Now, did you give someone in Admissions the name of another family member to contact?"

The patient nodded. She said she had given the name of her mother and father, and she'd had word from an ER nurse that her parents were coming to the hospital.

"That's wonderful," said Laura. "As soon as they arrive, we'll bring them to see you."

Reflective Questions

Reflect on the story that you've just read.

1. What is the name of the hospital unit to which Glory has been admitted?

 ____

2. Who is trying to find out more information about Glory's husband, Gilbert Loeppky?

 ____

3. What is an obstetrician?

 ____

For audio exercises, visit **http://www.MedicalLanguageLab.com.** 

Learning Objectives

After reading Chapter 8, you will be able to do the following:

- Recognize and use the language of pregnancy and the female reproductive system.
- Recognize and use the language of birth and delivery.
- Recognize diagnostic tools and procedures related to obstetrical care.
- Recognize and use medical terminology related to Cesarean section and premature birth.
- Recognize and use medical and anatomical terminology related to pregnancy and birth.
- Become familiar with the terminology used for surgical procedures and patient care.
- Recognize and use medical terminology related to blood.
- Recognize and use medical terminology related to newborn infants.
- Recognize and use medical terminology related to neonatal care and assessment.
- Recognize and use medical terminology related to pathological and physical risks to the child both prepartum and postpartum.
- Recognize and use medical terminology related to wound infection and care.
- Recognize and use terminology related to pharmacology.
- Appreciate the education and training of a medical social worker.
- Appreciate the education and training of a medical records technician.

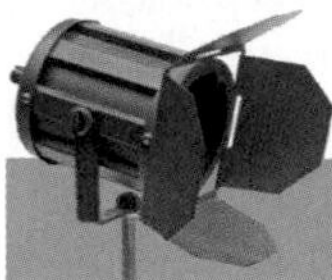

CAREER SPOTLIGHT: Medical Social Worker

The minimal entry level of education for a *social worker* is a bachelor's degree in social work (BSW). According to the Bureau of Labor Statistics,* however, a master's degree is the generally accepted level of education required for specialized fields of social work practice. This type of education includes study in the humanities: social work, sociology, psychology, social policy, and other coursework related to the study of the human condition. In the United States, licensure, certification, and registration may be required, depending on the state in which the social worker wishes to practice.

Social workers help people solve problems of daily living, advocate for the social and financial support of people in need or crisis, protect the care and custody of children, facilitate the maintenance or achievement of healthy relationships among people, and work with community groups to build healthy communities and environments. Many graduates go on to specialize in a particular field, such as child and family, schools and school-aged children, public service, or health care.

A medical or public health social worker is an integral part of the treatment team in many cases. This professional works with at-risk or vulnerable populations who face health challenges. The medical social worker assists not only individual clients (patients) but also families and groups of individuals with similar concerns or health issues. He or she helps with predischarge planning before a patient leaves hospital care. The social worker may help to arrange at-home care and other services in the community for the client. In care facilities, this team member may also help locate next of kin, assist with the establishment of financial support for the treatment, and facilitate group meetings with clients and their caregivers to help them cope

*Bureau of Labor Statistics, USA, Occupational Outlook Handbook, 2010-2011 Edition

with medical conditions and health crises such as grief and loss. Mental health and substance abuse social workers can be found working in hospitals, rehabilitation and detoxification centers, jails, and the community at large. (Note: A *medical social worker* is sometimes referred to as a *hospital social worker,* but please remember that a medical social worker can work at a variety of health-care sites.)

Right Word or Wrong Word: Does *MSW* Mean *Medical Social Worker*?

Do you think the abbreviation for a medical social worker is *MSW*? What else might this abbreviation mean?

The Language of the Female Reproductive System

Before you can learn more about Glory Loeppky's pregnancy, you need to understand the language of the female reproductive system.

Anatomy and physiology: female reproductive system

Basically, the female reproductive system consists of the breasts and the reproductive organs. However, anatomically and medically speaking, the reproductive system also includes the **hypothalamus** in the brain, which is responsible for the release of a number of growth hormones that lead to the development of the genital organs and the functioning of the reproductive system. The hypothalamus also coordinates the activities of the pituitary and adrenal glands, which produce small amounts of male and female sex hormones.

The major organs of the female reproductive system are the breasts, oviducts (also referred to as the fallopian tubes), ovaries, uterus, and the vagina.

The general term **genitalia** is used to describe the reproductive organs and the structures located in the lower abdomen and pelvis. The root of *genitalia* is *gen,* meaning *to be born or producing.* There are two parts to the genitalia: the external organs and the internal organs. The term **vulva** refers to the external genital organs of a female. In this case, the English word is exactly the same as its Latin root, which means *covering.* The **perineum** is the external area between the vulva and the anus. (For men, the perineum is the area between the scrotum and anus.) Although it is not specifically part of the reproductive system, the perineum is often involved in the symptoms, care, and treatment of reproductive conditions, disorders, and diseases.

Let's Practice

Name the part of the female reproductive system that fits each description.

1. situated anterior to the kidneys bilaterally ____________________
2. coordinates the growth and development of genitalia and the reproductive system ____________________
3. a canal-shaped organ that sits medially and internally in the lower abdomen ____________
4. located on the anterior of the chest bilaterally ____________________
5. the organ that produces eggs for reproduction ____________________

Learn the word parts: female reproductive system

A number of core terms related to the female reproductive system appear frequently when in the areas of health care that concern girls and women. It is important to recognize the combining forms of the roots of these terms to more efficiently recognize what is being said or written. Table 8-1 provides some examples.

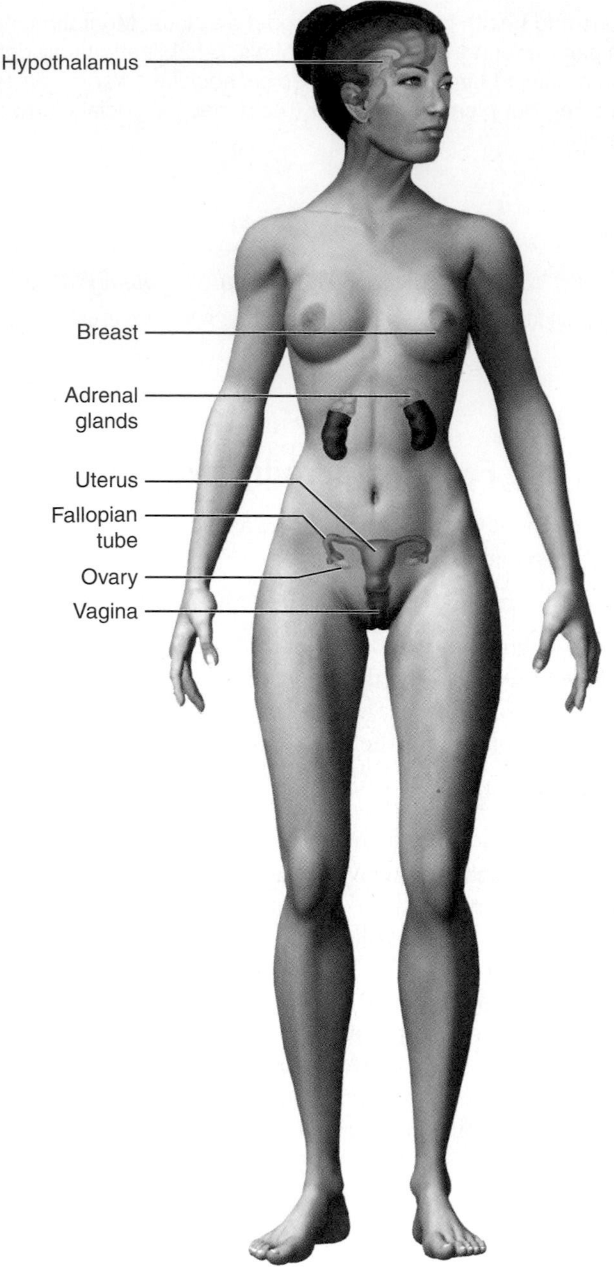

Figure 8.1: Female reproductive system and related glands (simplified)

TABLE 8-1: Combining Forms: Organs of the Female Reproductive System

Combining Form	Meaning	Combining Form	Meaning
uter/o hyster/o metr/o	womb; of or pertaining to the womb (the uterus)	ova/i	eggs; the root is found in the words ovaries, which produce eggs, and oviducts, which release one egg or more per month
vagin/o vagin colp/o	vagina	oophor/o	ovary

Name the Suffix

This exercise tests your memory of the suffixes that you have learned in previous chapters. The more often you see and use them, the more likely you are to recognize and remember them in the future, even if you do not understand the root of a new term right away. Recognizing suffixes will help you begin to break down and interpret the meanings of new terms. Read the meaning given and then identify the appropriate suffix.

1. to form ______________________________
2. inflammation or swelling ______________________________
3. pain ______________________________
4. removal ______________________________
5. to make ______________________________
6. the study or science of ______________________________
7. to perform an action related to the root ______________________________
8. the state of ______________________________

The female breasts

An integral part of the female reproductive system, the female breasts develop in response to the hormonal changes of puberty. They are what are known as *secondary sexual characteristics,* which means that they are present but not fully developed for their function until puberty. Their function is to produce nourishment for offspring, and this ability is set in motion by the hormonal changes that occur in response to conception. At approximately 8 weeks into the pregnancy, the hormone prolactin is released, and the process of milk production begins; this peaks with the birth of the child. You will learn much more about the anatomy of the breasts in Chapter 17 as we connect again with Glory Loeppky postnatally.

Fill in the Blanks

Consider all that you have learned about the language of the reproductive system so far. Use this knowledge to complete these sentences.

1. A fetus sits *in utero.* This means that the fetus is located in the ______________________.
2. When something is inflamed, the medical suffix for this is ______________________.
3. The patient had a ______________________ to remove her uterus.
4. The ______________________ coordinates hormone production for the growth of the reproductive organs and for the stimulation of sexual impulse and drive.
5. ______________________ is a broad term that refers to the reproductive organs internally and externally that are located in the pelvic area.
6. Cleanliness of the ______________________ is an important aspect of caring for the patient who may not be able to attend to this area by himself or herself at this time.
7. The entrance to the uterus is called the ______________________.
8. Ova are produced in the ______________________.
9. A ______________________ does not deliver babies, although he or she is very concerned about women's reproductive health and the diseases of the reproductive system.

Female genitalia and reproductive organs

Key terms: external female genitalia

The external or surface portion of the female genitalia includes the labia majora and labia minora, clitoris, the opening of the vagina, the hymen, and Bartholin's glands. **Bartholin's glands** are located near the vaginal opening, at the base of the labia majora. These are mucous glands that keep the vagina lubricated.

Table 8-2 defines these terms and breaks them down into their component parts to help you understand them better.

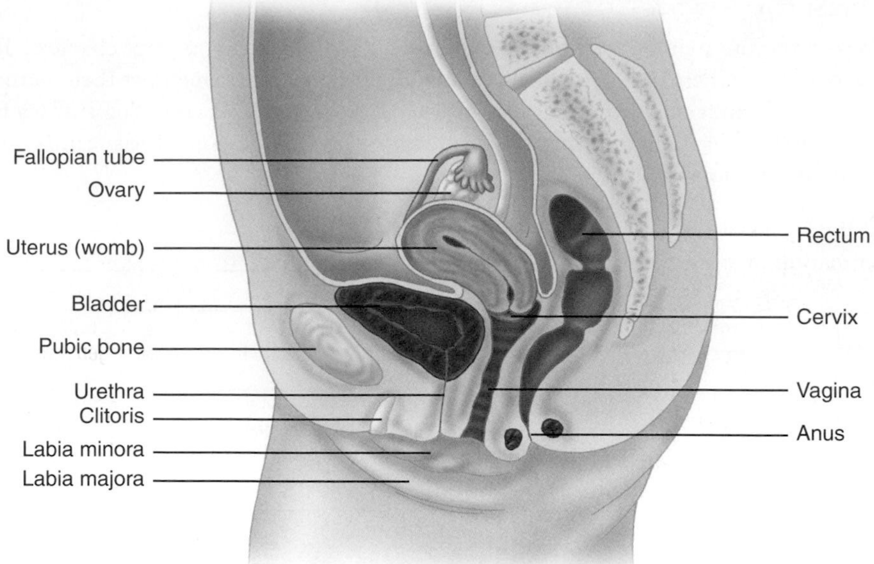

Figure 8.2: Female reproductive system: sagittal view (detailed)

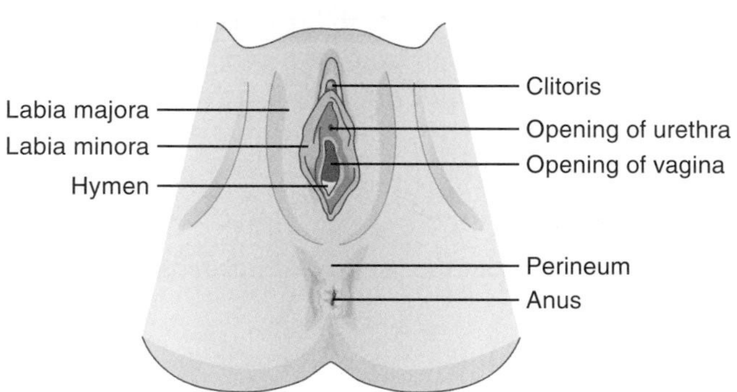

Figure 8.3: External female genitalia

TABLE 8-2: Terms and Word Parts: External Female Genitalia

Term	Word Parts	Meaning
labia majora	labium (root meaning *fleshy border or lips*) labia (plural form of *root*) major/a (prefix meaning *greater or larger*)	two major, large folds of skin and adipose tissue located near the vaginal opening
labia minora	labia (see above) minor/a (prefix meaning *smaller or less than*)	two minor, thin folds of skin located between the labia majora, closer to the vaginal opening
clitoris	kleitoris (root referring to this structure) clit- (the combining form of the root)	name of a small structure located at the anterior but beneath the labia minora; the clitoris is composed of nerve endings, which make it highly sensitive; it is connected internally to the reproductive organs
vagina	vagin vagin/o	the passageway between the vulva and the cervix; the vagina is composed of musculomembranous tissue
hymen	hymen/o (combining form of root meaning *skin or membrane*)	a mucous membrane that partly occludes the entrance to the vagina; most often found in young females before sexual or reproductive activity; the purpose of the hymen is to protect the internal reproductive organs before puberty occurs

Anatomical terms: internal female genitalia

The internal portion of the female genitalia includes the vagina, ovaries, oviducts (fallopian tubes), uterus, cervix, fundus, and ligaments.

Table 8-3 defines these terms and breaks them down into their component parts to help you to understand them better.

TABLE 8-3: Terms and Word Parts: Internal Female Genitalia

Term	Root or Combining Form	Meaning of Term
ovary	ovari/io combining form of *ovary,* from the root *ova,* meaning *eggs*	a gland that produces eggs for reproduction, as well as the hormones estrogen, progesterone, and inhibin; there are two ovaries in the female body
fallopian tubes or oviducts	fallopian The term *fallopian* is an eponym; the tubes were named after Gabriel Fallopius, a 16th-century anatomist ovi combining form of root *ova,* meaning *eggs* + duct root meaning *path*	tubes that extend bilaterally from the uterus and that end near the ovary; the fallopian tubes carry ova from the ovary to the uterus and sperm from the uterus toward the ovary
uterus or womb	uter/o combining form of root meaning *womb*	the function of this organ is to sustain a developing fetus; the uterus is divided into three parts: the cervix (neck), the fundus (upper part), and the corpus (main body)
fundus	fundus root meaning *base*	the largest part of a hollow organ or the part of an organ that lies farthest away from its opening into something else or externally

Naming uterine tissue

As you have seen, there are three medical roots that mean *uterus.* However, one root in particular is used in its combining form to name different types of uterine tissue; that combining form is *metr.* There are three main tissues of the uterus, and each name uses a prefix and a suffix. The prefixes are as follows:

endo- meaning *within*

myo- meaning *muscle* (a root that sometimes functions as a prefix)

peri- meaning *around or surrounding*

The suffix used is *-ium,* which means *tissue or structure.*

Proceed to the exercise to discover how these word parts combine to create anatomical terms.

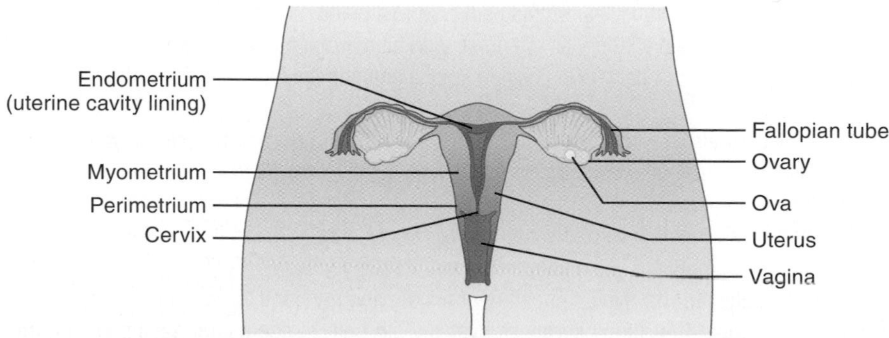

Figure 8.4: Internal female genitalia

Let's Practice

Read each description. Combine word parts related to the uterus to name each type of tissue described. Use a prefix, a combining form of the root *metr,* and a suffix.

1. the smooth muscle layer of the uterus; this tissue is the largest component of this organ

   ____

2. a membranous lining of the uterus that protects and separates it from other internal organs

   ____

3. inside the uterus, this tissue changes over the monthly reproductive cycle

   ____

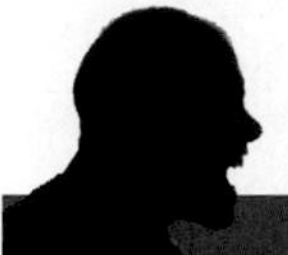

PRONUNCIATION PRACTICE

Say these words aloud to a friend or classmate if you can. You are given the phonetic pronunciation. Your instructor can help you with pronunciation, or visit **http://www.MedicalLanguageLab.com.** 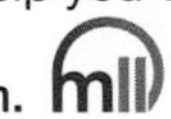

adrenal	ăd-**rē**´năl	labia	**lā**´bē-ă
cervix	**sĕr**´vĭks	myometrium	mī-ō-**mē**´trē-ŭm
endometrium	ăn-dō-**mē**´trē-ŭm	obstetrician	ŏb-stĕ-**trĭsh**´ăn
fallopian	fă-**lō**´pē-ăn	perimetrium	pĕr-**mē**´trē-ŭm
genitalia	jĕn-ĭ-**tāl**´rē-ă	uterus	**ū**´tĕr-ŭs
gynecology	gī″nĕ-**kŏl**´ō-jē	vagina	vă-**jī**´nă
hypothalamus	hī″pō-**thăl**´ă-mŭs		

The Language of Obstetrics

Now you're ready to follow Glory Loeppky's treatment in the antepartum unit.

Patient Update

RN Laura asked Glory's permission to examine her abdomen. When Glory agreed, Laura began the inspection, using Leopold's maneuvers to determine fetal position and presentation. Visually, Laura also assessed for bruising, lacerations, and contusions. Nothing adverse was noted.

"Is everything okay?" asked Glory as the nurse worked through the assessment.

Laura nodded. "Yes, your baby is in position, and everything seems to be fine at the moment. How are you feeling?"

"Well, my belly feels . . . sore. It feels a little sore. I didn't notice it before. Maybe I didn't notice it because my leg was hurting so bad. I got a really nasty gash to my thigh where I cut it on some metal or something," said Glory.

"Yes, I understand that you've had some sutures to close that wound. Is your leg giving you any pain right now?" the nurse inquired. "How about your hand? I see you have a spica cast on."

"No, it's not really hurting. Well, I'm aware of my leg and my hand all the time, but I can live with the slight pain. What about that funny soreness over my big belly?" she asked as she smiled and ran her hands lovingly over her abdomen. She stopped a moment to consider and then said, "It's probably just from the baby moving around so much today. He . . . or she . . .," Glory laughed quietly, "had a pretty rough afternoon being in that car accident. Are you sure my baby's okay, nurse?" Glory suddenly looked frightened again.

"Your baby seems fine," the nurse said calmly. "We're going to keep an eye on things just to make sure. And I want you to help, too. I want you to let us know immediately if the pain or discomfort in your abdomen increases, okay?" The patient nodded. "Now, let's do a little more checking. I'm going to start a nonstress test now. We call it an *NST*." Laura went on to explain the test. "I understand that you had a fetal monitor in the ER. Well, I'm going to attach a fetal heart monitor again. I'm going to place a belt around your abdomen, and, as you'll see, the machine electronically monitors your baby's well-being. You can see the readings on the monitor. We're going to record fetal movement, heart rate, and reactivity, which show how and when the baby's heart rate changes related to any movement," she explained. "Just like us, the baby's heart rate should increase with movement. These evaluations are performed for 20- to 30-minute periods." She paused for a minute to let Glory process the information.

"Why is it called a *nonstress test*?" Glory asked. The nurse explained that the term arises from the fact that the monitor's sensors do not cause any stress or discomfort to the fetus.

"The monitor does something else, too," Laura added. "It assesses uterine irritability or contractions. One of these belts monitors the baby, and the other monitors your uterus." The nurse noticed a confused look on Glory's face. "Let me explain this a little more. The monitor assesses the response of your uterus, something we refer to as uterine activity. In other words, it assesses whether your uterus is contracting or not. The monitor also detects something that we call *uterine irritability*. Do you know what that means?" Glory nodded.

"Yes, my doctor told me about that. It has something to do with contractions, but they don't lead to labor, right?"

Laura nodded. "Yes, this means that your uterus may be contracting, but there are no changes in your cervix, and you're not actually going into labor. So, to do this part of the test, I'm going to slip another belt around your abdomen, just for this purpose." The RN went on to explain that the treatment team would be using the fetal heart monitor again within the next 24 hours, so if any changes in the baby's condition arose or if evidence of labor occurred, the team would be ready to take the appropriate actions. Finally, Laura asked Glory to participate in the monitoring.

"Each time you feel the baby move while this NST is being done, I want you to press this button." She handed Glory a small device like a call bell that attached to the monitor. We want to see how often the baby moves in an hour, okay?" Glory nodded. Finally, the nurse pointed out the call bell nearby, and a small pitcher of water that Glory could use to stay hydrated. Then she left.

The antepartum unit

Antepartum means *before birth*. The prefix *ante-* means *before*. The root *partum* is the English form of the Latin *partus*, meaning *to bring forth*, *to bear*, or *to produce*. An **antepartum unit** is part of a hospital's obstetrical unit. Although it may be part of a maternity, labor, and delivery department, the antepartum unit is designed specifically for expectant mothers who are experiencing high-risk complications. One of the most common reasons for admission to an antepartum unit is the condition called **hypertension of pregnancy**. This is a recently introduced term. Previously, this condition was referred to as **preeclampsia** or **pregnancy-induced hypertension (PIH)**. Expect to hear all three medical terms if you are working in this field.

Patients in an antepartum unit may have a variety of other needs as well. For example, women who are expecting multiple babies and those with diabetes or other health conditions might be admitted to an antepartum unit during the last stages of their pregnancy. In addition, pregnant women who are at risk for other reasons will also be admitted. These risks may include recurrent pregnancy loss and risk for or history of preterm delivery. Glory Loeppky arrived in the antepartum unit as an assessment precaution related to her involvement and injury in the motor vehicle accident. She is what's referred to as an "at-risk patient."

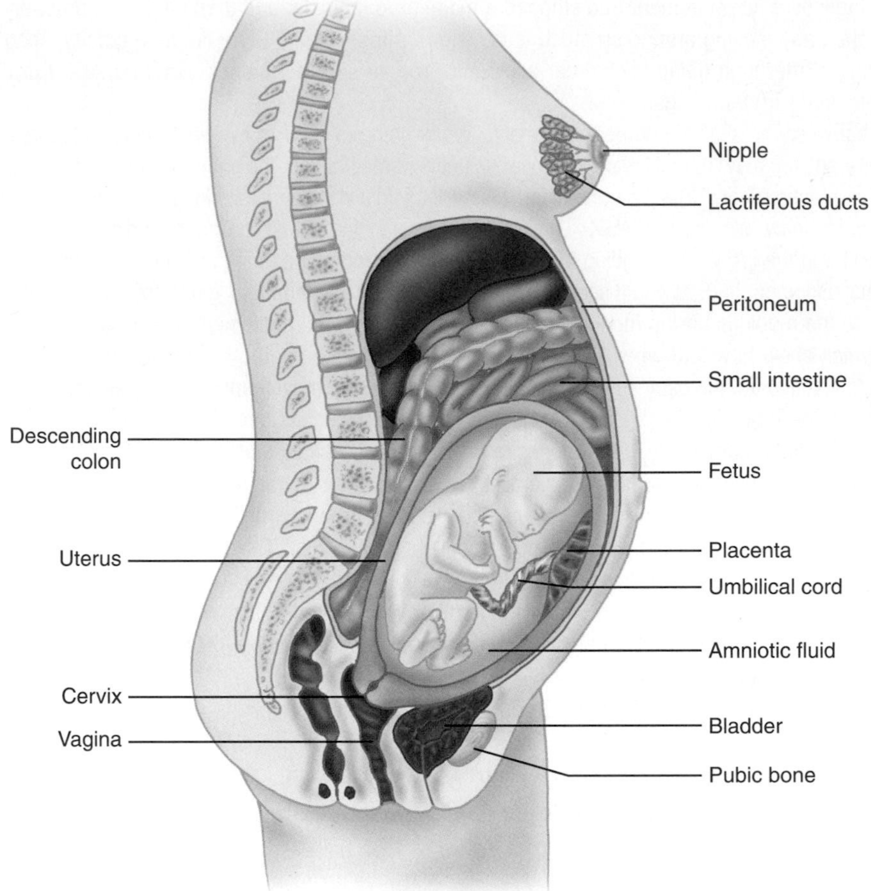

Figure 8.5: Pregnant female at 6 months' gestation (sagittal view)

Key terms: obstetrics

As the registered nurse, Laura, introduced Glory Loeppky to the antepartum unit, she used terminology related to obstetrics and patient care specific to that unit. Key terms and phrases from the dialogue are examined here to introduce you to these new terms and their meanings.

"... using *Leopold's maneuvers* ..."

Leopold's maneuvers: methodical movements used in the processes of palpation and evaluation of the position of the fetus in utero (in the uterus).

Maneuver A: While facing the patient, the upper abdomen is palpated with both hands. Toward the end of the pregnancy, the fetal bottom should be at the top, just under the rib cage.

Maneuver B: While facing the patient, both hands are moved to the abdomen to feel for the fetal back on one side and the extremities (i.e., legs and knees) on the other.

Maneuver C: While facing the patient, one hand is placed just above the symphysis pubis (the junction of the pubic bones in the pelvic area) to assess for the position of the fetal head.

Maneuver D: Change positions. While facing the patient's feet, both hands are placed on the lower abdomen and moved slowly downward toward the pubis to assess for the fetal brow of cephalic prominence (a distinction of the head).

". . . to determine the *fetal position* and *presentation.*"

fetal position: the relationship of the fetus's bony landmarks (which are found through palpation) with their location or position within the woman's abdomen. This is assessed through abdominal palpation.

fetal presentation: the determination of which part of the fetus is entering the birth canal first. The diagrams in Figure 8-6 depict different fetal presentations. Fetal presentation is discovered through vaginal inspection (the insertion of a finger into the vagina). *Fetal attitude* may also be determined during this assessment. The term **fetal attitude** refers to the posture of the fetus in utero during the last months of pregnancy (i.e., whether the fetus's head is tucked down on his or her chest or whether the neck is extended).

"Well, I'm going to attach a *fetal heart monitor* again."

fetal heart monitor (FHM): a machine designed to monitor the fetus's heartbeat in utero. It records the *fetal heart rate (FHR).* The FHM is composed of two sensitive electrodes that are placed on the abdomen; these are attached with stretchy elastic belts. The FHM also detects the presence and duration of uterine contractions, which you will learn more about later in this chapter. However, because the FHM cannot discern the strength of the contractions or how the fetus is tolerating them, a nonstress test would be the next step in the care of the patient if more frequent contractions occur.

"I'm going to start a *nonstress test* now. We call it an *NST.*"

nonstress test (NST): an external and noninvasive method of monitoring the fetus. It is not usually performed until after the 27th week of pregnancy. The NST is used to assess fetal heart rate and movement.

". . . response of your uterus, something we refer to as *uterine activity* . . ."

uterine activity: contractions and any changes in the sound and frequency of the fetal heartbeat.

". . . your *cervix* . . ."

cervix: the narrow passage that leads from the uterus into the vagina. It becomes part of what is known as the *birth canal* or *birth passage.* The cervix widens during delivery.

". . . the nurse pointed out the *call bell* nearby . . ."

call bell: a device found in hospitals and care facilities that is used to summon the care staff to the patient's bedside. There are standards and protocols that require easy access for patients to call bells. For example, these devices should never be placed where the patient cannot reach them. The call bell may set off a light or sound above the doorway to the patient's room, or it may simply ring on the desk at the nurses' station. For reasons of safety and for legal, ethical, and moral care, all call bells should be answered.

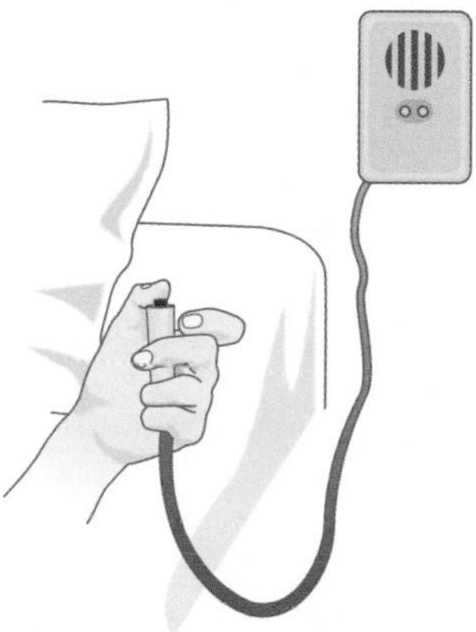

Figure 8.7: Hospital call bell

Eponyms: Leopold's maneuvers

Christian Gerhard Leopold was an eminent German gynecologist at the turn of the 20th century. Leopold practiced medicine and taught midwifery at a number of schools and colleges in Austria, Scotland, England, and Germany. During his later years, he was the director of the school of midwifery at Dresden Royal Gynecological Infirmary in Dresden, Germany. He is remembered today for his four now classical maneuvers that are used for the assessment of the position and the presentation of the fetus in utero.

TABLE 8-4: Fetal Presentations

Name	Description
cephalic presentation	the head of the fetus is completely flexed onto the chest, and the occipital portion of the head is presenting; this presentation occurs with most births
vertex presentation	the vertex (top or apex) of the head is presenting
sinciput presentation	part of the skull and forehead are presenting
brow presentation	the brow or forehead is facing first into the birth canal
face presentation	the fetus's face is presenting first
breech presentation	the buttocks or feet are presenting
shoulder presentation	a fetal shoulder or arm presents first; this position is also referred to as a *transverse lie*

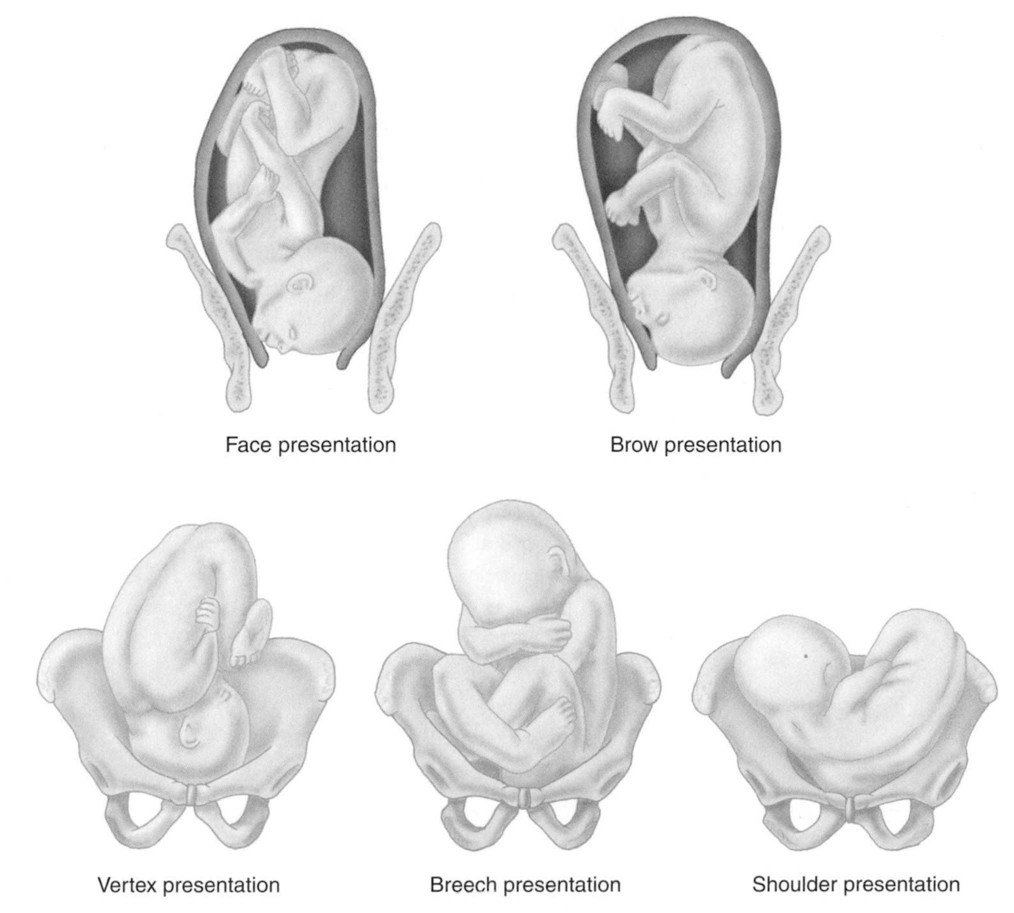

Figure 8.6: Fetal presentations

Fill in the Blanks

Fill in each blank with the most appropriate medical term.

1. ______________________ are a series of step-wise moves in which a fetus is assessed through palpation of the mother's abdomen.
2. The insertion of a finger intravaginally can help with the assessment of the ______________________ presentation.
3. The term ______________________ is used to determine whether the baby's feet are presenting into the birth canal first.
4. The specialty obstetrical unit mentioned in the opening scene of this chapter is the ______________________ unit.
5. Another medical way to say "the apex of the head is presenting" is to say that "the ______________________ is presenting."
6. A breech is an abnormal presentation. Another way to say this is to say that it is a ______________________.

Right Word or Wrong Word: *Hospital Unit* or *Hospital Ward*?

Are these two terms synonymous? Where might you hear either one?

The Language of Pregnancy

Chapter 3 introduced some of the basic language of pregnancy as Glory Loeppky was given an initial physical assessment in the emergency room. As we continue to monitor Glory's pregnancy and health status, you will need to expand your understanding of the terminology related to pregnancy.

You will recall that our patient is 7½ months pregnant, which means that she is in the third trimester of her pregnancy. Medically, Glory is referred to as *gravid* or *gravida,* and her gestation is estimated at 30 to 32 weeks. She has not been pregnant previously, so to be even more precise, she is **primigravida**, which means that she is pregnant for the first time. By the same token, she has never given birth before; the term for this condition is **nullipara**. The suffix *-para* means *birth.*

This is the first child for Glory and Gil, and they are happy and excited about his or her arrival. They have planned for a normal vaginal birth, and they have taken classes to prepare for this. Gil plans to be in the delivery room with his wife for the birth. Now, as a result of a motor vehicle accident, Glory finds herself alone in an antepartum unit undergoing assessment for both maternal and fetal health.

TABLE 8-5: Prefixes: Maternity and Obstetrics

BEGIN with a Prefix	ADD the Root *Gravida* or the Suffix *-para*	CREATE a New Medical Term	Meaning
nulli-	gravida	nulligravida	no pregnancies
nulli-	-para	nullipara	no births
multi-	gravida	multigravida	multiple pregnancies
multi-	-para	multipara	multiple births
primi-	gravida	primigravida	first pregnancy
primi-	-para	primipara	first birth

Key terms: pregnancy

gravid: pregnant; heavy with child.

gravida: a pregnant woman; a woman's status regarding pregnancy. (See Table 8-5 for prefixes that are commonly used with this word.)

maternity: motherhood. This is also the typical name for the obstetrical unit in a hospital.

maternal health: the health of the mother during pregnancy, childbirth, and the postpartum period.

gestation: the length of time from conception to birth. The average *gestational period* for humans is 40 weeks. The status of a pregnancy is usually identified by how many weeks of gestation (gestational weeks) have occurred.

fetus: the medical term for the stage of human development from 8 gestational weeks until birth. (See Chapter 3 for a detailed discussion of the terms *embryo, fetus,* and *baby.*)

uterus: a reproductive organ. The uterus provides a safe, protective, and nourishing environment for the growing embryo and fetus. The uterus is also known as the *womb.*

placenta: an organ of reproduction that attaches the embryo or fetus to the inside of the uterine wall and, by doing so, is able to provide nutrients, remove waste products, and provide vital gas exchanges that promote healthy growth. These processes occur through the flow of *amniotic fluid,* which is produced by the placenta and later by the fetus' kidneys in utero. After delivery, when the placenta is expelled, it may be referred to as the *afterbirth.*

labor: the process of giving birth. Labor begins with uterine contractions that are repetitious and that become more frequent and forceful as birth becomes imminent. Labor is synonymous with the terms *parturition* and *childbirth.* Labor is divided into 3 stages:

First stage *dilation:* contractions begin and the cervix dilates (expands)

Second stage *expulsion:* the process of birth occurs

Third stage *placental:* the placenta is expelled

delivery: the end point of labor, including expulsion of the placenta and its membranes.

birth: the act of being born. Medically, birth occurs when the child passes through the uterus into the world. The word *birth* is a proper medical term.

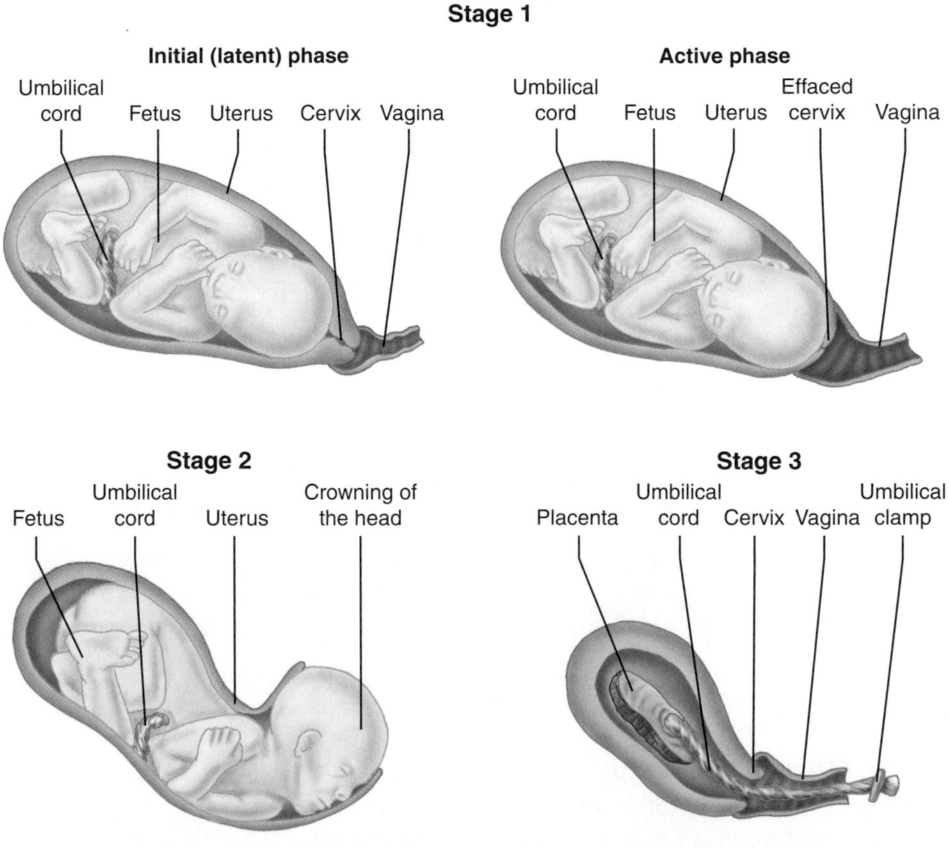

Figure 8.8: The three stages of labor

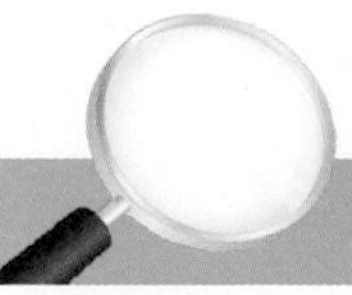

FOCUS POINT: The Placenta

The placenta is an organ of the endocrine system (see Chapter 7), and it produces hormones called *gonadotropics.* When these hormones are detected in a urine specimen, pregnancy is confirmed. The hormones estrogen and progesterone are also secreted by the placenta.

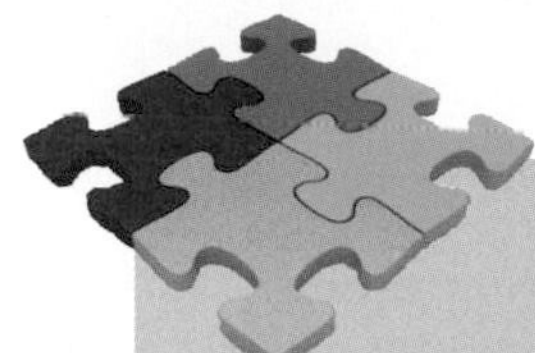

WORD BUILDING: Formula for Creating Words with the Combining Forms *Parturi* and *Uter/o* and the Root Word *Embryo*

1. parturire = Latin root meaning *to be in labor or to give birth.* The combining form is *parturi.*

parturi + ent = *parturient*

Definition: concerning childbirth; about to give birth; at the time of childbirth. *adjective or noun*

Examples: The *parturient* woman was taken to the delivery room.
The *parturient* was taken to the delivery room.

parturi + tion = *parturition*

Definition: the act of giving birth; childbirth. *noun*

Example: *Parturition* occurred at 1900 hrs., after 5 hours of labor.

parturi + facient = *parturifacient*

Definition: inducing labor. (The second root derives from the Latin *facere,* meaning *to make.*) *adjective*

Example: As the ninth month of the pregnancy came to an end, a *parturifacient* medication was administered to bring on labor.

peri + parturient = *periparturient*

Definition: around the time of giving birth. *adjective*

Example: Some *periparturient* women may develop thrombocytopenia, which is a low platelet count in the blood.

intra + part + al = *intrapartal*

Definition: during pregnancy. (The prefix *intra-* means *within or during.* The root word *parturient* becomes *part.* The suffix *-al* is added to create an adjective.) *adjective*

Example: During pregnancy, women are screened for *intrapartal* risk factors such as abnormal presentation or multiple gestations.

post + parturient = *postparturient*

Definition: concerning the period immediately after delivery or childbirth. *adjective*

Example: If the mother's uterus does not return to its normal size after delivery, a *postparturient* pathology may occur.

2. uterus = womb. The combining form is *uter/o.*

intra + uterine = *intrauterine*

Definition: within the uterus. *adjective*

Example: *Intrauterine* infections during pregnancy can be dangerous to both the mother and the fetus.

Continued

utero + otomy = *uterotomy*

Definition: incision of the uterus. *noun*

Example: A Cesarean section involves a *uterotomy.*

utero + pexia = *uteropexia*

Definition: fixation of the uterus to the abdominal wall. (The suffix *-pexia* means *fixation.*) *noun*

Example: *Uteropexia* is a surgical procedure that is performed to correct a displaced uterus. More common terms for the procedure are *hysteropexy* and *uterofixation.*

utero + placent + al = *uteroplacental*

Definition: referring to both the uterus and the placenta. *adjective*

Example: A trauma to the abdomen of a pregnant woman may cause *uteroplacental* injuries.

3. embryo = from the Greek root *embryon,* meaning *something that swells in the body*. The root word *embryo* refers to the stage of human development during the first 7 weeks after conception; this stage begins on the fourth day after the fertilization of an ovum.

embry + ology = *embryology*

Definition: the science of the origin and development of embryos. *noun*

Example: Human *embryology* is the scientific study of fertilization of the ovum and the creation and development of the embryo through to the fetal stage.

embryo + scopy = *embryoscopy*

Definition: the direct visualization of the embryo or fetus through a small incision in the abdominal wall. *noun*

Example: Diagnostic *embryoscopy* occurs during the first trimester of pregnancy for those families at risk for genetically inherited fetal abnormalities.

embryo + troph = *embryotroph*

Definition: a maternal fluid that nourishes the embryo. (The second word part stems from the root *trophe,* meaning *nourishment.*) *noun*

Example: *Embryotroph* is a mixture of maternal blood and other nutrient material from which an embryo is formed and nourished.

Name the Term and Break It Down

Write the term that fits each definition or description. Next, break down the term into its separate word parts, and then write the meaning of each part.

1. any disease of the embryo
   Term: ______________________ Word parts: ______________________
2. around the time of giving birth
   Term: ______________________ Word parts: ______________________
3. pain in the womb
   Term: ______________________ Word parts: ______________________
4. referring to the uterus and the vagina
   Term: ______________________ Word parts: ______________________
5. during pregnancy
   Term: ______________________ Word parts: ______________________
6. inflammation of the uterus
   Term: ______________________ Word parts: ______________________

Let's Practice

Write the meaning of each prefix (see Table 8-5).

1. nulli- ______________________________
2. multi- ______________________________
3. primi- ______________________________

Mix and Match

Draw a line to connect the synonyms.

1. parturition	afterbirth
2. dilates	pregnant
3. placenta	womb
4. gravid	apex
5. -para	birth
6. maternity	after the birth
7. obstetrics	expands
8. vertex	labor
9. uterus	motherhood
10. postpartum	management of childbirth; pregnancy

PRONUNCIATION PRACTICE

Say these words aloud to a friend or classmate if you can. You are given the phonetic pronunciation. Your instructor can help you with pronunciation,

or visit **http://www.MedicalLanguageLab.com.** 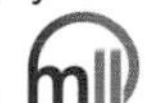

embryo	**ĕm´** brē-ō	parturifacient	păr-tū-rĭ-**fā´**shĕnt
embryopathy	ĕm″brē-**ŏp´**ă-thē	parturition	păr-tū-**´rĭsh´**ŭn
embryoscopy	ĕm″brē-**ŏs´**kō-pē	placenta	plă-**sĕn´**tă
embryotroph	**ĕm´** brē-ō- trōf	uteralgia	ū″tĕr-**ăl´**jē-ă
gestation	jĕs-**tā´**shŭn	uteroplacental	ū″tĕr-ō- plă-**sĕn´**tăl
gravida	**grăv´** ĭ-dă	uterus	**ū´**tĕr-ŭs
intrapartal	ĭn″-tră-**păr´**tăl	womb	woom
parturient	păr-**tū´**rē-ĕnt		

Diagnostics and monitoring: antepartum unit

Glory Loeppky had a number of diagnostic tests during her assessment in the emergency department at Fayette General Hospital; these were discussed in Chapter 3. The results have now come in. It is the responsibility of the obstetrician and the nurses who are caring for this patient to review the results, and RN Laura is doing so now. Study the "On the Job: Lab Report" on page 306 for this patient. How many terms and abbreviations do you recognize from earlier chapters? How many new terms do you see?

Fayette General Hospital
Labs

Today's Date: *June XX, 2015* Date of Specimen Collection: *June XX, 2015*

Submitting Physician's Name: *Dr. Abrams*

Physician's Contact Information: *Fayette General Hospital, Emergency Department*
(may be stamped)

Name: *Glory Loeppky* Date of Birth: *XX/XX/XXXX* Age: *32 years*

Gender: ✓ Female ___ Male Hospital Admission # *2928*

Hematology:
CBC with platelets

Hematrocrit: *40%*
(normal range 39–37%)

RBC: *4.6/mm³*
(normal range 4.2–5.4 million/mm³)

WBC: *5,200/mm³*
(normal range 4,500–11,000/mm³)

Platelets: *300,000/mm³*
(normal range 150,00–400,000/mm³)

HGB: *14 g/dL*
(normal range 12–16 g/dL)

Prenatal Serology:
ABO
Anti-A negative
Antib-B negative
Type 0

Rh factor

Rh+ fetus

Rh- female
(normal)

Microbiology:
Urinalysis
Ketones: ___ positive ✓ negative (normal)
Glucose: ___ positive ✓ negative (normal)
Proteins: ___ positive ✓ negative (normal)
WBC: ___ positive ✓ negative (normal)

Biochemistry:
Glucose: ___ random ✓ fasting
85 mg/dL (normal range 70–99 mg/dL)

Let's Practice

The following abbreviations used in the "On the Job: Lab Report" (shown above) should already be familiar to you. Write the meaning of each one.

1. HGB ______________________________
2. WBC ______________________________
3. INR ______________________________
4. CBC ______________________________
5. RBC ______________________________
6. PTT ______________________________

New key terms: lab report

The "On the Job: Lab Report" for our patient introduces a number of new abbreviations and terms:

ABO: antibody screen. This blood test is performed during the last trimester of pregnancy. It identifies antibodies in the mother's blood that react with antigens in the fetus's blood. This test is particularly important to determine if the mother's antibodies are attacking the fetus's red blood cells, which would be a life-threatening situation for the fetus. The letters in the abbreviation *ABO* denote three human blood groups: A, B, and O (see "Focus Point: Blood Groups").

Antibodies are also known as *antiglobulins* or *immunoglobulins.* They are specialized proteins produced in response to foreign antigens being introduced into the body. The production of antibodies is a major function of the immune system.

Antigens are proteins, glycoproteins, carbohydrates, or glycolipids (organic compounds that are not soluble in water) that are found on the red blood cells. They cause antibodies to react. Antigens are often at the core of allergic responses.

Rh factor: a classification system used to type blood for transfusion purposes. **Rh** is a type of antigen (protein) found on the membranous surface of red blood cells. There are actually five subtypes of Rh antigen, but the most important is antigen D. Antigen D can trigger an immune system response in the other four Rh antigens, which leads to a medical crisis for the fetus. Incompatibility between the mother and the fetus leads to *hemolytic disease of the newborn (HDN)* (see "Focus Point: Hemolytic Disease of the Newborn" as well as Figure 8-9).

ketones: water-soluble compounds in the body that are byproducts of the breakdown of fatty acids. Usually the body uses glucose and carbohydrates to produce energy; however, when these are not in sufficient supply, stored fat is burned for energy. This latter process produces ketones, which are excreted in the urine. Ketone levels are tested during pregnancy to assess for gestational diabetes (see Chapters 3 and 7).

proteins: essential elements at all levels of the body. These organic compounds are composed of amino acids, and they provide nourishment and energy. Protein levels are tested during pregnancy to rule out urinary tract infection in the mother, as well as the potential for maternal kidney disease. At a later point during pregnancy, protein tests can also identify maternal high blood pressure, a serious but treatable symptom called *preeclampsia (hypertension of pregnancy).*

Metric measurements: lab report

You will notice that many of the numbers on the "On the Job: Lab Report" (see page 306) are given in metric measurements. This is standard procedure in laboratories and in science in general. There is no need for you to learn each metric measure now, but be aware that these terms and abbreviations are common in health care and that you are likely to encounter them in your future work. Here are some examples from Glory Loeppky's lab results.

mm^3: cubic millimeters; synonymous with μL, meaning *microliters*

Conversion: 1 liter is equivalent to 0.33 (⅓) of an American gallon
3 American ounces are equivalent to 0.9 liters

mg/dL: milligrams per deciliter

Conversion: 3 grams are equivalent to 0.9 ounces
1 milligram is equivalent to 0.001 gram
1 liter is equivalent to 0.33 (⅓) of a gallon
1 deciliter is equivalent to 0.03 of a gallon or 3.38 of an ounce

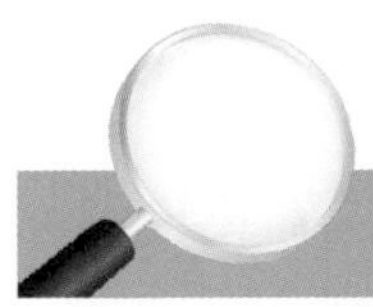

FOCUS POINT: Blood Groups

Group A blood contains group A antigens.

Group B blood contains group B antigens.

Group AB blood contains both A and B antigens. This person is a *universal recipient,* which means that he or she can successfully receive blood transfusions from any other blood group.

Group O blood contains neither A nor B antigens. This person can be a *universal donor,* which means that he or she can donate blood to people of any blood group.

Eponyms: Rh Factor

The Rh factor is actually named after rhesus macaque monkeys, in whose blood the antigen was first discovered in the 1940s. Working with fellow researcher Alexander Weiner, Karl Landsteiner—who had earlier discovered the A, B, AB, and O blood groups that made transfusions safe—discovered the Rh antigen. The researchers used the blood of rhesus monkeys to develop an anti-Rh serum, which is now injected into Rh-negative mothers who are carrying Rh-positive babies.

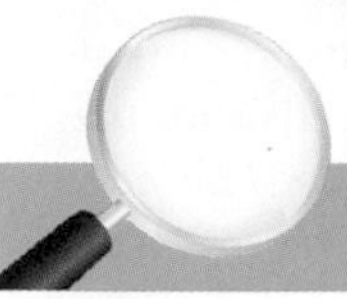

FOCUS POINT: Hemolytic Disease of the Newborn

Hemolytic disease of the newborn (HDN) is a life-threatening condition for the fetus and newborn and a major cause of fetal loss (stillbirth) and death in newborns. The cause is related to the fetus's red blood cells coming under attack by maternal antibodies as a result of the incompatibility between their Rh blood types (see Figure 8-9.) HDN can also be caused by an incompatibility of the ABO blood groups; however, this type of incompatibility is usually less severe than the Rh incompatibility condition.

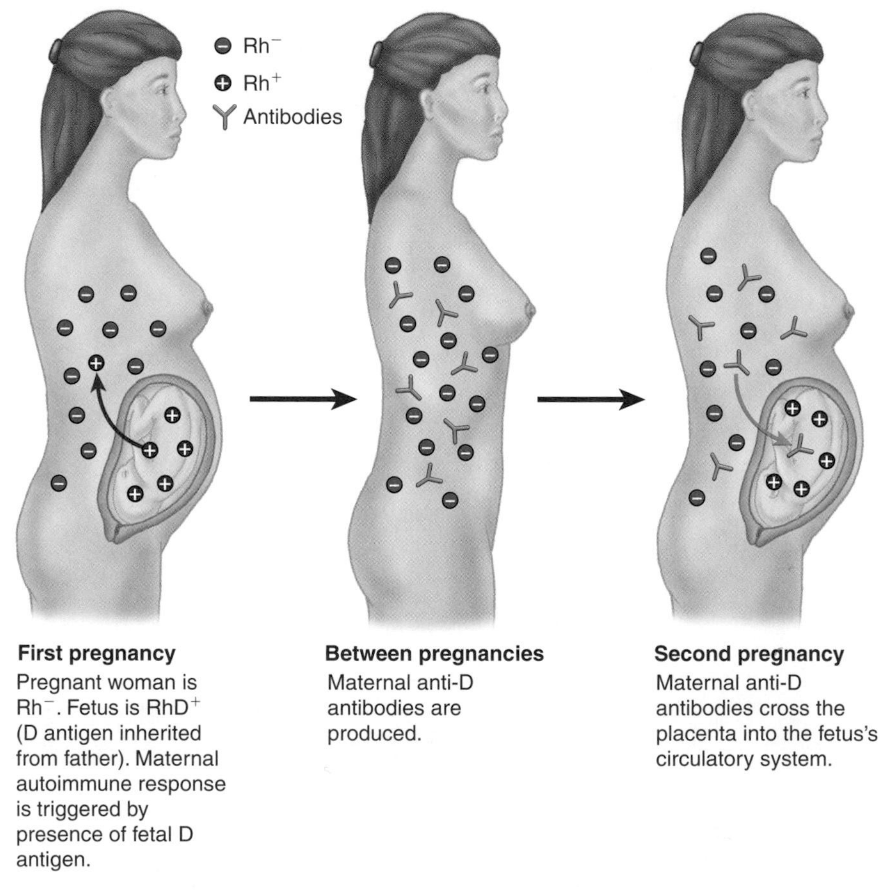

Figure 8.9: Development of hemolytic disease of the newborn

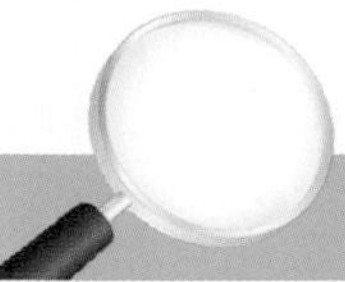

FOCUS POINT: Hemolytic Anemia and the Rh Factor

Hemolytic anemia is a rare disease in the 21st century. With the advent of immunization of the mother right after birth, subsequent pregnancies are protected from this condition. The condition develops when the waste product bilirubin (a yellow pigment) is not removed from red blood cells and the bilirubin overwhelms the fetus's system (see Figure 8-10). High levels of bilirubin can cause the newborn's skin to turn yellow. In severe cases, brain damage is a possibility, but this is rare and may be preempted by a blood transfusion.

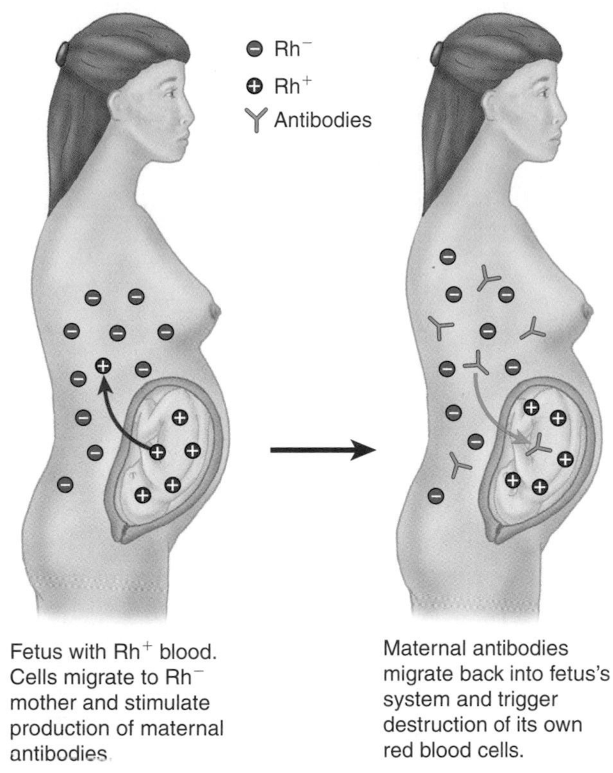

Figure 8.10: Development of hemolytic anemia

The Language of Vital Signs and Baselines

In addition to studying the laboratory test results for Mrs. Loeppky, the treatment team has begun to record the patient's vital signs. The vital signs on her initial tests provide the staff with **baselines** or measurements that they can use to compare any changes in the patient's status while she is being observed and treated. Study the "On the Job: Vital Signs Record" on page 310. You should already be familiar with the terms and abbreviations shown on this form. How many of them do you remember?

Vital Signs Record

Patient Name: *Glory Loeppky* Hospital Admission # *2928*

Unit: *AP*

Blood Pressure	Vital Signs
Date: *June XX, 2015*	Date: *June XX, 2015*
Time: *1330 hrs*	Time: *1500 hr*
On admission to ER: *(anxious)*	On admission to ER: *(anxious)*
Systolic: *138*	Temp: *96.8 °F*
Diastolic: *64*	Pulse: *95*
	Resp: *20*
	o_2 sats: *94%*
	Baseline FHR: *150 bpm*
On admission to Antepartum: *(mildly anxious)*	On admission to Antepartum: *(mildly anxious)*
Systolic: *132*	Temp: *96.8 °F*
Diastolic: *60*	Pulse: *80*
	Resp: *18*
	o_2 sats (SO_2): *98.2%*
	Baseline FHR: *146 with moderate variability, accelerations present, no decelerations noted. Normal NST*

TABLE 8-6: Normal Ranges for Vital Signs: Adults

Normal Ranges for Vital Signs: Adults	Vital Signs Using Medical Abbreviations
Temperature: 97.8°F to 99.1°F (average 98.6°F)	Temp 97.8–99.1° T 97.8–99.1°
Pulse rate: 60 to 80 beats per minute at rest	P 60–80 P 60–80 bpm
Respirations or breath rate: 12 to 19 breaths per minute	Resps 16–20 R 16–20
Blood pressure: 120/80 mm/Hg	BP 120/80 BP 120/80

Mix and Match

Match each abbreviation from the lab report and the vital signs record with its full term. Draw a line to connect them. Be careful! There are a couple of review terms here for which you must be on the lookout. This is designed to keep previously learned terms fresh in your mind.

1. ABO	partial thromboplastin test
2. PTT	a blood group system based on antigens, especially D
3. HGB	antibodies screen
4. ABG	fasting blood sugar
5. Rh	oxygen saturation level
6. BP	arterial blood gases
7. SO2	blood pressure
8. FBS	hemoglobin

Free Writing

Use new terminology to write sentences. You are given some clue words to help you. Use these words in your sentence, although you might have to change them slightly. Of course, you will also need to add a number of your own words to make a logical sentence.

EXAMPLE: shouldn't blood eat glucose 12 hours test

Sentence: To prepare for a fasting glucose test, a person shouldn't eat anything for 12 hours beforehand.

1. groups important compatible tests pregnancy determine

 ____

2. antibodies antigens trigger

 ____

3. measure glucose g/dL hemoglobin levels

 ____

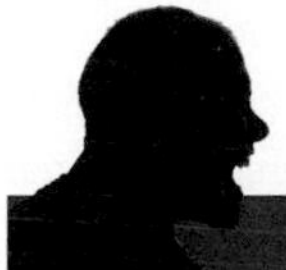

PRONUNCIATION PRACTICE

Say these words aloud to a friend or classmate if you can. You are given the phonetic pronunciation. Your instructor can help you with pronunciation, or visit **http://www.MedicalLanguageLab.com.** mll

antigen	**ăn**´tĭ-jĕn	mm^3	cubic **milli**meters
hemolytic	hē˝mō-**lĭt**´ĭk	mg/dL	milligrams per **deci**liter

Patient Update

Glory's mother and father have arrived at the antepartum unit of Fayette General Hospital. The nurse, Laura, has not yet fully informed them of Glory's condition because she has not yet sought the patient's permission to share confidential information with anyone. Instead, she accompanies the parents to Glory's room, and she will stay for a few moments to be involved in the conversation.

"Glory? Glory, I have someone here to see you," the nurse called quietly from the doorway when she noticed that the patient was sleeping. Glory opened her eyes just as Laura stepped away from the door. She saw her parents, and she broke into a huge smile that quickly disintegrated into tears.

"Oh, Mama, there's been an accident. We were in an accident," Glory wept. Her mother crossed quickly to her side and hugged her. Her father joined them.

"Yes, honey, we've heard. Are you all right?" Glory's mother asked as she released her daughter and stood up, holding her hand. Glory nodded quickly through the tears and then hugged her father fiercely.

"Yes," she whispered, "I'm okay, I think." She looked quickly at the nurse.

Laura said, "Glory's doing fine right now. She's had a very stressful day, and we are monitoring her health and the baby's." Laura was quiet then, allowing time for Glory to talk.

Glory explained that she had some tenderness in her abdomen and was using the nonstress test monitor to record fetal movement. She told her parents that she had received a gash on her left thigh during the accident, and she explained that she'd had stitches for that. Then she broke into a loud sob, "Oh, Mama, Daddy, where is Gil? I can't stand it. I haven't heard. I'm supposed to stay calm but I just can't help worrying about Gil. Oh, please, tell me that you know something about Gil!"

Her father said that he'd heard from Gil's parents, who were going to see him at Okla Trauma Center. He tried to reassure her that Gil was okay and that his parents would make sure that he was receiving good care. This didn't satisfy his daughter.

"What is it, Daddy? You're not really telling me anything. What is it?" Glory looked anxiously from mother to father and back. "I know it's something serious. I can tell. Oh, tell me! I can't stand it!"

Reluctantly, her father began, "Well, honey, Gil's been hurt." Glory gasped, and her eyes filled with tears again. "Whatever happened in that accident, he hit his head on the windshield, and he has a head injury. He was unconscious at the scene." Again, Glory gasped, and her eyes went wide. "Wait, wait, don't panic," her father said. "Nobody said it was a really bad head injury, so I don't want you to jump to that conclusion. They'll be keeping a pretty close eye on him at Okla. It's a good hospital, honey." Glory cried softly and held on tightly to her parents' hands. Her father went on to explain that her husband had also suffered a fractured thighbone and injuries to his knee and ankle.

"Excuse me, Laura?" The unit clerk was at the door. "There's a phone call for you. Dr. Bedard. Can you come?" The nurse nodded and left the room.

"Laura Sherman here," she said as she picked up the phone at the nursing station.

"Hi, Laura, it's Ricki Bedard here. I've just finished looking at Mrs. Loeppky's ultrasound. It looks like there is a tear in her placenta, and there appears to be a hematoma under the distal edge. We'll need to keep a sharp eye on that for hemorrhage. How is she doing?" The nurse explained that the patient and the fetus were stable at the moment and that Glory's parents had just arrived and were with her.

"Good. What does the nonstress test show?" asked Dr. Bedard.

"She's only been on it a short while, but it looks okay. The baseline is about 148 with good accels. There are no decels and only moderate variability. Her vitals are stable. However, she has complained about some generalized tenderness across her abdomen. I checked, and her uterus is soft. There's no vaginal discharge, either." The doctor was quiet while Laura reported, and then she asked about the patient's urine. "The urine dip is negative for everything," said Laura.

"Okay, that's good. Listen, I've got another patient to see in the ER, but I'll be on my way up to see her shortly. However, I want you to page me STAT if anything changes, anything at all. I'm very worried about abruptio placentae. We may be looking at a C-section." Laura agreed. "In the meantime, I've got a few more orders for you . . ."

Reflective Questions

Reflect on the dialogue you've just read as you answer these questions.

1. Where have Glory Loeppky's parents located their daughter?

____

2. What current test is Glory undergoing?

____

3. What has the obstetrician identified on the patient's ultrasound that worries her?

____

4. What is causing the patient to become increasingly anxious?

____

Critical Thinking

Consider all that you've read and learned about Glory Loeppky's state of health post-MVA, then consider that she was admitted to an antepartum unit. Think about her condition as you answer these questions, and use medical terminology whenever possible.

1. How did Mrs. Loeppky qualify for admission to the antepartum unit?

____

2. When Mrs. Loeppky was admitted to the unit, was she stable?

____

3. Is the patient at risk for anything now? If so, what and why?

____

4. What effect do you think increasing anxiety may have on the unborn child and the mother?

____

Key terms: antepartum care

During her phone call with the obstetrician, RN Laura used a combination of medical terminology and other medical language that is common in the context of maternal and child care. Study this language now, and keep the context in mind as you learn to "translate" the jargon and terminology.

"... a *tear in her placenta* ..."

tear in her placenta: a **placental abruption** (also referred to as *placenta abruptio* or *abruptio placentae*): a detachment of the placenta from the uterus. This occurs when blood collects between the placenta and the uterus; as the pressure and volume of blood increase, the placenta eventually tears away from the uterus. Hemorrhaging is also likely to occur.

"... appears to be a *hematoma under the distal edge.*"

hematoma under the distal edge: a mass of blood in the tissue located under the distal edge of the placenta (see Chapter 2 for terms that refer to direction).

"... *baseline* is about 148 ..."

baseline: in this context, this term refers to the baseline fetal heart rate. A normal fetal heart rate is 110 to 160 beats per minute. During early gestation, the rate is usually toward the top end of the scale; toward the end of gestation, the rate is usually lower. The fetus's baseline is seen on the fetal heart monitor. Glory's baby's baseline fetal heart rate is 148 beats per minute and therefore normal.

"... good *accels.*"

accels: a term referring to **accelerations** or increases in the fetal heart rate as compared with the baseline. This normally occurs when the fetus moves, and it is to be expected.

"... no *decels* ..."

decels: decelerations in the fetal heart rate as compared with the baseline that occur in relation to contractions and that are not normal in a non-laboring patient. Decelerations require prompt attention and can indicate fetal distress. This is usually related to some form of compression or compromise of the umbilical cord, a critical internal lifeline.

"... moderate *variability*."

variability: baseline variability. This is a measure of the difference in the beat-to-beat intervals of the fetal heart rate. It's read on the FHR tracing (readout). Normal variability in a term fetus is 6 to 25 beats per minute. This indicates a normally functioning central nervous system.

"Her *vitals are stable*."

vitals are stable: the vital signs are within the normal range and are not fluctuating greatly.

"... her *uterus is soft.*"

uterus is soft: the normal state for the pregnant uterus. When the uterus is hard to the touch, contractions are occurring.

"There's no *vaginal discharge*, either."

vaginal discharge: secretions from the vagina. In Glory Loeppky's case, the nurse is referring to her observation that there is no vaginal bleeding or leaking of the amniotic fluid in which the fetus floats in the womb.

"The *urine dip* is *negative for everything* ..."

urine dip: a urine test in which a dipstick is inserted into the patient's urine. The stick, which is usually made of plastic, is coated with a number of colored patches. When this stick is exposed to the various composites of urine, the colors brighten or change. This test is a quick way to assess the patient's condition. A urine dipstick test identifies the following elements and characteristics of urine: protein (albumin), glucose, ketones, blood, leukocytes, bilirubin, nitrite, pH, and specific gravity. See Chapters 5 and 9 to learn more about the composition of urine.

negative for everything: the results of the urine dipstick tests show no abnormalities.

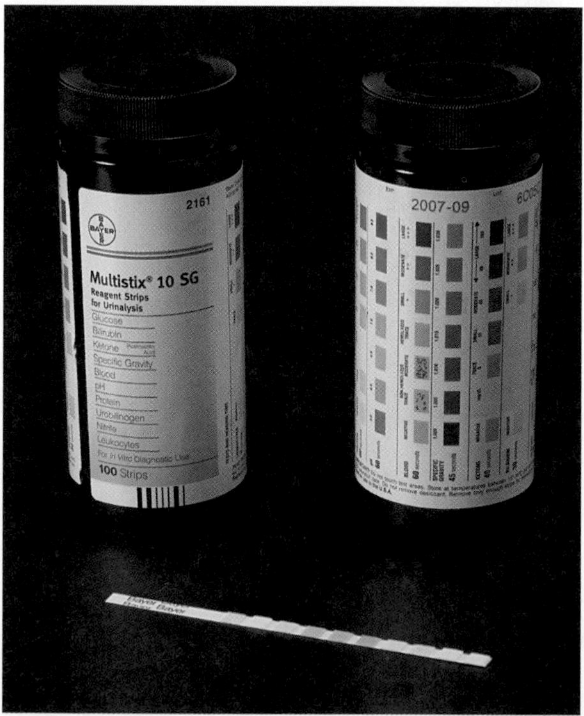

Figure 8.12: Urine dipstick test (From Eagle S, Brassington C, Dailey C, Goretti C: *The Professional Medical Assistant: An Integrative, Teamwork-Based Approach.* Philadelphia: FA Davis, 2009, p. 924. With permission.)

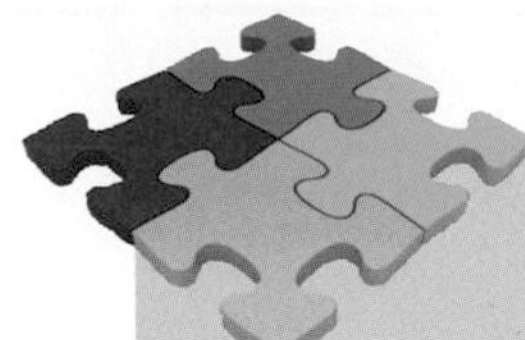

WORD BUILDING: Word Building with the Root Word *Placenta*

placenta = the oval structure in the uterus of mammals from which a fetus derives oxygen and nutrients. The combining form is *placent/a.*

placenta + tion = *placentation*

Definition: the process of the formation of the placenta and its attachment to the uterine wall. *noun*

Example: The process of *placentation* begins within the first week after conception.

placent + itis = *placentitis*

Definition: inflammation of the placenta. *noun*

Example: *Placentitis* can be the result of intrauterine infection and infection of the amniotic fluid.

placent + o + graphy = *placentography*

Definition: radiographic examination of the placenta. *noun*

Example: Ultrasonic *placentography* requires the injection of a radiopaque contrast medium (dye); it is considered a safe procedure.

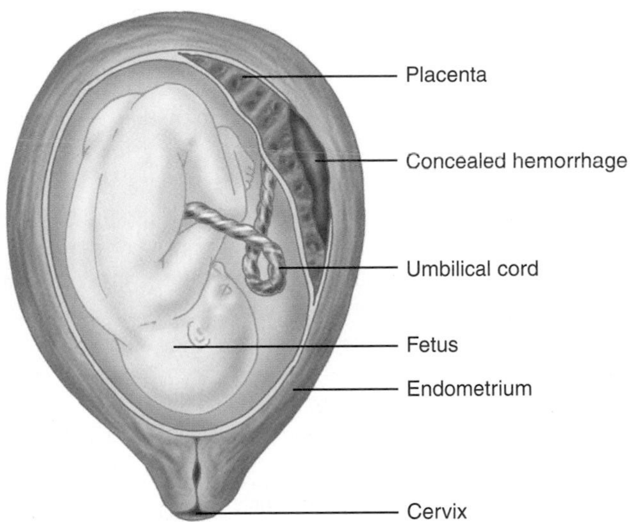

Figure 8.11: Placental abruption

Patient Update

On the antepartum unit, some of the nurses are taking advantage of a quiet moment to catch up on charting and other duties at the desk. Other staff members are busy with patient care. It's late in the afternoon now, and visitors are beginning to arrive.

"Nurse, nurse, come quick!" called Glory Loeppky's mother from the doorway of her daughter's room. The call light went on above her at the same time. She glanced back to see her husband, Glory's father, pushing the call bell. "Nurse!" she called again, and then she saw Laura and another nurse come from behind the main desk on the run. She stepped aside as they entered the room.

"Oh, hi . . . um . . . my belly hurts," groaned Glory as the nurses approached.

"What sort of pain are you having?" asked Laura when she saw the pinched look on Glory's face.

"Ooh," came the only reply. Laura gently reached over to palpate the patient's uterus. It was hard. Laura looked up across the bed to her colleague, Brenda, and nodded. "UC," she said. "I'm going to take another nonstress test." The nurse worked quickly to complete another fetal monitor check and immediately noticed that the baseline had now increased. She noted a definite increase in uterine pressure and some subtle decelerations in the fetal heart as the uterus began to relax a bit. "Brenda, please take care of Glory. I'm going to page Dr. Bedard." Laura then turned and abruptly left the room. The second nurse, an LPN, took the patient's vital signs and noted a shift in the patient's pulse and BP. She knew that this could mean hemorrhage. Brenda spoke calmly to the patient and her parents.

"Well, Glory, it looks like you're having some changes happening here. Laura's gone to get Dr. Bedard to come see you. In the meantime, I'll stay here with you. Are you feeling any pain or discomfort anywhere else?" Brenda asked and pulled the sheets back gently to observe for any vaginal bleeding or the presence of amniotic fluid.

"Why does she need the doctor?" interrupted Glory's mother. "What's happening to Glory and the baby?" she asked anxiously, reaching out to hold her husband's hand. "Glory, are you okay?" Glory looked frightened and rubbed her hand over her belly.

"I . . . I don't know, Mama. I suddenly don't feel so well. It sort of hurts here, but . . . well . . . I don't know what it is, but I just don't feel well," Glory said in a worried voice. Brenda attempted to calm the family and encouraged the patient to take some deep, relaxing breaths. She then asked the mother to pitch in and to encourage her daughter to do some deep breathing with her. Glory's mother complied. In the background, the elevator doors opened, and the sound of feet coming quickly down the hallway could be heard. Laura and another woman were talking and moving closer to Glory's room.

"Hello, I'm Dr. Bedard," the obstetrician said as she entered the room. "Hello, Mrs. Loeppky. We haven't met yet, but I'm going to be looking after you." Dr. Bedard smiled and touched Glory's hand gently. She then reached over to read the FH monitor strip. Afterward, she palpated the patient's abdomen. As she finished, she gave orders to the nurses. "We'll need an ultrasound STAT. Do it here. Get the OR on standby for a possible STAT C/S, too," she said calmly. As Brenda turned to leave to complete the orders, Dr. Bedard added, "Say, Brenda, see if Frank Jasper's around, will you? Ask him if he'd like to scrub in."

Brenda nodded and went on her way to ask the unit clerk to make the arrangements. Laura remained with the doctor and the patient. "Mrs. Loeppky, when I looked at your ultrasound a short while ago, I found evidence of placental tearing; this means that the placenta is coming away from the wall of the uterus. There is a hematoma forming under the placenta where it is separating from the uterine wall. This can cause internal bleeding, and it is unsafe for the fetus. It looks like we may have to deliver your baby."

"What?" came the family's joint response of disbelief. Their eyes went wide as they stared at the doctor. Brenda came back and advised the doctor that OR was standing by.

"In the case of a placental abruption, which I think is what we have here, the fetus's life may be in jeopardy. A Cesarean section is the only answer."

A sonographer arrived then, bringing with him a portable ultrasound machine. Dr. Bedard stood beside him and watched as the examination proceeded. At its conclusion, Dr. Bedard said, "All right. It's confirmed. There is an abruption of the placenta. We'll prepare for OR. Don't worry, Mrs. Loeppky. You're in good hands, and we're going to do everything we can to make sure you and your baby have a healthy delivery." She smiled and touched Glory's arm gently again. The patient was crying. Her mother moved closer to her as the doctor left the room, but Glory pushed her away. Her father stepped out into the hallway, following Dr. Bedard for more information.

"Laura? Is my baby going to be okay? Brenda?" Glory asked nervously. The nurses tried to reassure her that the treatment team would do everything they could to achieve the best results for everyone involved. "But my baby isn't old enough! I'm only 7½ months pregnant. That's too soon, it's too early! I'm afraid," she cried and reached out to touch the nurse beside her.

"Babies can be born preterm, Glory. Your baby is about 30 to 32 weeks old now. It will be small, but we have a wonderful modern neonatal intensive care unit here at Fayette General. After the birth, your baby will receive extra special care while he or she continues to grow and develop," Laura said reassuringly.

Glory was still unnerved, and she asked about the possibility of disabilities like cerebral palsy, cystic fibrosis, spina bifida, and mental retardation, which were conditions that she had heard or read about or seen on television. Together, Laura and Brenda explained the unlikelihood of these conditions occurring, because she had told them she'd had routine checkups with her physician all through her pregnancy and was taking very good care of herself and the baby. As they talked, they helped ready Glory for the OR. Glory's father returned to the room and stood quietly off to one side as the nurses worked.

"But . . . but . . . what about Gil?" Glory said, and her eyes brimmed with tears. "What about Gil? Wait, we can't go. Gil has to be here! We planned this together. He wanted to be here. I want him here. Oh, please! I want him here. This is not the way it's supposed to be. Mama, Daddy, what about Gil?"

Reflective Questions

Reflect on the dialogue that you've just read as you answer these questions.

1. What is the medical term that is used to describe how Glory's uterus feels to the touch when the nurse and the obstetrician palpate it? ____________________
2. What is the status of this patient's placenta? Use the proper medical term.
____
3. What do the initials *OR* stand for in the context of this patient update? ____________________
4. Who books (reserves) the OR for the antepartum unit? ____________________
5. What type of procedure or surgery is Glory going to have? ____________________
6. What will be the result of that surgery? ____________________

Critical Thinking

Based on all that you've read and learned from this most recent patient update, think deeply about the situation and the patient before answering this question.

Does Mrs. Loeppky want to deliver her child today? Explain why or why not.

____

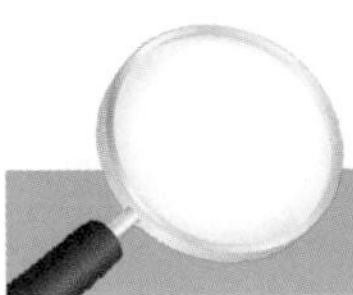

FOCUS POINT: The Abbreviation *UC*

Context is important when deciphering medical terminology. The abbreviation *UC* can mean *unit clerk,* but it can also mean *uterine contractions*!

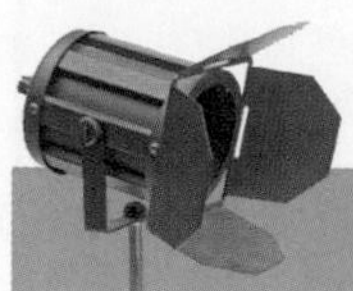

CAREER SPOTLIGHT: Unit Clerk

A *unit clerk (UC)* is an essential member of the treatment team in any hospital or medical facility, even though he or she is not—strictly speaking—a health-care professional. The UC is part of a medical facility's *support staff,* which supports the care staff and assists with the day-to-day operations of the unit, clinic, or medical department. The UC is often known as the *hub* or heart of the unit.

The UC's support role includes many responsibilities. For example, he or she is responsible for the maintenance of patient-care records. The UC also coordinates patient activities, such as diagnostic appointments and OR bookings. He or she requisitions and schedules services and supplies that directly relate to patient care. The UC is also responsible for communication in the workplace, including phone calls, call bells, paging, and the intercom. In addition, the UC prepares notices of patient discharge for administrative and billing purposes, directs visitors to patient rooms, and keeps a running census of patients who are housed in the facility or visiting the clinic. The UC must be skilled with regard to computer functions and the basics of information technology. Training involves the achievement of a certificate or diploma as a hospital UC, a medical UC, or a ward clerk. Learning medical terminology is part of that training.

Key terms: labor and delivery emergency

Explore the meaning of key terms used in this recent patient update:

"'*UC,*' she said."

UC: uterine contractions; the actions of the uterine muscles tightening and shortening.

"*. . . uterine pressure . . .*"

uterine pressure: pressure exerted onto the pelvis by the expanding uterus. When uterine contractions occur, they push or exert force on the fetus.

". . . uterus began to *relax a bit.*"

relax a bit: the action of the uterine muscle going into a relaxed state (i.e., not tight, cramped, or contracted).

". . . *vaginal bleeding* or the presence of *amniotic fluid.*"

vaginal bleeding: a type of bleeding that is not expected in a pregnant woman. During the first trimester, it may indicate miscarriage. Throughout the rest of the term, it can indicate placentae previa (i.e., the cervix or opening to the womb is blocked by the placenta, and some placental blood vessels may rupture) or abruptio placentae.

amniotic fluid: a fluid that gathers in the *amniotic sac* that surrounds the fetus, particularly by the second trimester. The fetus floats in this fluid, and he or she breathes and swallows it. The amniotic fluid provides a cushioning function, helps with the development of the lungs, prevents fetal heat loss, and allows for movement that enhances bone growth. The fetus excretes amniotic fluid in its urine. Amniotic fluid is released just before birth, when the amniotic sac bursts. This release of fluid is commonly referred to as "the water breaking."

". . . where it is separating from the *uterine wall.*"

uterine wall: the outer edge of the uterus that separates it from the other organs in the abdomen (i.e., bladder, rectum).

"... *internal bleeding* ..."

internal bleeding: bleeding that occurs within the body as a result of damage to an artery or vein. Internal bleeding generally cannot be seen. However, there are usually accompanying symptoms of fever. Intra-abdominal bleeding may cause pain, weakness, lightheadedness, and decreased blood pressure. (Recall that Glory seemed unsure about what was happening to her when she was discussing her abdominal pain; this could be because of the symptom of lightheadedness.)

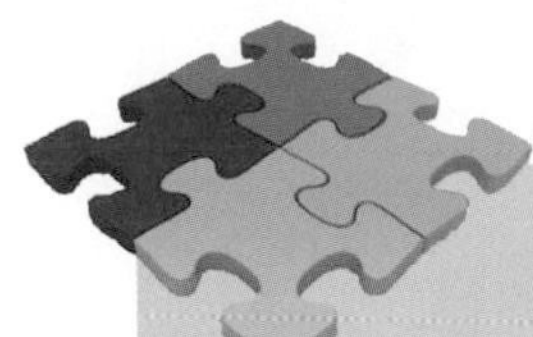

WORD BUILDING: Formula for Creating Words with the Combining Form *Amni/o*

amnion* = the innermost fetal membrane. The combining form is *amni/o.

amnio + genesis = *amniogenesis*
Definition: formation of the amnion. *noun*

Example: *Amniogenesis* occurs within the first weeks after the fertilization of the ovum.

amnio + rrhea = *amniorrhea*
Definition: flow of amniotic fluid. *noun*

Example: *Amniorrhea* normally occurs when a woman's "water breaks" as she is preparing to deliver a child.

amnio + centesis = *amniocentesis*
Definition: an assessment test of amniotic fluid obtained through abdominal puncture. (The word part *centesis* means *puncture.*) *noun*

Example: *Amniocentesis* is used to detect genetic and biochemical disorders, as well as to determine the compatibility of the maternal and fetal blood supplies.

TABLE 8-7: Possible Complications Related to Childbirth

Disease, Disorder, or Disability	Etiology [or Cause]	Symptoms or Results	Time of Onset
cerebral palsy	for preterm infants: bleeding while in utero or respiratory distress (insufficient or no oxygen at birth or shortly thereafter)	abnormality of motor function	higher risk in premature and low-birth-weight infants
cystic fibrosis	genetic a disease of the exocrine glands (see Chapter 8)	impaired respiration	genetic inheritance at conception
spina bifida (meningomyelocele)	a congenital malformation (birth defect)	part of the spinal cord is exposed (not protected by the vertebral column); involves learning disabilities, mobility impairments, and bowel and bladder incontinence	embryonic development during first trimester
mental retardation	may be caused at time of birth by lack of oxygen; may be caused during pregnancy by genetic influences, diseases, substance abuse, malnutrition, and other things	impaired cognitive and intellectual abilities: limited cognition, communication skills, self-care skills, and social skills	various trimesters and at birth

Continued

TABLE 8-7: Possible Complications Related to Childbirth—cont'd

Disease, Disorder, or Disability	Etiology [or Cause]	Symptoms or Results	Time of Onset
hydrocephalus	abnormal buildup of cerebrospinal fluid in the brain; may be caused by intraventricular hemorrhage in the ventricles of the brain; may be caused by infection, head injury, tumor, and other things	pressure on the brain causes brain damage; abnormally large head in infants; irritability, fatigue, and drowsiness	before birth or any time afterward
hypoxic-ischemic encephalopathy	result of a combination of brain hypoxia (lack of oxygen) and ischemia caused by reduced cerebral blood flow	neuronal damage, learning difficulties, developmental delay, cerebral palsy, and mental retardation	during the third trimester or at the time of full-term birth
severe neonatal encephalopathy	lack of oxygen at birth	seizures, coma, lethargy, respiratory problems, irritability, and jitters	second or third trimester

Let's Practice

Write the term or terms that best identify what is being described.

1. bleeding in the ventricles of the brain ____________________
2. abnormally large head of a newborn or infant ____________________
3. genetic condition that results in the impairment of respiratory function and ability ____________________
4. seizures, nervous behaviors, and respiratory problems are some of the symptoms of this condition ____________________
5. the actions of the uterine muscle contracting and expanding ____________________

Break It Down

Break down the following terms into their word parts, and then identify what each part means.

1. amniorrhexis ____________________ Meaning: ____________________
2. amnioscopy ____________________ Meaning: ____________________

Fill in the Blanks

Begin to use new terminology by choosing terms to complete the following sentences. By doing so, you will become more familiar with these terms in their proper context.

1. Lack of oxygen at birth can cause the conditions of ____________________, ____________________, and ____________________.
2. ____________________ is inherited from the genes of at least one of the parents.
3. The most prominent symptom of ____________________ is motor impairment.
4. A condition that can be diagnosed during the embryonic stage of human development is ____________________.
5. Another way to say "lack of oxygen" is to say "____________________."
6. Another way to say "an inadequate supply of blood" is to say "____________________."

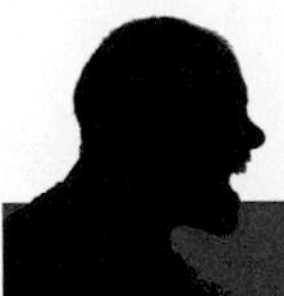

PRONUNCIATION PRACTICE

Say these words aloud to a friend or classmate if you can. You are given the phonetic pronunciation. Your instructor can help you with pronunciation,

or visit **http://www.MedicalLanguageLab.com.** 

abruptio	ă-**brŭp**´shē-ō	hypoxia	hī-**pŏks**´ē-ă
amnion	**ăm**´nē-ŭn	ischemia	ĭs-**kē**´mē-ă
cystic fibrosis	**sĭs**´tĭk fī-**brō**´sĭs	meningomyelocele	mĕ-nĭng″gō-**mī**´ĕ-lō-sēl″
encephalopathy	ĕn-sĕf″ă-**lŏp**´ă-thē	radiopaque	rā-dē-ō-**pāk**´
hydrocephalus	hī-drō-**sĕf**´-lŭs	spina bifida	**spī**´nă **bĭf**-ĭd-ă

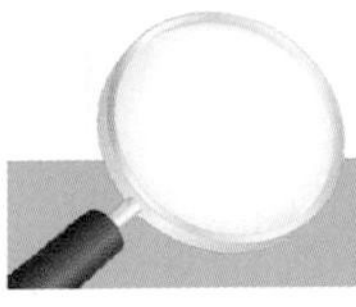

FOCUS POINT: The Umbilical Cord

The umbilical cord is a structure that connects the embryo—and, later, the fetus—to the placenta, thereby connecting it to the mother. The cord contains one large umbilical vein and two small arteries that spiral around the vein, thereby giving the umbilical cord its strength. Oxygen and nutrients are passed to the fetus through the vein, whereas waste products and deoxygenated blood are carried away from the fetus through the two arteries.

The umbilical cord also consists of stem cells. These are generic cells that can either become specialized cells in the body or that can remain unspecialized. Stem cells are responsible for the growth and development of the embryo and the fetus, and they also play an enormous role in the repair of damaged organs and tissues. Recently, umbilical cord stem cell research has opened up the possibility of replacing or regenerating damaged or diseased cells in the human body.

The language of Cesarean section

A **Cesarean section** is a surgical procedure in which the birth occurs through an abdominal and uterine incision. This is common practice in cases of placenta previa, placental abruption, problems with the umbilical cord, failure to progress during labor, active genital herpes, and other conditions that may make a vaginal birth problematic. Generally, an anesthetic and an analgesic (pain medication) are both given. Read the "On the Job: Surgical Report" on page 322 that describes Glory Loeppky's Cesarean section.

Fayette General Hospital
Surgical Report

Patient Name: GLORY LOEPPKY Hospital Admission # 2928

Unit:

Date of Surgery: JUNE XX, 2015 DOB: XX/XX/XXXX

Time: 1500 HRS

Time In: 1830 Time Out: 1920 Obstetrician: DR. R BEDARD

PATIENT TRANSFERRED TO OR FOR STAT C. SECTION FOR TRAUMATIC PLACENTAL ABRUPTION AT 30–32 WEEKS GESTATION. GENERAL ANESTHETIC PERFORMED BY DR. WONG. MATERNAL VITALS NORMAL. FETAL HEART RATE PRIOR TO C. SECTION 138 BPM. PATIENT POSITIONED IN SUPINE WITH LEFT LATERAL TILT. INDWELLING FOLEY CATHETER PLACED TO OPEN DRAINAGE. STERILE PREP AND DRAPE WITH LEFT LATERAL TILT. PFANNENSTIEL INCISION. ABDOMEN OPENED THROUGH LAYERS, UNCOMPLICATED ENTRY INTO PERITONEAL CAVITY. TRANSVERSE INCISION INTO THE LOWER UTERINE SEGMENT, EXTENDED MANUALLY. AMNIOTIC FLUID BLOODY. FEMALE INFANT DELIVERED VERTEX WITH EASY DELIVERY OF THE HEAD OUT OF THE PELVIS AND ATRAUMATIC DELIVERY OF HEAD, TRUNK, AND LIMBS. CORD CLAMPED AND SEPARATED, INFANT HANDED OVER TO PEDIATRICIAN FOR CARE. CORD GASES OBTAINED. PLACENTA DELIVERED BY CONTROLLED CORD TRACTION AND APPEARS COMPLETE. EVIDENCE OF ABRUPTION OF DISTAL THIRD OF PLACENTA.

Key terms: Cesarean section

"*. . . general anesthetic . . .*"

general anesthetic: an **anesthetic** is a drug that causes a lack of sensation or a lack of feeling. The root is **anesthesia,** meaning *a total or partial loss of the sensation of pain; causing numbness.* A general anesthetic causes a complete lack of consciousness; in other words, it "knocks the patient out." (See Chapter 3 for information about local anesthesia.)

"*. . . left lateral tilt . . .*"

left lateral tilt: a position in which the patient's right hip is slightly elevated on the operating table. For pregnant women, this position facilitates the maintenance of blood pressure and maternal-fetal blood gas exchanges.

"*Indwelling Foley catheter . . .*"

indwelling catheter: a urinary catheter inserted through the urinary meatus into the bladder (see Chapter 5).

Foley: A trade name of a thin, sterile urinary catheter.

"*Sterile prep* and *drape* . . ."

sterile prep: preparation of the patient for surgery with the use of disinfecting agents and the creation of a sterile environment or sterile field from which to work.

drape: A sterile sheet made of fabric or paper. Sterile drapes provide a sterile surface next to the patient. The sheets are draped onto the patient.

"*Pfannenstiel incision* . . ."

Pfannenstiel incision: an incision that transverses the lower abdomen, including the rectus abdominis muscle (see Chapter 3). The incision takes a semicircular shape just above the mons pubis.

". . . *extended manually* . . ."

extended manually: opened by hand.

". . . delivered *vertex* . . ."

vertex: the normal presentation for a fetus, with the head tucked down on the chest and the crown of the head facing the birth canal (vagina).

"*Cord clamped* and *separated* . . ."

cord clamped: the umbilical cord shared by the mother and baby is clamped off to stem the flow of blood through it.

cord separated: the umbilical cord is severed, and the newborn and mother have their first physical disconnect.

"*Cord gases* obtained."

cord gases: a blood test performed on specimens that are taken from the umbilical cord. This test helps to identify the newborn's pH balance and also detects neurological complications and hypoxia at birth. **Hypoxia** means *lack of oxygen.* Any prolonged length of time (measured in seconds and minutes) that the fetus or newborn is deprived of oxygen can result in brain damage.

". . . *controlled cord traction* and *appears complete* . . ."

controlled cord traction: the placenta (including the umbilical cord) is removed from the mother through a controlled procedure. This is particularly so in the case of a Cesarean section, when the procedure is performed manually. However, there is less chance of infection occurring when the woman is given oxytocin (see Chapter 7) and when external massage of the abdomen is used to ease the removal of the placenta. This combination causes the placenta to detach, and the placenta is then pulled from the womb with the help of gentle traction being placed on the umbilical cord.

appears complete: medical jargon to indicate in a chart that the procedure was completed. It is necessary to record this.

Eponyms: Cesarean Section

Experts disagree about the origin of the term *Cesarean section.* Some say it derives from the fact that Roman emperor Gaius Julius Caesar was delivered surgically, whereas others say that it derives from the Latin word *caesus,* which is the past participle of *caedere,* meaning *to cut.* Another possible origin of the term stems from the old Roman law known as *Lex Caesarea,* which permitted a baby to be cut out of a mother's womb if she were to die before the child was born. Gaius Julius Caesar was born in 100 BC and died in 44 BC. It is undetermined if Lex Caesarea became law before or after his birth. His mother did not die during childbirth.

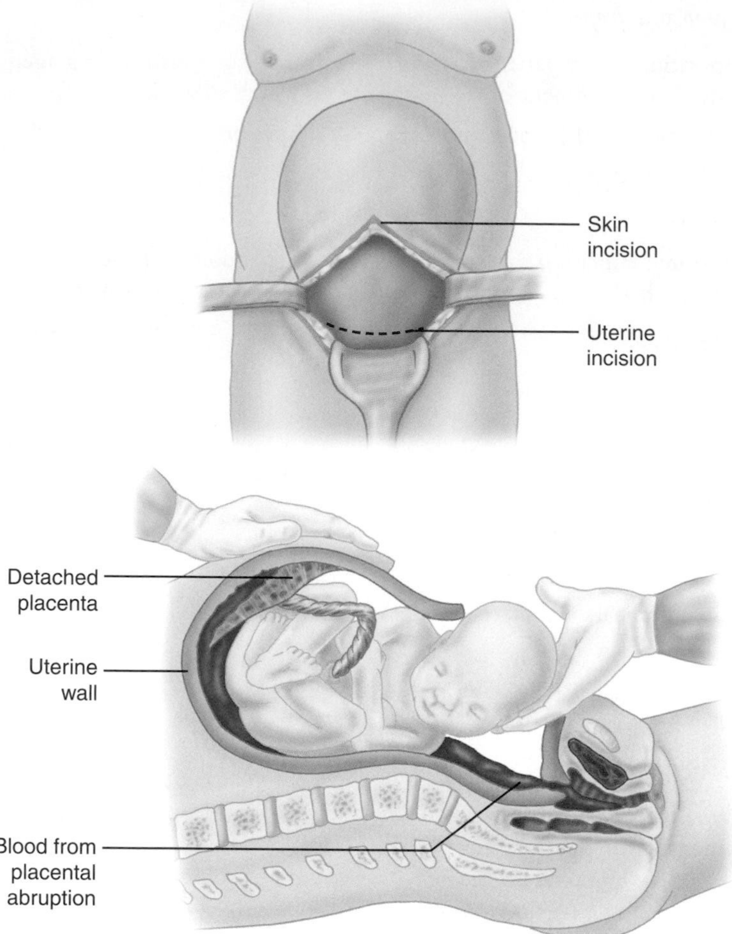

Figure 8.13: Emergency Cesarean section with placental abruption

TABLE 8-8: Medical Terms for Birth

Original Medical Term	Modern English Term	Meaning
natus	natal	pertaining to birth or day of birth
natalis	natality	birth rate per a specific population
nascens	nascent	just born; born

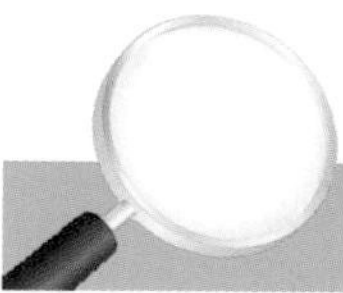

FOCUS POINT: Natal

Be very careful about using medical language in context. For example, the word *natal* has been used in this chapter to mean *pertaining to birth.* However, the term *natal* can also mean *pertaining to the buttocks.* In that context, it derives from the root *nates,* meaning *buttocks.*

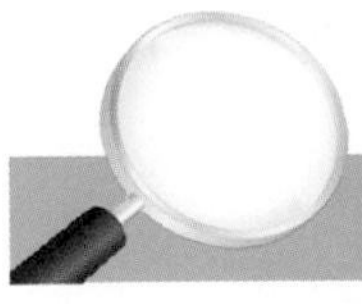

FOCUS POINT: Natimortality

If you are working in a research hospital or a facility that is interested in birth rates, the term *natimortality* will be common. This is a measure of the rate of stillbirths as compared with live births for a given population. This information is helpful for planning, prevention, and health promotion in both maternal and child health care. This medical term breaks down as follows: *nati* (a combining form of *natal*) + *mortality* (a word meaning *death.* The root of this word is *mort*. The second part, *-ality,* is a combination of two suffixes *-al* and *-ity*, both meaning pertaining to.).

The language of postnatal recovery

After the infant is born, the period of *postnatal recovery* occurs. The nurse completes an Apgar score (see page 328) and a full head-to-toe assessment of the baby. An infant identification band is placed on both the baby and the mother (as well as on the father, a significant other, or an identified person of support). Whenever possible, the infant is presented to the mother on her chest for bonding. Nurses evaluate and care for the mother postpartum until she is recovered sufficiently to be left on her own for increasing periods from 15 minutes to 2 hours and more.

In the case of a preterm baby such as Mrs. Loeppky's, the infant will be cared for, evaluated, and quickly placed in an incubator to keep him or her warm and secure. Although it may not be possible for the baby to be placed in the mother's arms or on her chest, the nurses will show the mother her baby, and, if at all possible, let her touch it, even momentarily. They will also give a complete running report to the mother while they are cleaning and evaluating the baby to give the mother a sense of connectedness and participation. In a day or so, the parents may very well be able to hold their baby. If this is still not possible, they will be able to reach into the incubator to stroke their child.

TABLE 8-9: Prefixes Related to Birth

BEGIN with a Prefix	ADD a Root or Combining Form	CREATE a New Term	Meaning
ante-	partal	antepartal	before birth
pre-	natal	prenatal	before birth
intra-	partal	intrapartal	during birth
post-	natal	postnatal	occurring after birth
post-	partum	postpartum	occurring after birth
post-	partal	postpartal	just after birth
neo-	natal	neonatal	newly born; beginning

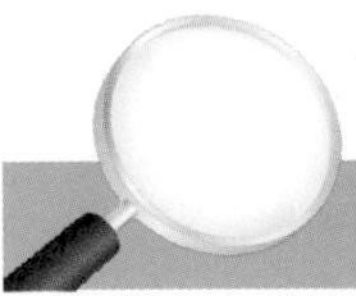

FOCUS POINT: Incubator

An *incubator* is an apparatus that is designed to provide a safe, secure, health- and growth-promoting environment for newborns with special needs. Many premature babies face the challenge of maintaining body heat: they cannot *thermoregulate* (regulate their body temperature) or produce enough heat from the energy that their bodies receive. Heat loss is a great concern. An incubator provides a neutral thermal environment in which the baby is not stressed by changes in temperature. Incubators are made of transparent plastic, and they surround the infant. The incubator also protects the infant from infection. Incubators have *ports,* areas in which the family and care team can insert their hands to fondle the baby and care for him or her. As the baby stabilizes, short times outside of the incubator may be permitted for more human contact, which is also essential for the infant's well-being and survival.

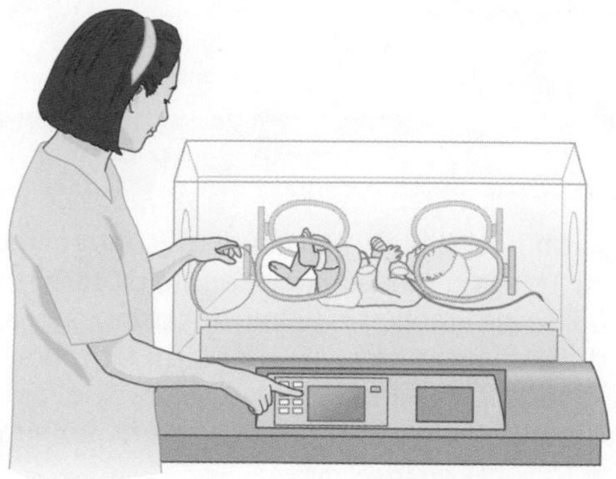

Figure 8.14: Incubator

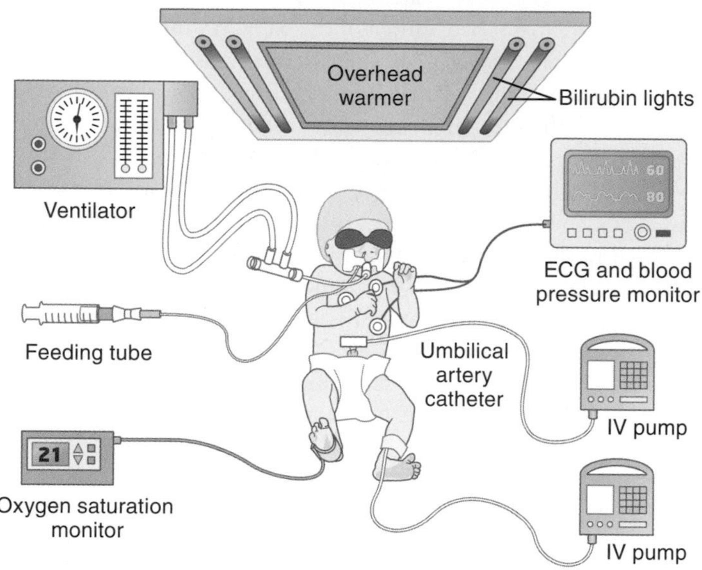

Figure 8.15: Equipment and devices used in an incubator

Right Word or Wrong Word: *Postpartal* or *Postpartum*?

Are these two words synonymous? Are they interchangeable?

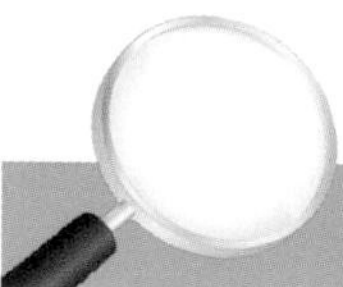

FOCUS POINT: *Baby, Neonate, Newborn,* and *Infant*

These terms can be used interchangeably when referring to the newborn.

Patient Update

Baby Emily Grace Loeppky was born to Glory and Gil Loeppky at 1900 hours, with her maternal grandparents in attendance. She was delivered preterm, which means that she was born at less than 36 or 37 weeks' gestation. The pediatrician assisting with surgery was Dr. Jasper. He determined that the infant had a gestational age of 31 weeks.

Emily Grace is healthy and stable. However, as a preemie (a preterm baby), her body systems are not fully developed. For example, she is at particular risk for respiratory problems because her lungs are not fully mature.

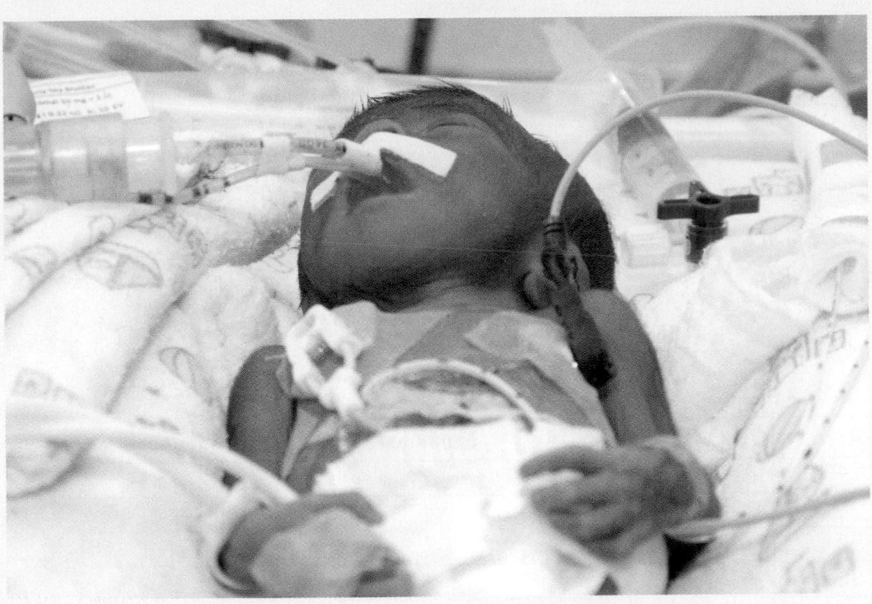

Fayette General Hospital
Pediatric Report of Birth

Patient Name: Glory Loeppky
Hospital Admission # 2928
Unit: AnTeparTum

Date of Delivery: June XX, 2015
Pediatrician: Dr. F. Jasper

Time of Delivery: 1900 hr
Anesthetist: Dr. A. Wong

Newborn: Sex ✓ Female ___ Male
Obstetrician: Dr. R. Bedard

Weight: 3 lb, 6 oz

Female infanT delivered aT 1900 hr by STAT C. secTion for placenTal abrupTion. IniTial resusciTaTion and assessmenT compleTed, sucTioned for bloody fluid, sponTaneous respiraTory efforT noTed by 1 minuTe. PosiTive pressure venTilaTion x 3 minuTe. APGAR scores of 4, 6, and 7. Transferred To special care nursery for observaTion.

APGAR Score

APGAR	1 minute	5 minutes	10 minutes
Heart Rate	2 (1006 pm)	2	2
Resp. Effort	1	1	1
Muscle Tone	1	1	1
Response to Stim	0	1	2
Color	0	1	1
Score:	4	6	7

The Apgar score

Study the "On the Job: Pediatric Report of Birth" (shown above) for Glory Loeppky's newborn, Emily Grace. At the bottom of the form, you will see a section labeled "Apgar Score." The **Apgar test** is a screening tool that is used to determine whether or not a newborn (NB) requires medical attention to stabilize his or her heart and his or her breathing functions.

Apgar scores are determined using values of 0, 1, or 2 for five specific criteria: heart rate, respiratory effort, muscle tone, skin color, and response to stimuli. Scores of less than 8 indicate that the neonate needs assistance and cannot function on his or her own. A baby with a complete set of scores that show low scores at the first reading at 1 minute after birth but with a normal score at 5 minutes after birth should not expect any long-term health problems.

Healthy normal scores are determined as follows:

Heart rate: >100 beats per minute

Respiratory rate: the newborn cries well

Muscle tone: active motion by newborn

Response to stimulation/grimace response: infant grimaces, coughs, sneezes, or cries vigorously in response to an irritant; this is a measure called **reflex irritability**

Color: skin color is entirely pink

Eponyms: Apgar Score

Virginia Apgar was an American anesthesiologist (1909-1974). She received a number of honors and awards for her work with anesthesiology, children, and public health. Through her long years of work in obstetric anesthesiology and her concern for neonatal status at birth, she developed a scoring system to assess neonatal health, which soon became known as the Apgar score. In 1994, Apgar was pictured on a U.S. postage stamp as part of the Great American series, and, in 1995, she was posthumously inducted into the National Women's Hall of Fame in New York.

Key terms: pediatric report of birth

Notice the language in the "On the Job: Pediatric Report of Birth" on page 328. It is full of medical jargon rather than strict and formal medical terminology. This is quite common.

"... *STAT C section* ..."

STAT C section: immediate Cesarean section.

"... initial *resuscitation* ..."

resuscitation: process of reviving or bringing to life by providing air.

"... *suctioned for bloody fluid* ..."

suctioned for bloody fluid: the neonate's nose and mouth are suctioned with the use of a hand-held device to clear the airways of bloody fluid from birth and to promote independent breathing.

"... spontaneous *respiratory effort* ..."

respiratory effort: breathing effort. For the Apgar score, this is scored as follows: 0 = not breathing, 1 = breaths are slow or irregular, or 2 = the baby cries and breathes well.

"... *positive pressure ventilation* ..."

positive pressure: forcing air into the lungs.

ventilation: circulation and supply of air.

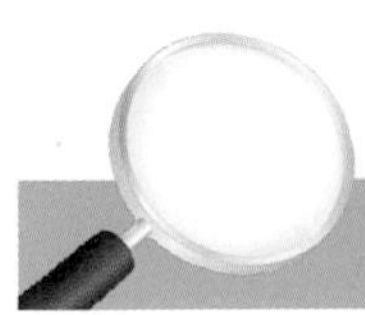

FOCUS POINT: Assessment of Color

Do not be confused about what is meant by *assessment of color* for a newborn. This term refers only to the infant's cardiopulmonary functioning: circulation and oxygenation. It has *no* association with race or ethnicity. All skin types will "pink up" when they are properly oxygenated and when good circulation is present.

The language of birth weights

Newborns are often weighed using the grams or kilograms of the metric system rather than ounces or pounds. This may depend on the standards of measurement used in a particular place of work. Metric conversions that apply to birth weights include the following:

1 ounce = 28 grams

1 pound = 454 grams

1000 grams = 1 kilogram

1 kilogram = 2.2 pounds

Some newborns may be identified as being of *low birth weight (LBW),* but this determination must be made within the context of the baby's ethnicity, because some groups of people have lower weights and smaller overall statures in general as compared with others. It is important to consider ethnicity before concluding that a newborn is less than normal with regard to weight or height.

A healthy birth weight is a significant factor for decreasing the risks of complications after birth, for both premature and full-term babies. For example, even though Emily Grace Loeppky was born prematurely, her birth weight of 3 pounds and 6 ounces is high enough to help her immensely as she continues her development over the next month.

TABLE 8-10: Weights for Full-term and Preterm Newborns

Age of Newborn	Weight in Kilograms (kg) and Pounds (lbs)	Weight in Grams (gm)
full term	2.041 to 3.2 kg 4.5 to 7 lbs	2041 to 3200 gm
preterm (30 to 32 weeks' gestation)	0.9 kg to 1.81 kg 2 to 4 lbs	900 to 1810 gm
preterm (<29 weeks' gestation)	<1 kg <2.2 lbs	<1000 gm

Critical Thinking

Review Emily Grace Loeppky's Apgar scores on the "On the Job: Pediatric Report of Birth" (see page 328), and answer the following questions.

1. Which indicators of the Apgar score identified the fact that Emily Grace needed immediate assistance after her birth? ______________________
2. Based solely on her Apgar score at birth, what is the likelihood that this baby will have any long-term health problems? Explain.
____
3. Convert Emily Grace's birth weight of 3 lbs, 6 oz to kilograms.
____
4. Emily Grace Loeppky has a gestational age of 31 weeks. What is the gestational age in weeks of a full-term baby? ______________________

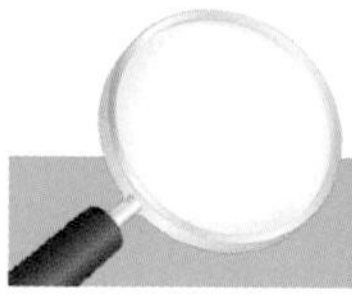

FOCUS POINT: Premature and Prematurity

In the context of obstetrics and maternal care, the terms *premature* and *prematurity* refer to any infant who is born before the 37th week of gestation.

Potential complications for preterm newborns born at less than 37 weeks' gestation

As noted previously, preterm newborns are at risk for a number of health challenges, particularly related to the immaturity of their body systems. The third trimester of pregnancy is almost solely focused on the final growth and development of a fetus to promote its viability (the ability to sustain life on its own).

Digestive system complications

Nutrition and growth are the major focus of the third trimester of pregnancy. After they are born, preterm babies grow at a faster rate than full-term babies, but their digestive systems are still immature. As a result, they may have difficulties with digestion, sucking, and swallowing.

To resolve these issues, preemies are often fed through **gavage:** nutrients are administered either through **nasogastric** (nose to stomach) or **orogastric** (mouth to stomach) tubes. Because breast milk is the healthiest form of nutrition for these babies and because it provides a number of essential antibodies to strengthen the infant's immune system, it can be fed to the baby by gavage. Breastfeeding, however, is not entirely ruled out. By 32 to 34 weeks' gestation, the preterm baby can usually suck from a breast or a bottle.

Respiratory system complications

Respiratory distress syndrome (RDS) is one of the most common problems that affects preterm infants, and its onset can be immediate and life threatening. During respiratory distress, the lungs suddenly stop functioning. RDS occurs when the lungs lack the ability to produce a substance called **surfactant**. This substance is needed to allow the lungs to expand properly after birth. To prevent this respiratory complication, most pregnant women are given medication just before delivery to speed the production of surfactant in the baby's lungs, and surfactant is often given to the baby directly after birth as well. Surfactant-deficient babies who cannot be treated in this manner will require *ventilation or continuous positive airway pressure (CPAP)* until they mature sufficiently to breathe on their own. Setting the pressure level of these airway-assisting devices helps to keep the premature lungs open so that the infant can breathe.

Ventilation, in a medical context, means the use of a ventilator machine that pumps continuous oxygenated air for a patient who cannot breathe on his or her own. In an incubator, ventilation may be accomplished with the use of an endotracheal tube inserted into the lungs. Oxygen will be given via positive pressure at a rate deemed appropriate by the physician.

A **continuous positive airway pressure (CPAP)** machine blows oxygenated air into the patient at a prescribed pressure through nasal prongs. It is increasingly becoming the preferred medical intervention for premature babies.

Bronchopulmonary dysplasia (BPND) is a chronic lung disease that is caused by injury to the immature lungs. It is more common in very premature babies (i.e., 24 to 26 weeks' gestation and weighing less than 2.2 pounds). Medication and oxygen are used to treat this condition, although there is some debate in medical circles about whether it is the ventilation process itself that might cause the injury.

Neurological system complications

Neurological problems—including difficulty achieving basic motor skills such as grimacing, smiling, and moving the head, arms, and legs—may be an issue for a premature baby. Variation in muscle tone is another possible complication. This complication is the result of immature muscle development, as well as of the immaturity of the coordination centers of the brain and the neuropathways that elicit motor movement. Cerebral palsy (see Table 8-7) is one example of motor and muscle tone complications that can occur.

Muscle tone refers to the amount of tension or resistance present in a muscle at any given time. **Muscle tension** is the continuous partial contraction of a muscle (i.e., when the arm is naturally bent at the elbow).

Apnea of prematurity is yet another common problem for preterm babies. The term **apnea** means *without breath;* it is a brief pause in breathing. However, *apnea of prematurity* is not a respiratory complication; it is the result of neurological immaturity, particularly in the medulla oblongata of the brainstem (see Chapter 4). Apnea spells are more frequent among premature babies who are born before 30 weeks' gestation. As the infant ages, the frequency of these spells decreases. The condition is not generally life threatening.

Arterial ischemic stroke is a rare event, and it is most often seen in premature babies who are born before 31 weeks' gestation. However, it is possible in all premature infants. The stroke and the arterial bleeding occur in the brain. This complication is life threatening, and it can also lead to brain damage.

Cardiovascular system complications

Anemia of prematurity occurs because the premature neonate lacks the appropriate number of red blood cells necessary to carry adequate oxygen to the body. The potential for anemia is monitored through blood tests.

Patent ductus arteriosus (PDA) is a condition in which a short blood vessel that connects the main blood vessels that support the lungs and the aorta has not closed during fetal development. This condition can lead to heart failure. It is **congenital**, which means that it is present at birth, and it may require surgery to correct, although it can also be treated with ibuprofen (see Chapter 7) and indomethacin (a similar drug) to close the ductus arteriosus.

Intraventricular hemorrhage (IVH) is an acute, critical event. In this situation, a blood vessel in the brain bursts and floods the ventricles of the brain, which normally house cerebral spinal fluid, as well as the surrounding tissues. Ultrasound during pregnancy and CT of the infant at birth can detect this problem before the hemorrhage occurs. Uncontrolled hemorrhage can lead to hydrocephalus (see Table 8-7), developmental delay, and brain damage. This condition is rare among full-term babies.

Visual complications

Retinopathy of prematurity (ROP) is also known as *retrolental fibroplasia.* This is a condition in which the eyes of premature infants are vulnerable to injury after birth. It is more prevalent among preterm newborns who are born at less than 30 weeks' gestation or weighing less than 2.76 pounds (1250 grams). It is the result of the incomplete or abnormal growth of the blood vessels in the fetus's or newborn's eyes, particularly those blood vessels that feed the **retina,** the organ in the back of the eye that senses light and sends impulses to the brain that enable us to see. Symptoms of ROP can include crossed eyes, abnormal eye movements, and severe nearsightedness. Premature babies receive eye examinations in the neonatal intensive care unit. The prognosis for a baby with ROP can vary widely, from no long-term visual problems to mild visual problems (i.e., nearsightedness and the need for glasses) to, in extreme cases, blindness.

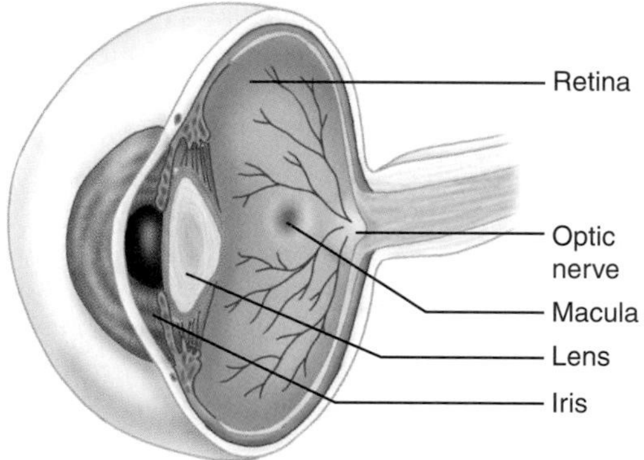

Figure 8.16: Anatomy of the eye

Critical Thinking

Demonstrate your comprehension of medical terminology. Review the section of this chapter entitled "Potential Complications for Preterm Newborns Born at Less Than 37 Weeks' Gestation," and apply what you've read to little Emily Grace Loeppky, who was born at 31 weeks' gestation.

1. Which medical term describes the potential for the development of a vision problem? __________
2. What is the likelihood or level of risk regarding whether or not Emily Grace will develop vision problems? __________
3. From the reading about patent ductus arteriosus, consider the terms *ductus* and *arteriosus.* To what do these terms refer? __________

Let's Practice

The following medical abbreviations apply to possible complications of premature birth. Write the meaning of each abbreviation.

1. BPND ______________________________
2. ROP ______________________________
3. RDS ______________________________
4. IVH ______________________________
5. PDA ______________________________

Break It Down

Break down the following terms into their word parts, and then write the meaning of each term.

1. retinopathy ____________ Meaning: ____________
2. hypoxia ____________ Meaning: ____________
3. prematurity ____________ Meaning: ____________
4. intrapartal ____________ Meaning: ____________

Right Word or Wrong Word: *Neonate* or *Preemie*?

Are all preemies neonates? Are all neonates preemies (preterm babies)?

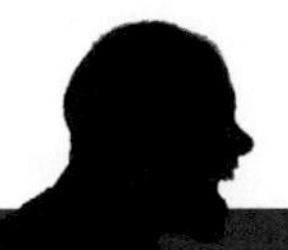

PRONUNCIATION PRACTICE

Say these words aloud to a friend or classmate if you can. You are given the phonetic pronunciation. Your instructor can help you with pronunciation,

or visit **http://www.MedicalLanguageLab.com.** 

anesthetic	ăn″ĕs-**thĕt**′ ĭk	neonate	**nē**′ō- nāt
Apgar	**ăp**′ găr	postpartal	pōst-**păr**′ tăl
apnea	**ăp**-nē′ă	patent	**păt**′ĕnt or **pā**′tĕnt
bronchopulmonary	brŏng″kō- **pŭl**′ mō-nă-rē	Pfannenstiel	**făn**′ĕn-stēl
dysplasia	dĭs-**plā**′ zē-ă	retinopathy	rĕt″ĭn-**ŏp**′ă-thē
incubator	**ĭn**′kū-bā″tŏr	umbilical	ĭm-**bĭl**′ ĭ-kăl
natimortality	nā″tĭ-mor-**tăl**′ ĭ-tē		

Patient Update

Glory Loeppky is resting comfortably in her room at Fayette General. She is 4 hours postpartal. Her parents have gone off to watch the baby through the nursery room window. Glory continues to have an IV in situ, but it is on the dorsal surface of her right hand. Her left hand remains in a spica cast.

She and her parents have met with Dr. Bedard and Dr. Jasper to discuss baby Emily's health status and prognosis. Her prognosis is good. Glory has been reassured that, with the advent of many recent advances in neonatal care, more than 90% of premature babies in the United States who weigh 800 grams or more survive. The doctors reminded her that her baby weighed much more, coming in at a healthy 3.6 pounds, or 1632 grams. Glory was also keen to learn that, although her baby remains at risk for respiratory problems because she is premature, the injection of surfactant that Glory was given prior to birth has likely lessened Emily's risk considerably.

Even so, the baby will stay in the neonatal intensive care unit for some time, probably a month or more. Glory waxes and wanes between disappointment over not being able to take her baby home and relief that Emily is healthy and well taken care of. In 20 minutes, Glory will be assisted into a wheelchair, and her parents and the nurse on duty will accompany her down the short hallway to see her baby again. When she thinks of the joy that she experienced when she was able to touch Emily's little hand after delivery, she starts to cry. She then hears footsteps in the corridor, and moments later her mother pops her head into the room.

"Glory, honey," her mother begins, "your dad and I have a surprise for you." She is smiling broadly. Glory's father peeks around the corner and then comes into the room with one hand behind his back. Glory smiles, thinking that he's bought the baby her first teddy bear. Her father stops near the bedside and smiles. From behind his back, he pulls out a cell phone. "Honey," he says, "it's for you." She looks at her father, not clearly understanding, but she takes the phone. Her parents step quietly out into the hallway.

"Hello?" Glory says softly. Then she gasps and begins to cry.

"Hello, sweetheart, it's Gil," says a soft, masculine voice at the other end of the line.

"Gil, Gil! Oh my God, Gil, where are you? Are you okay? Oh, Gil, we had the baby! Gil, she's beautiful. But honey, where are you? What's happened? Are you okay?" Glory's questions come rapidly through her tears of joy and relief.

"Listen, Glory," comes Gil's reply. "I'm not so good, but I'll be okay. I broke some bones and banged my head, but I should be okay. I'm over here at Okla Trauma Center. I'll have to stay here for a week, I think. I need an operation on my hip." Gil's voice is hoarse, and he hesitates sometimes as he speaks. "Honey . . . Glory . . . are you there?" There is silence on the other end of the line as his wife processes the information.

"Yes, yes, Gil, I'm here. I'm so sorry to hear about what's happened to you. Gil, oh, I love you so much! I want to be with you there," Glory says through tears.

"Honey, tell me about the baby, about our baby," Gil says, distracting her from the topic of himself. She tells him about how tiny but how beautiful Emily is and how much she knows he will love her the minute he lays eyes on her. She can hear his happiness and pride as he makes short affirming comments while she talks. Glory can't keep the tears from her eyes or the smile from her lips.

"Are you okay, Glory?" Gil asks finally. She explains her own injuries then. "Gil, I have to stay here another day or two, and then I'm coming to see you immediately." She pauses, as if thinking. "I can't bring Emily, though. She has to stay here for a few weeks."

"I know, honey, it's all right. As soon as I'm well enough, I'll come to see her myself," he says reassuringly. "Meanwhile, can you send me some pictures on your cell phone? I'd love that!"

"Oh, yes, yes, I can do that!" says Glory. "That's a great idea! I'll do it soon. I'm going to see our baby again in just a few minutes. She's in an incubator, you know, but I can reach in and touch her a bit right now. It's so wonderful!" They decide to end the call then so that she can prepare for her visit with the baby and so that he can rest. Glory hangs up, lies back on the pillow, looks up at the ceiling, and sighs happily.

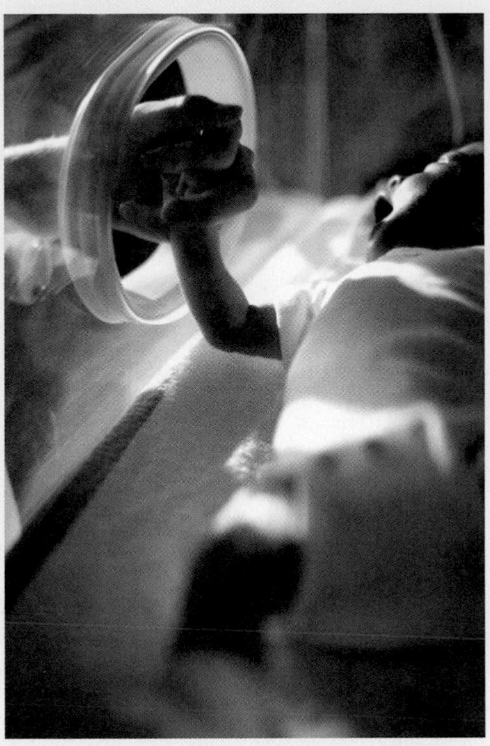

CHAPTER SUMMARY

Chapter 8 has introduced many new terms related to the female reproductive system, obstetrics, labor, and delivery as it followed our patient, Glory Loeppky, through the delivery of her child. It introduced the terminology for Cesarean section and provided some new surgical terms. In the context of premature birth, vocabulary for potential complications of birth and the assessment of newborns was provided. The careers of unit clerk and medical social worker were explored.

See How Much You've Learned

For audio exercises, visit **http://www.MedicalLanguageLab.com.** 

Chapter 8 also introduced many new abbreviations. A number of them appear again here in a concise table to promote study.

TABLE 8-11: Abbreviations in Chapter 8

Abbreviation	Meaning	Abbreviation	Meaning
ABO	antibody screen	lb(s)	pound(s)
BSW	bachelor of social work (degree)	mg	milligram
BPD	bronchopulmonary dysplasia	NB	newborn
CPAP	continuous positive airway pressure	oz	ounce
dL	deciliter	PIH	pregnancy-induced hypertension
FHR	fetal heart rate	RDS	respiratory distress syndrome
gm	gram	SW	social worker
kg	kilogram	UC	uterine contractions or unit clerk

Key Terms

ABO
accelerations (accels)
amniotic fluid
anemia of prematurity
anesthesia
anesthetic
antepartum
antepartum unit
antibodies
antigens
Apgar test
apnea
apnea of prematurity
arterial ischemic stroke
Bartholin's glands
baseline/baselines
birth
bronchopulmonary dysplasia (BPND)
call bell
cervix
Cesarean section
congenital
continuous positive airway pressure (CPAP)
controlled cord traction
cord gases
decelerations (decels)
delivery
drape
fetal attitude
fetal heart monitor (FHM)
fetal position
fetal presentation
fetus
gavage
general anesthetic
genitalia
gestation
gravid
gravida
hematoma
hypertension of pregnancy (pre-eclampsia)
hypothalamus
hypoxia
indwelling catheter
internal bleeding
intraventricular hemorrhage (IVH)
ketones
labor
left lateral tilt
Leopold's maneuvers
maternal health
maternity
mg/dL
mm^3 (μL)
muscle tension
muscle tone
nasogastric
nonstress test (NST)
nullipara
orogastric
patent ductus arteriousus (PDA)
perineum
Pfannenstiel incision
placenta
placental abruption
positive pressure
pregnancy-induced hypertension (PIH)
primagravida
proteins
reflex irritability
respiratory distress syndrome (RDS)
respiratory effort
resuscitation
retina
retinopathy of prematurity (ROP)
Rh
Rh factor
sterile prep
surfactant
UC
urine dip
uterine activity
uterine pressure
uterine wall
uterus
vaginal bleeding
vaginal discharge
variability
ventilation
vertex
vulva

CHAPTER REVIEW

Critical Thinking

Reread the "Career Spotlight" feature about social workers at the beginning of this chapter. In your own health-care career, you may find yourself working with an at-risk or vulnerable population. With that in mind, answer the following questions by thinking deeply about the people who are helped by social workers.

1. What does the term *at risk* mean in the context of what you've read about social workers?

____

2. What does the term *vulnerable population* mean?

____

Label the Diagram

Write the names of the organs in the female reproductive system on the blank lines provided here with the diagram.

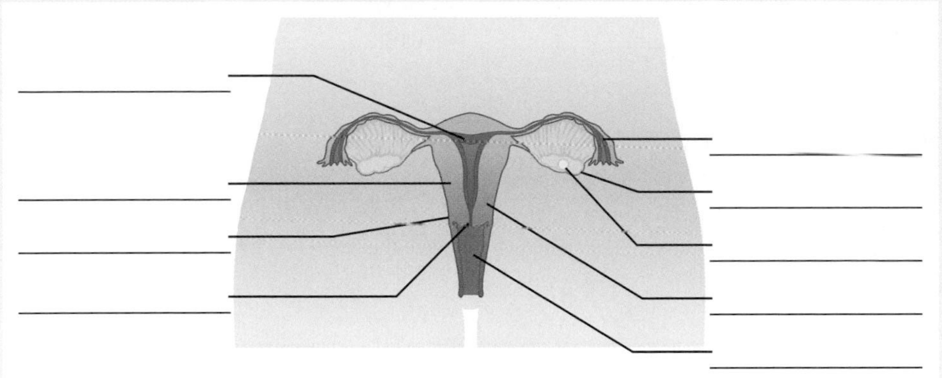

Name the Term

Write the term that names each part of the reproductive system that is described below.

1. external area of the lower part of the abdomen, where the genitalia, anus, and rectum are located ______________________________
2. a term that refers to the reproductive organs and structures on the outside of the body ______________________________
3. a hollow muscular organ located within the abdomen ______________________________
4. the narrow passage that leads from the uterus into the vagina ______________________________

Critical Thinking

Consider all that you have learned about the antepartum unit. In some hospitals, this 21st-century term may not yet be in use. What other names might be used for a unit on which pregnant women and postpartum women may be admitted and cared for? (Hint: All of these terms have appeared in this chapter.)

____

True or False?

Answer the following by writing either *true* or *false.*

1. The assessment of color in a neonate is done to identify the racial origins of the child. ______
2. A Cesarean section is a type of surgical operation. ________
3. The term *gavage* is an adaptation of a French term meaning *garbage or debris.* ________
4. Apnea of prematurity is a respiratory condition. ________

Right Word or Wrong Word: *Premature* or *Preterm*?

What is the difference, if any, between the terms *premature* and *preterm* in the context of pregnancy and delivery?

Break It Down

Break down the following terms into their word parts, and then write the meaning of each part.

1. orogastric ______________________ Meaning: ______________________
2. nasogastric ______________________ Meaning: ______________________
3. antepartal ______________________ Meaning: ______________________

Prefixes

Write the meaning of each prefix.

1. nulli- ______________________
2. ante- ______________________
3. intra- ______________________
4. post- ______________________
5. neo- ______________________

True or False?

Review the "Career Spotlight" features in this chapter, and then read each statement about the career fields of social work and unit clerk. Write *true* or *false* to describe each statement.

1. Social workers only work with poor children and families. ____________
2. Medical social workers are medically trained and can only work in hospitals. ____________
3. A unit clerk counts units and inventory only. ____________
4. Unit clerks study medical terminology. ____________
5. A hospital unit clerk is an essential part of the health care team who supports the team's work and patient care. ____________

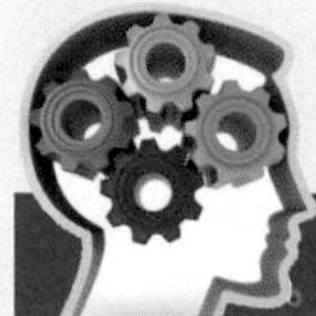

MEMORY MAGIC

You may find the following memory tips helpful:

Here is a mnemonic that identifies possible reasons for early cord clamping: RAPID CS

R = Rh incompatibility
A = asphyxia (fetus is unable to obtain oxygen)
P = premature delivery
I = infections
D = diabetic mother
CS = Cesarean section has been done previously

Here is another mnemonic for remembering components of the Apgar score: SHIRT

S = skin color (pink or blue)
H = heart rate (below or above 100 beats per minute)
I = irritability of newborn (grimace, cry, or none)
R = respirations (good or irregular)
T = tone of muscles (some flexion or activity)

CHAPTER NINE

Medical Records, Test Results, and Referrals

Focus: Male Reproductive System and Respiratory System

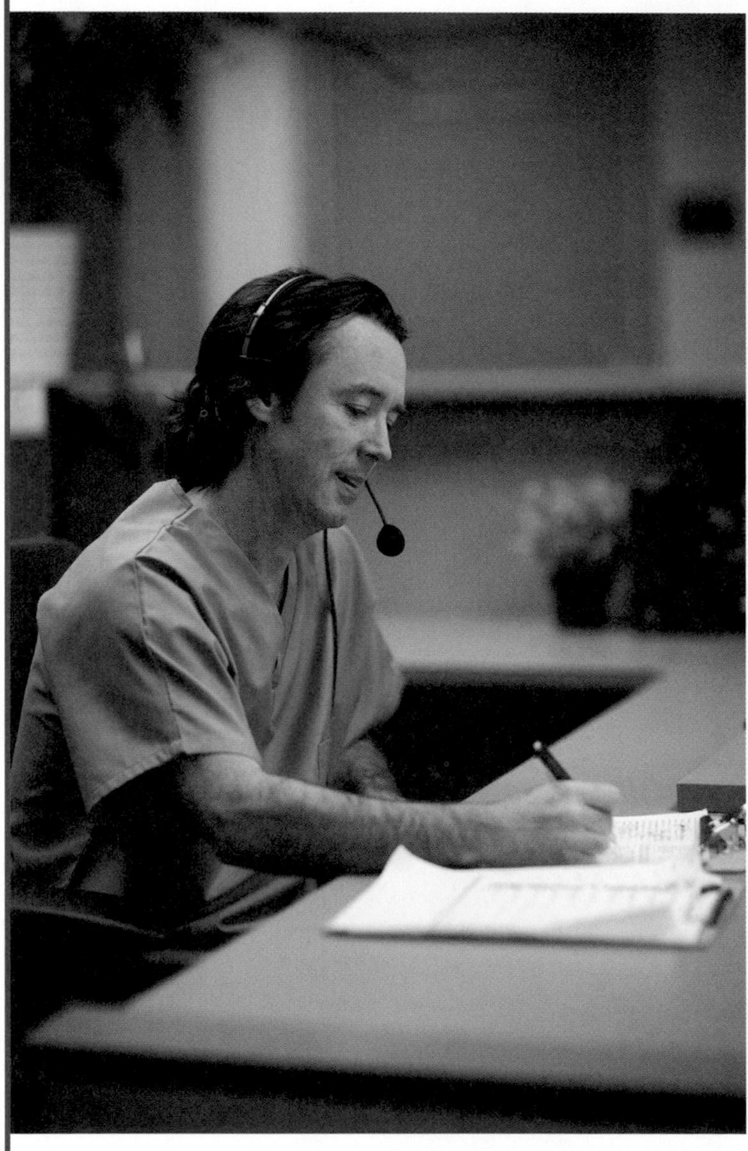

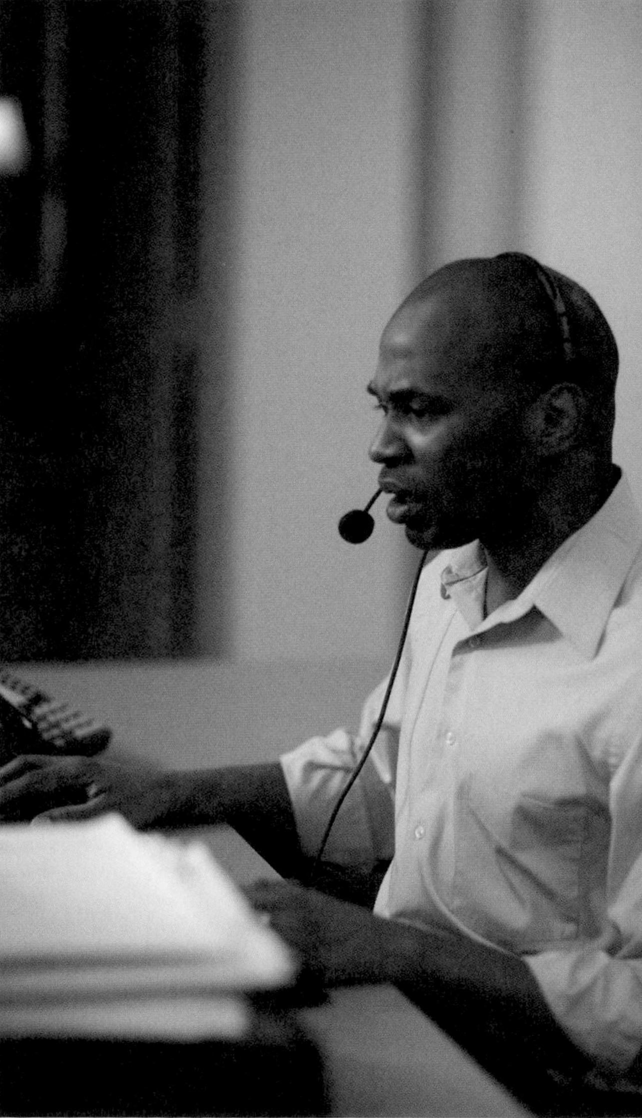

In Chapter 5, our patient, 74-year-old Zane Davis, presented as confused in the ER at Okla Trauma Center. He was rushed there by Rescue Unit 155 from the scene of a motor vehicle accident; it remains unclear if he was the driver of one of the vehicles. Mr. Davis did not appear to sustain any overt traumatic injury; however, he was transported to Okla Trauma on suspicion that he may have been having a cerebrovascular accident (CVA). In the ER, he was triaged, and the physician explored the possibility that the patient had just had one or more transient ischemic attacks (TIAs). The treatment team members were concerned that Mr. Davis's suspected TIA could be the precursor to a CVA, and there was even some speculation that he may have had a CVA en route to the hospital. Mr. Davis was given a computed tomography (CT) scan to determine this. The results confirmed that the patient had coronary artery disease (CAD), but they did not reveal any blockages or ruptures of blood vessels. Mr. Davis was also referred to a cardiologist and given further testing to completely rule out the possibility that he had experienced a stroke. At the time of his arrival at Okla Trauma, Mr. Davis had also been incontinent of urine, and the cause of his incontinence is also a concern to the team. A urinary catheter was inserted as an intermediary precaution related to the incontinence but also because of the patient's level of confusion (see Chapter 5).

As the treatment team awaits the results of the patient's diagnostic reports and continues to monitor his condition, Mr. Davis has been admitted to the intensive care unit (ICU) as a standard protocol for cardiovascular emergencies (see Chapter 5). His confusion has lifted, and he is now oriented × 3. He remains in bed. His heart, pulse, and respirations are being monitored frequently, as are his O_2SATs (see Chapter 5).

Patient Update

To complete the intake data for Mr. Davis, Victor, the medical unit clerk in the ICU, is now speaking with Larry from the Admissions Division of Medical Records at Okla Trauma Center. Victor will review some of the patient's basic biographical data, confirm a variety of orders that have been given for the patient's diagnosis and treatment, and determine if lab work has been completed for the patient.

"Hi, this is Victor in the ICU. We've just admitted a Zane Davis, 74 years old. Is there someone there I can speak to about this patient?" The voice on the other end of the phone identified himself as "Larry in Admissions" and confirmed that he would be able to assist. Victor thanked him and began the process of reviewing, confirming, and adding to the admission record for Mr. Davis. First, he confirmed the spelling of Mr. Davis's name, his date of birth, and his address, and he then confirmed Mr. Davis's insurance information. He also asked about the patient's next of kin.

"We have here that Mrs. Stevie-Rose Davis is his wife, and I see a note that says that she was transported to Fayette General Hospital, so someone in ER got a second name. Do you have that?" When Victor said that he did not, Larry filled him in. "Okay," Larry said. "He has a couple of sons and a daughter, but it says here that Social Work was able to contact a son named Quincy Davis. Do you want that number?" he asked. Victor did, so Larry gave him the contact phone number.

"What about the consents?" asked Larry. "Do you have the originals with you in the chart?" Larry heard his colleague shuffling through pages.

"Yes, here it is," said Victor. "I have a signed consent for treatment from Mr. Davis, but I can't see the TAR. Do you have that?" Now, Victor waited while the medical records technician searched the patient record. In a moment, Larry confirmed that he did indeed have the TAR. "What's the status of that, Larry?" asked Victor. "Are his admission, lab work, and treatments approved by the VA?" Larry confirmed that all three had been approved.

Then Larry said, "I'm looking at the TAR right now, and there are a couple of diagnoses here that went in. I'm wondering if these are still valid or if someone in Medical Billing needs to follow this through? That's often what happens when a patient comes through the ER with some sort of trauma." Victor agreed that following up with Billing might be wise; he noted that the patient was stable, but he was unsure of the current diagnosis, because the physician, Dr. Fillmore, had not yet been on the unit.

"Before I go, Larry," said Victor, "do you know if there are any previous records on Mr. Davis with us here at Okla? I can't see any when I enter the name on my computer, but that's not always 100% accurate, so while I have you on the phone, perhaps you could just check for me? It really helps if there are some old records around. Our patient was confused when he arrived, and we don't have a full history on him yet. One of the nurses is in with him now, trying to complete the medical history and the nurse's admissions form. But if you've got more data, this could help her out. It would help Dr. Fillmore with the diagnosis, too."

Victor waited as Larry looked through his own database. Victor could hear the clicking of the keys on Larry's computer keyboard as Larry searched for records. Finally, RMT answered that there had never been a patient by the name of Zane Davis at Okla Trauma Center in the past and that this looked like the patient's first admission. Victor thanked Larry for his help, and they said their goodbyes.

Reflective Questions

Reflect on the story that you've just read.

1. In Chapter 8, you were introduced to the job of unit clerk. In this chapter, what task is the unit clerk, Victor, involved in?

   ____

2. The unit clerk reports that a document included in the chart has been signed by the patient. What is that document?

   ____

3. The opening scenario uses a number of abbreviations that you have learned through your work in previous chapters. What are the meanings of the following: TIA, CVA, ICU, and CAD?

   ____

Critical Thinking Questions

1. Larry, the medical records technician, is concerned about a document called a *TAR*. You have not yet learned what these initials mean. Based on the context of the conversation, what do you think is the purpose of this document?

   ____

2. Mr. Davis's care seems to be covered by his medical insurance through the VA. What do you think the abbreviation *VA* stands for?

   ____

For audio exercises, visit **http://www.MedicalLanguageLab.com.** 

Learning Objectives

After reading Chapter 9, you will be able to do the following:

- Recognize and use medical and anatomical terminology related to the respiratory system.
- Recognize and use medical and anatomical terminology related to the male reproductive system.
- Understand the education and training of a medical records and health information technician.
- Recognize and use medical terminology related to pathology of the respiratory system.
- Recognize and use medical terminology related to the pathology of infection in the urinary tract.
- Recognize and use medical terminology related to pathology and diagnostics of the male reproductive system.
- Interpret diagnostic results for the cardiovascular, respiratory, and urinary systems.

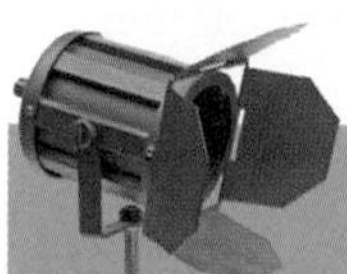

CAREER SPOTLIGHT: Medical Records and Health Information Technicians

Medical records technicians and *health information technicians* are responsible for the creation and maintenance of patients' medical records. An integral part of the health-care team, they consult with physicians, nurses, and other staff to ensure that records are always up to date and that all documents from the various members who are caring for the patient are in the record. They keep records and patient information in both written and electronic forms. Their records become essential to the monitoring of medical histories, patterns of disease, patterns of treatment, and care visits. These medical records may be used for direct patient care and, where applicable, for the gathering of health-information data for public health purposes and research.

Training and education for these careers may vary, but the standard is an associate's degree in medical records or health information technology. Courses generally include medical terminology, anatomy and physiology, clinical classification and coding systems, health data standards and requirements, and database management and security. Many medical records and health information technicians register to obtain a credential of Registered Health Information Technician (RHIT).

The Language of Admissions and Medical Records

In the opening dialogue, the ICU unit clerk and a medical records technician were consulting about our patient, Zane Davis. They were ensuring that the patient's records were accurate and complete. These two health careers are invaluable to the care of patients and the work of treatment teams: accuracy with regard to patient records and medical record management are of paramount importance. Take a look now at some of the words and phrases that were used in the dialogue. Notice how much of it is medical language rather than strict medical terminology. How much of this language did you understand when you first read it?

Key terms: admissions and medical records

"... *biographical data* ..."

biographical data: information regarding the patient's name, address, age, family, health history, and employment or financial status (i.e., ability to pay for treatment).

"... confirm a *variety of orders* ..."

variety of orders: the physician's orders for diagnostic tests and treatment as recorded on the patient's medical record, which accompanied the patient to the unit.

"... *lab work* ..."

lab work: results and requisitions pending for any laboratory tests ordered by the physician.

"... to the *admission record* ..."

admission record: the patient's biographical information, as well as his or her immediate assessment and treatment at the time of admission to hospital.

"... *next of kin*."

next of kin: the patient's closest family member. The next of kin for Mr. Davis is his wife, Stevie-Rose Davis. Because she is unavailable to be there for this patient, the next of kin are now identified as Mr. Davis's children. In some cases, a brother or sister may also be identified as next of kin. The person who is listed as the patient's next of kin is legally entitled to give permission for the treatment of a patient who is unconscious or otherwise incapacitated.

"... so someone in ER *got a second name*."

got a second name: an employee in the emergency department obtained the name of another family member who could be considered next of kin.

"'What about the *consents*?'"

consents: signed documents in which the patient or next of kin gives approval for specific diagnostic tests, treatments, and health-care interventions. These consents are legal requirements and must be part of every medical record.

"... I can't see the *TAR*."

TAR: **treatment authorization request**. This document is a request that an insurance company or health maintenance organization (HMO) make payment for the tests, procedures, or other care identified by the health-care provider.

"I'm looking at the TAR right now, and there are a couple of *diagnoses here that went in*."

a couple of diagnoses here that went in: preliminary possible diagnoses that the attending physician entered on the treatment authorization request document. On the original TAR for Mr. Davis, his final diagnosis had not yet been confirmed because the physician was still working through the process of ruling out a number of possible diagnoses. (See Chapter 5 to review Mr. Davis' admitting diagnoses and Chapter 7 to review the process of ruling out.)

"... we don't have a *full history* on him yet."

full history: a complete medical history, including a list of the medications that the patient is currently taking.

"... and *their own admissions* ..."

their own admissions: nursing admissions forms.

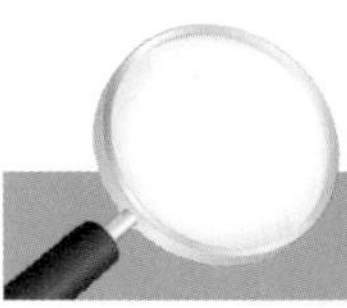

FOCUS POINT: *Next of Kin* vs. *Significant Other*

The term *next of kin* generally refers to the person who is most closely related to the patient by blood, legal adoption, or marriage. It does not include individuals who are identified as "domestic partners" or step-family members. For States in which these relationships are honored, the term *significant other*—rather than *next of kin*—is used. The patient is usually required to identify the person to be named as his or her significant other. This is a safety precaution so that care and support are provided for the patient by the person whom he or she believes will act in his or her best interests. More specific information about who fits the criteria for next of kin or significant other should be sought from your workplace.

Right Word or Wrong Word: *Diagnosis* or *Diagnoses*?

Is there a difference between these two words? Look very carefully at the spelling of each as you consider your answer.

Okla Trauma Center

Admissions Form

Date: June xx, 2010 Admitting service: Emergency

Patient Information

Last name: Davis First name: Zane Middle: C.

DOB: XX/XX/XXXX Age: 74 Gender: Male

Address: XXXXXXXXXXXXXXXXXXXXXXXXXX
XXXXXXXXXXXXXXXXXXXXXXXXXX

City: XXXXXXXXXXXXXXXXXXXXXXXX State: XXXXXXXXXXXXXXXXXXXX Zip: XXXXXX

Phone: XXX-XXX-XXXX Cell: N/A Work: N/A (retired)

Email: XXXXXXXXXXXXXXXXXXXXXXXXXXXXXXXXXXXXXX Social security #: XXX-XX-XXXX

Marital status: Married Next of kin/significant other: Stevie-Rose Davis, wife

Contact number(s) for next of kin/significant other: 555-XXX-XXXX

Emergency contact person and number: Quincy Davis, 555-XXX-XXXX
(not living with patient)

Relationship to patient: Son

Occupation: Telecommunications technician Employer: Retired

Health Insurance Information

Insurance Plan: Veterans Health Agency Effective date: XX/XX/XXXX

Personal insurance ID #: XXXXXXXXXXXXX Group #: XXXXXXXXXXX Plan #: XXXXXXXXXXX

Address of insurer: Department of Veterans Affairs

Policy Holder Information

Last name: Davis First name: Zane Middle: C.

DOB: XX/XX/XXXX Age: 74 Gender: Male

Treatment Authorization Request

Provider name and address: OKLA TRAUMA CENTER XXXXXXXXXXXXXXXXX

Provider phone #: ______________

Patient's authorized representative (if any) ______________________________

Type of service requested: ☐ Drug ☐ Other: ______________________

Retroactive claim: ☐ Yes ☐ No

Medicare eligible? ☐ Yes ☐ No

Patient Information

Last name: ______________________________

First name: ______________________ Middle: ______

DOB: ______________ Age: ______ Gender: ________

Approved as requested: ☐ Yes ☐ No

By medical consultant:

____

Date: ______________

Comments: ______________

Description of diagnosis: ______________________

Medical justification: ______________________

ICD Diagnostic Code

Specific Services Requested

Authorized	Specific services requested	Units of service	Procedure or drug code	Quantity	Code
☐ Yes ☐ No					
☐ Yes ☐ No					
☐ Yes ☐ No					
☐ Yes ☐ No					
☐ Yes ☐ No					

Physician signature: ______________________________ Date: ______________

TAR authorization for dates: ______________ to ______________ TAR #______________

Patient Label

Okla Trauma Center

General Consent for Treatment

The undersigned patient and/or responsible relative or person hereby consent to and authorize Okla Trauma Center's physicians and medical personnel to administer and perform medical examinations, investigations, medical treatments, outpatient procedures, vaccinations, and immunizations during the course of the patient's care, as an outpatient, as deemed advisable or necessary.

The undersigned also consents to the use of medical information for research purpose or for insurance coverage.

The undersigned also consents to the Hospital contacting him/her by telephone if needed regarding appointments and follow-up needs.

Witness: ______________________________ Date: ____________

Signature of patient: ______________________________ Date: ____________

Let's Practice

Study the "On the Job" forms: Admissions Form, TAR Form, and Consent Form (pages 345-347). Next, answer these questions by referring to the appropriate forms.

1. Who makes the TAR request? ______________________
2. Who approves the TAR request? ______________________
3. What important health information must be listed on a TAR for consideration for payment? ______________________
4. Which form requires the patient's signature or that of a next of kin or significant other? ______________________
5. On which form are data such as vital signs and allergies noted? ______________________
6. Of all of the medical record forms that you have now seen, which will the patient be actively involved in completing? ______________________

Let's Practice

Identify each statement about hospital admissions and medical records as true or false.

1. To qualify as a significant other for medical or health-care purposes, you must be a blood relative. ______________________
2. The nursing admissions form and the hospital admissions form are the same. ______________________
3. The hospital and the physician are unable to treat a patient if the TAR (or elements of the TAR) are rejected. ______________________

Patient Update

Mr. Davis was resting comfortably in the intensive care unit. He had been there for approximately an hour after having undergone a series of tests. He was fatigued from the events of the day and still mulling them over, trying to put the pieces of the accident together in his mind. As he did so, his son Quincy arrived.

"Hi, Dad, I got here as soon as I could," said Quincy as he rushed over to his father's bedside. His father opened his eyes and smiled at him. Quincy noted that Mr. Davis looked pale and tired. To Quincy, it seemed that he had never seen his father look this old before, and it worried him.

"How ya' doin', son?" Mr. Davis said softly. "Quite a pickle we all got ourselves into today, your mom and me. Have you seen your mom? They won't tell me too much about her. Is she okay? And Clay? What about Clay? I heard he's here, too, but because I'm just his grandpa, I haven't heard much. Is he okay? Help me get up and let's go find out what's going on," Mr. Davis said with some urgency. He started to sit up and reached to pull off the leads of his heart monitor, coughing as he did so. Quincy stopped him. He also saw that his father had an IV in his left arm.

"Dad, stop! You'll pull out that IV!" Quincy warned. His father, surprised, stopped a moment to collect his thoughts. He looked around as if seeing his situation for the first time. His coughing subsided.

"My gosh, son, I really have had a day, haven't I?" Mr. Davis asked, once again sounding tired and worn. "What the heck happened?" He looked at his son for answers and reassurance. Quincy shared all that he knew about the accident and his father's injuries.

"I'm not clear on any of this yet, either," said Quincy. "I just know what they told me on the phone: that you'd been in an accident and were admitted to the intensive care unit. They wouldn't give me a whole lot of details, something to do with confidentiality or something. And when I asked, they told me that they thought Mom was at Fayette. I jumped in my car and headed over here." He explained that he had then called his sister, Angie, from his cell phone as he was getting into his car to come to see his father. That's when Quincy found out Angie had been reached by the other hospital. He tried to call his brother, too, but there was no answer at the home phone, and he didn't have his brother's cell phone number. "It didn't quite dawn on me at the time that Clay was with you. I forgot that you had Clay staying over for a week," Quincy added.

"Quincy, tell me about your mom and about little Clay," his father said with apprehension. Quincy explained he'd been in phone contact with his brother, Steve, who was downstairs with Clay. "He's got a lot of injuries, Dad. They say he broke his jaw. He's going to have surgery any minute now. And Mom's over at Fayette General. Angie's on her way over there. She might even be there by now. She said she'd call me as soon as she finds out what's going on."

"Yes, but what did they tell Angie? They must have told her something. Is Stevie-Rose hurt?" interrupted Zane. Quincy explained that their mother was supposed to be physically okay according to the hospital, but that she was certainly confused. As he spoke, he resettled Zane back onto the bed.

"Are you okay, Dad? What about you?" Quincy asked worriedly, noticing the IV, the monitors, and a urinary catheter bag hanging from the bottom of the bedrail. "What happened?"

"I don't really remember much about what happened, son. We were at home having coffee on the back deck, and then Clay came bouncing out of the kitchen, you know, like he always does. So full of energy. He crashed right into your mother. She was carrying the coffee pot and was going to fill up my cup." He paused for a moment to let this sink in for Quincy, and his son's eyes widened. Zane nodded and went on. "We were taking Clay to Fayette because he got scalded. Then, I don't know what happened. Next thing I know, they're wheeling me in here. I heard them say I had a stroke." Zane paused again, trying to collect his thoughts. "Did I?"

"I'm not sure, Dad," said Quincy

"What about the other vehicle, son? What about those people? Are they okay?" asked Zane.

"I don't know, Dad," Quincy sighed. "I have no idea."

Critical Thinking Questions

Based on what you've just read, answer the following questions.

1. What new symptom has Mr. Davis developed? ______________________________
2. Using medical terminology, describe Mr. Davis's color. ______________________________
3. Mr. Davis doesn't quite remember the accident, although he can now recall parts of the day preceding it. What is the medical term for this type of short-term memory loss? (See Chapter 7.) ______________________________
4. How did the child, Clay Davis, get burned? ______________________________

Interpreting Diagnostic Test Results

Patient Update

The story continues. Mr. Davis and his son are together as a physician arrives.

Suddenly, a deep voice from behind Quincy said, "Hello, I'm Dr. Fillmore, cardiologist here at Okla." A young man about 35 years old appeared, wearing a white lab coat over green scrubs and carrying a clipboard. He reached out to shake hands with Quincy and his father.

"At first, some of your symptoms suggested that you might have suffered a stroke, Mr. Davis," continued Dr. Fillmore. "But we've now ruled that out." Quincy let out an audible sigh of relief. The physician then explained the results of Zane's blood work while he referred to the chart in his hand.

"Your CBC and platelet levels are just fine," he said. "And since we wanted to rule out the likelihood of a CVA—a stroke—we did some tests to see if your blood was clotting or maintaining a balance between thrombus formation and hemorrhage. It's a delicate balance, so we ran a PTT and an INR. Those results were within normal range as well." Dr. Fillmore paused for a second to scan the page that he was reading. "Let me see what else I can tell you.... Your cardiac enzymes, CK, and CPK-MB were okay. We weren't suspecting cardiac arrest, but we ran those tests just to be sure."

Dr. Fillmore paused momentarily and looked at both the patient and his son for confirmation that they understood what he was saying. Then he went on: "Here's what's interesting. Your electrolytes are normal, except for potassium. Your potassium level is somewhat lower than usual, but that may be an indicator of dietary changes related to living with coronary artery disease. Finally..." Suddenly Dr. Fillmore was cut off by Mr. Davis coughing harshly. The doctor waited and listened. When the coughing spasm subsided, he continued.

"Finally, we do know that you have been diagnosed with coronary artery disease, so we wanted a CT scan to ensure that your blood vessels were not blocked or at risk for blockage. It appears that you have some plaques on your arteries, but nothing that would require surgical intervention at this time. I wonder what you've been told about this and if you've been taking care of this condition?"

"Yup," said Mr. Davis. "I've had that diagnosis for about 6 years now. I've been taking some—oh, what do you call that, umm, oh yes!—a statin drug for that. My doctor says it's working. I also make sure to eat a lot of oatmeal. I've heard that eating oatmeal regularly can really help to keep your arteries clear," he explained, using a tone that was almost as if he was asking a question. Dr. Fillmore nodded. "I also take my dog for a walk every morning and evening, so I make sure to get some exercise." The cardiologist nodded and went on.

"We've done a number of other tests, too, Mr. Davis," Dr. Fillmore said directly to Zane. "Your O_2SATs were low, and the nurses noticed that you had some shortness of breath, so we drew some blood to measure your arterial blood gases. Results show some borderline normals. That's another reason why we took a CT and both posteroanterior and lateral x-ray films of your chest. You don't have any broken or cracked ribs from the accident, but we're going to want to learn more about your respiratory health.

Mr. Davis suddenly changed the subject. "Say, doctor, what about this...this...this tube?" he asked, reaching down to indicate his catheter. "I'm okay now. Can't I get this thing out? Why the heck do I have this thing?" Dr. Fillmore explained to Mr. Davis that he'd had a fever when he was admitted and that he was put on antibiotics and an antipyretic to treat the condition when the first STAT urinalysis, a dipstick test, indicated a urinary tract infection. Subsequently, a urine specimen was collected via catheter, and those results confirmed the diagnosis.

"I see from your chart that your fever has resolved, so we're on the right track." The doctor explained how the urinary tract infection may have contributed to Mr. Davis's presentation at the scene of the MVA and also while he was being transported to the hospital. He described Mr. Davis's symptoms of restlessness, confusion, and urinary incontinence. However, he also cautioned Mr. Davis that these symptoms may be related to low oxygen and high carbon dioxide levels in the body. Finally, the doctor said, "Yes, I think that we can remove the catheter now. I'll let the nurse know. She'll do that for you."

"Good. Then when can I get out of here? I know what you've just said about tests, but my wife's over at Fayette General. I need to get there. She needs me, you know! And I've got to see my grandson. He's here, and he's not doing so well. I can't lie around here all day," Mr. Davis said impatiently.

"Sir, I know you've got a lot on your plate today, but you're going to have to let your family help you as much as they can," said Dr. Fillmore. "You need to stay with us here until all of your test results come back and we can clear you medically for discharge. I may want to talk to you again, too. I'm still concerned about the potential for a TIA related to your coronary artery disease. Are you currently seeing a cardiologist?"

"Nope. I went to a cardiologist once. He told me I had hardening of the arteries, but if I took care of myself and followed his advice, I wouldn't really need to see him again," replied Mr. Davis.

"Okay," said Dr. Fillmore. "But I think you should follow up with your own doctor when you're discharged. We'll send him the report of your stay and treatment here, if you like." Mr. Davis nodded. I'll get one of our respiratory specialists to take a look at you, too, while you're here. "In the meantime, I'm going to leave orders that you can be transferred over to a medical unit. You no longer need ICU care, and you don't need a cardiologist, so you'll be assigned a new physician," Dr. Fillmore informed Zane and Quincy as he wrote a few notes on the chart in his hand. Then, he looked up, put his pen in his pocket, thanked them for their time, and suddenly took his leave. Quincy and Zane, caught off guard, simply watched Dr. Fillmore as he departed.

Reflective Questions

Reflect on the story that you've just read.

1. What medical conditions have now been ruled out for Mr. Davis? ______________________
2. What was the cause of Mr. Davis's fever? ______________________
3. What does Mr. Davis want removed? ______________________
4. X-rays were taken of the patient's chest and lungs. What angle was used? ______________________
5. Why does Dr. Fillmore want a respiratory specialist to examine Mr. Davis?

____

Okla Trauma Center

Diagnostic Laboratory

Today's date: *June XX, 2015*　　Date of specimen collection: *June XX, 2015*

Submitting physician's name: *Dr. Crowchild*

Physician's contact information: *Okla Trauma Center, Emergency Department*
(*may be stamped*)

Name: *Zane Davis*　DOB: *XX/XX/XXXX*　Age: *74*　Allergies: *None*

Gender: ☐ Female ☑ Male　Hospital admission #: *D793015*

Presenting Complaint/Diagnosis:

? TIA, CVA, r/out MI　*History of CAD*　*? UTI*

***star means abnormal findings

Hematology	Hematology Normal Values	Microbiology
CBC: **14.5** with platelets: **300,000** Hematocrit: **45** RBC: **4.6** ***WBC + diff: **18,000** HGB: **14 g/dL**	**CBC:** 13.5–16.5 male Platelets: 100,000–400,000 **HTC:** 41–50 **RBC:** 4.5–5.5 **WBC/diff:** 4,500–10,000 **HGB:** 12–16 g/dL	**Urinalysis:** Ketones: **Negative** (normal) Glucose: **Negative** (normal) Proteins: **Negative** (normal) WBC: **Positive** Bacteria: **Positive**
Other: (please write in)	**Other:** (corresponding normals)	**Biochemistry**
MB-CK: *not present* Troponin 1: *not present* Troponin 2: *not present* Serum Electrolytes: ***Potassium (K): *3.1* ***LDL: *190 mg/dL* HDL: *40 mg/dL*	**MB-CK:** 0–3.9% **Troponin 1 and Troponin 2:** Elevated within 4–6 hr of cardiac event **Serum Electrolytes:** **Potassium:** 3.5–5 mmol/L **LDL:** 65–180 mg/dL **HDL:** 30–70 mg/dL	**Glucose:** _____ random FBS _____ (fasting) _____ mg/dL (normal range 70–99 mg/dL)
Arterial Blood Gases	**ABG – Normal Values**	
pH: **7.4** pCO_2: **35** pO_2: **68** HCO_3: **19** O_2: **88**	**pH:** 7.35–7.45 **pCO_2:** 35–45 **pO_2:** 70–100 **HCO_3:** 19–25 **O_2:** 90–95	

Key words: diagnostic test results

In the Patient Update dialogue, Dr. Fillmore reviewed the results of various diagnostic tests that he had ordered to rule out cardiovascular or cerebrovascular causes of Mr. Davis's symptoms. In addition, because Mr. Davis had been in a motor vehicle accident, the doctor checked the patient's cardiac enzyme levels in case Mr. Davis had suffered a chest injury, which would have put stress on his heart muscle. Key terms from the dialogue are italicized in the example and highlighted below with the explanation.

"... *cardiac enzymes, CK, and CPK-MB* ..."

cardiac enzymes: essential proteins released by the heart muscles into the bloodstream that are essential to the healthy functioning of the heart. They also serve as biochemical markers of heart disease, malfunction, or injury.

CK and CPK-MB: two tests that measure the patient's levels of creatinine, a substance found in blood, urine, and muscle that can indicate kidney dysfunction. These tests are ordered when patients present with symptoms of fatigue (exhaustion), confusion, or problems with urination.

"... your *electrolytes* are normal ..."

electrolytes: substances that conduct electrical impulses in the cells of the body (see Chapter 5).

"... a *statin* drug ..."

statin: a type of medication proven to reduce levels of low-density cholesterol and to lower the risk of heart attack. Cholesterol is a solid compound that is waxy or fat-like and found throughout the body. There are two types of cholesterol: Healthy cholesterol or *high-density lipoprotein (HDL)* cholesterol is necessary for the health of cell walls, and it is involved in the creation of bile and the production of hormones. Alternatively, *low-density lipoprotein (LDL)* cholesterol can increase the risk of cardiovascular disease. LDL has the ability to adhere to the walls of arteries and to form plaques or waxy buildups. The number and size of the plaques can impair circulation.

"... help to keep your *arteries clear* ..."

arteries clear: keep arteries clear or free of plaque buildup.

"Results show some *borderline normals*."

borderline normals: a descriptive term identifying that the results of a test are right at the top or bottom of the normal and acceptable range for that test.

"... and an *antipyretic* ..."

antipyretic: a medication used to clear a fever. Recall that the prefix *anti-* means *against,* and **pyretic** means *fever.*

"... a *dipstick test* ..."

dipstick test: a biochemical test that uses a **reagent strip** (a dry, plastic strip with tiny microfiber pads attached) to identify the following elements and characteristics of urine. The reagent strip is dipped into a urine specimen. Although a table in Chapter 5 identified some of the common tests that are included as part of urinalysis, the following notes contain additional information about the results of a urine dipstick test. Notice that it is possible to identify which subtest on the dipstick (reagent strip) indicates disease as opposed to infection.

albumin: a protein found in blood that helps to maintain blood pressure and blood volume. Its presence in the urine may indicate kidney disease rather than a simple infection.

ketones: byproducts or waste products that are the end result of the body burning stored fat for energy. An example of a ketone is acetone. Should they occur, ketones are excreted in the urine. They can be an indicator of insufficient insulin rather than infection.

bilirubin: the yellowish pigment found in bile (a fluid secreted by the liver that reduces fats and oils). Bilirubin is the result of the natural breakdown of red blood cells over time and does not indicate infection.

nitrates: inorganic compounds that are composed of nitrogen and oxygen. The chemical name is NO_3. Nitrates inhibit the ability of hemoglobin to carry oxygen, and they are therefore detrimental to health. *Escherichia coli* bacteria can lead to the presence of nitrates in the urine, so the presence of nitrates can indicate infection.

specific gravity: a measurement that identifies how concentrated the urine is. This is measured against a standard volume of water. Water has a specific gravity of 1.000, and normal urine has a specific gravity of 1.020 to 1.028. More highly concentrated urine can indicate the presence of dehydration, heart failure, and kidney disease. A decreased specific gravity of urine can indicate pyelonephritis (severe kidney disease). Some specific brands of urine dipsticks can measure specific gravity, but a laboratory test is preferred.

"'I see from your chart your *fever has resolved*, so we're *on the right track*.'"

fever has resolved: the fever is now gone.

on the right track: the physician is confirming that the medication administered has found its target and is working to help the patient recover.

TABLE 9-1: Commonly Prescribed Statin Drugs

Generic Name	Trade Name (name by which the medication is sold)
rosuvastatin	Crestor
atorvastatin	Lipitor
simvastatin	Zocor
fluvastatin	Lescol
lovastatin	Mevacor
pravastatin	Pravachol

TABLE 9-2: Cardiac Enzyme Tests

Cardiac Enzyme (Abbreviation)	Where and When the Enzyme Is Present	Normal Levels
alanine aminotransferase (ALT or SPGT)	found in a variety of muscles; an elevation in the levels of this enzyme can indicate congestive heart failure, myocardial infarction, or kidney disease, among other conditions	20 to 30 units per liter of blood
aspartate aminotransferase (AST) or serum glutamic oxaloacetic transaminase (SGOT)	found in a variety of muscles and tissues, including the liver, heart, kidney, and brain; it is released into the bloodstream when one of these organs is damaged; the test for this enzyme is often referred to as a *liver function test*	20 to 30 units per liter of blood
creatinine kinase (CPK-MB)	released from muscle tissue when the heart is injured or damaged; however, levels do not begin to rise until 12 to 24 hours after the event	CPK-MB 0 to 5 IU/dL (international units/deciliter) or 0% to 6% of total CPK (0.00 to 0.06)
creatinine phosphokinase (CPK)	present in all muscles of the body	CPK 30 to 150 IU/dL (international units/deciliter)
Total creatinine kinase (CK)	released into the bloodstream 4 to 6 hours after heart damage has occurred	Men: 38 to 174 IU/L (international units per liter) Women: 26 to 140 IU/L
Troponin T (TnT or TnI)	found only within the cardiac muscle, this enzyme is released into the bloodstream 2 to 6 hours after a myocardial infarction and at the time of death	TnI = <0.2 mcg/L TnT = <0.2 mcg/L

Let's Practice

Write the medical term that fits each description.

1. an enzyme released after a myocardial infarction or at the time of death ______________
2. might be referred to as a "liver function test" ______________
3. high levels in the blood could indicate a heart attack, congestive heart failure, or kidney disease ______________
4. an overwhelming sense of exhaustion and an inability to function ______________
5. given to reduce or resolve fever ______________
6. chemicals that inhibit hemoglobin from carrying oxygen through the body ______________
7. a method of examining urine for ketones, bilirubin, and albumin ______________
8. a type of waxy substance found in the body that is important for maintaining cell membranes, as well as for producing bile and hormones ______________
9. proteins released by the heart, particularly in the presence of physical stress or trauma ______________
10. prescribed to decrease LDL levels ______________

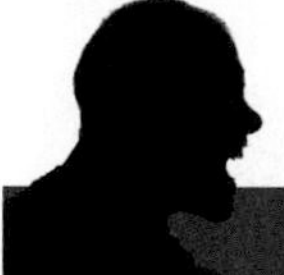

PRONUNCIATION PRACTICE

Say these words aloud to a friend or classmate if you can. You are given the phonetic pronunciation. Your instructor can help you with pronunciation,

or visit **http://www.MedicalLanguageLab.com.**

alanine	ă**l**´ă-nēn
creatinine	krē-ă**t**´ĭn-ĭn
lipoprotein	lĭp˝-**prŏ**tēn
nitrate	**nī**´trāt
statins	**stă**´tĭnz
troponin	**trō**´pō-nĭn
transaminase	trăns-**ăm**´ĭn-ās
transferase	**trăns**´fĕr-ās

Interpreting the results of urinalysis

Mr. Davis has been transferred to Unit 8B-Medical at Okla Trauma Center. His status continues to be one of observation, and he is still awaiting news of the results of some diagnostic tests. He knows that the cardiologist had some questions about his respiratory system, but the details were not made clear.

Patient Update

"Hello, Mr. Davis, I'm Jenny, your nurse here on 8B. How are you feeling?" inquired a young woman with a friendly demeanor.

Mr. Davis smiled. "Honestly, I feel like I've been hit by a bus, nurse. I don't know why. I'm not injured. I just feel beat. Pooped right out. Maybe it's all the excitement and worrying about my family. But I'm not sick. And I'm not injured," he insisted.

Jenny reflected on what Mr. Davis said, and then she began to speak with him about his urinary tract infection. She asked if he had a history of this or any other urinary, bladder, or kidney problems that he could remember.

"No, nothing like that. How'd I get an infection anyway?" he asked. "How does a person get a ... what do you call it?"

"A urinary tract infection, sir. We call it a 'UTI' for short," replied the nurse. "Bacteria is the cause of this type of infection. It enters your urethra and travels up it, blocking the flow of urine out of your body. That's when you'll notice difficulty urinating or pain when you urinate. Any time that urine cannot flow out of the body, the system backs up and the bacteria multiplies, which causes the infection to get worse or to spread upward into your kidneys and bladder." Jenny paused for a moment. "On the other hand," she added, "sometimes something like a kidney stone or an enlarged prostate can impede the flow of urine. Have you ever suffered from anything like that?"

"No, not that I'm aware of," came Mr. Davis' reply.

Jenny then asked Mr. Davis about the fact that he had been incontinent of urine at the time of admission. "Has that ever happened to you before, Mr. Davis? Urinary incontinence?" He looked at her in silence. "Urinary incontinence is nothing to be ashamed of, Mr. Davis. It can happen to anyone. But I need to know if this is a pattern for you or a one-time event. It may have something to do with your infection, or it may not." Jenny paused then, waiting for Zane to reply.

"Oh, for heaven's sakes," Mr. Davis said in exasperation. "Yes ... well ... oh ... You know, I'm 74 years old. For the last couple of years, I have had to go a lot, if you know what I mean."

"Go a lot, sir? Do you mean that you have had urinate frequently?" Jenny inquired non-judgmentally, putting Mr. Davis at ease. He nodded in the affirmative. "Well, urinary frequency can be a normal part of aging for people, that's true. But urinary incontinence is something a little different. Let's talk about that for a minute," the nurse invited. Mr. Davis continued. He told her that he'd "almost" been incontinent a number of times over the past year or so. He explained that he had to be careful how much liquid he drank each day so that he wouldn't have to worry about not making it to the bathroom in time. He added that the need to urinate woke him up during the night more and more often lately as well.

Jenny asked, "Do you ever have difficulty starting a urine stream? Or stopping it? Or do you ever find that you dribble a bit when you think you've finished urinating, but you actually haven't?" Zane nodded. "Well, Mr. Davis, these are symptoms that you should talk to your physician about, and they should be assessed so that they can be treated. I'm going to tell Dr. Jackson about them on your behalf. In the meantime, have you experienced any pain while urinating during the last couple of days?" Mr. Davis nodded. "Well, you are being treated for a UTI," Jenny said. "The doctor has ordered an antibiotic to relieve the infection, and you can also have some ibuprofen if you need it. It has anti-inflammatory and analgesic properties that can alleviate some of that pain for you and make you more comfortable."

Jenny went on to talk with Mr. Davis about the effects that a UTI can have on a person's body and mind, noting that confusion in the older adult was not an uncommon symptom. Mr. Davis was surprised to hear this, and he wondered if that was why he hadn't felt clear-headed since he got up that morning. Jenny confirmed that the infection may indeed be the reason and that it could also explain why Mr. Davis felt so tired and worn out. At this point, Jenny made sure that Mr. Davis understood all that they had talked about, and she then continued on her rounds.

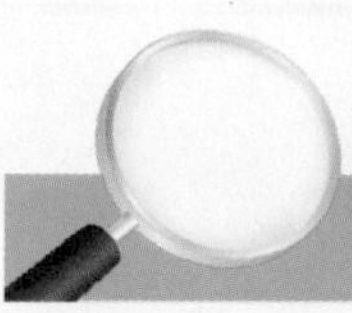

FOCUS POINT: Antibiotics and Bacteria

Antibiotics are antibacterial medications that are designed to eradicate bacterial infections; they do *not* treat viruses. *Bacteria* is the plural form of *bacterium.* Bacteria are a specific type of single-celled microorganisms. There are good (essential) bacteria and bad (unhealthy or infection promoting) bacteria. See Chapter 5 for more information.

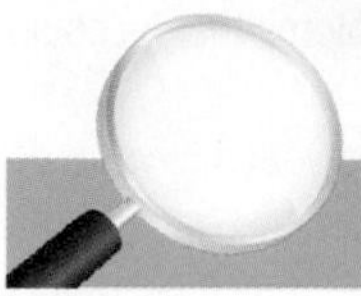

FOCUS POINT: Urinary Tract

Urinary tract is a medical term that is used to describe all parts of the urinary system. The word *tract* refers to a group of organs that form a pathway. The urinary tract consists of the ureters, the bladder, and the kidney. See Chapter 5 for more information.

Causes and types of urinary tract infections

Urinary tract infections are extremely common. Bacterial and viral infections of the urinary tract can cause a number of unpleasant symptoms that can become **systemic,** which means that they can cause reactions not only in the urinary system but also in other systems of the body as the immune system mobilizes to defend the body against the infection. For example, fever is an immune response of the body to deal with the invasion of a pathogen such as a bacterium or virus. Although most UTIs are caused by the bacteria *Escherichia coli (E.coli),* which is usually found in the colon (bowel), you will recall from Chapter 5 that other pathogens can also cause infections.

Common types of urinary tract infections include the following:

Cystitis is a bladder infection.

Pyelonephritis is an infection of the kidneys that includes inflammation of the kidney and renal pelvis. This condition can result if cystitis is not treated promptly.

Chlamydia is an infection of the urethra and the reproductive system. It is a sexually transmitted infection.

Mycoplasma is an infection of the urethra and the reproductive system.

Other infections related to the urinary tract

Infections of the male genitalia can mirror urinary tract infections or lead to them. For example, it will be important to check the male patient who seems to have a UTI for the following:

Epididymitis

Epididymitis is an inflammation and infection of the **epididymis,** the internal tube-like structure that contains sperm. This can be caused by urinary infections and by mumps, syphilis, or tuberculosis. The laboratory diagnostics for this condition include urinalysis, a urine culture, and a white blood cell count.

Remember that our patient, Mr. Davis, does not know exactly what type of UTI he has yet. Although he may have a common form of this condition, note that he has been in recent close contact with his young grandson. We do not yet know if that young person has had the mumps or been in contact with someone with the mumps or if Mr. Davis has ever had the mumps before. Should epididymitis be diagnosed, these questions would need to be answered. We also have no knowledge of whether Mr. Davis has a diagnosis of syphilis or tuberculosis. The physician will need to speak to him about the lab results when he sees him.

Orchitis

Orchitis is the inflammation or infection of the testes. This condition can also be caused by the mumps, but it may also result from a bacterium, a virus, or a trauma. The laboratory diagnostics for this condition include urinalysis, a urethral culture, and a urine dip.

To further understand the pathology of a urinary tract infection, it will help to expand your vocabulary related to the kidneys. (See Chapter 5 for an introduction to the kidneys and the urinary system as a whole.) Figure 9-1 helps to set the context for word building related to kidney function.

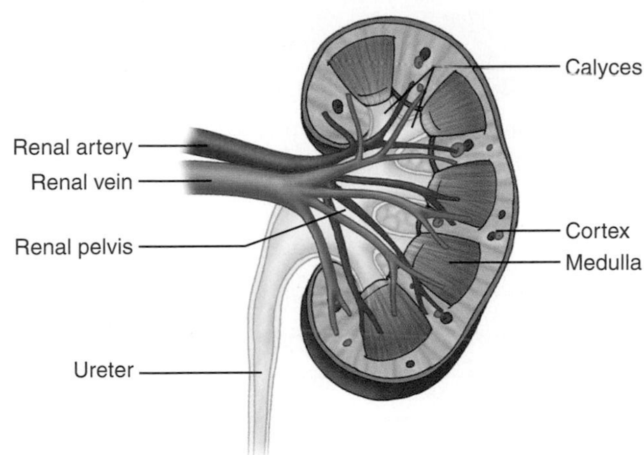

Figure 9.1: Anatomy of the kidney

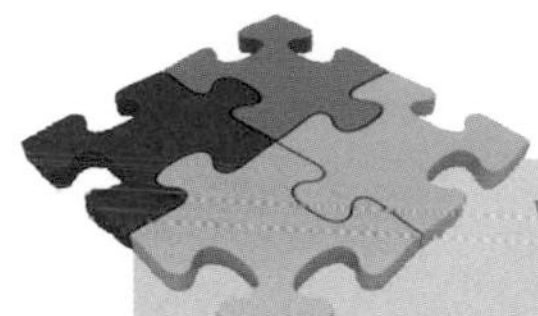

WORD BUILDING: Formulas for Creating Words from the Combining Forms *Pyelo* and *Nephro*

1. pyelos = pelvis; renal pelvis. The combining form is *pyelo-*.

pyelo + cyst + itis = *pyelocystitis*

Definition: inflammation of the bladder and the renal pelvis. *noun*

Example: The bacteria *Shigella* can cause *pyelocystitis.*

pyelo + gram = *pyelogram*

Definition: a radiograph of the renal pelvis and ureter(s). *noun*

Example: Mr. Davis is not suspected of having a kidney infection, so he will not be getting a *pyelogram.*

pyelo + nephr/o + osis = *pyelonephrosis*

Definition: disease of the kidney. (The second root is *nephr/o,* meaning *kidney,* and the suffix *-osis* means *condition.* A synonym is *pyelopathy.*) *noun*

Example: Acute renal failure can result from untreated *pyelonephrosis.*

2. nephros = kidney. A nephron is the structural and functional unit of the kidney. The combining form is *nephr/o-*.

nephr + ectom + y = *nephrectomy*

Definition: the surgical removal of a kidney. *noun*

Example: After a *nephrectomy,* a person can live quite well with only the remaining kidney.

Continued

nephr + itis = *nephritis*

Definition: inflammation of the kidney as a result of bacteria, toxins, or disease. *noun*

Example: *Nephritis* is a serious autoimmune disorder of the kidney.

nephro + lith + iasis = *nephrolithiasis*

Definition: the presence of kidney stones (calculi in the kidneys). The second root is *lithos,* meaning *stone. noun*

Example: *Nephrolithiasis* is not an infection; however, if it is left untreated, the urinary tract can become inflamed, and infection can set in.

Build a Word

Use your knowledge of root words and their combining forms to build words from the word parts that are given. You will need to change the word parts to make the proper term and then provide a definition of each new term.

1. pyelo graph nephr/o y ______________ Meaning: ______________
2. rrhapy nephr/o ______________ Meaning: ______________
3. toxin nephr/o ______________ Meaning: ______________
4. -tomy pyel/o ______________ Meaning: ______________
5. ology nephro ______________ Meaning: ______________
6. lithos nephro tome ______________ Meaning: ______________
7. pathos nephros ______________ Meaning: ______________

Mix and Match

Match the name of the infection or condition with its description.

1. nephritis	infection of the testes that affects the flow of urine
2. cystitis	an x-ray or CT image of the renal pelvis and the ureters
3. nephrectomy	surgical removal of a kidney
4. orchitis	bladder infection
5. pyelogram	inflammation of the kidneys

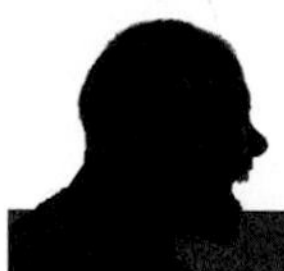

PRONUNCIATION PRACTICE

Say these words aloud to a friend or classmate if you can. You are given the phonetic pronunciation. Your instructor can help you with pronunciation,

or visit **http://www.MedicalLanguageLab.com.** 

cystitis	sĭs-**tī**´tĭs	nephritis	nĕf-**rī**´a tĭs
chlamydia	klă-**mĭd**´ĕ-ă	orchitis	or-**kī**´ tĭs
epididymitis	ĕp″ĭ-dĭd″ĭ-**mī**tĭs	pyelocystitis	pī″ĕ-lō-sĭs-**tī**´tĭs
mycoplasma	mī″kō-**plăz**´mă	pyelonephritis	pī″ĕ-lō-nĕ-**frī**´tĭs
nephrolithiasis	nĕf″rō-lĭth-**ī**´ă-sĭs		

The Language of the Male Reproductive System

Assessments of the male urinary system and reproductive system are often co-occurring. This is because of the close proximity of the prostate gland to the urethra and also because the penis serves not only as a sexual organ but also as the conduit for the passage of urine (see Figure 9-2). For men, therefore, an examination of one system generally includes both systems. This becomes even more likely as men age and as the prostate gland enlarges.

The *prostate gland* is responsible for blocking off urine flow through the urethra during sexual activity. It also produces *seminal fluid* to protect *sperm* and to facilitate its movement in the process of *ejaculation*. An enlarged prostate can lead to urinary symptoms of hesitancy (slow initiation of urination, even though there is an urge to void), a weak urine stream when it does start, and some dribbling. (Recall that the nurse, Jenny, spoke with Mr. Davis about these symptoms earlier in this chapter.)

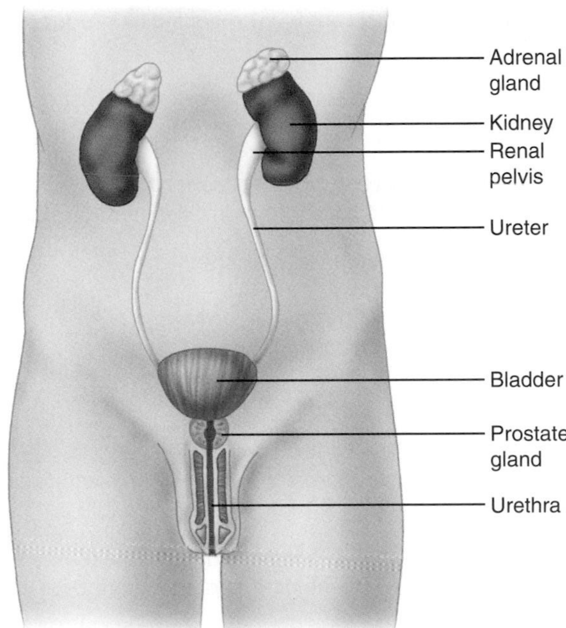

Figure 9.2: The male urinary system

The field of science and medicine involved in male reproductive health is called **andrology**. In this discipline, the focus is on male sexual health, family planning, fertility, and impotency.

Key terms derived from andro

Study the following terms that include the root *andro:*

android obesity: a type of obesity in which the bulk of the weight and fatty tissues are situated around the waist and the abdominal area.

android pelvis: a male or masculine-shaped pelvis.

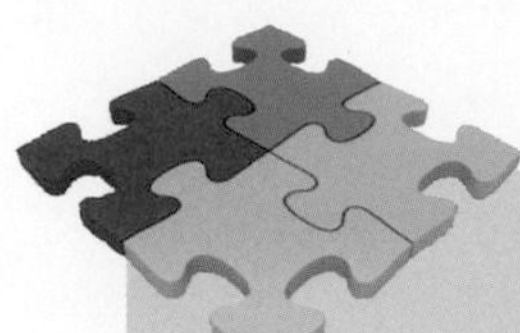

WORD BUILDING: Formula for Creating Words with the Combining Form *Andr/o/os-*

andros = male or man

andro + oid = android

Definition: 1) resembling a male; 2) manlike or almost human, when used in the context of technology; 3) a robot. (The root *eidos* is altered to *oid* in English, meaning *shape or form.*) *adjective* or *noun*

Example: A male skeleton has a distinct *android* pelvis.

andro + gen + s = *androgens*

Definition: male sex hormones. (*Gen* is a root word meaning *to produce or arising from.* The suffix -*s* connotes a plural form.) *noun*

Example: *Androgens* stimulate the development of male characteristics and include testosterone and androsterone.

pre + andro + gens = *preandrogens*

Definition: biochemical compounds that lead to the development of male hormones. *noun*

Example: The levels of *preandrogens* decrease with age.

andro + pathy = *andropathy*

Definition: any disease specific to males. *noun*

Example: Benign prostrate hypertrophy is a type of *andropathy;* it occurs only in men.

andro + sterone = *androsterone*

Definition: one of the androgens; a male steroid hormone. (The root *sterone* indicates a steroid.) *noun*

Example: *Androsterone* is a steroid hormone supplement that is taken by some athletes to make them stronger and huskier, but it may be harmful to the natural hormonal balance of the body.

andro + stenedione = *androstenedione*

Definition: male hormone; one of the androgens. (The root *stenedione* identifies that the substance is a steroid hormone. Synonyms are *androstenediol* and *stenediol.*) *noun*

Example: *Androstenedione* is a male steroid hormone that is used by some athletes as a performance enhancer.

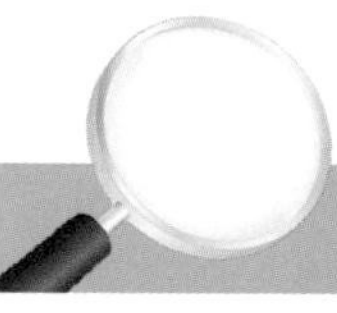

FOCUS POINT: More About Androgens

Androgens are male sex hormones that are essential to the determination of sexual identity. The presence of androgens is required for masculinization in utero to promote the development of a penis, testicles, and scrotum in the fetus. When a boy reaches puberty, the production of androgens increases, along with increasing levels of follicle-stimulating hormone (FSH) and luteinizing hormone (LH). Together, these hormones produce overt male characteristics such as a deepening voice, the strengthening and thickening of the musculoskeletal systems, and the development of the secondary sexual characteristics of facial and pubic hair.

During adulthood, androgens and FSH continue together to regulate sexual drive and aggression. They also promote sperm production in the testes. Higher levels of aggression in males are thought to be partially the result of higher levels of androgens in males than females. Testosterone is one of the most commonly known androgens.

Fill in the Blanks

Use new language and terms in a meaningful way. Complete these sentences by filling in the blanks

1. ________________ is a field of medicine that focuses on the male reproductive system.
2. ______________ is a male sex hormone that is particularly active during puberty.
3. A term that suggests disease of a male reproductive organ is ________________________.

Critical Thinking Exercise

Work with a partner or in a small group to answer the following questions.

1. The male urinary and reproductive systems are often considered together because they share two organs. What are those two organs? ____
2. What changes occur in a man's urinary and reproductive systems during later life? ____
3. What organ or structure of the male reproductive system is of interest to the doctor who is diagnosing Mr. Davis? ____

Anatomy and physiology: male reproductive system

Basically, the male reproductive system consists of the *penis, testes, epididymis, urethra, vas deferens* (also known as the *ductus deferens*), *seminal vesicles*, and the *prostate gland*. These will be the focus of this section. However, don't forget that, anatomically and medically speaking, the reproductive system also includes the hypothalamus and the pituitary gland in the brain, as well as the adrenal glands (see Chapter 8). The function of the male reproductive system is to produce and secrete male hormones and to produce and transport male reproductive cells (sperm) to be discharged into the female reproductive canal (the vagina).

Male hormones include the following:

androgens: hormones produced in the testes and adrenal glands.

testosterone: a specific androgen related to the sex drive (although it is important to realize that the sex drive and sexual interest require the external stimuli of sight, sound, and touch as well.)

estrogens: female sex hormones; their purpose in males has not been determined. However, increased levels of estrogen can lead to a decrease in a man's sex drive, a worsening of erectile dysfunction, and the development of secondary female characteristics (i.e., breast enlargement and the loss of some body hair.)

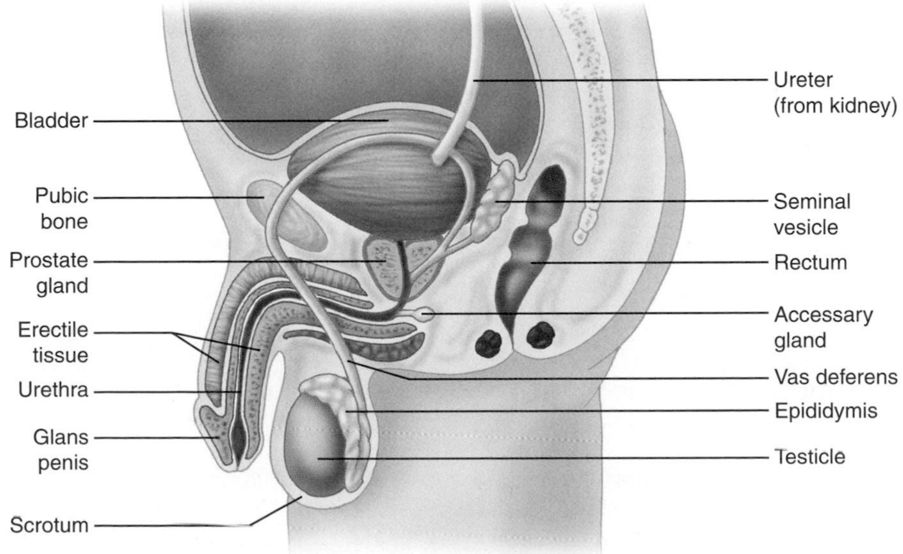

Figure 9.3: The male reproductive system

Fill in the Blanks

Use Figure 9-3 to help you fill in the blanks about the organs of the male reproductive system.

1. The _____________ sits dorsally and somewhat superior to the testes.
2. The testes are located internally in the _____________.
3. An organ called the _____________ is anatomically located in the scrotal, inguinal, and peritoneal areas and is androgen dependent.
4. The _____________ is a canal-shaped organ that sits medially in the penile shaft.
5. The _____________ are situated inferior to the penis bilaterally.

Word parts: male reproductive system

A number of core terms related to the male reproductive system appear frequently when working in health care with male clients. It is important to recognize the combining forms of the roots for these terms. Table 9-3 identifies a number of these. Table 9-4 shows common suffixes that are used to form terms related to this system.

TABLE 9-3: Male Reproductive System: Roots and Combining Forms

Roots and Combining Forms	Meaning
ur	urine
urethr/o/a	urethra
vas/o	vascular; a fluid-carrying vessel or duct
vesicul/o	a bladder or bladder-shaped container; a vesicle
prostat/e/o	prostate
test/o	testes; testicle
testicul/o	testes
orch/o orchid/o orchid/o	testes
didymis	testicle; can also mean *twin* or *double*
balan/o	penis
pen/o	penis
duc	to lead

TABLE 9-4: Suffixes Used with *Test/o, Testicul/o, Pen/o,* and *Erect/o*

BEGIN with a Root or Combining Form	ADD a Suffix	CREATE a Medical Term
test/o	-icle (very small)	testicle
test/o	-es	testes (plural)
testicul/o	-ar	testicular
pen/o	-ile (relating to)	penile
erect/o (to stand)	-ile	erectile
erect/o	-ion (action or condition)	erection

Build a Word

Refer to Figure 9-3. Combine the word parts to form a term that is related to the male reproductive system.

1. the prefix *epi-* (on) + a combining word meaning *testicle* ________________
2. a short word meaning *vascular* + *deferens* ________________
3. a root meaning to *lead* + *deferens* ________________
4. a combining form meaning *seed* + the suffix *-al* ________________

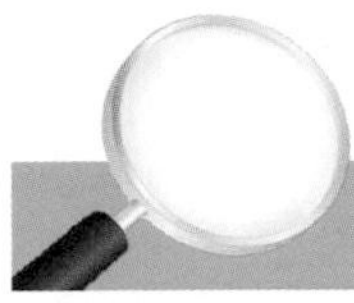

FOCUS POINT: Epididymis

In some text references, the epididymis is considered an internal organ, whereas in others it is identified as an external one. As a student of language, it is not necessary to enter this debate, as long as you know what the word means.

Male genitalia

Recall from Chapter 8 that *genitalia* is the term used to identify reproductive organs and structures located in the lower abdomen and pelvis. In addition, recall that the genitalia are made up of both external and internal organs.

Key terms: external male genitalia

The external or surface portion of the male genitalia includes the penis and the *scrotum*. The scrotum contains the *testicles*. The structures of the penis include the *shaft*, the *glans*, and the *foreskin*.

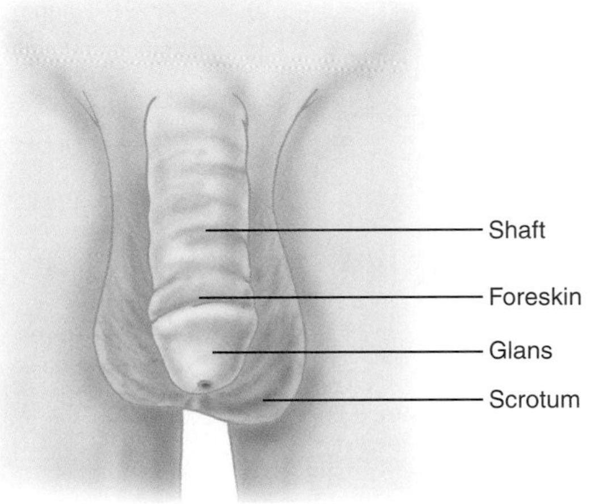

Figure 9.4: External male genitalia

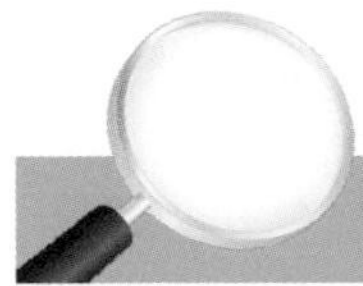

FOCUS POINT: Testes and Scrotum

Although the testes are considered internal reproductive organs, they are actually external to the body. The testes are situated within the scrotum, which is a pouch-like sac made of skin. The testes are internal to the scrotum; however, both the scrotum and the testes are external to the body.

Key terms: internal male genitalia

The internal portion of the male genitalia includes the following organs and glands. Refer to Figure 9-5 to discover where each is located.

vas deferens: a duct (a narrow channel or tube-shaped vessel) that carries sperm from the epididymis to the ejaculatory duct in the urethra.

urethra: a tube-like structure that extends from the bladder to the outside of the body. In males, the urethra exits at the distal end of the penis, the **glans penis.** (In females, this exit point is located between the clitoris and the vagina.)

seminal vesicles: two sac-like glands that sit below the bladder in males. They produce a substance that enhances the viability and motility (movement) of sperm.

ejaculatory duct: the duct that conveys sperm from the vas deferens into the urethra.

prostate gland: a gland that secretes a substance that forms part of the semen.

bulbourethral glands (also known as **Cowper's glands**): two small glands on either side of the prostate that are similar in function to Bartholin's glands in females (see Chapter 8). The bulbourethral glands secrete a substance called *pre-ejaculate* to help lubricate the urethra. (Note: *Bulb/o* is a combining form meaning *bulb-shaped.*)

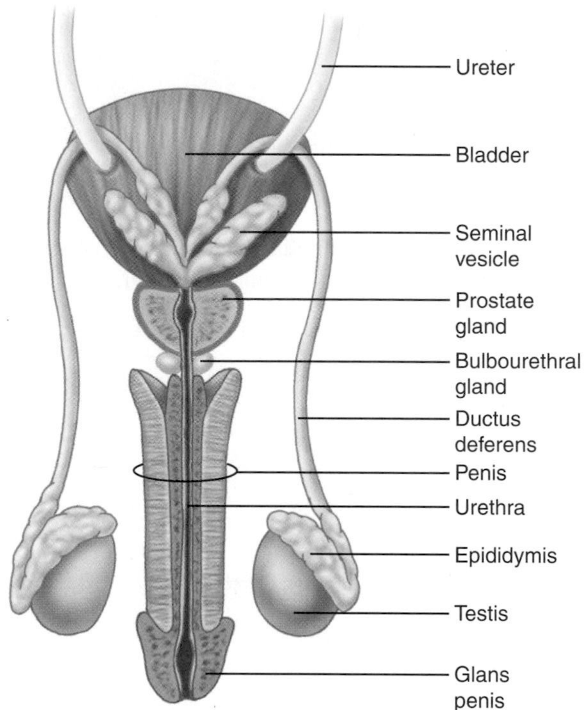

Figure 9.5: Internal male genitalia

The prostate gland

The prostate is a small gland in the male reproductive system. The fluid produced by this gland contributes to the production of semen. **Semen** is a secretion that is discharged through the urethra of a male at the time of ejaculation. It is composed of the products of the prostate and bulbourethral glands, plus spermatozoa. **Spermatozoa** is the plural form of *spermatozoon,* meaning *a mature male sex cell.* Spermatozoa are produced in the testicles and stored in the seminal vesicles.

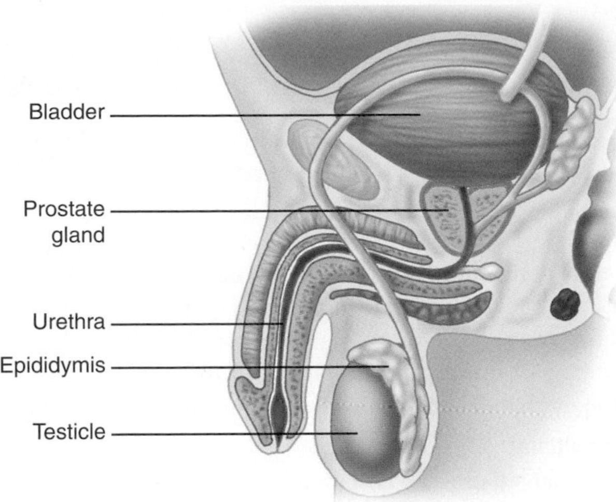

Figure 9.6: The prostate gland

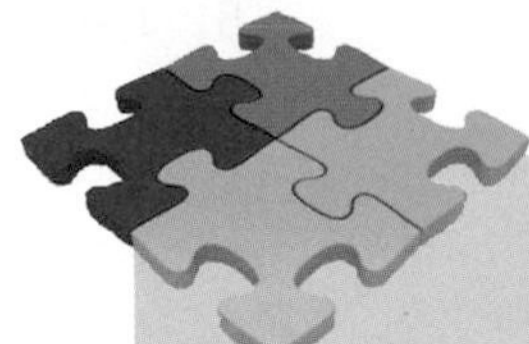

WORD BUILDING: Formula for Creating Words with the Combining Forms *Sperma* and *Spermat/o*

sperma = spermatozoa; semen. The combining forms are *sperma* and *spermat/o.*

spermati + cide = *spermaticide*

Definition: something that destroys sperm. (The second root derives from *cidus,* meaning *to kill.* A synonym is *spermicide.*) *noun*

Example: Some birth control products are designed as *spermaticides.*

sperma + cysto + tomy = *spermatocystotomy*

Definition: drainage of the sperm from the seminal vesicles by surgical incision. (The root *cysto-* means bladder [and, in this case, *vessel*]. The suffix *-tomy* means *incision.*) *noun*

Example: A condition of seminal vesicle enlargement may be a case for *spermatocystotomy.*

spermato + logy = *spermatology*

Definition: the study of seminal fluid. *noun*

Example: *Spermatology* includes the sciences of embryology, physiology, and histology.

Build a Word

Use your knowledge of word parts and word construction to create terms that may be new to you. Combine the word parts given, and then write the meaning of each new term.

1. uria spermat/o ____________________ Meaning: ____________________
2. pathy spermat/o ____________________ Meaning: ____________________
3. genesis spermat/o ____________________ Meaning: ____________________

Right Word or Wrong Word: *Sperm* or *Semen*?

Are these two words interchangeable? Are they synonymous? Think about your answer before referring to the Answer Key.

Prostate pathologies

In the dialogues with our patient Zane Davis, you've learned that the changes in the prostate gland over a lifetime can cause changes in urinary health. The prostate is also very vulnerable to cancer. Figure 9-6 shows the anatomical location of this gland and how its proximity to the urethra and bladder can impede the flow of urine. Notice that the prostate gland sits inferior to the bladder, where it empties into the urethra. The prostate also sits just anterior to the rectum.

Benign prostatic hyperplasia

The technical term for an enlarged prostate is **benign prostatic hyperplasia (BPH)**. The enlargement of the prostate is a natural occurrence in the male body that results from the presence of testosterone, which triggers the prostate's growth over a man's life span. The most common symptoms of BPH include the following urinary problems: hesitancy, frequency, urgency, and **nocturia** (the need to urinate during the night). To diagnose BPH, prostatic cancer must first be ruled out, because the symptoms of BPH and the more serious condition of cancer are almost identical. In cases of BPH that significantly impede the passage of urine, surgery may be necessary to correct the problem.

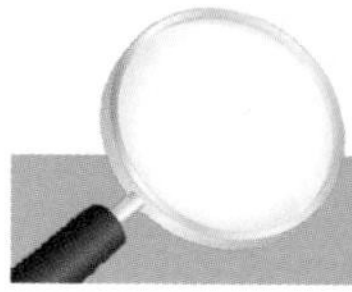

FOCUS POINT: Benign Prostatic Hyperplasia

The medical diagnosis of benign prostatic hyperplasia (BPH) identifies a condition in which the prostate gland enlarges. It is *not* a type of cancer. BPH usually occurs as men reach their senior years. It is also known as *benign prostatic hypertrophy* (enlargement).

Right Word or Wrong Word: *Prostate* or *Prostrate*?

Do these two terms refer to the same thing? Are they both related to the male reproductive system?

Prostate cancer

The incidence of prostate cancer (carcinoma of the prostate gland) is on the rise in the United States and in much of the world. One reason for this may be that men are living much longer lives, and, as the prostate gland ages and enlarges, it becomes more vulnerable to cancer-producing agents.

As noted previously, the symptoms of prostate cancer can mimic those of benign prostatic hyperplasia. When these symptoms occur, a blood test called a *PSA* (prostate-specific antigen) is used to rule out cancer. Assessment also includes a digital rectal examination (DRE) because the prostate lies so close to the rectum that the enlargement of the prostate gland can be felt through the rectum. Should both of these preliminary examinations prove to be negative, the chance of prostate cancer is determined as very low. Even so, the physician or health care provider will want to follow the patient's prostate health more frequently in the future. Prostate cancer can be life threatening if it is not caught early. Available treatments include hormone therapy, radiation, chemotherapy, and the removal of the prostate gland (prostatectomy).

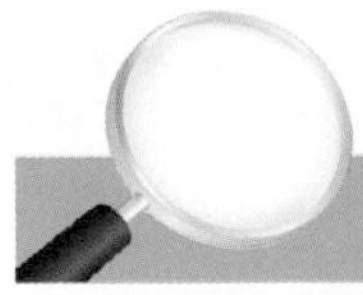

FOCUS POINT: Cancer and Oncology

Oncology is the field of medicine and science that is dedicated to cancer research, treatment, and care. *Carcinoma* is the medical term for cancer.

Diagnostic tests: prostate gland

Acid phosphatase and the prostatic acid phosphatase (PAP) test: Acid phosphatase is an enzyme found mostly in the prostate gland. It is assessed by a blood test. Increased levels of this enzyme in the blood can indicate that prostatic cancer has **metastasized** (spread to the rest of the body).

Prostate-specific antigen (PSA) test: This blood test detects glycoprotein in cells of the prostate gland. PSA levels increase in the presence of prostate cancer, with higher levels indicating more advanced stages of cancer.

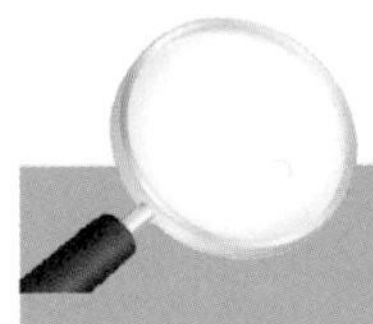

FOCUS POINT: PAP and Pap: Diagnostic Examination for Men or Women?

As a health care professional, you must listen carefully and be attuned to the context of where and when you hear or see the initials *PAP or Pap.* There is a PAP/Pap test for both men and women, but they are distinctly different:

Prostatic acid phosphatase (PAP): a blood test for men that measures acid phosphatase from the prostate gland.

Papanicolaou test (Pap test): a test for cervical cancer in women that is performed by taking a Papanicolaou (Pap) smear, which is a collection of cellular material from within the cervix, and then analyzing the cells in the laboratory.

Fill in the Blanks

Consider all that you've learned about the language of the male reproductive system so far. Use this knowledge to complete these sentences.

1. An ________________ is a necessary condition of the penis before ejaculation.
2. Glands ________________ substances such as hormones.
3. The attending physician in the ER wants a diagnostic assessment of Mr. Davis's ________________ ________________ to determine if its condition has led to the patient's incontinence.
4. The ________________ are located within the scrotum.
5. As a man ages, the ________________ can be impeded by the enlargement of the prostate gland.
6. Male sex hormones are called ________________.
7. The epididymis is external to the main body but internal to the ________________.
8. The urinary meatus (opening) of the male is located on the ________________
9. A ________________ is the removal of the prostate gland through surgery.
10. A researcher who is interested in cancer works in the field of ________________.

Let's Practice

Name the part of the male reproductive system that fits each description.

1. This organ surrounds the urethra and can impair the passage of urine. ________________
2. This organ has two functions and is located externally on the body. ________________
3. The ________________ coordinates the growth and development of the genitalia and the reproductive system.
4. Spermatozoa are stored in this organ. ________________

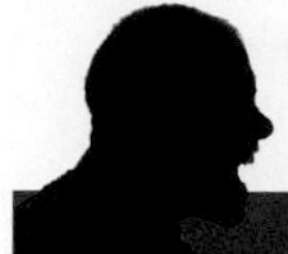

PRONUNCIATION PRACTICE

Say these words aloud to a friend or classmate if you can. You are given the phonetic pronunciation. Your instructor can help you with pronunciation,

or visit **http://www.MedicalLanguageLab.com.** 

andrology	ăn-**drŏ**´lō-gē
androstenedione	ăn-drō-stēn″**dī**´ōn or ăn-dr_-**stēn**´dē-ōn″
benign	bē-**nīn´**
preandrogens	prē-**ăn**´drŭ-jĕnz
spermatocystotomy	spĕr″mă-tō-sĭs-**tŏt**´ō-mē
spermatozoa	spĕr″mă-t-ō-**zō**´ ă
testes	**tĕs**´tēs

The Language of the Respiratory System

Patient Update

Dr. Jackson on Unit 8B at Okla Trauma center has reviewed Mr. Zane Davis's medical chart. He has identified some worrying signs and symptoms of possible respiratory problems, including abnormal levels of oxygen in the blood, shortness of breath, and the sound of crackles in the lungs. These prompt him to interview and examine the patient.

"Good afternoon. I'm Dr. Jackson. Are you Zane Davis?" the physician asked as he entered the patient's room. When the patient confirmed his identity and this safety precaution was taken care of, the physician explained his presence. He said that he would be taking over Mr. Davis's care for now and attending to his health needs. The doctor paused a moment, taking his stethoscope from around his neck and preparing to use it.

"I have a few questions for you, and I'd like to examine your chest, Mr. Davis." The patient agreed. "Are you having any shortness of breath now, sir?" Mr. Davis indicated that he was not. "Good. Please sit up for a moment. I'd like to listen to your lungs." Dr. Jackson reached over and began the exam. He placed his stethoscope over the intercostal spaces of the patient's rib cage. He asked the patient to breathe in and out and then to hold his breath. The patient had difficulty filling his lungs completely, and the doctor mentioned this to him. He also told Mr. Davis that he heard some dry, crackling sounds. "Do you smoke, Mr. Davis?" Dr. Jackson inquired as he took the patient's hands one at a time to examine the fingertips and nailbeds. At the same time, Mr. Davis's son, Quincy, returned to the room. Zane introduced his son and then replied to the doctor's question.

"Yes, sir, I've smoked all my life. Started in the Navy when I was about 18," Mr. Davis replied, a bit defiantly. "Been all over the world," he said. "Fourteen years in the Navy. Saw action, too." Dr. Jackson nodded and continued with the interview.

"In the Navy, you say. Mmm-hmm. And how old are you again?" Mr. Davis said that he was 74 years old. Again the doctor nodded, as if thinking to himself. Then he asked, "Have you ever been diagnosed with any lung disorders?" Quincy looked worried, but his father did not. Mr. Davis told the doctor that he was prone to bronchitis and that he'd had pneumonia a few times over the years. He added that he sometimes now felt a strain on his lungs when he was doing something quite physical, but he chalked that up to "old age."

"Uh-huh, I see," said the doctor. "Well, since your lab tests have come back with some abnormal results that look like they are respiratory in nature, I'd like to pursue this with you for a bit before we release you from the hospital. I'm just headed down to Radiology now to consult with Dr. Krenshaw about your x-ray and CT results. When I learn more, I'll get back to you, and we can make some plans." With that, Dr. Jackson said his farewells and departed.

Reflective Questions

Reflect on the story that you've just read.

1. Why does Dr. Jackson ask this patient if he smokes?

 ____

2. Which one of Mr. Davis's body systems is now of more concern to the doctor?

 ____

Critical Thinking Question

Answer this question based on the scenario.

Dr. Jackson used a safety precaution when he first met with Mr. Davis. This is standard practice for health professionals. What was the safety precaution, and why did he do it?

____

____

Key terms: respiratory assessment

The following passages from the dialogue between Dr. Jackson and Mr. Davis show some of the processes used to assess a patient's respiratory health. Key terms, phrases, and abbreviations are italicized in the example and highlighted below with the explanation.

"... *abnormal levels of oxygen* in the blood ..."

abnormal levels of oxygen: this finding indicates that gas exchanges in the respiratory system are not functioning normally.

"... the sound of *crackles* in the lungs."

crackles: a crackling sound that occurs within the lungs when the lungs are inflamed or when they are congested with mucous or other fluids.

"... over the *intercostal spaces* ..."

intercostal spaces: the spaces between the ribs.

"... to *examine the fingertips* and *nailbeds*."

examine the fingertips: the doctor is looking at the shape of the patient's fingers, particularly the fingertips. **Clubbing** or club-shaped fingers can be a sign of chronic **hypoxemia** (low levels of oxygen in the blood over a long period).

nailbeds: the parts of the fingers that are covered by fingernails; examining the color of the nailbeds and their ability to quickly return to normal color after being pressed for a second or two helps the doctor to diagnose the patient's cardiac output and whether he suffers from hypoxia. A bluish color to the nailbeds signals cyanosis, and the slow return of color signals poor circulation and capillary refill. Recall that the prefix cyano- means blue (Chapter 2).

"... he was *prone to bronchitis* ..."

prone to: susceptible; likely to get.

bronchitis: inflammation of the bronchi (the air passageways in the lungs).

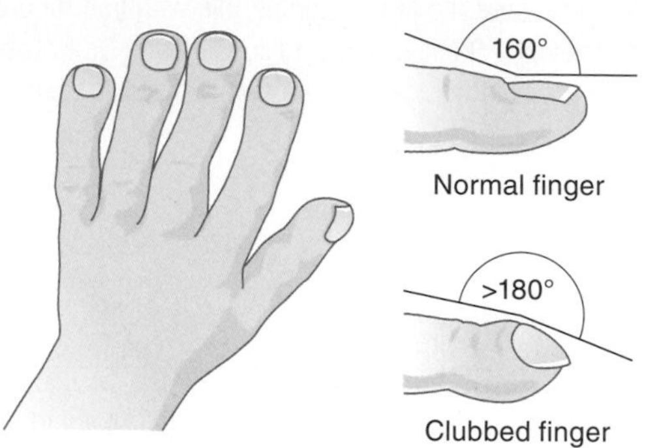

Figure 9.7: Clubbing of the fingers

Anatomy and Physiology: Respiratory System

All of the doctors who have examined Mr. Davis have been concerned about his respiratory status. To understand Mr. Davis's condition, you need to be familiar with the anatomical terminology of the respiratory system. The term *respiratory* derives from the root word *respire.*

Respire is a root word meaning *to breathe oxygen and expel carbon dioxide.*

Respiration means *the act of breathing.*

Respiratory means *related to breathing.*

TABLE 9-5: Medical Terms Using the Word Respiratory

BEGIN with *Respiratory*	ADD Another Term	CREATE a New Term	Meaning
respiratory	failure	respiratory failure	any impairment in ventilation or oxygenation; during respiratory failure, arterial oxygen amounts decrease, and carbon dioxide amounts increase
respiratory	distress	respiratory distress	severe impairment of respiratory function with the potential for death
respiratory	therapy	respiratory therapy	any treatment that preserves or improves respiratory function

The respiratory system consists of the major organs of the *lungs, pharynx, larynx,* and the *trachea.* Recall from Chapter 6 that *pharynx* is the anatomical term for the throat and that *larynx* is the anatomical term for the voice box.

Generally, the respiratory system is associated with the *thorax* or chest; however, it is actually much more extensive than that. The respiratory system extends from both the nasal and oral cavities (see Chapter 6), down through the pharynx, and into the lungs (see Figure 9-8.) The major muscle of the respiratory system is the *diaphragm,* which is situated just below and behind the lower ribs, inferior to the heart.

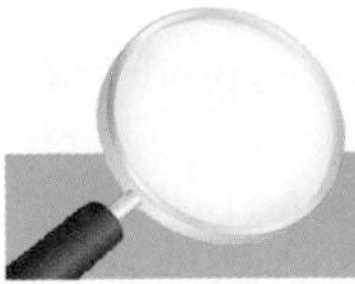

FOCUS POINT: Anatomical Location of the Thorax

Recall from Chapter 2 that the thorax or chest is located on the transverse (axial) plane of the body. This plane divides the body horizontally into superior (upper) and inferior (lower) halves. Also recall that the combining form of the word *thorax* is *thorac/o.*

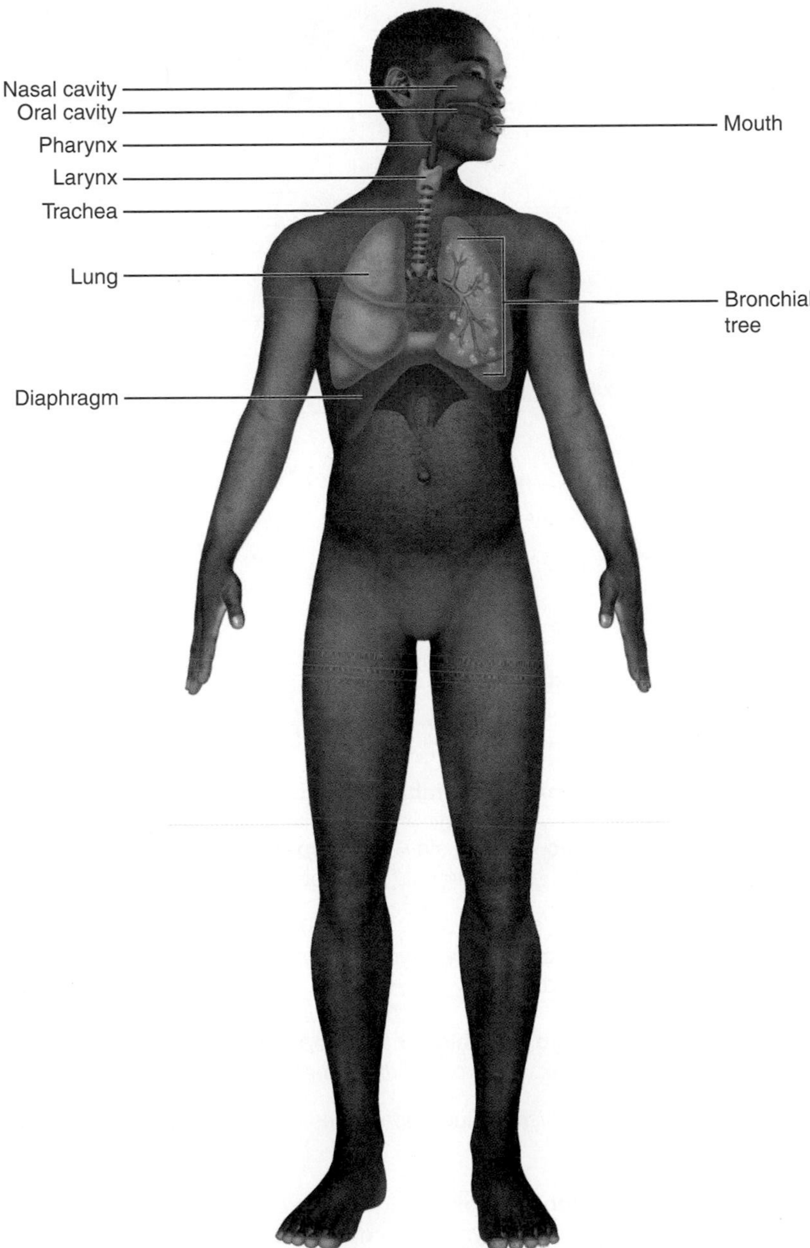

Figure 9.8: The respiratory system

The larynx

The **larynx** or voice box is an organ that is essential to the processes of breathing, voice production (*phonation*), and swallowing (*deglutition;* see Chapter 11). Anatomically, the larynx sits at the entrance to the esophagus. As air passes across the larynx during the process of expiration (exhaling), the vocal cords within it change position and tension, vibrate, and are able to create sound and voice.

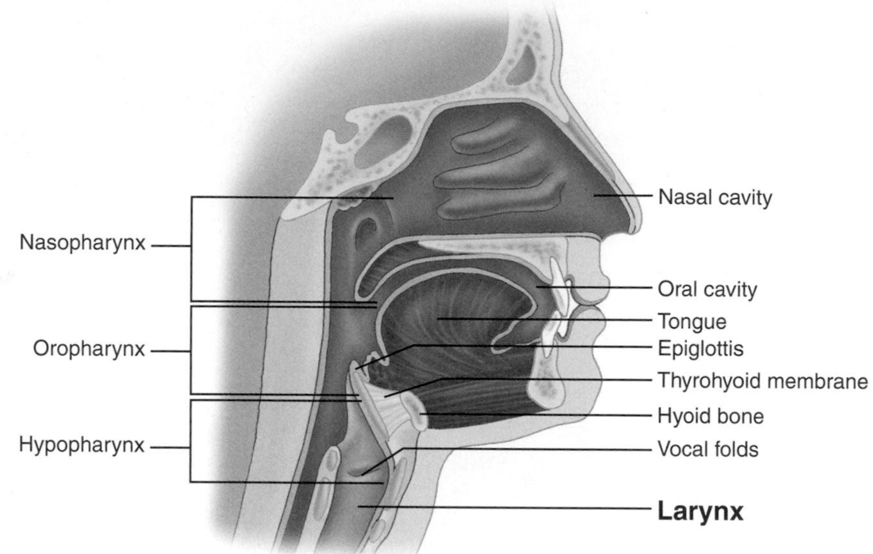

Figure 9.9: The larynx

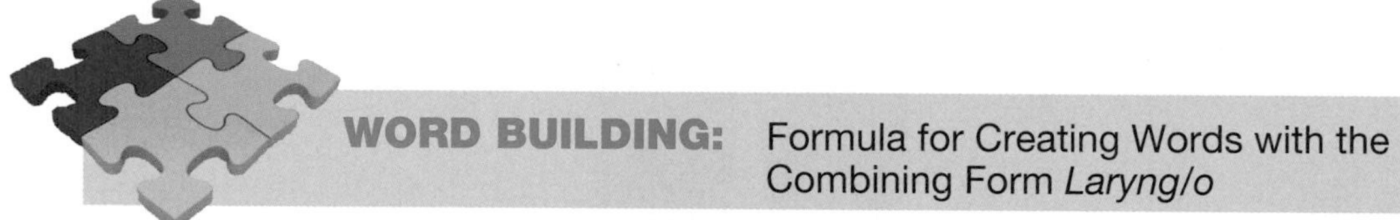

WORD BUILDING: Formula for Creating Words with the Combining Form *Laryng/o*

larynx = upper windpipe; voice box. The combining form is *laryng/o.*

laryngo + paralysis = *laryngoparalysis*
Definition: paralysis of the muscles of the larynx. (The root word *paralysis* means *to disable. noun*

Example: *Laryngoparalysis* can be caused by physical trauma, toxins, infection, or it may be an adverse reaction to some medications.

laryngo + phthisis = *laryngophthisis*
Definition: tuberculosis of the larynx. (The root *phthisis* means *wasting.*) *noun*

Example: Symptoms of *laryngophthisis* include hoarseness, cough, and the formation of an ulcer (sore) on the larynx.

laryngo + xeros + is = *laryngoxerosis*
Definition: an abnormal dryness of the larynx. (The root *xeros* means *dry.*) *noun*

Example: *Laryngoxerosis* may occur as a result of dehydration or of any illness that impairs the production of sufficient mucous to coat and protect the larynx.

Build a Word

Use your knowledge of word parts and word construction to create terms that may be new to you. Combine the word parts given, and then write the meaning of the new term.

1. -itis laryng/o ______________ Meaning: ______________
2. -ectomy laryng/o ______________ Meaning: ______________
3. parhyng/o -itis laryng/o ______________ Meaning: ______________
4. scope laryng/o ______________ Meaning: ______________

The trachea

The **trachea** or windpipe is a cartilaginous organ that permits the flow of air into and out of the respiratory system; it connects the oral and nasal cavities to the lungs. The trachea is situated in the neck. It sits anterior to the sixth cervical vertebra of the spine and immediately inferior to the larynx. The trachea extends down through the throat to a place where it ends near the fifth thoracic vertebra. It lies anterior to the esophagus (see Figure 9-10). The trachea eventually divides into two main branches called the *bronchi*. (Recall from Chapter 4 that cartilage is a specific type of connective tissue. Focus Point: Cartilage explains even more.)

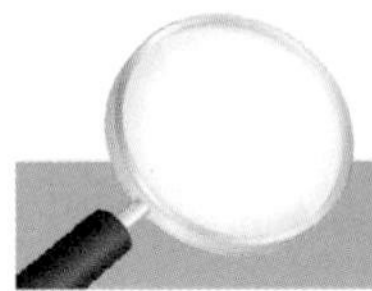

FOCUS POINT: Cartilage

Cartilage is a stiff yet flexible type of connective tissue that does not contain blood vessels.

Hyaline cartilage is found between bones, within the ribcage, and within the discs of the spinal column. It is also found in the nasal septum and the trachea.

Elastic cartilage is found in the ear, the nose, and the trachea.

Fibrous cartilage is found in the meniscus at the end of a bone, where that bone meets another bone in a joint (i.e., in the joints of the ankle, knee, and elbow).

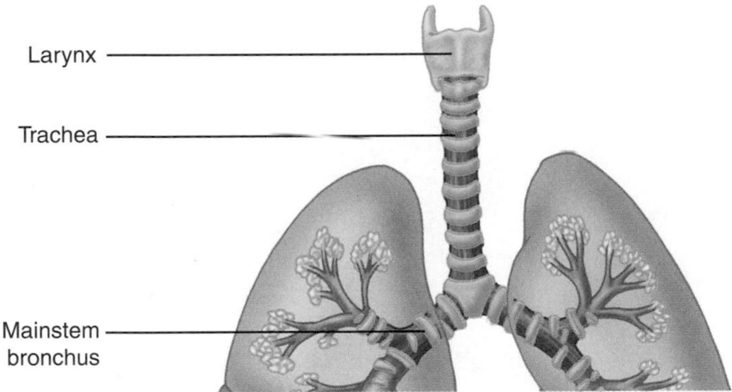

Figure 9.10: The trachea

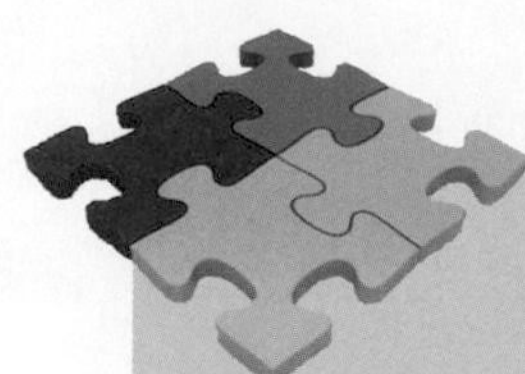

WORD BUILDING: Formula for Creating Words with the Combining forms *Trache/o* and *Trachelo-*

trachea = originally meant *rough;* now means *windpipe.* The combining form is *trache/o. Trachelo-* is a combining form meaning *neck.*

tracheo + stom + y = *tracheostomy*
Definition: an incision into the trachea to open the airway passage when it is blocked. (The second root is *stoma,* meaning *mouth or opening*. A synonym is *tracheotomy.*) *noun*

Example: A *tracheostomy* is an emergency procedure that can save a person's life.

tracheo + broncho + megaly = *tracheobronchomegaly*
Definition: a condition in which the trachea and the bronchi are larger than normal. (The root *bronchus,* meaning *windpipe,* appears in its combining form.) *noun*

Example: *Tracheobronchomegaly* is also known as *Mounier-Kuhn syndrome,* and it is associated with respiratory infections.

trachel + ismus = *trachelismus*
Definition: a spasm of the neck in which the neck is thrown backward. (The suffix *-ismus* means *condition.*) *noun*

Example: *Trachelismus* can sometimes be observed just before an epileptic seizure.

Bronchi and bronchioles

The **bronchi** consist of two bronchial tubes that branch off from the trachea as it reaches the lungs. They transport air directly into the lungs. Often referred to as the *primary bronchi*, these air tubes further divide into branches within the lungs called *secondary bronchi* or *intrapulmonary bronchi*. As they approach the lungs, the secondary bronchi become smaller and smaller. At this stage, they are called **bronchioles**.

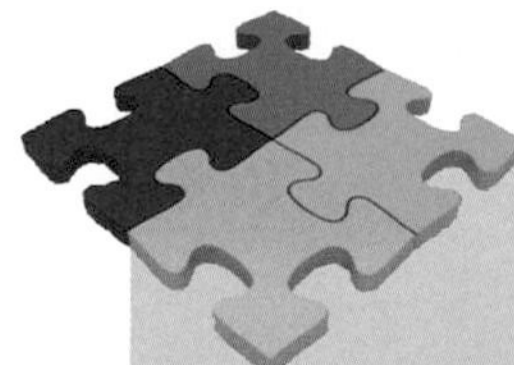

WORD BUILDING: Formula for Creating Words with the Combining forms *Bronch/i/io/o* and *Bronchiol/io/o*

bronchus = windpipe. The combining forms are *bronch/i/io/o.*

bronch + itis = *bronchitis*
Definition: inflammation of the mucous membranes in the bronchi. *noun*

Example: *Bronchitis* produces a harsh, painful, recurring cough that produces sputum.

broncho + blenno + rrhea = *bronchoblennorrhea*
Definition: a type of chronic bronchitis in which there is an excessive production of sputum. (The second root is *blennos,* meaning *mucous.*) *noun*

Example: The sputum produced by a patient with *bronchoblennorrhea* is purulent (consists of pus).

bronchi + ectasis = *bronchiectasis*

Definition: a condition in which there is a chronic dilation of the bronchi, usually as a result of a longstanding infection. (The word part *ectasis* means *dilation.*) *noun*

Example: Left untreated for too long, tuberculosis can cause *bronchiectasis.*

bronchio + gen + ic = *bronchiogenic*

Definition: originating in the bronchi. *adjective*

Example: *Bronchiogenic* cancer is one of the most frequent types of malignant carcinomas.

broncho + pneumonia + *bronchopneumonia*

Definition: a complication of bronchitis in which one or more of the lobes of the lungs become plugged with mucous or exudate (waste). (The root word *pneumonia* indicates lung inflammation.) *noun*

Example: *Bronchopneumonia* is thought to be more common in children than in adults.

bronchiolus = air passage. The combining forms are *brochiol/o/io.*

bronchiol + itis = *bronchiolitis*

Definition: inflammation of the bronchioles. *noun*

Example: Although it is not common in adulthood, *bronchiolitis* occurs in infants and newborns, and it is noticed in the presence of sneezing, wheezing, runny nose, and rapid breathing.

Build a Word

Combine each set of word parts to create a medical term. Then, using your knowledge from previous chapters, define each term in your own words.

1. edema bronch/i/o/io ____________ Meaning: ____________
2. rrhagia bronchi/i/io ____________ Meaning: ____________
3. rrhaphy bronchi/o/io ____________ Meaning: ____________
4. trache/o tomy laryng/o ____________ Meaning: ____________
5. -algia trache/o ____________ Meaning: ____________

Let's Practice

Write the medical term that fits each description.

1. a medical condition in which two respiratory illnesses combine to form one and in which portions of the lungs may be plugged by mucus ____________
2. this condition produces frequent, painful, and loud coughing ____________
3. a respiratory infection that is not attended to for a long period can lead to this condition ____________
4. organs that sit bilaterally in the thoracic cavity ____________
5. a structure that is located inferior to the heart, lungs, and rib cage ____________
6. two hollow spaces that are important to the respiratory system and that are located within the cranium ____________
7. an air passage composed of a tough connective tissue ____________
8. a structure that is situated at the anterior of the pharynx and inferior to the oral cavity ____________
9. a structure that is involved in the production of sound and voice ____________
10. the sinuses are found here ____________

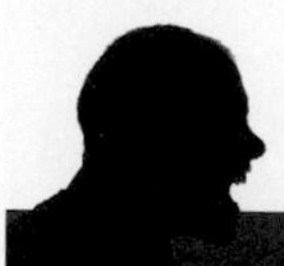

PRONUNCIATION PRACTICE

Say these words aloud to a friend or classmate if you can. You are given the phonetic pronunciation. Your instructor can help you with pronunciation,

or visit **http://www.MedicalLanguageLab.com.**

bronchi	**brŏng**´kī
bronchiole	**brŏng**´kē-ōl
bronchiectasis	brŏng″kē-**ĕk**´tă-sĭs
hyaline	**hī**´ă-līn
laryngoparalysis	lăr-ĭn″gō-păr-**ăl**´ĭ-sĭs
laryngophthisis	lăr″ĭng-**gŏf**´thĭ-sĭs
laryngoxerosis	lăr-ĭn″gō-zĕr-**ō**´sĭs
laryngopharyngitis	lăr-ĭn″gō-făr-ĭn-**jī**´tĭs
respiratory	rĕs-**pīr**´ă-tō-rē or **rĕs**´pĭ-ră-tō″rē
thorax	**thō**´răks
tracheostomy	trā″kē-**ŏs**´tō-mē
tracheotomy	trā″kē-**ŏt**´ō-mē
tracheobronchomegaly	trā″kē-ō-brŏng″kō-**mĕg**´ă-lē

The lungs

The **lungs** are at the core of the respiratory system, and they are crucial to life. They are cone-shaped organs that sit lateral to the heart in the pleural cavity of the thorax. Each lung is divided into lobes. Understanding the language of the anatomy, physiology, and function of the lungs is essential in most health care situations. Medical terms that relate to the lungs generally include the root word *pulmonary.*

Situated within the thoracic cavity, the *pleural cavity* is actually two cavities that are divided at a point near the mid sternum. Each cavity is lined with **pleura**, a type of **serous membrane** (membrane supplied by blood). The function of the pleural cavities is to protect the lungs from coming into direct contact with the thoracic wall and the diaphragm.

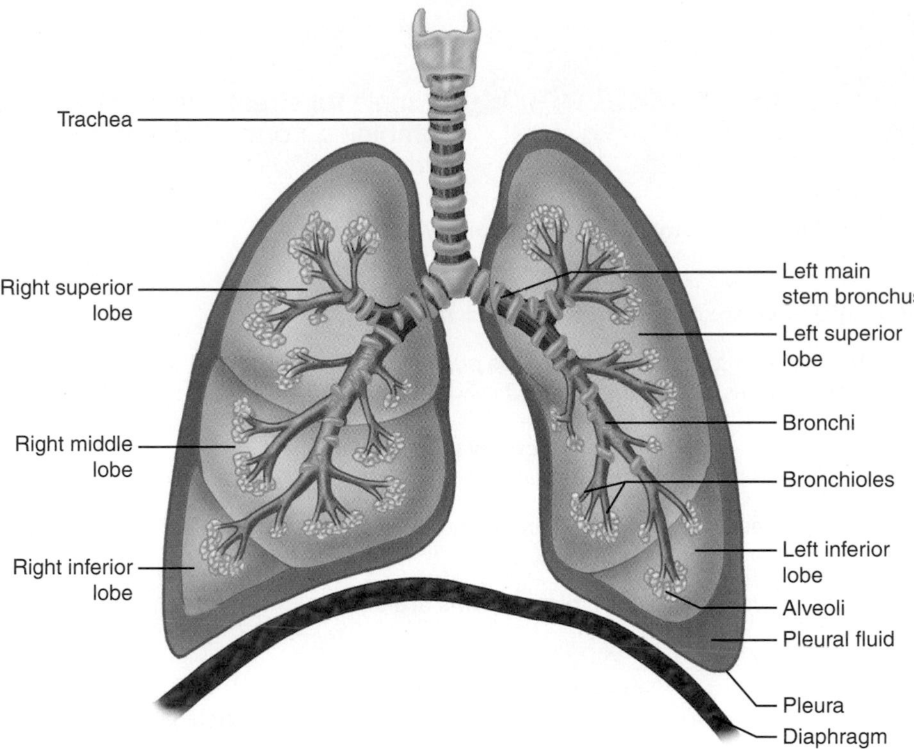

Figure 9.11: Anatomy of the lungs

Lobes of the lungs

The *lobes* of the lungs can be described by their shape. The top of each lobe is called its *apex*. The broader or lower portion of the lobe is referred to as its *base*.

Lobes are divided by gaps called **fissures**. The left lung is divided by an oblique fissure, which divides it into superior and inferior portions. The right lung is divided into three lobes: superior, middle, and inferior. An oblique fissure divides the inferior and middle lobes; a horizontal fissure divides the superior and middle lobes (see Figure 9-12).

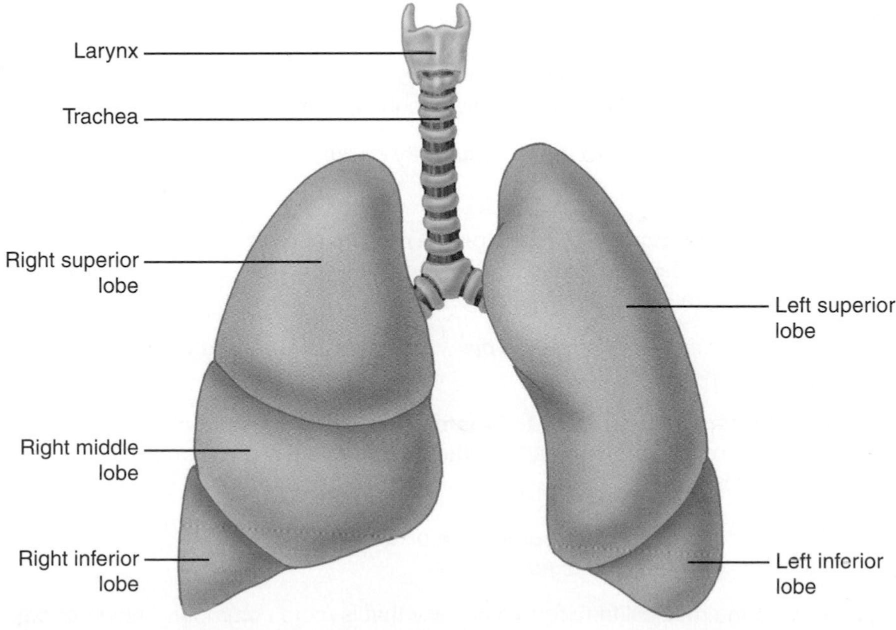

Figure 9.12: Lobes of the lungs

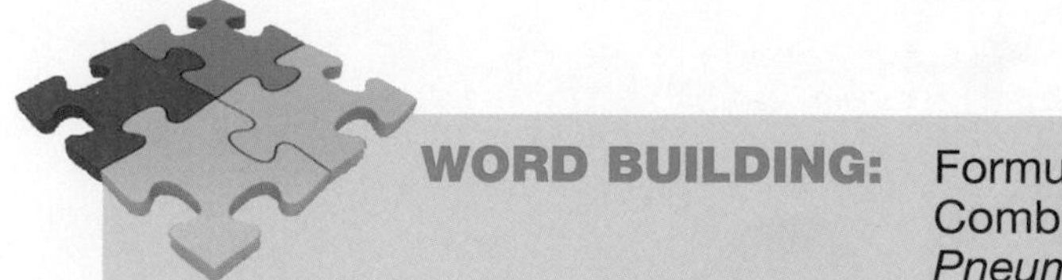

WORD BUILDING: Formula for Creating Words with the Combining Forms *Pulmon/o, Pulmo, Pneumo-,* and *Pleuro*

1. pulmonis = lung. The combing form is *pulmon/o* or *pulmo.*

pulmon + itis = *pulmonitis*
Definition: inflammation of the lung; pneumonia. *noun*

Example: The bacteria and viruses that cause *pulmonitis* infect the alveoli of the lungs and can overrun entire lobes of the lungs.

pulmon + ectomy = *pulmonectomy*
Definition: surgical removal of a lung. *noun*

Example: In some cases of pulmonary carcinoma (lung cancer), a *pulmonectomy* is the treatment of choice to save the patient's life.

2. pneuma = air or breath. The combining forms are *pneum/a/ato, pneum/o,* and *pneumono.*

pneumat + osis = *pneumatosis*
Definition: a condition of air or gas being found in the body where it should not be. *noun*

Example: *Pneumatosis* can occur if a lung is punctured and air escapes into the pleural cavity or the thorax.

pneumo + bulb + ar = *pneumobulbar*
Definition: referring to both the respiratory center in the brain (the medulla oblongata) and the lungs. *adjective*

Example: A *pneumobulbar* trauma can lead to the need for a ventilator to help the patient breathe.

pneumo + dynamics = *pneumodynamics*
Definition: the field of science, research, and treatment concerned with the force required to breathe. (The second root in this word is *dynamis,* meaning *force.*) *noun*

Example: Respiratory technicians work in the field of *pneumodynamics.*

pneumo + hydro + thorax = *pneumohydrothorax*
Definition: a condition in which fluid, gas, or air is found in the pleural cavity. *noun*

Example: Blood or air escaping into the pleural cavity causes the condition of *pneumohydrothorax.*

pneumono + melan + osis = *pneumonomelanosis*
Definition: a condition of black or blackening of lung tissue. (The second root is *melano,* meaning *black.* A synonym is *pneumomelanosis.*) *noun*

Example: *Pneumonomelanosis* is known as *black lung disease,* and it is the result of years of inhalation of coal dust.

3. pleura = side. *Pleura* is the term for the membrane that encases both lungs and separates them from the interior walls of the thorax and from the diaphragm. The combining form is *pleur/o.*

pleur + itis = *pleuritis*
Definition: inflammation of the pleura. *noun*

Example: *Pleuritis* is the medical term for the disease that is more commonly known as *pleurisy.*

pleuro + clysis = *pleuroclysis*

Definition: a process of injecting into and then removing fluid from the pleural cavity to clean it. *noun*

Example: The procedure of *pleuroclysis* may be indicated when foreign matter or fluids have been present in the pleural cavity.

Build a Word

Use your word-construction skills to make new medical terms from the following word parts, and then write the meaning of each term.

1. lithiasis pneumo ______________________ Meaning: ______________________
2. ectomy pneum/o/mono ______________________ Meaning: ______________________
3. rrhapy pneumono ______________________ Meaning: ______________________
4. peri- pleuro cardi/o -itis ______________________ Meaning: ______________________
5. pleuro pulmono -ary ______________________ Meaning: ______________________

Function of the respiratory system

Air is all around us. It is made up of a mixture of gases, including water in its gaseous state of vapor. Air is essential to the respiratory system. To understand the constituents of air more completely, see Tables 9-6 and 9-7.

TABLE 9-6: Composition of Inhaled Air

Composition of Inhaled Air
Nitrogen: 79%
Oxygen: 20%
Carbon dioxide: 0.04%

TABLE 9-7: Composition of Exhaled Air

Composition of Exhaled Air
Nitrogen: 79%
Oxygen: 16%
Carbon dioxide: 4%

The respiratory system is designed for gas exchange through the process of respiration, which is composed of inhalation and exhalation. The gases that are exchanged include oxygen, carbon dioxide, and nitrogen. The system is responsible for the oxygenation of the blood and for the removal of carbon dioxide. It also plays a critical role in communication because air passing through the trachea—and, more specifically, the larynx—produces sounds. Within the lungs themselves, gas exchange occurs between the *alveolar sacs* and the blood in the *pulmonary capillaries.*

Alveoli are tiny air sacs in the lungs with structures that accommodate gas exchange. The exchange of gases occurs by a process of diffusion across the alveoli and the cell membranes of the pulmonary capillaries. *Alveoli* is the pleural form of *alveolus,* meaning *a small, hollow pocket or sac.* **Alveoli pulmonis** are the air sacs of the lungs.

The combining form of *alveolus* is *alveol/i/o.*

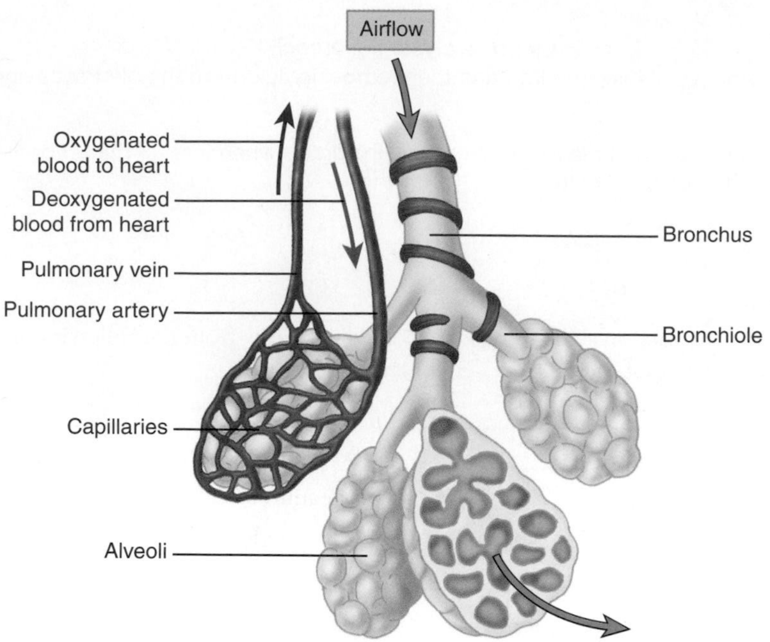

Figure 9.13: Alveoli in the lungs

Physiology of breathing

The process of respiration is more commonly known as *breathing*. Air is inhaled through the mouth and the nasal cavity. In the nasal cavity, it is met by thick mucous membranes that are covered with **cilia**, which are fine, hair-like projections that trap dust, allergens, and other foreign particles and prevent them from entering the respiratory system beyond that point. Next, the air moves into the trachea, down through the bronchi, and into the lungs, where it finishes its journey at the alveoli. When gases are exchanged in the alveoli, used air is then forced out through the system during the reverse process of exhalation.

To inhale and exhale, muscles must contract and expand. The muscle that is most important to breathing is the **diaphragm**. This dome-shaped muscle sits inferior to the lungs. For inhalation, the diaphragm contracts, flattens, and pulls downward toward the abdomen. During exhalation, the diaphragm expands to reduce the amount of space that is available to the lungs, thereby forcing the air within to vacate. The **intercostal muscles**, which are located around the chest wall and between the ribs, assist with the breathing process by allowing the rib cage to expand as the lungs take in air.

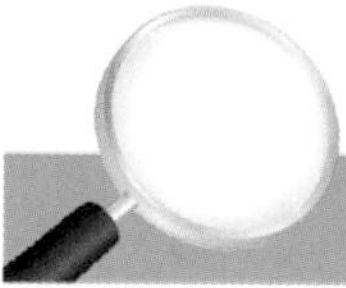

FOCUS POINT: Diaphragm: Organ or Muscle?

There are two schools of thought regarding the diaphragm. In structure, the diaphragm is a muscle, but its importance to respiratory function is so crucial that it is also considered an organ. This is similar to how we refer to the heart.

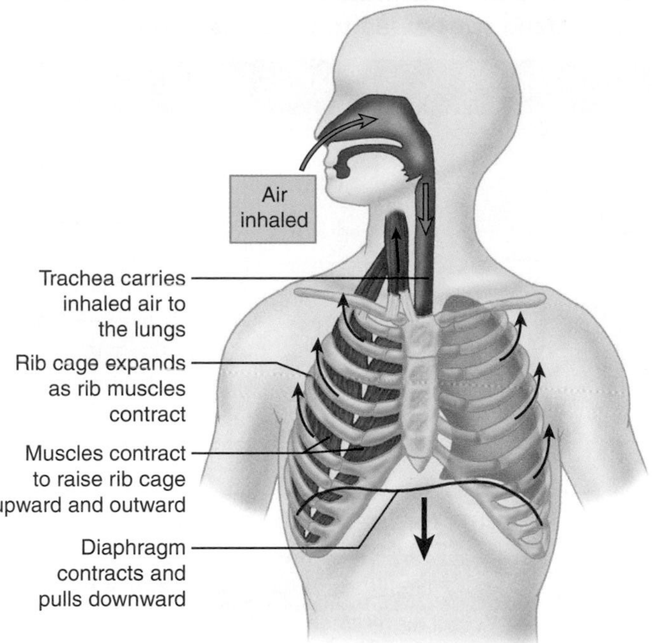

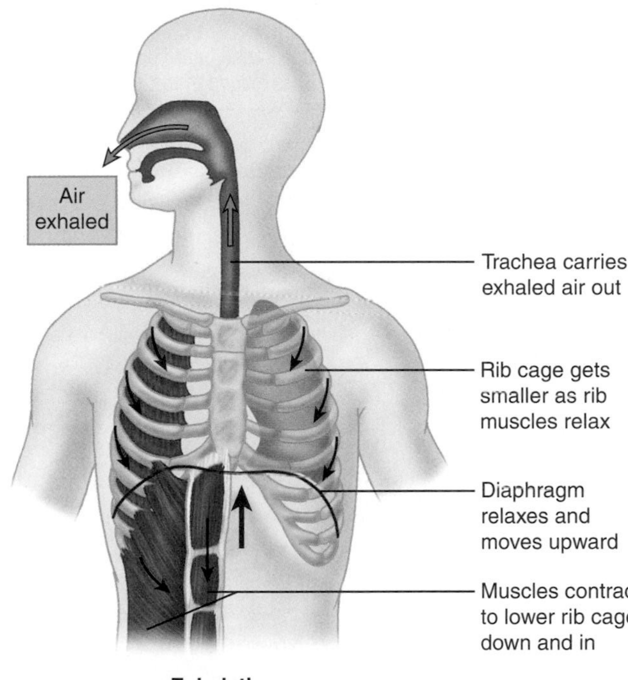

Figure 9.14: Physiology of breathing

TABLE 9-8: Prefixes Used with *-pnea* to Describe Breathing

Prefix	Suffix	New Term and Its Meaning
a-	-pnea	apnea not breathing; breathing has stopped
dys-	-pnea	dyspnea difficulty breathing
eu-	-pnea	eupnea normal breathing
tachy-	-pnea	tachypnea rapid rate of breathing
brady-	-pnea	bradypnea slow rate of breathing

TABLE 9-9: Descriptive Terms for Breathing

Descriptive Term for Breathing	Meaning
Kussmaul's breathing	a very deep, gasping type of breathing that is usually associated with coma or diabetic acidosis
wheezing	a musical, almost whistling sound that occurs on inhalation and exhalation; it signifies an airway obstruction and is often heard in asthmatic patients
stridor	a very loud, harsh sound heard on inspiration (inhalation); it indicates that an object is lodged in the airway

Eponyms: Kussmaul's Breathing

Adolph Kussmaul was a German physician who lived during the nineteenth century. He was also a prolific writer who documented the steps of medical diagnostics and procedures, many of which he also developed. Examples include respiratory diagnostic tests, gastric lavage (washing out of the stomach), and his work on aphasia, which is the inability to use or understand speech. He identified the symptomatic pattern of gasping breaths that is now known as *Kussmaul's breathing.*

Critical Thinking

Consider what you've been learning about the inner workings of the respiratory system as you answer these questions.

1. What is the function of the alveoli pulmonis? ____________________
2. Mr. Davis's oxygen saturation levels were low. Knowing that, which parts of the respiratory system would need to be assessed? ____________________
3. What is the combining form of the word *alveolus*? ____________________
4. If our patient Mr. Davis has difficulty fully expanding his lungs when he tries to take a deep breath and he doesn't have any broken ribs, what organ in the respiratory system needs to be assessed? ____________________
5. What is air? ____________________
6. Sometimes people stop breathing momentarily when they are sleeping. What is the medical term that describes the cessation of breathing? ____________________

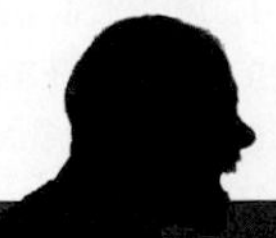

PRONUNCIATION PRACTICE

Say these words aloud to a friend or classmate if you can. You are given the phonetic pronunciation. Your instructor can help you with pronunciation,

or visit **http://www.MedicalLanguageLab.com.**

alveoli	ăl-vē´**ō**-lī
apnea	**ăp**-nē´ă
bradypnea	brăd″ĭp-**nē**´ă
dyspnea	**dĭsp**´nē-ă
eupnea	ūp-**nē**´ă
cilia	**sĭl**´ē-ă
diaphragm	**dī**´ă-frăm
pulmonary	**pŭl**´mō-nĕ-rē
pulmonitis	pŭl-mō-**nī**´tĭs
pulmonectomy	pŭl″mō-**nĕk**´tō-mē
pneumonectomy	nū″mōn-**ĕk**´tō-mē
pneumatosis	nū″mă-**tō**´sĭs
pleuritis	ploo-**rī**´tĭs
pleuroclysis	ploo-**rŏk**´lĭ-sĭs
tachypnea	tăk″ĭp-**nē**´ă

Patient Update

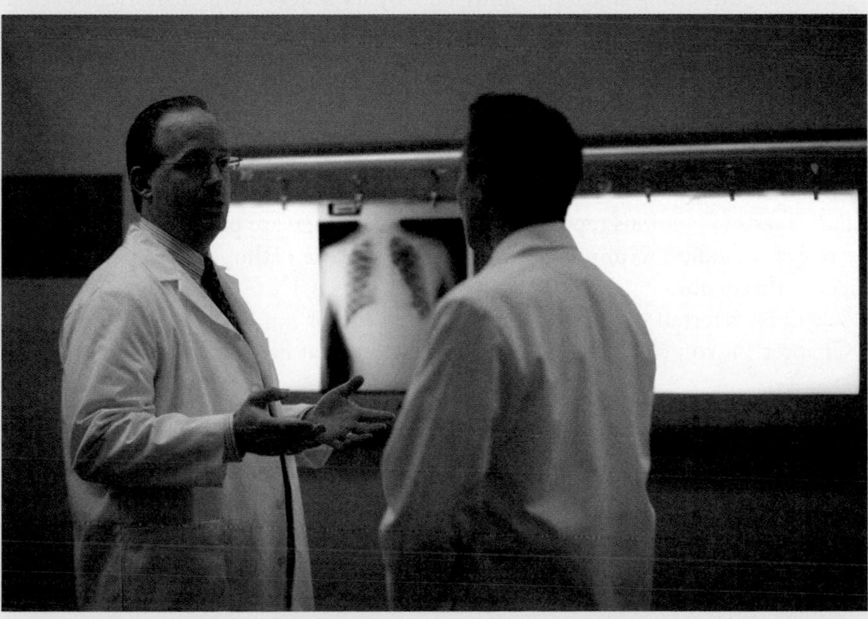

Dr. Jackson has gone to consult with Dr. Krenshaw, the radiologist at Okla Trauma Center. Together, they have reviewed Zane Davis's x-rays and CT scans. They understand from their own assessment—as well as the learned opinion of their colleague, Dr. Fillmore, in cardiology—that the patient's health concerns at the moment are not the result of any injury or of the motor vehicle accident and that Mr. Davis has not suffered any cardiovascular or cerebrovascular trauma. They all concur that, in addition to having a urinary tract infection that is responding well to antibiotic treatment, Mr. Davis also has some respiratory concerns.

Dr. Krenshaw pointed out that there are some unusual shadows on the patient's lung x-rays. Dr. Jackson told his colleague that the patient was a lifelong smoker and that he had a medical history of some bouts of bronchitis and pneumonia. They talked for a while about the possibility of chronic obstructive pulmonary disease and lung cancer. Together, they wondered whether the shadows on the patient's lungs were scars, tumors, or even evidence of pneumonomelanosis. Dr. Jackson added that the patient had some clubbing in his fingertips and that his color was generally pale if not slightly cyanotic in appearance. The radiologist in turn reported that the CT scan, in combination with the blood and urine tests, had at least preliminarily ruled out cancerous tumors in the lungs. However, more tests were certainly warranted to explain the shadows and the reasons for the other physical symptoms of pulmonary dysfunction that were being exhibited by the patient.

"You know, Mr. Davis was in the Navy for many years, and a good deal of that time was spent aboard a ship," said Dr. Jackson. "I wonder if he might have been exposed to asbestos there?" The other physician nodded slowly, thinking about that possibility.

"That's a good point, Bob. I hadn't thought of that. Hmm . . . yes, pneumonoconiosis or asbestosis might be something to look for. That's a definite possibility for a Navy man. I haven't encountered that condition yet, but I am beginning to hear about more and more cases of it." The doctors sat for a moment in silence, thinking about the implications of what they were saying.

"All right, then, I'll follow that up," said Dr. Jackson as he arose from his chair. "I hope for the patient's sake that the shadows are not an indication of mesothelioma. That's an awful diagnosis to have to present to someone." He sighed.

Critical Thinking Questions

Answer the following questions on the basis of what you have just read.

1. Dr. Jackson and Dr. Krenshaw have decided that one lung disease is not likely but that another lung disease is a possible diagnosis. What are the two medical terms for these diseases? ____________________
2. What disease does Dr. Jackson hope to rule out for Mr. Davis? ____________________
3. The patient is not exhibiting signs of healthy pulmonary functioning; instead, he is exhibiting signs of pulmonary ____________________.

Pathophysiology of the respiratory system

In the most recent Patient Update, Doctors Jackson and Krenshaw interpreted patient Zane Davis's diagnostic test results and considered a number of possible diagnoses to explain his symptoms. To fully understand their reasoning, you need to know the language of pathophysiology of the respiratory system. Various types of respiratory pathology are presented here to familiarize you with the relevant medical terminology and some of the core pathophysiologic concepts related to the physicians' discussion.

Mr. Davis will be referred out to respiratory specialists for a more comprehensive diagnostic workup. In Chapter 14, you will learn more about the steps that need to be taken to reach his final diagnosis.

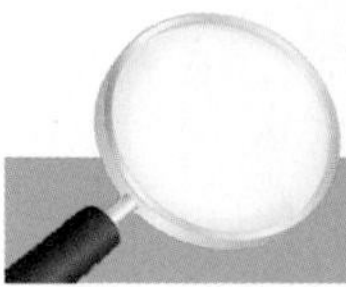

FOCUS POINT: *Referred Out*

The medical term *referred out* means to be referred out of the service or care of one physician, facility, or clinic and into the care of another. Most medical referrals (but not all) require a letter of referral or a request for consultation from one physician to another.

Chronic obstructive pulmonary disease

Chronic obstructive pulmonary disease (COPD) is the medical term for a group of disorders that include asthma, chronic bronchitis, emphysema, and others. In each case, the lungs are the focus of the illness.

Asthma is a chronic inflammatory disease of the airways in which they are particularly sensitive to irritants and allergens (triggers). It is a chronic condition that develops when the bronchi and the bronchioles become inflamed and mucous production increases. Over time, the muscles that permit the passage of air into the lungs can narrow or close. Symptoms of asthma include shortness of breath, wheezing, coughing, and a sense of tightness in the chest. During an acute asthmatic attack, wheezing and gasping occur. The word asthma derives from the early Greek and means *to gasp*.

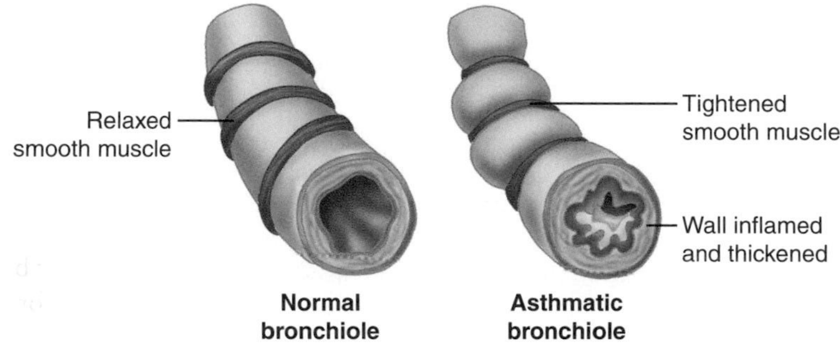

Figure 9.15: The pathology of asthma

Emphysema is a chronic disease of the lungs that is related to smoking and chronic bronchitis. The inability of the lungs to expel air is the key diagnostic criterion for this serious disease; this means that gas exchange is impaired. Emphysema results from the inflammation, damage, or death of alveoli. It is a progressive disease. Emphysema can be treated to stop its progression, but it cannot be cured. Symptoms include shortness of breath and wheezing. The term *emphysema* derives from two early Greek words meaning *to inflate or swell* and *to blow or breathe*.

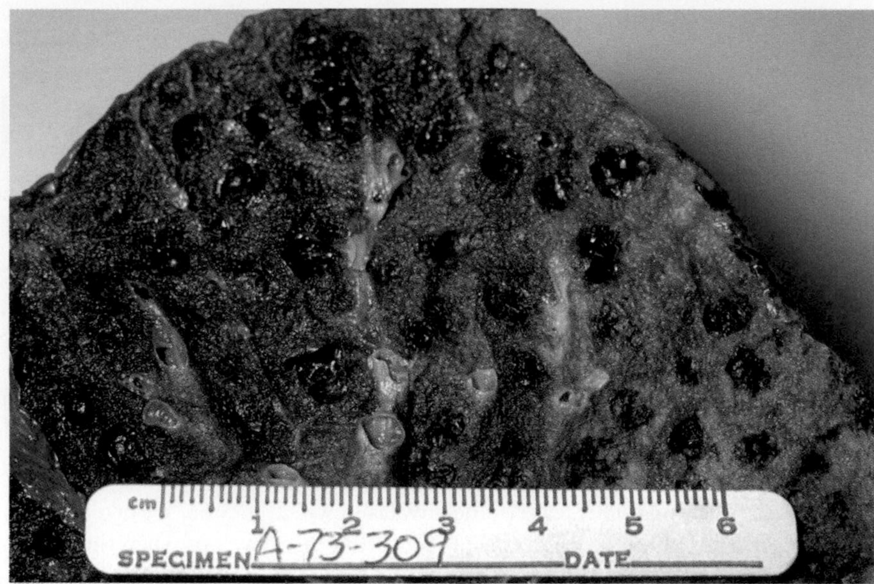

Figure 9.16: An emphysemic lung (Courtesy of the Centers for Disease Control and Prevention and Dr. Edwin P. Ewing, Jr, 1973.)

Asbestosis

Asbestosis is a chronic disease of the lungs that stems from exposure over time to asbestos particles. When it is inhaled, asbestos penetrates the bronchioles and the alveoli and causes inflammation. The body's response is to try to dissolve the foreign particles by secreting a defensive acid. Unfortunately, this defensive maneuver does not work, and the acid itself causes scarring deep within the lungs; this condition is referred to as **diffuse interstitial fibrosis**, and it cannot be reversed after it has occurred.

Asbestosis progresses over time because the foreign particles remain in situ. Because it develops slowly, the condition is not generally diagnosed until 25 to 40 years after exposure to asbestos has occurred. Smoking worsens the condition. Eventually, the use of a portable oxygen machine may be necessary to assist the patient who suffers from asbestosis. Symptoms can include coughing, hoarseness, pain in the chest on exertion (dyspnea on exertion), shortness of breath, and fatigue.

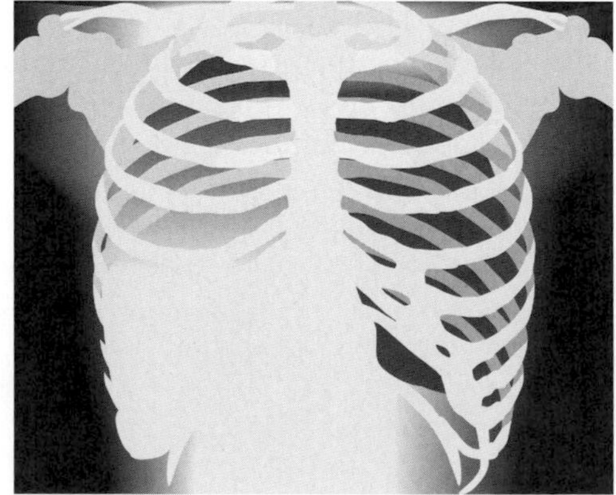

Figure 9.17: X-ray of a lung showing asbestosis damage

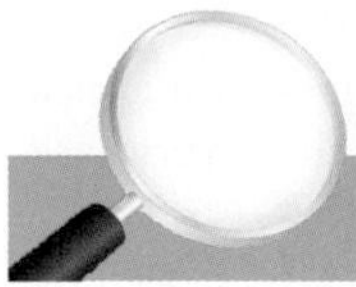

FOCUS POINT: Asbestos

Asbestos is a mineral. For many years, it was used as an insulator and fire retardant in homes, buildings, and ships. As asbestos naturally deteriorates with age or is exposed to air for any length of time, it disintegrates into a powdery form that can be inhaled. In that form, it can also be ingested if it appears on the hands, on dishes, or in foods. When large amounts of asbestos are inhaled or ingested, it causes scarring on the lungs; this is known as *asbestosis.* It can also lead to a form of lung cancer known as *mesothelioma.* The use of asbestos in new housing and commercial construction was banned in the United States in 1978; however, asbestos can still be found in many older structures, including ships.

Mesothelioma

Mesothelioma is a form of lung cancer that affects the **mesothelial cells**, which are the cells that form the surface layer of the pleura, the peritoneum, or the pericardium. Mesothelioma derives from asbestosis, and it is the worst form that this disease can take. Mesothelioma can take 30 to 40 years to manifest itself (to become apparent). It is a malignant and untreatable disease that seems to progress quickly to destroy the lungs. However, this is not exactly what occurs. Early signs and symptoms of asbestosis and mesothelioma are often disregarded by patients, who tend to dismiss changes in their respiratory patterns. When symptoms get worse or interfere with daily living, mesothelioma may have already taken hold in the mesothelial cells of the lungs.

The word *mesothelioma* is formed from the following word parts:

meso: a combining form meaning *middle*

thelio: a combining form that originally meant *nipple* but that now means *nourishing or feeding.*

-oma: a suffix meaning *tumor*

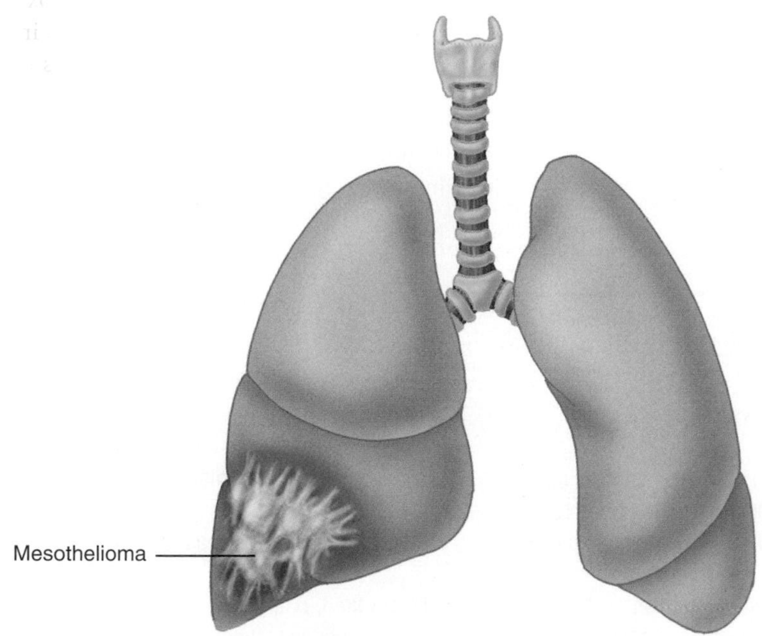

Figure 9.18: A lung with mesothelioma

Mix and Match

Match each respiratory condition with its description. Notice that the descriptions do not appear all that different when you first read them. To succeed at this exercise, you need to think very carefully and use your critical-thinking skills before answering.

1. asthma	a malignant condition of the cell membranes in the lung
2. emphysema	a chronic condition that affects the bronchioles
3. mesothelioma	a chronic condition of the bronchioles and the alveoli
4. asbestosis	a chronic condition that affects the alveoli
5. COPD	any chronic pulmonary condition that adversely affects breathing

Let's Practice

Provide the correct medical term for the description given.

1. difficulty breathing when active or working ____________________

2. originally referred to the processes of inflation and blowing ____________________

3. means *gasp* in its original form ____________________

PRONUNCIATION PRACTICE

Say these words aloud to a friend or classmate if you can. You are given the phonetic pronunciation. Your instructor can help you with pronunciation,

or visit **http://www.MedicalLanguageLab.com.**

asbestosis	ăs″bĕ-**stō**′sĭs
asthma	**ăz**′mă
emphysema	ĕm″fĭ-**sē**′mă
cyanotic	sī-ăn-**ŏt**′ĭk
mesothelioma	mĕs″ō-thē-lē-**ō**′mă
pneumonomelanosis	nū″mō-nō-mĕl″ăn′-**ō**′sĭs
pneumonoconiosis	noo″mă-nō-kō″nē-**ō**′sĭs

Patient Update

Dr. Jackson has returned to see Mr. Davis on Unit 8B to discuss treatment plans with him.

"Hello, Mr. Davis," Dr. Jackson said pleasantly as he entered the room. "Hello, Quincy," he added, nodding in recognition of the patient's son. "How are you feeling now, sir?" he asked, turning his attention back to the patient.

"Well, better, yes. Better, but not great. I still feel tired, but, you know, it's been a heck of a day." He paused a moment. The doctor nodded, and Mr. Davis continued. "I got a hold of my wife, you know."

Dr. Jackson said he had not known this and asked if all was well. "She's over at Fayette General," said Mr. Davis. "She's had some troubles over there; some confusion and such. My daughter Angie's with her. Angie says Stevie-Rose is okay, and I don't need to rush right over there this minute." Zane looked at Quincy for confirmation and received it. "So, what's going on here? Are all my tests back? When can I go?"

Dr. Jackson sat down then and went over the patient's case. He explained the discovery of shadows on Mr. Davis' lungs and said that, in the light of the additional physical signs that he'd seen—Mr. Davis's inability to get a good deep breath, some crackling in his lungs, and other symptoms—some follow-up tests would be necessary. Quincy and his father looked at each other and then back at the doctor, not sure about what to say.

"What do you mean by *follow-up*?" replied the patient. "What are you trying to tell me, doctor? Don't beat around the bush, please." Dr. Jackson explained how important further respiratory assessment would be to rule out chronic obstructive pulmonary disease. Mr. Davis coughed a bit while he listened. Quincy watched his father, clearly making the connection to what Dr. Jackson was saying.

"It is possible, sir, that some of your confusion during and after your MVA today were related to low levels of oxygen in your system. This could be a sign of lung disease," said Dr. Jackson.

"Lung disease?" said Quincy incredulously. "I know he smokes a lot. Are you going to tell me Dad has lung cancer?"

"We've seen no indication of cancer at this point," said Dr. Jackson, "but a very strong potential for asbestosis exists. Asbestosis is a very serious and chronic lung disease that doesn't appear until years after exposure to the material." The doctor went on to explain that many sailors may have been exposed to asbestos in ships and shipyards before the mid 1970s. Since this group included Mr. Davis, more tests were warranted. Dr. Jackson waited for the patient and his son to consider this, and then he added, "This testing can be done on an outpatient basis, Mr. Davis. I can refer you for a toxicology screen to be done by any lab of your choice. That test can show us if you have been exposed to high levels of asbestos. I'd also like to refer you to a respiratory specialist for pulmonary function tests, or perhaps VHA has some suggestions for respiratory follow-up for you. But I cannot stress enough the importance of taking care of this, sir."

Both Mr. Davis and Quincy asked a few questions about the testing involved and discovered that it could also include another CT scan, blood tests, and a bronchoscopy.

"I would also like to talk to you about your urinary health, Mr. Davis," said Dr. Jackson. "As you know, you have a UTI, and I would also like to suggest that you see a urologist about that, too, just to be on the safe side."

"A urologist? Whatever for?" came the patient's response.

"On the safe side of what?" asked Quincy, with a touch of fear in his voice.

Dr. Jackson explained the problems that aging men often encounter with the prostate gland. He informed them that Mr. Davis had been given a PSA test when he was admitted. It had come back negative for cancer, but benign prostatic hyperplasia was still a possibility. The doctor said that this condition could be contributing to Mr. Davis's difficulties with urination. "I can refer you to a urologist for follow-up tests for this condition as well," said Dr. Jackson. He reassured Mr. Davis that he was not at any immediate risk for prostate problems but that these tests would be health-promotion activities: in other words, he would be being proactive about his prostate health rather than reactive. The patient and his son agreed.

"So, Doc, what are you saying in the end here? Can I go home today?" asked Mr. Davis. "I'd like to go home with my son, and I'd like to see my family, too." Zane looked at Quincy. "I need to see my grandson. Oh, it's really awful. He got burned at our house, and we were bringing him here when we got in that accident," he said forlornly. "If I could just get out of here."

"Well, sir, I can hear your need. I was going to suggest that you stay overnight because it's getting late now, but I can see that you'll be in good hands with your son. I'm going to agree to discharge you now, but I want you to agree to take my referrals for respiratory assessment very seriously in return. Will you do that?"

"Yes," pledged the patient and his son in unison.

Critical Thinking Question

1. Why is Dr. Jackson so insistent that Mr. Davis follow through with his referrals for further pulmonary assessment? ______________________________
2. In a medical context, what does this phrase mean: "being proactive about his prostate health rather than reactive"? ______________________________

CHAPTER SUMMARY

In Chapter 9, you continued to build language skills related to cardiac and urinary assessment. You were also introduced to terminology related to male reproductive and respiratory assessment and care. Mr. Davis received the results of diagnostic tests that were begun in Chapter 5. You followed his progress from his hospital admission to the point of his discharge from Okla Trauma Center and his referral to other medical services. You learned to identify and interpret important medical records associated with hospital admission and diagnostic test results. Exercises reinforced your learning by providing you with opportunities to use new vocabulary, terms, and concepts related to the identified systems and processes. The career field of medical information technology (medical records) was also introduced.

See How Much You've Learned

For audio exercises, visit http://www.MedicalLanguageLab.com.
Chapter 9 also introduced new abbreviations. A number of them appear again here in a concise table to promote study.

TABLE 9-10: Abbreviations in Chapter 9

Abbreviation	Meaning	Abbreviation	Meaning
BPH	benign prostatic hyperplasia	CK	creatinine
DRE	digital rectal examination	T	troponin
PSA	prostate-specific antigen	K	potassium
COPD	chronic obstructive pulmonary disease	NO_3	nitrogen
		CO_2	carbon dioxide
RHIT	registered health information technician	0_2	oxygen

Key Terms

admission record
albumin
alveoli
alveoli pulmonis
androgens
andrology
antipyretic
asbestosis
asthma
benign prostatic hyperplasia (BPH)
bilirubin
bronchi
bronchioles
bronchitis
bulbourethral glands (Cowper's glands)
cardiac enzymes
chronic obstructive pulmonary disease (COPD)
cilia
clubbing
consents
crackles
diaphragm
diffuse interstitial fibrosis
dipstick test
ejaculatory duct
electrolytes
emphysema
epididymis
epididymitis
estrogens
fissures
glans penis
hypoxemia
intercostal muscles
intercostal spaces
ketones
lab work
larynx
lungs
mesothelial cells
mesothelioma
metastasized
mycoplasma
nailbeds
next of kin
nitrates ($N0_3$)
nocturia
orchitis
pleura
prostate gland
pyelonephritis
pyretic
reagent strip
respiration
respiratory
respire
semen
seminal vesicles
serous membrane
specific gravity
spermatozoa
statin
systemic
testosterone
trachea
treatment authorization request (TAR)
urethra
vas deferens

CHAPTER REVIEW

What Do You Know?

Use your new knowledge of medical terms to answer these questions.

1. What is the prefix that means *normal*? ______________________
2. In the strictest sense of the word, what does *pneumonia* mean? ______________________
3. Which hormone is specifically related to the male sex drive? ______________________
4. Which suffix means *breath or breathing*? ______________________

Label the Diagram

Write the correct anatomical term for each part of the male reproductive system indicated in the diagram.

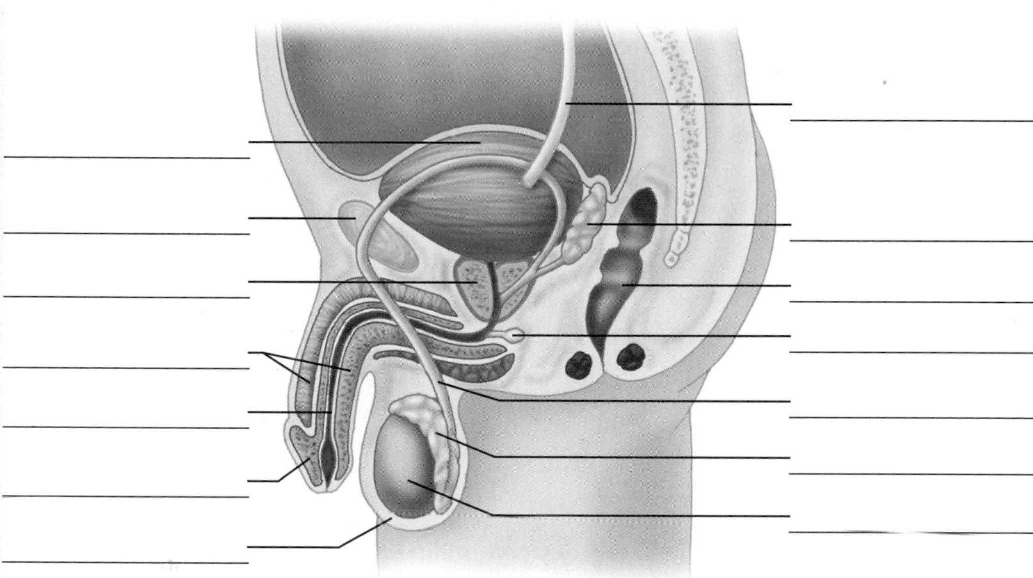

Name the Term

Read the description given, and identify the correct medical term.

1. an external organ essential to both the male reproductive system and the urinary system

____

2. a reproductive system hormone that is found in both men and women

____

3. the science and medicine of male reproductive health

____

4. a very serious infection of the kidneys

____

5. a condition in which renal calculi (calculus) is present

____

Break It Down

Break these words into their component parts of prefix-root-suffix, as applicable. Name each element.

1. pneumothorax ______
2. cardiopulmonary ______
3. lobectomy ______

Translate the Terminology

Rewrite each sentence in your own words.

1. Mr. Davis suffers from dyspnea.
______
2. For some people, periods of sleep apnea can be a chronic condition.
______
3. When you are running, you may develop tachypnea.
______

Mix and Match

Draw a line to connect the synonyms that appeared in this chapter.

1. pyelopathy	pyelonephrosis
2. windpipe	pneumomelanosis
3. tracheostomy	hydropneumothorax
4. voice box	tracheotomy
5. throat	larynx
6. pneumonomelanosis	trachea
7. breathing	respiration
8. pneumohydrothorax	pharynx

Label the Diagram

Write the correct anatomical term for each part of the respiratory system indicated in the diagram.

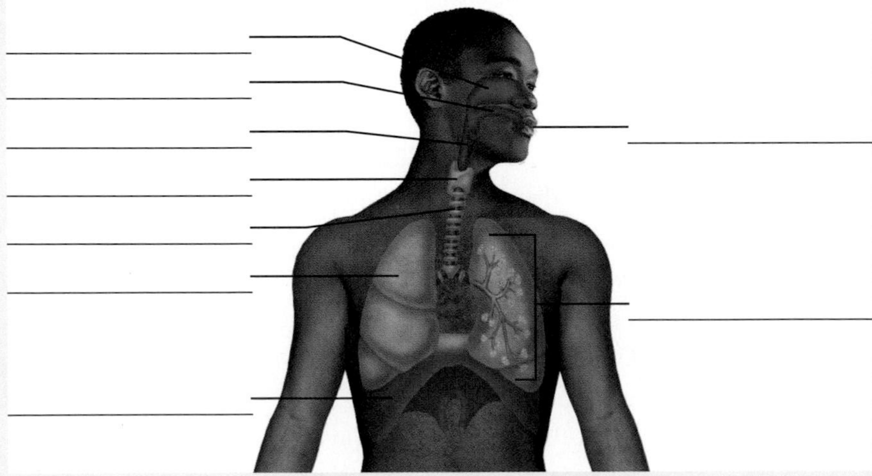

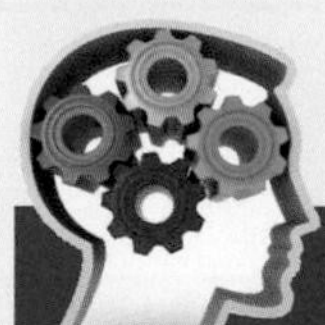

MEMORY MAGIC

If you are interested in remembering information about the respiratory system, you will find these mnemonics helpful.

To remember the names of air passages, try this one:

"Mouthy People are Loud Talkers."

M = mouth

P = pharynx

L = larynx

T = trachea

To remember some signs and symptoms of pulmonary disease, remember this one:

"The 4 Cs of Pulmonary Disease"

Clubbing

Cyanosis

Crackles

Cough

CHAPTER TEN

Orthopedics and Brain Injuries

Focus: Musculoskeletal and Neurological Systems

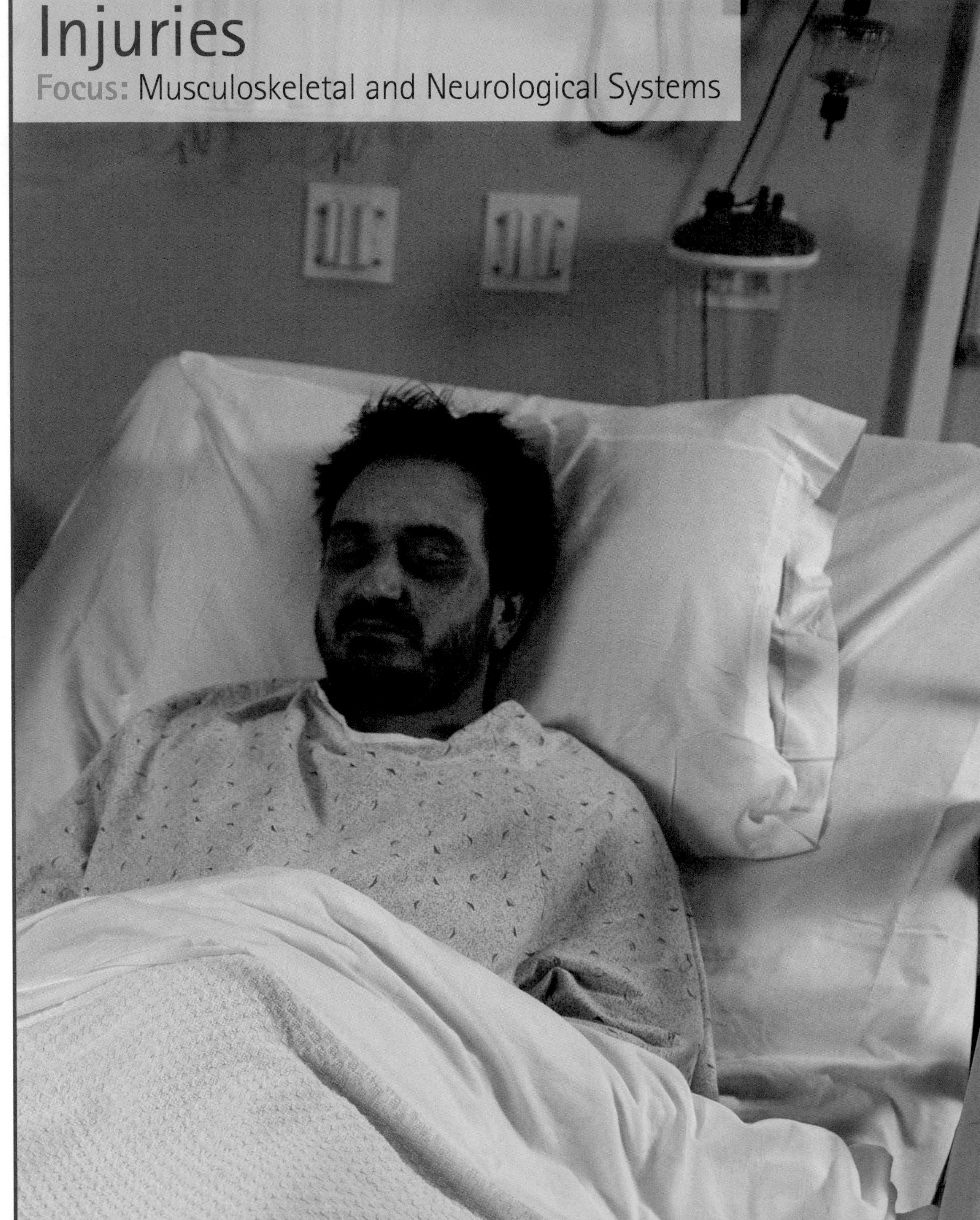

Mr. Gilbert Loeppky (or "Gil," as he prefers to be called) was admitted during the early evening to the Surgical Unit of Okla Trauma Center from the ER. As a victim in a motor vehicle accident that same day, Gil incurred a blunt force head injury and was unconscious at time of arrival at Okla Trauma; he gained consciousness approximately 2 hours after admission (see Chapter 4). Diagnostics determined that there was no internal hemorrhaging within the cranial cavity. However, Gil remains on close monitoring and is receiving neurovital sign checks every 30 minutes, a precautionary measure for all patients with head injuries. In addition, Gil suffered fractures and injuries to his right leg. Although he has yet to speak with a physician in any detail about these injuries, he knows that he is scheduled for surgery to repair them. Gil's parents, Pat and Pearl Loeppky are with him now, awaiting a visit from the surgeon.

In the midst of all of this trauma, Gil has become a new father. His wife, Glory gave birth to a little girl prematurely over at Fayette General Hospital, where she was admitted after the motor vehicle accident (see Chapter 8). Gil and Glory have spoken by telephone.

Patient Update

"Good evening, I'm Dr. Elaine Karras, orthopedic surgeon," announced a tall woman in light-blue scrubs as she strode confidently into Gil's room. She stretched out her hand to the patient and said, " Gilbert Lop... Lop-key, I presume?" She smiled.

Gil shook her hand and politely corrected her. "Lep-key. Gil Loeppky. Call me Gil. How do you do?" Gil replied in a raspy voice. "These are my parents," Gil added, nodding stiffly in their direction.

"Hello, I'm Pat Loeppky, and this is my wife, Pearl," Gil's father said as an introduction. The doctor shook hands with Pat and Pearl as well, and then she returned her attention to the patient.

"Well, Gil, as you know, you've broken a number of bones in your right leg. I'll be performing the surgery to repair them tomorrow afternoon around 5 pm. I wanted to pop in this evening before I go off duty to talk with you a bit and to answer any questions that you might have." Dr. Karras paused to wait for Gil to consider what she was saying.

Gil's mother interjected: "Tomorrow afternoon! Why so long? That sounds awful to make him wait in pain for so long!"

The surgeon explained that, because Gil had sustained a concussion, it was not wise to administer anesthetic medications to him until he had been monitored for neurological, cognitive, and vital signs over a period of at least 12 full hours. She said to Gil, "Although anesthesia is generally safe for someone who, like you, has had a moderate concussion, there are some risks involved as you emerge from it postoperatively. When you wake up, you might exhibit behaviors similar to delirium or changes in brain functioning. As a result, we want to be sure that your neurological status is stable before we put you in that position. I also must tell you that, under anesthesia, a patient who has sustained a head injury may also be at risk for hypoxia; this involves decreased levels of oxygen in the tissues, particularly in the brain, when respirations are slowed for a surgical procedure. We do not expect this in your case because your head trauma was not to the respiratory centers located at the posterior base of the skull, but we like to be cautious just the same."

"I'd like to take a moment to go over your injuries with you," Dr. Karras continued. She waved to the chairs nearby, and Pat and Pearl took a seat. "You have two fractures that require surgical reduction. It seems that you have a pilon fracture of the distal end of the right tibia. We call this a 'high-energy fracture,' and you likely received it when you hit the brakes during the MVA. Although it looks at first blush like an ankle fracture, your x-rays have shown that the bones of the ankle remain intact. We'll be more certain of that after we surgically incise the area and take a better look. Sometimes small bone chips can be found that may not have been apparent at the time of x-ray but that have detached themselves during the interim. We won't be surprised if we find this.

"Pilon fractures occur when the talus—an ankle bone—is actually driven into the bottom of the tibia, shattering one end of the tibia and causing multiple displaced fracture fragments. These fragments can embed themselves in tissue and cause a great deal of grief, including tissue swelling and so on." Dr. Karras paused to let this information sink in. "When we go in, we will assess the damage. It is likely that we are going to perform a reduction of the tibia, ensure that the fibula is unharmed, and also stabilize the ankle by fixating it. In other words, we will use some lag screws and K-wires to hold the joint of the ankle together where the tibia, fibula, and talus meet. This is a surgical procedure called an *anteromedial joint arthrotomy.*"

"Fixating? What does that mean?" Gil inquired. Dr. Karras explained that this meant that there would be reduced movement in Gil's ankle. He wouldn't be able to rotate the ankle in a normal way in the future. The ankle would feel stiff, and he would no longer be able to point his toes as he does now. Gil groaned in frustration.

The surgeon continued: "In the meantime, I can appreciate that tomorrow afternoon seems like a long time to wait. For now, we've placed an air cast around the ankle to protect it from any movement and to stabilize it. That should provide a modicum of pain relief, too. I've ordered an analgesic prn every 4 to 6 hours to help you with the pain. I believe that the nurse has administered that to you. Is that correct, Gil?" Gil nodded in the affirmative.

"And how you would rate your pain right now, say, on a pain scale of 1 to 10, with 10 being the worst pain imaginable?" Dr. Karras waited while Gil thought about this question. Gil reported his pain level as a 6 on the pain scale. "And is that manageable for you?" She asked. Gil nodded again. "Good. I want you to know that if it goes up anywhere from 7 to 10, you are to immediately notify the nurses, and they will see what they can do to help alleviate that. However, just like I was saying about the anesthetic, because of your head injury, we cannot give you anything stronger than what you are receiving right now. We don't want to cloud the results of your neurovital monitoring.

"Gil, you also have a complex spiral fracture of the hip; this is a fracture at the distal end of the femur where it impacted with the acetabulum. This, too, probably occurred when you hit the brakes or as you came to a sudden stop in your vehicle. The high-energy impact not only forced the talus into the tibia, but it also forced your femur or thigh bone into your pelvis. Because the connection between the femur and the pelvis is a ball-and-socket joint, some rotation occurred." Dr. Karras took out a pen and paper and drew a diagram of this for Gil and his parents to explain the situation in more detail.

"For this injury, we have to straighten—or reduce—your hip. Afterward, you'll be in traction for a while. This will be necessary because of the high density of musculature in the thigh area and the potential for the muscles to contract and stay contracted after realignment. Because you aren't going to surgery until tomorrow, we've applied a temporary splint to stabilize that hip. Surgically, we are going to put a pin into the bone to stabilize it. You'll have a cast postoperatively and after discharge as well." Dr. Karras paused and looked at Gil. His brows were knit in consternation. "I know it's a lot to take in right now, sir, but you will recover from this and be able to work again, if that is what concerns you."

"Yes," Gil rasped, "but after how long? How long is this recovery going to take? My wife and I just had a baby today, Doctor. A baby. Our first. My wife will be off work for a while. I have to get back to work," Gil said, pleadingly. Dr. Karras empathized, but she could not offer a quick solution for him. Gil's parents, Pat and Pearl, joined in to reassure their son that they would step in to offer any help that they could. They chatted for a moment or two before the surgeon continued.

"Finally, Gil, I must also tell you that your right knee is injured as well. That is quite understandable with such a high-energy injury to your leg. The knee injury may also have occurred if your knee came into direct contact with the dashboard of your vehicle. Do you know if that happened?"

Gil said that he couldn't remember the details of the accident at all. "Well," Dr. Karras said, "I am happy to tell you that this injury doesn't require my services. An acute patellar injury heals quite well if you rest it and take care of it. While you're in the hospital, an orthopedic technician will help you with your traction, casts, and so on. Then, we'll want to get you into physical therapy as quickly as possible once you've started to heal. You'll need to mobilize the muscles, joints, and ligaments in that right leg to keep it healthy and ready to return to weight bearing. I'll arrange that for you when the time comes." Dr. Karras smiled and looked at the patient and his family as she said this.

"Why is his voice so raspy, Doctor?" asked Mrs. Loeppky. Dr. Karras explained the symptom. When Gil had first been attended to, he had been intubated to ensure that an airway remained open. Intubation, the doctor clarified, involved the insertion of an artificial airway into the trachea through the mouth. "This procedure, although necessary, can cause a drying of the mucosal lining of the throat and mouth, and it can irritate the tissues," said Dr. Karras. "We removed the airway as soon as we deemed it safe to do so and started Gil on oxygen via nasal prongs instead. You'll see that he no longer has those, either." Then the doctor turned back to the patient. "Although we must keep you NPO before surgery tomorrow, Gil you are able to have some clear fluids this evening until midnight. That will help to alleviate the dryness in your throat. Ice chips are also here at the bedside, I see. Sucking on a few of those from time to time will help." Dr. Karras paused again to let Gil and his parents consider all of the information that she had given them.

"You have a urinary catheter in situ as well, Gil. Are you having any difficulties with that? Any pain?" asked the surgeon. Gil shook his head "no." Dr. Karras said, "Good. We'll need to keep that in for another couple of days at least. You won't be able to get up and walk to the bathroom for a while yet." Gil nodded in reply, sparing his voice. "All right, then. Do any of you have any questions?" asked Dr. Karras.

"Yes, just one last thing," answered Pearl. "Did Gil hit his nose on the steering wheel or something? It doesn't look like his nose is broken, but his eyes are so swollen and black and blue. I asked him, but he doesn't remember much about the accident." Dr. Karras told them how Gil had likely received the black eyes and assured them that his nose had not been broken (see Chapter 4) .

"I'll leave you then, Gil, and see you tomorrow," said Dr. Karras. "I'll pop in again before your surgery. In the meantime, if you have any questions about that or about your care, please just ask the nurses. They're wonderful here on the surgical floor. They're very helpful and extremely knowledgeable regarding these types of surgeries." Dr. Karras then said goodbye and left the room.

Reflective Questions

Reflect on the story that you've just read.

1. What type of surgeon has come to visit Gil? ______________________________

2. How many fractures need to be repaired during surgery? Name them.

   ____

3. Why does the patient have to wait until almost 24 hours after his injury to have surgery?

   ____

4. In the future, Gil won't be able to perform dorsal flexion or extension with his right foot and ankle. Why not? ______________________________

Critical Thinking Question

What is causing the most stress and anxiety for this patient? Is it pain, the thought of surgery, the inability to have free range of motion in his right ankle, or something else? Identify the major cause of his stress.

____

For audio exercises, visit **http://www.MedicalLanguageLab.com.** 

Learning Objectives

After reading Chapter 10, you will be able to do the following:

- Recognize, define, and use terminology related to orthopedic surgery.
- Have a basic understanding of terminology related to intravenous administration of medications and solutions.
- Enhance recognition and use of terminology related to the neurological system.
- Recognize the subdivisions of the neurological system, beginning with the central nervous system.
- Recognize, define, and use terminology related to emergency neurosurgery and recovery.
- Recognize and use terminology related to brain injury and disease.
- Name the meninges.
- Explain the second-impact syndrome as it relates to patients with concussions.
- Recognize the terminology and assessment language related to intracranial pressure and increased intracranial pressure.
- Have an introductory understanding of magnetic resonance imaging related to the central nervous system.
- Recognize the process of calling an emergency code, as well as the language that is used.
- Appreciate the education, training, and work of orthopedic surgeons and orthopedic technicians.

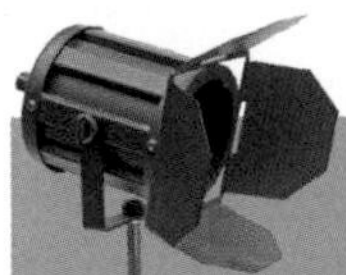

CAREER SPOTLIGHT: Orthopedic Surgeons and Technicians

A physician who practices in orthopedics is an *orthopedist.* He or she may be a generalist or a specialist. Examples of orthopedic specialties include hands, ankles, and feet. There are two main types of orthopedics: surgical and nonsurgical. Examples of nonsurgical orthopedics are practices in sports medicine and physical medicine in which surgery is not part of the work.

Orthopedic technicians assist orthopedic physicians with surgical and nonsurgical muscle and skeletal system therapies. Working directly under orthopedists, these technicians care for patients who are undergoing orthopedic procedures and some physical therapies. They are often found in the "cast room" of clinics and hospitals, where they apply and remove casts, dressings, and splints. To qualify for this work, they have studied radiology interpretation so that they can understand the injuries revealed by patients' x-rays and how to appropriately cast or splint these injuries. They are also qualified to care for and protect surgical bone pins and related wound beds, as well as to assist patients with mobility devices such as canes, crutches, and walkers. Orthopedic technicians are also qualified to maintain traction devices. Orthopedic technicians generally earn a 1- to 2-year certificate from a technical school or a community college. Their studies must include clinical practicum experience. They may also be required to seek certification by the National Board for Certification of Orthopaedic Technologists, Inc (NBCOT). Their education and training should occur in an institution that has been accredited by the National Association of Orthopaedic Technologists (NAOT).

The Language of Orthopedics

Orthopedics is the field of medicine that deals with the musculoskeletal structures of bones, ligaments, muscles, and joints. The language of orthopedics includes terms related to the prevention of disorders of the musculoskeletal system, as well as to the correction of injuries, pathologies, or abnormalities in this system.

Right Word or Wrong Word: *Orthopedic* or *Orthopaedic*?

Are these two terms the same? Is one of them a spelling mistake?

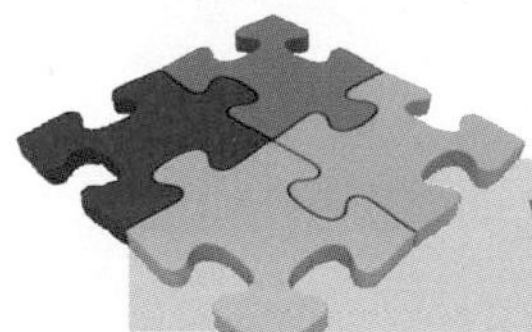

WORD BUILDING: Formula for Creating Words with the Combining Form *Orth/o-*

orthos = root meaning *correct, straight, or in the proper order.*

ortho + kinetics = *orthokinetics*

Definition: techniques that are used to stimulate the muscles and tendons for rehabilitation. The second root derives from the word *kinesis,* meaning *motion. noun*

Example: *Orthokinetics* may be part of Gil Loeppky's rehabilitation after surgery.

orth + osis = *orthosis*

Definition: a device or devices used to straighten, stabilize, or immobilize a body part. *noun*

Example: Types of *orthosis* include splints and traction devices.

orth + otics = *orthotics*

Definition: the science of devising and using orthopedic appliances. The second word part, *-otics,* is a suffix meaning *of, affected with, or producing. noun*

Example: Orthopedists must keep up to date with the latest developments in *orthotics.*

ortho + static = *orthostatic*

Definition: pertaining to a condition caused by standing erect. *adjective*

Example: *Orthostatic* hypotension is a sudden drop in blood pressure that occurs upon standing; dizziness may ensure.

ortho + de + ox + ia = *orthodeoxia*

Definition: decreased arterial oxygen while in an upright position. Two prefixes are used before the combining form *ox,* meaning *oxygen. noun*

Example: A patient with *orthodeoxia* must be kept in a supine position.

Key terms: orthopedic surgical prep

In the opening scenario, Dr. Karras, an orthopedic surgeon, arrives to discuss Gil Loeppky's upcoming surgery with him. This is standard procedure. In medical language, this meeting is referred to as one facet of *surgical prep:* preparing the patient by teaching, providing information, discussing possible outcomes, and providing an opportunity for the patient to ask questions.

Take a look now at some of the words and phrases that Dr. Karras used to prepare Gil Loeppky for orthopedic surgery. Notice that the surgeon uses a combination of formal medical terminology and everyday speech to connect with the patient. This technique is important for building a professional interpersonal relationship between any health provider and patient. It establishes trust and rapport, both of which are conducive to better patient outcomes.

"... as you *emerge from it postoperatively.*"

emerge from it: regain consciousness as the effects of anesthesia wear off.

postoperatively: after the surgery.

"... *respirations are slowed* for a surgical procedure."

respirations are slowed: the rate of breathing is decreased.

"... two fractures that require *surgical reduction*."

surgical reduction: the fractured bone is straightened and returned to its natural state by way of surgical intervention (i.e., opening of the skin to reach into and treat the bone).

"... we *surgically incise* the area ..."

surgically incise: cut into the tissue with the use of surgical procedures and equipment.

"... small *bone chips* can be found ..."

bone chips: fragments of bones or cartilage that come loose.

"... causing multiple displaced *fracture fragments*."

fracture fragments: bone chips that are the result of injury rather than of bone pathology.

"... we will use some *lag screws* and *K-wires* to hold the joint of the ankle together ..."

lag screws: specific types of stainless steel screws that are used in orthopedic surgery; they can be tightened to keep pressure on the bone to stabilize and support it.

K-wires: Kirschner wires, which are sharp, stainless steel pins that are used to hold bone fragments in place.

"... a surgical procedure called an *anteromedial* joint *arthrotomy*."

anteromedial: in front and toward the center.

arthrotomy: cutting into a joint.

"... we've placed an *air cast* around the ankle ..."

air cast: an alternative to a plaster or fiberglass cast, an air cast is a supportive brace-like device that encircles an injured or postoperative body part to stabilize it, promote healing, and reduce pain. The injury site is surrounded by an air-filled splint that is in turn supported and braced by a harder splint made of plastic resin. An air cast can be held in place by Velcro straps.

"... a *modicum* of pain relief, too."

modicum: a moderate amount.

"... an *analgesic prn every 4 to 6 hours* ..."

analgesic: pain-relief medication.

PRN every 4 to 6 hours: as needed, once every 4 to 6 hours. This is how a medication order is written and spoken. The abbreviation *prn* is a short form of the Latin phrase *pro re nata*, meaning *as necessary* or *as circumstances require.*

"... a *pain scale* of 1 to 10 ..."

pain scale: a common system of pain measurement in which the patient rates the intensity of his or her pain on a scale of 1 to 10, with 1 being pain free and 10 being very bad or unbearable.

"'And is that *manageable* for you?'"

manageable: in this context, the word is used to determine if the pain is controlled enough for the patient to be able to tolerate or manage it.

"... don't want to *cloud the results* ..."

cloud the results: an expression that means that the results of a test might not be clear because symptoms could be masked or heightened by the medication that the patient is taking.

"...you also have a complex *spiral fracture* of the hip..."

spiral fracture: a torsion fracture in which the bone has been twisted apart (see Chapter 4).

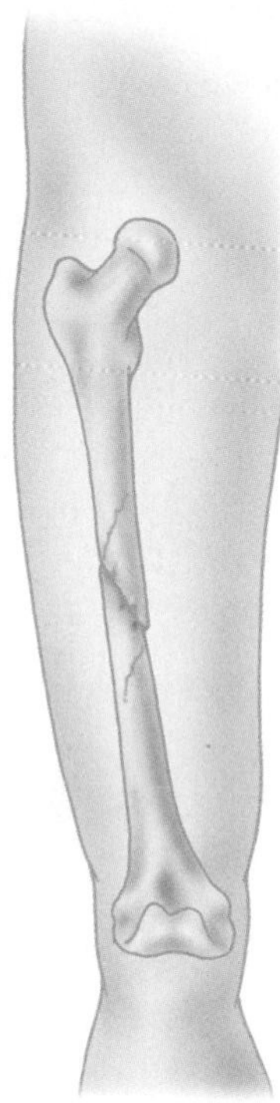

Figure 10.1: Spiral fracture of the femur

"...you'll be in *traction*..."

traction: a medical procedure in which a device called an *orthosis* is used to apply a pulling force on a bone to maintain its alignment. Traction helps to reduce pain, and it prevents the formation of a hematoma (see Figure 10-2).

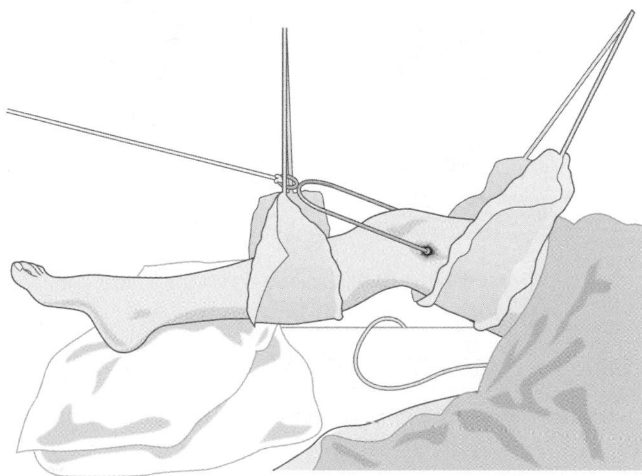

Figure 10.2: Patient in femoral traction

"...because of the *high density of musculature* in the thigh area..."

high density of musculature: a descriptive medical term that refers to the thickness of the muscle, tendons, and ligaments in a certain area.

"...we've applied a temporary splint to *stabilize that hip.*"

stabilize that hip: to keep the hip from moving to prevent more injury or pain.

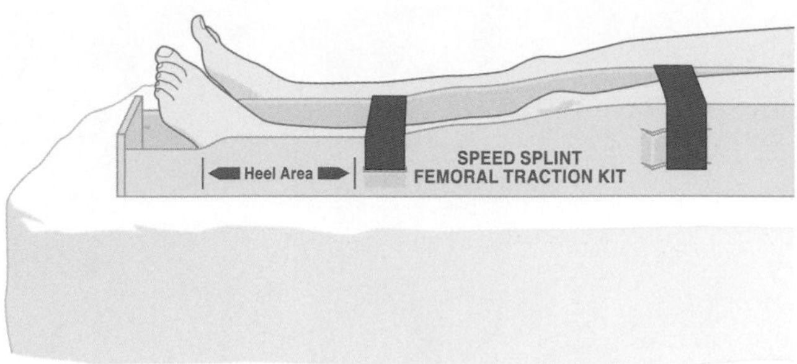

Figure 10.3: Temporary femoral splint

"...we are going to put a *pin* into the bone to stabilize it."

pin: a retrograde nail or a K-wire. (A retrograde nail is actually a screw. It is a sterile piece of steel that has threads that help to ease it into a bone to fixate the bone [hold it tightly and firmly in place].)

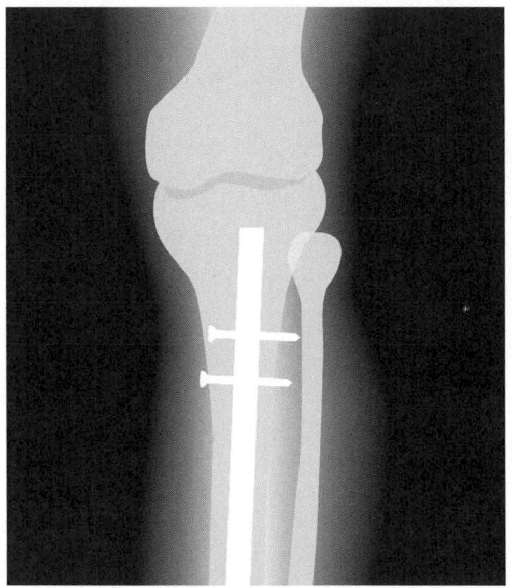

Figure 10.4: X-ray: pins in a fracture

"...we'll want to get you into *physical therapy*..."

physical therapy: treatment to restore or maintain the optimal functioning of the musculoskeletal system.

"You'll need to *mobilize* the muscles, joints, and ligaments..."

mobilize: to move or put into action so that muscle atrophy (wasting) does not occur and so that healthy circulation is maintained to tissues and bone.

"... ready to return to *weight bearing.*"

weight bearing: the ability to carry the load of one's own weight on a bone or joint.

"... we must keep you *NPO* before surgery tomorrow..."

NPO (or npo): a medical abbreviation meaning *nothing by mouth.* The abbreviation is the short form of the Latin phrase *non per os.* An NPO order is standard procedure before surgery so that the stomach, intestines, and bowel will have little or no solids or fluids within them. During surgery, an incision can accidentally spill the contents of these organs into the body cavity, thereby contaminating it. In addition, as patients recover from anesthetic, they may experience nausea and vomiting. Because they may be confused or because their gag reflexes may not be functioning, they are at risk for inhaling any gastric contents that have come up the esophagus.

"... you are able to have some *clear fluids*..."

clear fluids: liquids that leave no gastric residue (leftovers) and that are not likely to cause nausea and vomiting postoperatively. These include water, apple juice, ginger ale, tea, and clear broth. "Clear fluids" is a type of diet that is ordered preoperatively.

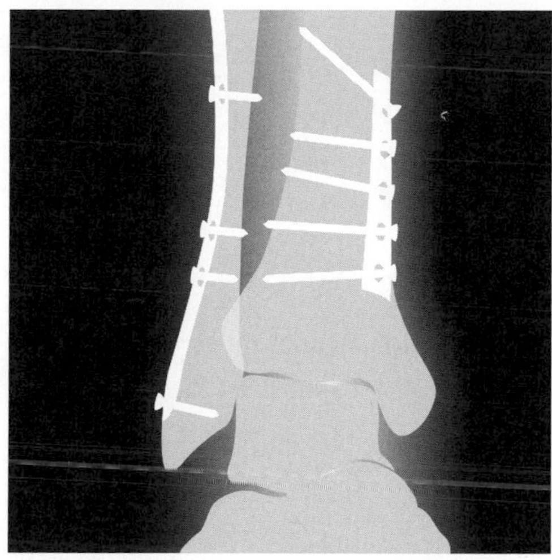

Pilon fracture nine months after surgical reduction

Figure 10.5: X-ray: surgical reduction of a pilon fracture

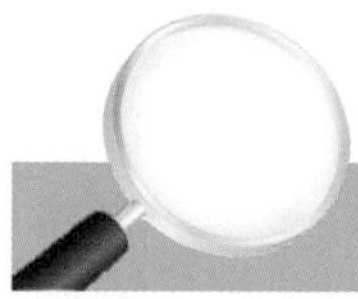

FOCUS POINT: *Pilon, Pylon, Pile,* and *Pillion*

These four words have something in common, but there are distinct differences among them. The similarities in meaning are described in the text below. Pay attention to the context in which you hear these words before you type or write them.

Pilon is a French word that means *pestle.* A pestle is an instrument that is used for crushing or pounding (i.e., using force to compress). Pestles are used in medicine to crush medications into powdered form.

A *pilon fracture* is a serious injury of the ankle joint. The fracture is in the tibia, where the tibia articulates with the talus bone. The distal end of the tibia is crushed by the force of the talus ramming up against and into it.

Continued

In medical English, *pilon* can also refer a wooden leg or a conical shape that, when the point is cut off, becomes a funnel.

In medical English, a *pylon* is a temporary artificial leg.

Pillion is a medical English term that also refers to a temporary artificial leg.

In the field of construction, the term *pile* refers to a heavy beam of timber, steel, or concrete that is driven with extreme force into the ground to form a foundation or to provide support for a structure.

In medical English, *piles* are hemorrhoids, which are swollen veins of the anus.

Let's Practice

Name the procedure using the new terminology that you have learned.

1. the use of weights to apply enough force to pull a bone straight or to keep it in that position ________________
2. the process of realigning a broken bone ________________
3. to insert a device into the endotracheal passage ________________
4. the medical specialty that deals with all aspects of the musculoskeletal system ________________

Mix and Match

Match the description with its medical term.

1. toward the center and front	fixate
2. nothing by mouth	arthrotomy
3. after the operation	analgesic
4. for pain management	post-surgery
5. move and use a body part	intubate
6. awaken from	anteromedial
7. prevent free movement	emerge from
8. incision of a joint	NPO
9. insert an airway	mobilize

Eponyms: Kirschner and K-wires

During the early 20th century, the German doctor Martin Kirschner pioneered a method of repairing fractures with the use of wires and splints. The procedure of drilling a hole in a bone and running a wire through it to stabilize it so that traction can be applied is called *Kirschner traction.* The term *K-wires* is short for *Kirschner wires.*

The Language of Neurological Emergency

Patient Update

"Dark, so dark," Gil Loeppky thought. "Why can't I move?" He tossed and turned and tried to free himself. "What's happening?" he wondered. He felt stifled and claustrophobic, like the world was closing in around him. It hurt so bad! His leg. Was it trapped? He couldn't be sure. He drifted off for a moment into the blackness. Visions swirled in his head.

"Glory," he muttered, thinking of his wife. He saw a flash of the truck—his truck. The pain sliced through him. Confusion enveloped him. He heard the sound of breaking glass, the crunch of steel on impact. "Car accident," he thought. He reached out for his wife, but he couldn't find her. He had to move, to help Glory. He felt trapped and powerless, and he struggled harder. The pain tore through his right leg and caused him to suck in a deep breath. He willed himself to move so that he could help his wife. "Got to get up," he told himself. He struggled in the darkness to free his trapped leg. He ignored the pain, although it was constant and fierce. He pulled and tugged, and, suddenly, the leg came free. He rolled out of the truck door and fell. Down, down into the darkness he fell, thinking only of his wife.

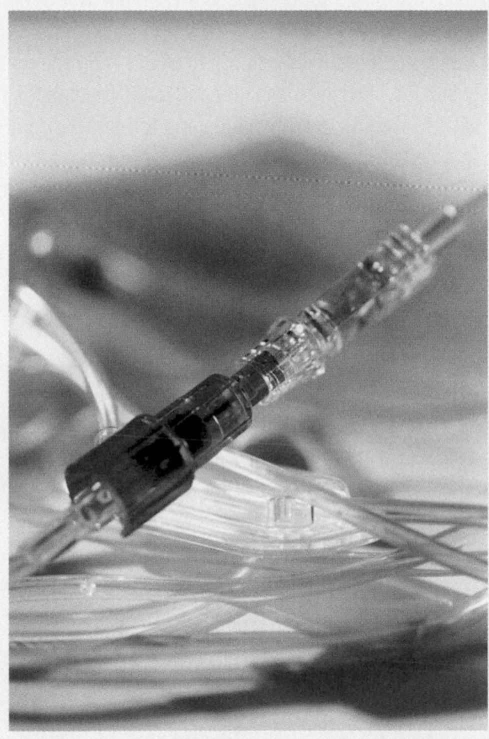

"Call a Code!" shouted the nurse, Franklin, from the doorway of Gil Loeppky's room on the Surgical Unit. "Call a Code!" he repeated, and then he turned abruptly and rushed to the patient's side.

Franklin had heard a loud crash just as he was doing rounds down the corridor, and he had come running. He found Gil lying in a contorted position on the floor beside his bed. The RN knelt down and quickly performed an ABC assessment. He attempted to rouse the patient by calling his name, but he did not shake him. There was no way at the moment to tell if a spinal cord injury had occurred. Franklin pulled out his penlight flashlight from his uniform pocket just as the Code Team arrived with the crash cart.

"Get a gurney," Franklin ordered. "Pupils sluggish, and the left one is slightly larger than the right. Airway open, breathing shallow but regular, pulse thready and rapid at 150. Limbs are pliant. He's unconscious," Franklin called out, as one of the other nurses grabbed the clipboard attached to the cart and began to record patient data. Another nurse announced that a physician was en route and would arrive momentarily. A third nurse unhooked the backboard from the back of the crash cart. Together, the team approached the patient, ready to slide the board into place when they were ordered to do so.

The nurses heard the sound of feet running down the hallway, and then two physicians appeared: Dr. Swanson from the ER night shift and Dr. Benjamin, the duty doctor for Medicine and Surgery. The doctors quickly moved in to assess the patient and provide direction. Franklin filled them in on the patient's history while they did so.

"Call the OR STAT," said Dr. Swanson. "And get someone from Neuro there. I want this man moved, now. Alert MRI and have them stand by for an emergency." She continued to confer with Dr. Benjamin as they completed a rapid but comprehensive physical assessment of the patient after his fall. Gil remained unconscious.

"Clearly he tumbled onto his upper body and face first," said Dr. Swanson. "Point of impact appears to be frontotemporal. These black eyes don't help; they complicate our visual inspection."

Dr. Benjamin nodded affirmatively as he palpated the patient's nose, brow, and orbital sockets as a precaution. Behind them, a nurse picked up the fallen IV pole. Another nurse unhooked the patient's catheter bag from where it was hung on the side rail of the bed, and she moved it closer to the patient. Franklin, who remained on the floor with the patient and the physicians, checked to see that both the IV of normal saline and the indwelling catheter were still in place. After he confirmed that they were still connected, he reported his findings to the team.

"The nose is intact," said Dr. Benjamin. "No leakage of CSF there or from the ears. I agree with you, Dr. Swanson. It doesn't appear that his face struck the floor directly. I think we're at high risk here for a subdural hematoma. Increased intracranial pressure is a real likelihood, especially based on the current diagnosis of head injury."

"Agreed, Dr. Benjamin. But we can't rule out second-impact syndrome just yet, either. If that's the case, we've got to move extremely quickly." Dr. Swanson stepped aside then as the nurses brought the backboard nearer. She and Dr. Benjamin assisted them with positioning the patient on it.

"Bag him," Dr. Benjamin directed, as they lifted the patient onto a stretcher. Franklin complied. "MRI STAT," the doctor ordered. The team rushed away with Gil, headed for Radiology.

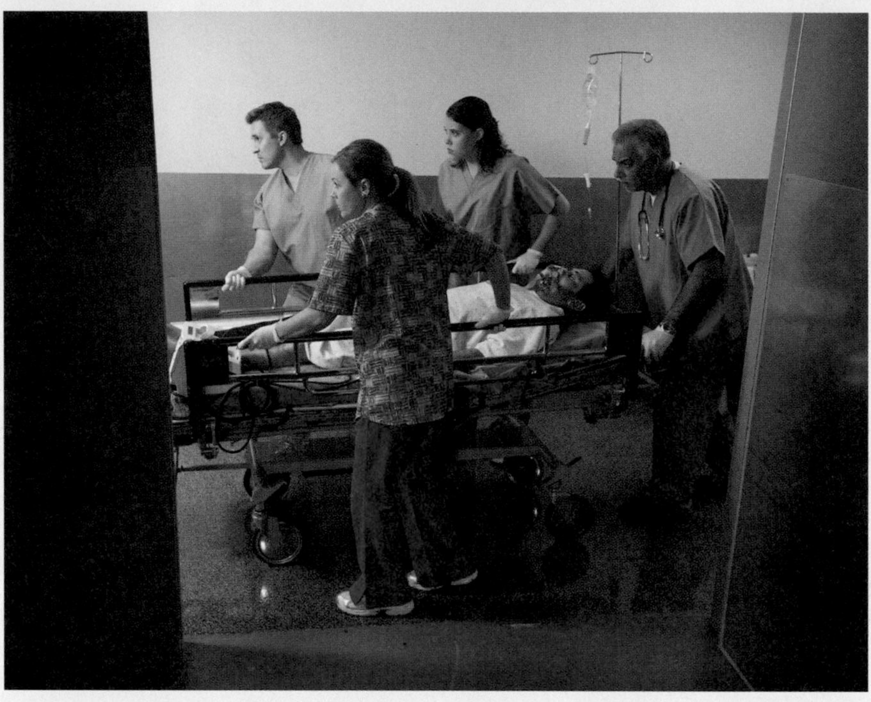

Reflective Questions

Reflect on the Patient Update you've just read as you answer these questions.

1. When is this emergency occurring? How do you know? ______________________________

2. What two medical complications are new potentials for this patient? ______________________

3. One of the physicians palpates Gil's nose. Why? ______________________________

Critical Thinking

Consider Gilbert Loeppky's emergent health crisis as you answer these questions.

1. Why did Franklin use the term *Code* instead of just calling out to the staff on duty that he had an emergency in Gil's room?

   ____

2. Why did Gil Loeppky try to get out of bed?

   ____

Key terms: neurological emergency

"'*Call a Code!*' shouted the nurse ..."

call a Code: medical jargon referring to the policy and protocol for responding to an emergency. (Refer to Chapter 5 for more details about different kinds of codes.)

"... as he was doing *rounds*..."

rounds: in the context of the Patient Update, the term *rounds* refers to a routine inspection of the unit, when a nurse sees all of his or her assigned patients. In this context, rounds are conducted quite frequently and routinely.

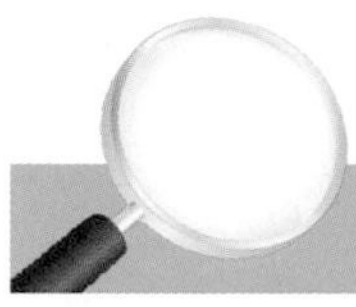

FOCUS POINT: More about Rounds

In a hospital, the word *rounds* is used in several different contexts:

Medical rounds occur when physicians check in with their patients to speak with them or assess them. This might happen only once per shift, depending on the patients' medical needs.

Nurses' rounds, in another context, might refer to the time when one shift is ending and another is starting. An incoming nurse may tour her patients with the outgoing nurse. Together, they speak with each patient about the day's health-care concerns.

The term *nurses' rounds* can also refer to a special meeting of a larger group of nurses than those on just one unit. At this meeting, there is an exchange of information and ideas that are pertinent to nursing care activities. This type of nursing rounds is not focused on individual patients. Similarly, *medical rounds* can also refer to a special meeting of a wider group of physicians working in the facility for the same purpose.

Grand rounds are presentations of medical information, case studies, and medical education to facility-wide groups of doctors, nurses, and other health-care professionals.

"...just as the *Code Team* arrived with the *crash cart*."

Code Team: in a large medical center, this is a group of doctors and nurses who are designated responders to any Code alert that occurs during a specific work shift. In smaller facilities, a Code Team may include all available nurses and doctors on site, as well as laboratory, respiratory, and electrocardiology staff members.

crash cart: a portable trolley that includes medication and equipment for the treatment of cardiac arrest, injury, and other emergencies. It is sometimes called the *Code cart* (see Figure 10-6).

"'Get a *gurney* ...'"

gurney: a synonym for *stretcher.*

"Limbs are *pliant*."

pliant: moveable, flaccid (not rigid), flexible, and bendable.

"... get *someone from Neuro* there."

someone from Neuro: in this emergency context, the doctor is referring to a neurosurgeon.

"*Alert MRI* and have them stand by..."

Alert MRI: in this context, this means that someone needs to notify the magnetic resonance imaging (MRI) technicians and radiologists that an emergency case of head trauma is coming to them in the very near future.

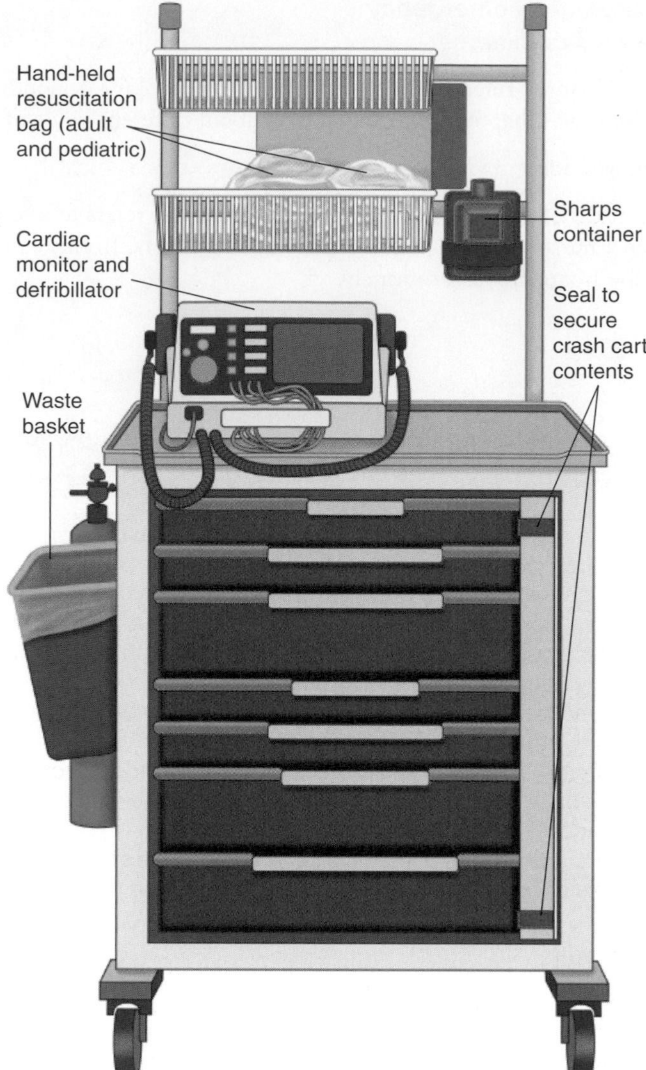

Figure 10.6: Crash cart (From Eagle S, Brassington C, Dailey CS, Goretti C: *The Professional Medical Assistant: An Integrative, Teamwork-Based Approach.* Philadelphia: FA Davis, 2009, p. 970. With permission.)

"Point of impact appears to be *frontotemporal.*"

frontotemporal: the front and side (near the temple) of the skull.

"... the *IV* of *normal saline ...*"

IV: intravenous, meaning *within a vein.* The patient, Gil Loeppky, has an intravenous line in place (in situ) to keep him properly hydrated. The body requires an adequate amount of hydration throughout the day to maintain homeostasis and to promote the effective functioning of organs. The term **dehydration** refers to increased fluid loss, which involves a water and sodium deficit. It is a serious condition that can be caused by trauma, fever, blood loss, infection, or disease. Gil Loeppky's IV will prevent dehydration, but it may also have been inserted to ensure that the care team has access to his veins in case they need to give the patient another type of IV solution or a blood transfusion. Intravenous infusion—the uptake of intravenous solution (and any medications or other substances that are within it)—is rapid.

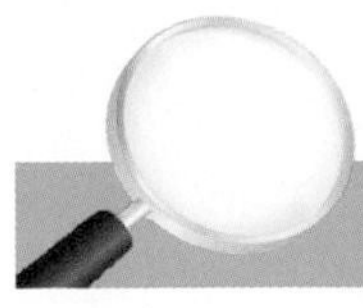

FOCUS POINT: Keep Vein Open: KVO

Access to a vein is a medical expression. When a patient is in the hospital, it is important to keep a vein "open" or ready for receiving fluids to avoid the complication of having to search for a useable vein in the midst of a crisis. For example, electrolytes and many medications are best given via the intravenous route. The medical abbreviation for maintaining access to a vein is *KVO,* which is short for the phrase *keep vein open.*

normal saline: a type of intravenous solution that consists of sodium chloride (NaCl; salt) and water. In the intravenous form, it is sterile. This is the most common type of intravenous solution that is used. It is hydrating, it mirrors the body's own fluids, and medications can be added to it through a port in the intravenous line. This solution is sometimes referred to as *NS* or *NS 0.9%.*

"No *leakage of CSF* there or from the ears..."

leakage of CSF: a critical situation in which cerebrospinal fluid (CSF) leaks into the cranium. Leakage occurs through the nose and ears. The cause is usually blunt force trauma to the head. Our patient, Gil Loeppky, has now suffered two incidents of blunt force trauma to the head, so looking for the leakage of CSF a significant factor during the emergency assessment performed by the Code Team.

"... a *subdural hematoma* ..."

subdural: below the dura mater; a layer of tissue that covers and protects the brain.

hematoma: swelling and an accumulation of blood that is caused by a break in a blood vessel.

"*Increased intracranial pressure* ..."

increased intracranial pressure: a rise in the normal pressure exerted within the cranium.

"...we can't rule out *second-impact syndrome* ..."

second-impact syndrome: an injury to the brain that happens after an original brain or head injury.

"'*Bag* him...'"

bag: medical jargon that refers to the use of an AMBU bag to force air into a patient's lungs to sustain brain vitality (life). The acronym **AMBU** stands for **air-shields manual breathing unit.** (The term *bagging* refers to the action of a health-care provider when he or she manually forces air into the patient's lungs by compressing and decompressing the AMBU bag that is attached to an airway valve placed over the patient's nose and mouth. The activity itself is called *forced ventilation.* When a person is found unconscious and not breathing, forced ventilation is used to oxygenate the lungs and prevent brain injury. There is an AMBU bag on every crash cart.

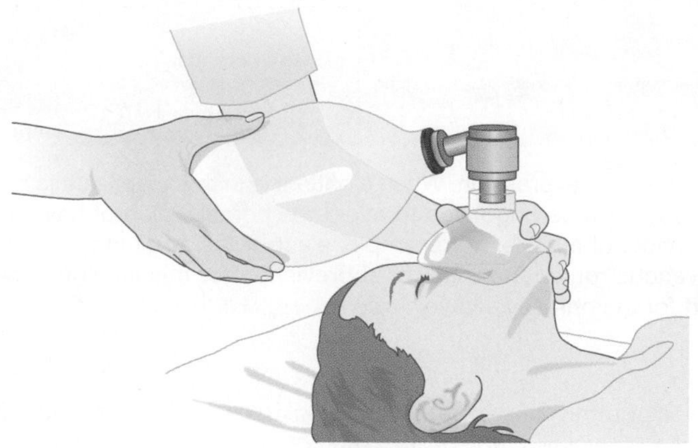

Figure 10.7: AMBU bag

Date/time	Nurse notes
XX/XX/XX 0315 hr	Pt. found on floor at 0300 hr moments after falling out of bed. Room lights up. ABC completed. Unconscious. Airway open and breathing. Pulse 150, thready and rapid. Code called. First aid for unconscious patient begun. Attended on floor. Head stabilized between two pillows. Body and limbs assessed. Reddened area approx. 1 inch circle, frontal-temporal skull, left side. Code team arrived at 0303 hr. Drs. Swanson and Benjamin in attendance. IV and urinary catheter in situ. Temporary leg splint in place. Backboard applied. Patient to OR at 0315 hr. Chart accompanying pt. —— M. Howell, RN

Critical Reflection Questions

Read "On the Job: Nurses' Notes: Code Team" (shown above), which describes Gil Loeppky's critical incident. To answer these questions, draw on the knowledge that you have gained in this and previous chapters to decipher what was written, and then answer these questions.

1. What does the abbreviation *ABC* stand for? ______________________
2. Franklin, the nurse, was concerned about the patient's spinal cord. What evidence do you see regarding that concern in the nurses' notes? ______________________

Mix and Match

Match each word, phrase, or abbreviation on the left with the correct medical term on the right.

1. stretcher	intracranial
2. type of bruise or swelling	Code
3. inside the skull	gurney
4. immediately	bagging
5. medical emergency	hematoma
6. CSF	cerebrospinal fluid
7. a form of forced ventilation	STAT

Brain anatomy and physiology

In Chapter 4, you were introduced to the neurological system and basic terms related to head injuries. With that strong foundation, you are now ready to expand your language and knowledge base by learning more terminology and more details about head injuries. To follow Gil Loeppky through his current crisis, you need to develop a more detailed knowledge of the brain.

The brain sits in the *cranial vault* (cavity). It is protected by the bones of the skull, the meninges, and the CSF.

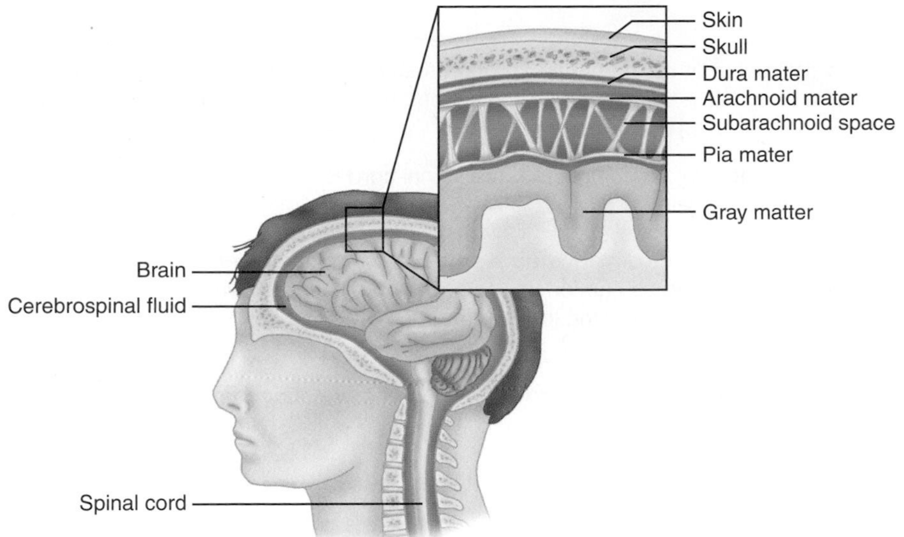

Figure 10.8: The covering of the brain: cross-sectional view

The meninges

The **meninges** are made up of specialized membranous connective tissues that surround the brain and the attached spinal cord. These layers of connective tissue are called *mater.* There are three different layers of mater: the *dura mater*, the *arachnoid mater,* and the *pia mater.*

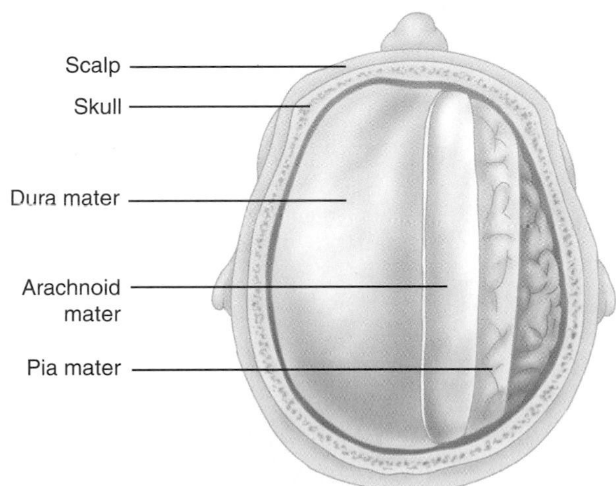

Figure 10.9: The meninges: topical view

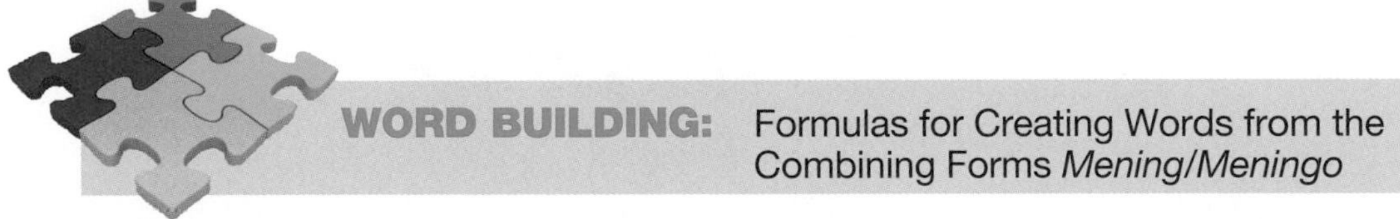

WORD BUILDING: Formulas for Creating Words from the Combining Forms *Mening/Meningo*

meninge = a root meaning *membrane.* The combining forms are *mening-* and *meningo-*.

mening + itis = *meningitis*

Definition: an inflammation of the spinal cord or brain. *noun*

Example: *Meningitis* can be viral, bacterial, or infectious.

Continued

meningo + cele = *meningocele*

Definition: a protrusion of the meninges through the cranium or through a rupture in the spine as a result of a congenital (birth) defect. (The second root is *cele,* which is derived from *kele,* the Greek word for *hernia.*) *noun*

Example: In a patient with a *meningocele,* the spinal cord is not damaged; therefore, neurological function is not impaired.

myelo + meningo + cele = *myelomeningocele*

Definition: an incomplete fusion (union) in utero of the spinal cord, which results in the spinal cord's protrusion through an opening in a vertebra. (The prefix *myelo-* means *spinal cord.* A synonym is *meningomyelocele.*) *noun*

Example: *Myelomeningocele* can lead to difficulties with urination, defecation, and walking.

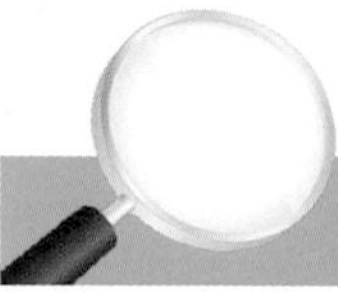

FOCUS POINT: Spina Bifida

The condition of *spina bifida* occurs before birth. It is a type of myelomeningocele in which the meninges protrude from the spinal cord. This occurs in an embryo when the fusion of the spinal cord is incomplete. The result is the underdevelopment or damage of the nerves that originate at the level of the spinal cord. Partial paralysis from that point downward is possible, as are problems with bladder and bowel control.

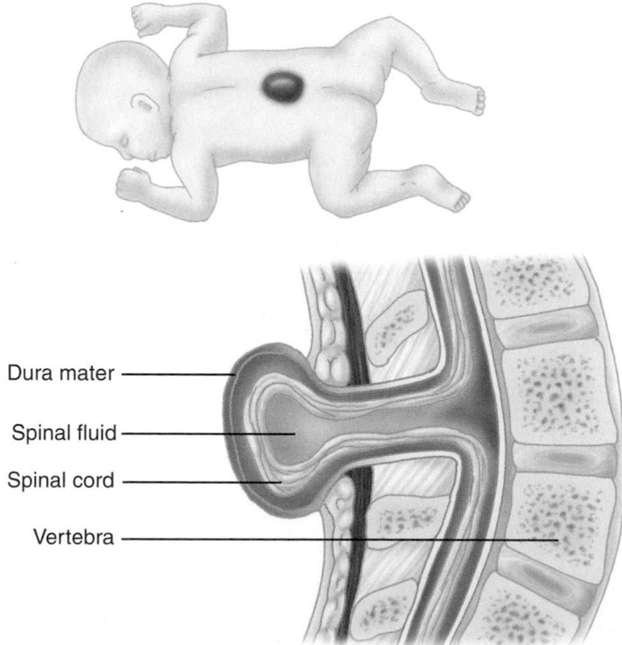

Figure 10.10: Infant with spina bifida

Let's Practice

Write the medical term that fits each description and that includes a combining form of *mening/meningo.*

1. This viral infection seems to target high school students. It causes swelling in the brain.

   ____

2. Protection is provided for the central nervous system by this group of specialized tissues.

   ____

3. Before birth, this condition results from a tear in the membranes that surround the spinal cord. It can result in the child's inability to walk properly.

   ____

Types of mater

Dura mater is the outermost membrane of the meninges. It is a strong because it is highly fibrous in nature. The dura mater (or dura) supports the larger blood vessels of the brain, which transport nutrients to and from the heart. Dura mater is also known as *pachymeninx* (singular) or *pachymeninges* (plural).

Dura means *hard.*

Pachy- means *thick.*

Arachnoid mater is a loose, sac-like membrane between the dura mater and the pia mater that covers the brain. *Arachnoid* is the scientific name for *spider.* The arachnoid mater is web-like in appearance (see Figure 10-11).

Pia mater is the meningeal membrane that adheres to the brain and the spinal cord. Blood vessels permeate it.

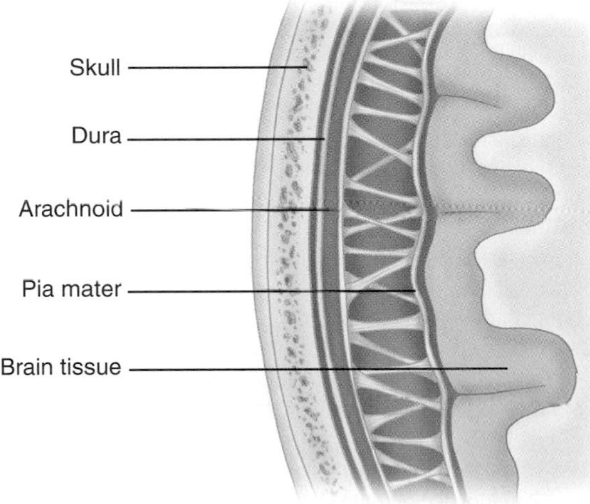

Figure 10.11: Meninges and mater: cross-sectional view

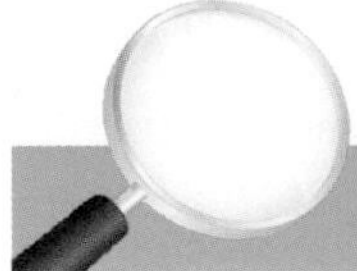

FOCUS POINT: Meningismus

Meningismus is a disorder of early childhood that presents as symptoms of meningitis. However, diagnostic testing determines that there is no pathology of the meninges present. The symptoms are thought to be caused by pneumonia.

Pathology of the meninges

Meningitis, which is the inflammation of the meninges, is the most common pathology of the meninges. It can be either infectious or non-infectious. When the strain of meningitis is contagious, it can cause brain damage and even death. There are four main types of infectious meningitis, which are classified by the type of organism that is responsible for the infection: bacterial, viral, fungal, and parasitic (see Chapter 5). Vaccination is available only for meningococcal meningitis, a bacterial form of the disease. Table 10-1 explains the types of meningitis in more detail.

Symptoms of bacterial and viral meningitis can include the following:

- fever
- severe headache
- nuchal rigidity (stiff neck)
- nausea and vomiting
- photophobia (sensitivity to light)
- confusion
- sleepiness and lethargy
- seizure

Noninfectious causes of meningitis include disease and the adverse effects of medication. Non-steroidal anti-inflammatory drugs and antibiotics can also be culprits (see Chapters 5, 7, and 9).

TABLE 10-1: General Types of Meningitis and Their Pathophysiology

Type of Meningitis	Pathophysiology, Symptoms, and Treatment Outcomes
Bacterial	The result of a bacterial infection that has colonized somewhere in the body. These bacteria enter the bloodstream and find their way into the cerebrospinal fluid. Bacterial infections in the ears, mouth, or sinuses can spread quickly to the brain and spinal cord The most severe of all the types of meningitis, it can cause brain damage and death Common pathogens: *Streptococcus pneumoniae, Neisseria meningitis* Treatment includes hospitalization with antibiotics given via the intravenous route
Viral	Often caused by enteroviruses (intestinal viruses); most common during the spring and fall months Spread through mucous, saliva, and feces Can also develop as a result of infection by the viruses that cause measles, polio, and chickenpox or can be the result of complications of the mumps Treatment includes rest at home with the use of minor analgesics for headaches and other pains
Fungal	Less common in the general population, this type of meningitis often strikes people with immunocompromised conditions such as human immunodeficiency virus/acquired immunodeficiency syndrome, lupus, leukemia, or diabetes Causative agents include *Cryptococcus neoformans* (found in soil and aged pigeon feces) and *Candida albicans* (yeast infections) Treatment includes intravenous and oral antifungal agents
Parasitic (amoebic/amebic)	Derives from tiny organisms found in hot springs/geothermal pools and improperly maintained pools and hot tubs Rare; cannot be passed from person to person as the other types of meningitis can; invades the host through the nose Treatment includes large doses of antifungal medications and antibiotics given intravenously; hospitalization is necessary

Name the Term and Break It Down

Write the term that fits each definition or description. Next, break down the term into its separate word parts, and write the meaning of each part.

1. inflammation of the three layers that cover the brain and the spinal cord
   Term: ______________________________
   Word parts: ______________________________
2. an adjective for the spinal cord and the brain together
   Term: ______________________________
   Word parts: ______________________________

Mix and Match

Draw a line to connect the synonyms.

1. deleterious	meningomyelocele
2. dura mater	stiff neck
3. nuchal rigidity	harmful
4. myelomeningocele	pachymeninx

Ventricles and cerebrospinal fluid

The **ventricles** of the brain are the four main cavities within it. Each ventricle connects to the canal of the spinal cord. The ventricles are filled with CSF, which is created from structures in the roofs and walls of the ventricles. Capillaries extend into the ventricles and carry blood plasma that, once filtered, will become one of the constituents of the CSF.

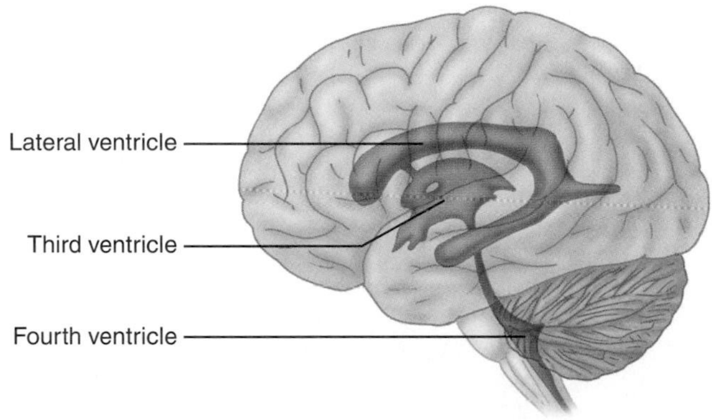

Figure 10.12: Ventricles of the brain

Cerebrospinal fluid is a clear, colorless liquid that circulates in the ventricles and the spaces around the brain and spinal cord. It is found in the *subarachnoid space* between the arachnoid mater and the pia mater. It is formed within the ventricles and then reabsorbed into the blood there.

The functions of CSF include the following:

- *Protective:* Physically, the CSF provides lubrication for the brain, the spinal cord, and the accompanying bones. It provides buoyancy for support, and it acts as a protective cushion in case of injury, thus distributing the force of any impact. CSF also assists with the maintenance of a constant level of intracranial pressure (ICP).
- *Nutritive:* The CSF transports hormones, magnesium, sodium and chloride ions, and minute quantities of other elements to the brain and provides a chemically stable environment for the brain and the spinal cord.

- *Cleansing:* The CSF carries waste materials such as metabolites, drugs, and other substances away from the brain.
- *Communicative:* The CSF acts as a chemical messenger to the central nervous system, particularly with regard to levels of interstitial fluid. **Interstitial fluid**, which surrounds cells and is found between cells, allows nutrients to enter the cells. It absorbs metabolic wastes from the cells and transports these away. It is also known as **intercellular fluid**.

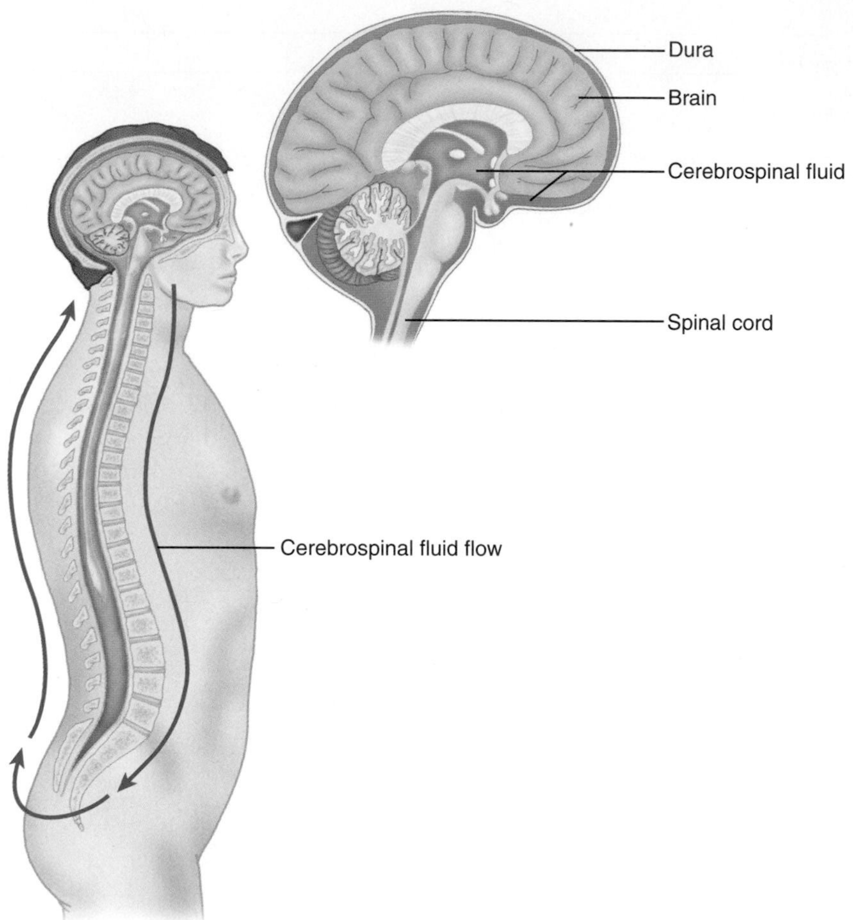

Figure 10.13: Cerebrospinal fluid

Break It Down

Break each word down into its component parts. Identify prefixes, roots, and suffixes.

1. subdural ______
2. hematoma ______
3. intracerebral ______
4. subarachnoid ______

PRONOUNCIATION PRACTICE

Say these words aloud to a friend or classmate, if you can. Here you are given the phonetic pronunciation. Your instructor can help you with pronunciation,

or you can visit **http://www.MedicalLanguageLab.com.**

arachnoid	ă-**răk**´noyd	nuchal	**nū**´kăl
dura	**dū**´ră	permeate	**pĕr**´mē-āt
decerebrate	dē-**sĕr**´ĕ-brat	pia	**pē**´ă
mater	**mā**´tŭr	myelomeningocele	mī″ĕ-lō-mĕn-**ĭn**´gō-sēl
meninges	mĕn-**ĭn**´jēz		

Intracranial pathology

Increased ICP and intracranial hemorrhage can have devastating effects on the functional abilities of the central nervous system (i.e., the brain and spinal cord). As ICP increases, it pushes down on the brain, and it can eventually push hard enough to impair or destroy the brainstem (see Figure 10-14). The brainstem descends just under the cerebellum to meet and join the spinal cord. Any trauma to the brainstem can be life threatening because this structure is the center of control for respiration and the beating of the heart.

The physicians at Okla Trauma Center are concerned that our patient, Gil Loeppky, has incurred the second-impact syndrome of a concussion, developed an intracranial hematoma, or both. Each of these conditions has the potential to cause increased ICP with an additional risk of an intracranial bleed or hemorrhage. The quicker the medical team works to diagnose and intercept any trauma that is occurring in the patient's brain, the better the chances for his full recovery.

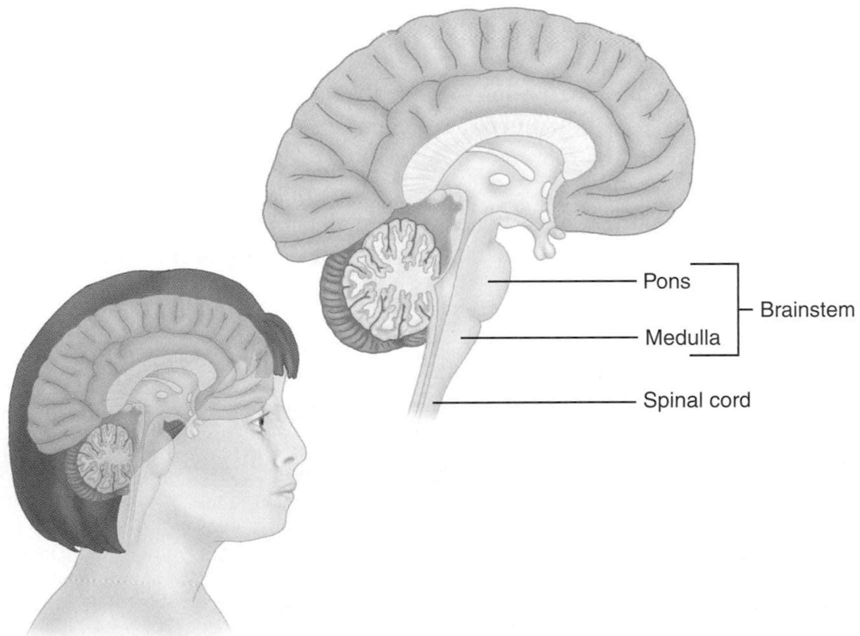

Figure 10.14: The brainstem

Increased intracranial pressure

The brain is encased in the skull. Under normal conditions, the pressure level of CSF within the skull remains constant and unchanging. However, any trauma or disease that causes inflammation of the brain or bleeding into the skull cavity causes an increase in the pressure in that small space. When this occurs, the CSF is unable to circulate, yet it continues to be produced, thereby creating even more pressure. The increased **intracranial pressure (ICP)** compresses the brain, and brain damage or death may be the result. Relief can be provided by emergency surgery or by a variety of other medical interventions and medications.

Symptoms of abnormally high ICP can include the following: headache, nausea, vomiting, alterations in pupil size, seizures, increased fatigue and drowsiness, memory loss, and changes in levels of consciousness (see Chapter 4). ICP is measured in millimeters of mercury (mm Hg), a standard measure of atmospheric pressure.

Intracranial pressure ranges

0 to 10 mm Hg: normal

>20 mm Hg: abnormal

>40 mm Hg: indicates neurological dysfunction, with a poor prognosis for full recovery of mental or neurological function

>60 mm Hg: fatal

Intracranial hemorrhage

Intracranial hemorrhage is bleeding within the cranium. This can occur as the result of a head injury that causes a jostling and tearing of the brain and its blood vessels. It can also be the result of blood disorders, blood clots, and other factors. If it is not treated immediately, this condition is always critical. Facts about one type of intracranial hemorrhage appear in Table 10-2.

Head injuries can also have deleterious (harmful) effects on the meninges. With or without a skull fracture, the patient is at risk for intracranial hematoma or hemorrhage. Arteries and veins run above, through, and below the meninges, and they can be pierced, stretched thin and tight, and ruptured. In each case, blood flow is interrupted, and it may leak into the cranial vault and the ventricles of the brain.

Intracranial hematoma

As you know, a **hematoma** is a collection of blood under the skin or within an organ or muscle. It is composed of either partially clotted or fully clotted blood. The blood clot of an intracranial hematoma may sit within the cranium for some time undetected while it exerts pressure on the brain. Symptoms of neurological dysfunction may appear over time (see Table 10-3). Permanent damage and neurological deficits can occur as a result of hematomas that develop in response to head injury.

The dura mater attaches itself to the bones of the skull at points where the bones meet. These points are called **suture lines**. Should an injury cause a hematoma to develop in any of

TABLE 10-2: Example of an Intracranial Hemorrhage

Example	Location	Etiology and Development	Symptoms	Treatment
Subarachnoid hemorrhage (SAH)	Under the arachnoid mater	Begins as an aneurysm (bulge in an artery) that finally ruptures	Headache and vomiting; meninges will be irritated by the presence of blood, which can result in low back pain, bilateral leg pain, and neck stiffness	Use of the diuretic mannitol to reduce intracranial pressure; use of antihypertensive medications; surgery is not always necessary

these tight spaces, the increase in ICP will be swift, and the hematoma itself will exert pressure against brain tissue. Brain damage is a strong potential in this situation. Treatment is indicated to remove the offending hematoma and to relieve the pressure. The most serious risk presented by an intracranial hematoma is its potential to rupture, thereby causing intracranial hemorrhage.

There are three main types of intracranial hematoma: epidural, subdural, and intracerebral.

Epidural hematoma

An **epidural hematoma (EDH)** is a buildup of blood between the dura mater and the bone. This can occur in the brain or the spinal cord. An intracranial EDH is extremely serious and requires immediate surgery. An EDH occurring at the site of the temporal bone of the skull (just above the ear) is especially dangerous. A meningeal artery runs just below that bone, so bleeding may be rapid and profuse.

Subdural hematoma

In the case of a **subdural hematoma (SDH)**, the collection of blood occurs between the brain tissue and the dura mater. This medical situation can be caused by a stretching or tearing of the veins that bridge between the dura mater and the brain. SDHs are classified as acute or chronic. With an acute SDH, symptoms appear suddenly after an injury. With a chronic SDH, symptoms appear gradually, and a small, slow bleed may be occurring in the cranium without anyone's knowledge. A reinjury or second-impact injury could be immediately life threatening.

Intracerebral hematoma

Intracerebral hematoma (ICH) is usually the result of severe head injury, which is known as *cerebral contusion* (see Chapter 4). It does not include the meninges. Instead, with an ICH, fluid accumulates in the brain itself. This is the most common reason for death after a head contusion. Surgery is not recommended for these patients, and associated brain damage cannot be reversed. ICHs are detected by CT or MRI.

Details about one type of intracerebral hemorrhage appear in Table 10-3.

Is it a hematoma or a stroke?

When there is a loss of blood to the brain, a cerebral infarction or stroke (cerebrovascular accident) can occur. Table 10-4 compares the potential symptoms of a cerebral infarction and an intracranial hematoma. It suggests the difficulties doctors may have when diagnosing these conditions. For example, you will notice that both conditions may involve patients that present with symptoms of *anisocoria*, **vertigo**, *dysphasia*, *paralysis*, *hemiparesis*, and *paresthesia* (see definitions on Table 10-4), as well as visual impairment, memory loss, headache, difficulty concentrating, and loss of consciousness. The importance of attaining CT and MRI scans before diagnosing either condition cannot be overlooked.

TABLE 10-3: Example of an Intracerebral Hemorrhage

Example	Location	Etiology and Development	Symptoms	Treatment
Intraparenchymal hemorrhage (bleeding within the tissues) caused by cerebral contusion	Tissues of the brain	Bleeding into the brain, where the blood pools; caused by trauma	Dependent on where the pool of blood occurs and exerts pressure	Minor bleeding may stop on its own; more significant bleeding may require surgery

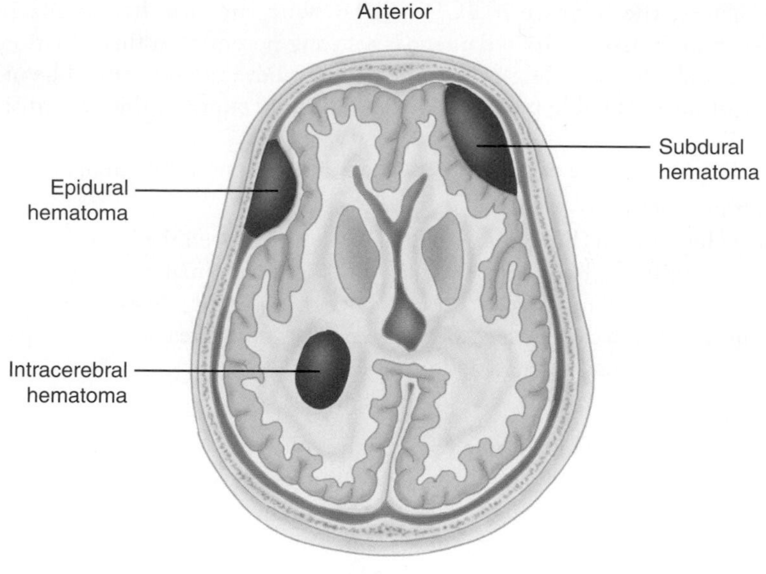

Figure 10.15: Types of hematoma

TABLE 10-4: Comparison: Potential Symptoms of Cerebral Infarction and Intracranial Hematoma

Potential Symptoms	Present with Cerebral Infarction	Present with Intracranial Hematoma
Anisocoria (unequal pupil sizes)	√	√
Vertigo (dizziness; a sense of whirling and loss of balance)	√	√
Dysphasia (impairment of language function; difficulty understanding language)	√	√
Aphasia (lack of language function or ability)	√	No
Dysarthria (impairment of clarity of speech; inability to articulate words)	√	No
Changes in cerebrospinal fluid levels	Moderate to severe increase in levels	No change
Paralysis (loss of muscle strength in the limbs, which leads to a loss of motor function [the ability to move and control one's muscles])	√	√
Hemiparesis (paralysis on one side or plane of the body)	√	√
Hemianesthesia (sensory disturbances)	√	No
Paresthesia (a stinging, burning, or prickling sensation or a feeling of numbness as a result of nerve injury)	√	√
Visual impairment or blindness	√	√
Seizures	No	√
Memory loss	√	√
Headache	√	√
Difficulty concentrating	√	√
Anxiety	No	√
Drowsiness or lethargy	No	√
High body temperature	Should not occur; if it does, the reduction of body temperature is critical	May occur; attempts will be made to reduce body temperature and to keep it slightly lower than normal
Loss of consciousness/coma	√	√
Potential for death	√	√

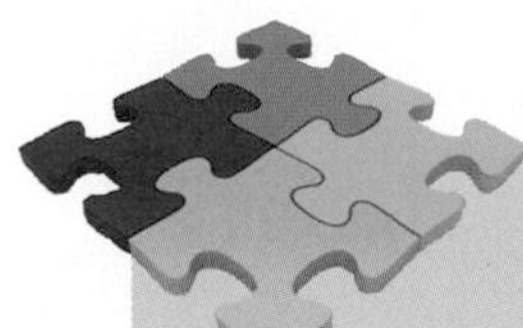

WORD BUILDING: Formula for Adding the Prefix *Par-* or *Para-*

The Prefix *Par-* or *Para-*

The prefix *par/a-* has numerous meanings. The ability to interpret a word that begins with this prefix requires knowledge of root words, combining forms, and even suffixes, as well as strict attention to the context of the sentence.

***Par/a-* can mean *beside, at or to one side, by, near, beyond, or past.* It can also mean *resembling, apart from, or abnormal.* Here are some examples:**

para + nas/o + al = *paranasal*

Definition: situated beside or along the nasal cavities; beside the nose. *adjective*

Example: Complications of *paranasal* sinus trauma from a facial injury can include hemorrhage, unconsciousness, meningitis, and the leakage of cerebrospinal fluid.

para + hypn/os + osis = *parahypnosis*

Definition: a condition resembling sleep; abnormal sleep that may include a state of hypersuggestibility. (The root *hypnos* means *sleep.*) *noun*

Example: A state of *parahypnosis* can be induced by anesthesia or hypnosis, and the patient may be aware of what is said around him or her during a medical procedure.

para + somnia = *parasomnia*

Definition: an abnormal event that occurs during sleep. (*Somnia* is a combining form of the root *somnus,* meaning *sleep.*) *noun*

Example: Two types of *parasomnia* are night terrors and sleepwalking.

para + paresis = *paraparesis*

Definition: partial paralysis that affects only the lower limbs. The root word is *paresis,* meaning *weakness and partial loss of motor function. noun*

Example: Tropical spastic *paraparesis* is a progressive disorder of the neurological system that is generally found in people who live in tropical regions near the equator.

para + profession + al = *paraprofessional*

Definition: an occupation that is ancillary or subsidiary to a professional; a person with some training and expertise who works beside a professional. *noun*

Example: A paramedic is a *paraprofessional.*

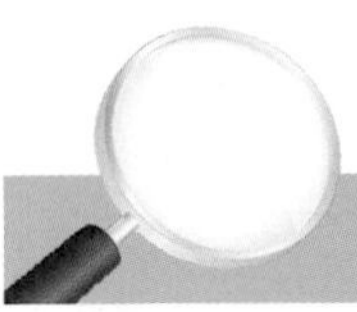

FOCUS POINT: *Para-* and *Parallel*

Parallel is a root word that includes the meaning of the prefix *para-* within it. The word *parallel* means *side by side.*

Right Word or Wrong Word: *Paresis* or *Paralysis*?

Study these two words. They are similar, but not the same. What is the difference in meaning?

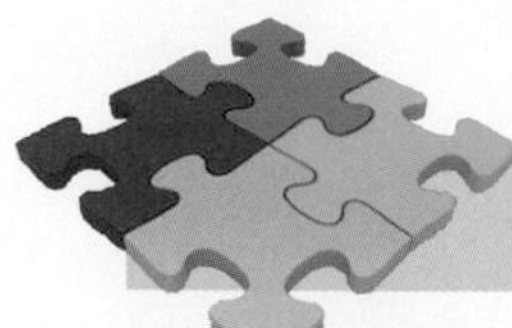

WORD BUILDING: Formula for Adding the Prefix *Dys-*

The Prefix *Dys-*
Recall from Chapter 8 that *dys-* can mean *difficult, impaired, or painful.* It can also mean *lack of, inability,* or *bad.* The ability to interpret a word that begins with *dys-* requires knowledge of root words, combining forms, and any suffixes that may be attached. Here are some examples:

dys + bas + ia = *dysbasia*
Definition: difficulty walking as a result of a disease of the central nervous system. (The second word part is a combining form of the root *basis,* meaning *step.*) *noun*

Example: *Dysbasia* is a neurological symptom that often originates in the spine.

dys + lexia = *dyslexia*
Definition: impairment in the ability to read or write words. *noun*

Example: *Dyslexia* is a learning disorder that is more common among males but that can also occur in females.

dys + kines + ia = *dyskinesia*
Definition: difficulty of movement or uncontrolled movement. (The second word part is the combining form of *kinesis,* meaning *motion.*) *noun*

Example: Damage to the central nervous system can lead to symptoms of *dyskinesia.*

dys + phor + ia = *dysphoria*
Definition: a state of long-lasting altered emotion. (The second word part is derived from the root *pherein,* meaning *to bear.*) *noun*

Example: *Dysphoria* is a mood disorder.

Let's Practice

Identify the prefix in each word, and then write its meaning. Although you have seen most of these words before, learning is reinforced when you use new terms, knowledge, and skills frequently.

1. epidural Prefix: ____________ Meaning: ____________
2. intracranial Prefix: ____________ Meaning: ____________
3. aphasia Prefix: ____________ Meaning: ____________
4. parasomnia Prefix: ____________ Meaning: ____________
5. dysphasia Prefix: ____________ Meaning: ____________
6. subdural Prefix: ____________ Meaning: ____________
7. hemiplegia Prefix: ____________ Meaning: ____________
8. leukemia Prefix: ____________ Meaning: ____________
9. photophobia Prefix: ____________ Meaning: ____________
10. reinjury Prefix: ____________ Meaning: ____________
11. neoformans Prefix: ____________ Meaning: ____________
12. enteroviruses Prefix: ____________ Meaning: ____________

Critical Thinking

On the basis of what you've been learning about ICP and other brain pathology, review the Patient Update that told the story of when Gilbert Loeppky fell out of bed.

1. Write the symptoms identified by RN Franklin here.

   ____

2. Is Gil suffering from an intracranial hematoma, an intracranial hemorrhage, increased ICP, meningitis, or cerebral infarction? How can you tell?

   ____

Fill in the Blanks

Use the new medical terminology that you have learned to complete these sentences.

1. A term that means *a bleed within the cranium* is ____________________.
2. A collection of blood under the dura mater is called a(n) ____________________.
3. Another way to say that "pressure is exerted on the brain" is to say that "the brain is ____________________."
4. The medical term for bleeding is ____________________.
5. A hematoma that occurs above the dura mater is referred to as a(n) ____________________.
6. In neurology, millimeters of mercury (mm Hg) are used as measurements of ____________________.
7. ICP is the abbreviation for ____________________.
8. The proper medical term for the skull is the ____________________.

Mix and Match

Match each medical term with its description.

1. nuchal rigidity	cavity
2. arachnoid	three layers of mater
3. vault	stiff neck
4. photophobia	harmful
5. meninges	spider
6. deleterious	sensitivity to light

Let's Practice

Study Table 10-4, and then write the medical term that fits each description.

1. inability to use language ____________________
2. partial inability to move ____________________
3. difficulty experiencing sensation on one side of the body ____________________
4. trouble articulating words ____________________
5. loss of balance as a result of a sense of spinning ____________________
6. unequal pupil sizes ____________________

Right Word or Wrong Word: *Intercranial* or *Intracranial*?

Are these two words the same or different? Do they differ in meaning?

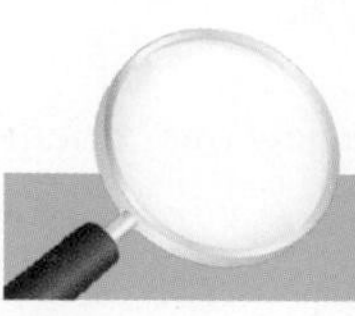

FOCUS POINT: Ataxia

Ataxia is an important clinical sign of neurological impairment. It is a signal of pressure on the brain or brain damage. *Ataxia* means *lack of coordination.* To understand the term, deconstruct it as follows:

a: without

taxis: root meaning *order or coordination*

Patient Update

Recall from Chapter 4 that Gil Loeppky had originally been assessed for concussion and contusion. After his fall from the bed in this chapter, his doctors were afraid that he might have acquired second-impact syndrome as a result of a second concussion (i.e., a second insult to the brain). However, Gil did not have the full symptoms of this syndrome, so the physicians decided that they had sufficient time to transport him to surgery. As you read the next section about the second-impact syndrome of concussion, refer to the previous Patient Update to confirm the reasons that the health-care staff have for making their decision.

Second-impact syndrome of concussion

Second-impact syndrome occurs when a second blow to the head—for example, when Gil fell out of bed and hit his head on the floor—causes a loss of *autoregulation* of the blood supply of the brain, thereby leading to increased ICP. There is also risk for the *herniation* of the brain. Should that occur and if the brainstem is thus compromised, respiratory failure and death are likely. If the patient lives after such an occurrence, severe brain trauma may be evident. The average time from a second impact to brainstem failure can be as little as 2 to 5 minutes. The trauma team must react with precision and promptness to mitigate the damage and the risk to the patient's life.

autoregulation: the body's ability to keep blood flow constant, even though blood pressure may vary. Autoregulation can happen at the level of the organs and tissues, which are able to autoregulate their required levels of blood supply. Autoregulation is homeostatic.

respiratory failure: the cessation of breathing, which occurs when the respiratory center in the cerebellum has failed.

herniation: a term derived from *hernia,* meaning *the protrusion of a bodily structure through a wall that normally contains it.* (The term is most frequently heard in reference to an abdominal hernia, a condition that is more common in men and that is often the result of heavy lifting.) **Cerebral herniation** refers to a downward displacement of the brain into the brainstem.

Symptoms of second-impact syndrome include dilated pupils, stupor, irregular respirations, **hemiplegia** (weakness on one side of the body), and decerebrate rigidity. **Decerebrate rigidity** is an abnormal posture in which there is a rigid extension of the extremities. In other words, the limbs and the hands are turned down and back. It is often referred to informally as *posturing* (see Figure 10-16).

de + cerebr + ate = decerebrate

Definition: showing signs of the loss of brain functioning

The prefix *de-* means *removal of.*

The combining form *cerebr/o* means *brain.*

The suffix *-ate* means *showing the characteristics of.*

The assessment and treatment of suspected second-impact syndrome include airway management with intubation and neurosurgery. However, the prognosis for a patient with this condition is not good.

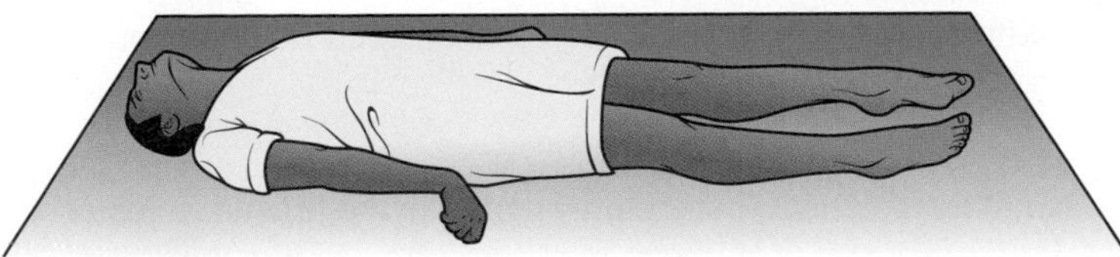

Figure 10.16: Body displaying decerebrate rigidity (From Eagle S: *Diseases in a Flash!: An Interactive, Flash-Card Approach.* Philadelphia: FA Davis, 2012, p 160. With permission.)

Mix and Match

Match each word part on the left with one on the right to create a proper medical term. Draw a line to connect your choices.

1. para-	normal
2. intra-	dural
3. epi-	coccal
4. cerebro	spinal
5. meningo	anesthesia
6. entero-	virus
7. hemi-	venous

Right Word or Wrong Word: *Cerebro-* or *Cephalo-*?

These two word parts seem similar, but they are not the same. How do they differ with regard to meaning?

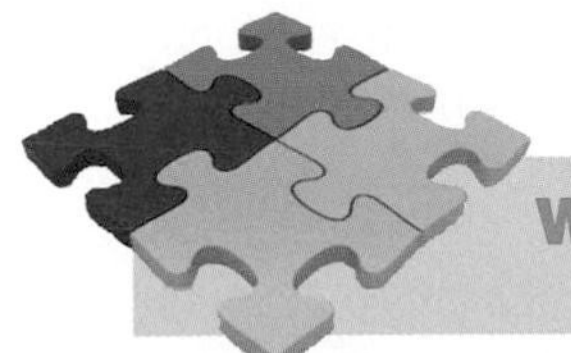

WORD BUILDING: Formula for Adding the Prefix *En-* and the Combining Form *Cephalo-*

As you know, the prefix *en-* means *in.* The combining form *cephalo-* means *cranium.* You should now also be familiar with the other word parts that compose the following examples.

en + cephalo + gram = *encephalogram*

Definition: a radiograph of the brain. *noun*

Example: Today, CTs and MRIs have largely replaced the taking of *encephalograms.*

electro + en + cephalo + gram = *electroencephalogram*

Definition: a device that is used to record brain wave activity. *noun*

Example: An *electroencephalogram* is used to help diagnose epilepsy, brain damage related to trauma or disease, and brain death.

en + cephal + oma = *encephaloma*

Definition: a tumor of the brain. *noun*

Example: An encephaloma is a cancerous tumor that grows within the skull.

Continued

en + cephalo + mening + itis = *encephalomeningitis*

Definition: the inflammation of the brain and the meninges. (A synonym is *meningoencephalitis.*) *noun*

Example: Patients with *encephalomeningitis* have an increased potential for seizures, tremors, and paralysis.

en + cephal + itis = *encephalitis*

Definition: the inflammation of the white and gray matter of the brain as a result of a virus. *noun*

Example: *Encephalitis* often accompanies meningitis and may also include the inflammation of the spinal cord.

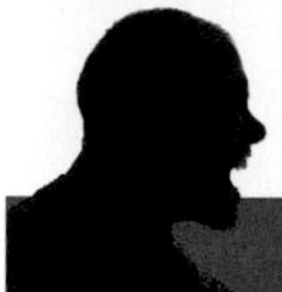

PRONOUNCIATION PRACTICE

Say these words aloud to a friend or classmate, if you can. Here you are given the phonetic pronunciation. Your instructor can help you with pronunciation,

or you can visit **http://www.MedicalLanguageLab.com.**

dysbasia	dĭs-**bā**´zē-ă	encephalitis	ĕn-sĕf″ă-**lī**´tĭs
dyskinesia	dĭs″kĭ-**nē**´sē-ă	encephalomeningitis	ĕn-sĕf″ă-lō-mĕn″ĭn-**jī**´tĭs
dysphoria	dĭs-**fō**´rē-ă	paresis	**păr**´ĕ-sĭs or pă-**rē**´sĭs

The Language of Neurological Function

In Chapter 4, you were introduced to basic terminology for the neurological system. Now, you will expand your vocabulary as you learn about the anatomy and physiology of this system and also explore two very important subsystems: the central nervous system (CNS) and the peripheral nervous system (PNS). The **central nervous system** consists of the brain and the spinal cord. The **peripheral nervous system** is the network of nerves that carry messages to and from the CNS to the rest of the body.

Anatomy and physiology: neurological system

Key terms

The **neuron** is the basic unit of nervous tissue. Each neuron consists of a *nucleus*, an *axon,* and *dendrites*. A neuron generally has only one axon but many dendrites (see Chapter 4).

Nerves are bundles of axons and dendrites. Some nerve tissue contains both sensory and motor nerves. When a stimulus is received from anywhere inside or outside of the body, a nerve is stimulated. This occurs when the stimulus is detected by the dendrites as an electrical impulse. With the help of the axon, the electrical impulse travels up the dendrite into the neuron.

A **stimulus** is a motivator, something that causes a response. The plural form is *stimuli.* In the CNS, a stimulus becomes a nerve impulse. Once a stimulus is perceived, it is encoded into a neurotransmitter.

Neurotransmitters are chemicals that allow a stimulus to be transported across neurons to eventually stimulate muscles, glands, hormones, and other bodily responses.

Dendrites are the receptors of nerve impulses. There are many dendrites on a neuron.

An **axon** is the long projection that stems from the neuron. It sits on the outer edges of the neuron. An axon functions to conduct nerve impulses away from the cell body and outward to the next receptor.

A *synapse* is any place where an axon of one neuron comes into contact with a dendrite from another neuron. At these junctures, electrical impulses can be passed from nerve cell to nerve

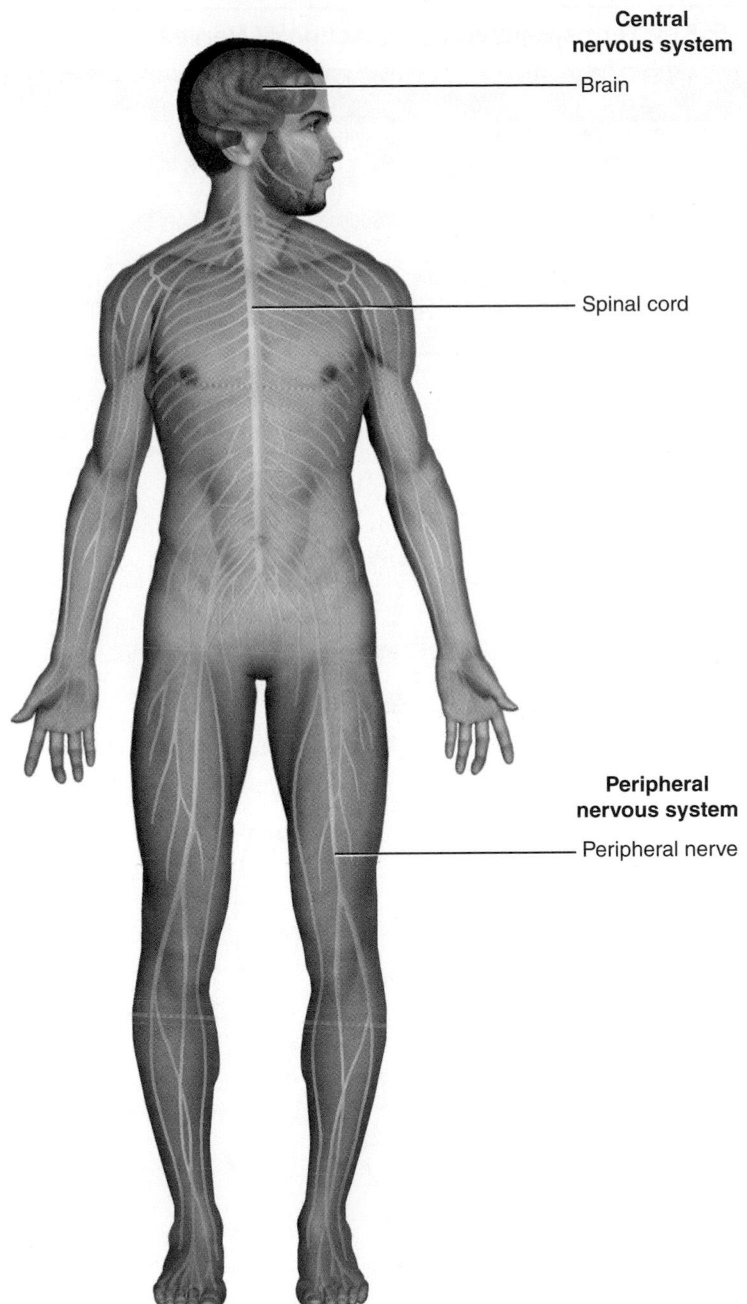

Figure 10.17: Central and peripheral nervous systems

cell with the help of neurotransmitters. Impulses are transmitted from neuron to neuron to the spinal cord and then up into the brain, where they will be interpreted.

Nervous tissues are specifically responsible for sensing stimuli and transmitting impulses about stimuli to appropriate parts of the body

Neuroglial cells (or glial cells) are not actually nerve cells, but they do support the neurons. Neuroglial cells do not have a synapse or dendrites. They function to preserve the electrochemical balance of the nerve cells and to form the myelin sheaths that protect neurons.

Myelin sheaths are fine protective tissues that insulate (cover) nerve axons and that promote the transmission of nerve impulses. (The word *myelin* is derived from the early Greek *myelos,* meaning *marrow.*)

TABLE 10-5: Key Terms Related to the Action of Nerves

Term	Definition
innervation	the process of stimulating or causing an organ, muscle, or body part to act; this happens in response to an action taken by a nerve or nerves; in this context, the prefix *in-* means *in, into, or toward*
enervation	the process of weakening the response to a nerve action; the prefix *en-* means *in or bring into*
denervation	the process of blocking either an afferent or efferent nerve as a result of an incision, an excision, or another blockage of the blood supply to it; in this context, the prefix *de-* means *remove or reverse*

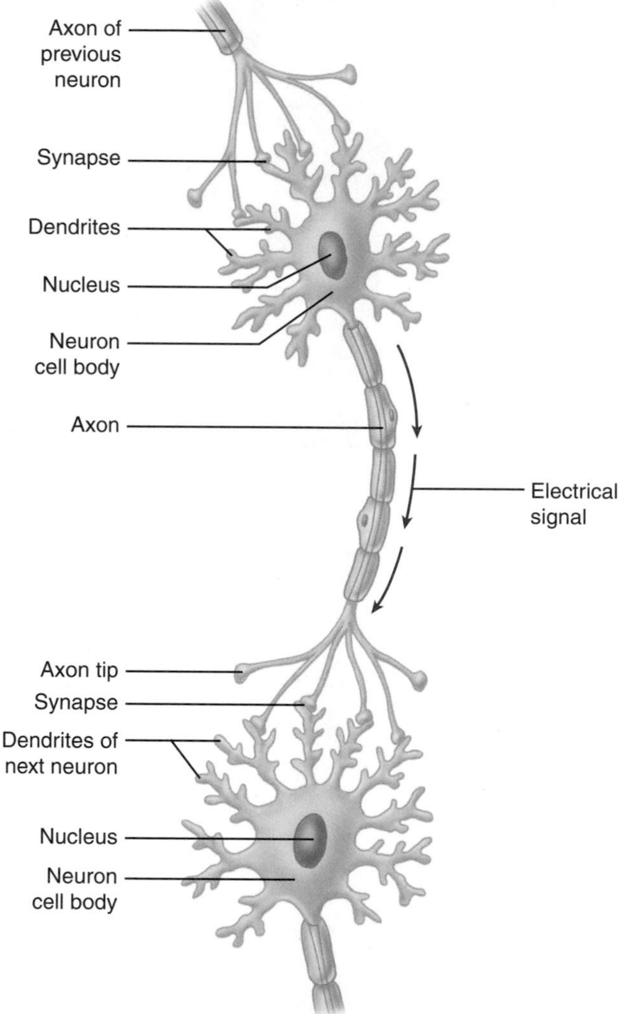

Figure 10.18: Neurons and stimulus conduction

The central nervous system

The CNS is responsible for processing and interpreting information from every other part of the body and then responding appropriately to these stimuli. That is why any damage to the brain or spinal cord impairs a person's sensory and motor functions.

Axon damage in the brain

Diffuse axonal injury (DAI) is a great risk with cerebral trauma, and it is not uncommon. This condition contributes to loss of consciousness, and it can be the cause of profound coma and brain damage. If DAI is caught and surgically treated in time, recovery will occur but there may be residual impairments in motor function; the patient may have acquired disabilities.

Gil Loeppky suffered a closed head injury during a motor vehicle accident. With a *closed head injury,* the CNS is not exposed through an opening in the skin and skull. For this and other injuries, Gil was admitted, and he is being monitored at Okla Trauma Center. After his admission, he incurred another closed head injury. It is quite possible that brain damage may have occurred if axons were damaged as a result of either of these injuries. Refer to Figure 10-19 to see how this damage to the axons might look.

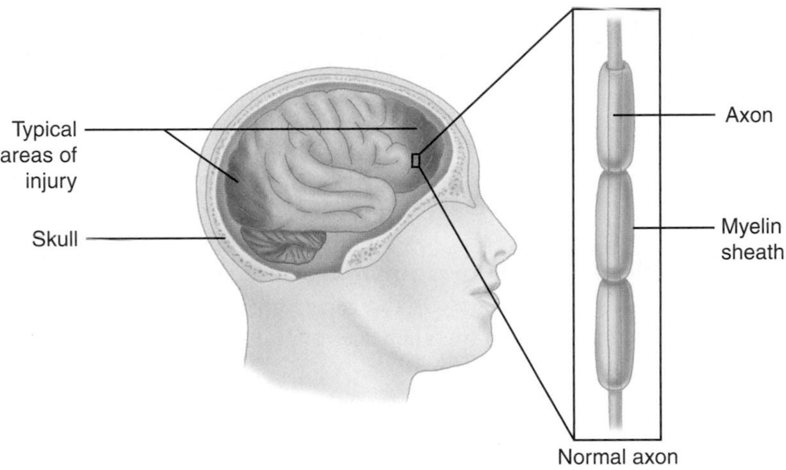

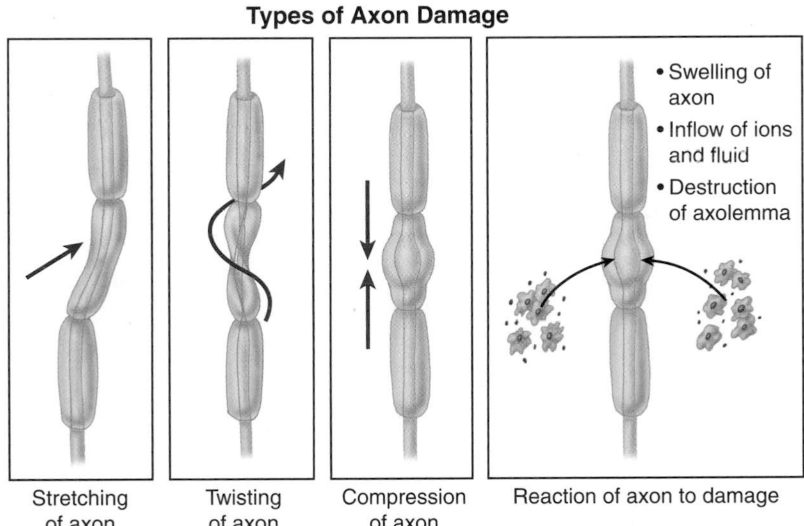

Figure 10.19: Closed head injury: damage to axons

Let's Practice

Name the part of the neurological system that fits each description.

1. cells that receive impulses ______________________________
2. support and protect neurons ______________________________
3. bring impulses into the neuron ______________________________
4. a collection of nerve cells ______________________________

5. bundles of axons and neurons ____________________
6. space between an axon and a dendrite from another nerve cell ____________________
7. a product of glial cells that protects nerve cells ____________________

Critical Thinking

On the basis of your new understanding of the CNS, answer the following questions.

1. If Mr. Loeppky has axon damage in his brain, what will this mean for him?

____

____

2. Imagine that Mr. Loeppky is trying to step down on his broken leg and ankle before they are surgically repaired. His nervous tissue would perceive the pain stimuli through dendrites. If he has had axon damage in his brain, what will happen next? Why?

____

____

Build a Word

Use the new terminology that you have learned. Apply your knowledge of how word parts combine. Consider when you need to drop or add vowels and consonants. Combine each set of word parts below to create a medical or anatomical term. Then use your knowledge of word parts to define the term you've written.

1. in- -able operar/ia Term: ____________ Meaning: ____________
2. cephal/o/a en- algia Term: ____________ Meaning: ____________
3. compress/i/o de- -ion Term: ____________ Meaning: ____________
4. cele cephalo Term: ____________ Meaning: ____________
5. myelin -ate de- Term: ____________ Meaning: ____________

Right Word or Wrong Word: *Nerve* or *Nerve Cell*?

Is there a difference between a nerve and a nerve cell?

The peripheral nervous system

The PNS carries messages to and from the CNS. It involves the nerves that extend from the spinal cord to the body's periphery (see Figure 10-20). Nerves that originate in the spinal cord are found in pairs and extend to the right or left of the spinal cord. The point of origin of a nerve is referred to as the *nerve root.* The PNS also includes the 12 cranial nerves. The PNS is further divided into two subdivisions: the **autonomic nervous system (ANS)** and the **somatic nervous system.**

The autonomic nervous system

The ANS functions, without our conscious awareness or control, to monitor conditions in the body and to help the body to keep functioning. Two of its most important functions are to preserve life through the initiation of the fight-or-flight response (i.e., self-protection that occurs during emergency or highly stressful situations) and to initiate the rest-and-digest response function for healing and nutrition.

A third critical function of the ANS is the role that it plays in homeostasis (maintaining of the internal environment of the body in a steady state). The ANS plays a vital role in returning the body to a homeostatic state after trauma.

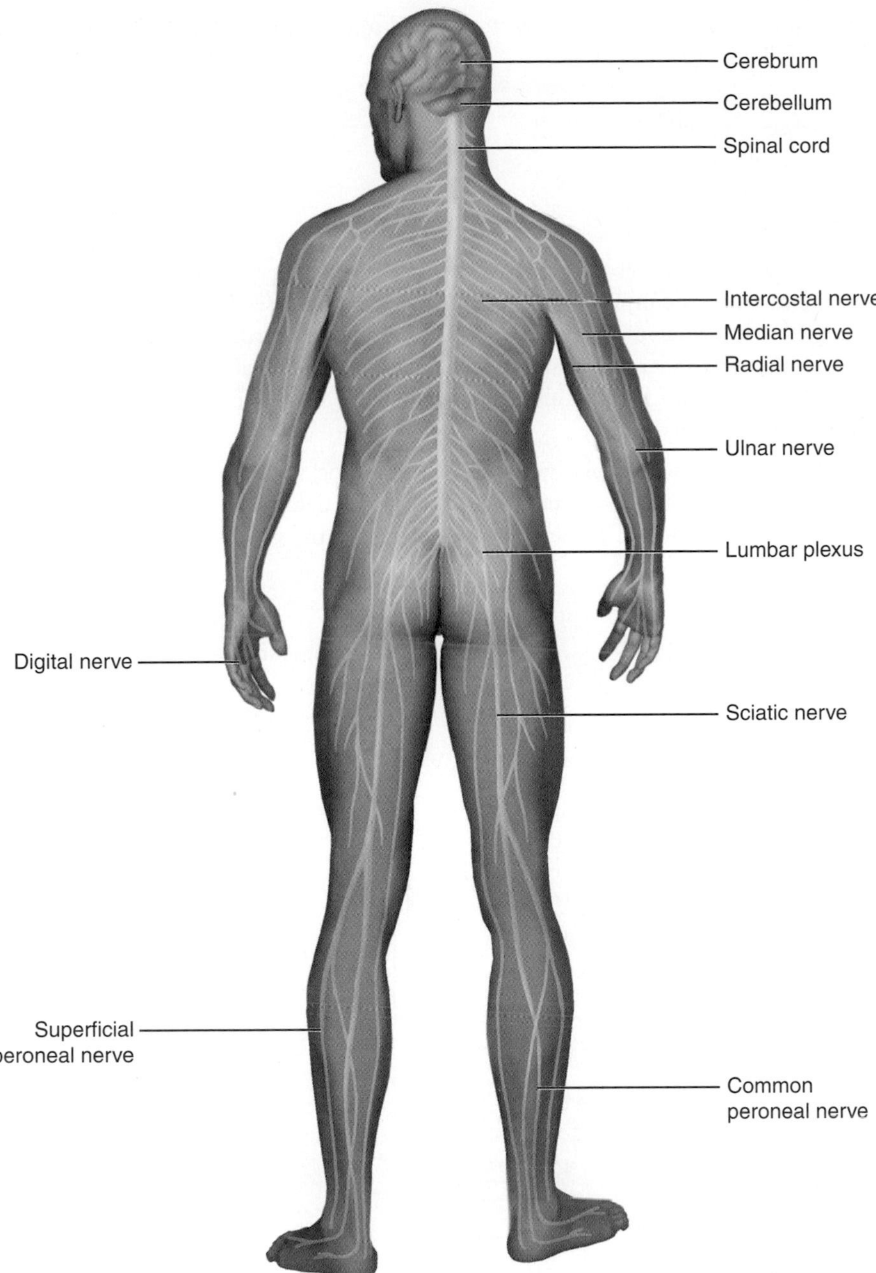

Figure 10.20: Peripheral nervous system

The ANS is further divided into the *parasympathetic* and *sympathetic* branches. See Figure 10-21 to learn more about the functions of each of these. Note that diagnostic imaging cannot be used for the assessment of the ANS.

The somatic nervous sysem

The somatic nervous system are sometimes referred to as the *voluntary nervous system*. There are two main types of somatic nerves: sensory nerves and motor nerves.

Sensory nerves are also called *afferent nerves*, and *they consist only of dendrites*. Afferent nerves carry sensations from the periphery of the body to the CNS. Some of the sensations that are perceived are the awareness of one's own body (i.e., temperature), as well as of pain, touch, taste, and impressions are drawn from these. Sensory nerves relay information from the senses to the CNS, where the brain decides how to respond to the stimuli. Medical terms for the senses include the following:

- olfactory: sense of smell
- tactile: sense of touch
- gustatory: sense of taste
- vision: sense of sight
- auditory: sense of hearing

Motor nerves or *efferent nerves* consist only of axons. These nerves carry nerve impulses from the CNS to the muscles and other tissue. All voluntary muscles (see Chapter 6) are controlled by motor nerves. Motor nerves are nerves of motion. In other words, they are nerves that stimulate muscles that are under our voluntary control. These nerves allow us to consciously react to external stimuli by smiling, frowning, running, walking, raising our arms, and performing dozens of other motions.

Diagnostically, MRI is particularly useful for examining somatic nerves. An MRI can to see the minute details of the body to the point that it can even determine the precise location of nerve root pathology. In addition, MRI can also help to detect the causes of muscle denervation and nerve disorders.

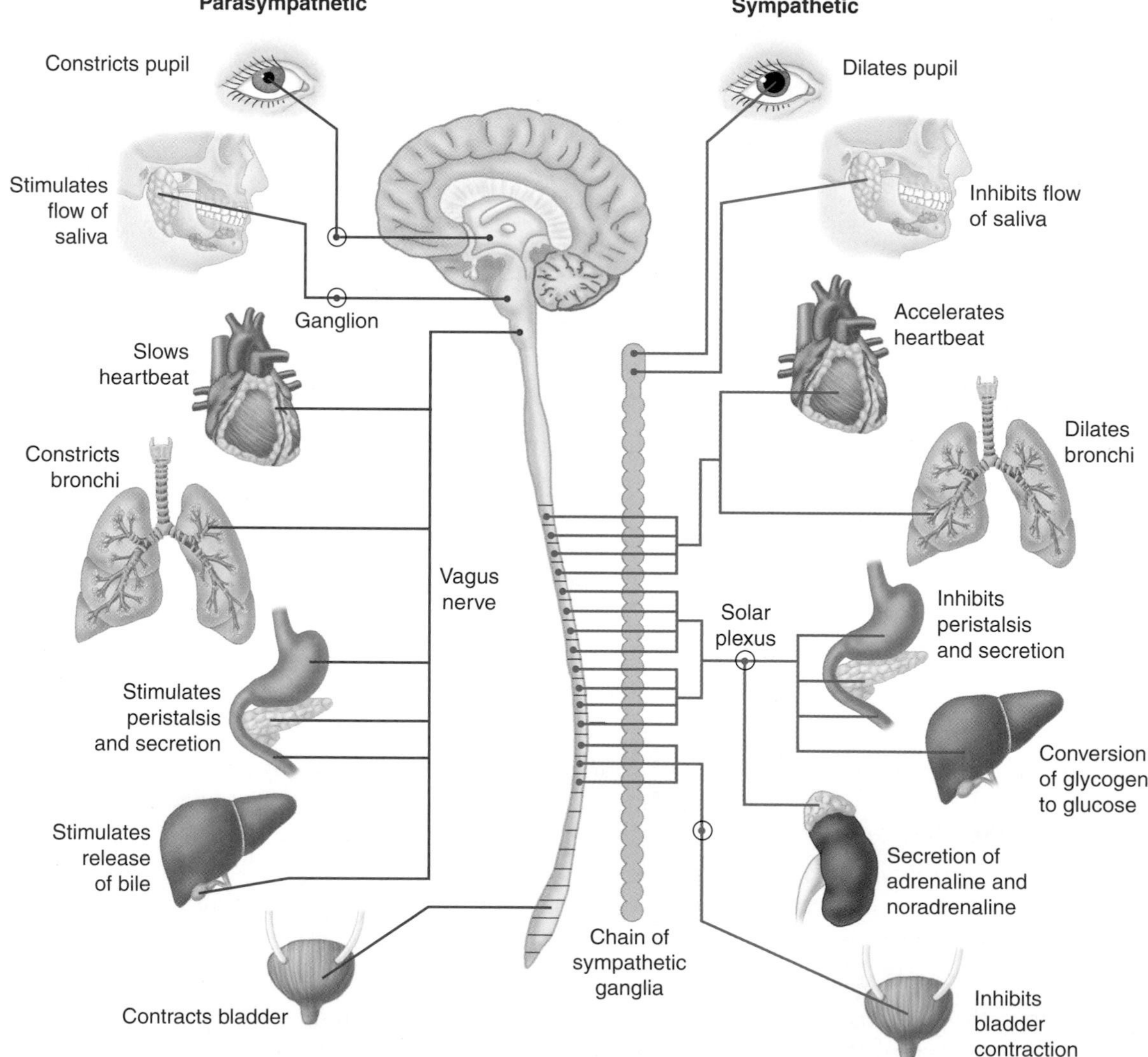

Figure 10.21: Autonomic nervous system: sympathetic and parasympathetic branches

Critical Thinking

Answer the following questions with the use of your new medical terminology and knowledge.

1. Which nervous system *cannot* be studied with MRI scanning?

____

2. Which nervous system receives the most input and sends messages about input to the spinal cord, which then sends it to the brain for interpretation and processing?

____

Build a Word Using Suffixes

Throughout this chapter, you have been working with words that include suffixes that pertain to neurological functioning. Study the suffixes in Table 10-6, and then complete this exercise.

Combine each set of word parts to create a medical term, and then define each term in your own words.

1. -kinesia cyto
   Term: ______________ Meaning: ______________
2. -phasia dys-
   Term: ______________ Meaning: ______________
3. -paresis hemi-
   Term: ______________ Meaning: ______________
4. -esthesia kine-
   Term: ______________ Meaning: ______________
5. -algesia an-
   Term: ______________ Meaning: ______________
6. -lepsy epi-
   Term: ______________ Meaning: ______________
7. -taxia a-
   Term: ______________ Meaning: ______________
8. -sthenia neur
   Term: ______________ Meaning: ______________
9. -plegia quadri-
   Term: ______________ Meaning: ______________
10. -esthesia an-
    Term: ______________ Meaning: ______________

TABLE 10-6: Suffixes That Pertain to Central Nervous System Function

Suffix	Meaning	Suffix	Meaning
-algesia	sensitivity or pain	-phasia	speech
-esthesia	sensation or feeling	-plegia	paralysis
-kinesia	movement	-sthenia	strength
-lepsy	seizure	-taxia	muscle coordination
-paresis	weakness		

Fill in the Blanks

Complete the following exercise to ensure that you are clear about what you have just read. Fill in the blanks with the appropriate medical terms.

1. The __________________________ receives, interprets, and makes decisions about how to respond to sensory input or stimuli.
2. Surgery, such as the one that our patient Gil Loeppky is about to undergo, can cause nerve damage. This is because an incision can result in ______________________________
3. The __________________________ branch of the ANS has the ability to dilate the pupils (see Figure 10-21).
4. MRI scans can be helpful for examining the __________________________ and __________________________ nervous systems.
5. __________________________ occurs when a nerve sends an impulse into a muscle.
6. Sensory information is received and transmitted through __________________________.
7. The __________________________ nervous system ensures that our heart keeps beating.
8. The __________________________ subsystem is able to slow the heart rate down.
9. The medical term for the sense of smell is ______________________________________.
10. The medical term for the sense of taste is ______________________________________.

Mix and Match

Match the medical term on the left with the descriptors on the right.

1. gustatory	stinky or pleasant
2. vision	soft or scratchy
3. auditory	salty and sweet
4. olfactory	loud or soft
5. tactile	blurry or clear

The Language of Neuroimaging

Before proceeding, recall that Mr. Loeppky underwent neuroimaging via CT scan (see Chapter 4). Now, Dr. Swanson has sent Gil for emergency MRI assessment. Although CT scans are generally good for detecting acute hemorrhages, they can fail to discern smaller hemorrhages. MRIs are much better at detecting brain trauma and soft-tissue damage. Gil Loeppky is having an MRI because he has not shown acute signs of intracranial hemorrhage, but he may be showing signs of a much smaller bleed.

MRI scans are the preferred diagnostic assessment tool for the examination of the central nervous and musculoskeletal systems. The reason for this is that an MRI can pick up even the most subtle internal and external abnormalities in the brain, spinal cord, bone marrow, and the organs in the abdomen. MRI scans can see very deep into the body and produce minutely detailed images and slides. They can detect even the smallest brain lesions.

To obtain a picture using MRI technology, the body is bombarded with a combination of radio waves and a magnetic field while the patient, lying flat and unmoving, enters the MRI scanning machine (see Figure 10-22). Because the MRI does not involve the use of direct radiation, it is considered the safest type of diagnostic scan.

An MRI of the cranium can also detect any compression of the brain and any impairment of its electrical activity. Increased ICP tends to compress and deform the brain by pushing on its tissues. The deformity occurs when the brain is pushed to make way for a hematoma, bleeding, or swelling. This shifting of the brain's position is called a *midline shift.* When a midline shift is detected, a physician can conclude that increased ICP is present. MRI scans can also detect meningeal disease, blood clots (i.e., aneurysm or thrombosis), hemorrhages, and infarctions (lack of blood supply).

MRI machines are usually housed in a hospital's radiology department. Some of the larger hospitals have access to portable MRIs, which are stationed in or near the operating theaters (operating rooms) to save time and lives. An intraoperative MRI is used in a surgical suite (operating room).

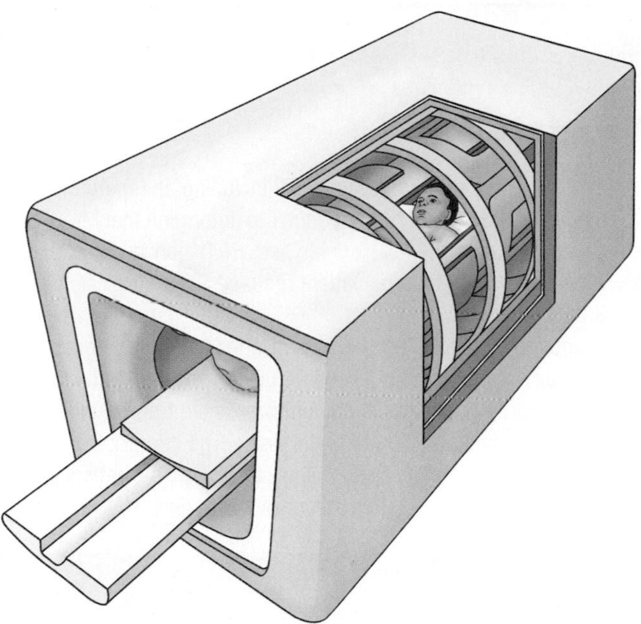

Figure 10.22: MRI machine (From Eagle S, Brassington C, Dailey CS, Goretti C: *The Professional Medical Assistant: An Integrative, Teamwork-Based Approach.* Philadelphia: FA Davis, 2009, p. 457. With permission.)

Fill in the Blanks

Use medical terminology to fill in the blanks.

1. An MRI uses ______________ and ______________ to obtain images of the inside of the body.
2. To obtain clear images with an MRI, the patient must ______________.
3. An MRI scan can help physicians assess the ______________ that cover the brain.
4. MRI is also used to scan the CNS and the ______________ systems of the body.

The Language of Neurosurgery

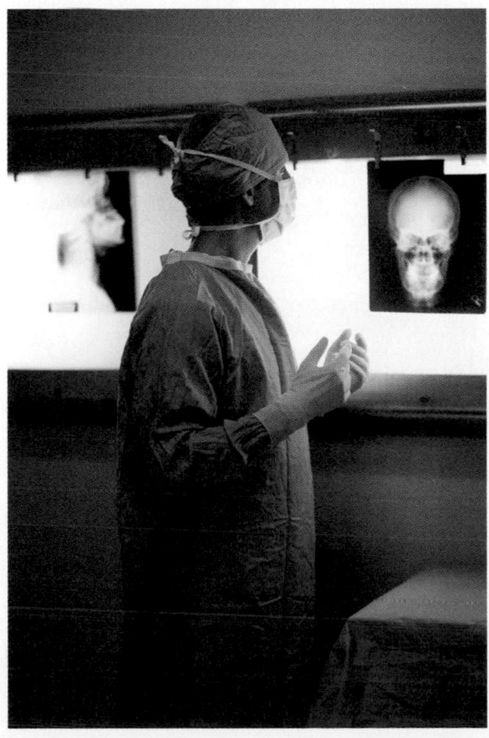

Patient Update

Results of the MRI and other emergency investigations (including an emergency CT, at the neurosurgeon's request) helped the medical team at Okla Trauma Center to determine that Mr. Gilbert Loeppky had acquired a subdural hematoma as a result of the fall from his bed. He began to show signs of ICP. The Code Team had moved quickly. They understood that the patient required STAT surgical intervention. Mr. Loeppky was rushed into the OR at 0330 hrs.

Dr. Hamidi, the neurosurgeon, awaited the patient after having scrubbed in with his surgical team. Dr. Hamidi then performed a craniotomy to evacuate blood from the patient's cranium. The patient also received the anticonvulsive drug phenytoin to prevent a possible trauma-induced seizure and the diuretic mannitol to reduce any further inflammation of brain tissue. The surgery took 4 hours and was successful (see "On the Job: Surgical Report" on page 437). Following surgery, the patient spent one hour in PAR. When he was deemed stable, he was transferred to the intensive care unit.

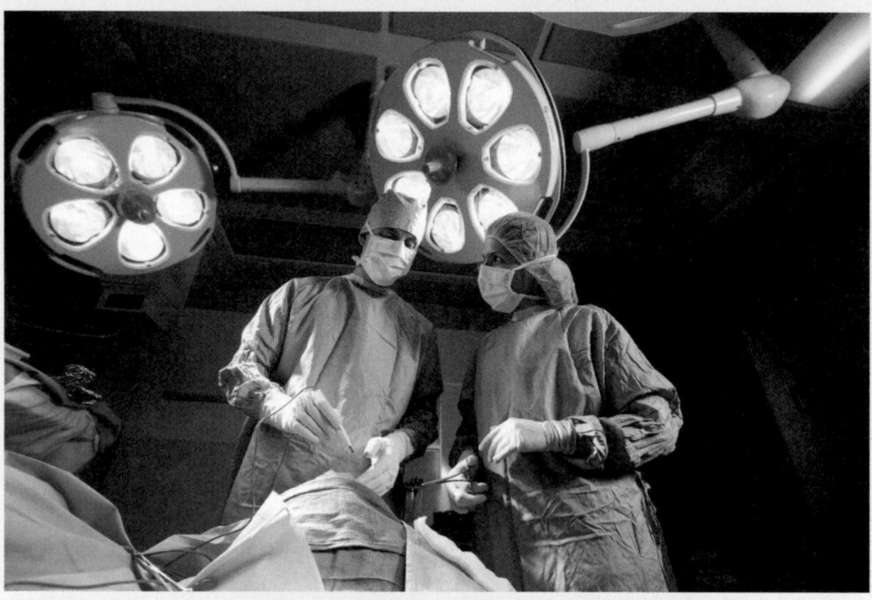

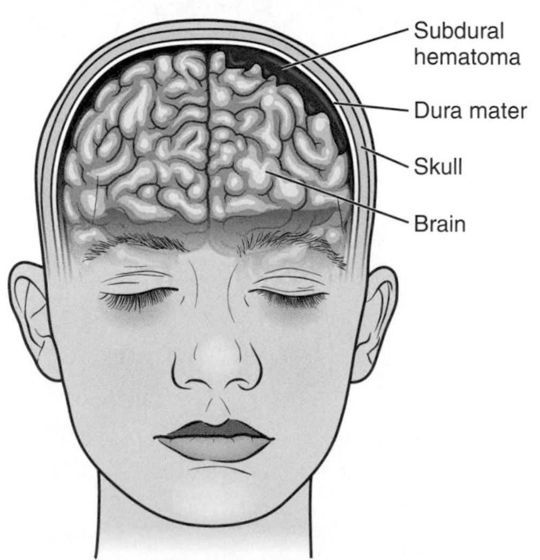

Figure 10.23: Subdural hematoma (From Eagle S: *Diseases in a Flash!: An Interactive, Flash-Card Approach.* Philadelphia: FA Davis, 2012, p 160. With permission.)

Okla Trauma Center
Surgical Report

Patient Name: *Gilbert Loeppky*
Hospital Admission # *4567*
Unit: *ICU*
DOB: *XX/XX/XXXX*
Date of Surgery: *June XX, 2010*
Surgeon: *Dr. Hamidi*
Anesthesiologist: *Dr. Jenzen*
1st Assisting: *Dr. Jackson*
Time In: *0330 hr* Time Out: *0730 hr*
2nd Assisting: *Dr. Havermore*
Reason for Surgery: *Craniotomy*
History: *Fall post-MVA. Head Trauma. ↑ ICP with loss of consciousness.*

Patient transferred to OR subsequent to MRI and CT scans indicating acute phase of a small subdural hematoma, crescent-shaped extra axial collection with increased attenuation. Pt. received unconscious and unresponsive. Intubated for oxygenation and ventilation. IV in situ running Mannitol. Anesthesia per Dr. Jenzen. Surgical evacuation commenced via craniotomy. Moderate amount of blood evacuated at site. No interruption of cerebrovascular flow noted.

Key terms: neurosurgery

The Patient Update and the "On the Job: Surgical Report" (shown above) included important medical language related to neurosurgery. Key terms from the update and the surgical report are highlighted and explained below.

"…having *scrubbed in*…"

scrubbed in: medical jargon that means that the surgeon completed the sterile protocols required before entering the operating room. Together, these protocols are known as **surgical asepsis**. The protocols include scrubbing the hands and forearms with a sterile brush and an antimicrobial solution. The term **asepsis** refers to the state of being free of pathological microorganisms (germs).

"…performed a *craniotomy* to *evacuate* blood…"

craniotomy: a procedure in which an incision is made in the skull through which blood can exit. In more severe cases of increased ICP, a craniectomy may be required. During a **craniectomy**, a section of the skull is actually removed to expose the brain and relieve pressure. Because Gil Loeppky received emergency treatment immediately after his fall, he did not require a craniectomy; he was a good candidate for craniotomy.

evacuate: remove.

"…received the *anticonvulsive* drug phenytoin to prevent a possible trauma-induced *seizure* …"

anticonvulsive: referring to a medication that is used to prevent seizures.

seizure: a medical condition in which the electroconductivity of the brain is abnormal; there are abnormal electrical firings of neurons occurring. The brain temporarily dysfunctions, and there may be some degree of loss of consciousness of one's surroundings (see Chapter 4).

"…and the *diuretic* mannitol…"

diuretic: a medication that increases urine output to prevent the buildup of excess fluid in the body.

… spent one hour in *PAR*…

PAR: post-anesthetic recovery. This is a room adjacent to the operating rooms of hospitals. Patients are transferred to PAR immediately after surgery, where they are monitored by nurses as they recover from anesthesia. Vital signs and levels of consciousness as the patient arouses are assessed frequently. When these are stable, the patient is then transferred to the next hospital unit for ongoing care. Mr. Loeppky will be transferred to the intensive care unit from PAR.

"...he was *deemed stable*..."

deemed stable: determined to have stable vital signs.

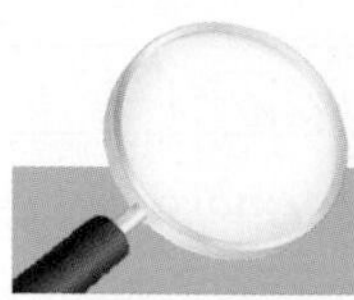

FOCUS POINT: Phenytoin

Phenytoin (trade name: Dilantin) is an antiepileptic (antiseizure) medication that may be used prophylactically (preventatively) in the case of head injury, when the possibility for seizure activity exists. It can be given to the patient orally, intramuscularly, or intravenously.

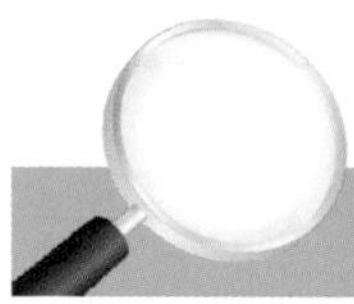

FOCUS POINT: Mannitol

Mannitol is an intravenous solution that is given to patients who present with intracranial pressure, intraocular pressure (pressure within the eyeball), or acute renal failure. It is a diuretic, which means that it inhibits or blocks the reabsorption of water or sodium back into the cells. Mannitol is used to assist the body with the flushing out of toxins. It does this by causing diuresis (increased urinary output).

Mix and Match

Match the term with its descriptor.

1. hematoma	anticonvulsant
2. subdural	incision into the skull
3. cerebral	collection of blood under the skin
4. craniotomy	pertaining to the brain
5. phenytoin	germ free
6. asepsis	beneath the dura mater

Build a Word with the Combining Form *Crani/o*

Use the new terminology that you have learned. Apply your knowledge of how word parts combine, and consider when to drop or add vowels and consonants. Combine each set of word parts given to create a medical or anatomical term, and then use your knowledge of word parts to define the term you've written.

1. crani/o cerebr/o -al

Term: ______________________ Meaning: ______________________

2. cele crani/o

Term: ______________________ Meaning: ______________________

3. ology crani/o

Term: ______________________ Meaning: ______________________

The Language of Postoperative Care and Recovery

Mr. Loeppky entered surgery in a state of unconsciousness, and he was given anesthesia during surgery to keep him in that state. After surgery, he will be kept in a medically induced coma for at least 24 hours to control any further increase in ICP. The mere act of opening the cranium to relieve a buildup of ICP is a trauma, and this trauma can itself cause inflammation to occur. In essence, a medically induced coma is used therapeutically to put the brain to sleep and to keep it asleep so that a period of healing and recuperation can occur. This is commonly achieved with the use of barbiturate medications.

There are some medical risks associated with the use of medically induced comas, so the patient's neurovital signs will be monitored frequently by the attending nurses and via electroencephalogram (EEG). The medication used to induce the coma will be a central nervous system depressant, and the risks involved with this kind of drug include the slowing of the heart and breath rates. The shorter the amount of time that a patient is kept in this type of coma, the better that patient's prognosis will be.

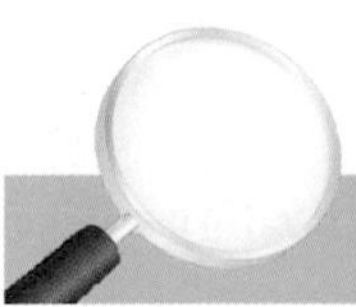

FOCUS POINT: Barbiturates

Barbiturates are a class of medications that depress (slow) the function of the central nervous system. In other words, they are sedating. They have the ability to reduce normal brain activity and to decrease cerebral blood flow. As a result, the blood vessels in the brain begin to narrow. This reduces the potential for swelling in the brain, which in turn decreases the potential for more brain trauma.

Some examples of barbiturates include the following:

Secobarbital (trade name: Seconal): prescribed for insomnia that is difficult to treat; also used preoperatively to decrease fear and anxiety

Phenobarbital (trade name: Luminal): prescribed for seizure disorders or for sedation

Butalbatil (trade name: Fiorinal): prescribed for very severe headaches

Barbiturates can be taken orally or intravenously. They are highly addictive, and they should be used sparingly in treatment. Barbiturates require a prescription.

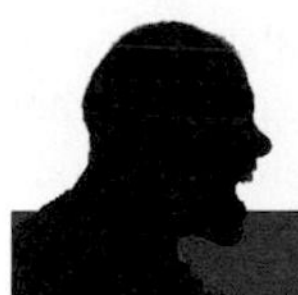

PRONOUNCIATION PRACTICE

Say these words aloud to a friend or classmate, if you can. Here you are given the phonetic pronunciation. Your instructor can help you with pronunciation,

or you can visit **http://www.MedicalLanguageLab.com.**

ataxia	ă-**tăk**´sē-ă	kinesthesia	kĭn″ĕs-**thē**´zē-ă
cephalocele	**sĕf**´ă-lō-sēl	myelin	**mī**´ĕ-lĭn
cytokinesis	sī″tō-kĭ-**nē**´sĭs	neuroglial	nū-**rŏg**´lē-ăl
craniotomy	krā-nē-**ŏt**´ō-mē	neurasthenia	nū″răs-**thē**´nē-ă
demyelinate	dē-**mī**´ĕ-lĭ-nāt	olfactory	ŏl-**făk**´tō-rē
encephalalgia	ĕn-sĕf″ăl-**ăl**´jē-ă	phenytoin	**fĕn**´ĭ-tō-ĭn
gustatory	**gŭs**´tă-tō-rē	peripheral	pĕr-**ĭf**´ĕr-ăl
hemiparesis	hĕm″ē-păr´ĕ-sĭs	quadriplegia	kwŏd″rĭ-**plē**´jē-ă

Patient Update

Although subdural hematomas do not usually have a fully favorable prognosis, the sooner they are detected, the better the patient outcomes. In Mr. Loeppky's case, RN Franklin was on the scene immediately and began the patient's assessment and treatment. In particular, Franklin knew not to move the patient, so he avoided the risk of incurring further trauma to Gil's head, brain, and spine. The Code Team began a neurological assessment immediately and provided pertinent data for the physicians when they arrived. The patient was then treated with forced ventilation through an AMBU bag to ensure the presence of oxygen flow to the brain. Mr. Loeppky's prognosis was further enhanced when he was sent STAT to MRI, CT, and surgery. These steps saved his life, and his prognosis to recover full functioning is very good at this time.

Mr. and Mrs. Pat Loeppky have arrived at ICU after having received an urgent phone call in the middle of the night advising them of their son's situation.

"Mr. and Mrs. Loeppky?" asked an older man in green operating room scrubs and cap. They nodded. "I'm Dr. Hamidi." They all shook hands, and Dr. Hamidi continued: "I'm a neurosurgeon, and I've been working on your son, Gilbert." They nodded expectantly, and Pearl was clearly shaken; her color was pale, and her eyes were wide.

"Is he all right? Is he going to be okay?" Pearl asked in a frightened voice. Pat took her hand in his. It was Dr. Hamidi who nodded this time.

"Yes, he's going to be fine. Please, sit for a minute," offered the surgeon. Gil's parents did, and Dr. Hamidi joined them on a settee. "I'm afraid that your son suffered a head injury again tonight. We're not sure of the details, but he fell on the floor. The way he fell seems to indicate that he was trying to get up."

Pearl gasped. "Get up? What in the world would possess him to do something like that?" She looked inquiringly at both men. "Surely he was aware of his broken leg?" she asked the doctor.

"It is quite possible that he awoke confused and disoriented," said Dr. Hamidi. "It's not unheard of in patients with concussions. His room was not totally dark because of his condition, but the lights were dim, and he may just not have had enough time to process where he was and why. He may have been dreaming about something or felt an urge to go somewhere. We won't know unless he remembers, and that is quite unlikely."

"What do you mean 'quite unlikely,' Doctor?" asked Pat, his brow wrinkled with concern now. "What exactly is going on with our son? Is he going to be all right?"

"Yes, his prognosis for full recovery is good. However, I don't want you to get your hopes up too high right now. The brain is quite unpredictable. There was some bleeding into the cranial cavity, which caused a hematoma to form. The cranium is only so large, and any swelling within it causes pressure to bear down on the brain itself." The surgeon paused while Gil's parents thought about this for a moment, and then he continued. "We performed a craniotomy, which means that we opened the skull to relieve the pressure from the hematoma. I believe that we moved quickly and efficiently enough to prevent any permanent brain damage. However ..."

Again, Pearl gasped and reached out to clutch the sleeve of her husband's shirt.

"However," the doctor continued, "I have to be honest with you. Your son may have some impairments. It's impossible to tell for the moment."

"Impairments?" questioned Pat. "Do you mean brain damage?" He paused for a quick moment while he thought. "Do you mean he won't be able to talk or walk or feed himself?"

"No, no sir, nothing that severe. It is likely that Gilbert will have some memory loss associated with this trauma, in addition to that of the motor vehicle accident that occurred earlier. He may have some dysphasia, which means that he may have trouble pronouncing certain words. He may also show some evidence of ataxia, which involves problems with the coordination of muscle activity." The Loeppkys looked at each other in anguish. "I'm hoping that this will be temporary," added the surgeon. The Loeppkys' eyes immediately reverted to the doctor's and held fast.

"Temporary? He won't be permanently disabled?" asked Pearl.

"There are no guarantees here that he won't have some form of minor disability arising from the traumas he's experienced over the past 24 hours," answered Dr. Hamidi, "but I believe that they will be, for the most part, temporary impairments. He's going to need time in the hospital and time for rehabilitation, though, for both his leg and his neurological recovery."

"Oh, my goodness!" said Pearl, suddenly remembering, "I had forgotten about that leg. He's supposed to have surgery later today. What about that?"

"No, ma'am, he won't be having surgery today," said Dr. Hamidi. "It's not safe to subject a head-injury patient to another bout of surgery so soon. We'll need to be sure that he's stable and strong enough to undergo such a procedure. That will take a few days at least." Gil's parents looked at each other in dismay.

"What about his pain, then?" asked Gil's mother. "How's he going to cope with the pain of his leg and, I suppose, his head, too?" The doctor explained that they were keeping Gil in a state of chemically induced coma for now to reduce the chance of movement and reinjury. This, he said, would also help with pain management. Dr. Hamidi went on to explain that Gil would receive constant monitoring in the ICU, and his neurovital signs would be taken frequently to assess his progress. He would also receive medications and oxygen to promote brain health and to decrease intracranial swelling. Dr. Hamidi reassured Gil's parents that there were methods of assessing the progress of Gil's healing even when Gil was unconscious.

"Can we go see him, doctor?" asked the anxious mother. "Please?"

Dr. Hamidi nodded. "You can see him for a moment or two, but I'd like to keep the stimulus around him very quiet for the next few hours. Just a few minutes, all right?" Pat and Pearl agreed. "When you are with him, please speak to him softly. But do feel free to speak to him and perhaps to touch his arm or hand if you like. We believe that an unconscious patient has some awareness. At some level, he'll be aware that the people who care about him are nearby." Pearl started to cry softly then; the emotion was too much for her now. The surgeon rose and said goodnight, leaving the Loeppkys to go see their son in the ICU.

Suddenly, Gil's mother looked up at her husband and whispered, "What about Glory?"

Critical Reflection Question

According to Dr. Hamidi, what is Gil's prognosis for recovery?

___

CHAPTER SUMMARY

Chapter 10 has introduced the language of surgical preparation within the context of Gil Loeppky's pending orthopedic surgery. It also provided new language that applies to the emergent neurological crisis of a subdural hematoma. Key medical and anatomical terms were used to explore both subjects, and terms related to pathophysiology were included. Opportunities for using and enhancing vocabulary and word-building skills were provided, including exercises that highlighted key prefixes.

See How Much You've Learned

For audio exercises, visit **http://www.MedicalLanguageLab.com.** 

Chapter 10 also introduced new abbreviations. A number of them appear again here in a concise table to promote study.

TABLE 10-7: Chapter 10 Abbreviations

Abbreviation	Meaning	Abbreviation	Meaning
AMBU	air-shields manual breathing unit	KVO	keep vein open
ANS	autonomic nervous system	NS	normal saline
CNS	central nervous system	PNS	peripheral nervous system
CSF	cerebrospinal fluid	SAH	subarachnoid hemorrhage
DAI	diffuse axonal injury	SDH	subdural hematoma
EDH	epidural hematoma	SIS	second-impact syndrome (of a concussion)
EEG	electroencephalogram		
ICP	intracranial pressure		

Key Terms

air-shields manual breathing unit (AM BU)
analgesic
anteromedial
anticonvulsive
arachnoid mater
arthrotomy
asepsis
autonomic nervous system (ANS)
autoregulation
axon
central nervous system
cerebral herniation
cerebrospinal fluid
clear fluids
Code Team
craniectomy
craniotomy
crash cart
decerebrate rigidity
dehydration
dendrites
diffuse axonal injury (DAI)
diuretic
dura mater
epidural hematoma (EDH)
evacuate
fracture fragments
frontotemporal
gurney
gustatory
hematoma
hemiplegia
herniation
increased intracranial pressure
intercellular fluid
interstitial fluid
intracerebral hematoma (ICH)
intracranial hemorrhage
intracranial pressure (ICP)
intravenous (IV)
Kirschner wires (K-wires)
lag screws
manageable
meninges
meningitis
midline shift
mobilize
nerves
nervous tissues
neuron
neurotransmitters
normal saline
NPO (npo)
orthopedics
pain scale
peripheral nervous system
physical therapy
pia mater
pin
pliant
postoperatively
PRN
respiratory failure
rounds
second-impact syndrome
seizure
somatic nervous system (SNS)
stimulus
subdural
subdural hematoma (SDH)
surgical asepsis
surgical prep
surgical reduction
suture lines
traction
ventricle
vertigo
weight bearing

CHAPTER REVIEW

Critical Thinking

1. Which type of surgeon will perform the surgery for Gil Loeppky's leg fractures?

____

2. Which type of surgeon performed the surgery for Gil Loeppky's intracranial hematoma?

____

3. Who will have the postoperative responsibility for setting up and maintaining the traction devices on Gil's injured leg? ______________________________

4. Our patient, Gil Loeppky, suffered an injury to his meninges, rather than a disease. What is the general term for disease of the meninges? ______________________________

Prefixes

Write the meaning of each prefix.

1. intra- ______________________________
2. dys- ______________________________
3. epi- ______________________________
4. myelo- ______________________________

Right Word or Wrong Word: *Meningocele* or *Myelomeningocele*?

Are these two words the same? Do they name the same condition or two conditions with different etiologies?

Abbreviations

The following abbreviations should now be familiar to you. Write the meaning of each one.

1. CSF ______________________
2. SAH ______________________
3. CNS ______________________
4. SIS ______________________
5. LOC ______________________

Label the Diagram

Write the name of each part of the nerve cell on the correct line.

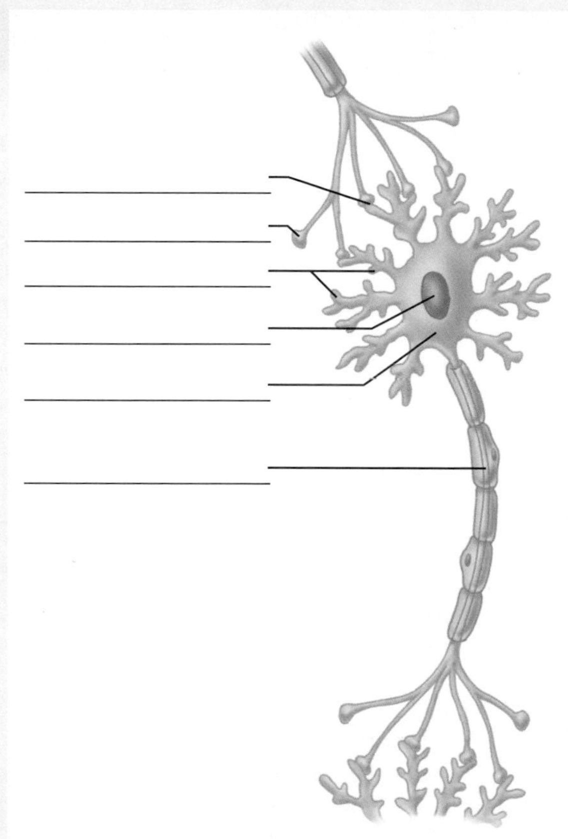

Sentence Scramble

The following scrambled sentences contain new terminology and medical language. Rearrange the words in each sentence so that they make sense.

1. Detect the can even the within bones minute MRI abnormalities an body within.

____

2. Useful MRI peripheral help diagnose imaging of is disorders and broad nerve range a particularly nerves for can examining.

____

3. Tissue neuroglial contains body cells neurons and nervous the.

____

4. Neuroglial not but them of supporters the cells actually cells are nerve.

____

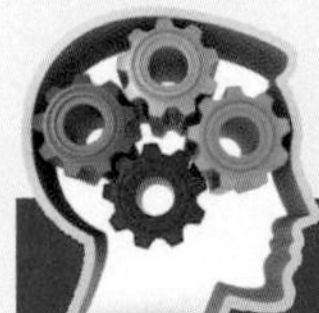

MEMORY MAGIC

Take the Word-a-Day Challenge

To enhance your memory for new terms, follow these simple strategies:

1. Adopt one difficult or challenging word from the chapter, and write it down. Do not write the definition.
2. Say this new word aloud at least 10 times over the next 24 hours. Use it in a silly sentence, use it in a proper sentence, tell it to a friend, rhyme it, or sing it. The choice is yours.
3. At the end of the 24-hour period, log your success. Next to your chosen word, make a personal prediction regarding whether you think you'll remember this word in the future.
4. On the second day, chose a new word, and repeat steps 1, 2, and 3.
5. Do it all again with a fresh word on the third day.
6. On the fourth day, review your word list aloud. As you go through the three chosen words, orally define them.

How Did You Do?
Congratulate Yourself for Improving
Your Medical Terminology Vocabulary.
Now…
What Do You Think about Repeating the Exercise
for Another Three Days
with Three New Words?
Take a Chance!
Enjoy!

CHAPTER ELEVEN

Postoperative Nutrition and Healing

Focus: Digestive and Integumentary Systems

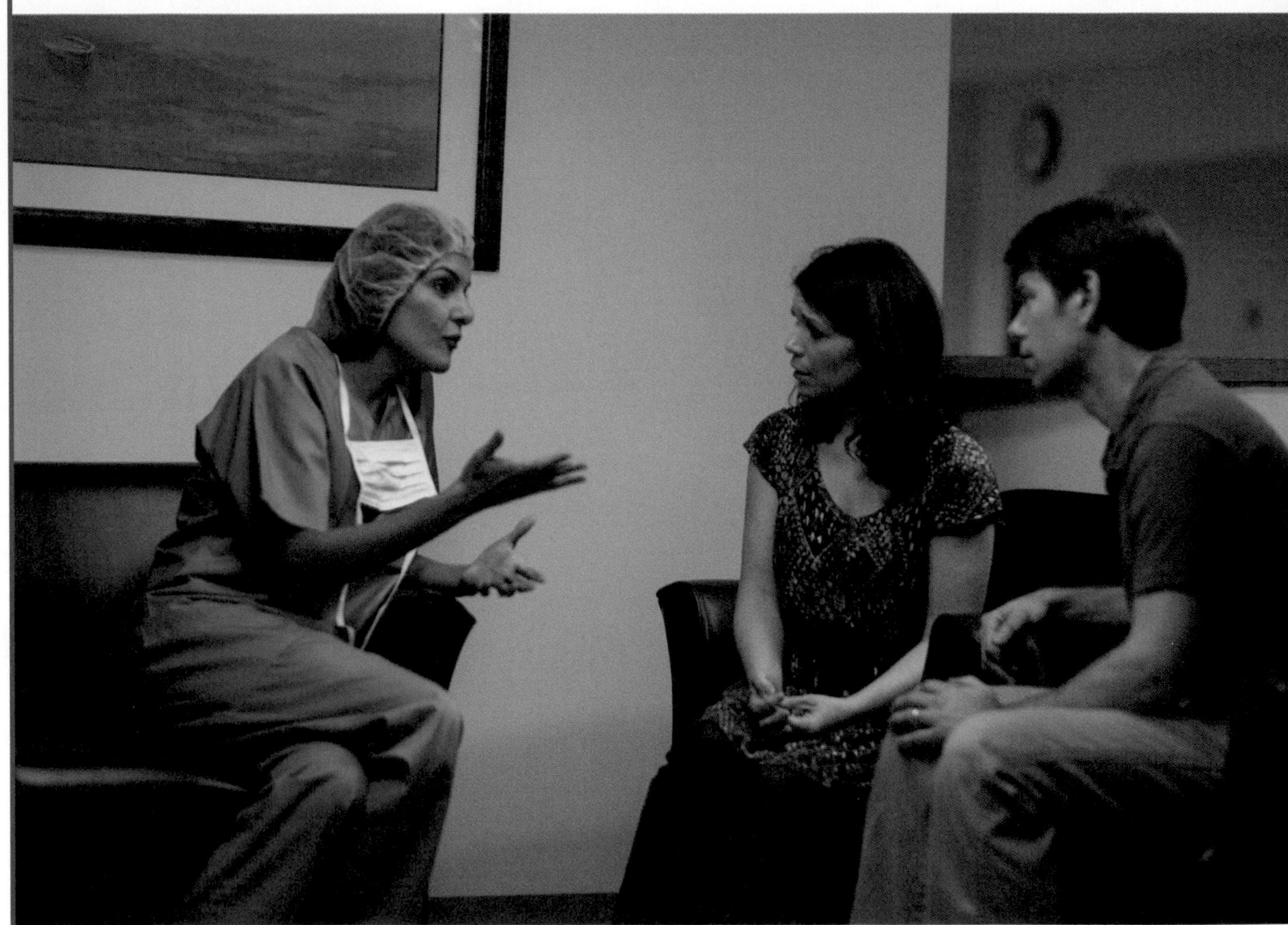

Seven-year-old Clay Davis is now recovering from maxillofacial surgery for a symphyseal fracture midline on the lower mandible (see Chapter 6). Because of the instability of this type of fracture, Clay's fracture was surgically reduced and fixed with titanium mini-plates to achieve rigid fixation. There was no need to wire his upper and lower jaws. The oral and maxillofacial surgeon, Dr. Sandor, has left the operating room to speak with Clay's parents, who are nervously awaiting the results in the OR patient waiting room.

Patient Update

"Mr. and Mrs. Davis?" inquired a surgeon who was wearing blue scrubs. Mrs. Mickey Davis extended her hand. Clay's father, Steve Davis, stood up from where he had been sitting on a settee and shook the doctor's outstretched hand. "We met downstairs in ER," the doctor added. "I'm Dr. Sandor, an oral and maxillofacial surgeon here at Okla." Mickey Davis came to her husband's side. Both parents greeted Dr. Sandor with worried, nervous looks. "Your son is fine," Dr. Sandor calmly asserted, in a voice that was both confident and compassionate. "It's been a long operation for a child, but he's doing just fine." She paused for a moment to let this information sink in. The parents sighed in unison, and the surgeon could see them both relax some of the tension that they'd been holding in their shoulders.

"Can we see him?" Clay's mother asked eagerly.

Dr. Sandor shook her head. "Not just yet. Clay is still in PAR recovering from the anesthetic, and we need to leave him there with the nurses for about another hour, I'd say. Then he'll be moved to Pediatrics and back to Dr. Lincoln's care. That's up on the fourth floor, in the west wing." Mickey looked confused. "I believe you met Dr. Lincoln earlier today in the ER?" Dr. Sandor asked. The Davises confirmed that they had, but said that they didn't know where the pediatric unit was. "Don't worry about that right now," Dr. Sandor replied. "One of the nurses will come out to speak with you when the time comes, and he or she will tell you how to get there."

"Doctor, what exactly is happening with Clay?" asked Steve. "We don't have a lot of information. When we got here, our son was already being rushed up to surgery."

"As you know, your son was in a motor vehicle accident, and he received a traumatic injury to his lower jaw," explained Dr. Sandor. "His injury is called a symphyseal fracture." With her finger, Dr. Sandor drew a line down the middle of her jaw from top to bottom to illustrate what she meant. "To stabilize and repair that, we attached a titanium metal mini-plate across the fracture line."

"A plate," said Clay's father. "I thought he was going to have his jaw wired shut. How long will he have a plate in his mouth?"

Dr. Sandor smiled and continued. "Your son's lucky," she said. "His jaws were not broken or dislocated at the condylar region, the joints. If that had been the case, we would have had to do a maxillomandibular fixation using wires, and he would not have been able to open his mouth for at least 2 weeks. Since the injury was only to the symphyseal region, we did not have to wire the jaws in place to stabilize them." She paused a moment, as Mr. and Mrs. Davis let out a sigh of relief in unison. She smiled and went on.

"Even so, Clay won't be able to speak or eat for 5 to 7 days as we wait for the healing to begin. He will be able to open his mouth ever so slightly in the meantime, but that will be quite uncomfortable for him for a while yet. In the meantime, he'll have a feeding tube for nutrition. We'll remove the tube in a few days, if all goes well," Dr. Sandor said, reassuringly, to Clay's parents.

"We'll have a dietician consult with the treatment team and with you as well so that you, too, can support Clay through this difficult time. Your help is going to be very important to his recovery. The dietician will be able to tell you more about how we're going to feed Clay to ensure that he receives adequate nutrition. We'll get a speech pathologist in here, too, to help Clay with chewing and swallowing." Mr. and Mrs. Davis looked at each other with concern on their faces. Dr. Sandor went on. “Usually, the NG tube is removed in 5 to 7 days as well, after primary healing of the surgical wound has begun. The plate itself could possibly be removed in about 6 months. We'll talk about that much later in his recovery, all right?” Mr. and Mrs. Davis nodded.

“And his teeth? Are his teeth okay?” asked Mickey.

Dr. Sandor nodded and told the parents that their son had been lucky in this respect, too. None of his teeth had been damaged or knocked out by the impact. “He did have some movement in the central and lateral incisor teeth of the lower jaw,” Dr. Sandor added. “The plate will help to stabilize those, too, and we will keep an eye on them to ensure that nothing untoward occurs.”

“We'll also be monitoring his airway,” she continued. “You'll notice when you see him that we have him propped up in the bed. He is in this position to prevent any impediment of the airway.” Both parents looked at Dr. Sandor, waiting for her to continue. “After an accident like this and surgery, it's possible that Clay's tongue will become inflamed or swell up in response. We don't want it to block the air passage at the back of his oral cavity. With his altered levels of consciousness postoperatively, we don't want to risk laying him flat to avoid the risk of the tongue falling back into the pharynx and impeding his airway. Finally, we want to avoid the risk of pulmonary aspiration. That means accidentally sucking things into his lungs. This can happen when the tongue is not able to move materials toward the throat correctly, and fluids, mucus, or foods are suddenly moved into the trachea and lungs rather than into the esophagus and stomach.” Clay's parents nodded to show that they understood.

“And his burn, Doctor? What about that?” asked Steve. “We have no idea what's happening with that, either. We only know that he has a scald on his chest. What can you tell us about that?”

“Yes, that's correct. He has a second-degree scald burn across his chest, more prominently on the left upper torso near his collarbone. We had that covered with a special dressing while we were operating. The burn will now be taken care of by the nurses and the pediatrician assigned to your son's case. We've had Dr. Lincoln assessing and consulting on this burn, and you will be able to speak with him over on Peds.”

“Thank you, Doctor. You've been very helpful,” said Mickey. “We can't thank you enough for what you've done.” Steve shook the surgeon's hand again, and Mickey gently touched her arm in acknowledgment.

“You're very welcome,” said Dr. Sandor. “I'll be checking in on Clay tomorrow, and of course, because I'm his surgeon, the nurses have my pager number and will contact me if they need me to look in on him sooner for any reason.” She smiled warmly and turned to leave, and then she stopped and turned back. “Oh, by the way,” she said, “I noticed that your son has as appendectomy scar. When was his appendix removed?”

Steve and Mickey explained that Clay had suffered from acute appendicitis and had his appendix removed when he was 5. Dr. Sandor nodded and left them then. Steve and Mickey Davis sat down on the settee together to wait to see their son. They held hands.

Reflective Questions

Reflect on the story that you've just read.

1. Where is Clay while the surgeon is speaking with his parents?

   ____

2. Why will Mr. and Mrs. Davis need to speak with a dietician?

   ____

3. Where is Clay going to be moved to when he leaves PAR?

   ____

Learning Objectives

After reading Chapter 11, you will be able to do the following:

- Recognize, define, and use terminology related to the digestive/gastrointestinal system.
- Expand your vocabulary and use terminology related to the integumentary system.
- Recognize and understand terms related to burn care.
- Identify prefixes and suffixes that are common to the vocabulary of the digestive/gastrointestinal system.
- Understand the terms for different types of feedings.
- Differentiate between swallowing and gagging.
- Identify and use terms related to the functions and processes of the digestive tract.
- Recognize terms of pathology related to the digestive and integumentary systems.
- Enhance your vocabulary related to the care and treatment of tissue damage, including scald burns and second-degree burns.
- Differentiate among different types of catheters.
- Understand the role of dietetics and nutrition in health and healing.
- Recognize pediatric pain assessment scales.
- Recognize and appreciate the education, training, and treatment role of a dietician.
- Recognize and appreciate the education, training, and treatment role of a speech therapist.

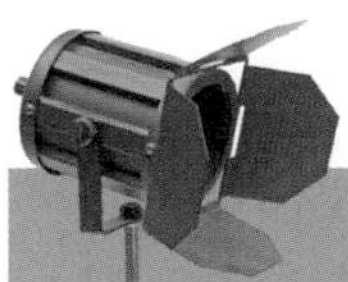

CAREER SPOTLIGHT: Dietician

Dieticians play an important role in the maintenance and restoration of health because good nutrition is essential to support life and the healing processes. Dieticians promote healthy eating through education with health colleagues and with clients and their families. In care facilities and schools, dieticians may manage food services. Some dieticians also have careers in research.

Clinical dieticians are part of the multidisciplinary care team. They assess their patients' nutritional needs and then develop and implement nutritional treatment plans and programs. They also evaluate the effects of nutritional treatment and report the results to the other members of the treatment team. In medical and other care facilities, the dietician will attend to the normal dietary requirements of patients while assessing for, designing, and implementing medical diets in consultation with the physician.

Community dieticians work in a wide variety of settings, from public health clinics and community organizations to home care. These individuals provide nutritional counseling for health promotion and illness prevention.

Education for dieticians includes, at a minimum, the completion of a baccalaureate degree. Courses of study include dietetics, foods and nutrition, and food service management. There are graduate and doctoral degrees available in these fields as well. In the United States, most states have laws that govern dieticians, and approximately two thirds of the states require licensure.

Critical Thinking Question

Why would a dietician confer with a physician before implementing a diet for a patient?

Right Word or Wrong Word: *Dietician* or *Dietitian*?
Are these two words the same? Are they homonyms?

The Language of Postoperative Care

Key terms: postoperative update

In the opening scenario, Clay Davis's surgeon, Dr. Sandor, sat with Clay's parents to discuss Clay's health status postoperatively. Key terms from the conversation are italicized in the example and highlighted below with the explanation.

"... in still in *PAR* recovering from the *anesthetic*..."

PAR: post-anesthetic recovery room. This is a specialized hospital unit adjacent to the operating room, where patients are closely monitored as they recover from anesthesia.

anesthetic: a type of medication that is used to induce a loss of sensation and thereby reduce or eliminate a sense of pain.

"Because of the *instability of this type of fracture*..."

instability of this type of fracture: a phrase that refers to the fact that the jaw is naturally moveable and that a fracture of the jaw is susceptible to movement. Such movement has the potential to delay bone healing, which involves the ability of the bone to set and of bone cells to regenerate.

"... *surgically reduced* and *fixed* with *titanium mini-plates* to achieve *rigid fixation*."

surgically reduced: a surgical procedure is used to reset a bone.

fixed: held firmly in place to prevent movement.

titanium mini-plates: small strips of titanium metal that are placed along the fracture to support bone healing. They allow the two sides of the fracture to come together and to remain in exceptionally close proximity until new tissues and bone are able to fill the gaps caused by the break. These metal plates are held in place by screws. Titanium is a lightweight, corrosion-resistant metal (see Figure 11-1).

rigid fixation: a surgical technique in which tiny screws or plates are attached directly onto the fractured section of the jawbone (see Figure 11-1).

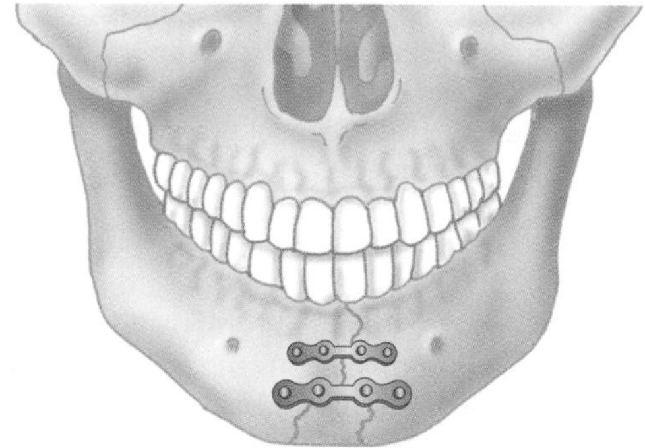

Figure 11.1: Repair of a symphyseal fracture

"... *across the fracture line*."

across the fracture line: an expression that means that a plate has been laid over the top of and across the line of the fracture (see Figure 11-1).

"... his *jaw wired shut*."

jaw wired shut: a common expression that refers to mandibular fixation. This surgical procedure keeps the jaws from moving and aligns and stabilizes the bones while they heal. This procedure can be performed only by a maxillofacial surgeon (see Figure 11-2).

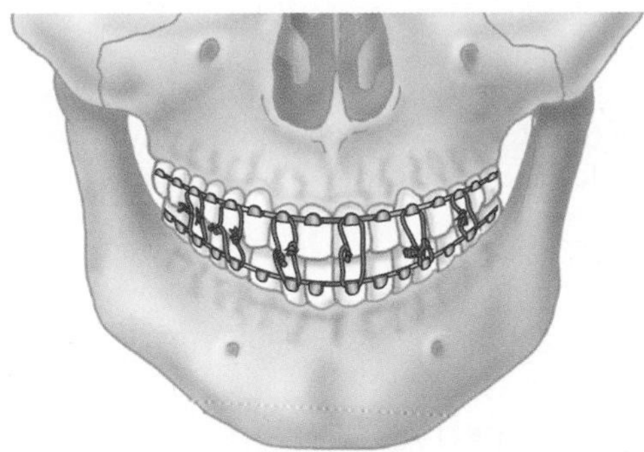

Figure 11.2: Wired jaws

"... or *dislocated* at the *condylar region,* the joints."

dislocated: displaced. In the context of joints, a dislocation means that the ends of the bones in the joint are no longer articulating or connecting with each other and that movement is either impaired or impossible until this condition is corrected. Jaw articulation occurs at the temporomandibular joint and involves both bones and muscles. (You'll learn more about this injury later in this chapter, as well as in Chapter 13.)

condylar region: the area at and around the temporomandibular joint in the mouth (see Figure 11-3 and Chapter 6).

"... a *maxillomandibular fixation* using *wires* ..."

maxillomandibular: pertaining to both the maxilla (the upper jaw) and the mandible (the lower jaw).

fixation: a state of being held firmly in place to prevent movement. In this context, the word *fixation* refers to a process of binding the jaw shut.

wires: stainless steel wires used in dentistry to hold the jaws in place.

"... the central and lateral *incisor* teeth ..."

incisor: one of the teeth at the front of the mouth (see Chapter 6).

"... *monitoring his airway* ..."

monitoring his airway: observing and assessing to ensure that the airway passage in the throat remains open and unblocked.

"... *altered levels of consciousness* ..."

altered levels of consciousness: in and out of consciousness; sometimes alert and aware and other times semi-stuporous or completely unaware (see Chapters 4 and 10).

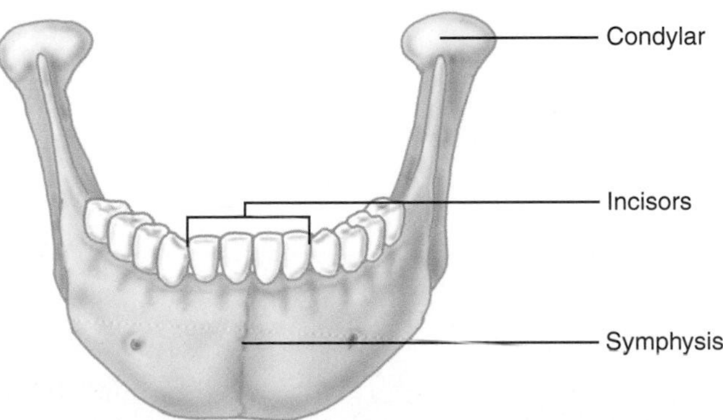

Figure 11.3: Simple anatomy of the lower mandible

"... *acute appendicitis* when he was 5 ..."

acute appendicitis: an emergency situation in which the appendix is inflamed and may burst. This condition can be life threatening. Appendicitis is fairly uncommon among children who are younger than 5 years old. The appendix is an organ that is attached to the large intestines; it is part of the digestive system.

"... he'd had his *appendix removed.*"

appendix removed: the surgical removal of the appendix is known as an **appendectomy**.

The Language of the Digestive System

The digestive system is also known as the gastrointestinal (GI) system. It is equally common to hear the terms *digestive tract* and *GI tract* as well. The anatomical term *gastrointestinal* can be understood as follows: *gastro* (stomach) + *intestinal* (referring to the intestines or bowels).

Key terms: digestive system

Ingestion means taking in a substance by mouth and then swallowing it; it refers to oral consumption. Although Clay Davis can still swallow, he will be unable to consume anything by mouth for some time yet because of his jaw injury. Later in this chapter, you will learn about the medical procedures and treatment initiatives by which he will be fed.

The *alimentary canal* is the anatomical term for the digestive or GI tract. The word **alimentary** derives from the Latin root *alimentum,* meaning *food, nutrition,* or *the digestive tract itself.* The word **tract** means *pathway.* The alimentary tract is a canal-like structure that extends from the mouth to the anus. After food is ingested, all solid matter and fluids are pushed along the tract by a process called *peristalsis.*

Peristalsis refers to a wave-like motion caused by the muscular contractions of the digestive tract. These contractions are naturally occurring phenomena. Peristalsis is critical to a well-functioning digestive system, and it ensures that what is ingested is metabolized (processed). Normal, natural waves of peristalsis are under the control of the central nervous system. Swallowing and peristalsis in the esophagus are under voluntary control; the remainder of the digestive tracts falls under involuntary control (see Chapter 10).

PRONUNCIATION PRACTICE

Say these words aloud to a friend or classmate if you can. You are given the phonetic pronunciation. Your instructor can help you with pronunciation,

or visit **http://www.MedicalLanguageLab.com.**

alimentary	ăl″ĭ-**mĕn**′tăr-ē
appendicitis	ă-pĕn″dĭ-**sī**′tĭs
gastrointestinal	găs″trō-ĭn-**tĕs**′tĭn-ăl
incisor	ĭn-**sī**′zor
ingestion	ĭn-**jĕs**′shŭn
peristalsis	pĕr-ĭ-**stăl**′sĭs

Anatomy and physiology: digestive system

The organs of the digestive system include the following, from top to bottom: the mouth (see Chapter 6); esophagus, stomach, small intestine (which is divided into the *duodenum, jejunum,* and *ileum*); the large intestine (which includes the ascending, descending, transverse, and sigmoid *colons*); rectum; and the anus (see Figure 11-4).

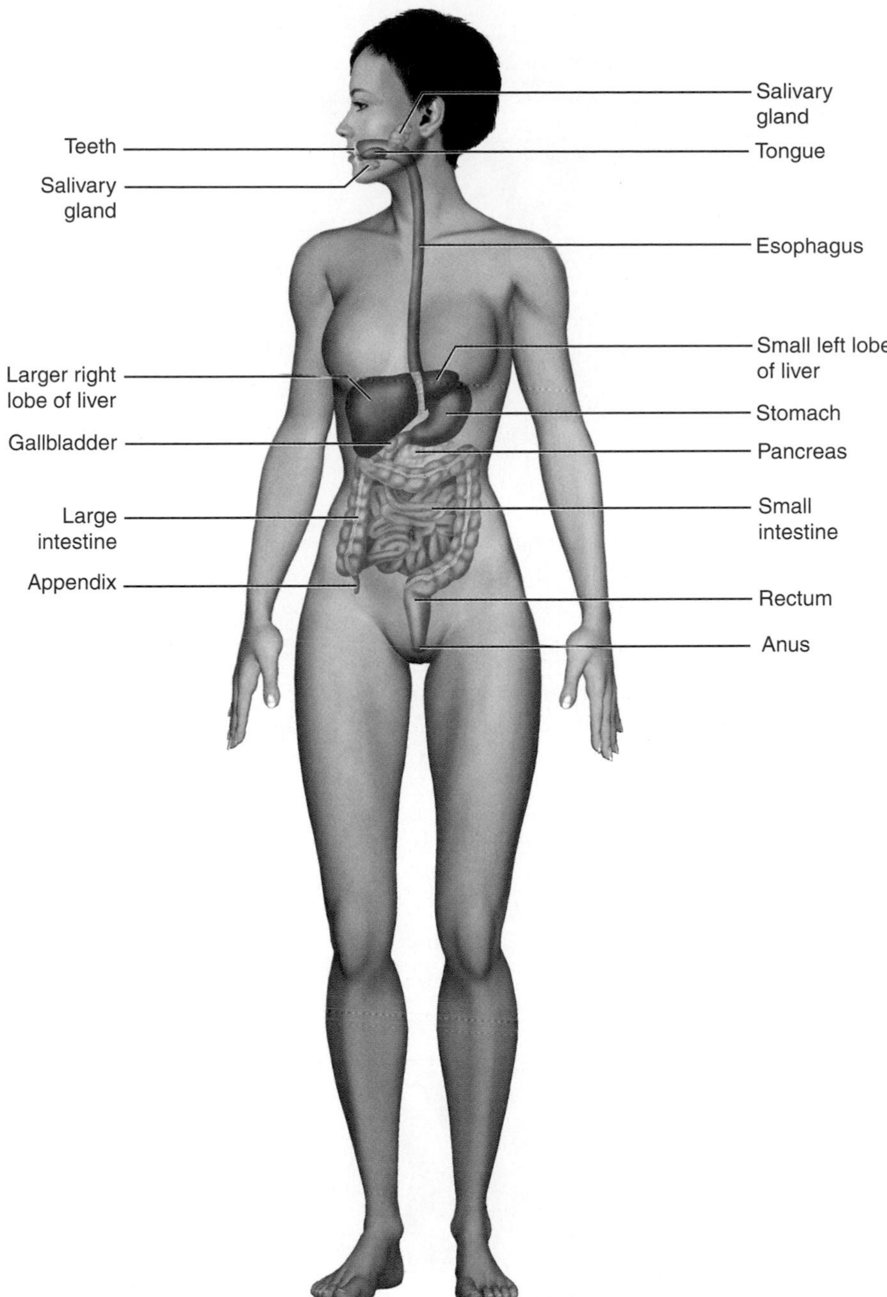

Figure 11.4: The digestive system

Organs of the digestive system

In Chapters 6 and 7, medical terms for the mouth, the salivary glands, and the pharynx were explored. Now, learn more language and facts about the rest of the digestive system.

Tongue

The **tongue** is essential to the digestive system; it is the organ that propels food through the oral cavity into the esophagus. A group of muscles within the tongue and associated with the tongue in the mouth also help to position matter for **mastication** (chewing) and then swallowing. Trauma to the mouth can adversely affect the tongue and cause inflammation or dehydration (drying). The tongue is covered with mucus to keep it moist. **Taste receptors** (taste buds) are located laterally along the surface of the tongue (see Figure 11-5). The word *tongue* is a root word.

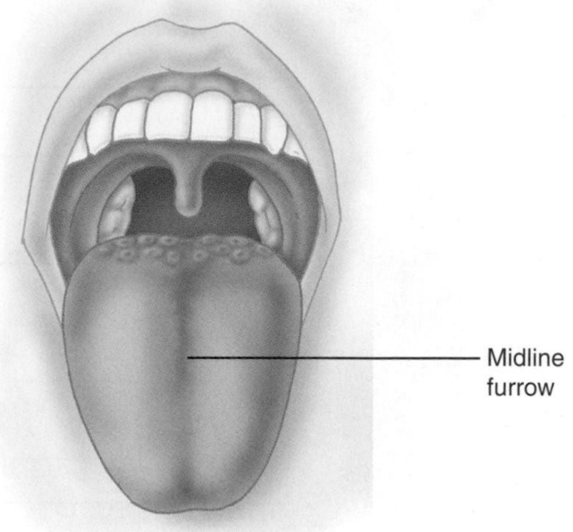

Figure 11.5: The tongue

Esophagus

The esophagus sits within the pharynx, and it runs parallel but posterior to the trachea. The aorta runs up the pharynx and alongside it (see Figure 11-6). The esophagus is designed to permit the flow of solids, liquids, and saliva from the oral cavity into the stomach.

Esophagus is a root word.

Esophageal is the associated adjective.

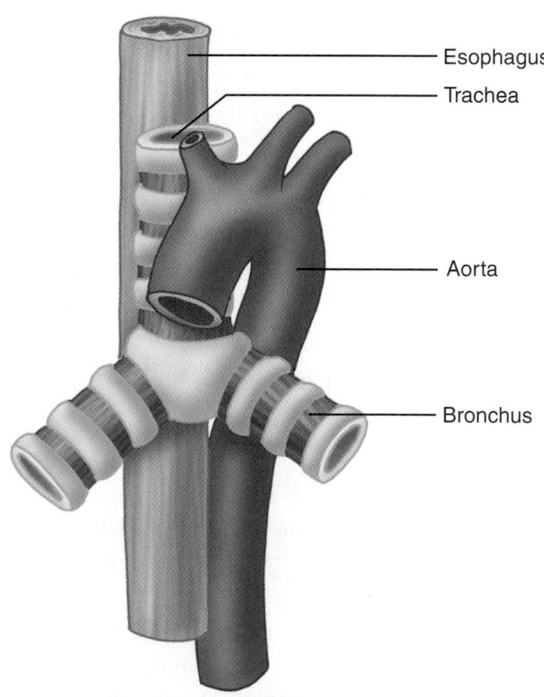

Figure 11.6: The esophagus and trachea

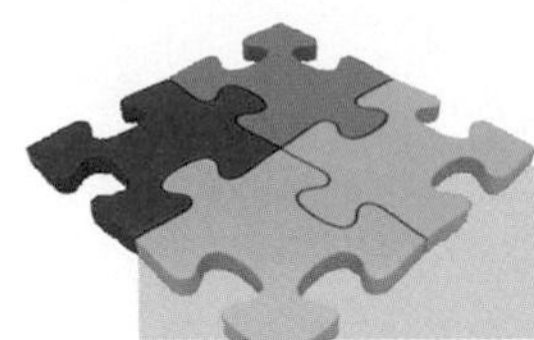

WORD BUILDING: Formula for Creating Words with the Combining Form *Esoph/ag/o*

Esophagus = The part of the body designed to permit the flow of solids, liquids, and saliva from the oral cavity into the stomach. The combining from is *esoph/ag/o.*

esophag + eal = *esophageal*

Definition: relating to the esophagus. (The suffix -*eal* turns the word into an adjective.) *adjective*

Example: A cancer in the esophagus is called *esophageal* cancer.

esophag + ectomy = *esophagectomy*

Definition: the surgical removal of all or part of the esophagus. *noun*

Example: In cases of esophageal cancer, an *esophagectomy* may be necessary.

esophago + enter + ostomy = *esophagoenterostomy*

Definition: the surgical creation of an opening between the esophagus and the intestine after the stomach has been removed. (The second root, *enteron,* is used in its combining form. It means *intestine.*) *noun*

Example: After his gastrectomy, the patient received an *esophagoenterostomy.*

esophago + myc + osis = *esophagomycosis*

Definition: a fungal infection of the esophagus. (The combining form, *myc-,* means *fungus.*) *noun*

Example: The fungal (yeast) infection candidiasis can cause *esophagomycosis.*

Right Word or Wrong Word: *Esophagus* or *Oesophagus*?

Are these two words the same? They are spelled differently, but are they pronounced the same? Do they mean the same thing?

Stomach

The **stomach** sits inferior to the esophagus and on the left side of the abdomen. It is divided into three regions: the pyloris, the body, and the fundus. The stomach is a temporary storage unit for solids and fluids during the process of digestion (see Figure 11-7).

The *fundus* is the uppermost portion of the stomach. The esophagus empties into it.

The *body* of the stomach is the main or central portion.

The *pyloris* is the lowest portion of the stomach. It opens into the duodenum.

The combining form, *pyle-*, means *gate, orifice, or opening.*

The combining form, *pylor/o,* means *gatekeeper.*

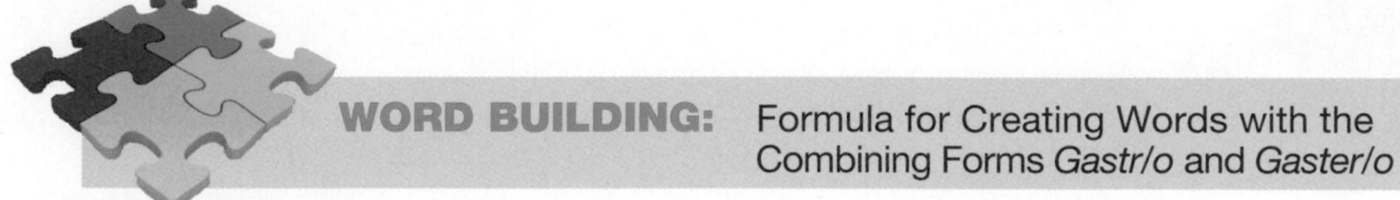

WORD BUILDING: Formula for Creating Words with the Combining Forms *Gastr/o* and *Gaster/o*

gaster = root meaning *stomach.* The combining forms are *gastr/o* and *gaster/o.*

gastr + esophagag + eal = *gastroesophageal*

Definition: pertaining to the stomach and the esophagus. (The suffix *-eal* turns this word into an adjective.) *adjective*

Example: *Gastroesophageal* reflux disease is a common condition in adults in which the stomach contents flow back up into the esophagus and cause a burning sensation.

gastro + enter + algia = *gastroenteralgia*

Definition: pain in both the stomach and the intestines. (The second root is *enter/o,* a combining form that refers to the intestines. The suffix *-algia* means *pain.*) *noun*

Example: For some people, *gastroenteralgia* can be caused by eating very spicy foods, particularly when they are not used to such foods.

gastro + gavage = *gastrogavage*

Definition: feeding done through an opening into the stomach or through a tube that is inserted into the stomach. (The second root is *gavage,* meaning *cramming.*) *noun*

Example: After jaw surgery, some patients must be fed by *gastrogavage.*

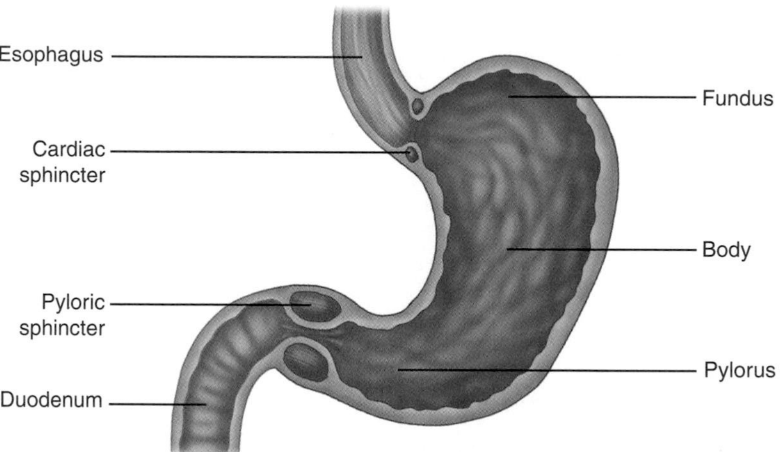

Figure 11.7: The stomach

Intestines

The intestines are composed of two distinct parts: the *small intestine* and the *large intestine*. Each plays an essential role in digestion by distinguishing the nutrients and water needed by the body and absorbing them. The intestines also identify the waste products of digestion and propel them along so that they can be expelled from the body. The intestines sit in the abdomen, just below the stomach and the liver. The word **intestine** derives from the Latin word *intestinum.*

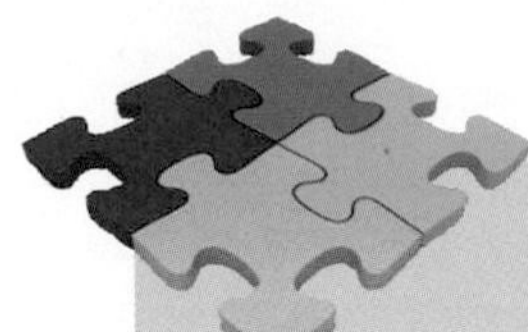

WORD BUILDING: Formula for Creating Words with the Combining Form *Enter/o*

enteron = Greek root meaning *intestine.* The combining form is *enter/o.*

entero + patho + gen = *enteropathogen*
Definition: any microorganism that causes disease of the intestines. *noun*

Example: *Enteropathogens* such as *Escherichia coli* almost always cause diarrhea.

entero + spasm = *enterospasm*
Definition: painful intermittent muscle contractions of the intestines. (The root word *spasm* means *contraction, seizure, or cramp* [i.e., of a muscle].) *noun*

Example: *Enterospasms* are often accompanied by diarrhea.

entero + toxin = *enterotoxin*
Definition: a toxin (poison) that is found in the contents of the intestines. *noun*

Example: Usually caused by bacteria in food, *enterotoxins* cause nausea, vomiting, and diarrhea.

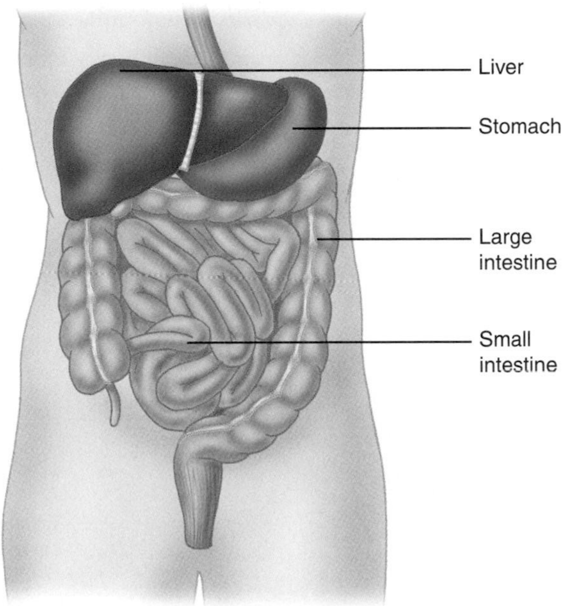

Figure 11.8: The intestines

Small intestine: also known as the *small bowel,* the small intestine is divided into three parts: the *duodenum*, jejunum, and ileum (see Figure 11-9).

The **duodenum** is the first part of the small intestine; it begins at the pylorus and ends at the jejunum. As partially digested matter and fluids are released intermittently into the duodenum from the stomach, digestive enzymes from the liver and pancreas are also released into the duodenum by way of the common bile duct (see the information about the gallbladder later in this chapter). *Duodenum* is a root word; the combining form is *duoden/o.*

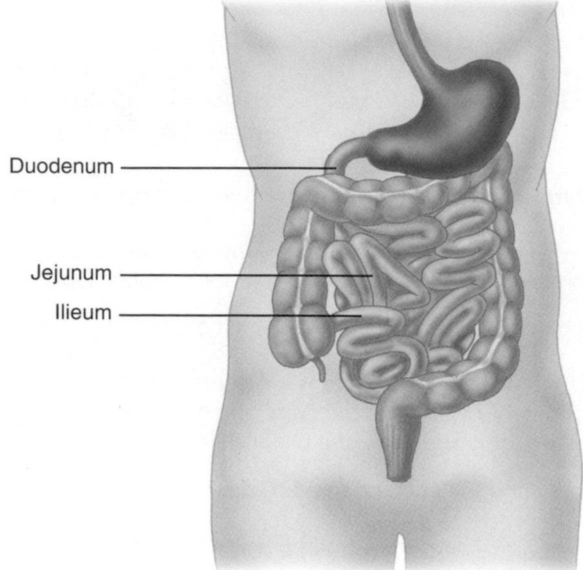

Figure 11.9: The small intestine

The **jejunum** is the second section of the small intestine. It is partially responsible for the absorption of nutrients such as carbohydrates, fats, proteins, and vitamins A and D into the bloodstream. The root word *jejunum* means *empty.* The combining form is *jejun/o.*

The ileum is the last part of the small intestine, as well as the longest. Here, vitamin B_{12} is absorbed for storage in the liver. Water and bile salts also pass through the membranes of the ileum and into the bloodstream.

Large intestine (colon): The large intestine is more formally referred to as the **colon** or the *large bowel.* It consists of four sections: the *cecum, ascending colon, descending colon*, and the *transverse colon*. The large intestine is located along the upper and outer walls of the abdomen and inferior to the stomach (see Figure 11-10).

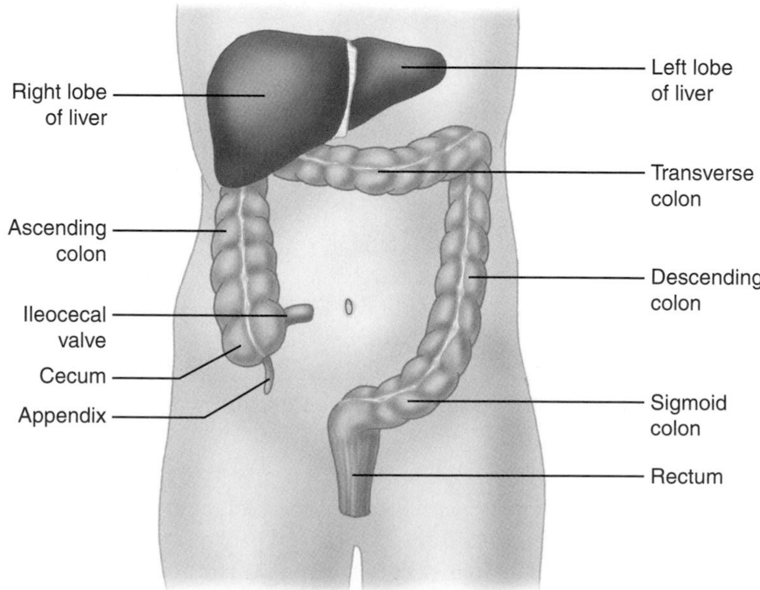

Figure 11.10: The large intestine

The large intestine begins at the distal end of the small intestine and functions to complete the digestion and elimination process, with a particular focus on the extraction and absorption of water and electrolytes (see Chapter 9). The large intestine terminates at the *anus*. The reabsorption of any water left in digested matter has a drying or solidifying effect on the digested matter, which becomes the waste product of feces. **Feces** are solid waste materials that, through continued peristalsis, move through the large intestine to the anus and that are eliminated during the process of defecation. Feces are composed of food wastes and bacteria. Certain types of bacteria are essential to the function of the large intestine; they process wastes, and they also protect the body against harmful bacteria (see Chapter 9). Feces are also referred to as *stool*.

The **cecum** is a pouch-like structure that is located at the very beginning of the large intestine, in the lower right quadrant of the abdomen. Because much of it is covered by the peritoneal area, the cecum can be described as sitting in the *retroperitoneal* region of the abdomen (behind the peritoneum; see the information about the peritoneum in Chapters 2, 3, and 9). The cecum receives partially digested matter from the small intestine and holds it temporarily for disbursement into the ascending colon. It functions as a receptacle (container) for liquids and for the salts and electrolytes that are contained within liquids. The cecum then absorbs these materials through its membranes to replenish the body. It also targets plant material (cellulose fibers) and completes their digestion. The cecum is lined with a thick mucus to help propel feces into the ascending colon. The combining form of the word *cecum* is *cec/o*.

The **appendix** is a tube-like structure that is attached to the cecum; it is more formally known as the *vermiform appendix* or the *cecal appendix*. The appendix seems to serve no known purpose in the human body, although pathology of the appendix can be life threatening.

The *ascending colon* is located along the right side of the abdomen, where it travels upward (ascending) to meet the transverse colon. It is found just posterior to the right lobe of the liver, and it is near the right kidney.

The *transverse colon* is located across the upper abdomen at the level of the 10th and 11th ribs, adjacent to the diaphragm. It sits in the intraperitoneal region of the abdomen.

The *descending colon* is located along the left side of the abdomen along the lateral border of the left kidney. It begins at the distal end of the transverse colon and continues downward (descending) to meet the sigmoid colon. The descending colon is parallel to the ascending colon, and much of it is covered by the peritoneum. As a result, it too may be referred to as sitting in the retroperitoneal region of the abdomen.

The *sigmoid colon* is located at the distal end of the descending colon, where it attaches to the rectum. It, too, sits intraperitoneally. The combining form of *sigmoid* is *sigmoid/o*.

Rectum

The **rectum** is a repository for feces, which is also known as *fecal matter*. It continues from the sigmoid colon through to the anus. The rectum sits at a mid-sacrum point (between the two femurs, at a point that originates near the base of the spine [the sacrum]). When feces enter the rectum, they are held until sensors alert the brain that the rectum and bowels need to be evacuated. These same sensors are able to distinguish between solid matter, liquids, and gases. When the urge to evacuate is recognized on a conscious level, we decide whether or not to do so; we have voluntary control of this function. The muscles of the rectum initiate what is called the *defecation reflex*. The word *rectum* is a root word, and the combining form is *rect/o*.

Anus

The anus is an organ attached to the rectum. It is a circular muscle and canal through which wastes are excreted (evacuated). The anus contains two *sphincters* (described later in this chapter). Sensory nerves distinguish solids, liquids, and gases in this part of the colon as well.

The word *anus* is a root word. Its combining form is *an/o*.

The combining form *proct/o* refers to both the anus and the rectum.

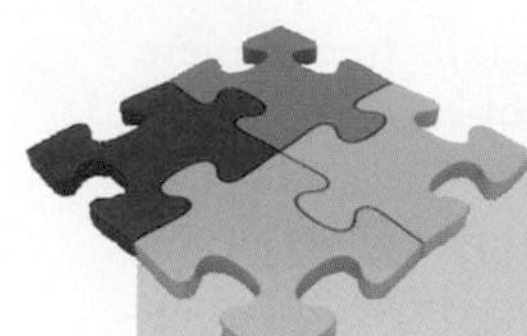

WORD BUILDING: Formula for Creating Words with the Combining Forms *Col/o* and *Colon/o*

Colon is a root word. The combining forms are *col/o* and *colon/o.*

colon + ic = *colonic*

Definition: relating to the colon. *adjective*

Example: A constipated person is said to suffer from *colonic* inertia.

col + itis = *colitis*

Definition: inflammation of the colon. *noun*

Example: *Colitis* is one cause of diarrhea.

col + ostomy = *colostomy*

Definition: a surgical connection that is made between the colon and the skin in which the rectum and the anus are bypassed and feces are transported out of the body through this stoma (opening). *noun* (An adjective that is used to describe this procedure is *colocutaneous.*)

Example: A *colostomy* may be necessary when the colon is severely damaged or diseased or when the colon and rectum require surgical removal as a result of bowel cancer.

colono + scopy = *colonoscopy*

Definition: a diagnostic procedure in which a tube-like endoscope is inserted into the rectum and up through the colon for examination. (A synonym is *coloscopy.*) *noun*

Example: A *colonoscopy* is a highly effective diagnostic test for detecting bowel or rectal cancer.

Build a Word

Practice using combining forms to create medical terms. Your repertoire of word parts should be sufficient now to accomplish this task. Create the term, and then provide its meaning. Remember, you may have to change some of the word parts slightly to create a new term.

1. jejun/o stoma col/o Term: ____________ Meaning: ____________
2. ectomy pylor/o Term: ____________ Meaning: ____________
3. col/o itis enter/o Term: ____________ Meaning: ____________
4. duoden/ al gastro Term: ____________ Meaning: ____________
5. itis enter/o gastr/o Term: ____________ Meaning: ____________
6. pathy colon/o Term: ____________ Meaning: ____________
7. scope sigmoid/o Term: ____________ Meaning: ____________
8. sigmoid rect/o Term: ____________ Meaning: ____________
9. ectomy gastr/ Term: ____________ Meaning: ____________
10. an/o rect/o -al Term: ____________ Meaning: ____________

Let's Practice

Identify the term or prefix that indicates each direction or location.

1. across ____________
2. upward ____________
3. downward ____________
4. within or toward the middle ____________
5. occurring behind ____________

PRONUNCIATION PRACTICE

Say these words aloud to a friend or classmate if you can. You are given the phonetic pronunciation. Your instructor can help you with pronunciation,

or visit **http://www.MedicalLanguageLab.com.**

anus	**ā′** nŭs
colostomy	kō-**lŏs′** tō-mē
colonoscopy	kō″lŏn-**ŏs′** kō-pē
cecum	**sē′** kŭm
duodenum	dū″ō-**dē′** nŭm or dū-**ŏd′**ē-nŭm
enteropathogen	ĕn″tĕr-ō-**păth′**ō-jĕn
esophagus	ē-**sŏf′**ă-gŭs
esophagectomy	ē-sŏf″ă-**jĕk′** tō-mē
fundus	**fŭn′** dŭs
feces	**fē′** sēz
gavage	gă-**văzh′**
gastroenteralgia	găs″trō-ĕn″tĕr-**ăl′** jē-ă
ileum	**ĭl′**ē-ŭm
intraperitoneal	ĭn″tră-pĕr″ĭ-tō-**nē′**ăl
jejunum	jē-**jū′** nŭm
pylorus	pī-**lor′**ŭs

Other structures of the digestive system

Valves

The epiglottis is a valve-like structure at the back of the oral cavity, strategically situated to discriminate between air and other matter. It opens and closes to direct solids and liquids down the esophagus to the stomach, and it prevents them from traveling into the trachea and the lungs. Conversely, the epiglottis can detect air and facilitate its transport into the trachea. The opening and closing of the epiglottis is, for the most part, involuntary, which means that it is controlled by the autonomic nervous system. However, the epiglottis can also be controlled voluntarily. For example, a person can make a conscious effort to swallow, gulp, or burp.

The **ileocecal valve** is situated at the base of the ileum, where it meets the cecum of the large intestine. It prevents the contents of the ileum from passing into the cecum too rapidly, and it also prevents any backflow from the cecum into the ileum.

Sphincters

Sphincters are circular bands of muscle that control the flow of matter through body orifices or openings.

The *external anal sphincter (EAS)* is more formally known as *the ani externus sphincter* or the *sphincter ani externus.* It is located at the opening of the anus. This striated muscle is under our voluntary control. The EAS allows feces to be expelled from the body during the act of defecation.

The *internal anal sphincter (IAS)* consists of smooth muscle. We do not have voluntary control over the IAS. It remains closed until it is signaled by the body that it is time to have a bowel movement. The IAS allows feces to enter the anus in anticipation of the act of defecation. The feces are stored there until the EAS is opened.

The *pyloric sphincter* keeps material in the stomach. It is located at the pyloris, which is the opening between the stomach and the intestines.

The *cardiac sphincter* or *cardioesophageal sphincter* sits near the heart at the entrance to the stomach. It opens to let in matter that has been swallowed and that has moved down through the esophagus.

Accessory organs

Accessory organs are those that help with the work of major organs or organ systems. In the digestive system, these include the salivary glands (Chapter 6), the pancreas (Chapter 7), the liver, and the gallbladder.

The liver

The **liver** is a major organ in and of itself. It is located in the upper right quadrant of the abdomen, just below the diaphragm and under the lower ribs. The liver is composed of two lobes and two main blood vessels (see Figure 11-11). The *hepatic artery* receives oxygenated blood from the aorta. The *portal vein* receives blood from the small intestine. A central function of the liver is to remove toxins from the blood; in this way, it is not unlike the kidney. In essence, the liver cleans the blood, and it also assists with the blood-clotting process.

The liver is an accessory organ of the digestive system because it is instrumental in the metabolism of the products of digestion (see "Focus Point: Metabolism, Catabolism, and Anabolism"). The liver produces **bile**, which is a thick, yellow-green substance that is stored in the gallbladder. Bile is used to digest fats. In addition, the liver creates urea by chemically altering parts of proteins that the body does not need. Urea is then transported from the liver to the kidney, where it is filtered and expelled as urine. Proteins are also used by the liver to create amino acids. In addition, the liver processes glucose from ingested carbohydrates, stores some of it, and releases the rest into the bloodstream for use as energy in the body. Finally, this accessory organ of the digestive system also stores certain types of vitamins.

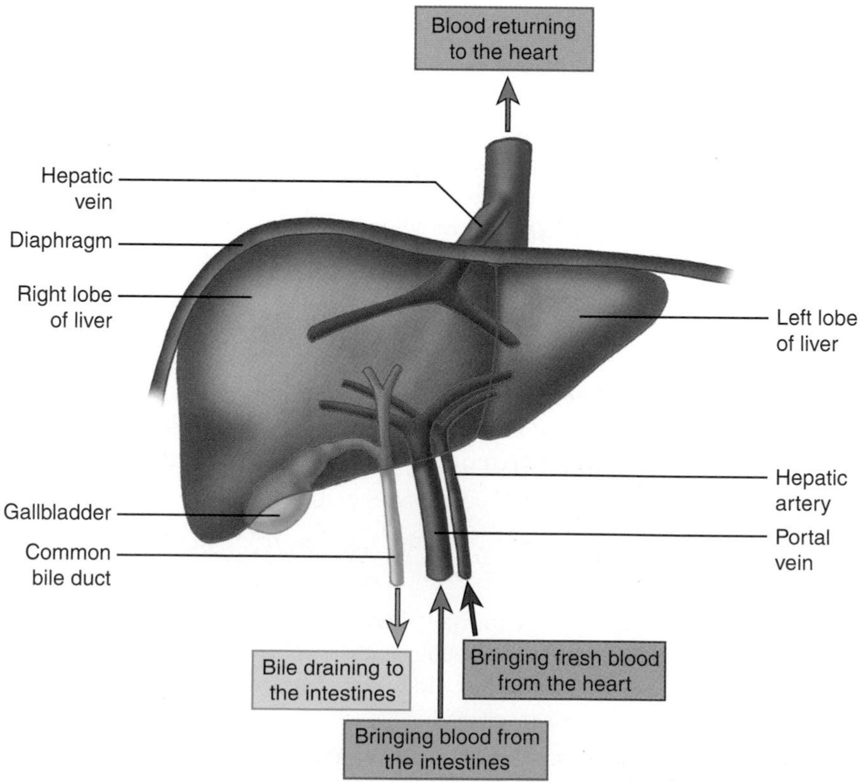

Figure 11.11: The liver

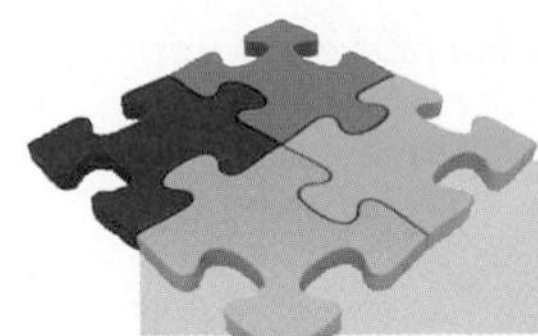

WORD BUILDING: Formula for Creating Words with the Combining Form *Hepat/o*

hepar = liver, from the Greek root *hepatos.* The combining form is *hepat/o.*

hepat + ic = *hepatic*

Definition: pertaining to the liver. *adjective*

Example: The *hepatic* vein carries blood from the liver.

hepat + atrophia = *hepatatrophia*

Definition: wasting away of the liver. (*Atrophia* is a derivative of the root word *atrophy,* meaning *wasting away or degenerating.*) *noun*

Example: *Hepatatrophia* can be expected in patients with chronic hepatic disease.

hepato + carcin + oma = *hepatocarcinoma*

Definition: cancer of the liver. (The combining form *carcin* means *cancer.*) *noun*

Example: Most types of *hepatocarcinoma* originate within the liver cells themselves. In this case, a synonym is *hepatocellular carcinoma.*

hepato + blast + oma = *hepatoblastoma*

Definition: an aggressive and malignant tumor of the liver. *noun*

Example: *Hepatoblastoma* is typically found in children who are 3 years old or younger.

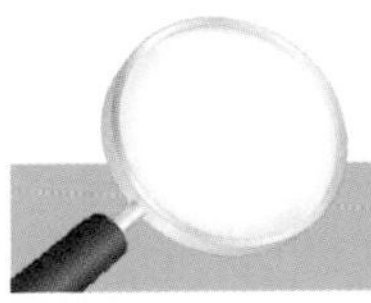

FOCUS POINT: Metabolism, Anabolism, and Catabolism

Metabolism is the general term for a number of biochemical processes in the body that convert food sources into energy for growth, healing, bodily responses to changes in the environment (i.e., the need to suddenly run or lift), and activities of daily living. During the process of metabolism, one compound is chemically altered to form another. Enzymes provide the catalysts for this process to occur. The term *metabolism* is derived from the Greek root *metaballein,* meaning *to change.* Metabolism includes anabolism and catabolism.

Anabolism is also known as *constructive metabolism* or *biosynthesis.* This process makes effective use of the products of digestion to enhance and maintain the size and strength of cells, tissues, organs, and bones. The root word *ana* is derived from the Greek word *anabole,* meaning *to build up.*

Catabolism is also known as *destructive metabolism.* During this process, the products of digestion are further broken down. As this process occurs, energy is released into the body. Catabolism provides the energy that allows physical activity to occur. The general function of catabolism is to provide the materials that are necessary for anabolic reactions. The root word *cata* is derived from *katabole,* a Greek word meaning *to cast down.*

The gallbladder

The gallbladder and the bile duct (the common bile duct) are attached to the liver (see Figure 11-11). The **gallbladder** is a small, sac-like structure that is located on the underside of the liver and on the right side of the abdomen. This sac functions as a reservoir, and it stores bile that is produced by the liver. When food enters the small intestine, a hormone called *cholecystokinin* is released. This signals the gallbladder to release the needed bile.

Chole: bile or gall.

The combining form is *chol/e.*

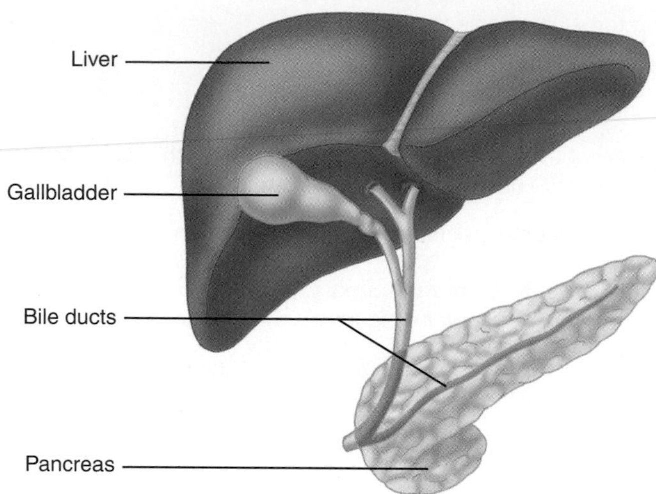

Figure 11.12: The gallbladder

Ducts

As you learned in Chapter 7, a duct is a narrow tube or passageway through which fluids can be secreted. There are a number of ducts involved with the liver, the pancreas, and the gallbladder. These include the *pancreatic duct, cystic duct,* and the *hepatic ducts,* all of which feed into the *common bile duct* (see Figure 11-13). Each of these ducts contributes to the process of digestion and metabolism.

The *common bile duct* is a tube-like structure that connects the liver to the duodenum. Bile that is produced by the liver is also transported through it. When the common bile duct is blocked by disease or scarring, bile backs up into the bloodstream. This leads to a condition called **jaundice**, which involves a yellowing of the skin and of the sclera of the eyes. In this situation, the patient becomes severely itchy (see Figure 11-14).

The *pancreatic duct* empties into the common bile duct from the pancreas (see Chapters 7 and 12). It secretes enzymes in the form of pancreatic juices.

The *cystic duct* connects the gallbladder to the common bile duct.

The *hepatic ducts* are branches of the common bile duct as it enters and leaves the liver. They drain bile into the common bile duct.

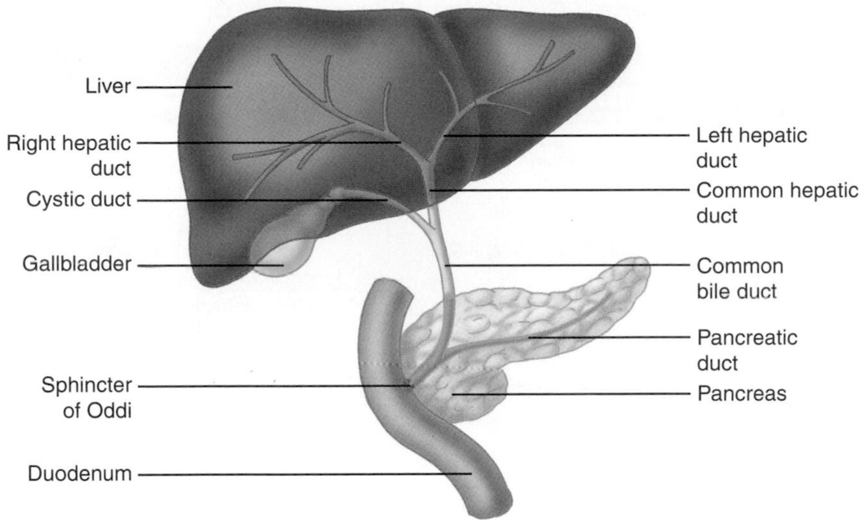

Figure 11.13: The bile ducts

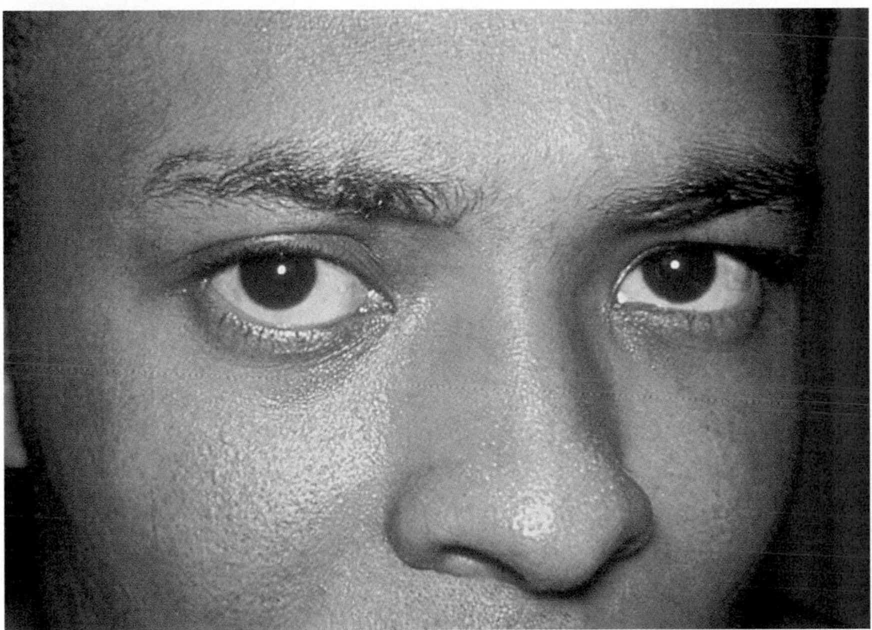

Figure 11.14: A jaundiced eye (Courtesy of the Centers for Disease Control and Prevention, Dr. Thomas F. Sellers, and Emory University, 1963.)

Word Parts for Ducts: There are several different combining forms for words that are used to refer to bile and the bile duct, including the following:

The combining form *choledoch/o* derives from the archaic medical term *choledochos,* meaning *to contain bile* or *bile duct.*

The combining form *cholangi/o* means *bile vessel.* This word form derives from the early Greek roots *chole,* meaning *bile,* and *angeion,* meaning *vessel.*

The combining form *cholecyst/o* derives from the early Greek roots *chole,* meaning *bile,* and *kystis,* meaning *bladder.* The modern translation of *kystis* is *cyst,* meaning *sac, vessel, or bladder.*

Refer to Table 11-1 to learn about word parts related to the gallbladder and bile ducts and to see how they combine for the creation of new medical terms.

TABLE 11-1: Medical Terms: Gallbladder, Bile, and Bile Ducts

BEGIN with the Root or Combining Form	ADD Another Word Part	COMBINE to Create a New Word
cholecysto/o	+ itis (inflammation)	cholecystitis (inflammation of the gallbladder, usually related to a blockage in the bile ducts)
cholecysto/o	+ lithiasis (condition of having a stone)	cholecystolithiasis (the presence of a stone in the gallbladder; gallstones)
choledocho/o	+ ectasia (distention, swelling, or enlargement)	choledochectasia (distention of the common bile duct)
choledocho/o	+ lithiasis (condition of having a stone)	choledocholithiasis (the presence of a calculi [stone] in the common bile duct)
cholangi/o	+ carcinoma *carcin,* meaning *cancer* + *oma,* meaning *tumor* (cancer)	cholangiocarcinoma (cancer of the common bile duct)
cholangi/o	+ tomy (incision)	cholangiotomy (surgical incision of one of the bile ducts to remove a gallstone)

Mix and Match

Match each word with its definition or description.

1. hepatitis	rupture of the liver
2. hepatogastric	inflammation of the liver and kidneys
3. hepatocystic	poisonous to the liver
4. hepatonephritis	referring to the stomach and the liver
5. hepatorrhexis	inflammation of the liver
6. hepatotoxic	pertaining to the gallbladder and the liver

Break It Down

Break down each term into its component parts. Define each part, and then define the term.

1. cholecystitis ______________________ Meaning: ______________________

2. cholecystopathy ______________________ Meaning: ______________________

3. cholangiography ______________________ Meaning: ______________________

4. cholangioma ______________________ Meaning: ______________________

PRONUNCIATION PRACTICE

Say these words aloud to a friend or classmate if you can. You are given the phonetic pronunciation. Your instructor can help you with pronunciation,

or visit **http://www.MedicalLanguageLab.com.** 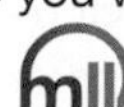

anabolism	ă-**năb**´ō-lĭzm
catabolism	kă-**tăb**´ō-lĭzm

cholangiocarcinoma	kō-lăn″jē-ō-kăr″sĭ-**nō**′mă
cholecystokinin	kō″lē-sĭs″tō-**kīn**′ĭn
cholecystitis	kō″lē-sĭs-**tī**′tĭs
cholecystolithiasis	kō″lē-sĭs″tō-lĭ-**thī**′ă-sĭs
choledocholithiasis	kō-lĕd″ō-kō-lĭ-**thī**′ă-sĭs
epiglottis	ĕp″ĭ-**glŏt**′ĭs
hepatatrophia	hĕp″ăt-ă-**trō**′fē-ă
hepatocarcinoma	hĕp″ă-tō-kăr″sĭn-**ō**′mă
hepatogastric	hĕp″ă-tō-**găs**′trĭk
hepatonephritis	hĕp″ă-tō-nĕ-**frī**′tĭs
hepatorrhexis	hĕp″ă-tō-**rĕks**′ĭs
ileocecal	ĭl′ē-ō-**sē**′kăl
metabolism	mĕ-**tăb**′ō-lĭzm
sphincter	**sfĭngk**′tĕr

Functions of the digestive system

There are three main functions of the digestive system: the digestion of food, the absorption of nutrients, and the elimination of wastes.

Digestion is the conversion of substances (foods) in the stomach and intestines into **soluble** or diffusible (able to pass through membranes) products that can be absorbed into the bloodstream.

Absorption refers to the movement of the products of digestion into the circulatory and lymphatic systems. This occurs through the process of diffusion through the membranes of the intestines.

Elimination refers to the removal of solid wastes through the process of defecation and the removal of fluids through the kidneys, the lungs, and the skin.

The word *digestion* is derived from the early Latin word *digestio,* meaning *to take apart.* That is exactly what occurs during the process of digestion: solid and liquid substances are taken apart, and their nutrients are extracted. Elements that the body does not need or that can be harmful (toxic) are eliminated.

The combining form of *digestio* is *gestio.*

Suffixes that refer to eating, ingesting, and digestion are *-phagia* and *-phagy.*

A number of key prefixes are often used with the word *digestion.* Refer to Table 11-2 to learn more about them.

Right Word or Wrong Word: *Egestion, Excretion,* or *Elimination*?

Are these terms interchangeable? Do they mean the same thing? Think carefully.

TABLE 11-2: Word Building with *Digestion* and *Gestio-*

BEGIN with a Prefix	ADD Digestion or Combining Form	Create a New Term
in-	+ gestion	ingestion (the process of taking matter or substances into the body, usually through the mouth)
e-	+ gestion	egestion (the process of voiding or eliminating undigested material through the anus)
in-	+ digestion	indigestion (the condition that results from the failure to properly or adequately digest food or other substances in the digestive tract)
un-	+ digest + ed	undigested (pertaining to substances in the digestive tract that have not been fully digested or that cannot be digested; undigested substances will still pass through the digestive tract to be eliminated, and this may or may not cause some physical discomfort)

Digestive enzymes

Enzymes are essential to the digestive system. Essentially, enzymes turn what is ingested into energy for immediate use or stored energy for use later when the body needs it. Every cell and every organ in the body requires the assistance of enzymes. They are biological **catalysts**. This means they are chemicals that regulate most of the biochemical reactions in the body. These include digestion, absorption, transportation, metabolism, and the elimination of nutrients and wastes. To learn more about three types of digestive enzymes, see Table 11-3.

Right Word or Wrong Word: *Excretion* or *Secretion*?

You have been reading about excretion, but you have also seen the term *secretion* in this and previous chapters. Is there a difference in meaning between these two terms?

TABLE 11-3: Types of Enzymes

Types of Enzymes	Locations and Functions
Digestive enzymes Examples: pepsin, lipase, protease, ptyalin, trypsin, and amylase	• secreted all along the digestive tract • break down foods into nutrients that the body can use for energy
Metabolic enzymes	• produced by the pancreas, the cell walls, and certain organs (see Chapter 7) • produce energy • help with breaking down fat • lower cholesterol and triglyceride levels • essential to cell production of muscle, nerve, blood, lung, and bone tissue • detoxify the body by helping to eliminate those waste products that are harmful to us
Food enzymes	• ingested via raw foods; organic • designed specifically to help digest the particular food product that has been eaten

Patient Update

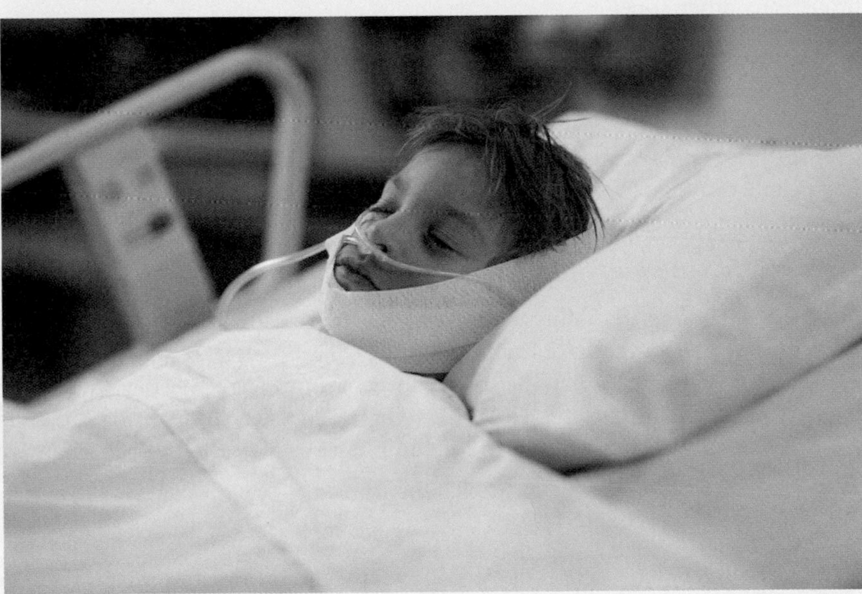

It is late evening, and young Clay Davis has been moved from PAR into a four-bed room in the pediatric unit (Peds) at Okla Trauma Center after his maxillofacial surgery. He is in and out of consciousness as the anesthesia continues to wear off and in response to the analgesia (pain medication) that he is receiving by IV. He is receiving oxygen via nasal prongs, and he has a tube inserted into his right nostril for feeding purposes. His parents are with him.

Upon the patient's arrival in Peds, a nurse was able to spend some time with Mr. and Mrs. Davis. She gathered more information for the medical history for Clay's chart. She discovered that Clay has special dietary needs because he is lactose intolerant. He had his appendix removed when he was 5, and he has no known allergies. He has never broken any other bones besides the one he broke during the motor vehicle accident. Mrs. Davis reported that Clay is an active 7-year-old boy who plays baseball on a team, enjoys riding his bike and swimming, and has been learning some carpentry from his father as a hobby. Mrs. Davis proudly noted that her son had recently won a competition for building a high-rise birdhouse.

The nurse then talked with Mr. and Mrs. Davis about Clay's treatment plan. She informed them that, although Clay had a urinary catheter in place for the duration of the surgery, this had now been removed; Clay was now wearing an incontinence pad. She explained that Clay would be able to void and defecate into the pad, if necessary. This greatly dismayed his mother, who was worried that Clay wouldn't feel comfortable doing this. She was afraid that he would see it as a setback and that he might think that people considered him "a little baby." The nurse acknowledged Clay's possible embarrassment but explained that this was simply a precautionary measure until Clay was able to sit up on his own and be assisted onto a bedside commode. The treatment team expected Clay to be able to do this within the next 24 hours, although he would require their assistance to do so. In the meantime, the nurses and aides would pop in frequently to offer the child a bedpan. Clay's mother was relieved to hear this. The nurse also reassured Clay's mother that keeping the patient dry, comfortable, and free from any embarrassment related to toileting were priorities for the nursing staff. Finally, the nurse told the parents that they would soon be able to speak with a dietician, who would be very helpful with regard to planning and guiding them through the process of nutritional care and the reestablishment of Clay's ability to eat by mouth.

Reflective Question

When is it likely that Clay will be able to sit up in bed on his own and possibly use the toilet?

____

Let's Practice

Reword the following phrases from the patient update into more formal medical terms.

1. "appendix removed" ______________________________
2. "a tube inserted into his right nostril" ______________________________
3. "never broken any other bones" ______________________________
4. "in place" ______________________________

Key terms: medical history and postsurgical condition

Although the nurse working with Clay and his parents generally used medical language that many people without medical training can understand, a few terms in the Patient Update are not so easily understood by people who don't work in health care. These are italicized in the example and highlighted below with the explanation:

"... he is *lactose intolerant.*"

lactose intolerant: not having the ability to digest lactose or digesting it only with difficulty. **Lactose** is a sugary product that is found in milk and milk products. However, lactose intolerance is not an allergy to milk. The condition arises in the patient's digestive system, where the enzyme lactase is not sufficiently able to break down the lactose in foods and beverages. Some medications in solid form contain lactose as filler, so it is important for the treatment team to be aware of this condition.

"... he has *no known allergies.*"

no known allergies (NKA): this is a critical piece of inquiry and information that all health-care providers gather whenever they first meet a patient or client. It is never assumed that just because it says "no known allergies" on a medical record or because this section on the record has not been filled in that the patient is actually free of allergies. Each health-care provider will ask the question again to ensure that the patient is protected from any odors, products (i.e., latex), foods, and medications that could cause an adverse reaction, possibly one that could lead to a medical crisis or death.

"... wearing an *incontinence pad.*"

incontinence pad: a hygiene product designed to catch any substances or liquids voided from the body. It is made of multiple layers of material that are permeable to liquids and that trap and hold liquids to prevent leakage beyond the pad.

"... assisted onto a bedside *commode.*"

commode: any container that can be used as a toilet. A bedside commode is a portable toilet that looks much like a chair on wheels. It can be brought to the patient's bedside so that he or she may defecate or void in a manner that is more familiar and comfortable to him or her.

Let's Practice

Unscramble these sentences to practice using medical terms in full sentences.

1. incontinence of needs child pad use immobile to is the incontinent urine and an.

   ____

2. no admission the patient shows record allergies the known has.

   ____

3. patient's arrived staff is shellfish to mother allergic when later she the told the her child.

   ____

The Language of Nutrition and Diet

Patient Update

It is early morning, and Mickey Davis is sitting at her son's bedside, where she spent the night. She'd sent her husband home around midnight so that he could contact his brother and sister to find out how his parents were doing and so that he could also make arrangements for his absence at work. Clay had been awake for short periods during the night, but he was very groggy. He tried to speak, but of course he could not; his lips are swollen from the trauma that he endured. His lips are also very dry; throughout the night, his mother gently applied a lip balm to keep them from drying out completely. Clay's jaw remains swollen and bruised. His left upper torso is not covered with blankets, but with a light gauze dressing to protect his fragile, scalded skin. Clay's mother made sure to tuck the light flannel blanket on the bed snuggly up around his right shoulder to keep him warm as he slept. Mickey spent the night crying off and on. She still wants to cry. When Clay opened his eyes occasionally during the night, Mickey did her best to remain strong so that she could comfort and reassure him. However, when he drifted back off to sleep, his mother cried softly again.

Both parents are present now. Clay's father is holding Mickey in his arms as she cries. He, too, is trying to remain strong, but he has tears in his eyes. "Mickey, it's going to be all right," Steve says softly into her ear as he holds her. "The doctor said everything went well last night in surgery, and Clay's going to be all right." Mickey nods her agreement into his shoulder.

"I know, Steve, I know. It's just that I can't stand to see him like this. My poor Clay. Oh, Steve, it must hurt so much," she whispered back to her husband. They turned together to watch their son sleep. A knock came at the open door.

"Hello... Mr. and Mrs. Davis?" They nodded and turned to face the speaker, a woman in her 30s who was dressed professionally in a skirt and blouse and holding a clipboard in her hand. "I'm Takeisha Cameron, a registered dietician here at Okla Trauma. How are you doing today?" Ms. Cameron paused before going on. "I've come to talk with you about Clay's nutritional status and whatever needs he may have as he recovers from his jaw surgery." She paused for a moment again. "Please, please sit down." She smiled as she waved her hand toward the chairs at Clay's bedside as an invitation.

"As you can see," the dietician began again, "your son has an intravenous line running there, in his arm, and a couple of tube-like devices inserted into his nostrils. I'm wondering if you know what all of these are for?" Takeisha paused to give the Davises time to answer. Mr. Davis replied that he and his wife both understood the purpose of the IV and the nasal prongs, but they only knew a little about the other tube. He said that the nurse had referred to it as an "NG tube" and that it was supposed to feed their son, but that was really all they knew. He also mentioned they had been very much looking forward to speaking with Takeisha.

"Thank you. And you are correct: Clay is receiving oxygen through those little nasal prongs that are inserted just to the inside of his nostrils. You are also correct in saying that the other tube, going into this right nostril, is an NG tube. That stands for *nasogastric.* The tube extends through the nose and the nasal cavity, down the esophagus, and into the stomach. That is how your son is going to be receiving his daily nutrition for a while. His status is NPO: nothing by mouth." Takeisha paused again to allow Clay's parents some time to process this information.

"I thought it was possible to feed people intravenously," commented Clay's father. "Wouldn't that be easier for him?" Takeisha nodded. She went on to explain that this was indeed possible but that this type of IV feeding was not as effective as the method that the doctor had chosen for Clay.

"Parenteral nutrition is designed only to supplement what a patient is able to ingest by mouth. As you can see, Clay is not able to ingest anything by mouth. Although this complicates his care, the insertion of a nasogastric feeding tube allows us to supply most of his daily requirements of vitamins, carbohydrates, and dextrose, a type of sugar, through a highly specialized formula that the nurse administers into the tube on a scheduled basis. Nasogastric intubation is a type of enteral nutrition that involves feeding directly into the stomach or intestines. It is not always possible when the face is injured, because access to the nose and throat are necessary. However, in Clay's case, his nose and the supporting bones of the cheeks did not suffer any trauma."

"What would you have done if you could not have put the tube down into his stomach this way, through his nose and throat?" asked Clay's mother.

"That's a very good question, Mrs. Davis. We may have reverted to something we call *total parenteral nutrition.* In that case, a new intravenous line would be started, perhaps in a large vein in the chest, with a larger-sized tube and an intravenous catheter to facilitate the administration of nutrition by that route. Then again, for cases in which longer periods of assisted feeding are required, the doctors may even decide to surgically create an opening called a *stoma* directly into the stomach or jejunum of the small intestine to create a port through which a feeding tube can be inserted." Mr. and Mrs. Davis suddenly looked quite concerned. Noticing this, the dietician quickly said, "Not to worry; this is not going to happen with your son. The surgery that he had to repair his jaw is quite standard, and we all expect a good recovery." Takeisha paused again to be sure that the child's parents felt reassured.

"So you're saying that Clay will have to be tube fed for awhile but that this will be through that NG tube only?" Mr. Davis paraphrased. The dietician nodded. "How long can we expect that to continue?" Mr. Davis then asked with concern.

"Your son is going to receive his nutrition by NG tube for about a week. Then, if the swelling has receded in his mouth and along the site of the surgery and if he is able to open his jaw even a little bit on his own, we will be able to start him on a liquid diet by mouth. He'll need to stay on a liquid diet for about another week, and then we can move on to soft foods. We don't want to risk reinjuring that fracture line by having him chew down on something." The parents nodded their understanding.

"Oh," lamented Mrs. Davis, "This is going to be so hard on our little guy. He's going to be so hungry!" The dietician smiled warmly and reassured them that Clay would be receiving sufficient nutrition to not truly be hungry; however, because hunger is also related to smell and to the routines associated with eating, Clay may still feel hungry. Takeisha talked with the Davises then about ways to distract Clay from that feeling and to help him cope with his frustration. She also suggested that Mr. and Mrs. Davis refrain from bringing any food or beverages into Clay's room for the time being. Finally, Takeisha advised Clay's parents that she would be checking on their son daily. She reassured them that she would be there with them when it was time for Clay to begin his liquid diet and have the NG tube removed. She pointed out that a speech therapist would make an assessment of Clay's ability to move food from the front to the back of his mouth and to swallow. Finally, Takeisha gave them her hospital business card and invited them to contact her anytime if they had any questions.

Steve and Mickey Davis got up to say goodbye to the dietician. They then resettled into their chairs, one on each side of the bed, where they could hold their son's hands and watch him. They sat quietly like that for some time. Then Mickey asked, "Did you speak with your parents? Your brother and sister? Is everyone okay? Oh, Steve, how did all of this happen?" And he began to tell her.

Reflective Questions

1. How will nutrition be supplied to our patient, Clay Davis? ______________________

2. An enteral feed involves the use of a tube that is inserted into the digestive tract (alimentary canal) at some point. How is a parenteral nutrition tube inserted? ______________________

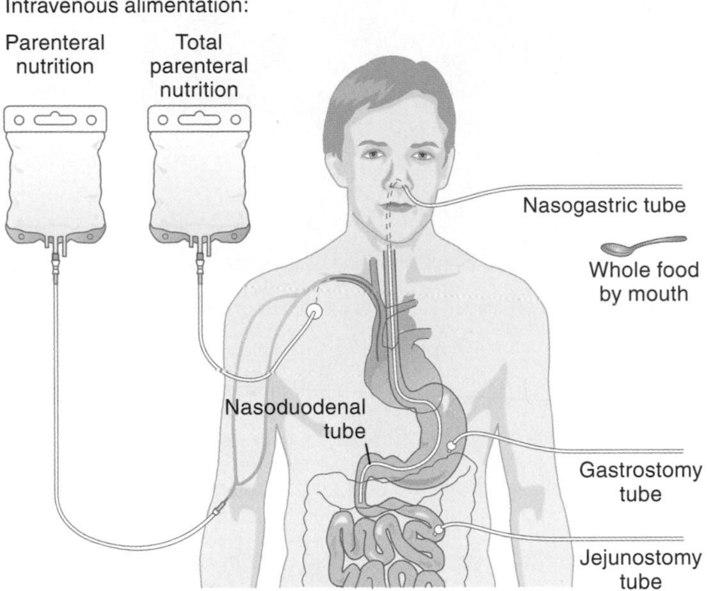

Figure 11.15: Methods of feeding

Key terms: nutrition

This patient update demonstrates once again that, when speaking with clients, health professionals choose words and phrases that facilitate the ability of patients and their families to take part in the conversation. Key terms from the dialogue italicized in the example and highlighted below with the explanation:

"... talk with you about Clay's *nutritional status...*"

nutritional status: the balance between the intake of nutrients and the expenditure of energy from nutrients; the extent to which the nutrients available are able to meet a person's metabolic needs.

"Parenteral nutrition..."

parenteral: inside the body but bypassing the digestive tract.

"Nasogastric intubation..."

nasogastric: from the nose to the stomach or intestines.

intubation: the condition of having a tube inserted and in place in the body. The opposite of *intubation* is **extubation,** which means *the removal of a tube;* however, this term is rarely used.

"... enteral nutrition..."

enteral: into the digestive/GI tract. Enternal nutrition refers to how nutrition is delivered to the body.

"... total parenteral nutrition..."

total parenteral nutrition (TPN): the administration of all nutrition through an intravenous line into the vena cava and the bloodstream.

"... an intravenous *catheter...*"

catheter: a hollow, flexible tube that is inserted into the body either to keep a passage open or to administer or withdraw fluids. An intravenous catheter is inserted directly into a vein and then connected to intravenous tubing (see Figure 11-16).

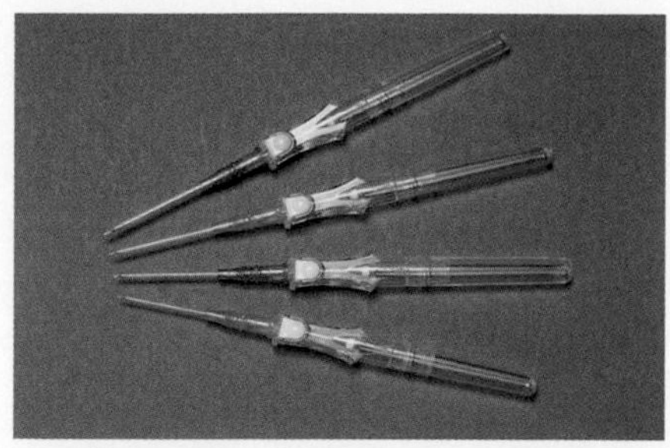

Figure 11.16: Intravenous catheters (From Rutherford CJ: *Differentiating Surgical Equipment and Supplies.* Philadelphia: FA Davis, 2010, p 195. With permission.)

"... to *facilitate the administration of nutrition by that route.*"

facilitate the administration of nutrition: medical jargon meaning *to make easier or to assist with the process of feeding.*

by that route: medical jargon that refers to a pathway of delivery: orally, intravenously, subcutaneously (below the skin), topically (on the skin), and so on.

"... *assisted feeding* ..."

assisted feeding: a common term in health care that implies that the patient needs help to eat and cannot feed himself or herself.

"... *a stoma* ..."

stoma: an opening. In the context of feeding and nutrition, a stoma is a surgical opening made from the stomach or intestine to the outer wall of the abdomen. Through this opening, a feeding tube can be inserted and nutrition administered.

"... a *feeding tube* ..."

feeding tube: latex or plastic tubing through which liquid nutrition is delivered.

"... have to be tube *fed* for a while ..."

tube fed: medical jargon that refers to the process of feeding someone via a tube.

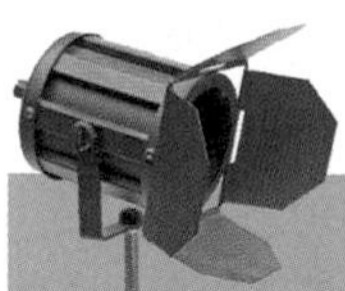

CAREER SPOTLIGHT: Speech Therapist

Speech therapists are more properly known as *speech and language pathologists.* Most often prepared at the master's degree level, these health professionals assess, diagnose, treat, and work to prevent disorders of speech, language, communication, voice, and swallowing. On the multidisciplinary health care team, these individuals work closely with physicians, nurses, and others. When dieticians are part of the treatment team, speech therapists confer and consult with them to recommend types of diets for patients with impairments or deficits of speech, language, or swallowing. Speech therapists also work closely with patients and clients for the restoration, rehabilitation, and recovery of these abilities.

Education for speech and language pathologists includes graduation from an accredited school with a course of study that includes a clinical practicum. After graduation, candidates must pass a national licensing examination and successfully complete a period of postgraduate clinical experience.

Critical Thinking Questions

Think carefully about all that you've learned about Clay Davis's treatment at Okla Trauma Center and about the members of his care team, and then answer the following questions.

1. Clay Davis has had two types of catheters placed since his arrival at the hospital. Name them.
   ____

2. Why will a speech therapist be involved in Clay's care, even though he cannot speak and won't be able to speak for some time yet?
   ____

Break It Down

Study the following terms. Identify the prefix in each term, and state what that prefix means. You have encountered these prefixes in previous chapters.

1. parenteral Prefix: ______________ Meaning: ______________
2. intravenous Prefix: ______________ Meaning: ______________
3. intubation Prefix: ______________ Meaning: ______________
4. extubation Prefix: ______________ Meaning: ______________

Fill in the Blanks

Review the key terms from the Patient Update, and then fill in the blanks using medical terminology.

1. Clay is going to be receiving ______________ nutrition.
2. Nutrition is going to be supplied or administered to Clay Davis via a ______________.
3. NG tubes extend from the ______________ down through the ______________ and into the ______________.
4. ______________ supplements nutritional intake by mouth, whereas ______________ provides all nutritional intake.

Nutrition

Nutrition is the study of the nutrients in food and of how the body makes use of those nutrients. This field includes the research and study of the relationships among health, illness, and diet. Good nutrition is the body's ability to consume, digest, absorb, and fully metabolize adequate supplies of the nutrients that are needed to maintain health and promote healing.

The term **dietetics** refers to the dissemination of nutritional information. The goal of dietetics is health promotion by means of providing information through teaching and learning strategies that enable individuals to make healthy nutritional choices.

As you learn the language of nutrition, consider the challenges that are faced by our young patient, Clay Davis, who is 7 years old. In his current postoperative medical state, he will not be able to take any foods by mouth for up to a week. His nutritional status can be compromised by this fact. **Compromised** is a medical term meaning *impaired or complicated by a factor such as injury or disease;* in other words, the patient is not able to function normally or optimally.

Nutrients

Nutrients are substances that provide nourishment for the body. These include carbohydrates, proteins, lipids, water, vitamins, and minerals. Nutrients play important roles in the health and healing of the body. Refer to Table 11-4 for an overview, and then read on to learn more about each category of essential nutrients.

Carbohydrates or *saccharides* are organic compounds. They consist of starches, fiber, and sugars. They function as sources of energy, particularly for the neurological system. Carbohydrates are classified as *simple* or *complex,* depending on their chemical makeup and how quickly they can be digested and absorbed by the body.

The term **saccharide** refers to a category of carbohydrates that contain sugars. They are named by their chemical makeup and specifically for the number of sugar molecules that are contained within them. The prefixes *mono-, di-, oligo-,* and *poly-* are added to the root *saccharide* to create the names *monosaccharide, disaccharide, oligosaccharide,* and *polysaccharide.*

TABLE 11-4: Essential Nutrients and Their Functions

Essential Nutrients	Role in Health Promotion and Maintenance	Role in Healing
Carbohydrates	Provide a source of energy (from glucose), fiber, and vitamins A factor in the construction of organs and nerve cells, as well as the control of body weight	Energy source Protective: a balanced intake of carbohydrates prevents the body from using the protein tissue of the muscles as a source of energy (glucose); prevents the breaking down of muscles for fuel Lack of sufficient carbohydrates can lead to malnutrition and the body's abnormal use of proteins for fuel
Proteins	Necessary for growth and as a source of strength and energy; carry oxygen in the blood	Produce antibodies and enhance the immune system Repair body tissue and cells, especially the muscles and the vital organs Support maternal tissue and the production of milk postpartum Insufficient levels of proteins can lead to an inability to build new tissues, as well to disorders such as anemia; the body also becomes more vulnerable to infection
Lipids	Facilitate the absorption and transportation in the intestines of vitamins A, D, E, and K Cushion and protect the heart, kidneys, and liver Insulate the body from cold Prevent heat loss through the skin	Protection: the storage of lipids in the body is a natural protective function when the body senses or anticipates a state of starvation An insufficient supply of lipids can cause the body to search for and use proteins as a fuel source
Water	Released as sweat to maintain body temperature as sweat evaporates, it cools the skin Lubricates the joints and the eyes Forms the basis of amniotic fluid to protect a growing fetus (see Chapter 8)	Role in maintenance of pH balance: if the balance is too acidic or alkaline, cells can die When the pH balance is acidic, the body cannot absorb the vitamins and minerals that are essential to health and healing When the pH balance is more alkaline, oxygen intake and distribution are enhanced, which contributes to an enhanced immune system and better healing outcomes

Protein is a naturally occurring compound of amino acids (see Chapters 8 and 9). Proteins are actually chains or **polymers**. Each link of the chain is an amino acid. There are 22 amino acids, 8 of which are *essential.* This means they cannot be made outside of the body. The others are obtained through diet. Proteins are present throughout the body.

Lipids are molecules that consist of fats, oils, and waxes. They are **insoluble** (i.e., they do not dissolve or break down) in water, and they are derived from plants and animals. Lipids provide more energy for the body than carbohydrates and proteins do, and they are essential components of cell membranes. The lipid cholesterol is a major component of cell membranes (see "Focus Point: Cholesterol" in Chapter 9).

The combining form of *lipid* is *lip/o.*

Water is an essential nutrient. Its chemical structure of two parts hydrogen and one part oxygen (H_2O) affects the natural pH balance of the body (see Chapter 5). Water is also a natural solvent for other nutrients, and it provides the means of delivery of these nutrients throughout the body.

The Greek root for forming words related to water is *hydro.*

Water is a key element in *sweat,* which is secreted by the integumentary system onto the surface of the skin. The formation of sweat is called *hidropoiesis.* (*Hidro* means *sweat,* and *poiesis* means *formation.*)

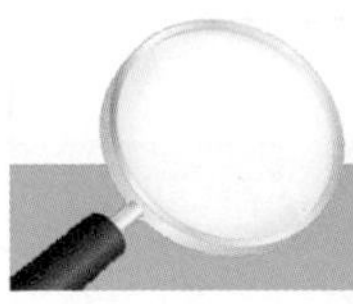

FOCUS POINT: Sweat

The medical term for sweating is *hidrosis.* The combining forms for words relating to sweat are *hidr/o-* and *sudor/o.* Excessive sweating may be referred to as *hyperhidrosis, sudoresis,* or, more commonly, *diaphoresis. Diaphoresis* is the term that is used in particular reference to the process of sweating that occurs as a result of fever. An antiperspirant is more technically known as an *antisudorific.*

Vitamins are essential substances that promote growth, development, and normal cell function in the body. They also boost the immune system. Vitamins are *organic,* which means that they originate in plants or animals. There are two main categories of vitamins: fat soluble and water soluble. There are 13 essential vitamins, and each one has its own distinct functions (see Table 11-5).

Minerals are *inorganic* compounds from soil and water that are eaten or absorbed by plants and animals. They are essential to growth and development, and they are constituents of the cells and bones. Minerals play key roles in regulating the permeability of the cell membranes and the capillaries, allowing muscle contraction, and facilitating the metabolism of water to regulate blood volume. There six minerals that are essential for human life: calcium, iron, magnesium, phosphorus, potassium, and zinc (see Table 11-6).

TABLE 11-5: Functions of Essential Vitamins

Essential Vitamin	Function
A (retinol)	facilitates the formation and maintenance of the teeth, bones, cell membranes, and skin
B_1 (thiamine)	facilitates the changing of carbohydrates into energy
B_2 (riboflavin)	assists with the growth of the body and in the production of red blood cells
B_3 (niacin)	assists with maintaining or restoring healthy skin and nerve cells and with the lowering of cholesterol levels
B_6 (pyridoxine)	responds to proteins and facilitates their metabolism; participates in the development of red blood cells and the maintenance of brain function
B_{12} (cobalamin)	assists with the maintenance of the central nervous system; facilitates metabolism and the formation of red blood cells
C (ascorbic acid)	promotes the health of the gums and teeth; facilitates the absorption of iron; promotes wound healing
D (calciferol)	promotes the absorption of calcium for teeth and bones; assists with the maintenance of calcium and phosphorus
E (tocopherol)	participates in the formation of red blood cells; facilitates the use of vitamin K; promotes wound healing
biotin	participates in the production of hormones and cholesterol; metabolizes carbohydrates and proteins
folate	essential to the development of DNA (genetic material) related to cell function and tissue development; cooperates with vitamin B_{12} to create red blood cells
pantothenic acid	metabolizes food; assists with the production of hormones and cholesterol
K	Special Note: Vitamin K is not always listed as an essential vitamin, but it is essential to the coagulation (thickening and clotting) of blood, and it is implicated in the promotion of bone strength among elderly patients.

TABLE 11-6: Functions of Essential Minerals

Essential Mineral	Function
calcium	facilitates the development of strong bones and teeth
iron	enables the hemoglobin of red blood cells to carry oxygen
magnesium	facilitates muscle and nerve function; maintains regular heart rhythm; contributes to bone strength
phosphorus	participates in metabolism and digestion as well as the formation of teeth and bones
potassium	assists with neurological function; regulates water balance in the blood and tissues
zinc	contributes to normal growth and development, enhances the immune system, and promotes wound healing; when used topically (on the skin), it provides protection to the skin from the rays of the sun

Let's Practice

Review the material about nutrition and nutrients, including Tables 11-4, 11-5, and 11-6, and then write the definition of each term given here.

1. vitamin ____________________
2. saccharide ____________________
3. compromised ____________________
4. polymer ____________________
5. ascorbic acid ____________________

Mix and Match

Match each term with its definition.

1. ascorbic acid	assists with muscles, nerves, and heart rhythm
2. water	causes a cooling effect on the skin
3. magnesium	promotes the health of the gums and teeth
4. lipids	strengthens the teeth and bones
5. calcium	provide a cushion for some major organs

Build a Word

Use each set of word parts to create a new term, and then define each term. You have studied these word parts in this and previous chapters.

1. -ation hydro- ____________________ Meaning: ____________________
2. phagi/a/o dys ____________________ Meaning: ____________________
3. -gen adipo -ci ____________________ Meaning: ____________________
4. suction lipo ____________________ Meaning: ____________________
5. -tic hidr/o- ____________________ Meaning: ____________________

Let's Practice

Write the common name of the vitamin that is identified by each term below.

1. thiamine ____________________
2. tocopherol ____________________
3. ascorbic acid ____________________
4. pyridoxine ____________________
5. retinol ____________________

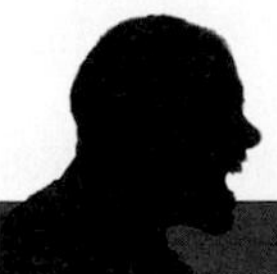

PRONUNCIATION PRACTICE

Say these words aloud to a friend or classmate if you can. You are given the phonetic pronunciation. Your instructor can help you with pronunciation,

or visit **http://www.MedicalLanguageLab.com.** 

appendectomy	ăp″ĕn-**dĕk**′tō-mē	lactose	**lăk**′tōs
cholesterol	kō-**lĕs**′tĕr-ŏl	parenteral	păr-**ĕn**′tĕr-ăl
commode	kŏ-**mōd**′	pyridoxine	pĭ-rĭ-**dŏks**′ēn
diaphoresis	dī″ă-fō-**rē**′sĭs	retinol	**rĕt**′ĭ-nŏl
enteral	**ĕn**′tĕr-ăl	stoma	**stō**′mă
enzyme	**ĕn**′zīm	thiamine	**thī**′ă-mĭn
hidropoiesis	hī″drō-poy-**ē**′sĭs	tocopherol	tō-**kŏf**′ĕr-ŏl
lipid	**lĭp**′ĭd		

Patient Update

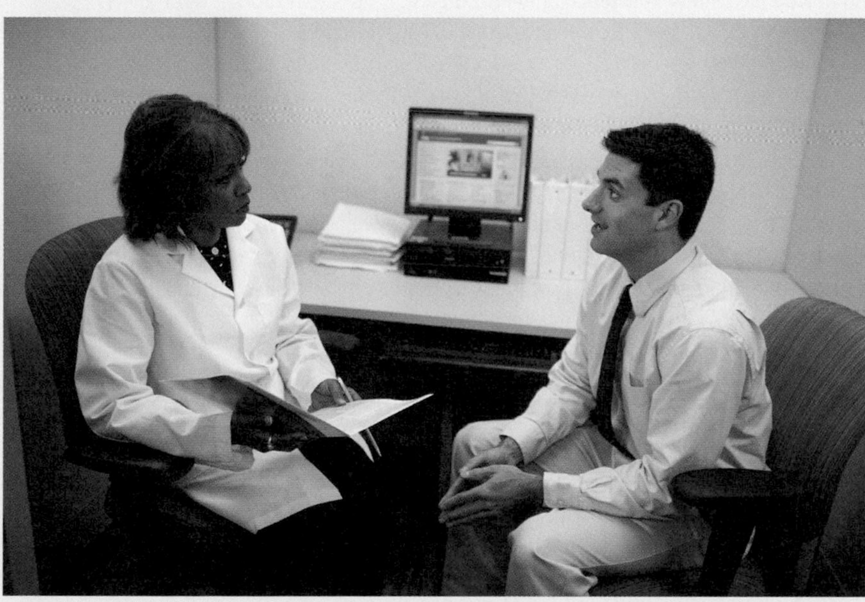

The dietician, Takeisha Cameron, is meeting with her colleague, speech pathologist Simon Rosenblum, early in the morning just after meeting with the Davises. Takeisha and Simon have come together to discuss the nutritional treatment plan for Clay Davis.

"Hi, Simon, good to see you," said Takeisha, as her colleague walked into the meeting room in the pediatrics unit.

"Hey, Takeisha, good to see you, too," said Simon, as he pulled up a chair beside her at the table. "I see we have a child with a recent repair of a symphyseal. Have you seen him yet this morning?" The dietician nodded and explained that she'd also done some preliminary teaching with his parents.

"Excellent. I'll go see them, too, in a few minutes, or you could come see them with me, if you like. Then they could see that we're a team. What do you think?"

"Well, I'd love to do that, and normally I would," Takeisha responded, "but today I am just swamped. You don't mind seeing them on your own, do you?"

"No, of course not, not at all," Simon said collegially, and he smiled. "I know how it goes around here. Sometimes we're so busy, and then it's suddenly quiet for a few days." They both laughed. "All right, so, our young man is going to be fed by NG for awhile, and that tube is in place, right?" Simon began. Takeisha nodded and confirmed that the NG tube had been placed during the final minutes of Clay's surgery, before the child went into PAR. "We'll need to set a schedule for feeding. Standard times, I suppose. That's pretty basic until he is allowed anything by mouth. I can't really see that you'll need me much until then?" the speech pathologist asked.

"Correct, but I wanted to set that up with you right now. Clay Davis will, we hope, be able to start on a liquid diet in about 6 or 7 days. I know the unit clerk will alert you to when that's going to be done, after Dr. Lincoln lets her know. The nurses and I will teach the family how to manage the NG tube and feedings in the interim, but I'd like to confirm an entire nutritional treatment plan with them prior to discharge." Takeisha paused a moment. "So, as you know, in cases of jaw fractures like this, the patient is to have nothing solid by mouth for 2 to 3 weeks, and we begin with a liquid diet of clear and then thickened fluids."

"Yes, that's where I come in for sure," said Simon. "I'll need to see the child when he has his NG tube removed and is assessed during follow-up by Dr. Lincoln. I'll be there for that, and I'll assess the condition of his oral cavity. I'll need to be absolutely sure that he can move a bolus of liquid food along the midline furrow of his tongue toward his pharynx. To do this, he'll need to be able to move the tongue muscle in an upward and downward motion against the hard palate. I'll want to see that. Next, it will be critical to assess whether or not he can swallow and if his gag reflex is intact. By placing my hands gently on his throat, I'll be able to feel his ability to swallow and to feel the contractions of the circular muscles of the pharynx. I'll do all of that without putting anything into his mouth. When I'm sure that these mechanisms are functioning, I'll introduce just a very small amount of minced food into his mouth and observe what happens as he tries to swallow it." Simon paused for a minute. "Of course, this assessment of swallowing begins right now, here on the unit." Takeisha nodded in agreement. Simon continued, "Like you, I will be checking routinely on the patient's ability to swallow and on the status of his gag reflex. We both know that he will still be swallowing saliva and mucus, despite the presence of the NG tube."

"Yes, that's a crucial part of his care: assessment of swallowing and of the gag reflex," agreed Takeisha. "We'll be monitoring that frequently. We don't want to risk any complications of inflammation of the tongue and it impeding the airway, nor do we want to risk any chance of his choking on his natural secretions. We've also got the patient propped up in bed in a semi-Fowler's position to help prevent any risk of choking. The secretions are able to drain down the esophagus and not pool in the back of his throat." The speech pathologist concurred and added that, without a fully functioning epiglottis, there is also a risk for the aspiration of secretions into the lungs, thereby causing further medical complications.

"Okay," continued Simon. "I can appreciate that once the NG tube is removed and the patient is able to open his mouth a bit more than he can now that his jaw movement will be stiff and possibly painful for him. I'll help with that rehab. I'll speak with his parents then, too, so that they can participate with their son in getting his full range of motion back. We'll cross that bridge when the time comes."

Takeisha then confirmed the next stages of the process. "So, if he can swallow on his own, the next step will be to start him on clear fluids and then to progress to full fluids and so on, correct?" Simon nodded, and Takeisha continued. "I'll help the family to preplan the types of foods and fluids that are suitable for this and explain why those foods are appropriate. I want to get started on this ASAP so that the family has plenty of lead time to prepare." Again, Simon nodded his support. Simon and Takeisha each took notes and got out their cell phones to use the calendar functions. Together, they worked out target dates for changes in the patient's diet, and they developed a nutritional treatment plan.

"Where are you off to next, Simon?" asked Takeisha.

"I've got a call for ICU for a patient with a post-op subdural hematoma. Apparently, he already had a concussion, and then he fell out of bed last night and received a secondary brain injury. He'll need a full assessment for swallowing and so on."

When they were done, both colleagues went to the nursing station to discuss the plan with the nursing team and to document it in their patient's medical records. (See "On the Job: A Dietician's Charting" on page 481.)

Reflective Questions

Consider what you've just read to answer the following questions.

1. Why does the dietician want to confer with the speech pathologist?

____

2. What type of foods will Clay be able to eat after the NG tube is removed?

____

3. Which anatomical structures require close assessment before allowing this patient to try to ingest anything by mouth? _______________

Right Word or Wrong Word: *Dietician* or *Nutritionist*?

Is there a difference between a dietician and a nutritionist? Are the two titles synonymous?

Critical Thinking

Keep in mind what you've just read, and answer the following questions.

1. Why is Clay Davis at risk for choking right now, even though he's not taking in anything by mouth? _______________
2. Who is the speech pathologist going to see next? Name the patient.

____

Date/time	Dietician's notes
June XX 10 am	First visit with 7-yr-old male patient with potential for daily imbalance and inadequate nutrient intake related to repair of mandibular fracture and insertion of NG tube. Also suffering from second-degree burn (scald) to upper chest area, left side. PLAN: due to age and medical status, will require enteral feeding six times per day with possible supplements of vitamin-enhanced liquid to promote bone and skin healing and sustain normal growth and development. Ensure head of bed is elevated during feeding. Use pediatric enteral formula XXX for a concentration of 1900 calories in 24 hours. Use gravity assist delivery over a 30-60 minute period. Flush tubing with 30 mL normal tap water at room temperature pre- and post feed as per doctor's orders. Nurses are aware of dietary plans. Nurses will feed, monitor intake and output, and assess patient responses. Dietary to visit once per shift to assess progress. ——— T. Cameron, RD

Key terms: nutritional treatment plan

Study the following terms and phrases to ensure your complete understanding of what you've just read.

"... to set a *schedule for feeding.*"

schedule for feeding: just as with normal eating, maintaining feeding routines is important to a patient's sense of physical and mental well-being. In this case, Clay has grown up with set meal times, and his body and his mind will prepare for these. Scheduling feedings helps to decrease any anxiety that the patient may have about being fed and any hunger that he or she may begin to experience.

"*Standard times,* I suppose."

standard times: tube feeding is generally performed every 4 to 6 hours throughout the waking day.

"... on a *liquid diet* ..."

liquid diet: a diet of fluids only.

"... *manage* the NG tube and feedings ..."

manage: medical jargon meaning *to adequately perform a task.*

"... *nutritional treatment plan* ..."

nutritional treatment plan: a detailed plan of action to provide nutrition that is relevant to the patient's medical condition, needs, and desires.

"... move a *bolus* of *liquid food* ..."

bolus: a small, round, soft mass; liquid entering the esophagus has the potential to form a bolus in the throat if the patient's swallowing mechanisms are not working properly and if too much fluid enters the throat at the same time.

liquid food: food that has been liquefied, such as broth and clear fruit juices.

"... along the *midline furrow of his tongue* ..."

midline furrow of his tongue: a longitudinal furrow or crease down the center of the tongue that is slightly depressed or lower than the rest of the tongue. The midline furrow is able to hold foods sufficiently so that the tongue can wrap itself around the materials and move them around in the mouth.

"... against the *hard palate.*"

hard palate: roof of the mouth (see Chapter 6).

"... he can *swallow* ..."

swallow: to pass ingested material from the mouth to the esophagus; swallowing is also known as **deglutition**.

"... if his *gag reflex* is *intact.*"

gag reflex: an automatic response to the presence of matter touching the soft palate at the back of the mouth, this reflex is not under voluntary control. Triggering (stimulating) the gag reflex can cause retching and lead to vomiting. It is technically referred to as the **pharyngeal reflex**.

intact: whole; not compromised; fully functioning.

"... these *mechanisms* ..."

mechanisms: processes.

"... on the *status* of his gag reflex."

status: condition.

"... chance of his *choking* ..."

choking: a blocking of the airways to the lungs.

"... not *pool* in the back of his throat."

pool: collect.

"... a *fully functioning epiglottis* ..."

fully functioning epiglottis: medical language that, in this context, refers to the ability of the epiglottis to serve its purpose of distinguishing between solids and liquids that should be directed down the esophagus to the stomach versus air. The epiglottis remains closed when there is an intake or expulsion of air to or from the lungs; it opens for other substances.

"... for the *aspiration* of secretions into the lungs ..."

aspiration: a situation in which a foreign material or substance has been sucked or drawn into the lungs.

"I'll help with that *rehab.*"

rehab: rehabilitation.

"... get started on this *ASAP*..."

ASAP: as soon as possible.

"... plenty of *lead time*..."

lead time: time before an event during which to prepare.

"I've *got a call for* ICU..."

got a call for: medical jargon meaning that another unit has requested a visit from a health professional for one of its patients. In this case, the request is from the ICU for the speech pathologist to come and assess a patient.

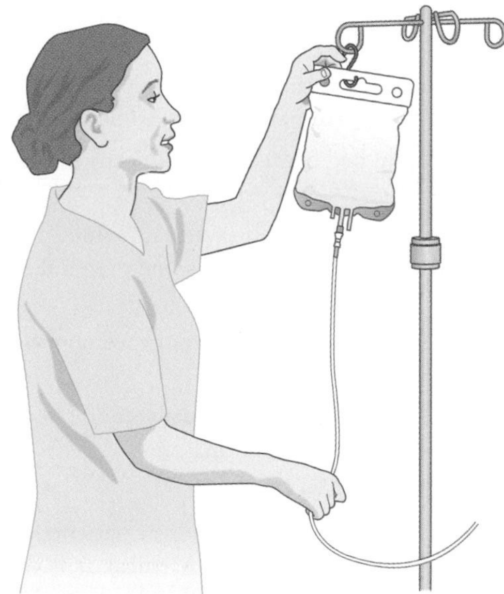

Figure 11.17: Delivery of enteral nutrition by gravity

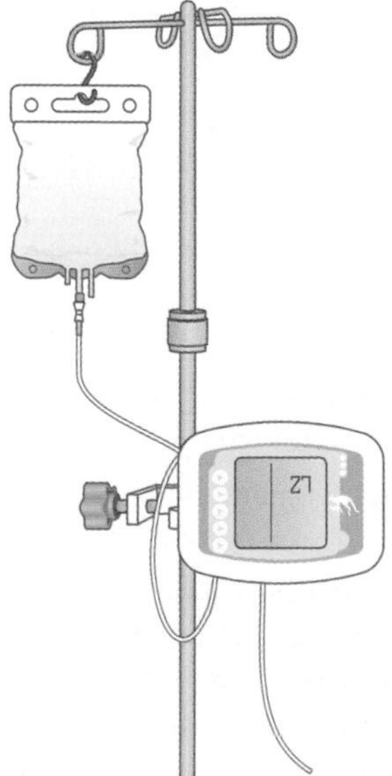

Figure 11.18: Delivery of enteral nutrition by pump

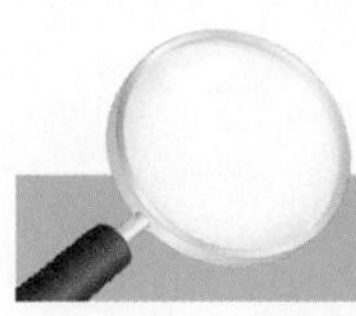

FOCUS POINT: "Swallowing Your Tongue"

It is impossible to actually swallow your tongue. The expression "swallowing your tongue" refers to the possibility of the tongue slipping back into the opening of the pharynx, where it may block the airway. This may occur when the tongue muscle relaxes to the extreme (i.e., in the case of unconsciousness) and slips back in the mouth, thus impeding or completely restricting the airway. In simpler terms, it blocks breathing and can cause death. Patients who are at risk for "swallowing their tongues" are placed on their sides or in Fowler's or semi-Fowler's positions in bed; see Chapter 2 for illustrations of these positions.

Let's Practice

Use the new vocabulary that you have learned to complete these sentences.

1. In a hospital or another care facility, the dietician may supervise all ______________ ______________ ______________ for patients and residents.
2. Clay Davis has been propped up in bed because his epiglottis is not yet ______________ ______________.
3. When a person starts to choke and sputter and says that "something went down the wrong pipe," they mean that they have ______________ some material into the trachea or the lungs.
4. The ______________ or process of chewing requires movement of the jaw and tongue and the use of the teeth.
5. The ______________ ______________ is not under voluntary control; it is a protective mechanism to prevent the swallowing of certain materials.

Medical diets

Medical diets are designed to meet the nutritional needs of patients with health challenges. This process is sometimes referred to as *medical diet therapy.* Medical diets vary on the basis of the needs of the individual client. They must be prescribed by a qualified health care professional, who is usually (but not always) a physician in consultation with a dietician or another nutritional expert. There are several commonly prescribed types of medical diets:

Restricted diets: those diets that restrict the daily intake of calories or that eliminate certain foods from the general diet. A vegetarian diet is a restricted diet.

Progressive diets: those diets in which the patient is gradually allowed more and more variety in the diet as he or she can tolerate it. At each stage, the person's ability to ingest and digest is evaluated.

Enteral and parenteral formulas: Although these are not generally referred to as *diets,* parenteral and enteral nutrition employ highly specific formulas to meet the nutritional needs of each individual client. Examples include the following:

Complete or standard formulas are designed for patients with normal digestion. These formulas include proteins, lipids, carbohydrates, vitamins, and minerals.

Elemental formulas include predigested matter and are designed for people who have little or no ability to digest.

Home-prepared formulas are made with the use of a blender. Because they are made at home, they may lack adequate nutrition from time to time, so supplements may be necessary. They may also vary in consistency from one feeding to another. They are generally administered only through gastrostomy tube, because they may clog NG tubes.

Modular formulas contain specific nutrients that may, from time to time, be added to home-prepared formulas to enhance nutrition.

Specialized formulas can be created for individuals with highly specific nutritional needs and health conditions. For example, because Clay Davis is lactose intolerant, each tube feed that he receives will have to be screened to ensure that there are no products in it that contain lactose.

Parenteral formulas (parenteral solutions) bypass the digestive system and provide nutrition directly into the bloodstream. These formulas can provide up to 2000 calories per day for an adult, and more than half of these calories are provided by lipids. Parenteral solutions also contain proteins, electrolytes, vitamins, and minerals. Carbohydrates, particularly dextrose (a sugar), provide energy.

Diets by consistency

In the Patient Update, the dietician and speech therapist talked about the consistency of the foods that their patient will be able to have as he recovers. Table 11-7 explains the types of diets that are prescribed for patients who cannot chew or swallow. Study this table in preparation for some exercises.

TABLE 11-7: Consistency and Medical Diets

Consistency and Type of Medical Diet	Description and Rationale
Clear fluids	consists of transparent liquids only; designed to keep the stomach and intestines clear of undigested residue
Full fluids	consists of fluids and foods that are normally found in liquid form or that turn to liquid at room temperature; designed for easy digestion, especially pre- or post-operatively or in preparation for medical diagnostics or other procedures
Soft diet	a transition diet from fluids toward the eating of solid food; designed for post-operative care and recovery from illnesses
Thickened fluids	a form of modified-texture diet that is used to prevent the patient from swallowing too quickly; designed for people with swallowing difficulties (dysphagia)
Minced or mashed diet	all food is minced (finely chopped), mashed, or pureed; designed for persons who have difficulty chewing and swallowing and who are at risk for choking on solids
Modified texture diet	consists of foods that are minced, mashed, pureed, and liquid; designed to assist with chewing and swallowing development or rehabilitation, by providing variety in the mouth that the client must learn to discern and process

Let's Practice

Name each type of medical diet described below.

1. slows the habit of swallowing in rapid succession to avoid the risk of choking or aspiration

   ____

2. given via NG tube to patients who are not able to digest completely or at all

   ____

3. designed to keep the stomach and the bowels free of waste matter preoperatively

   ____

4. designed to supplement nutritional intake while bypassing the digestive tract

   ____

Diets by medical condition

Table 11-8 identifies a number of medical diets that are designed to enhance the nutrition and health of patients or clients with specific medical conditions. Many of these diets are self-explanatory. Study this table in preparation for an exercise.

TABLE 11-8: Types of Medical Diets

Types of Medical Diets	Features
Lactose free	removes foods and beverages that contain lactose
Diabetic	high in dietary fiber; controlling the intake of sugars and carbohydrates
Gluten free	removes foods that contain gluten, such as wheat, barley, rye, and malt
Restricted fiber (low fiber)	limits the intake of fiber foods that can cause the blockage of the large intestine when it is susceptible to irritation and disease
High fiber	includes foods that are high in fiber, which softens and gives bulk to stool (feces), thus promoting bowel movements
Exclusion (elimination)	removes certain foods or food groups from the diet
Allergen free	removes identified food allergens from the diet
Bland	a diet that includes foods that are not irritating to the stomach
Cardiac	reduces the intake of saturated fats, red meats, eggs, and dairy products to reduce levels of "bad cholesterol" and to maintain a healthy weight
High calorie	ensures a sufficient calorie intake to provide energy and other nutrients in the presence of illness or physical fragility
Low calorie	used for weight reduction
High protein	indicated for patients with protein loss as a result of illness or disease
Low residue, surgical soft	prevents constipation or the accumulation of bulk waste products in the intestines; important for patients who have had abdominal surgery
BRAT: bananas, rice, applesauce, and toast	a type of elimination diet that is used to assess for food allergens: it is followed for a short period and then, one by one, other foods are introduced and the response to them is assessed; this simple diet is also used for children and some adults who are recovering from diarrhea
Low sodium	restricts the amount of sodium intake daily; important for patients with kidney, heart, and liver disease

Critical Thinking Questions

Recall the patients that you have been working with in this textbook. Review the information about the different types of medical diets, and then identify which diet or diets you think will be appropriate for each patient.

1. Gilbert Loeppky ____________________
2. Stevie-Rose Davis ____________________
3. Zane Davis ____________________
4. Clay Davis ____________________
5. Baby Emily Grace Loeppky ____________________
6. Glory Loeppky ____________________

Mix and Match

Match the description with the type of medical diet.

1. BRAT	restricts or eliminates spices and other irritants
2. High fiber	controls the levels of glucose and carbohydrate intake
3. Low sodium	for patients with liver, kidney, or heart disease
4. Diabetic	eliminates possible sources of food allergies
5. Bland	promotes bowel elimination

Right Word or Wrong Word: *Dysphagia* or *Dysphasia*?

Look carefully at these two words. Do they have the same meaning? Are they pronounced the same?

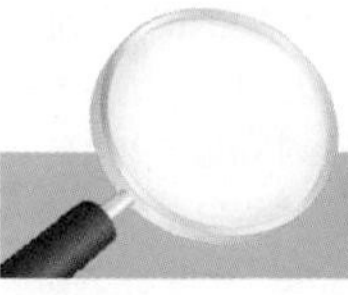

FOCUS POINT: The Fractured Jaw Diet

The term *fractured jaw diet* is medical jargon. The foods included in this diet do not require chewing. Patients like Clay Davis will be started on this type of diet as soon as it is possible for them to move liquids or pureed foods past the teeth and into the mouth. At that time, the patient will continue to have small feedings six to eight times per day. Because it is difficult or impossible for such patients to open their mouths very wide, it is extremely important that the temperatures of the foods that are ingested be monitored to prevent a sudden spontaneous response to substances that are too hot or too cold. This response would require opening the mouth too wide to gasp or spit out the food.

PRONUNCIATION PRACTICE

Say these words aloud to a friend or classmate if you can. You are given the phonetic pronunciation. Your instructor can help you with pronunciation, or visit **http://www.MedicalLanguageLab.com.**

aspirate	**ăs**´pĭ-rāt
aspiration	ăs-pĭ-**rā**´shŭn
dysphagia	dĭs-**fā**´jē-ă
dysarthria	dĭs-**ăr**´thrē-ă
dextrose	**dĕks**´trōs
gluten	**gloot**´ĕn
gastrostomy	găs-**trŏs**´tō-mē

The Language of Pain

Patient Update

Pediatric patient Clay Davis is awake and in the company of his parents. Nurse Miranda has been in to see them all. She assessed Clay's ability to swallow, checked his NG and IV tubing to ensure they were patent (open and unobstructed), and took his vital signs. She spoke directly to Clay about his situation, and she reassured the little boy that he was safe and that the team was looking out for him. Nurse Miranda then gave Clay a pencil and paper and pulled the bedside table up in front of him, over the bed. She talked to him about writing down anything that he wanted to say on the paper and cautioned him to try not to speak for a couple of days yet. She also talked to him about pain and pain management in terms that a child could understand. Clay rated his pain as a 4 on a pain-scale diagram that she put in front of him. Miranda nodded and then turned to speak to Clay's parents.

"Clay is indicating that he has some pain but that it is manageable at the moment," Nurse Miranda said. "We are giving him analgesics to keep the pain as minimal as possible. He gets that through his IV line routinely, but if he has any breakthrough pain, we want to know so that we can give him a little something extra for that. It is most important that his discomfort is limited, and we are proactive about this. You can rest assured of that," she said, looking directly at both parents, one by one. Miranda showed Clay's parents the diagram of the pain scale that she'd given Clay and explained how they might use it with their son. "Mr. and Mrs. Davis, you know your son's mannerisms best, and if you think at any time that he is showing signs of increasing pain and discomfort, I want you to come and let one of us know at the nurses' desk," she invited. They assured her that they would. Miranda continued: "I'd like to teach you a little bit about something that we call the FLACC scale. We use this as a pain assessment with children who are unable to speak to us. Even though Clay can open his mouth just ever so slightly, he may hesitate to do so. Using a pain scale like this can help us all to care for him in the best way possible. I'd like you both to use it, too." She paused for their reply, and, when they agreed, she taught them how to assess behavioral cues in Clay's facial expressions, leg movements, cries, and ability to be consoled. She provided examples of each and then asked Clay's parents to summarize what they had learned.

"Thank you, Miranda, that's very helpful," said Steve Davis, and they all turned their attention to Clay once again. He had begun to moan.

Critical Reflection Questions

Consider what you've just read in this most recent Patient Update to answer the following questions.

1. What is the name of the nurse who is attending Clay? ____________________
2. What does the nurse want Clay's parents to help her with?

   ____
3. How does Miranda evaluate Clay's pain? ____________________

Key terms: pain management

Key terms from the Patient Update are italicized in the example and highlighted below with the explanation.

"... a *pain-scale diagram* ..."

pain-scale diagram: a cartoon-like depiction of pain rated from 1 (very bad and intolerable) to 10 (not evident or not discomforting). In pediatric care, diagrams, colors, puppets, and dolls are often used to communicate with children who have limited vocabulary, who have difficulty with speech, or who are unable to speak (see Figure 11-19).

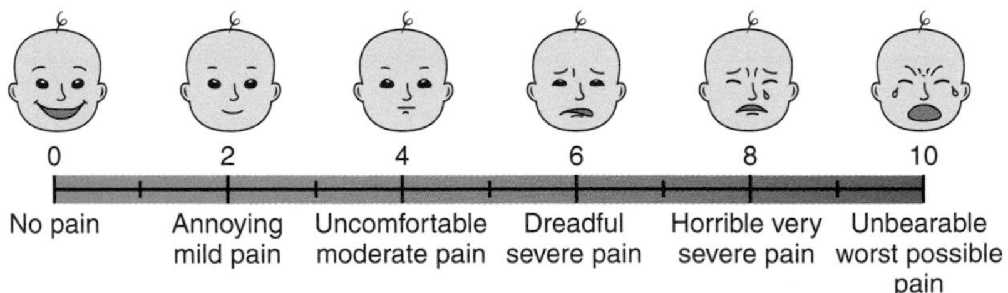

Figure 11.19: A pediatric pain scale

"... has any *breakthrough pain* ..."

breakthrough pain: pain that breaks through the barrier imposed by analgesic medication or other pain-reducing and pain-numbing treatments. This is usually a sign that the medication or treatment is wearing off.

"... at the *nurses' desk* ..."

nurses' desk: medical jargon that refers to the nursing station or the desk area where nurses and other health and allied health professionals gather to work and communicate about patients and their care.

"... something that we call the *FLACC* scale."

FLACC: a mnemonic for the elements of behavioral assessment related to a pain response in children: **F** = face, **L** = legs, **A** = activity, **C** = crying, and **C** = consolability. Each of these areas is given a score of 0, 1, or 2. Pain is rated by scoring each criterion, finding the total, and then multiplying it by 10. The higher the number, the more severe the pain (see Figure 11-20).

Categories	Scoring		
	0	1	2
Face	No particular expression or smile	Occasional grimace or frown, withdrawn, disinterested	Frequent to constant frown, quivering chin, clenched jaw
Legs	Normal position or relaxed	Uneasy, restless, tense	Kicking or legs drawn up
Activity	Lying quietly, normal position, moves easily	Squirming, shifting back and forth, tense	Arched, rigid, or jerking
Cry	No cry (awake or asleep)	Moans or whimpers; occasional complaint	Crying steadily, screams or sobs, frequent complaints
Consolability	Content, relaxed	Reassure by occasional touching, hugging, or being talked to; distractible	Difficult to console or comfort

Figure 11.20: FLACC pain scale (From Merkel SI, Voepel-Lewis T, Shayevitz JR, Malviya S: The FLACC: A behavioral scale for scoring postoperative pain in young children. *Pediatr Nurs* 1997;23(3):293-297.)

Critical Thinking Questions

Study the pain scales, and then answer the following questions.

1. The post-surgical child cannot be reassured or comforted by his mother. Which scale would be used to rate his pain? ______________________
2. Clay Davis moans from time to time and occasionally grimaces. Rate each of these signs on the FLACC scale. ______________________
3. A 5-year-old child circles this picture on a pediatric pain scale of 1 to 5. What does it mean, and to which number does it refer? ______________________

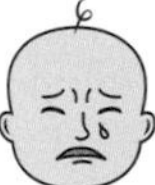

4. A 3-year-old child circles this picture on a pediatric pain scale of 1 to 10. What does this tell you? ______________________

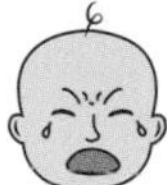

More Language of the Integumentary System

Patient Update

RN Miranda and the Davises were still with Clay when Dr. Lincoln arrived on his morning rounds. He shook Mr. Davis's hand, smiled at Mrs. Davis, and immediately moved forward so that he could stand close to Clay. The doctor then spoke directly to the patient.

"Hello, young man. It's very nice to see you awake." Dr. Lincoln smiled at the boy. "I'm your doctor, Dr. Lincoln. I'm going to be taking care of you while you're here with us in the hospital. Miranda, I and a whole crew are going to take very good care of you," he reassured the child. Clay moaned in response, with his eyes wide as if he wanted to speak. "It's all right," said Dr. Lincoln calmly and gently, "you don't need to talk right now. You've had some surgery on your mouth—your jaw, actually—and it's going to be hard for you to speak for a couple of days yet, but we're all here to help you get through this tough time. Your mom and dad have been here every minute with you, too." He smiled again and touched Clay gently on the hand. The child grasped Dr. Lincoln's hand tightly, as if for reassurance, and tears came to the boy's eyes. "I know, I know, it's pretty darn scary for you right now," said the doctor, "but it's going to get better. You have my word on that." He squeezed the boy's hand to reinforce the reassuring message.

Dr. Lincoln then turned to the nurse. "Miranda, what's the status of his NG tube? Have you been able to feed him through it yet?" The nurse confirmed that she had and that the child had tolerated the procedure well. The doctor then turned to Clay's parents and discussed the need for tube feeding for the rest of the week; he occasionally glanced at Clay to include the patient in the discussion.

"Clay, I'm going to take a look at that burn you have on your chest right now," announced Dr. Lincoln as he walked around to the left side of the bed and gently pulled back the covers. As he did so, he explained to the parents and the nurse, "This is a second-degree burn. It's quite common in children. The outer layer of the skin, the epidermis, has been damaged, and the burn—a scald from a hot liquid, in this case—has penetrated down into the next layer of tissue, the dermis. Our goals here in the hospital are to manage the pain and to prevent infection at the site."

Dr. Lincoln paused for a moment and waved the parents over to look at the burn. "You'll see here that your son has some blisters on his skin. They are all intact, and we will let these run their natural course right now. To open them runs the risk of inviting infection, so we'll avoid that. In the meantime, you'll see that the nurses are keeping the wound bed clean and dry by keeping it covered with a sterile gauze dressing that is lightly applied to the affected area." He nodded at Miranda to acknowledge this. "The dressing is kept quite loose to permit air to circulate across the wound. As the blisters begin to deteriorate, we'll gently apply some antibiotic cream to protect the exposed tissues."

"How long is this burn going to need treatment?" asked an anxious Mrs. Davis. "Will there be a scar?"

Dr. Lincoln explained that most scalds of this type begin to resolve after 24 to 48 hours and that they are fully resolved after 3 to 4 weeks if no complications occur. Scarring, if any, is expected to be quite minimal, and it should fade over time.

Mrs. Davis took her son's hand in hers and consoled him. "Did you hear that, honey? The doctor says your burn won't take long to heal." The child merely blinked at his mother, squeezed her hand tightly, and moaned. His swollen lips parted ever so slightly, and he whispered, "Momma."

"I know, I know, honey. This is all very painful, and I wish I could make it all go away for you. But I'm here, Daddy's here, and we're going to be right here for you every minute till you're better. And you're going to get better, mister, I promise you that!" Mrs. Davis spoke in a voice that sounded strong and confident. She reached over and stroked her son's hair gently. Clay watched her closely and began to relax under her soothing touch. Dr. Lincoln asked if the Davises had any more questions; he took his leave when they did not.

The nurse came to the bedside then and ran a hand quickly under the patient's bed sheets. "Mr. and Mrs. Davis, you'll have to excuse us for a minute. Clay's been incontinent of urine, and I'm going to ask the care aide to come and help me freshen him up. I wonder if you could step into the hallway while we do that so that we can have a little more room to work. They nodded and did as they were asked. Clay responded immediately by thrashing his legs a little and trying to call out "Momma." Mrs. Davis went back to him and reassured him that she and his dad would be just outside in the hallway for a few minutes while the nurse helped him with something. He relaxed again, feeling safe and assured of their proximity.

Out in the hallway, Mrs. Davis spoke to the nurse, again about something that was bothering her. "Miranda, this must just be awful for Clay to have to pee and poop in his bed. I just can't imagine how he must feel about this," she lamented.

"Yes, I know that is very embarrassing for most of our pediatric patients," she said gently. "The staff here try not to make anything of it and to treat it as just a routine part of our daily tasks. In that way, we don't embarrass or frustrate the child. You'll notice that I used the term *incontinent of urine* in his presence and mentioned freshening him up?" Mr. and Mrs. Davis nodded that they had. "Well, we do that for exactly that reason: it is unlikely that a child will know immediately what those words mean, and in that way we are able to prevent him from feeling embarrassed by a normal body function occurring in an unusual circumstance." The parents nodded and thanked her for this sensitivity and compassion. "This is only temporary, Mr. and Mrs. Davis. We hope to have him up onto a commode by tomorrow or the next day at the latest." Miranda left them to find a care aide to assist her.

Critical Reflection Questions

Consider what you've just read in this most recent Patient Update, and answer the following questions.

1. What is the status of Clay's burn blisters? ______________________________
2. What are the treatment goals for a second-degree burn? ____________________
3. Will Clay Davis have any scarring from the burn? _________________________
4. How long will Clay be unable to use the toilet? ___________________________

Anatomy and physiology: skin

In Chapter 6, you were introduced to the basic anatomy and physiology of the integumentary system. Our patient's skin—the outermost layers of the integumentary system—has been damaged. The epidermal and dermal layers of his skin were exposed to high temperatures when coffee spilled on him, and the protective functions of those layers was lost (see Chapter 6). Dr. Lincoln spoke to the Davises about the effects of the burn on the layers of Clay's skin tissue. He explained that the scald has left the child's underlying tissues vulnerable to infection from pathogens. Burns also leave patients at risk for fluid loss and imbalance.

Skin is *cutaneous* membrane. The skin provides insulation, acts as a sensory organ, and assists with thermoregulation (the temperature control of the body). It consists of the epidermis, the dermis, and the subcutaneous tissues. With a second-degree burn such as Clay's, the subcutaneous tissue remains unaffected.

The root of *cutaneous* is *cutis,* which is Latin for *skin.*

Recall that the epidermis is the outermost layer of the skin. It serves to protect the inner body, and it functions as the first line of defense against infection. It is responsible for fluid balance, and it prevents excessive fluid loss from the internal tissues. Under normal circumstances, the epidermis sloughs off and regenerates every 2 to 3 weeks.

The **dermis** is a thick layer of connective tissue just below the epidermis. It contains proteins, carbohydrates, plasma, blood vessels, and much more. The dermis provides flexibility for the skin and contains all of the elements that are needed to replicate and repair both itself and the epidermis. The dermis is also a conduit for the delivery of nutrients across the body. In young children and the elderly, the dermal layer of tissue is much thinner than that of adults. The dermis also regenerates itself (see Chapter 6).

In the case of a burn trauma, this cycle of skin regeneration is impaired. The deeper or larger a burn, the more likelihood that the skin will not regenerate as it should and that the skin may have to be replaced or repaired with surgery.

Blisters

Second-degree burns cause blistering of the skin. A **blister** is a bubble-like skin formation. The medical term for a blister is *vesicle* or a *bulla*. Burn blisters contain a serous fluid, and they are formed as part of the body's reaction to heat and nerve damage. These types of blisters should be left to heal on their own; breaking them open prematurely can lead to infection. The skin beneath the blister is raw and unprotected, so a protective sterile covering is advised for all stages of the blister.

Scars

Scars or scar tissue can occur in response to a trauma such as a burn, an injury, or a surgery. Their formation is part of the natural process of wound healing. **Scars** consist of fibrous tissue that replaces injured tissue, and they are initially red and swollen. Over time, scar tissue shrinks, and it may disappear almost entirely from view. Clay Davis has an old appendectomy scar on his abdomen that is still visible but that has healed. His mother now worries that he will have burn scars on his chest. If so, they will be minimal because his burn did not go deep into the muscles and the underlying tissues. The medical term for a scar is *cicatrix*; the plural form of this word is *cicatrices*.

Types of scars

Contracture scars: these scars are the result of burn injuries, when the healing skin tightens over the affected area. This new skin does not ever look quite like the surrounding skin. This over tightening of the skin over the wound bed can lead to restricted movements.

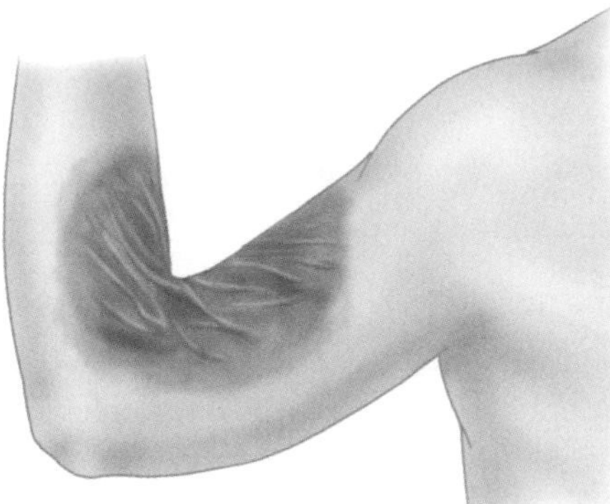

Figure 11.21: Contracture scar tissue

Keloid scars: these scars extend beyond the original injury. An overgrowth of fibrous tissue makes the scar look thicker, and it is raised from the surface of the skin.

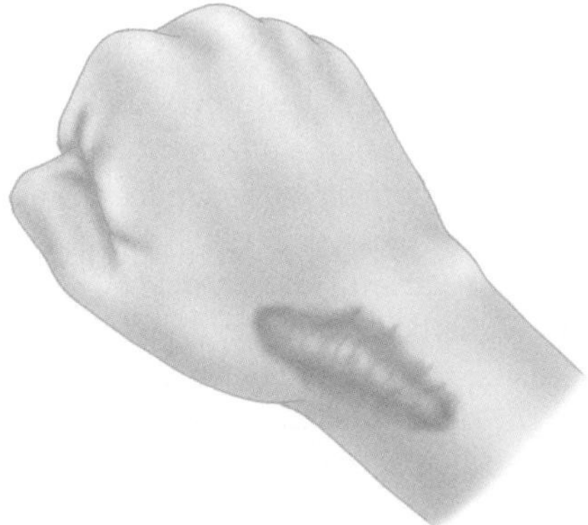

Figure 11.22: Keloid scar tissue

Hypertrophic scars: these raised, red scars are somewhat like keloid scars, but they do not go beyond the boundaries of the original injury, and they are not as thick and fibrous.

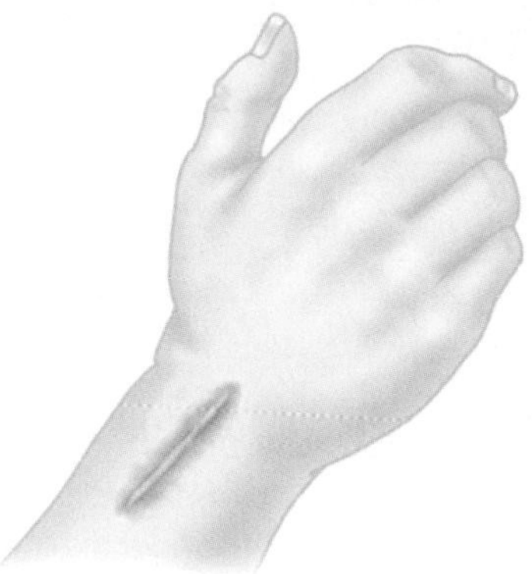

Figure 11.23: Hypertrophic scar tissue

Fill in the Blanks

Use vocabulary related to the integumentary system to fill in the blanks.

1. ____________ commonly occur as a result of a second-degree burn.
2. ____________ scars can occur after a severe burn that penetrates below the epidermis and the dermis.
3. Skin is a ____________ membrane.
4. The ____________ is vascular, and it facilitates the transport of nutrients.
5. Second-degree burn ____________ and ____________ should be covered with loose, sterile, gauze dressings.
6. When the ____________ is damaged or destroyed, the potential for infection increases significantly.
7. In the case of a burn, ____________ loss may occur rapidly when tissue is exposed to the air.
8. Skin ____________ itself every 2 to 3 weeks on average.

PRONUNCIATION PRACTICE

Say these words aloud to a friend or classmate if you can. You are given the phonetic pronunciation. Your instructor can help you with pronunciation, or visit **http://www.MedicalLanguageLab.com.**

cutaneous	kū-**tā**´nē-ŭs	contracture	kŏn-**trăk**´chūr
cicatrices	**sĭk**´ă-trĭks or sĭk-**ā**´-trĭks	keloid	**kē**´lŏyd
cicatrix	sĭk´ă-**trī**´sēz or sĭk**ā**´trĭsēz		

CHAPTER SUMMARY

Chapter 11 has introduced the language of the digestive system. Medical terms were explored that refer to the anatomy and physiology of the system, and medical language related to postsurgical nutrition and diet were highlighted as they were used in conversations between health professionals and the patient's family. The integumentary system was revisited to explore the language of skin, burn healing, scars, and blisters. Opportunities were provided to construct medical terms, use prefixes, and identify suffixes. Terminology was introduced and used in a patient-care context, and pediatric pain scales were introduced as well.

See How Much You've Learned

For audio exercises, visit **http://www.MedicalLanguageLab.com.** 

Chapter 11 has introduced you to some medical abbreviations. These have been organized into a study table here for quick reference. Some of them you will recognize immediately, and some will reappear throughout the following chapters with more explanation and application.

TABLE 11-9: Abbreviations

Abbreviation	Meaning	Abbreviation	Meaning
PAR	post-anesthetic recovery room	H_2O	water
TPN	total parenteral nutrition	NKO	no known allergies
NG	nasogastric	NPO	nothing by mouth

Key Terms

absorption
acute appendicitis
alimentrary
altered levels of consciousness
anesthetic
appendectomy
appendix
ASAP
aspiration
assisted feeding
bile
blister
bolus
breakthrough pain
carbohydrates
catalysts
catheter
cecum
choking
colon
commode
compromised
condylar region
deglutition
dermis
dietetics
digestion
dislocated
duodenum
elimination
enteral
extubation
feces
feeding tube
fixation
fixed
FLACC
gag reflex
gallbladder
hard palate
ileocecal valve
incisor
incontinence pad
ingestion
insoluble
intact
intestine
intubation
jaundice
jejunum
lactose
lactose intolerant
lead time
lipids
liquid diet
liver
mastication
maxillomandibular
mechanisms
minerals
nasogastric
nutrients
nutrition
nutritional status
pain-scale diagram
PAR
parenteral
peristalsis
pharyngeal reflex
polymers
pool
protein
rectum
rigid fixation
saccharides
scars
soluble
sphincters
status
stoma
stomach
surgically reduced
swallow
taste receptors
titanium mini-plates
tongue
total parenteral nutrition (TPN)
tract
vitamins
water
wires

CHAPTER REVIEW

Critical Thinking

Consider what you've learned in the Patient Updates and the rest of the chapter to answer the following question:

Why is a speech pathologist involved in Clay Davis's care?

____

What Do You Know?

Use medical terminology to answer these questions.

1. Where are the salty taste receptors located? ______________
2. What is the medical term for a scar? ______________
3. What is the purpose of the appendix? ______________
4. What substance or material is found within the colon? ______________
5. Which layer of skin contains nutrients? ______________
6. Where is the cecum located? ______________
7. What is the medical term for a blister? ______________
8. Which layer of the skin is the first line of defense against infection? ______________
9. What is the difference between enteral and parenteral nutrition? ______________
10. What is the name for the procedure of feeding through a tube that empties into the stomach or the intestines? ______________

Label the Diagram

Label the parts of the large intestine.

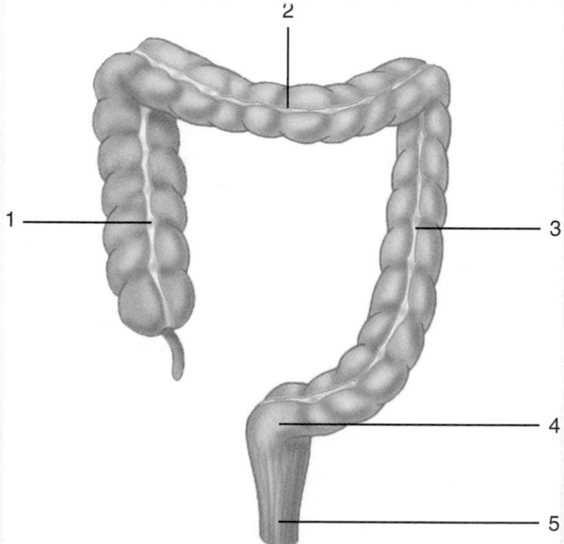

1. ______________
2. ______________
3. ______________
4. ______________
5. ______________

Right Word or Wrong Word: ***Milk Allergy*** **or** ***Lactose Intolerance*****?**

Is a milk allergy the same thing as lactose intolerance?

Mix and Match

Match the synonyms by drawing a line to connect them.

1. feces	water
2. colon	chain
3. enteron	ascorbic acid
4. polymer	large intestine
5. nutrient	nourishment
6. H_2O	colonoscopy
7. coloscopy	stool
8. vitamin C	intestines

Build a Word

Use each set of word parts given to create a proper medical term. These terms haven't actually appeared in this chapter, but many of their word parts have, and you have knowledge of the other word parts from previous chapters.

1. nutri mal- -tion ____________________
2. rrhag/i/a colon/o ____________________
3. patho derma/to logy ____________________
4. ur fecal -ia ____________________

True or False

Answer the following questions by choosing true or false.

1. Muscles can contract, but skin cannot. T___ F ___
2. Appendicitis is quite uncommon among children who are younger than 5 years old. T___ F ___
3. A symphyseal fracture is the same as a condylar fracture. T___ F ___
4. Scalds are not generally likely to cause long-lasting scars. T___ F ___
5. Parenteral nutrition is necessitated in the case of mandibular fixation. T___ F ___
6. A speech pathologist is also known as a *speech therapist.* T___ F ___
7. A medical diet does not require a prescription or a physician's approval. T___ F ___
8. The term *pediatric* refers to children. T___ F ___
9. *Gastrointestinal* and *digestive* are interchangeable names for the same system. T___ F ___
10. The gag reflex is under voluntary control. T___ F ___

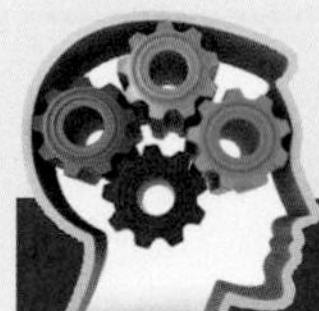

MEMORY MAGIC

Mnemonics are strategies that help you to remember important information. If you need to remember information about vitamins, try these three mnemonics.

1. Vitamins that are fat soluble (i.e., that dissolve in fat rather than water):

   That **FAT** cat is in the **ADEK**.

   (pronounced *attic*)

   FAT = fat soluble

   ADEK = vitamins A, D, E, and K

2. A different mnemonic for vitamins that are fat soluble:

   KADE

   Vitamins K, A, D, and E

3. The names of the B vitamins:

   The **r**hythm **n**early **p**roved **c**ontagious.

   T = thiamine (B_1)

   R = riboflavin (B_2)

   N = niacin (B_3)

   P = pyridoxine (B_6)

   C = cobalamin (B_{12})

CHAPTER TWELVE

Diagnoses and Medication Administration

Focus: Endocrine System: Diabetes and Post-Traumatic Stress Disorder

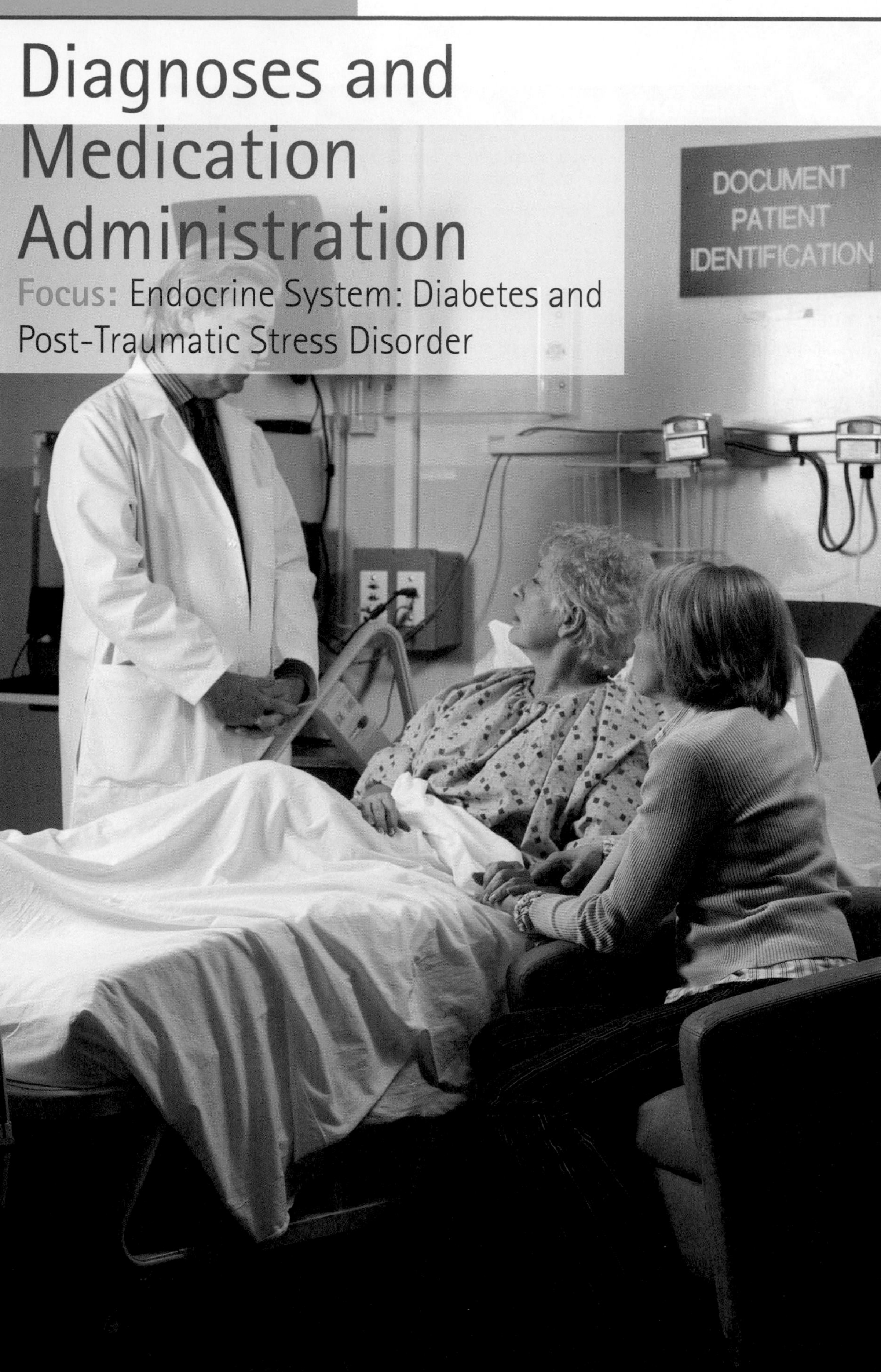

When we left Mrs. Stevie-Rose Davis in Chapter 7, she was struggling with some bouts of confusion. Specifically, she was not oriented to time and place. Dr. Jensen in the emergency room (ER) ordered a battery of tests to determine if the patient's state of confusion had a medical cause. As evening approached, Mrs. Davis's daughter Angie arrived and was able to remain with her mother until she settled down. The patient was kept in the ER overnight for further assessment. She was given PRN lorazepam (10 mg PO) at 2100 hours to promote relaxation and reduce symptoms of anxiety. This medication was effective, and its calming effect enabled the patient to sleep.

The patient was scheduled for blood glucose testing at 1900 and 2300 hours last night and again at 0600 hours this morning. Mrs. Davis was alert and oriented before she received sedation. Her neurovital signs were taken routinely until 2100 hours, when Dr. Jensen called in to assess the patient and discontinued these orders. He also ordered the nurses to do a urine dip for ketones on Mrs. Davis each time she voided and to continue with scheduled glucose testing with the use of a glucose monitor; the nurses have done so.

Dr. Jensen has arrived for his morning rounds. He has spoken with the nurses caring for Mrs. Davis, and he is aware that her glucose levels have been erratic since her admission. A pattern is emerging that concerns him, and he worries that the patient may no longer be able to manage her diabetes without medication. He is going to speak to Mrs. Davis about this, as well as about her lab work and her other assessment results.

Patient Update

"Good morning, Mrs. Davis," said Dr. Jensen as he entered her room. He noticed a family member at her side and nodded to her. "Do you remember me?" he asked the patient. She nodded and confirmed that she did by using his name. "And who is your guest, Mrs. Davis?"

"This is my daughter, Evangeline." Mrs. Davis smiled and waved her hand toward her daughter in a gesture of friendly introduction.

"Please call me Angie," came the equally pleasant response. "Everyone does, even my mother, from time to time," she laughed. "Pleased to meet you, Doctor . . . Doctor . . . ." She paused for a moment, awaiting the doctor's reply.

"Dr. Jensen," the physician added warmly. "Now, Mrs. Davis, how was your night? Were you able to get any sleep?" The patient reported that she had and was aware that he had ordered her sedation to help with that. The patient also explained that she'd gotten out of bed to void at least five times during the night and that she had felt quite dizzy and unsure of herself at those times. She also noticed how thirsty she felt and wondered if that was from the medication he'd prescribed. The doctor listened attentively.

"Mrs. Davis, it seems that you are quite clearheaded this morning. You have just given me a very clear account of your activities overnight, you're able to recall my name, and you remember that you were given some mediation to promote sleep." The patient nodded. "When we admitted you yesterday, you had some bouts of confusion. Do you recall any of that?"

"Vaguely," she replied. "I remember that I was in an accident with Zane and Clay. We were bringing Clay to the hospital because of a scald. My daughter says that Clay's at Okla Trauma Center and that he may have a broken jaw!" She paused for a moment. "And my husband has been released home. But Angie told me all of that stuff. While I was here in the ER, though, well, I have to admit it was kind of a blur for awhile, although I do remember speaking to a nurse who did some sort of mental or psychiatric assessment on me, I think." Dr. Jensen nodded in affirmation. "What was that all about?"

"You did incur a mild concussion in that car accident yesterday, and we wondered for awhile if that was causing your confusion," said Dr. Jensen. "Because of your concussion, I asked the nurses to monitor your mental and neurological status until around 9 p.m. But what I'm really referring to is something else that happed. There was an incident last evening where you were disoriented to time, place, and person. Do you recall that?"

"Not really," said Mrs. Davis, looking at her daughter and then back to the physician. "What did I do?"

"You thought that you were a nurse in a combat zone who was about to receive casualties. You wanted to organize a couple of the staff to prepare for that." Dr. Jensen paused and watched Mrs. Davis's response to this information. Her eyes widened, and she gasped slightly. "What can you tell me about that, Mrs. Davis?" he inquired gently. She explained then that she had been a military nurse serving in Vietnam years ago, and she quickly rationalized that she must have been dreaming or sleepwalking.

"Mrs. Davis, I am quite concerned that you may be experiencing the effects of post-traumatic stress disorder from your days in the military and from any traumatic events that may have occurred in Vietnam. Have you sought any counseling for that?" Dr. Jensen noticed that Angie suddenly sat straight up in her chair and was very alert.

Mrs. Davis scowled at him. "I do not have anything mentally wrong with me," she said angrily. "I just have some bad memories, that's all. They come and go from time to time. I don't need any help. So let's drop that right now!" She crossed her arms across her chest. Her breath became audible, and her chest rose in anger. She also broke eye contact with the physician. Dr. Jensen stood in silence, waiting for the patient to calm herself.

"Mom," interjected Angie plaintively. "Mom, please hear the doctor out."

"Evangeline! We will not discuss this. Leave it be," commanded her mother. They sat in silence then for a moment.

"Well, Mrs. Davis, I can see how sensitive you are about this subject. This tells me that you are indeed bothered by some of your bad memories. However at this time, I can only offer you encouragement to seek some help, if you'd like—counseling or other therapies. You do not have to carry this trauma with you all of your life; there is a way to deal with it when you're ready," he said kindly. At that point, Mrs. Davis refused to look the doctor in the eyes. He waited another moment. "I wonder if you'd be willing to discuss the option of medication?" She looked up at him then, quite angrily. "Mrs. Davis, post-traumatic stress disorder can manifest many years after a trauma. Anti-depressant medications can relieve some of the symptoms that you might be experiencing."

"Like what? I don't need any medications like that," said Mrs. Davis. "I'm not crazy, and I'm not depressed. How dare you!" came her quick retort.

"PTSD is a disorder that is well researched and well treated. I wonder if you ever have difficulty falling asleep or staying asleep? Do you have problems with concentration?" Mrs. Davis did not reply. Angie leaned in even closer to the conversation and nodded in affirmation to the physician. Dr. Jensen noticed this and went on, "Perhaps you experience irritability or mood swings?" He paused and waited. No answer came from the patient.

"Mom . . .," encouraged Evangeline, as if pleading with her mother to accept the doctor's advice and counsel. Mrs. Davis shot her a withering look that told Angie she had better stop the conversation.

"All right, then, I can see that this is a conversation you are not ready to have," said Dr. Jensen. "Let's go on to other things." Angie sat back in her chair again and sighed. Mrs. Davis did not return the doctor's gaze.

"An x-ray ruled out any neurological injuries for you. That meant we could give you just a little bit of medication last evening, an anti-anxiety drug to help relax you. You were quite restless." He paused to let her think about this. "I ordered a rather wide battery of tests so that we could get a better picture of your condition."

Dr. Jensen continued: "The results of your lab tests are quite good." He explained that a glucose test had been done on admission, and it was determined that the patient was slightly hypoglycemic at the time. The team was able to remedy that in a short time, especially after they learned that she had type 2 diabetes. "We found out that you were taking ibuprofen and glucosamine. Since we weren't sure what other medications you might be taking, I ordered a drug screen and toxicology test to rule out the influence of any adverse medication interactions that may have contributed to your confusion. These tests were negative." Mrs. Davis nodded confidently. "We also learned that you were taking levothyroxine, so we ran a thyroid function test. That was normal." The physician paused again.

"And so," interrupted Mrs. Davis, "what have you decided, Doctor? I was under a good deal of stress from that accident. Was it simply my diabetes giving me trouble? Is that why you kept me here overnight?"

"Perhaps," said Dr. Jensen. "Your blood glucose levels have been quite erratic since you've been with us. For reasons that are not yet clear to me, you have had more evidence of high serum glucose levels than of moderate or low levels. This concerns me. I've ordered a few more tests for you this morning, but I want you to prepare yourself for the possibility that you may need to take some diabetic medication or insulin to control your condition." Mrs. Davis looked directly up at him then.

"Insulin?" she asked incredulously. "But I'm able to manage my diabetes by watching my diet and getting the right amount of exercise," she asserted. Dr. Jensen explained that, although this is effective treatment for many people who are diagnosed with type 2 diabetes later in life, there is no guarantee that the disease will not progress. He also explained that a period of medication or insulin use could be temporary, just until they could determine exactly what was happening to Mrs. Davis physiologically. Finally, Dr. Jensen said that he had asked an endocrinologist to stop by to see her that day.

"Mom," said Evangeline, "I thought you said you were just a borderline diabetic." She looked at her mother inquisitively, then up at the physician. "My mother has type 2 diabetes?"

"Yes, it does seem that way," commented Dr. Jensen. "It may be that her condition requires much closer monitoring than it has received in the recent past." Dr. Jensen nodded at Mrs. Davis as he said this, conveying that she needed to consider this possibility.

"Phooey," she said in exasperation. "Just what I need!"

Reflective Questions

Reflect on the story that you've just read.

1. Who is Mrs. Davis's physician while she is at Fayette General Hospital?

____

2. A specialist may come to assess the patient today. What is his or her specialty?

____

3. In Chapter 7, when Mrs. Davis arrived in ER, her blood glucose level was low. Has it remained low? Explain.

____

4. Mrs. Davis was given medication to relax her last night, but it wasn't a sleeping pill. What was it?

____

Critical Thinking Question

1. Why do you think Angie sat up in her chair when Dr. Jensen began talking about post-traumatic stress disorder with her mother?

____

For audio exercises, visit **http://www.MedicalLanguageLab.com.** 

Learning Objectives

After reading Chapter 12, you will be able to do the following:

- Use enhanced language skills related to the results of diagnostic tests.
- Understand the terminology and concepts related to post-traumatic stress disorder.
- Use an enhanced level of terminology related to the endocrine system.
- Understand the results of particular diagnostic tests and their relationship to the endocrine system.
- Understand the context and language of glucose monitoring.
- Identify the role of an endocrinologist in relation to diabetes.
- Identify the different types of diabetes.
- Understand the medical terms related to the pathology of diabetes.
- Use enhanced language skills related to the symptoms of hyperglycemia.
- Understand the connection between nutrition and diabetes.
- Appreciate the relationship between pharmacology and medication administration.
- Interpret the terms and abbreviations related to medication administration.
- Interpret the terms related to diabetic medications and insulin.
- Appreciate the education and training of endocrinologists and research technicians.
- Interpret and use the language of referrals and consultation with multiple health disciplines.

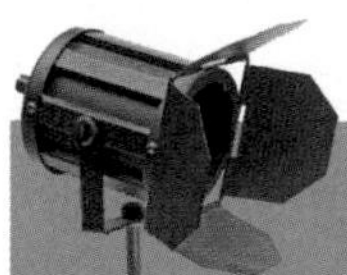

CAREER SPOTLIGHT: Endocrinologists and Research Technicians in Endocrinology

Endocrinologists are physicians who specialize in the treatment of patients with metabolic or hormonal disorders and diseases. After the completion of medical school, internship, and residency, a physician who wishes to specialize in endocrinology completes additional education and clinical training. Finally, he or she must pass a state licensing examination before beginning to practice independently as an endocrinologist. Endocrinologists often focus their careers on a subspecialty area, such as diabetes or thyroid disorders, but they are qualified to treat all kinds of hormonal disorders. Many work with clients to help address their hormonal changes across the life span. Endocrinologists are also medical scientists. Many work in research to explore the causes of human diseases while searching for cures and treatments.

Research technicians in endocrinology have degrees in biochemistry. They study various aspects of the endocrine system, as well as its interrelationship with the rest of the body. They may also be part of a research team that is studying medications and other interventions for endocrine pathology.

The Language of Diagnosis

In the opening scenario, Dr. Jensen explains the results of a battery of physical, mental, radiographic, and laboratory assessments that have been completed for Mrs. Stevie-Rose Davis. From these results, he has been able to make determinations about the patient's medical status. With the use of the clinical decision-making process of ruling out, he has been able to determine the patient's diagnosis. Even so, he would like the patient to be seen by at least one more specialist, an endocrinologist, to confirm what he suspects: that the patient's diabetes has worsened and requires more rigorous intervention. This process is standard procedure during a comprehensive assessment of diabetes.

Key terminology and jargon from the dialogue are explained below.

Key terms: diagnosis

"... some *bouts of confusion.*"

bouts of confusion: episodes of confusion; periods of not being fully oriented, which may include memory impairment.

"... ordered a *battery of tests* ..."

battery of tests: a series of tests.

"She was given *PRN lorazepam* (10 mg *PO*) at *2100 hours* ..."

PRN (prn): administer as needed; give as necessary.

lorazepam: a common anti-anxiety medication of the benzodiazepine family of drugs. This quick acting medication is highly effective, but it should be used sparingly because it is highly addictive.

PO: the abbreviation for the Latin phrase *per os,* meaning *by mouth.*

2100 hours: 9 p.m. on the 24-hour clock (see Chapter 7).

"... scheduled for *blood glucose testing* ..."

blood glucose testing: measurements of the concentration of glucose in the bloodstream. Under normal circumstances, when a specimen is tested before a meal, it provides a measure that is low; when it is tested after a meal, it provides a measure that is higher. Blood glucose is also referred to as *plasma glucose* or *serum glucose.*

"... before she received *sedation.*"

sedation: medicating a patient to induce a state of calm or relaxation.

A medication with the primary purpose of calming a patient is called a **sedative**, although other types of medication also have sedative properties. For example, lorazepam is not classified as a sedative, but it does have sedative or sedating properties.

The root word of *sedation* is *sedatio,* meaning *to calm, quiet, or settle.*

"... each time she *voided* ..."

voided: emptied the bladder; urinated.

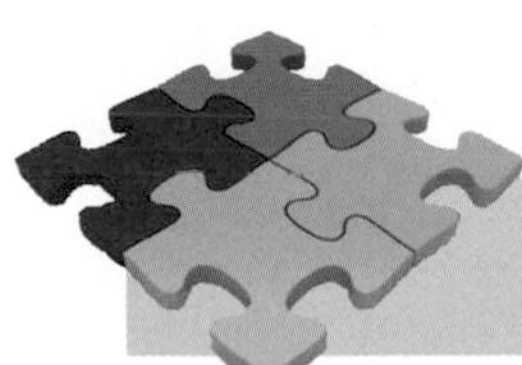

WORD BUILDING: Formula for Creating Words with the Root *Ketone*

ketone = a root word that describes the products of metabolism that are created from the breakdown of fat for energy. Ketones are usually derived from carbohydrates, but they can come from stored body fat as well (see Chapter 9). (Urine dip and dipstick tests are explained in Chapter 8.) The combining forms are keto/n.

keto + plasia = *ketoplasia*

Definition: the formation and excretion of ketones. (The second root is derived from the Greek root *plasis,* meaning *molding.*) *noun*

Example: Insulin depresses *ketoplasia;* it inhibits the production of ketones.

keton + ur + ia = *ketonuria*

Definition: the presence of acetone in the urine. (A synonym is *acetonuria;* see "Focus Point: Acetone.") *noun*

Example: *Ketonuria* may be a symptom of diabetes.

Continued

keto + acid + ur + ia = *ketoaciduria*

Definition: the presence of keto acids in the urine. *noun*

Example: A cause of mental retardation and possibly death in small children, branched-chained *ketoaciduria* is sometimes referred to as *maple syrup ketoaciduria* because the urine of affected individuals smells like maple syrup.

keto + acid + osis = *ketoacidosis*

Definition: a state of acidosis (an increase or excess of acid in the blood and body fluids) as a result of the excessive presence of ketones. *noun*

Example: *Ketoacidosis* is a sign of very high blood sugars, and it is potentially life threatening.

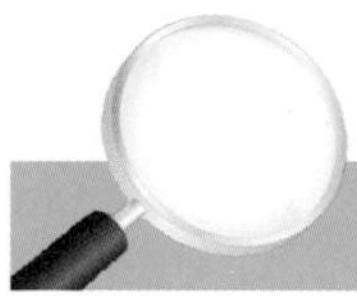

FOCUS POINT: Acetone

Acetone is a type of ketone. It is a chemical that is produced by the body when body fat is converted to energy in the absence of glucose. The production of acetone indicates that insulin is either not being produced or that it is being insufficiently produced.

Fill in the Blanks

Use one of the new terms from this chapter to fill in each blank.

1. The body can produce ____________ from fat stored in the body.
2. Rather than saying "a series of diagnostic tests," you can say "a ____________ of diagnostic tests."
3. Mrs. Davis has the symptom of urinary frequency. She needs to ____________ often.
4. It is possible to have ____________ of confusion, anger, depression, or diarrhea.
5. When a person is not oriented to time, place, and person, they are ____________.
6. Using the 24-hour clock, ____________ is 10 p.m.
7. ____________ ____________ are two Latin words that mean *by mouth.*
8. In the hospital, people who have difficulty falling asleep may receive a ____________.

Build A Word

Use your word-building skills to create medical terms from the following word parts, and then define each term in your own words.

-emia keton	Term: ____________	Meaning: ____________
-emia aceton/e	Term: ____________	Meaning: ____________
-pathy endocrin/o	Term: ____________	Meaning: ____________

Post-traumatic stress disorder

Dr. Jensen has tried to speak with Stevie-Rose about her mental state. He believes that she has demonstrated symptoms of an anxiety disorder called **post-traumatic stress disorder (PTSD).** Post-traumatic stress disorder is caused by a severe psychological trauma with which the individual is unable to cope. This disorder can occur immediately, shortly after the event, or years later.

Diagnostic criteria for PTSD include flashbacks or nightmares of the event, as well as the avoidance of incidents that remind the person of the traumatic event and that may trigger a dissociative state. Insomnia is common in these patients, and it contributes to an inability to concentrate or function. Withdrawal from friends, family, and other forms of intimacy are symptoms of emotional numbing. For some patients, PTSD can also be accompanied by a sense of overwhelming guilt for surviving or for not acting the way they believe they should have during the event. This guilt can lead to aggression and poor control of their anger and other impulses.

PTSD can also include **transient dissociative states**, which are periods of re-living or re-experiencing an event as if it were still occurring. Stevie-Rose Davis exhibited this symptom the day she was admitted, when she thought she was still in Vietnam working in a mobile army surgical hospital (MASH) unit. It is possible that the new trauma of the motor vehicle accident triggered this response.

Some people who suffer from PTSD seek treatment, whereas others avoid it. The thought of revisiting the traumatic event is so anxiety provoking for some victims that they are unable to face the idea of describing their condition to a professional. The defense mechanism of denial unconsciously exerts itself to protect the individual from this overwhelming state of anxiety. In a state of denial, patients with mental health problems cannot recognize or accept that they need help. Our patient, Stevie-Rose, exhibits both denial and avoidance. Notice that, whenever the possibility of PTSD is mentioned, she becomes irritable and defensive; however, she is pleasant and cooperative when discussing other subjects.

The most effective treatment for PTSD is individual or group therapy with a health professional who has specialized education and training in this field. Medications may also be helpful. Although PTSD is considered an anxiety disorder, anti-depressant medications are the drugs of choice, and they have proven to be most effective for reducing some of the long-term symptoms of the disorder.

PTSD is sometimes referred to as **occupational stress disorder (OSD)** when it is job related; this term is used in reference to workers in police, emergency, and military occupations. Our patient, Stevie-Rose Davis, is a veteran. When she is ready to seek help, she can consult the U.S. Department of Veterans Affairs, which offers free counseling to veterans and their families.

Key terms: post-traumatic stress disorder

"*. . . anxiety disorder . . .*"

anxiety disorder: any mental disorder that involves recurring feelings of uneasiness and dread when no real danger exists.

"*. . . flashbacks . . .*"

flashbacks: unexpected recurrences of images or sensations specific to a traumatic event. Flashbacks may occur as the result of a mental disorder or from the use of a hallucinogenic drug. They have a hallucinatory quality, and they are very vivid.

hallucinations: sensations and images that are either not based on reality or that are the result of a sensory misperception of reality. Hallucinations appear very real to the person who is experiencing them.

"*Insomnia* is common . . ."

insomnia: the inability to fall asleep or the inability to stay asleep for a sufficient period to attain necessary rest for the mind and the body.

". . . symptoms of *emotional numbing.*"

emotional numbing: protective mechanisms that are adopted to avoid experiencing emotional pain. This numbing process is not a conscious decision; rather, it is a form of self-protection that is frequently found among patients with PTSD. A synonym for *emotional numbing* is *emotional detachment.*

". . . can also include *transient dissociative states . . .*"

transient: temporary or fleeting.

dissociative states: experiences during which a person feels disconnected from himself or herself or from his or her surroundings, as if watching or dreaming his or her experiences. The person usually has no memories of what occurs around him or her during a dissociative state. A simple and normal example of this is daydreaming. However, prolonged periods of dissociation can be symptoms of PTSD or other abnormal mental conditions. Synonyms include depersonalization and, less commonly, derealization.

"*. . . mobile army surgical hospital (MASH) . . .*"

mobile army surgical hospital (MASH): A MASH unit is a combat support unit in the field. Its main purpose is to provide emergency medical, trauma, and surgical care for military personnel.

"The *defense mechanism of denial . . .*"

defense mechanism: in this context, the term refers to a psychological defense mechanism, which is a method of coping that is unconscious in origin and that alleviates feelings of unbearable anxiety, fear, or other stress (see Table 12-1).

denial: a defense mechanism in which a person denies a painful truth that would cause anxiety if it was admitted to himself or herself.

"*. . . unconsciously exerts itself . . .*"

unconsciously exerts itself: the person is not aware that something is happening or that he or she is behaving, thinking, or speaking in a particular manner. Simply put, "it just happens."

". . . are the *drugs of choice . . .*"

drugs of choice: the best or preferred drug chemical agents for a particular condition or disease. The chosen drug will generally offer the best therapeutic outcomes with the lowest range and rate of side effects or risk of toxicity. Clinical, scientific research provides evidence of the efficacy of the medication.

drug chemical agent: a chemical agent that affects the functioning of a living organism. Medications are drug chemical agents. The term **agent** means *the means or the cause of something.*

therapeutic outcomes: results of a treatment.

efficacy: effectiveness or value.

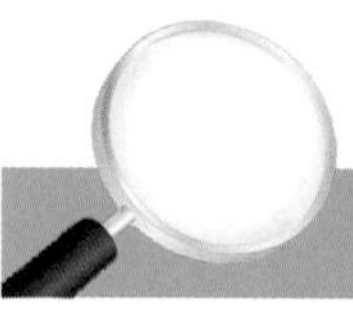

FOCUS POINT: Defense Mechanism

A defense mechanism is any action or interaction that defends the body. Defense mechanisms provide barriers from harm, and they can be physiological or psychological. An example of a physiological defense mechanism is the protection afforded by leukocytes: they protect against invasion by pathogens. An example of a psychological defense mechanism is the process of rationalization: explaining why something happened in a way that decreases the event's harmful emotional effects on yourself or others.

Remember that psychological defense mechanisms do not occur voluntarily; they are subconscious ways of coping that manifest (appear) in a person's thoughts and behaviors. Counseling and psychotherapy are excellent methods of treatment when defense mechanisms begin to interfere with everyday life.

TABLE 12-1: Common Psychological Defense Mechanisms

Psychological Defense Mechanism	Description
avoidance	refusal to participate in or enter into certain conversations, situations, or events
displacement	"dumping" on others: reducing anxiety by giving it or putting it onto others; sometimes referred to as *"kick the cat" syndrome*
denial	behaving as if the trauma or anxiety-provoking event or person has never occurred or existed
projection	blaming others or attributing negative characteristics to others instead of accepting responsibility for one's own thoughts and behaviors
rationalization	justification that makes one's actions look reasonable or logical; sometimes thought of as "making excuses"
regression	a return to the behaviors more typical of someone at a younger age in response to an anxiety-provoking situation; an example is curling up in a fetal position

Critical Thinking Questions

Answer the following questions about PTSD. Use new terminology that you have learned whenever possible.

1. Stevie-Rose Davis's mood shifts whenever anyone speaks to her about the possibility of PTSD, and she refuses to believe that she has this condition. What coping mechanism is she using? ______
2. What is the cause of PTSD? ______
3. Very basically, how is medication a chemical agent? ______

Let's Practice

Read each statement, and then state which defense mechanism each speaker is using.

1. "I failed my driver's license test today, but it wasn't my fault. The instructor didn't give me a fair chance and didn't seem to like me from the moment we met."

   This is the defense mechanism of ______.
2. "The only reason I didn't call you last night was because the battery in my phone was dead and then I couldn't find the charger."

   This is the defense mechanism of ______.
3. "I am not going to that science class where they are looking at spiders today. No way! Not a chance!"

   This is the defense mechanism of ______.

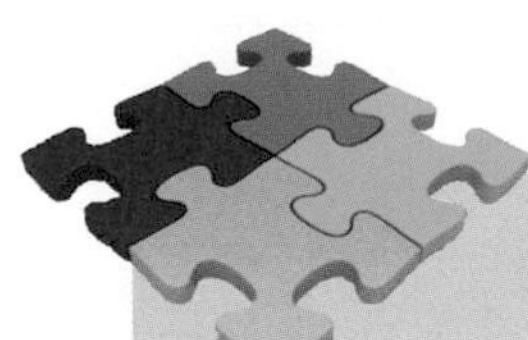

WORD BUILDING: Formula for Creating Words with the Root Word *Trauma*

trauma = a Greek root word meaning *wound.* The combining form is *traumat/o.*

traumato + logy = *traumatology*

Definition: a branch of surgery that deals with wounds and wound care. *noun*

Example: Physicians, surgeons, and nurses at Okla Trauma Center are experts in the field of *traumatology.*

Continued

neuro + trauma = *neurotrauma*

Definition: injury to the peripheral nerves of the central nervous system. *noun*

Example: Symptoms of *neurotrauma* can be physical and psychological, thus affecting both physical and mental functioning.

volu + trauma = *volutrauma*

Definition: a lung injury that can be caused by mechanical ventilation. (The combining form *volu-* is derived from the root word *volute,* meaning *rolled.*) *noun*

Example: Waves of air forced through the lungs by a breathing device roll in waves of inspiration and expiration, and these rolls can cause *volutrauma.*

baro + trauma = *barotrauma*

Definition: an injury caused by a change in atmospheric pressure between a closed space and the surrounding space. (The prefix *baro-* means *weight or pressure* and usually refers to atmospheric pressure.) *noun*

Example: A condition called "the bends" is a *barotrauma* that is sometimes suffered by deep-sea divers when they ascend back to the surface too quickly.

traumato + pnea = *traumatopnea*

Definition: air passing in and out of a wound in the chest wall. *noun*

Example: A chest wound through which air can pass causes the critical respiratory condition of *traumatopnea.*

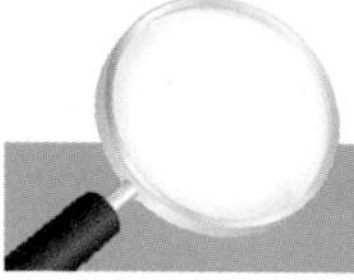

FOCUS POINT: The Plural Form of Trauma

There are two acceptable plural forms of the word *trauma: traumas* and *traumata.*

Build a Word

Use the word parts that you are given to create a medical term, and then define the term.

1. trauma/to -ic post- Term: ________________ Meaning: ________________
2. -therapy trauma/to Term: ________________ Meaning: ________________
3. -ic trauma/to Term: ________________ Meaning: ________________
4. path trauma/to -y Term: ________________ Meaning: ________________

The Language of Medication Administration

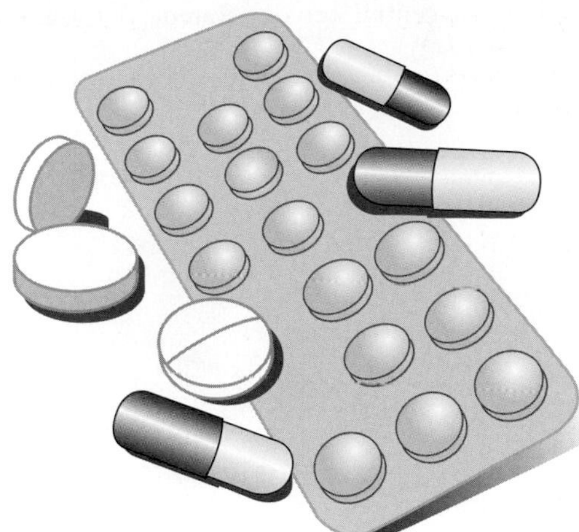

Figure 12.1: Medications

There are so many types of medication for so many disorders that this textbook cannot begin to introduce the terminology for all of them. However, discussing medications in the context of a particular illness or medical condition can shed light on the terminology and abbreviations that are often associated with medications and their administration. (Note: Chapter 8 introduced the language of pharmacology.)

Generic and trade names for medications

It is critically important to know the difference between generic and trade names. Each drug name *must* be unique to prevent mistaking one drug for another when it is ordered, dispensed, and administered.

The generic name of a medication is granted by the U.S. Food and Drug Administration when the drug is first approved. However, the name originates with the U.S. Adopted Names Council. The generic name of the drug is its official name, and it is usually more complicated and harder to remember than its trade names.

The **trade name** of a medication is given by a pharmaceutical company to brand or identify its product. This name can be chosen for marketing purposes, with the intent of that name coming first into the minds of consumers. On labels and in advertisements, trade or brand names are usually followed by the letters *TM*, which identify the names as trademarked or protected by patent (see the example later in this section). In health-care notations, the *TM* notice is not usually included.

There is also a third name for a drug: its chemical name. Although this name may appear on the label of a drug, in a formulary book for pharmaceuticals, or on the monograph (information handout) that comes with a prescription, the chemical name is rarely used in the field of medicine or by the public.

Here is an example of all of the names that can be used to identify the same drug:

2-p-isobutylphenyl propionic acid =	ibuprofen =	Advil™ or Motrin™
(chemical name)	*(generic name)*	*(brand names)*

Medication and post-traumatic stress disorder

Dr. Jensen has suggested that our patient, Stevie-Rose Davis, consider counseling or psychotherapy. This is the first-choice treatment for PTSD. However, he also suggested that she take an anti-depressant medication. Although Stevie-Rose refuses to acknowledge that she has a mental disorder, she has exhibited many of the symptoms of PTSD (see Chapters 2 and 7). Should the patient change her mind about treatment, a physician or psychiatric nurse practitioner might consider prescribing her an **anti-depressant** drug that influences the production, uptake, or reuptake of serotonin in the body.

Serotonin is a **neurotransmitter** (a neuroendocrine chemical that is produced in the brain). Its natural function is to control mood. It also affects bodily functions such as appetite and sleep. Serotonin neurons extend throughout the central nervous system. Serotonin can also be found in the gastrointestinal system (see Figure 12-2).

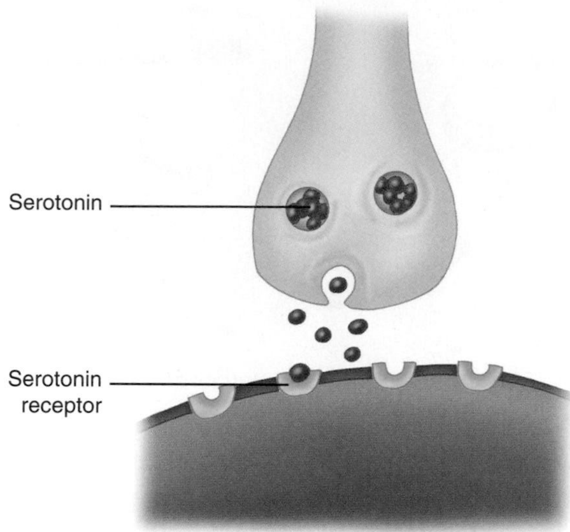

Figure 12.2: Serotonin neuron

After serotonin is released into the bloodstream, it eventually returns and is taken up again by the serotonin neurons. This process is called the *reuptake of serotonin.* It diminishes the level of serotonin that is available to the body. Low levels of serotonin are correlated with PTSD and diagnoses of depression, bipolar disorder, and anxiety. Another name for the neurotransmitter serotonin is 5-hydroxytryptamine (5-HT).

Selective serotonin reuptake inhibitors (SSRIs) are a class of drugs that inhibit or block the reuptake of serotonin in the brain. By doing so, they leave the serotonin circulating in the nervous system, thus maintaining a more stable and appropriate level for functioning. Treatment with an SSRI is a form of chemotherapy (see "Focus Point: Chemotherapy").

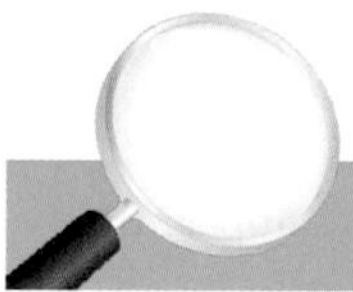

FOCUS POINT: Chemotherapy

The word *chemotherapy* means *drug therapy.* The combining form *chemo* means *drug.*

Although this term is often heard solely in relation to the treatment of cancer patients, this is a narrow use of the term. Anyone who is taking a medication for its therapeutic effects is being treated with a form of chemotherapy.

The U.S. Food and Drug Administration (USFDA) approves the use of all medications in the United States (see "Focus Point: The U.S. Food and Drug Administration"). In the case of PTSD, the USFDA has approved SSRIs as the drugs of choice for this disorder.

Explore the names and descriptions of some SSRIs in Table 12-2. Notice that both the trade and the generic names of the medications are given. It is important to recognize both types of names for drugs because they are frequently used interchangeably in health-care conversations and documentation.

TABLE 12-2: SSRIs – Generic and Trade Names

Generic Name	Trade Name (Brand Name)
Paroxetine	Paxil™, Aropax™, Seroxat™
Sertraline	Zoloft™, Lustral™
Citalopram	Celexa™, Cipramil™
Fluoxetine	Prozac™, Sarafem™

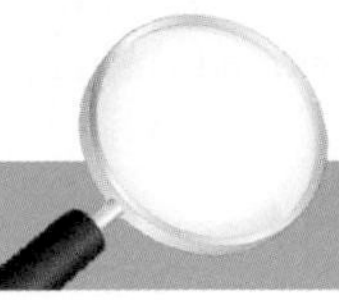

FOCUS POINT: The U.S. Food and Drug Administration

The U.S. Food and Drug Administration is an agency of the U.S. Department of Health and Human Services. Its mandate is to protect the public from the potentially harmful effects of chemical compounds, chemical agents, and radiation. It is concerned with the health and safety of the nation's food supply, cosmetics, and dietary supplements, and it also regulates tobacco products.

Medication administration

Anti-depressants such as SSRIs are dispensed in tablet or capsule form (see Figure 12-3) and taken orally (PO).

Tablet: a solid substance that contains medicinal compounds.

Buccal tablets dissolve when they are held between the cheek and the tongue.

Sublingual tablets dissolve under the tongue.

Enteric-coated tablets are those that dissolve in the intestines rather than the stomach.

The abbreviation *tabs* is frequently used to refer to tablets.

Capsule: a small soluble (dissolvable) container of medicine. A capsule is usually made of gelatinous (gel) material.

The abbreviation *caps* is sometimes used to refer to capsules.

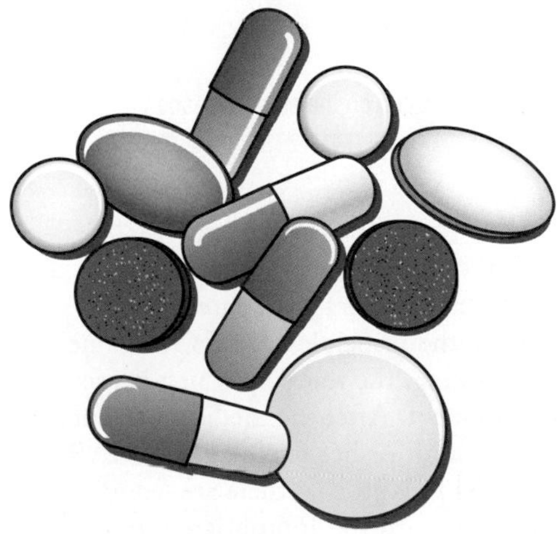

Figure 12.3: Anti-depressant tablets and capsules

Right Word or Wrong Word: *Pill, Tablet,* or *Capsule*?

Is a pill a tablet? Is it a capsule? What exactly is a pill?

Suffixes used in medication trade names

Manufacturers of medications are increasingly adding abbreviations as forms of suffixes to the trade names of their products. This usage has become common knowledge for the public. To help you learn to interpret what is meant by these suffixes, some examples are given in Table 12-3.

CAUTION: Although these suffixes are very popular, health-care and allied-health professionals should NOT use them. Instead, professionals should adhere to the guidelines mentioned earlier in this chapter.

TABLE 12-3: Suffixes Attached to Medication Trade Names

Abbreviation Used as Suffix	Full Term for Abbreviation Used as Suffix
A-D	anti-diarrheal
Allergy D	antihistamine and decongestant
CD	controlled delivery (The drug is released in a scheduled, controlled manner over an extended time period.)
CF	cold formula
DM	dextromethorphan (This is an anti-tussive [anti-cough] agent.)
ER SR XL	extended release or sustained release (The drug is released slowly into the body over time.)
FS	formulated with sucrose (The drug is made with a type of disaccharide, which is a combination of fructose and glucose.)
HCT	hydrochlorothiazide (This is a diuretic medication; see Chapter 9.)
HCL	hydrochloride (This is a salt component of a drug that helps makes to the drug into a solid. It also reduces the pH of gastric contents. See Chapter 11.)
LA	long acting
LQ	liquid
NS	nasal spray
T	topical (This medication is placed on the skin's surface.)

Medication administration: documentation

In all health-care settings, medication administration must be documented on a **medication administration record (MAR).** There is a strict procedure for doing so, and, although each employer may have a different MAR form, the principles remain the same. The name of the patient, the name of the drug, the amount of drug, the route by which it was given, and the time that it was given must all appear on the document. After the medication is actually administered, the person who has administered in must sign his or her name on the MAR (see "On the Job: Medication Administration Record" on page 513). Note that there are many types of MARs; the employer will be sure to acquaint a new employee with the appropriate form. Today, more and more hospitals are replacing the traditional paper forms with electronic MARs.

Medication Administration Record
Emergency Department - Fayette General Hospital

Name: Frasier McDxxx Age: 47 Doctor: Jensen

Date/time admitted: January 14, 2015 at 1400 hr

Date/time discharged: January 14, 2015 at 2300 hr

Admitting diagnosis: Respiratory infection

Medical History: Current diagnosis and treatment, depression

Allergies: Bee stings; none known for medications

Date	Medication + Dosage + Frequency	Time Given	Nurse's Initials
01/14/2015	Keflex 250 mg × 1 tab four times per day	1500 hr	MJ
01/14/2015	Citrolam 30 mg once per day at bedtime	2200 hr	EF
01/14/2015	Keflex 250 mg × 1 tab four times per day	2200	EF

The rights of medication administration

The term **rights of medication administration** is often used in medicine to identify safe practices for administering medications. Each right is checked before giving the patient the medicine. The word *right* means *correct* in this context. Some health-care staff will refer to the "five rights of medication administration," whereas others may mention six, seven, eight, or even nine rights. The basic "rights" include the following:

- Right patient
- Right drug
- Right dose
- Right route
- Right time
- Right purpose

Routes of medication administration

The term **route of administration** refers to how the medication is actually taken into or applied to the body. In other words, the route is the path. Possible routes include the following:

- Oral: by mouth (enteral)
- Topical: on the skin
- Enteral: by mouth, via tube feeding, or rectally into the gastrointestinal tract (see Chapter 11)
- Parenteral: by injection or infusion; this includes transdermal medicated patches (see Figure 12-4)
- Inhalation (aerosol): breathed into the respiratory system through the mouth or nose

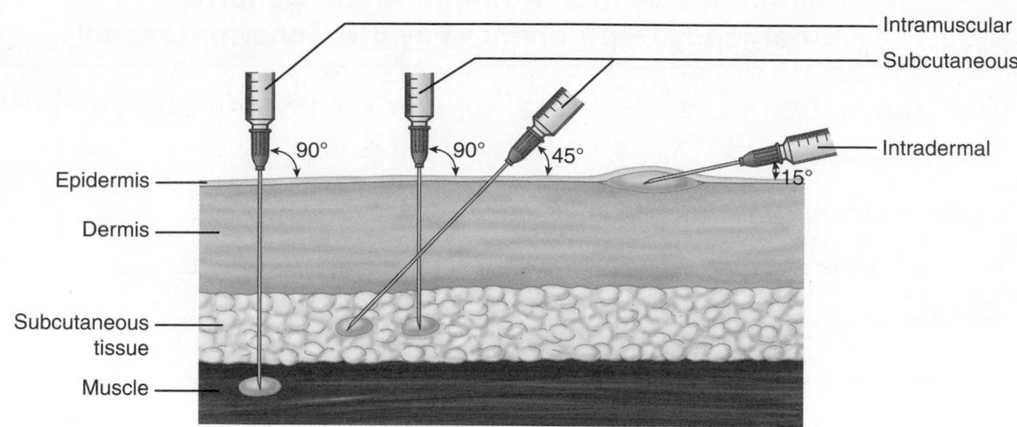

Figure 12.4: Parenteral routes of injection

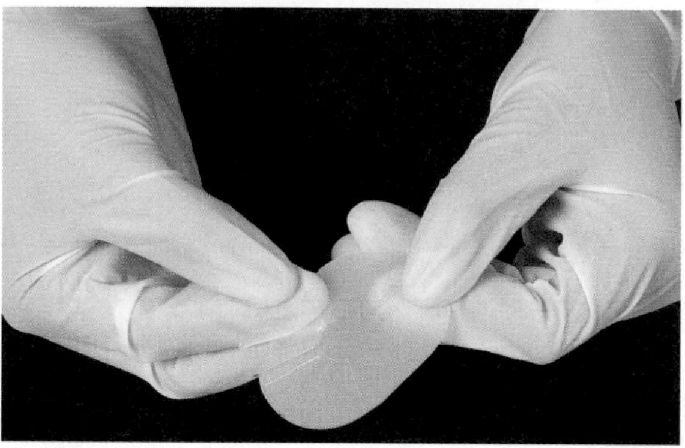

Figure 12.5: Transdermal patch (From Wilkinson HM, Treas LS: *Fundamentals of Nursing. Volume 1: Theory, Concepts, and Applications,* ed 2. Philadelphia: FA Davis, 2011, p 525. With permission.)

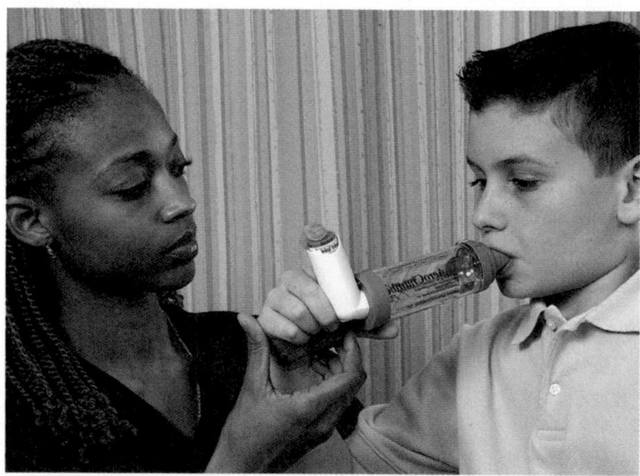

Figure 12.6: Inhaler (From Wilkinson HM, Treas LS: *Fundamentals of Nursing. Volume 1: Theory, Concepts, and Applications,* ed 2. Philadelphia: FA Davis, 2011, p 528. With permission.)

Prefixes: routes of medication administration

Although you will remember these prefixes from previous chapters, it is good to review them here, in another context. Common prefixes that are used to discuss medication administration are included in Table 12-4, along with examples.

TABLE 12-4: Common Prefixes Used in Medication Administration

BEGIN with a Prefix	ADD a Root Word or a Combining Form	CREATE a New Term That Refers to a Route of Medication Administration
sub-	lingual (lingu/o)	sublingual (a pill placed under the tongue, where it quickly dissolves)
sub-	cutaneous (cutane/o)	subcutaneous (an injection given just under the skin)
intra-	venous (ven/o)	intravenous (medication given by needle into a vein)
intra-	muscular (muscul/o)	within the muscle (an injection given deep into the muscle tissue)
trans-	dermal (derm/o)	transdermal (medication delivered via a patch that transports the drug across or through the skin)

Medication dosage and measurements

The prescribing physician or nurse practitioner will calculate a dosage for the patient on the basis of that patient's diagnosis, health status, and a variety of other criteria. Dosages for medications in tablet or capsule form are measured in milligrams or grams. For example, fluoxetine might be prescribed as 60 mg once per day at bedtime.

- Medications in *solid* form are measured in *grams* and *milligrams.*
- Medications in *liquid, elixir,* or *syrup* form are measured in *teaspoons, tablespoons or milliliters (mL or mLs).*
- Medications that are injected *intravenously* or *intramuscularly* are measured in *milliliters, units,* or *international units.*
- Medications that are delivered by *aerosol* are measured by *puffs.*
- Medications that are administered by *mask* or *nebulizer* are measured in *liters.*

A schedule of medication administration (times to take the drug) will be part of the prescription or medication order. This schedule will vary in accordance with the drug and the patient's needs. For example, anti-depressants are given at least once daily, often at bedtime. This specific time of administration is abbreviated as *hs.* Note that there are many abbreviations that pertain to medication administration and that not all of them are approved for or acceptable in health care. See "Focus Point: Approved Abbreviations for Medication Administration" to learn more.

Examples of medical abbreviations that identify times of day include the following:

a.m.: morning

p.m.: afternoon or evening

hs: at bedtime

The frequency of administration can be identified by abbreviations such as these:

bid: twice per day

tid: three times per day

PRN: as needed

Weights and measures related to medications must be documented in the correct form. This includes using capital and lowercase letters correctly. Abbreviations to be written in lowercase letters include the following:

mg: milligram

mcg: microgram

g: gram

kg: kilogram

Abbreviations to be written in uppercase letters include the following:

L: liter

Abbreviations to be written with a combination of uppercase and lowercase letters include the following:

mEq: milliequivalent
dL: deciliter
mL: milliliter

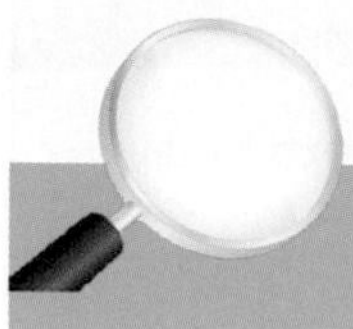

FOCUS POINT: Approved Abbreviations for Medication Administration

To provide the best and safest care during medication administration and documentation, only specific abbreviations are used. It is critical that you use only these approved abbreviations throughout your medical career.

To find a complete and current list of approved abbreviations for medication administration, you should frequently check the website of the Institute for Safe Medication Practices (www.ismp.org) and The Joint Commission's "Official Do Not Use" list of abbreviations (www.jointcommission.org; search the menu for "Topics," then choose "Patient Safety" and refer to the submenu "Safety Initiatives").

Let's Practice

You are given an abbreviation. Spell out the term, and then identify whether or not each abbreviation should be used by health-care and allied health-care providers.

1. DM Meaning: ____________ Appropriate to use? ____________
2. mg Meaning: ____________ Appropriate to use? ____________
3. tab Meaning: ____________ Appropriate to use? ____________
4. LQ Meaning: ____________ Appropriate to use? ____________
5. MAR Meaning: ____________ Appropriate to use? ____________

Critical Reflection Questions

Consider all that you've just learned about medications to answer the following questions.

1. What is the difference between a tablet and a capsule?

   ____

2. What is the term for the route by which a cream or ointment is applied to the skin?

   ____

3. A medication that goes into the digestive system uses which route?

   ____

4. In your career, you will be called upon to write or interpret abbreviations that pertain to the administration of medications. Where might you look for an approved list of abbreviations (or a "do not use" list of abbreviations)?

   ____

Mix and Match

Match the medical term on the left with its synonym on the right.

1. dissociation	means
2. serotonin	distribute or give
3. agent	detachment from emotions
4. dispense	a neurotransmitter
5. emotional numbing	depersonalization

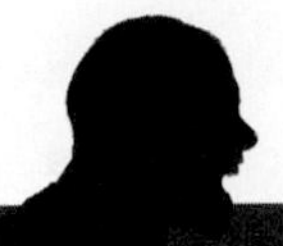

PRONUNCIATION PRACTICE

Say these words aloud to a friend or classmate if you can. You are given the phonetic pronunciation. Your instructor can help you with pronunciation,

or visit **http://www.MedicalLanguageLab.com.** 

barotrauma	băr″ō-**traw**′mă	neurotrauma	nū-rō-**traw**′mă
citalopram	sĭ-**tăl**′ō-prăm	paroxetine	păr-**ŏx**′ĕ-tēn
dextromethorphan	dĕk″strō-**mĕth**′or-făn	sertraline	**sĕr**′tră-lēn
enteral	**ĕn**′tĕr-ăl	subcutaneous	sŭb″kū-**tā**′nē-ŭs
fluoxetine	floo-**ŏks**′ĭ-tēn″	sublingual	sŭb-**lĭng**′gwăl
hydroxytryptamine	hī-drŏk″sē-**trĭp**′tă-mēn	trauma	**traw**′mă
ketone	**kē**′tōn	traumatology	traw-mă-**tŏl**′ō-jē
lorazepam	lō-**rā**′zĕ-pam	traumatopnea	traw″mă-tŏp-**nē**′ă
milliequivalent	mĭ″lē-ē-**kwĭv**′ă-lĕnt	volutrauma	**vŏl**′ū-traw″mă

Enhanced Language of Diabetes

Recall that the pathophysiology of the disease diabetes was introduced in Chapter 7, as were the three most common types of diabetes: type 1, type 2, and gestational. Key medical terminology related to the disease was also introduced. Refer to Table 12-5 now to expand that basic knowledge and to learn how to differentiate between the two main types of the disease.

The formal medical name for diabetes is **diabetes mellitus.**

The root word *diabetes* means *siphon or passing through a tube.*

The root word *mellitus* means *sweet.*

Derived from early Greek, the two words *diabetes* and *mellitus* together describe a symptom of frequent urination. The Greeks noticed that this frequent urination was often accompanied by the attraction of flies and bees to the urine and thus understood that something sweet must be contained within the urine.

TABLE 12-5: Differences Between Type 1 and Type 2 Diabetes

Type 1 Diabetes	Type 2 Diabetes
Juvenile (childhood) onset	Adult onset (mostly)
Body makes little or no insulin	Body makes insulin but cannot use it effectively
Cannot be prevented	Can be prevented
Dependence on insulin daily for survival	Diet, exercise, and medication controlled

Right Word or Wrong Word: *Mellitus* or *Melitus*?

Accurate spelling is essential in health care, and it is a core element of effective and accurate communication. With that in mind, are these two words the same or different? Is one a formal spelling and the other a newer and more common spelling of the same term?

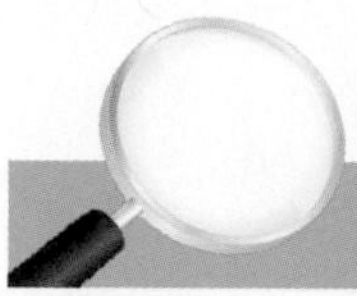

FOCUS POINT: Borderline Diabetic

Do *not* use this term. There is really no such thing as a borderline diabetic patient: diabetes is either diagnosed or not diagnosed. The term *borderline diabetic,* which is popular among the general public, has no real medical validity. It often arises from the results of an oral glucose tolerance test that indicates a state of prediabetes. The use of the term *borderline diabetic* can be misleading, and it minimizes the importance of follow-up testing, blood sugar monitoring, and other lifestyle, dietary, and glucose management strategies.

More about type 1 diabetes (IDDM)

Type 1 diabetes (IDDM) is also referred to as **insulin-dependent diabetes mellitus (IDDM)**. It is also sometimes referred to as *juvenile onset diabetes,* although this term is used less frequently today. Type 1 diabetes most often strikes during childhood, but there are some exceptions across the life span.

Type 1 diabetes is an *autoimmune disease*, which means that the body's own cells attack the insulin-producing cells. The pathophysiological result is that the pancreas does not produce insulin or does not produce enough insulin to control and maintain healthy blood glucose levels. With this ongoing, chronic disease, the *beta cells* of the pancreas are eventually completely destroyed, and insulin production ceases (see "Focus Point: Cells of the Pancreas"). The cardinal symptom of type 1 diabetes is a state of *hyperglycemia* (see Chapter 7). Some of the first signs of type 1 diabetes include fatigue, **polyphagia** (hunger), **polydipsia** (thirst), **polyuria** (frequent urination), weight loss, and **paresthesias** (tingling of the extremities); see Chapter 7 for more information.

Insulin is used to treat type 1 diabetes. However, the most appropriate amount of insulin per day must be individually set for each patient. No two people experience their diabetes in the same way. When type 1 diabetes is not well managed, serious consequences can arise.

Too much insulin can lead to *hypoglycemia* (see Chapter 7). Acute symptoms of hypoglycemia include headache, tachycardia or palpitations, diaphoresis (sweating), and hunger. Acute hypoglycemia requires the rapid delivery of an easily absorbed sugar such as candy, juice, or soda to elevate the person's glucose levels. For cases of chronic hypoglycemia, treatment involves the ingestion of complex carbohydrates throughout the day to keep glucose levels as stable as possible.

Too little insulin can lead to hyperglycemia, and acute hyperglycemia can be life threatening; this is a state of **diabetic ketoacidosis**. The cardinal symptoms are fruity-smelling breath (acetone breath), tachypnea (rapid breathing), flushed face, nausea, and vomiting. Emergency medical treatment includes the administration of insulin.

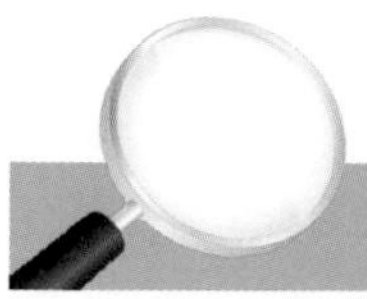

FOCUS POINT: Cells of the Pancreas

Chapter 7 introduced the pancreas and the islets of Langerhans, which are the sources of insulin. The islets of Langerhans actually contain three types of cells:

Alpha cells (A cells): these cells produce and secrete glucagon
Beta cells (B cells): these cells produce and secrete insulin
Delta cells (D cells): these cells secrete the hormone

Prognosis

There is no cure for type 1 diabetes, but there are many new surgeries being developed to treat the pancreas and to promote insulin production by surgically replacing the islets of Langerhans in this organ (see Chapter 7). In addition, an insulin pump may be surgically implanted in the abdomen. This pump releases a continuous and measured supply of insulin (see Figure 12-15).

Over a lifetime, type 1 diabetes can lead to the following:

- Kidney disease
- Neuropathy
- Circulatory impairments
- Cataracts, worsening of eyesight (diabetic retinopathy), and ultimately blindness
- Foot sores (ulcers) that could lead to amputation

More about type 2 diabetes (NIDDM)

At one time, type 2 diabetes was referred to as *non–insulin-dependent diabetes mellitus* (NIDDM). Although this term has begun to fade from the medical environment, it is still in use by older health-care providers and clients.

Our patient, Stevie-Rose Davis, has confirmed with the medical staff that she has **type 2 diabetes.** This means that her body is either unable to accept or unable to use naturally produced insulin in the body. Over time and if the condition is not well managed, the result of type 2 diabetes can be that less and less insulin is produced by the pancreas, thereby causing blood glucose levels to rise throughout the body. This increased level of insulin can be toxic to organs and cells and potentially fatal. For example, periods of extended high levels of glucose can cause blindness, heart disease, decreased circulation to the extremities, nerve damage (neuropathy), erectile dysfunction, and even stroke. Stevie-Rose Davis will require medical intervention in the form of some type of insulin replacement therapy, at least temporarily, until her blood glucose levels can be restabilized (see "Focus Point: Glucose and Impaired Glucose Tolerance").

There is no single cause of type 2 diabetes. The disease is believed to be the result of a genetic predisposition to the condition in combination with behavioral and environmental risk factors. Some risk factors include obesity, an age of more than 40 years, high blood pressure, and a history of gestational diabetes (see Chapters 3, 7, and 8). It has sometimes been called *adult-onset diabetes.* However, as more and more young people become overweight and lead sedentary lifestyles (without adequate exercise), type 2 diabetes is beginning to appear in younger people. As a result, the term *adult-onset diabetes* may soon become inappropriate. Treatment includes routine glucose monitoring and medication, if needed.

The prognosis for an individual with this condition is good, as long as the patient adopts healthy lifestyle habits and diet modifications, including limiting smoking and the drinking of alcohol, maintaining a healthy weight and an exercise regimen, and taking medications as prescribed. The self-monitoring of blood glucose plays a key role in the regulation of this condition as well.

Mix and Match

Match each medical term with the correct definition or description. Draw a line to connect the answers.

1. acetone breath	excessive acetone in the body; hyperglycemia
2. ketonuria	sweating
3. tolerance	sitting or minimal movement or activity
4. sedentary	the presence of ketones in the urine
5. neuropathy	tendency or potential to develop a disease or medical condition
6. diaphoresis	results or outcomes
7. consequences	capacity to endure large amounts without adverse effects
8. predisposition	nerve damage or disease

Build a Word

Read each definition, and then use the prefix *poly-* and an additional word part to create the medical term being defined.

1. excessive urination ______________________________
2. excessive hunger ______________________________
3. excessive thirst ______________________________

Diagnosing and monitoring diabetes

Diabetes is diagnosed through a variety of means, the most common of which is using blood tests to measure levels of glucose in the body (see Table 12-6).

Glucose is derived from carbohydrate foods. It is a common misperception that glucose (casually referred to as *sugar*) is derived only from foods and beverages that contain sugar or honey. In reality, carbohydrates such as bread, pasta, rice, potatoes, and cereal also increase glucose levels in the body.

Impaired glucose tolerance (IGT) is a condition in which blood glucose levels are high but not high enough for the patient to be considered to have diabetes. IGT is also referred to as *prediabetes,* and it can be a sign that the patient is vulnerable to type 2 diabetes, as well as to heart disease and stroke.

Blood glucose monitoring

Routine glucose monitoring facilitates the management of diabetes. Levels of blood glucose are checked throughout the day to assess and intervene for cases in which the levels are either too high or too low. In each of these circumstances, the person may feel lethargic or tired, and he or she may be experiencing a variety of symptoms that indicate hypoglycemia or hyperglycemia. When results are known, decisions can be made to intervene to adjust levels to normal or acceptable ranges.

All diabetics monitor their blood glucose levels, but the frequency of doing so depends on the degree of and stability of the diabetic condition. Many people are trained to **self-monitor blood glucose (SMBG).** This means that they are given instruction with regard to how to operate a glucose monitoring device, and they are able to follow a set routine for self-testing on their own. Others will have their levels taken at clinics, laboratories, or inpatient care facilities or by home care nurses. The most common device that is used for this assessment is the glucose meter or glucometer (see Chapter 7). The patient's finger is pricked with a lancet to draw a droplet of blood onto a glucose test strip (thin piece of coated paper). The test strip is then inserted into the glucometer, which measures the amount of glucose in the blood. Table 12-7 shows typical blood glucose levels obtained at different times throughout the day for patients with diabetes and for those with normal glucose levels.

Pricking a finger is a common medical expression that describes the procedure that is used to draw blood from a fingertip. This is achieved with the use of a tiny cutting instrument called a *lancet.* For the purposes of diabetic testing, a **lancet** is a sharp, pin-like device that punctures the skin no deeper than 0.75 mm (0.03 inches).

TABLE 12-6: Test Values for the Diagnosis of Diabetes

Test	Normal	Prediabetes	Diabetes
Fasting plasma glucose test	<100 mg/dL	≥100 and <126 mg/dL	≥126 mg/dL
Two-hour oral glucose tolerance test	<140 mg/dL	≥140 and <200 mg/dL	≥200 mg/dL

TABLE 12-7: Blood Glucose Ranges for Adults

Time Taken	Normal Blood Glucose Ranges for Adult	Blood Glucose Ranges for Adult
Fasting and/or before breakfast	<110 mg/dL*	80 to 130 mg/dL
After meals (postprandial)	<140 mg/dL	<180 mg/dL
Randomly	<140 mg/dL	>200 mg/dL
Before bed	<120 mg/dL	100 to 120 mg/dL

*Your employer may forbid the use of the symbols for greater than (>) and less than (<); you may be required to write out these words.

People who are living with diabetes and who are self-monitoring will keep a record of their daily food intake and blood sugar readings so that they may be aware of any changes in their blood sugar over time and so that they will know when to seek medical intervention (see "On the Job: Self-Monitoring Blood Glucose Record" below).

Daily Diabetes Record Page

Week Starting: ____________________ **Target blood sugar range:** ____________________

	Breakfast		**Lunch**		**Dinner**		**Bedtime**		**Other**
	Blood glucose	Insulin/ meds	Blood glucose	Insulin/ meds	Blood glucose	Insulin/ meds	Blood glucose	Insulin/ meds	Blood glucose
Monday	*109*				*122*		*115*		
Comments:									
Tuesday			*106*				*152**		
Comments: **Missed evening walk*									
Wednesday	*126*		*121*		*131*		*120*		
Comments:									
Thursday	*113*		*128*		*179*		*241**		
Comments: **Sick with flu*									
Friday	*159*		*147*		*162*		*150*		
Comments:									
Saturday	*127*				*152**				
Comments: **Had extra big snack in afternoon*									
Sunday	*119*		*121*				*140*		
Comments:									

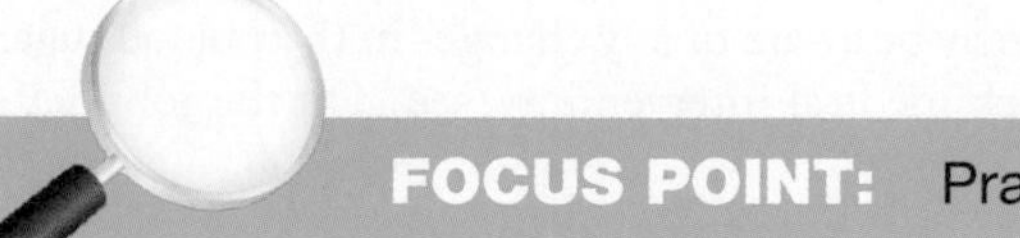

FOCUS POINT: Prandial

The word *prandial* is a medical term that means *breakfast or relating to a small meal.*

Blood glucose monitoring is done at very specific times of day to reflect the process of metabolism and the breakdown of carbohydrates, the production of insulin, and the changing levels of glucose in the body. Testing times are dependent on the person's pattern of blood glucose levels over a 24-hour period, any medication being taken for diabetes, and mealtimes. For the diabetic patient whose blood glucose levels are quite stable under these circumstances, monitoring is usually performed before meals (see Table 12-8).

The hemoglobin A1C test (HgA1C, A1C, or HbA1C)

This simple laboratory test measures the control of **glycemia levels** (blood glucose) that have occurred over a period of the previous 2 to 3 months. The results of the test demonstrate how well a person's diabetes is being managed. It measures the amount of *glycated hemoglobin* in the patient's blood.

The term **hemoglobin A1C** refers to hemoglobin A cells, which are the blood cells to which glucose binds. In simpler terms, hemoglobin A1C is a combination of red blood cells and glucose. The life span of hemoglobin cells is 3 months. Synonyms for hemoglobin A1C are *glycohemoglobin, glycated hemoglobin,* and *glycosylated hemoglobin.*

For the A1C test, blood is drawn in the physician's or nurse practitioner's office, or the patient draws his or her own blood and mails it in a self-test kit. A1C meters are currently being developed and marketed for self-monitoring purposes (see Figure 12-7). The higher the percentage of glycated hemoglobin found, the less controlled the diabetes is.

- A test result of 6.5% to 7% or more indicates poorly managed diabetes.
- A person who does not have diabetes will score around 5%.
- Prediabetic patients will score between 5.7% and 6.4%.

TABLE 12-8: Terms and Abbreviations Related to Glucose Testing Times

Time of Day	Medical Term for Time	Abbreviation*
Before meals	Antes comer	AC, a.c., or ac
After meals	Post comer	PC, p.c., or pc

*Check with your employer. You may be required to write out the words *before meals* and *after meals* and not allowed to use these abbreviations.

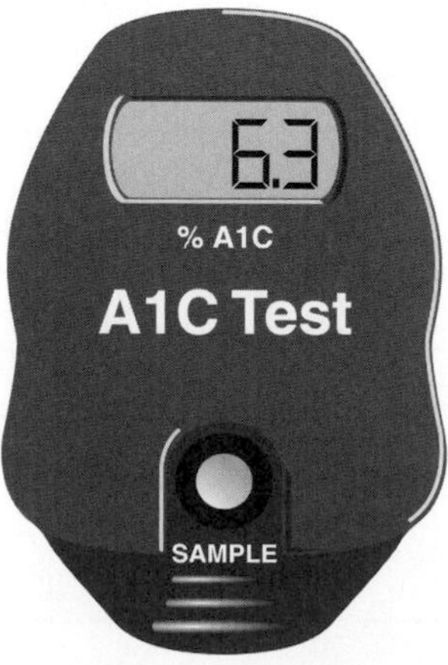

Figure 12.7: Self-monitoring with a portable hemoglobin A1C monitor

Mix and Match

Match the term on the left with its synonym on the right.

1. glycemia	blood glucose
2. facilitates	inactive, sitting, or settled
3. glycated hemoglobin	breakfast or a small meal
4. managed	assists
5. glycosylated hemoglobin	hemoglobin A1C
6. sedentary	glycohemoglobin
7. prandial	controlled

Fill in the Blanks

Use medical terminology to fill in the blanks.

1. Daily glucose monitoring at home requires ______________ the finger with a ______________ to obtain a ______________ of blood for testing.
2. In the context of diabetes, a urine ______________ test can determine if there are ______________ present.
3. Another term for *glycated hemoglobin* that uses almost all of the same word parts is ______________.
4. An HgA1C test score of more than 7% indicates ______________.
5. A formal term that is used in medical settings to mean *breakfast or a small meal* is ______________.
6. You can say ______________ *glucose* or *blood glucose;* these terms have the same meaning.
7. The term for voluntarily not eating for an extended period of time is ______________.
8. The abbreviation *SMBG* stands for ______________.
9. Another way to say "glucose meter" is "______________."
10. Fruity-smelling breath is called ______________, and it is indicative of ______________ in the ______________.

Critical Reflection Questions

Answer the following questions about diabetes.

1. What are the potential adverse outcomes of poorly managed type 2 diabetes?
____
2. Our patient, Mrs. Stevie-Rose Davis, has diabetes. Which type is it? ______________
3. Has Stevie-Rose Davis been using insulin to keep her blood sugar levels controlled? How do you know? ______________________________
4. Think back to our other patients. Someone was screened for gestational diabetes. Who was it, and why was the screening done? ______________________________

Blood glucose testing (BGT)

Blood glucose or serum glucose levels can also be tested in the laboratory with the use of a variety of tests. Because Stevie-Rose Davis's blood glucose levels have been erratic (unpredictable) since yesterday, she may be ordered a battery of blood glucose tests, including the ones described in the following sections.

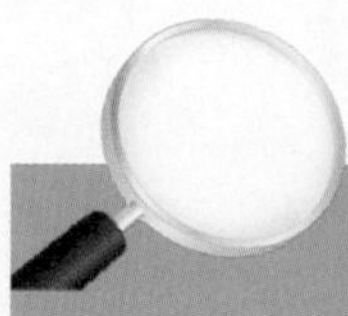

FOCUS POINT: Fasting Blood Sugar Test and the Diagnosis of Diabetes

Normal results of a fasting blood sugar test should show a level of 70 to 110 milligrams of glucose per deciliter of blood; this is also written as *70 to 110 mg/dL.* A diagnosis of diabetes is confirmed when abnormal results of 126 mg/dL or more occur on at least two tests given on two different days. A fasting blood sugar test is also sometimes referred to as the *fasting plasma glucose test.*

Random blood sugar (RBS)

This test measures serum glucose randomly throughout the day. Because normal levels do not vary widely during that time, this test is useful for determining variations. Should variations occur, they may indicate difficulties with insulin production and secretion or with the metabolism of glucose. Normal levels of blood glucose are less than 140 mg/dL.

A result of 200 mg/dL or more on an RBS test may suggest diabetes, but the diagnosis cannot be made simply by this test. Although a second RBS test might confirm a higher reading, fasting blood sugar and oral glucose tolerance tests are required for certainty.

Oral glucose tolerance test (OGTT)

An *oral glucose tolerance test* is used to diagnose a state of prediabetes or diabetes itself. The test begins with a fasting blood glucose test (FBS). After the FBS, the patient drinks a sweet glucose syrup. Beginning exactly 2 hours after that drink, a series of blood glucose measurements are taken, and up to four samples are taken in total. *For the person with diabetes, the levels of blood glucose rise rapidly after the drink and then fall slowly.* Diabetes is determined when the measurements show a level of 200 mg/dL or more.

Impaired glucose tolerance (IGT) test

The IGT test follows the same steps as the OGTT, but it is used to diagnose *impaired glucose tolerance,* which refers to a prediabetic state of *dysglycemia.* Dysglycemia can be a precursor to type 2 diabetes, as well as to cardiovascular disease. Impaired glucose tolerance is diagnosed when a measure of 140 to 199 mg/dL is achieved 2 hours after the ingestion of sweet glucose syrup.

2-Hour postprandial glucose test (PPGT)

The term **postprandial** means *after a meal.* This test measures blood glucose exactly 2 hours after a meal has been eaten. Excessive and prolonged increases in postprandial blood glucose levels are found in people with impaired glucose tolerance or type 2 diabetes. Their medical condition adversely affects their ability to secrete glucagon to release insulin appropriately or the ability to resist the effects of insulin when necessary (see Chapter 7). These problems cause an overall increase in the amount of glucose that is released into the bloodstream after a meal is eaten. The increase occurs within the first 2 hours after ingestion.

Before the 2-hour PPGT, an FBS is recommended. The FBS establishes a baseline measure of blood glucose after a long period of fasting (8 to 12 hours). After the FBS, the patient is given a high-carbohydrate meal. Then, exactly 2 hours later, the PPGT occurs. A normal serum postprandial glucose level should be less than 140 mg/dL.

Continuous blood glucose monitoring (CGM)

Continuous blood glucose monitoring is achieved via the insertion of a tiny sensor under the skin on the abdomen or the upper arm. The sensor is able to measure glucose levels in tissue fluids, and it then transmits this information to a wireless monitor (a pager-like device). CGM sensors need to be changed every week or more frequently. CGM is not as accurate as routine blood glucose monitoring, so the results need to be compared quite often with those obtained from a glucose meter (see Figure 12-8).

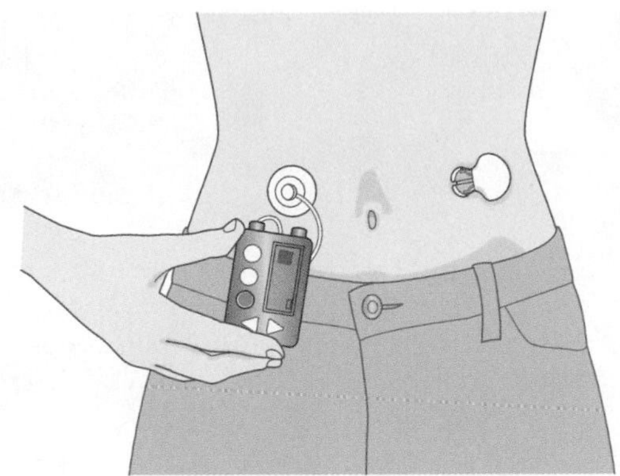

Figure 12.8: Continuous blood glucose monitor

Urine glucose testing (UGT)

Recall from Chapter 9 that a urine dipstick test is able to determine the presence or absence of glucose in the urine (and much more). **Urine glucose test strips** are paper strips that have been specially designed with small embedded pads that are glucose sensitive. When dipped in urine, these pads change color in the presence of glucose. Remember, glucose should *not* appear in the urine. The presence of glucose may indicate diabetes mellitus, renal glycosuria (glucose released from the kidneys into the urine), or pregnancy.

Urine test strips are also known as *reagent strips.*

The urine glucose test is also known as the *glucosuria test.*

Although UGT can be a simple way to identify glucosuria, it is not considered the best or most precise test for the measurement of blood glucose levels. For that reason, it is not used in every health care facility and it is not recommended for diabetic self-monitoring.

To collect a urine specimen for UGT, the patient is asked to void into a **urine hat**. The term *hat* is medical jargon for a plastic receptacle that has the appearance of a white hat. It is placed over the toilet bowl to collect specimens and for the measurement of urine output. Each hat is designed with volume calibration measures and a pouring lip. A wide variety of urine specimens can be collected in this manner. The urine glucose test can be accomplished simply by dipping the test strip into the hat after the patient has voided. A urine sample collected in a specimen bottle or another container designated for such use may also be used (see Figures 12-9, 12-10, and 12-11).

Volume calibration: markings that indicate standardized measurements of liquid. Urine hats and urine specimen bottles are marked with volume calibrations.

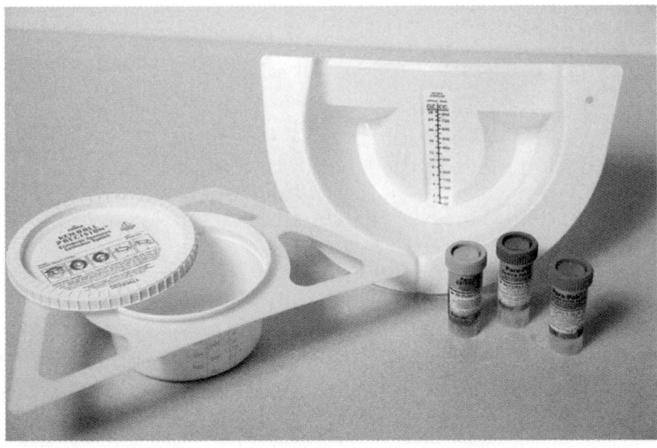

Figure 12.9: Specipan (hat) (From Strasinger S, Di Lorenzo M: *The Phlebotomy Textbook,* ed 3. Philadelphia: FA Davis, 2011, p 403. With permission.)

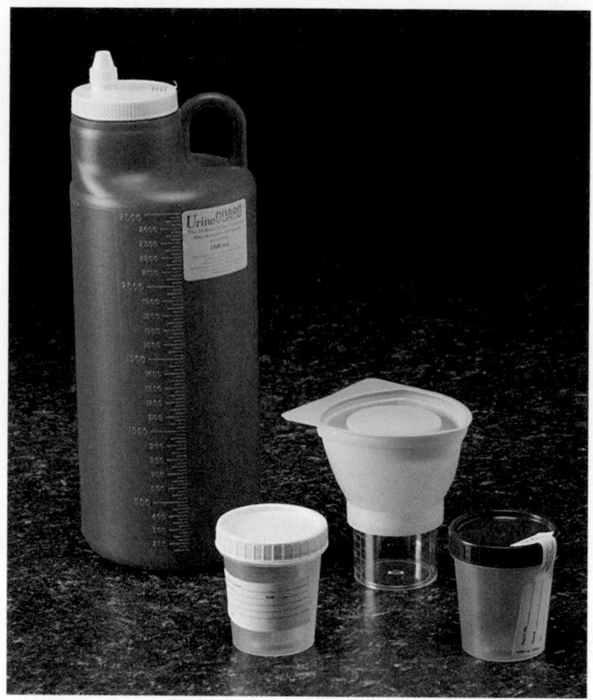

Figure 12.10: Urine specimen containers (From Eagle S, Brassington C, Dailey CS, Goretti C: *The Professional Medical Assistant: An Integrative, Teamwork-Based Approach.* Philadelphia: FA Davis, 2009, p 922. With permission.)

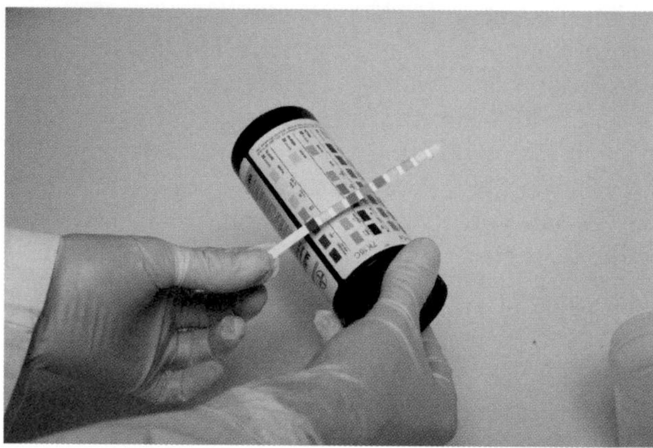

Figure 12.11: Urine glucose test strips (From Strasinger S, Di Lorenzo M: *The Phlebotomy Textbook,* ed 3. Philadelphia: FA Davis, 2011, p 383. With permission.)

Let's Practice

Read each description, and then identify the laboratory test being described.

1. A glucose syrup is ingested after an FBS specimen is taken.
   Test: ______________________
2. Nothing is taken by mouth for 8 to 12 hours before this test.
   Test: ______________________
3. A blood test is spontaneously given at different times of day to measure blood glucose levels.
   Test: ______________________
4. A blood specimen is drawn 2 hours after a small meal, usually the first meal of the day.
   Test: ______________________

Mix and Match

Match the abbreviation with the name of the test or type of diabetes to which it refers.

1. PPGT	non–insulin-dependent diabetes
2. DDM	impaired glucose tolerance (test)
3. IGT	urine glucose test
4. RBS	random blood sugar (test)
5. UGT	2-hour postprandial blood glucose test
6. NIDDM	insulin-dependent diabetes mellitus

Critical Thinking Questions

Consider what you have been learning, and then answer the following questions.

1. With which type of diabetes does the pancreas fail to produce insulin?

   ____

2. For many people, which type of diabetes can be controlled by diet, exercise, and lifestyle modifications? ______________________________

PRONUNCIATION PRACTICE

Say these words aloud to a friend or classmate if you can. You are given the phonetic pronunciation. Your instructor can help you with pronunciation,

or visit **http://www.MedicalLanguageLab.com.** 

acetone	**ăs**´ĕ-tōn
dysglycemia	dĭs-glī-**sē**´mē-ă
glycated	**glī**´kāt'd
glycohemoglobin	glī″kō-**hēm**´ă-glō-bĭn
lancet	**lăn**´sĕt
melitis	mĕl-**ī**´tĭs
mellitus	mĕl **ī**´tĭs or mĕl-**ī**´tus
paresthesia	păr″ĕs-**thē**´zē-ă
polydipsia	pŏl″ē-**dĭp**´sē-ă
polyphagia	pŏl″ē-**fā**´jē-ăl
polyuria	pŏl″ē-**ū**´rē-ă
postprandial	pōst-**prăn**´dē-ăl
prandial	**prăn**´dē-ăl
tachypnea	tăk″ĭp-**nē**´ă

Patient Update

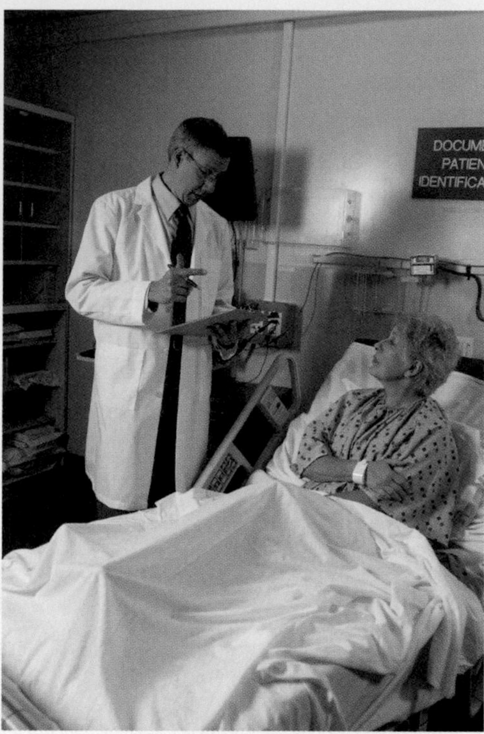

At mid morning, Stevie-Rose Davis received a visit from the endocrinologist, Dr. Shawshank. He confirmed for her that she needs to continue taking her thyroid replacement medication as prescribed by her physician, but he ruled out any thyroid involvement in the confusion that she had experienced on admission. He then spoke to her about his concerns regarding her fluctuating blood glucose levels. He showed her the blood sugar graph that the nursing staff had been plotting since her admission; he pointed out that she had arrived in a state of moderate hypoglycemia but that she had been experiencing hyperglycemia since that time (see “On the Job: Blood Sugar Level Report” on page 530). Mrs. Davis explained that she had been diagnosed with type 2 diabetes 3 years prior and that her condition was well maintained with a diabetic diet that restricted some of her carbohydrate and sugar intake. She told him that she likes to walk and that she and her husband have taken up square dancing as a hobby since they retired 5 or 6 years ago. She then laughed and said that they had both been considering taking up ballroom dancing now that it was so popular. The doctor, Mrs. Davis's daughter Evangeline, and Mrs. Davis all laughed.

“Well, Mrs. Davis,” said Dr. Shawshank, “It sounds as if you're doing all the right things to keep that blood glucose under control, so I can only wonder if there have been some changes in your lifestyle or if you have been under extra stress over the past few days and weeks. These things can contribute to changes in your ability to manage your diabetes as well as you have been.” He then waited for Mrs. Davis to reply.

“No, I can't really think of anything, Doctor, beyond what has just happened. You know that I was in a car accident yesterday, but that's not the half of it,” Mrs. Davis said. “We were in that accident when we were bringing my grandson, Clay, here to the hospital. Oh, what a disaster, Doctor!” She looked directly at him before continuing. “Do you know what happened? Oh, I feel just absolutely awful. Terrible. Dreadful. I'm an awful grandma!” Tears began to well up in her eyes, and her voice cracked. The physician waited for her to continue. “He's just a little boy!” She shook her head in sorrow and then continued.

“We were out on the terrace in the back of the house. Clay was there, he was staying over with us for a few days, like a little holiday. He was outside, and so was my husband. I was bringing Zane—that's my husband—another cup of coffee. I was bringing out the pot, actually.” She paused then, remembering, and she put her hand to her mouth in anguish. “I stepped outside and ran smack into Clay! Oh, Doctor, I burned him!" Mrs. Davis began to cry in earnest then. Evangeline, who was sitting nearby, stood up to comfort her. She put her hand on her mother's shoulder.

"From what I understand, Clay ran into Mom, and the hot coffee spilled on him," continued Evangeline. She gently patted her mom's shoulder. "It wasn't your fault, Mom. It was just an accident. Clay's going to be okay. Mickey tells me it was just a bad scald, but there won't be any scarring or anything." She looked back at the doctor.

"Okay? How can you say that, Angie! The burn is one thing, and I blame myself for that. I should have been watching more carefully. But Evangeline, the accident! Clay's not all right. He's badly injured, and it's all my fault!" Mrs. David cried and covered her eyes. "All my fault," she whispered into her hands. "If Steve and Mickey ever speak to me again, it will be a miracle," she sobbed. Angie continued the story.

"On the way to the hospital, Mom and Dad were in a car accident. Clay broke his jaw, and he had surgery last night. He's over at Okla Trauma Center. My Dad was also in the car. He's been released from the hospital; he didn't have any major injuries."

"Oh, I'm so sorry to hear all of this," said Dr. Shawshank. "I can see how truly distressing it all is for you, Mrs. Davis. And now, putting your symptoms in the context of these stressors, I think I can see how your diabetic symptoms may have been triggered." He paused for a moment, and Mrs. Davis looked up.

"Oh, please, I can't take any more bad news. Please don't tell me I have to go on insulin or medications or anything like that, please," Stevie-Rose pleaded.

"Mrs. Davis, you've been under an enormous amount of stress for the past 24 hours or more. Under extreme stress, the body needs to produce more energy to respond to it. When your body doesn't produce enough insulin or cannot readily use it, as in your case, glucose builds up in the blood, and a state of hyperglycemia ensues. You are most certainly experiencing this," Dr. Shawshank said. The patient and her daughter waited for the doctor to continue and to offer a prognosis.

Dr. Shawshank continued: "It seems to me that your condition may be quite situational, but I do not foresee a quick solution to alleviating some of the stress that you are under." Stevie-Rose looked up at him and raised her eyebrows in inquiry.

"Please, don't say it . . . I can't bear to hear it. Don't tell me that I have to take insulin injections now," Mrs. Davis said.

"What I am saying," Dr. Shawshank said, "is it that I can see that you will be carrying the stress of what has happened to your grandson for a while yet, until you come to terms with the facts of the accident. I'd like to start you on a low dose of medication to help you through this. I'll give you an anti-diabetic medication to help your body cope with the physical needs that this stress is causing you. You can see your own physician for follow-up on this, but I'd like to start you today. I think it will help."

"Oh, a medication for my diabetes?" the patient asked as her crying began to subside. "Well, that doesn't sound too bad. Would it be temporary? I'd like it to be temporary," Mrs. Davis said hopefully. The doctor nodded and explained that, if extreme stress was affecting the current fluctuations in the patient's blood glucose levels, then the treatment of this condition with the use of medication would likely be temporary.

"I cannot promise that, Mrs. Davis. You'll need to see your own physician and consult with him or her about this. Do not stop this medication on your own," said the doctor. Mrs. Davis nodded and said that she would follow his orders. "All right then," the doctor continued, "I'm going to order some Glucophage for you to start right now. Let's see how that works for you over the next 4 or 5 hours, okay? The nurse will continue to monitor and chart your glucose levels."

"Oh, the next 4 or 5 hours? Are you hinting that, if I stabilize, I might be able to go home today?" The doctor nodded, and Mrs. Davis smiled.

"Just one last thing, Mrs. Davis," said Dr. Shawshank. "You are facing a good deal of stress right now. Would you like me to order something to help you to cope with that, too? Perhaps a low dose of an anti-anxiety medication?"

"No, no more medication. I'd rather not, thank you," said Mrs. Davis. "I don't like to take a lot of medications. I take herbal teas for sleep and to calm me down. Walking in the park helps me, too. I learned meditation when I was in Southeast Asia years ago, and sometimes I practice that. I'll be okay." She smiled.

"Fine. We'll leave it at that," said the doctor. "I won't be back in to see you today, but I'll leave notes for Dr. Jensen about what we've talked about here. He'll be able to make further adjustments to your medication and help you set up some plans for discharge, if he deems you're ready when he comes by again this afternoon. Take care." At this point, Dr. Shawshank turned to leave.

"Just a moment, Doctor. I just have a question about Mom's medication, if you don't mind," said Evangeline. She followed Dr. Shawshank out into the corridor. As they took a few steps down the hall, she began to speak.

"Doctor, I'm worried about my Mom. I had really hoped she'd take you up on your offer of some anti-anxiety medication. She really needs it. What you don't know—and what she doesn't know—is that my Dad has just discovered he's quite ill. I don't know how Mom's going to cope when she hears this on top of everything else. The hospital told him that he may have lung disease or possibly even lung cancer!"

Blood Sugar Chart

Name: Stevie-Rose Davis Upper level: 120.00 Lower level: 80.00

Date	Time	Level	Notes
06/xx/2015	1430 hr	90	Arrived in ER; ambulant
06/xx/2015	1900 hr	210	1 hr after light supper; sitting up in bed
06/xx/2015	2200 hr	200	Lying in bed preparing for sleep
06/xx/2015	0300 hr	150	Sleeping; awakended for test
06/xx/2015	0630 hr	140	Sleeping; awakened for text. FBS collected as well. Hold breakfast for now.
06/xx/2015	0900 hr	130	Before meal. Given light, restricted diet.
06/xx/2015	1130 hr	180	Before lunch. Given glucophage Po now per doctor's orders.
06/xx/2015	1400 hr	110	2 hr after meal
06/xx/2015	1630 hr	100	Prior to meal. Dr. Shawshank aware. In to see patient now.

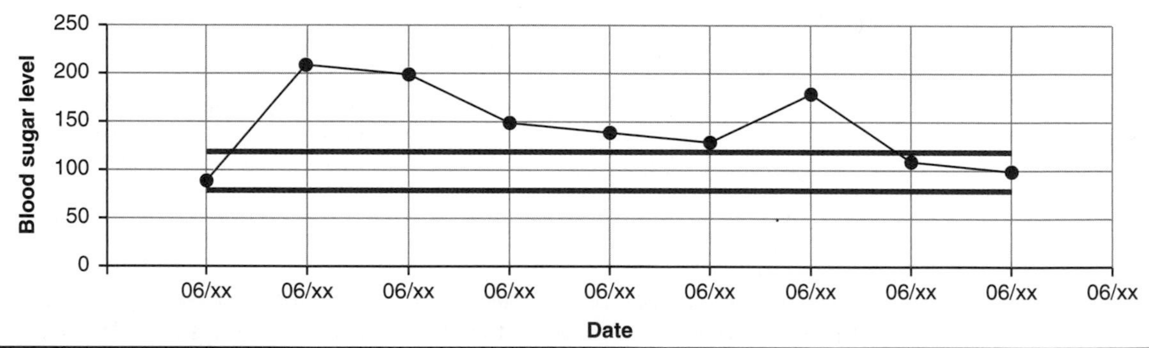

Critical Reflection Questions

Refer to the Patient Update to answer the following questions.

1. Stevie-Rose Davis was offered a type of medication that she declined. What was it?
____
2. What does the patient blame herself for? ____________________________
3. Does Stevie-Rose know about her husband's new diagnosis? __________________

Critical Thinking Questions

Consider all that you know about our patient, Stevie-Rose Davis, and then answer the following questions.

1. What major stressor is the patient about to face when she goes home?
____

2. What effect might this new stressor have on the patient's physical and mental health?
____

3. Stevie-Rose was afraid she might have to take a type of treatment that would include daily injections. What was it? ______________________________

Insulin and insulin replacement therapy

Insulin is a naturally occurring pancreatic hormone and a protein. Its function is to lower blood glucose levels by allowing glucose to leave the bloodstream and enter the cells of the body, where it becomes an essential source of energy. You will recall that, in patients with type 1 diabetes, the pancreas does not produce insulin. In patients with type 2 diabetes, the pancreas may produce insulin, but the body is unable to use it. For cases in which it is necessary to provide insulin from another source, *insulin replacement therapy* is instituted.

Insulin preparations, which are the substances that will be injected, are obtained from the pancreas of a pig or an ox. A preparation called *Humulin, insulin* is produced from bacteria in a laboratory, and it is almost identical to naturally occurring human insulin. Insulin is given by subcutaneous injection to bypass the gastrointestinal tract because it is a protein that would be broken down by the digestive juices. Patients who are receiving insulin replacement therapy are placed on a regimen of highly individualized and measured doses of insulin by injection. Glucose monitoring provides information about how well the therapy is working and whether the patient needs more or less insulin. The types of insulin preparations that are used are determined by a physician or an endocrinologist.

Different types of insulin vary with regard to their rapidity of onset, their peak time of effectiveness, and the longevity of their effect: in other words, how fast they act, when they are most effective, and how long they provide a benefit. Because of these differences, insulins are categorized into four classes. Table 12-9 explains more about the different types of insulin. The goal of this table is to familiarize you with the names of different classes of insulin and some of the more common brand names. Unless you are working directly with insulin, the data that address the onset, peak, and duration of effectiveness will be less important to you.

TABLE 12-9: Types of Insulin

Class	Example by Brand (Trade) Name	Onset	Peak	Duration
Rapid-acting insulin	Humalog NovoLog Lispro Aspart	Within 15 minutes	45 to 90 minutes	Up to 4 hours
Short-acting insulin	R or Regular Humulin (Novolin) Velosulin (for insulin pumps)	Within 30 minutes	2 to 5 hours	Up to 8 hours
Intermediate-acting insulin	NPH (N) Lente (L)	Within 2 hours	4 to 12 hours	Up to 24 hours
Long-acting insulin	Ultralente (U) Lantus	Within 3 hours	6 to 20 hours	Up to 36 hours
Premixed insulin (a combination of intermediate- and long-acting forms)	Humulin 70/30 Novolin 70/30 Humulin 50/50	Within 30 minutes	2 to 5 hours	Up to 24 hours

Insulin administration

Insulin is a protein rather than a drug. Even so, it is administered in the same manner as a medication and with the use of the same standard measures and protocols. It is most often injected subcutaneously with a very fine calibrated syringe.

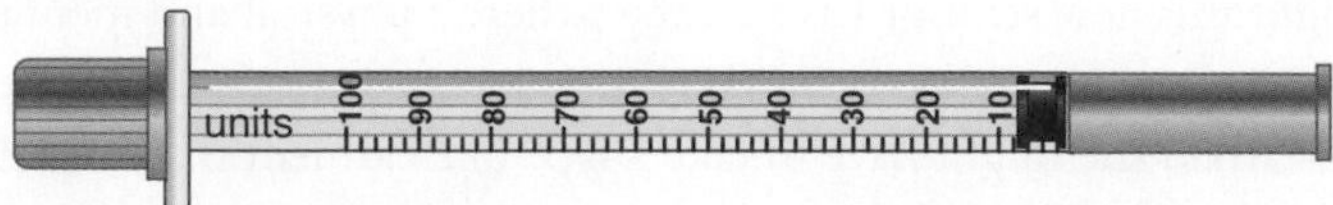

Figure 12.12: Insulin syringe (From Wilkinson HM, Treas LS: *Fundamentals of Nursing. Volume 1: Theory, Concepts, and Applications*, ed 2. Philadelphia: FA Davis, 2011, p 530. With permission.)

Other possible routes of administration include the following:

Insulin pen: A pen-like device into which an insulin-filled cartridge is placed for administration. At one end is a calibrated dial that can be rotated to the correct dosage; at the other end is a fine syringe (a pen needle) that delivers the dose when the apparatus on the pen is pushed to release it. Cartridges are removed and replaced after each use.

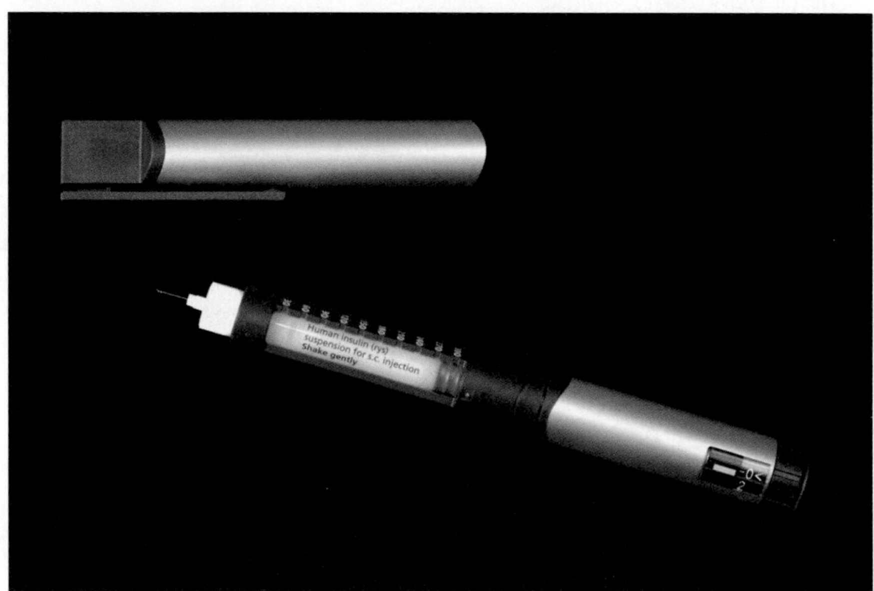

Figure 12.13: Insulin Pen (© Thinkstock)

Insulin inhaler: A device that involves the use of a powdered form of insulin, which is inhaled before meals. Insulin inhalers are very new to the market and offer a new form of treatment for diabetics.

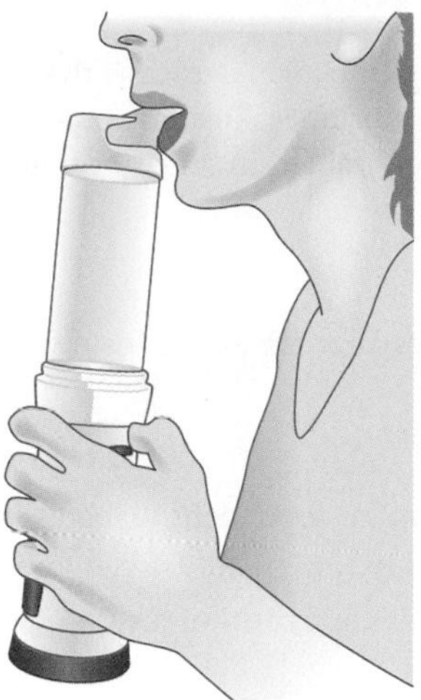

Figure 12.14: Insulin inhaler

Insulin pump: A continuous subcutaneous insulin infusion device. It consists of a number of parts: a battery-operated pump, an insulin reservoir (much like a disposable insulin cartridge), and an infusion set that consists of a **cannula** (a fine, soft, plastic needle) and tubing. The release of insulin is controlled by a computer chip to ensure a steady rate of flow. Short-acting insulin is used in the pump.

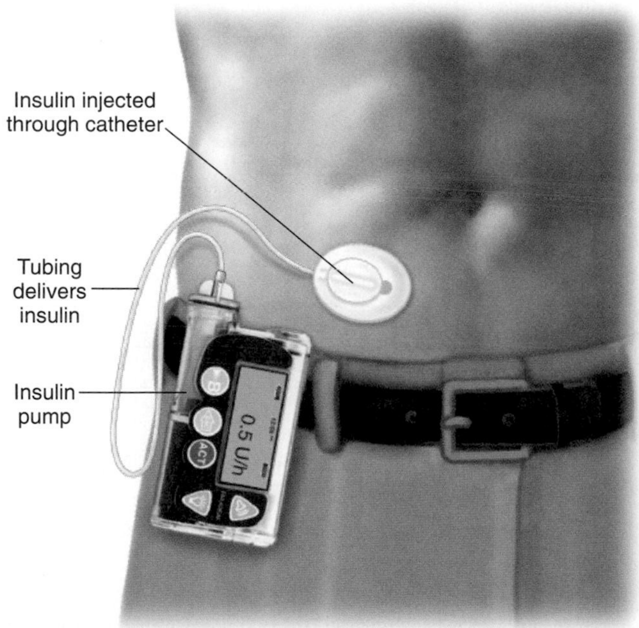

Figure 12.15: Insulin pump (From Eagle S, Brassington C, Dailey CS, Goretti C: *The Professional Medical Assistant: An Integrative, Teamwork-Based Approach.* Philadelphia: FA Davis, 2009, p 910. With permission.)

Insulin dosages

Insulins have standardized measurements, which means that all manufacturers use the same measures to identify the strength of the substance. Insulin is measured in units. For example, one type involves 100 units of insulin being contained in 1 mL of fluid; this is referred to as *U-100 insulin.* Insulin syringes use this calibration as well.

Fill in the Blanks

Fill in the blanks in these sentences that are about insulin and insulin administration. Use new terminology whenever possible.

1. Insulin syringes are ________________ by 100 units of insulin per milliliter of fluid.
2. A new form of treatment for insulin-dependent diabetes is the ________________ ________________.
3. Insulin ________________ provide a continuous flow of insulin into the body from the outside.

Name the Term

Identify the medical term that fits each definition.

1. take a breath in ________________
2. marks of measurement on a measuring unit ________________
3. a small container or casing that is loaded into a device ________________
4. variation or instability ________________
5. a blend or mixture ________________
6. life span or durability ________________
7. height or point of maximization ________________
8. needle ________________

Let's Practice

Practice your spelling. Unscramble the following letters to create medical terms.

1. g n e y s i r ________________
2. i i s l u n n ________________
3. p r t n o a i a e r p ________________
4. m i n l u h u ________________
5. r s o e v e r i ________________

Medication for diabetes

Oral anti-diabetic medication is effective only for patients with type 2 diabetes. Our patient, Stevie-Rose Davis, is being started on this type of medication. She is being prescribed Glucophage, a very common anti-diabetic medication that is designed to decrease the production of glucose and to improve insulin efficiency.

In general, oral anti-diabetic medications are used to lower blood glucose levels. In other words, they provide glycemic control when an individual's body is unable to do so. Some stimulate insulin production, whereas others perform like Glucophage (metformin). These medications are also known as *oral hypoglycemic drugs* or *oral anti-hyperglycemic drugs.*

Anti-diabetic medications come in tablet form. Some examples of these medications can be found in Table 12-10. Remember, the goal of this table is to familiarize you with just a few types of drugs. If your career leads you to work that involves medications, please seek out a medication guidebook.

Glucosamine and diabetes

In Chapter 7, it was discovered that Stevie-Rose Davis was taking glucosamine for her arthritis, and a question was raised about whether or not glucosamine might interfere with her glucose levels.

TABLE 12-10: Common Types of Anti-Diabetic Medications

Generic Name	Trade Name(s)	Generic Name	Trade Name(s)
metformin	Glucophage	tolbutamide	Aglicid, Butamide, Diabetol
acarbose	Prandase	glyburide	DiaBeta
repaglinide	GlucoNorm	rosiglitazone	Avandia
nateglinide	Starlix		

Research has found that glucosamine cannot be broken down into glucose. Therefore, it does not add glucose to the body, and it does not affect the secretion of insulin. Even so, many medical professionals are leery of the combination of glucosamine and diabetes because the research is quite new and limited. Therefore, diabetic and prediabetic patients are counseled to use this substance with caution.

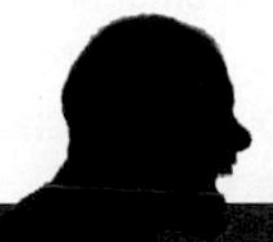

PRONUNCIATION PRACTICE

Say these words aloud to a friend or classmate if you can. You are given the phonetic pronunciation. Your instructor can help you with pronunciation,

or visit **http://www.MedicalLanguageLab.com.** 

acarbose	**ăk**´ăr-bōz
Glucophage	**gloo**´kō-fāj˝
glyburide	**glī**´bū-rīd
tolbutamide	tŏl-**bū**´tă-mīd

Patient Update

Late in the afternoon, Dr. Jensen returned on his rounds to see Stevie-Rose Davis. He found her in good spirits, oriented, and eager to go home.

"Hello again, Mrs. Davis," said Dr. Jensen. "You're looking much brighter this afternoon. How are you feeling?" he asked. Mrs. Davis smiled at him and reported that she felt very well, clearheaded, and energetic. She asked about discharge.

"Well, I've been reading your chart, and I see that your blood sugars have begun to stabilize since we've put you on a diabetic diet and given you a little Glucophage. I think the combination will work well to settle you." Mrs. Davis nodded, and Dr. Jensen went on. "I understand from the notes left by the nurses and Dr. Shawshank that this car accident was not the only stressor you were under yesterday." Again, Mrs. Davis nodded. "When you first arrived in ER, your blood glucose was low. What can you tell me about that?"

"Well, the accident with my grandson . . . I spilled the coffee on him," Mrs. Davis said while looking up at Dr. Jensen nervously, as if she was afraid that he would condemn her for this. When he did not show any signs of judgment, she continued. "It was morning, and I hadn't had any breakfast yet. I was too busy getting Clay's breakfast—that's my grandson—and feeding my husband. I was just going to give my husband another cup of coffee and sit down myself for something to eat. That's when this all happened. So, I didn't get my regular breakfast or even lunch. I'm usually careful to eat right to control my diabetes."

"I see. And then, of course, the accident occurred. Our initial treatment of providing some nutrition to you to bring your glucose levels up worked. However, it seems to have worked too well. After that initial intervention, your levels kept climbing. There were some lapses in there, but, until this afternoon, we weren't able to get your blood glucose down to an acceptable level, where we could be certain that you'd be able to manage again on your own. I expect that a good deal of that fluctuation and the high readings can be attributed to your series of stressors from yesterday." Dr. Jensen paused a moment for Mrs. Davis to think about this, and she nodded in affirmation. "Dr. Shawshank has started you on Glucophage tablets for now. I believe he spoke to you about this?"

"Yes," said Mrs. Davis. "He said that I should take this medication for a while, until I can see my primary care doctor or make some arrangements to see an endocrinologist. I have a very good relationship with my own doctor, so I'll just see her again after you release me from here," she said.

Dr. Jensen continued. "Very good. I can't stress enough the importance of making that follow-up appointment, Mrs. Davis. The goal here is to keep your diabetes at a manageable level and to prevent an escalation of symptoms or pathology."

"Yes, I hear you, doctor, and I totally agree," said Mrs. Davis. "I don't want my diabetes to get worse."

"And I think I need to add here that I do appreciate that you are under some circumstantial stress right now. I know how much you don't want to consider that this stress might also influence your mental health and any other symptoms that you might be experiencing." A cloud came over Mrs. Davis's face as Dr. Jensen spoke. "I'm not going to go there with you right now, Mrs. Davis. We don't need to talk about that issue. What I was going to suggest was that you take a very small dose of an anti-anxiety medication to help you through a stressful time right now. Short-term. What do you think about that?"

"Well, funny you should say that," said Mrs. Davis. "My daughter Evangeline and I had a long talk about that today. She made some very good points about my mood. She says that I have mood swings sometimes. And, you know, just between you and me, I think she's right. But maybe it's just because I don't sleep so well. I do have insomnia, and sometimes I have some pretty bad nightmares. I thought that this would pass in time, but it hasn't. So, I was wondering if, instead of anti-anxiety medication, might I be able to get a prescription for a sleeping pill?"

"I'm glad to hear you talking like this, Mrs. Davis. This conversation and the one we've just had about your diabetes show that you have good insight and that you are taking responsibility for your health." Dr. Jensen continued. "I'm not really an advocate for sleeping medication because some of these drugs can be quite addictive. I wonder if you would consider taking a low dose of anti-depressant medication at bedtime instead?" Instantly, a scowl came across the patient's face.

"Wait, wait," Dr. Jensen interjected, "I am not talking about anti-depressant therapy of any sort here. Certain anti-depressants are now used to promote relaxation and sleep. They have a sedative effect. An example of this is trazodone. We often use it on surgical units for preoperative patients for just this purpose. We give it only for a couple of days." Stevie-Rose's face and shoulders relaxed as she listened.

"Oh, I didn't know that," she said. "In my days as a nurse, we didn't do anything like that."

"It is quite common practice now, Mrs. Davis," said Dr. Jensen. "I'd like to suggest that you take a medication like trazodone for, say, 7 nights, and see how it works for you. This would give you time to see your primary care physician and to talk it over with her. Together, you could decide whether there were any benefits of the medication for you. Would you be interested in that?" Stevie-Rose thought it over for a few moments and then agreed.

"As long as it is on a trial basis, I'll do that," she said. "Who knows, maybe it'll work." She smiled.

"Very good then," said Dr. Jensen. "I'll write the order for you, and I'll also write the order for your discharge. How does that sound?"

"Oh, just wonderful," Mrs. Davis said. "Thank you so much. Can I phone my daughter now to come and get me?" The doctor nodded. "Oh, I've really got to go home and take care of my husband and make sure he's okay. And I just have to talk to Mickey and Steve, Clay's parents, and apologize and do whatever I can to make things right with everyone."

Dr. Jensen touched her arm gently then and said, "Mrs. Davis, you cannot be this stressed. It is very hard on your system. You've got to let the other family members pitch in as well during this difficult time. You, too, were in an accident. You, too, have health issues. You, too, need to rest and recover. Please promise me that you'll try to take it easy."

At this point, Mrs. Davis put her hand on the doctor's hand and thanked him for his kind and caring words.

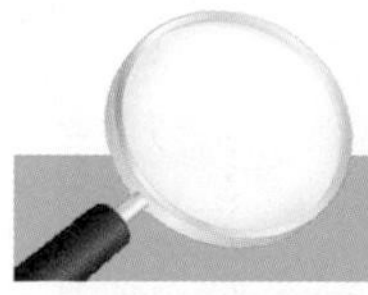

FOCUS POINT: The Anti-Depressant Trazodone

Trazodone is an oral anti-depressant that is also known by the trade names of *Desyrel, Desirel, Deprax, Trazorel,* and others. For patients who have been diagnosed with depression, doses range from 150 to 600 mg per day. However, trazodone is sometimes prescribed as a sedative. In that case, it is prescribed in doses of 25 to 75 mg once per day at bedtime. Trazodone has also been found to be effective for the treatment of panic attacks, agoraphobia, and cocaine withdrawal.

Critical Reflection Questions

You have come to the end of the chapter. Take a moment to think about what has occurred in this last Patient Update, and then answer these questions.

1. When can Stevie-Rose go home? ____________________
2. What type of prescriptions will the patient take home with her?
____
3. What arrangements for follow-up care (if any) have been made with and for this patient?
____
4. Types of diets and nutrition were introduced in Chapter 11. Stevie-Rose Davis follows one of these diets, which is mentioned in one of the Patient Updates in this chapter. Which diet is it? ____________________

Fill in the Blanks

Use a medical term to fill in each blank.

1. ____________________ is also known by the generic name *metformin.*
2. Depression is treated with an ____________________ type of medication.
3. Anti-anxiety medications can be ____________________, so it might be difficult to stop using them.
4. Sleeping medication is a type of ____________________.

CHAPTER SUMMARY

Chapter 12 has explored the language of diagnosis and medication administration by using the examples of PTSD and diabetes. Medical terminology related to medication and the treatment of these disorders was presented. Opportunities were offered to practice using new vocabulary through a variety of exercises that required critical thinking about context and word choices. The medical specialty of endocrinology was described to enhance your growing awareness of the wide variety of health-care careers that are available.

TABLE 12-11: Chapter 12 Abbreviations

Abbreviation or Acronym	Full Term	Abbreviation or Acronym	Full Term
5-HT	serotonin	FBS	fasting blood sugar (test)
ac	before meals	hr	hours
BGT	blood glucose test	IGT	impaired glucose tolerance (test)
DM	diabetes mellitus	IDDM	insulin-dependent diabetes mellitus
DM	dextromethorphan		

Continued

TABLE 12-11: Chapter 12 Abbreviations—cont'd

Abbreviation or Acronym	Full Term	Abbreviation or Acronym	Full Term
MASH	mobile army surgical hospital	PTSD	post-traumatic stress disorder
NIDDM	non–insulin-dependent diabetes mellitus	PRN	as needed; as necessary
		RBS	random blood sugar (test)
OSD	occupational stress disorder	SMBG	self-monitor blood glucose
pc	after meals	SSRIs	selective serotonin reuptake inhibitors
PPGT	postprandial glucose testing		
PO	per os (by mouth)	UGT	urine glucose test

See How Much You've Learned

For audio exercises, visit **http://www.MedicalLanguageLab.com.** 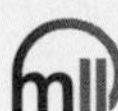

Key Terms

agent
anti-depressant
anxiety disorder
blood glucose testing
cannula
capsule
defense mechanism
denial
diabetes mellitus
diabetic ketoacidosis
dissociative states
drug chemical agent
drugs of choice
emotional numbing
flashbacks
glycemia levels
hallucinations
hemoglobin A1C
insomnia
insulin
insulin inhaler
insulin pen
insulin preparations
insulin pump
insulin-dependent diabetes mellitus (IDDM)
lancet
lorazepam
medication administration record (MAR)
mobile army surgical hospital (MASH)
neurotransmitter
occupational stress disorder (OSD)
paresthesias
PO
polydipsia
polyphagia
polyuria
post-traumatic stress disorder (PTSD)
postprandial
PRN
rights of medication administration
route of administration
sedation
sedative
selective serotonin reuptake inhibitors (SSRIs)
self-monitor blood glucose (SMBG)
serotonin
tablet
trade name
transient
transient dissociative states
type 1 diabetes
type 2 diabetes
urine glucose test strips
urine hat
voided
volume calibration

CHAPTER REVIEW

Critical Reflection Questions

Consider what you've learned in the Patient Updates and other readings to answer the following questions.

1. Who has non–insulin-dependent diabetes? ______________________________
2. What, specifically, may cause Mrs. Davis to have to take anti-diabetic medications for a while? Why? ______________________________
3. What is Dr. Shawshank's specialty? Is he a physician? ______________________________

Mix and Match

Match the synonyms by drawing lines to connect them.

blood glucose	temporary
PO	tingling
battery	means
ketonuria	series
transient	serum glucose
agent	by mouth
paresthesia	acetonuria

Build a Word

Use each set of word parts to create a proper medical term. These terms have appeared in this chapter.

1. pathy neur/o Term: ____________________ Meaning: ____________________
2. glyc/o dys -emia Term: ____________________ Meaning: ____________________
3. glycos/o uria Term: ____________________ Meaning: ____________________
4. pnea tachy Term: ____________________ Meaning: ____________________
5. phagia poly- Term: ____________________ Meaning: ____________________
6. pathy retin/o Term: ____________________ Meaning: ____________________

Critical Thinking Questions

Consider the patient who was discussed in this chapter to answer the following questions.

1. Although we do not know for certain what has caused it, Stevie-Rose Davis has a mental disorder. What is it? ____________________
2. Stevie-Rose Davis's behaviors and attitudes suggest that she was exposed to a number of serious emotional traumas when she was younger. Where and when might these traumas have occurred? ____________________

Name the Prefix

Write the prefix that fits each definition.

1. referring to pressure, particularly atmospheric pressure ____________________
2. after ____________________
3. above; above normal; in excess ____________________
4. below; below normal; diminished ____________________
5. excessive; many; multiple ____________________

Fill in the Blanks

Fill in the blanks with the missing word or words.

1. ____________ is a treatment for diabetes that is given by injections.
2. A ____________ of blood is smaller than a drop, and it is obtained by pricking the fingertip.
3. A ____________ is a small container that contains a dose of medication and that is taken orally.
4. When a medication is given by mouth, the MAR shows this route with the abbreviation ____________.

5. A ___________ can be either a tablet or a capsule.

6. A ___________ ___________ is a protective mechanism against intolerable anxiety, stress, or fear.

7. ___________ are vivid images of events that occurred in the past, but they are not quite the same as hallucinations.

8. The most effective treatment for PTSD is ___________, but this may be supplemented with medications.

Name the Device

Name each device that is described below.

1. used to prick a finger to elicit a droplet of blood

Device: ___________

2. looks like a pager and receives wireless transmissions from another device situated just under the skin

Device: ___________

3. reads a glucose strip

Device: ___________

4. comes color coded to detect ketones, glucose, and other elements in the urine

Device: ___________

True or False

Determine whether the following statements are true or false. Think very carefully before you choose "T" or "F."

1. Type 1 diabetics do not have to monitor their diets and lifestyles. T ___ F ___
2. Stress can lead to an insulin reaction. T ___ F ___
3. Type 2 diabetes begins during childhood. T ___ F ___
4. The use of defense mechanisms is a sign of mental illness. T ___ F ___
5. The defense mechanism of denial is the same as avoidance. T ___ F ___
6. Some types of anti-depressant medications can be used as sedatives. T ___ F ___

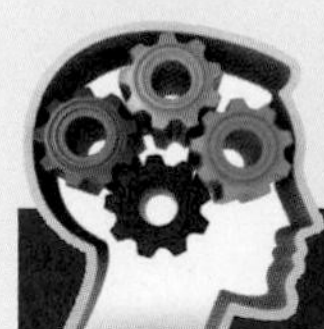

MEMORY MAGIC

If you need help remembering some important medical terms related to diabetes, try these simple memory devices.

1. the "2 ins" of insulin: insulin function

   INsul**IN** stimulates **two** things to go into cells: potassium and glucose.

2. the "3 Ps" of diabetes mellitus: signs and symptoms

   Polyuria (excessive urination)

   Polydipsia (excessive thirst)

   Polyphagia (excessive hunger)

3. **TIRED:** the signs of hypoglycemia

   Tachycardia

   Irritability

   Restlessness

   Excessive hunger

   Diaphoresis/**D**epression

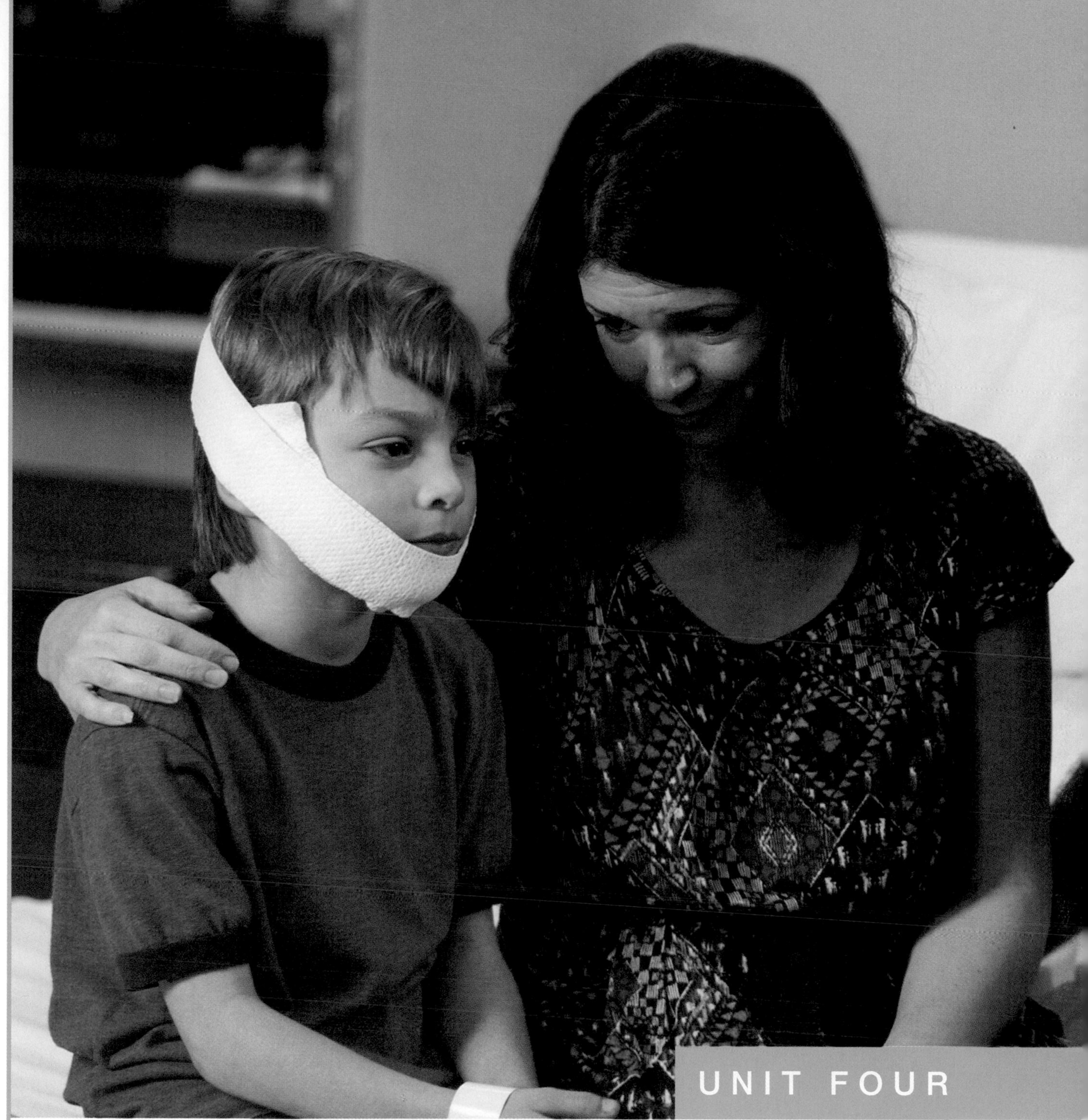

UNIT FOUR

The Language of Reparative, Restorative, and Rehabilitative Care

CHAPTER THIRTEEN

The Healing Process

Focus: Musculoskeletal and Integumentary Systems

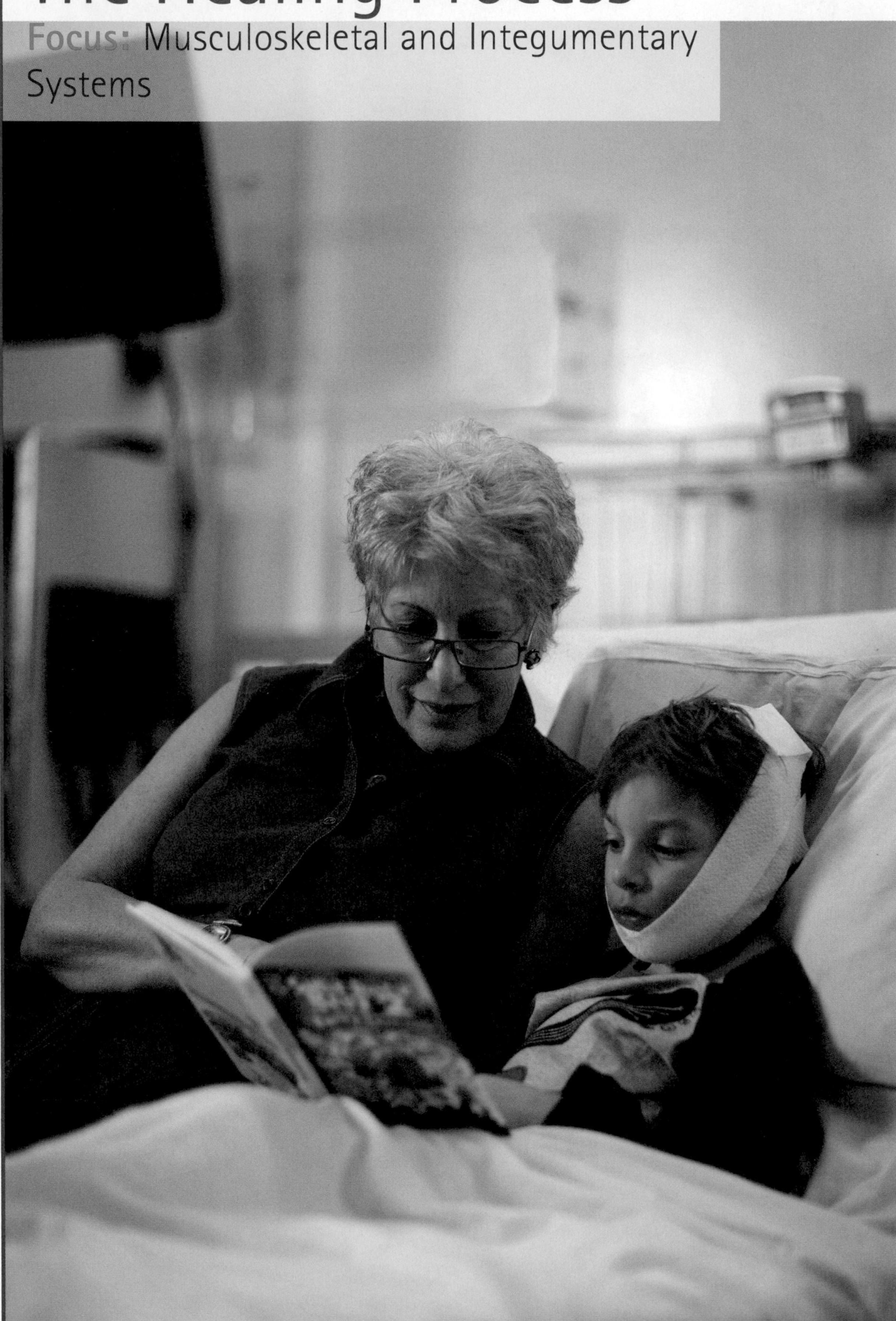

Clay Davis has been in the hospital for a week. The craniofacial surgery that he underwent to reduce the symphyseal fracture of the mandible at midline was successful, and the patient is healing well. His facial edema—particularly along the jaw lines—has begun to recede, although the swelling is still quite evident. His lower face is still somewhat discolored, but this bruising is also receding. His lips remain swollen. He is wearing a jaw wrap to maintain mandibular alignment and to apply pressure to reduce the possibility of further tissue swelling and pain.

During the past week, Clay has made steady progress. Within the first 48 hours post-op, he was able to ambulate PRN with the assistance of nurses and care aides. He has had bathroom privileges since that time, and incontinence has not been an issue. Clay's intravenous line was discontinued 48 hours ago, and his nasogastric tube was removed yesterday morning. The scald to his upper torso, which extends from the sternoclavicular joint leftward across to the upper deltoid of the left arm and down to the left nipple line, has also been healing. Skin discoloration is minimal; the redness has disappeared. Blisters have healed, and the damaged skin has begun to peel. There is no evidence to predict any residual scarring as a result of the burn.

Patient Update

Stevie-Rose and her grandson, Clay, sat together on his bed on the Pediatric Unit at Okla Trauma Center, reading Dev Pikey's *Captain Underpants.* Clay sat close to his grandmother, clearly appreciating the comfort of her presence, her soft voice, and her gentle touch. Stevie-Rose had been there when he woke up that morning, and she and his parents were taking turns being there for him. Now, after breakfast, Stevie-Rose was reading Clay a few chapters from the book. She'd been doing this for a number of days now. Clay put his hand on the book.

"Would you like me to stop for awhile, Clay?" Stevie-Rose looked down at her grandson. He nodded and attempted a little smile through his swollen lips.

"Walk around?" he asked, opening his lips just enough to express the words. Clay raised his eyebrows in hope as he did so. His grandmother smiled and stood up.

"Excellent idea, my boy. A little exercise is just what you need. Excellent for your circulation and excellent for your health!" Stevie-Rose laughed and pulled the wheelchair nearby closer to the bedside. "Hmm," she said, "I don't really think you need this anymore, but I am not a nurse working here, so I can't make that decision." She smiled at him. He pulled down his blankets and moved carefully to the edge of his bed. "Don't look down, Clay. It's not good to tip your face downward. It might hurt a bit if you do that," she cautioned warmly.

"I know, Grandma," he said. "Everyone keeps telling me that. I'm being careful." Stevie-Rose helped Clay into his robe and put on his slippers. Just as she was doing so, a nurse entered the room.

"Good morning, Clay," she said. "How are you today, my man?" Clay looked up at her and beamed. Stevie-Rose saw that her grandson clearly liked this person. "Up for your morning stroll? Well, I am happy to tell you that you don't really need this wheelchair anymore when your grandma or your mom or dad wants to walk you around. Today, you are back on your own two feet. I'm here just to stand by with you and your grandma while you start your walk together." The nurse looked up at Stevie-Rose then, confirming that her presence would be for the child's safety and that the two of them would work together. Clay's grandmother smiled back.

"You hear that, Clay? You're up and walking on your own today. That's just great!" applauded the grandmother. "This really means you're getting stronger."

The nurse lowered Clay's bed, and the two women took their positions on each side of the boy as he prepared to stand on his own.

"I can stand," he said. "I've been standing and walking this week already," he asserted proudly through slightly pursed lips. Clay stood up, and the nurse cautioned him to stand still for a moment.

"Wait now, Clay. Don't start yet. You need to stand for a minute to be sure you're not dizzy. Are you dizzy at all?" asked the nurse, leaning down to look at him directly.

"Oh, Marvane," said an impatient Clay through his slightly parted lips, "I'm 7 years old. I can stand up." His grandmother laughed.

"Yes, but you've had surgery," replied the nurse. "You've got to do things more slowly right now. You're not Superman, you know." Then she laughed, too. "Just one more thing now. When you start to ambulate—I mean walk—on your own, you've got to keep your chin up. Don't look down at your feet. Looking down will cause a feeling of pressure in your face, and that might cause it to hurt." Clay suddenly glanced at her, with his eyes wide. He jutted his chin way up, with his head tipped back, flexing the semispinalis capitis and other muscles in his neck. Marvane checked him quickly by putting a hand gently yet firmly on the top of his head. "Oops, be careful there, Clay. You shouldn't extend your jaw or neck so quickly like that. The muscles along the front of your neck and jaw will pull, and that might cause you some pain, too."

The boy stared at her with worry. "It's just a precaution, Clay," said Marvane. "Your face is still swollen, and I know it's sore. Bending your head down can put pressure on your wound and cause it to hurt. Tipping your head back quickly or too far can pull those darn muscles. You need to be careful."

Marvane looked at Clay's grandmother and nodded her head. "You see, Stevie-Rose, the accident, the jaw surgery, and even the burn across Clay's upper torso can all have an effect on the muscles beneath. You'll need to watch him for this." Clay's grandmother nodded in confirmation.

"Yes, Clay," his grandmother said firmly but kindly, "You listen to Marvane. For a while, you'll have to take everything a little more slowly than usual. Here, why don't you take my hand and we'll walk together—slowly—down to the play room?" Clay began to reach out but then suddenly withdrew his hand. With a very big smile on his face, Clay stepped tentatively and independently into the corridor.

For audio exercises, visit **http://www.MedicalLanguageLab.com.** 

Reflective Questions

Reflect on the story that you've just read.

1. What movements does the nurse, Marvane, caution Clay about because they may cause him pain?

   ____

2. According to Marvane, Clay can now walk on his own. Which term did the nurse use instead of the word *walk*?

   ____

3. The Patient Update mentions a major posterior neck muscle that is involved in tilting the head backward and looking up. Name that muscle.

   ____

Learning Objectives

After reading Chapter 13, you will be able to do the following:

- Understand and use medical terminology and language related to healing.
- Recognize, define, and use enhanced medical and anatomical terminology for the bones of the jaw and the neck.
- Recognize, define, and use medical and anatomical terminology for the musculature of the jaw and the neck.
- Interpret and use enhanced vocabulary related to tissue and tissue healing after a burn injury.
- Interpret and use terminology related to ossification (i.e., bone growth and bone regeneration).
- Recognize terms and concepts related to the stress response (i.e., flight or fight).
- Appreciate the education, training, and responsibilities of a physician assistant, particularly a pediatric physician assistant.
- Recognize and interpret the process of a clinical pathway (i.e., an algorithm).
- Recognize and understand concepts of discharge planning and follow-up care.
- Use enhanced language for body movements and directions.

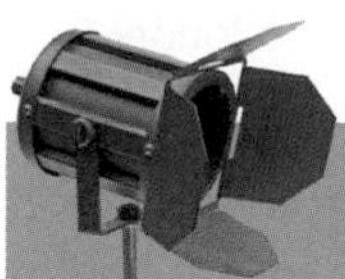

CAREER SPOTLIGHT: Physician Assistant/Pediatric Physician Assistant

A *physician assistant (PA)* is a medical practitioner who can perform most of the same tasks and duties as a fully qualified physician. Working under the supervision of a physician, the PA acts autonomously with patients but seeks consultation, guidance, and assistance from the physician, as required. The scope of practice for these health professionals includes the examination and treatment of patients, the diagnosis of illness, the requisitioning of laboratory tests and diagnostics, and the prescription of medication (in most states).

PAs study medicine in baccalaureate programs, graduate programs, or both, and they may take advanced specialty courses. They must receive their degrees in a program that is accredited by the American Medical Association, and they must pass a national certification examination.

Pediatric physician assistants (PPAs) are specialists who have undergone advanced education, training, and certification related to the health-care needs of children. These professionals may work in hospital pediatric units of all sorts (i.e., oncology, intensive care, burn wards) and in the offices of pediatricians or pediatric clinics.

Critical Thinking

Think carefully about the information in the Patient Update, and then answer the following questions.

1. Why are Clay's nurse and his grandmother staying close to Clay as he prepares to stand up and walk by himself? ____________________
2. At one point, Clay suddenly looks up at Marvane, with his eyes wide. Why do you think he does this? ____________________
3. What are the benefits of exercise for Clay as part of his postoperative recovery?

____

Key terms: postoperative healing

Key terms from the Patient Update are explained below.

"His *facial edema*..."

facial edema: fluid in the tissues of the face that causes swelling. In Clay's case, the edema is a natural response to facial trauma.

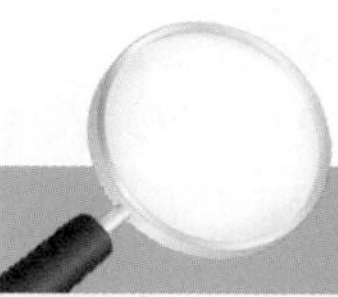

FOCUS POINT: Edema

Edema is a type of swelling that occurs in response to an influx of fluids into the intercellular or interstitial cells within the blood and the lymphatic vessels (see Chapters 3 and 5). It is not always the result of trauma. Under normal conditions, fluid levels in the blood vessels are held constant by two types of pressure: hydrostatic pressure and osmotic pressure. Working together, these two forces maintain fluid balance in the body.

Hydrostatic pressure filters fluids out of vessels, which are under high pressure, and into cells and tissues, which are low-pressure sites.

Osmotic pressure draws fluids from a place of low electrolyte concentration to one of a higher concentration (see Chapter 5).

The term *edema* is derived from a Greek root meaning *a swelling tumor,* but it no longer is indicative of a tumor. It simply means *swelling.* The adjective form is *edematous.*

- *Generalized edema* occurs throughout the body. It can be caused by organ failure, disease, pregnancy, menstrual cycles, and other factors.
- *Organ-specific edema* is located in one organ.
- *Peripheral edema* refers to the swelling of tissues in the limbs, particularly the lower limbs.
- *Localized edema* refers to edema that occurs at a specific site, which may or may not be an organ. The skin is often the site of localized edema, as in the case of an allergic reaction, a laceration, or a burn.

Table 13-1 provides examples of some of the many types of edema.

TABLE 13-1: Types of Edema

Type of Edema	Description
anasarca	severe generalized edema
pulmonary edema	edema within the lungs
pleural effusion	edema in the pleural spaces of the lungs
pericardial effusion	edema of the pericardial space around the heart
ascites	excessive fluid accumulation in the peritoneal cavity (this is often seen with severe alcoholism)
cerebral edema	edema within the brain (see Chapter 10)
lymphedema (Note that this is one word.)	excess fluid in the tissues that is localized to areas from which the lymph vessels cannot drain fluids; often seen after surgery involving the lymph nodes (i.e., mastectomy)
renal edema	edema in the tissues of the body because the kidneys are not functioning adequately; may lead to swelling of the legs and around the eyes
hepatic edema	edema in the tissues of the body because the liver is not functioning adequately; may lead to ascites and edema of the lower legs (i.e., peripheral)
cardiac edema	edema in the tissues of the body because the heart is not functioning adequately; can lead to edema of the legs and abdomen and pulmonary edema

"...wearing a *jaw wrap* to maintain *mandibular alignment*..."

jaw wrap: a type of compression bandage that fits over the head and under the jaw to reduce swelling, pain, and movement. (See the photo of Clay Davis at the beginning of this chapter.)

mandibular alignment: correct positioning of the two parts of the mandible (the lower jaw) on either side of the fracture line. When a fracture is reduced, the bones are realigned in their proper position. For healing, it is important that the bones remain in place. The metal plate that was used in Clay's surgery serves this purpose, but his jaw is still fragile at this stage of recovery.

"...able to *ambulate* PRN"

ambulate: to walk.

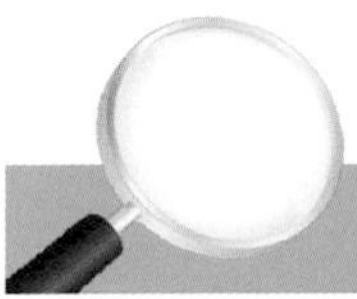

FOCUS POINT: Ambulate

The root word *ambulate* is derived from the Latin root *ambulare,* meaning *to move about.*

Derivatives include the following:

ambulance: a vehicle that is used to transport patients

ambulant: able to walk or move freely (i.e., not bedridden)

ambulation: the action of walking or moving about freely

ambulatory: able to walk or move freely

An *ambulatory care unit* is an outpatient medical care unit in which treatments (including minor surgical procedures) may be given without the full hospitalization of the patient. The term indicates that the patient comes in and goes out the same day.

"He has had *bathroom privileges*..."

bathroom privileges: medical permission given to a patient who is deemed medically well enough to get up to use the toilet and sink. Full bathroom privileges would mean that the patient can also shower on his or her own without supervision.

The term *privileges* in a medical context refers to permission granted to engage in an activity or an action.

"...extends from the *sternoclavicular joint* leftward..."

sternoclavicular joint: an anatomical point between the sternum (the breastbone) and the medial extremity of the clavicle bone; at the end of the clavicle, where it sits at a near mid-torso point (see Figure 13-1).

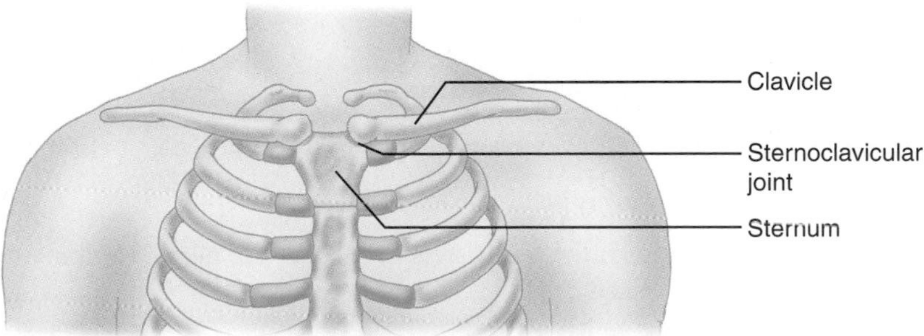

Figure 13.1: Sternoclavicular joint

"...across to the upper deltoid of the left arm and down to the left *nipple line*..."

nipple line: an imaginary horizontal line that crosses the chest through the center of both nipples. Note that the **mammillary line** is an imaginary vertical line that crosses through the center of a nipple (see Figure 13-2). These lines are used to pinpoint locations on the patient's chest.

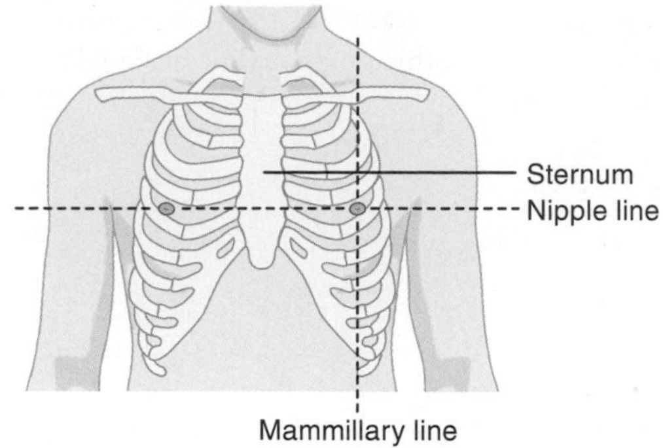

Figure 13.2: Nipple, showing the mamillary lines

Right Word or Wrong Word: *Mammillary* or *Mamillary*?

Are these two words the same? Do they have the same meaning? Are they synonyms or homonyms? Is one misspelled?

"*Skin discoloration* is minimal..."

skin discoloration: a change in skin color that is the natural result of a burn; it may be bright red (as a result of the inflammatory process) that lessens to pink and eventually turns back to the patient's normal skin tone. The epidermis produces the pigments *melanin* and *carotene*, both of which are responsible for skin color. A small amount of either leads to pale or pink skin that is colored only by the proximity of the capillaries beneath the surface. Pigments also protect deeper layers of dermis from sunburn by absorbing the sun's rays. A burn prevents the production of these pigments, and the result is a change in the pigmentation at the burn site as it heals.

carotene = a yellow or orange pigment that is found in plants. When we ingest carotene, it eventually becomes vitamin A (retinol). Too much carotene intake can cause the skin to turn yellow. This word is also sometimes spelled *carotin.*

Right Word or Wrong Word: *Carotene* or *Keratin*?

Are these two words the same? They sound very much the same. Is the difference simply a matter of spelling?

"...no evidence to predict any *residual* scarring..."

residual: remaining, lingering, or left over. (See Chapter 11 for more information about scars.)

"...confirming that her *presence* would be for the child's safety..."

presence: attendance. In this context, the term refers to the fact the nurse will remain close to the patient (i.e., within arm's reach or closer) should he faint, stumble, or suddenly face any difficulties standing or walking on his own.

"The nurse *lowered Clay's bed*..."

lowered Clay's bed: Hospital beds can be lowered or elevated by mechanical means. Whenever a patient is getting up and out of bed, the bed should be lowered so that the patient's feet can safely touch the floor before he or she attempts to stand up. This is a safety precaution to prevent slips and falls.

"...through slightly *pursed lips.*"

pursed lips: puckered lips. Clay may be pursing his lips to avoid stretching his sore lips and the tender tissues around his jaw. It may be a self-protective behavior that he may not even be aware that he is performing.

"...the nurse *cautioned him to stand still for a moment.*"

cautioned him to stand still for a moment: This phrase describes a standard procedure for ambulating a patient who has been in bed or sitting for a long period. The goal is to ensure that the patient is steady on his or her feet and not weak, dizzy, or experiencing postural hypotension before walking or being left to stand alone (see "Focus Point: Postural Hypotension").

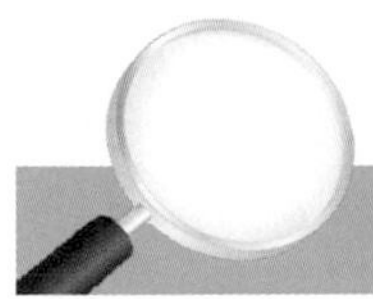

FOCUS POINT: Postural Hypotension

Postural hypotension, which is also known as *orthostatic tension,* is a transient medical condition in which there is a sudden decrease in the systolic and diastolic blood pressures to less than normal upon standing. The symptoms should recede within 1 minute.

"...will cause *a feeling of pressure* in your face, and that might cause it to hurt."

a feeling of pressure: **baresthesia**, meaning *a sense of weight or pressure.* In this case, the sensation would be caused by highly sensitive and traumatized tissue, bone, and muscle in Clay's face that have become inflamed. Recall that the body's first reaction to trauma is inflammation at the site (see Chapter 5 and 16 for more information about the inflammatory response). The term *baresthesia* is derived from the roots *bar/o,* meaning *weight,* and *esthesia,* meaning *sensation.*

"...flexing the *semispinalis capitis* and other muscles..."

semispinalis capitis: a longitudinal and deep skeletal muscle that is located in the posterior portion of the neck and that originates in the cervical spine and the thoracic spine (see Figure 13-3). It sits just under the trapezius muscle, and its movement allows for the rotation and extension of the head.

Note that the semispinalis capitis and trapezius muscles create the muscular column at the back of the neck. The semispinalis capitis muscle is just one of many muscles in the neck that promote movement and stability. For example, the sternocleidomastoid muscles, which sit bilaterally on the neck, permit the extension of the neck when the posterior muscles flex or contract (see Figure 13-4). More information about these muscles appears later in the chapter. (See Chapter 3 and 10 for a review of muscle terminology.)

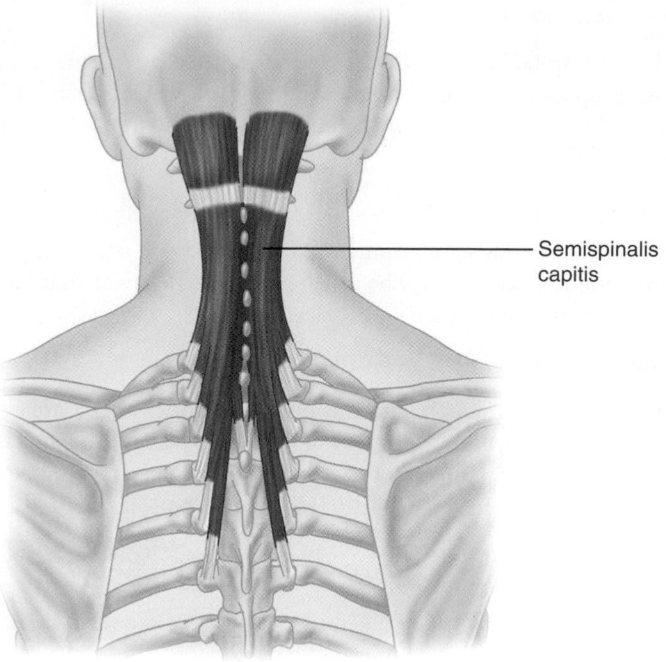

Figure 13.3: Semispinalis capitis muscle

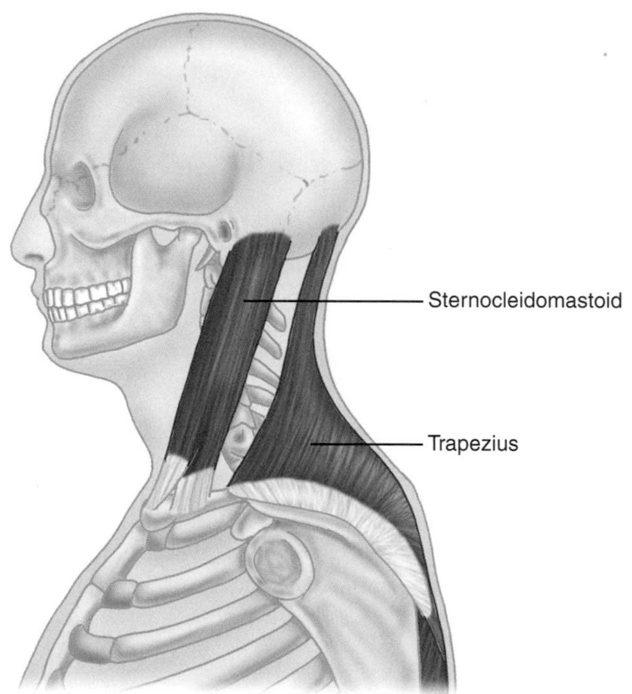

Figure 13.4: Sternocleidomastoid and trapezius muscles

Critical Thinking

Consider what you've learned about our patient, Clay Davis. You now know that he is experiencing some localized edema related to his facial trauma.

Is it likely that Clay will also experience some edema at the site of his burn? Explain your answer.

Let's Practice

Use words and phrases from the Patient Update to help you to answer these questions.

1. The nurse, Marvane, uses a synonym for the word *walk*. What is it?
   ____
2. What medical term does Marvane use to refer to the site of Clay's jaw injury?
   ____
3. What muscle did Clay extend when Marvane told him not to look down when walking?
   ____
4. What term is used to describe the situation when a wound has healed but there remains some visual evidence that it was there? ______________________________
5. Clay is wearing a bandage-like device that sits vertically along the lateral sides of his head, across the top of his head, and under his chin. What is it called, and what is its purpose?
   ____

Right Word or Wrong Word: *Postural Hypotension* or *Orthostatic Hypotension*?

Do these two terms mean the same thing?

Build a Word

Build medical terms using the word parts given, and then write the meaning of each term.

1. static hydro- Term: ______________ Meaning: ______________
2. spinal semi- -is Term: ______________ Meaning: ______________
3. -itis mammo Term: ______________ Meaning: ______________
4. current -ly con- Term: ______________ Meaning: ______________
5. tension hyper- Term: ______________ Meaning: ______________

Mix and Match

Match the word with its definition or description.

1. type of compression bandage	healthful
2. not bedridden	disfigurement
3. conducive to health	ambulant
4. action or state of walking	abnormal pigmentation
5. medical authority granted for action	privileges
6. alignment	jaw wrap
7. residual	position or placement
8. discoloration	ambulation
9. scar	enduring

Break It Down

Break down each of the following terms into its component parts: prefix, root, and suffix, as applicable. Each part has been taught in this chapter or in a previous chapter. Follow this example:

discoloration = dis + color + ation

1. sternalgia ______________________________
2. mandibulopharyngeal ______________________________
3. semispinalis ______________________________
4. baresthesia ______________________________
5. sternoclavicular ______________________________

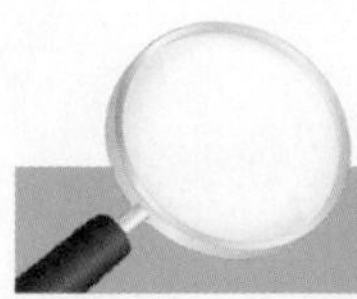

FOCUS POINT: Orthostasis and Orthostatic Intolerance

Orthostasis refers to the sensation of sudden dizziness when a person stands up too quickly.

Orthostatic intolerance is a condition in which a person cannot tolerate standing for any period of time without becoming dizzy. It is an autonomic nervous system disorder, and it is a type of *dysautonomia.* It is triggered by the change in the body's position. The symptoms of orthostatic intolerance will appear and remain unresolved for a longer period than those of postural hypotension.

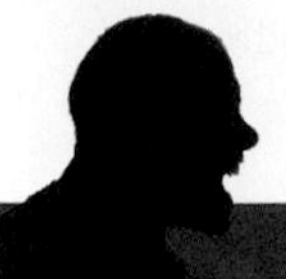

PRONOUNCIATION PRACTICE

Say these words aloud to a friend or classmate, if you can. Here you are given the phonetic pronunciation. Your instructor can help you with pronunciation,

or you can visit **http://www.MedicalLanguageLab.com.**

ambulate	ă**m**´bū-lāt	orthostatic	or″thō-**stăt**´ĭk
baresthesia	băr-ĕs-**thē**´zē-ă	semispinalis	sĕm″ē-spī-**năl**´ĭs
edematogenic	ĕ-dĕm″ă-tō-**jĕn**´ĭk	sternalgia	stĕr-**năl**´jē-ă
mandibulopharyngeal	măn-dĭb″ū-lō-fă-**rin**´jē-ăl	sternoclavicular	stĕr″nō-klă-**vĭk**´ū-lăr

The Language of Healing

As you work through the remainder of this chapter, be alert for key medical terms that are used to discuss and describe healing. Table 13-2 identifies and defines a number of these key terms. Although you will recognize a number of them, some may be new to you. Explore these—as well as their synonyms and antonyms—in preparation for the exercises that follow.

Right Word or Wrong Word: *Ameliorate* or *Meliorate*?

Which one of these words means *to make better or improve?* Do they both mean this?

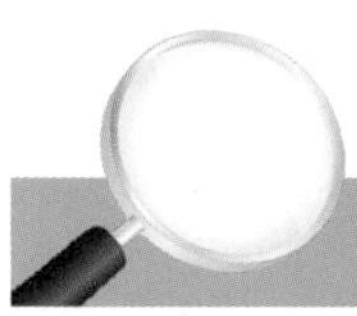

FOCUS POINT: *Heal* and *Health*

The root word *heal* originates in Old English and means *to cure or make whole.* Derivatives of this term include the following:

healer: someone who heals others

healing: the restoration of health

The root word *health* means *wholeness.* The World Health Organization defines *health* as *a state of complete physical, mental, or social well-being;* it specifies that health is not simply the absence of disease or infirmity. Derivatives of the word *health* include the following:

healthful: conducive to good health

healthy: exhibiting or promoting good health

TABLE 13-2: Medical Terms for Healing

Term and Derivatives	Meaning	Synonyms	Antonyms
alleviate alleviation alleviating	verb: to ease or reduce the intensity of (without curing)	verbs: lessen; relieve	verb: aggravate
ameliorate amelioration ameliorating	verb: to make better or more tolerable	verbs: improve, upgrade, help	verb: deteriorate
convalesce convalescing convalescence	verb: to improve	verbs: recover, recuperate, get better, pull through	verb: deteriorate
cure curative curing curable	noun: effective treatment verb: to heal	noun: remedy verb: restore to health, bring about recovery	verb: exacerbate
mitigate mitigating mitigation mitigative	verb: to alleviate	verbs: diminish, lessen, ease, relieve, dull, soften	verb: aggravate
palliate palliation palliative	verb: to soothe (without curing)	verb: soothe, relax, comfort, reassure	verb: irritate, aggravate
remedy remedial remediation	noun: cure verb: to cure; to resolve	noun: answer, resolution, treatment verb: improve, alleviate, solve, treat, fix	n/a
restore restoration restorative	verb: to fix, to bring back to a previous state	verb: re-establish, rebuild	n/a
reconstruct reconstruction reconstructive	verb: to rebuild	verb: restructure, reform, redo, repair	verb: destroy
recover recovery	verb: to get back, to get well	verb: regain, recuperate	verb: lose, deteriorate
recuperate recuperation	verb: to convalesce, to return to normal health	verb: get better, recover, get well, improve, build up strength, mend	verb: deteriorate
rehabilitate rehabilitative rehabilitation rehabilitating	verb: to restore, to return to an optimal level of functioning	verb: recover, mend, regenerate, repair, revitalize, re-establish, reintegrate, convalesce, recuperate	n/a
regenerate regenerating regeneration regenerative	verb: to renew, to reconstitute or reproduce	verbs: revive, restore, redevelop	verb: degenerate

n/a, Not applicable.

Fill in the Blanks

Use a word from Table 13-2 to complete each sentence.

1. Injured or damaged skin can ______________________ itself through a process of reconstitution.
2. Clay Davis will go home soon, where he will continue to ______________________ from his injuries.
3. Clay's nurse and his grandmother stood close to his side to ______________________ any chance of falling.

4. Initially, Clay Davis experienced a good deal of pain. He was given medication to ________________________ his pain.
5. If a patient is failing to ________________________, he or she is said to be deteriorating.
6. Burned skin is very sensitive to touch and temperature. In other words, touch and temperature ________________________ the patient's pain.

Mix and Match

Match the term on the left with its opposite on the right.

1. degenerate	recover
2. deteriorate	alleviate
3. deconstruct	recuperate
4. lose	construct
5. aggravate	regenerate

Stages of wound healing

Wound healing—including healing from a surgical wound—involves three stages: the *inflammatory phase,* the *proliferative phase,* and the *remodeling phase.*

Inflammatory phase: part of the inflammatory response to injury or infection. Monocytes (a type of leukocyte) migrate to the site to keep it free of harmful microorganisms.

Proliferative phase: begins when the wound is free of harmful microorganisms and continues until the wound site has filled with new tissue. The root word **proliferate** means *to grow by the rapid production of new cells.*

Remodeling phase: occurs when the wound is closed. Eventually, distortions and discolorations should minimize or disappear.

Assessment of healing

Patient Update

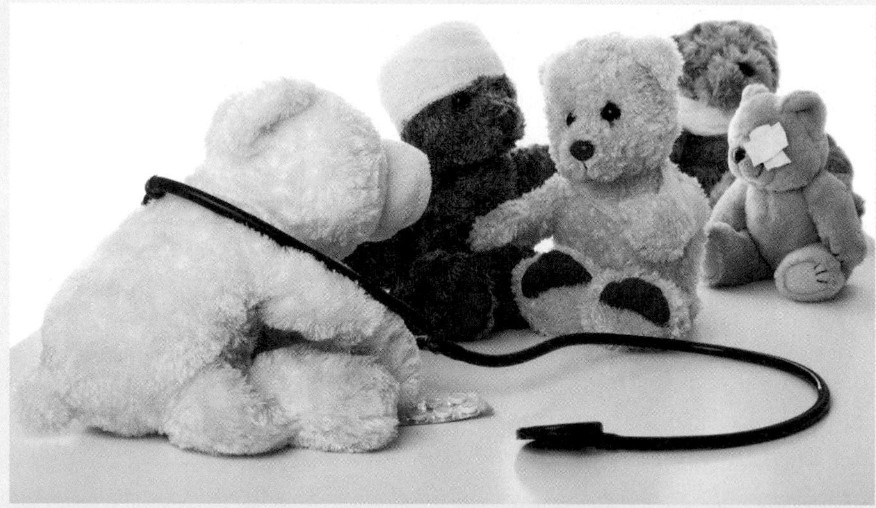

Clay enjoyed his freedom that morning at Okla Trauma Center. He was able to walk independently to the play area on the pediatric unit, where he could talk to some other children who were patients. He was playing a game with a couple of them when his parents walked in. He broke into a big smile, and he carefully got to his feet. He walked over to his parents for a big hug, but he was careful to keep his face away from direct contact with their bodies.

"I can walk on my own!" he said proudly through narrowly opened lips. "I can eat, and I can get up and down, and I can walk. Now can I go home with you?" Clay carefully peered up at his mom and dad with hope.

"Oh, I do hope so, Clay. We've just got to speak with the doctor today and find out. It should be soon now, son," said his mother, and she ran her hand through his hair gently.

"Hello, Steve and Mickey," said Stevie-Rose as she approached the couple. Mickey smiled and greeted her. Steve, on the other hand, was less cordial; he was more reserved and cool. His mother winced. "Clay's made wonderful progress, hasn't he?" she said as the four of them began to stroll back toward Clay's room. Her daughter-in-law agreed. They spotted Dr. Lincoln at the nurse's station as they passed and stopped. Mickey called out a greeting.

"Good morning, Mrs. Davis and Mr. Davis. I'm just starting my rounds here, and I'd very much like to speak with you both." Dr. Lincoln approached the four Davis family members. "Good morning, Clay," he said warmly. "Let's go down to your room, and we'll all have a talk, okay?"

When they were all settled and Clay was sitting back on his bed, Dr. Lincoln gave the family a progress report on the child. "We are very pleased with how quickly Clay's jaw is healing. You'll notice that the tissue is less inflamed and that its appearance is beginning to improve as well." Dr. Lincoln gestured toward the child's face, using both of his hands. Clay winced, wrinkling his brow as his eyes widened and his shoulders stiffened. "Don't worry, Clay, I won't touch your face without asking you first. I know it's quite tender to the touch." Dr. Lincoln turned back to Clay's parents.

"What about his lips being so swollen, Doctor?" asked Mickey.

"What about that bandage around his head? Does he have to wear that for a long while yet?" Steve asked at the same time.

"These are two very good questions. Let me answer them one at a time. Facial swelling from a jaw fracture or jaw surgery can take some time to recede. It's possible that Clay's face will seem a bit distorted and that it may be rounder and wider along the lower jaw line for another few weeks, perhaps even another month or so. But rest assured, the swelling will come down. It's caused by something we call the *inflammatory response.* This is quite normal. As you know, that jaw wrap is a device we use to keep the swelling down. It's a compression wrap that fits over the surgical area. By applying pressure to the tissue of the face, we are able to increase blood circulation to the site and to diminish swelling. By using the wrap, we accelerate the healing process and, of course, protect against the sudden jostling of the jaw as a result of coughing, sneezing, and so on. You'll recall that there are small pockets on either side of the wrap and that we inserted ice into them intermittently post-operatively for that very purpose as well." Clay's parents and grandmother nodded.

"Clay, I'd like to take a peek inside your mouth now. Let's take that wrap off for a little while." Dr. Lincoln undid the Velcro closure strips that held the jaw wrap in place over the crown of Clay's head, and he gently removed the wrap. He then put on gloves. "You're going to have to open your mouth, please, Clay. I'm going to touch your lips very gently so that I can take a look at how you're healing, okay?" Dr. Lincoln leaned over to inspect the child's mouth. Clay opened his mouth as wide as he deemed comfortable, but he seemed reluctant to open it more than an inch. "Try to open it just a little bit more, please, Clay," said Dr. Lincoln.

"Help the doctor, Clay. Open just a bit wider," coached his mother. Clay's fists clenched in fearful anticipation, and he opened his mouth wider. His fears were not realized: the action was not accompanied by excruciating pain. Clay's jaw was stiff, but, because no trauma had occurred to the temporomandibular joints, he was able to open his mouth much wider than he'd thought possible, although it was still not in a fully open position. Dr. Lincoln gently pulled Clay's lower lip away from the gums and inspected the intraoral space below. He inspected for color, which indicated circulation, and he also checked the status of the mandibular bone plating. Still gently pulling the lower lip out, Dr. Lincoln had the boy close his mouth slowly while he watched.

"Very good," said Dr. Lincoln, letting go of Clay's lip and taking off his gloves. "We have a united fracture with normal dental occlusion. This is just what we wanted, Clay," he said, as he threw his used gloves into a nearby trash basket. "I'm going to leave that wrap off you now for about an hour. I think it's time for you to begin using your jaw a bit more." Dr. Lincoln smiled, and Clay smiled back.

"Can I eat a hamburger?" the child asked, once again resorting to talking with his teeth close together and his lips open only slightly.

"Nope, no hamburger yet, young man," laughed the physician. "Maybe another two or three weeks for that yet." Clay glanced quickly at his mother for confirmation. She nodded that this was true, and Clay frowned. Dr. Lincoln turned to Clay's parents and said, "I'm going to order short periods without the wrap, about 30 to 60 minutes intermittently throughout the day. He'll need to keep it on for sleep for now. I want to get you a referral for physical therapy as well. It's important to get Clay using his jaw properly, through incremental steps. I can see already that he is favoring the injured area by trying to keep his lower jaw as still as possible. Although that is a good strategy for the early days after a trauma, it can become a habit, so it's important to nip that in the bud." Mickey and Steve nodded in agreement.

"So, Dr. Lincoln, are you saying that we can take Clay home soon?" asked Mickey.

"Yes, I think so," said Dr. Lincoln. "I'm going to go and speak with the nurses about setting up some discharge planning. They will also want to make some plans with you for Clay's care at home and to teach you some strategies that will help all of you through Clay's recovery and rehabilitation. Clay is also going to require follow-up care with a dental surgeon. Do you have one, or would you like me to refer you to one?"

"No, we don't know of one. A referral would be good, but our HMO probably has a list for us to choose from. I think we have to go that route," commented Steve. "What's going to happen with that metal bar... that plate in his mouth? Clay is still growing. Didn't Dr. Sandor say that plate would be coming out sometime?" Dr. Lincoln confirmed that the plate would be removed but stated that arrangements for this matter needed to be handled by the Davis's own health-care providers and in conjunction with their insurance plan. The parents looked at each other and nodded.

"And what about the burn, Doctor? It doesn't seem to be hurting him much at all now, and I can see that it's started to peel in places," said Clay's mother. Dr. Lincoln agreed. He explained that a pediatric physician assistant, Kuldeep Singh, was working closely on this aspect of their son's care and that Kuldeep was particularly skilled with regard to pediatric burns. The doctor further noted that he and Kuldeep were in close consultation and that they were both satisfied that the skin was healing well. He said that Mr. Singh would be in to speak with the family about how to care for Clay's wound after discharge.

"Clay," said the doctor, turning to look at the child again, "I'm going to let you go home today. What do you think about that?" Clay beamed from ear to ear, even while he was being careful to keep his lips sealed. "But you have to promise me that you'll follow all of the steps that your mom and dad will tell you about so that you can recover 100% from this accident. Will you do that?" Clay started to nod but he caught himself, and he put his hand up warily to his jaw. Instead, Clay smiled and gave the doctor a thumbs-up sign to show that he agreed. "Great," said Dr. Lincoln. "Now, do you have any questions for me, young man?"

"Can you tell my dad something?" Clay said in a soft, firm voice through parted lips. "I want you to tell my Dad that it's not Grandma's fault I got hurt," he said, tears welling up in his eyes. He reached out to touch the doctor. "Tell my Dad it's not her fault." Clay and Dr. Lincoln turned to look at Clay's parents and grandmother. Mickey had tears in her eyes and was looking at her husband, Steve. Stevie-Rose, Clay's grandmother, stood at the foot of the bed; she was silent and very pale. "Tell Dad that I was running and had an accident and that there was a bee in the car after that," Clay said, through tears and a stiff jaw. Looking up at the doctor, he whispered, "I'm afraid of bees."

"Yes, Clay, I'll do that," the physician said, reaching out to hold Clay's hand and squeeze it gently. Dr. Lincoln turned to Steve Davis and said firmly yet gently, "Sir, I know that this has been very difficult situation for everyone involved here, but the scald and the crash were accidents. Your son came to us through circumstances that were not predictable. No one is to blame, okay?" Stevie-Rose looked at her son, Steve, broke into tears, and fled the room. Dr. Lincoln smiled down at Clay reassuringly. "Clay's on the mend now. That should be everyone's focus. I'm going to write up the discharge orders, and the nurses will be in to speak with you about that shortly. I would suspect you can take your boy home sometime after lunch today." Dr. Lincoln turned, smiled at Clay, and winked, and then he walked over to the sink to wash his hands. When he was done, he said, "You take care of yourself, young man," and he waved to Clay as he left the room.

Reflection Question

Answer this question on the basis of what you've just read.

Why doesn't Dr. Lincoln speak with the family in depth about the patient's burn wound? Why does he defer this responsibility to Kuldeep Singh?

Critical Thinking

To answer these questions, you need make some inferences about what you've learned in the Patient Update.

1. Why does Dr. Lincoln wink at Clay before he leaves? Is his winking just about the discharge, or does he also have another reason for winking at the boy?
   ____

2. You have just been given another clue about what may have caused the motor vehicle accident that the Davis and Loeppky families have been involved in. What clue did Clay reveal? ______________________________

Key terms: healing assessment

Key terms and other important language from the Patient Update are italicized in the example and highlighted below with the explanation.

"...as his *eyes widened* and his *shoulders stiffened.*"

eyes widened, shoulders stiffened: symptoms of the human stress response (i.e., the fight-or-flight response) in which the body prepares to protect itself from real or perceived threats or *stressors*. For more information about the human stress response, see "Focus Point: The Stress Response" and Figure 13-5.

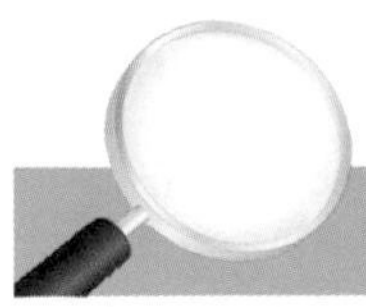

FOCUS POINT: The Stress Response

When a person is threatened or feels threatened, the body's homeostatic mechanisms take immediate action to try to regulate the body's internal environment and to ensure the individual's survival. An alarm reaction occurs within the body, which sets off the stress response; this is a series or syndrome of responses for dealing with the threat:

Real or perceived threat → Causes an alarm
↓
Physiological responses (autonomic nervous system arousal and neuroendocrine changes)
↓
Behavioral responses (fight or flight: aggression, avoidance, and disorganized activity)
↓
Cognitive responses (impaired concentration, misinterpretation, and memory difficulties)

During the alarm stage, the sympathetic nervous system (a subsystem of the autonomic nervous system) is activated. It releases a variety of hormones through the hypothalamus, the posterior pituitary, the anterior pituitary, the adrenal cortex, and the adrenal medulla (see Chapters 4 and 10). These hormones contribute to the body's ability to fight the threat or flee from it (i.e., flight). However, if the body is overstimulated, the threatened person may experience an inability to react, thereby seeming to freeze.

"...*tender to the touch.*"

tender to the touch: an assessment term that describes a hypersensitivity of the skin or its underlying structures so that the skin feels sore when touched. The tenderness or pain can be the result of damage or insult to the nerves in that area.

"...face will seem a bit *distorted...*"

distorted: altered in shape. Distortion of shape resulting from surgery or injury is most often a result of tissue inflammation and should remedy itself over time. In the case of our patient, Clay Davis, it is very likely that the lower portion of his face—particularly around the jaw line—will remain distorted for a few months. This condition will be exacerbated when the plate over the fracture line is removed. At that time, the tissue might once again become inflamed.

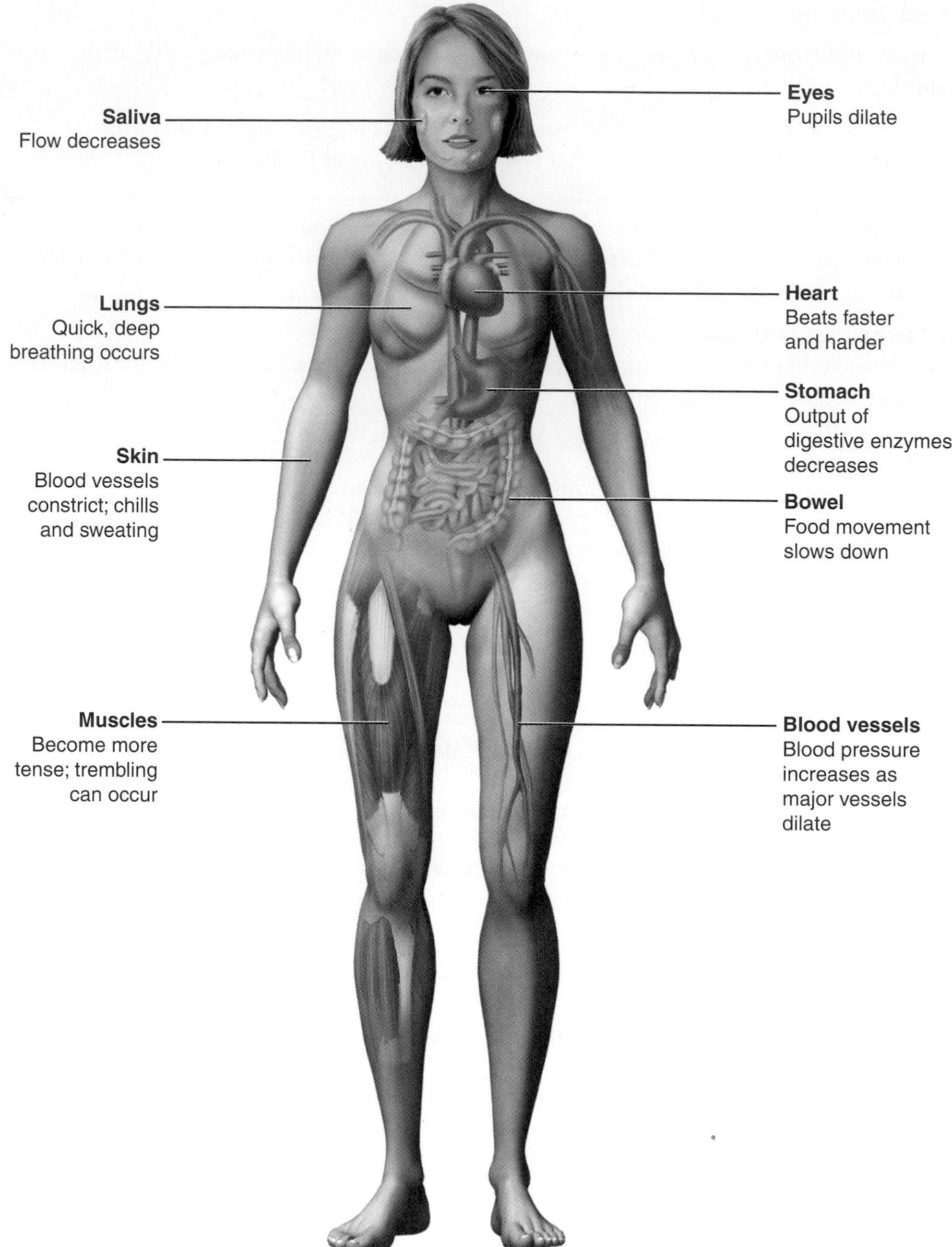

Figure 13.5: Physiology of the stress response

"... accelerate the *healing process* ..."

healing process: a natural process by which the body (or mind) heals or restores itself to health.

"... over the *crown* of Clay's head ..."

crown: the top, the uppermost part, or the highest point.

"He then *put on gloves.*"

put on gloves: a standard precaution to prevent the spread of microorganisms and pathogens when coming into contact with body fluids. (For more information about medical asepsis and infection control, see Chapter 5.)

"... not *accompanied by excruciating pain.*"

accompanied by: a medical expression that is used to describe how one symptom, illness, or process often includes or goes along with another; they are found together.

excruciating pain: pain that is unbearable. Excruciating pain requires medical or pharmacological intervention.

"Clay's jaw was *stiff*..."

stiff: inflexible or difficult to flex. In this context, the muscles of Clay's jaw are stiff as a result of a lack of use (i.e., he's holding them stiffly in place), blunt force trauma to his lower face that occurred during the accident, and surgical trauma.

"... inspected the *intraoral space* below."

intraoral space: in this context, the reference is to the surgical site within Clay Davis's mouth (see Figure 13-6).

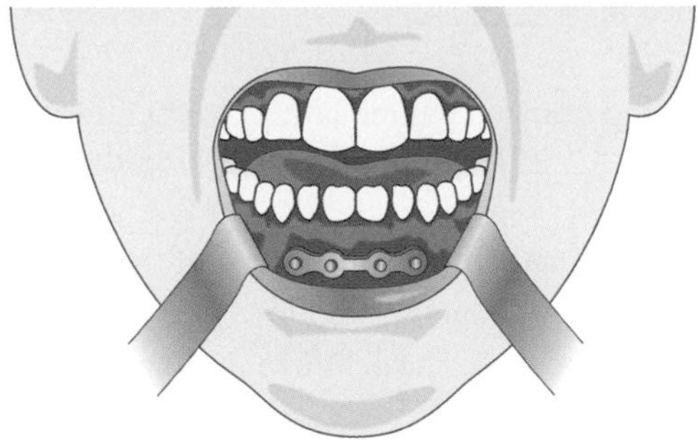

Figure 13.6: Jaw injury, with titanium plate in the intraoral space

"... *united fracture* with *normal dental occlusion.*"

united fracture: a fracture in which the broken bone is healing (i.e., becoming one again).

normal dental occlusion: a normal bite.

".... get you a referral for *physical therapy*..."

physical therapy: a field of health care that is dedicated to rehabilitation from a state of physical dysfunction to one of physical function (see Chapter 15).

".... through *incremental steps.*"

incremental steps: a process in which a goal is achieved one step at a time. Healing occurs in incremental steps. For an example, see "Focus Point: Stages of Wound Healing."

".... he is *favoring* the injured area..."

favoring: in medical context, this word means using extra caution when moving an injured part of the body.

"... the *early days* after a trauma ..."

early days: an expression meaning *the first few days.*

"... some *discharge planning.*"

discharge planning: a protocol and procedure in which health-care professionals work collaboratively with the patient and the patient's family to plan for follow-up care and a period of recovery. Discharge planning should always begin at the time of the first encounter with the patient. The discharge plans form part of the overall goals or *desired patient outcomes* throughout treatment.

"... our *HMO* probably has a list ..."

HMO: health maintenance organization. An HMO oversees the health plans and health needs of the members who subscribe to it. It is a form of health insurance.

"... that metal bar ... that *plate* in his mouth ..."

plate: in this context, this term refers to the steel plate that is screwed into Clay's mandible.

Fill in the Blanks

Use new terminology to fill in the blanks with the proper term.

1. In dentistry, braces are often used to reduce an abnormal dental ____________________.
2. The young woman seemed to be ____________________ her right foot when she walked, as if it might be injured.
3. When a patient is recovering from a fractured jaw, his or her diet begins with fluids and moves by ____________________ to soft foods, minced foods, and so on, until he or she can eat solid foods again.
4. An ankle swells when it is sprained. This is an example of the ____________________ response.
5. When a fracture is reduced, it begins to heal. When healing occurs, the bone becomes one again. In other words, it is ____________________ once again.
6. When faced with a real or perceived threat, the ____________________ system responds immediately.
7. A basic and highly effective procedure that helps to reduce the spread of infection is to wear ____________________ when coming into contact with ____________________.
8. ____________________ should begin when the patient or client first comes into care.

Critical Thinking

Refer to the features and diagrams in this section to answer the following questions. You will need to recall medical terms from previous chapters and apply them here.

1. During the stress response (i.e., the fight-or-flight response), does a person experience tachycardia or bradycardia? ____________________
2. What is the medical term for the type of breathing that occurs when a person is experiencing the alarm stage of the stress response? ____________________
3. Blood vessels constrict during the stress response. What is the medical term for this constriction of blood vessels? ____________________

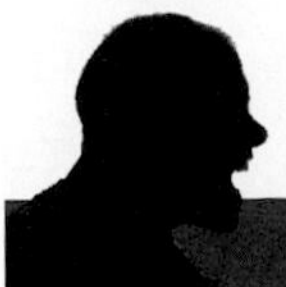

PRONOUNCIATION PRACTICE

Say these words aloud to a friend or classmate, if you can. Here you are given the phonetic pronunciation. Your instructor can help you with pronunciation,

or you can visit **http://www.MedicalLanguageLab.com.**

ameliorate	ă-**mēl**′yō-rāt	occlusion	ŏ-**kloo**′zhŭn
autonomic	aw-tō-**nŏm**′ĭk	tachycardia	tăk″ē-**kăr**′dē-ă
convalescence	kŏn″văl-**ĕs**′ĕns	tachypnea	tăk″**ĭp**′-nē′ă
meliorate	**mēl**′yō-rāt	vasodilation	văs″ō-dī-**lā**′shŭn
mitigate	**mĭt**′ĭ-gāt		

Bone healing

All fractures heal in three incremental yet overlapping phases that are very similar to those of wound healing; however, **bone healing** includes the phases of *inflammation, production,* and *remodeling.* The process in general takes 6 to 8 weeks, but this depends on the severity of the fracture, the health of the bone, and the overall health of the individual. *Bone regeneration* is another medical term that is used to refer to the healing process that occurs when a bone is traumatized. For children, bone healing can be much quicker, occurring in approximately 4 to 6 weeks.

The *inflammation stage* begins immediately at the time of fracture. Blood flow to the area increases rapidly and causes swelling, bleeding, and clotting at the site. These processes provide the foundation for healing to begin.

The *bone production stage* occurs as clotted blood is eventually replaced with fibrous tissue and cartilage. Together, these are called **soft callus**. Over time, the soft callus is replaced with **hard callus** (hard bone).

The *bone remodeling stage* can continue for several months. The bone itself becomes more compact and therefore stronger. It regains its original shape (or something very close to it). Blood supply to the site returns to normal.

As you know, Clay Davis has a fracture of his mandible, which is currently plated to hold the fracture in place long enough for bone regeneration to occur. The complication in this case involves the fact that, while the bone is growing to heal, the jaw is also growing as a normal function of childhood development. Because of this complication, it will be important for the dental surgeon to follow up with Clay Davis after his discharge from the hospital. The plate that has been surgically placed will need to be removed to allow the growth and development of the jaw to proceed. After Clay recovers from this injury, he may need to see an orthodontist to ensure that there are no faciolingual abnormalities or problems with the positioning of his teeth (see Chapter 6). Clay is 7 years old. By this age, he will have some of his permanent teeth (i.e., these teeth will have erupted), and his jaw growth will have become dynamic or active.

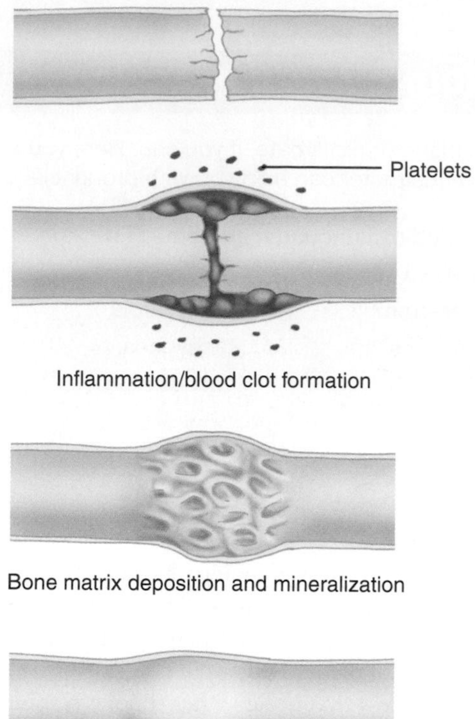

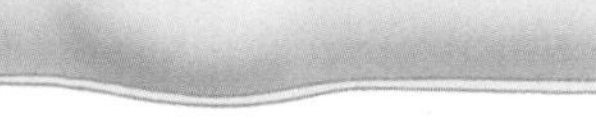

Figure 13.7: The bone healing process

Bone growth: ossification

Chapters 4 and 10 introduced key terms for the anatomy and physiology of the **ossa** (bones) and the medical field of orthopedics. It is also important to understand the medical terminology that pertains to bone growth and regeneration.

Ossification is the medical term for the process of bone creation (i.e., the process of the synthesis of bone from cartilage). A synonym for *ossification* is *osteogenesis*. Bones begin to form in the fetus as soft **cartilage**, a fibrous tissue. Throughout infancy and childhood, cartilage is transformed into bone through a process of **calcification** or hardening. There are two types of ossification, although bones are generally formed by a combination of the two:

Intramembranous ossification involves the cells of the embryo that are called **mesenchyme cells.** These cells are found within the mesoderm (an inner layer of a cell), and they eventually develop into connective tissues of either bone or blood.

Endochondral ossification is the process by which cartilage is replaced by bone, thus forming the skeleton. During this process, **osteoblasts** (primitive cells that make bones) develop into mature bone cells. These bone cells embed into the calcified portions of the evolving bone.

In the human embryo, the creation of bone and skeleton follows these steps: *morphogenesis* (growth) to *modeling* (shaping) and then *remodeling* (the final stage that identifies function).

Mature (fully developed) bone is a form of living tissue. It consists of *proteins, collagen, fibroblasts,* and an *extracellular matrix.* You will learn more about collagen later in this chapter.

fibroblasts: specialized cells that are capable of producing collagen and that are critical for wound healing and skin repair.

extracellular matrix: a substance that surrounds all cells found within the tissue. The structural support for them.

Ossification

Cartilage model forms

Blood vessel

Compact bone develops starting at primary ossification sites

Cavity

Spongy bone develops at secondary ossification sites

Cartilage growth plate

Compact bone containing osteocytes

Cartilage growth plate

The growth plates promote longitudinal growth until young adulthood

Fetus: first 2 months

Fetus: at 2–3 months

Childhood

Adolescence

Figure 13.8: The ossification process

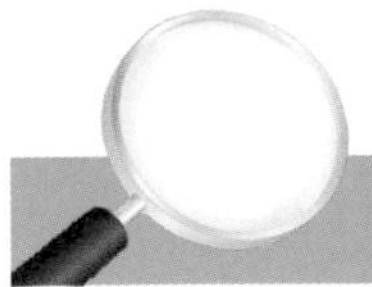

FOCUS POINT: Morphogenesis

Morphogenesis refers to a series of processes that enable body tissues and organs to grow and develop. Morphogenesis begins in the embryo, where it is referred to as *embryogenesis,* but it continues throughout life as body structures degenerate, regenerate, and maintain themselves.

The term can be broken down into the following roots:

morpho + genesis = morphogenesis
↓ ↓
(form) (birth)

A synonym for *morphogenesis* is *morphosis.*

Muscle healing

Our patient, Clay Davis, is recovering from trauma to the muscles and bones of his face. These injuries have a secondary impact on the muscles of the neck. Muscles of the neck do not simply connect to the head; they also connect to the spine and the shoulder. To completely understand the healing process that the patient will undergo, you need to understand the terminology for the musculature of the jaw and the neck. (To review other muscles and muscle terminology, see Chapter 3.)

The term **musculature** refers to the arrangement of muscles in the body. The root word is **muscle,** meaning *tissue composed of contractile cells and fibers that permit movement.*

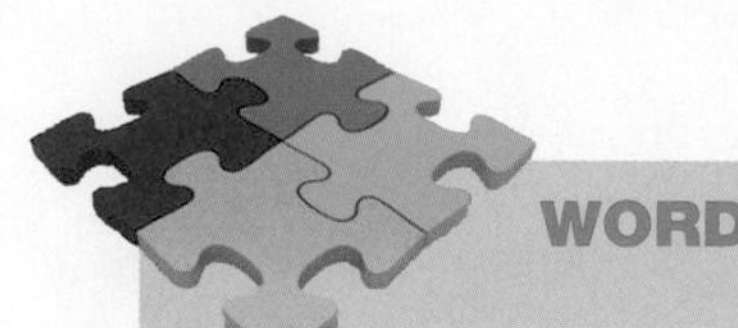

WORD BUILDING: Formula for Creating Words with the Combining Form *Musculo*

muscle = *tissue composed of contractile cells and fibers that permit movement.* The combining form of muscle is *muscul/o.*

musculo + tendinous = *musculotendinous*

Definition: pertaining to or containing both muscles and tendons. (The second root word, *tendinous,* means *resembling, pertaining to, or composed of tendons.*) *adjective*

Example: *Musculotendinous* stiffness can occur after a period of stretching or, conversely, after a period involving a lack of use of the muscles and tendons.

musculo + tropic = *musculotropic*

Definition: affecting or acting on muscle tissue, particularly with a stimulating effect. (The second root is *tropic,* meaning *turning.*) *adjective*

Example: Medications that reduce muscle spasm are *musculotropic* relaxants.

Musculature of the jaw

The function of jaw muscles is **mastication** or chewing, but the jaw muscles also play a significant role in craniofacial growth. They can affect the shape of the mandible by exerting pressure on it as it grows, and they can pull the mandible out of alignment with the maxilla bone. To review the anatomy of the jaw, refer to Chapters 6 and 11. For a quick visual review, see Figure 13-9.

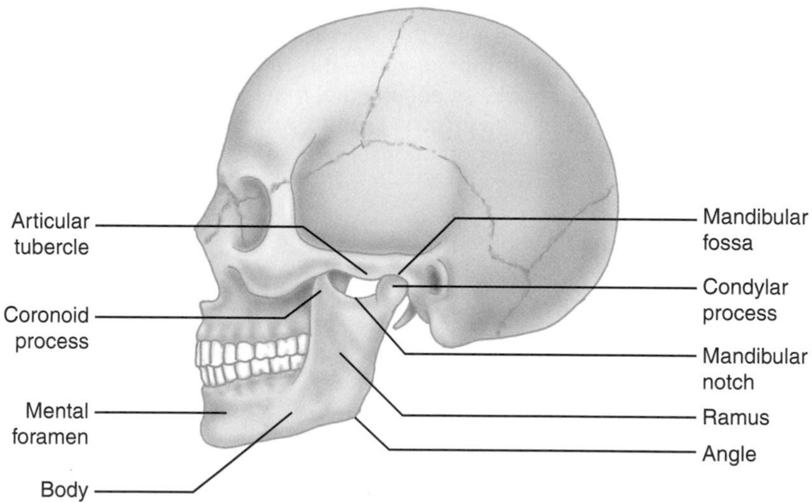

Figure 13.9: Review: anatomy of the jaw

Muscles of mastication

The process of chewing or masticating requires the muscles of the maxilla and the mandible to work cooperatively to open and close the mouth. These muscles will play a significant role in Clay Davis's recovery. In total, there are four core muscles of mastication: the *medial and lateral pterygoid*, the *masseter,* and the *temporalis* muscles. Table 13-3 describes the functions of these muscles. Figures 13-10 and 13-11 show where the muscles are located in the cranium.

TABLE 13-3: Core Muscles of Mastication

Muscle of Mastication	Origin and Insertion	Function and Movement
Temporalis	• originates along the temporal bones of the skull • inserts just above the mandible (see Figure 13-10)	• allows the mandible to be kept closed • facilitates the elevation (bringing a lowered mandible back up to normal position) and retraction of the mandible • assists with the grinding of food
Medial pterygoid	• originates at the maxilla and across the palate • inserts at the medial surface of the ramus and the angle of the mandible (see Figure 13-10)	• allows for jaw closing, protrusion (moving forward) and lateral movement (side-to-side motion)
Lateral pterygoid (LPM)	• originates at the pterygoid process and the sphenoid bone (the butterfly-shaped bone at the base of the skull) • inserts into the mandible and articular disk (see Figure 13-10)	• assists with mandible protrusion (moves the jaw forward and opens it) • a primary muscle of the temporo-mandibular joint
Masseter	• originates at the zygomatic arch (cheekbone) • inserts laterally on the mandible (see Figure 13-11)	• a series of three muscles: superficial, intermediate, and deep • elevates (opens) the jaw and extends and protracts it

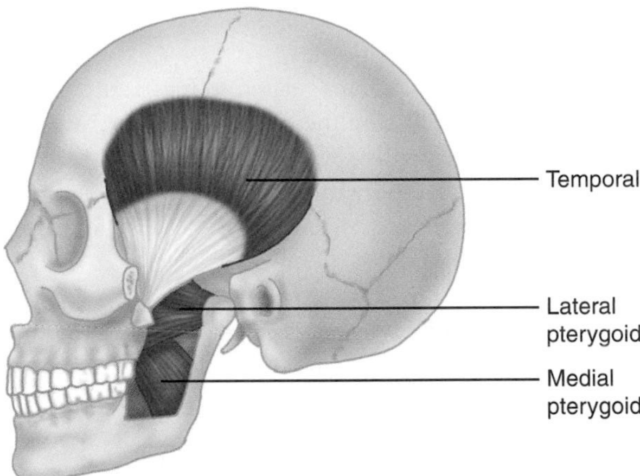

Figure 13.10: The muscles of mastication, part A

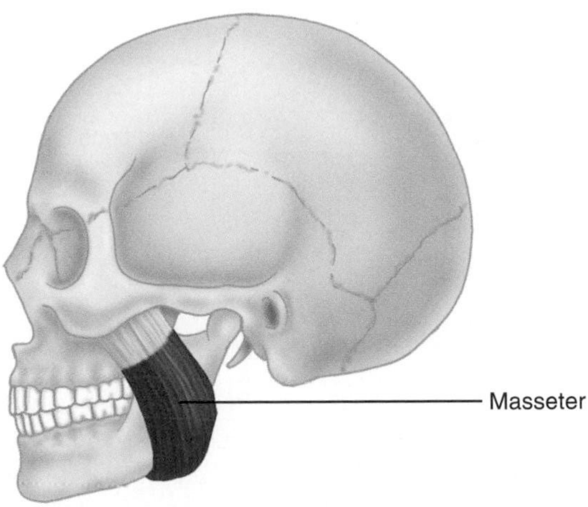

Figure 13.11: The muscles of mastication, part B

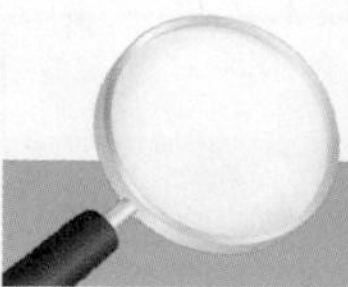

FOCUS POINT: Propalinal

The term *propalinal* describes movement that is backward and forward. The term can be applied to this movement of the jaw. The word deconstructs as follows:

pro +	palin +	al =	propalinal
↓	↓	↓	
(before)	(back)	(pertaining to)	

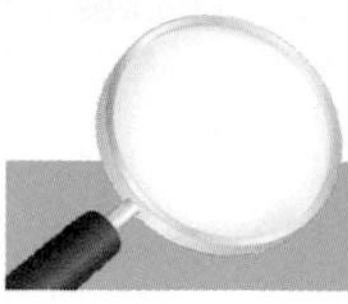

FOCUS POINT: Process

In anatomy, the term *process* refers to an appendage, outgrowth, or projection of tissue from a larger body of tissue. An example is the *pterygoid process* of the jaw. The pterygoid process consists of two long, bony plates that extend laterally down along the sphenoid bone.

In biology, the term *process* refers to any chemical reaction that causes a transformation.

Accessory muscles of mastication

Table 13-4 provides more terms and descriptions related to mastication and the jaw. It focuses on cheek muscles called **buccinators,** as well as on the neck muscles that are involved in chewing and swallowing. Many of these muscles are involved with the **hyoid bone** (see Figure 13-12). This bone sits at the anterior midline of the neck, and its function is to anchor the tongue. The terminology in Table 13-4 will be of particular interest to those who are studying for careers in dentistry, speech pathology, rehabilitation therapy, and physical therapy.

The term **hyoid** means *u-shaped.*

Note: There are many more muscles in the head, face, and neck. Only those that are relevant to our patient, Clay Davis, are explored here to help you understand his condition and to illustrate how complex his recovery from the symphyseal fracture may be.

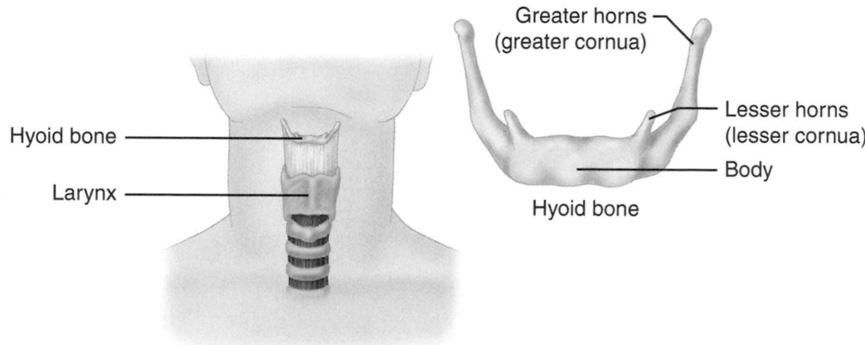

Figure 13.12: Hyoid bone

TABLE 13-4: Accessory Muscles of Mastication

Accessory Muscle	Origin and Insertion	Function and Movement
Digastric	• originates on the underside of the mandible (the digastric fossa), where it sits bilaterally to the symphysis menti (see Chapter 6) • inserts at the intermediate tendon connected to the hyoid bone (see Figure 13-12)	• depresses (lowers) the mandible
Mylohyoid (refers to both the molar region of the mandible and the hyoid bonc)	• originates inferior to the digastric muscle and spans the underside of the mandible • inserts at the hyoid bone from the underside and into the mental process (the chin) from above	• forms the floor of the mouth • supports the floor of the mouth when the mandible is depressed, particularly when swallowing or talking
Geniohyoid	• originates on the inner surface of the mandible • inserts into the hyoid bone	• depresses the mandible when talking or swallowing • elevates the tongue
Buccinators (situated between the maxilla and mandible along the cheek; the muscles of the cheek)	• originates on the buccinator ridge of the mandible, the alveolar process of the maxilla, and the pterygomandibular ligament (see Figure 13-13) • inserts at the angle of the mouth	• compresses the cheeks to prevent the accumulation of an excess of food in the oral cavity (the vestibule of the mouth) and to enable sucking; the action of sucking retracts the angle of the mouth
Orbicularis oris (a sphincter muscle; note that the term *orbicularis* means *surrounding an orifice*)	• originates at border of the maxilla and laterally to the midline on the mandible • inserts in a circumference around the mouth and into adjacent muscles	• helps with the opening and closing of the mouth • controls the movements of the lips and cheeks • permits the action of pursing and protruding the lips; this muscle is used when a person whistles

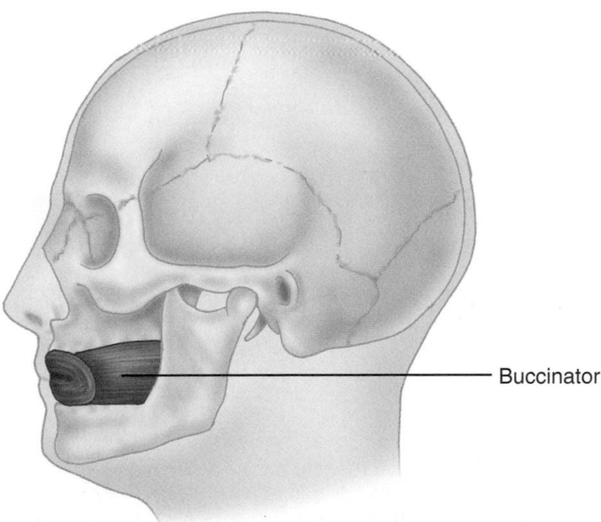

Figure 13.13: Buccinator muscle

Reflective Questions

Answer these questions on the basis of what you've learned about the four muscles of mastication.

1. Which muscles of mastication open the jaw? ____________________
2. Which muscle moves the jaw laterally? ____________________
3. Name the muscles of mastication that are responsible for closing the jaw.
____

Let's Practice

Read each description of a movement, and then write the correct medical term to identify each type of movement.

1. mandible extends forward, lower teeth become prominent ____________________
2. mandible is extended, chin is jutting out and then pulled into normal position
____
3. jaw is struck by a punch to the side of the face, mandible moves sideways
____
4. tongue is extended outside of the mouth and lips ____________________
5. small baby starts to cry, lips are still closed, bottom lip juts out ____________________
6. mandible moves back and forth, side to side: ____________________
7. temporomandibular joints open, roof of mouth seems to rise, mandible lowers, masseter muscle brings jaw back up to normal position ____________________
8. floor of mouth lowers to facilitate swallowing ____________________

Break It Down

Break down each of these names for muscles into their word parts (prefix, root, and suffix), and then write the meaning of each word part.

1. digastrics Word parts: ____________ Meaning: ____________
2. pterygomandibular Word parts: ____________ Meaning: ____________
3. mylohyoid Word parts: ____________ Meaning: ____________

FOCUS POINT: The Masseter Muscle

An interesting fact about the *masseter muscle* is that it is the strongest muscle in the human body.

Let's Practice

Read each description, and then name the muscle being described.

1. keeps jaw closed and helps with grinding food ____________________
2. forms the floor of the mouth and facilitates swallowing ____________________
3. muscles of the check ____________________
4. allows the jaw to move from side to side ____________________
5. allows you to purse your lips or smile, with the help of the buccinators ____________________

PRONOUNCIATION PRACTICE

Say these words aloud to a friend or classmate, if you can. Here you are given the phonetic pronunciation. Your instructor can help you with pronunciation,

or you can visit **http://www.MedicalLanguageLab.com.** mll

digastric	dī-**găs**´trĭk	morphogenesis	mor″fō-**jĕn**´ĕ-sĭs
endochondral	ĕn″dō-**kŏn**´drăl	mesenchyme	**mĕs**´ĕn-kīm
hyoid	**hī**´oyd	musculature	**mŭs**´kū-lă-chŭr
intramembranous	ĭn″tră-**mĕm**´bră-nŭs	musculotendinous	mŭs″kū-lō-**tĕn**´-dĭ-nŭs
mylohyoid	mī″lō-**hī**´oyd	musculotropic	mŭs″kū-lō-**trŏp**´ĭk
masseter	măs-**sē**´tĕr	orbicularis	ŏr-bĭk″yă-**lār**´ĭs
mastication	măs-tĭ-**kā**´shŭn		

Musculature of the neck

All of the muscles of the neck play a role in facilitating the motion of the neck (i.e., the cervical region of the spine), and they also aid in its postural control (i.e., keeping the head and neck erect).

Superficial muscles lie closest to the skin. The trapezius muscle is an example.

Deep muscles of the neck are farthest from the surface. These include all of the rectus and obliquus muscles.

Table 13-5 identifies the muscle groups of the neck and their functions. As you study this table and Figure 13-14, consider how these muscles may be affected when our patient, Clay Davis, attempts to mediate any pain and discomfort that he might experience as a result of moving his head up and down or from side to side. These are the muscles that will be involved. Favoring them (i.e., not using them to their full capacity) can lead to stiffness over time. This stiffness, in turn, can lead the patient to not want to use those muscles, even as his jaw heals. For this reason, physical therapy may be warranted as part of this patient's post-discharge follow-up care. For an example, see "Focus Point: The Trapezius Muscle."

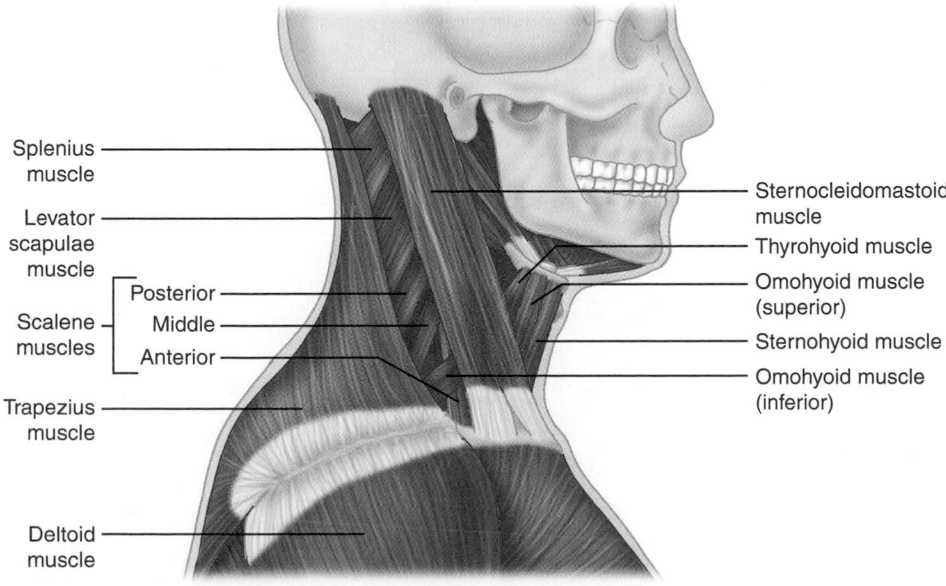

Figure 13.14: Musculature of the neck

TABLE 13-5: Muscle Groups of the Neck

Muscle Group	Muscles	General Function
Suboccipital (lying just below the occipital region of the skull [see Chapters 4 and 10]; running parallel to or oblique to the nuchal midline [the midline of the back of the neck])	obliquus capitis inferior, obliquus capitis superior, rectus capitis posterior major, rectus capitis posterior minor	rotation of the head; bilaterally extends and flexes the head
Prevertebral (lying at the base of the occipital bone and extending along the upper portion of the vertebral column [the spine])	longus colli, longus capitis and rectus capitis anterior, rectus capitis lateralis	flexion of the head and neck
Anterior (lying along the front of the neck)	sternohyoid, omohyoid, sternothyroid, thyrohyoid, stylohyoid, digastric, mylohyoid, geniohyoid	elevation of the ribs for respiration; rotation and flexion of the head and bilaterally of the neck; depression and elevation of the mandible to open and close the mouth
Anterolateral (lying along the sides of the neck and moving into the front of the neck)	superficial cervical, lateral cervical anterior vertebral, suprahyoid, infrahyoid, sternocleidomastoid, platysma (see "Focus Point: The Platysma Muscle"), trapezius, anterior scalene, scalenus minimus, middle scalene, posterior scalene (Note that *scalene* means *uneven* [i.e., a scalene triangle]. The term describes the shape of these muscles.)	depression of the hyoid and the larynx; some flexibility and rotation of the neck; depression of the mandible (pulls down the lower lip)

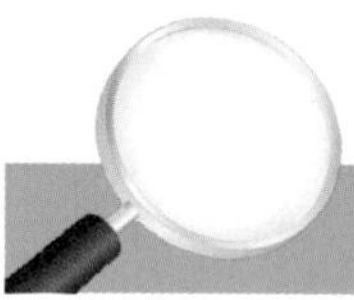

FOCUS POINT: The Trapezius Muscle

The *trapezius muscle* is a large superficial muscle of the posterior neck and the upper thorax. It originates at the occipital bone, and it inserts along the spine. Its functions include scapular elevation (i.e., moving the shoulder blades up and down) and scapular adduction (i.e., drawing the shoulder blades inward toward the spine). The longer that our patient Clay Davis holds his jaw and neck muscles still to prevent any pain, the greater the chance that his trapezius and other neck muscles will begin to stiffen and cause another form of discomfort for the child.

The term *trapezius* is indicative of the muscle's shape: it is a trapezoid, which is a four-sided figure with only one pair of parallel sides.

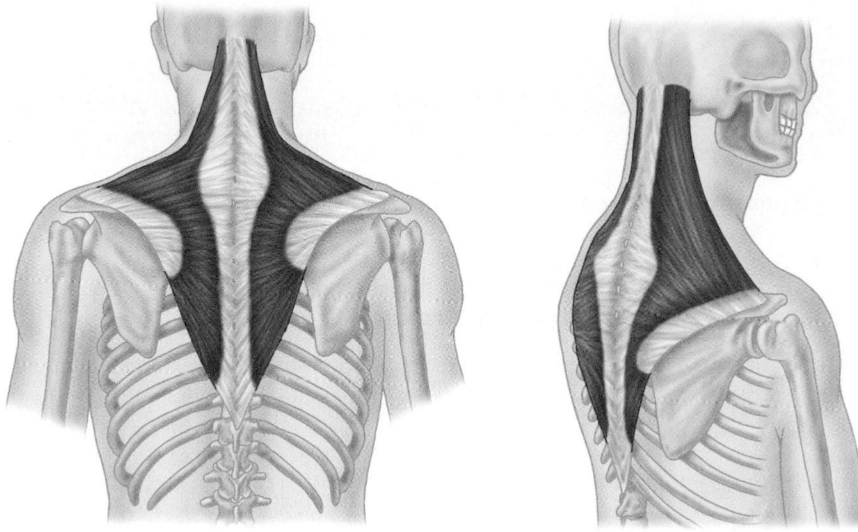

Figure 13.15: Trapezius muscle

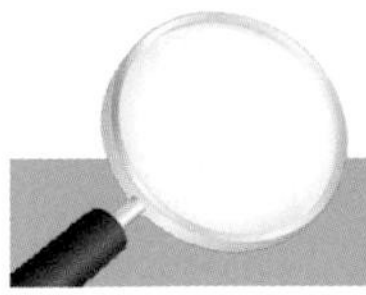

FOCUS POINT: The Platysma Muscle

The *platysma muscle* overlaps the sternocleidomastoid muscle, and it plays an important role in movement of the lips. It can move the lower lips and the corners of the mouth down or sideways, thus opening the mouth, and it exerts some influence on the mandible to do so. Interestingly, this is the muscle that is used to form a facial expression that indicates surprise.

The platysma muscle has a second and very important function: It assists with increasing the diameter of the neck to facilitate an increase in breathing during exertion (i.e., running, playing a sport).

The platysma muscle is a superficial neck muscle. During the process of aging, this muscle may become weaker and more flaccid, and it can contribute to what is commonly known as a *double chin.* Exercising this muscle can help to prevent the condition.

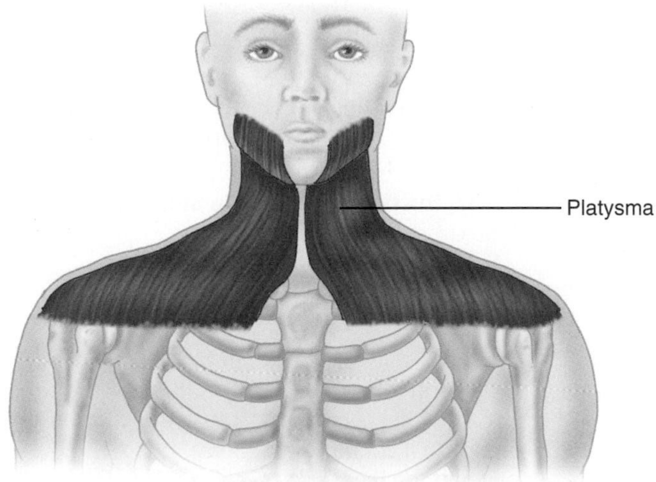

Figure 13.16: Platysma muscle

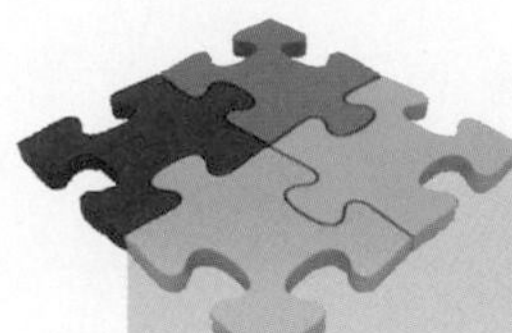

WORD BUILDING: Formula for Creating Words with the Combining Form *Sterno-*

sternum = the narrow, flat bone found at the midline of the anterior thorax. The combining form is *sterno-*.

sterno + clavicul/o + ar = *sternoclavicular*

Definition: pertaining to both the sternum and the clavicle. *adjective*

Example: The *sternoclavicular* joint is vulnerable to osteoarthritis, rheumatoid disease, infection, and injury.

sterno + costa + al = *sternocostal*

Definition: pertaining to the sternum and the ribs. (The second root is *costa,* meaning *rib.*) *adjective*

Example: The pectoralis muscle has a *sternocostal* head that originates in the sternum and the costal cartilage of the first through sixth ribs.

sterno + trypesis = *sternotrypesis*

Definition: perforation of the sternum. (The second root is *trypesis,* meaning *boring* [as in *boring a hole*]). *noun*

Example: *Sternotrypesis* may be the result of a surgical procedure or a penetrating injury.

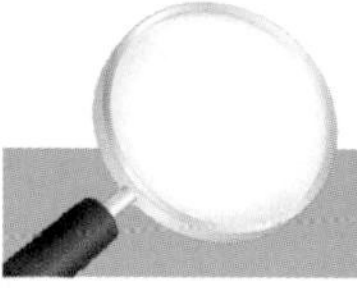

FOCUS POINT: Sternocleidomastoid Muscles

The *sternocleidomastoid muscles* (SCMs) are long, scalene muscles that are bilateral on the anterior portion of the neck. They allow for the rotation and flexion of the head and neck, and they support the weight of the head. The SCMs extend when the posterior muscles of the neck flex, thus tilting the head backward.

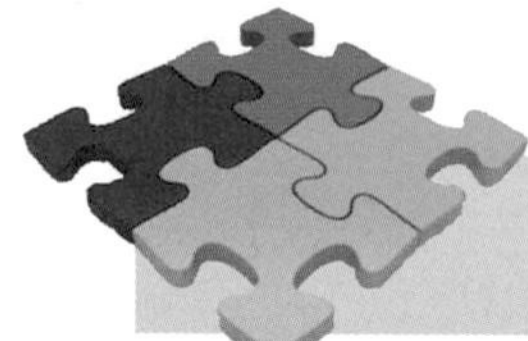

WORD BUILDING: Formula for Creating Words with the Combining Form *Occipit/o-*

occiput = the back part of the skull; the bone at the base of the skull. The combining form is *occipit/o.*

occipit/o + cervic/o + al = *occipitocervical*

Definition: referring to the occipital bone or region and the neck. (The second combining form is *cervic/o,* meaning *neck.*) *adjective*

Example: An *occipitocervical* injury (OCI) is usually fatal.

occipit/o + facial = *occipitofacial*

Definition: concerning the occiput and the face. *adjective*

Example: The *occipitofacial* circumference is a measurement of the head that is taken around the occiput and the anterior portion of the frontal bone of the skull.

occipit/o + mental = *occipitomental*

Definition: concerning the occiput and the chin. (In this context, the root *mental* means *chin.*) *adjective*

Example: Skull radiography can include an *occipitomental* x-ray.

Break It Down

Break down each term into its word parts (prefix, root, and suffix), and then write the meaning of each word part. Follow this example:

suboccipital = sub (beneath or under) + occipit (occiput bone at the base of the skull) + al (regarding or relating to)

1. prevertebral ______
2. sternalgia ______
3. anterolateral ______
4. suprahyoid ______

Build a Word

Use each set of word parts to create a medical or anatomical term.

1. hyoid sterno Term: ______ Meaning: ______
2. vertebr/a sterno -al Term: ______ Meaning: ______
3. temporal occipit/o Term: ______ Meaning: ______
4. tomy sterno Term: ______ Meaning: ______
5. odynia sterno Term: ______ Meaning: ______
6. frontal occipit/o Term: ______ Meaning: ______

Let's Practice

Write the term or terms that best identify what is being described.

1. This muscle group includes the obliquus and rectus muscles. ______
2. The scalene muscles are part of this group. ______
3. The capitis muscles belong to these two groups. ______

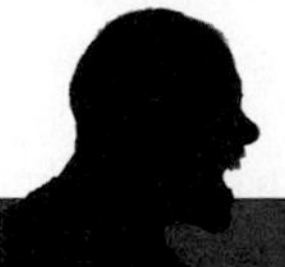

PRONOUNCIATION PRACTICE

Say these words aloud to a friend or classmate, if you can. Here you are given the phonetic pronunciation. Your instructor can help you with pronunciation,

or you can visit **http://www.MedicalLanguageLab.com.**

anterolateral	ăn″tĕr-ō-**lăt**′ĕr-ăl	sternodynia	stĕr″nō-**dĭn**′ē-ă
occipitofacial	ŏk-sĭp″ĭ-tō-**fā**′shăl	sternohyoid	stĕr″nō-**hī**′oyd
occipitofrontal	ŏk-sĭp″ĭ-tō-**frŏn**′tăl	sternotomy	stĕr-**nŏt**′ō-mē
occiput	**ŏk**′sĭ-pŭt	sternotrypesis	stĕr″nō-trī-**pē**′sĭs
prevertebral	prē-**vĕr**′tē-brăl	sternovertebral	stĕr″nō-**vĕr**′tē-brăl
scalene	**skā**′-lēn	suboccipital	sŭb″ŏk-**sĭp**′ĭ-tăl
sternocleidal	stĕr″nō-**klī**″dăl		

Burn healing

Patient Update

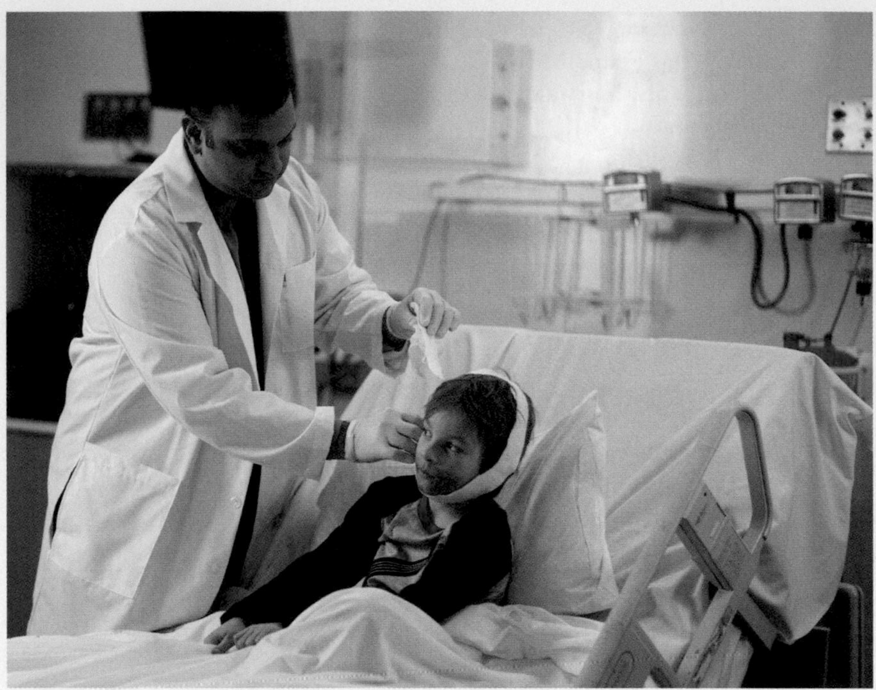

Kuldeep Singh, the physician assistant in Pediatrics at Okla Trauma Center, has come to speak with Clay Davis and his parents about Clay's burn. He has introduced himself and asked the family to call him by his first name. He explained his role at Okla Trauma and his experience with treating children who are recovering from a wide variety of burn injuries. At the bedside, he has donned gloves, and he is preparing to examine Clay's wound. He gently lifts the gown off of the child's shoulder, and he begins removing a very loosely taped piece of cotton gauze.

"As you know, Clay suffered a superficial partial-thickness burn across his upper torso," explained Kuldeep. Clay winced as he anticipated that the gauze would stick to the now-open blisters. He was relieved by how gentle the physician assistant was when baring the wound and that there was only very minor sticking. Clay carefully looked down at the site as the PA continued. "Burns are the result of the death of tissue that is caused by heat. We call that *tissue death necrosis,*" Kuldeep explained, throwing away the gauze. "You can see here," he said, pausing and pointing for the parents so that they could see, "how heat damages the cells of the skin. When that occurs, chemicals stimulate the nerve endings. That's what causes the pain. You can see where the outer layer of skin has burned away. That would be painful for the child." He stopped and looked down at Clay, waiting for affirmation. Clay put both of his thumbs up rather than nodding his head up and down to avoid causing his face to hurt.

The PA continued: "Burns begin to heal when new layers of skin begin to grow. That starts at the outer edges of a burn; see here and here." Kuldeep pointed to specific points along Clay's sternum and across the edge of his clavicle. "This is healing very well," he commented, as if to himself. "Superficial partial-thickness burns, like your son's, are often painful, and they are accompanied by painful blisters that must naturally rupture or degrade as part of the healing process. "

"Oh," said Mickey, "I can see that all but one or two of the very small blisters have gone and now they're just like flat, empty balloons." She smiled at Clay as she said this.

"Yes, and others have broken open and are peeling with the rest of the skin," said Steve.

Kuldeep nodded in confirmation. He explained that these types of burns usually heal over a period of 3 or 4 weeks. "We have been keeping the burn site covered very lightly to protect that raw tissue and the dermis from any risk of infection. Without the epidermis to protect it, this layer of skin—the pink skin that you can see in spots—is very vulnerable to infection. As you can see, we have successfully preventing that." Kuldeep smiled at the parents and the child.

"His skin does look so raw in some places. Are you saying that's normal and that it will eventually be covered by a new layer of skin in the next few weeks?" asked Mickey. The PA nodded. "Will there be any scars?" Mickey asked. "And what about the color? Will some of the color be off? Dark or pink or even white?"

Kuldeep explained that he didn't foresee any visible scars resulting from the burn, but he noted that some pigment changes in the skin might be possible. This, he advised, would depend on how deep the burn was at various sites and whether the melanin and carotene cells were still producing pigment. He cautioned the family to keep this new skin and the entire wound site out of direct sunlight for at least the next 6 months to ensure that healing and pigmentation would recover to the optimum level.

"Did you hear that, Clay? You're going to have to wear a t-shirt when you're out in the sun and even when you're in the pool or at the lake this summer," said his mom. Clay groaned in acknowledgement, and they all laughed.

"Lastly," said the physician assistant, "you'll want to keep an eye on the healing tissue itself. As time goes by, the wound area will start to shrink in size. A complication called a 'contracture of tissue' might occur." Mickey looked concerned. "It might not happen, Mrs. Davis, but I just want to be sure you are aware of this possibility. If the skin begins to tighten or pull a bit as it heals, you should tell your family physician or pediatrician as soon as you can. He or she can make some suggestions regarding how to keep the skin moist and pliable as it recovers. Of course, gentle exercise involving that area, such as moving the shoulder and neck a bit, will help to maintain healthy circulation in the area and to promote tissue regeneration and pliability."

"Oh, okay," said Clay's mother. "Could I put some aloe vera gel on it to help it along?" Kuldeep confirmed that she could but that she should do so sparingly. What was paramount, he explained, was keeping the wound site as clean as possible and free from further injury. He turned to the patient then and said, "Clay, this burn might start to itch now and then. I don't want you scratching it. That could tear that new, fragile skin, and an infection could set in." He paused to be sure that Clay was listening. "You won't scratch at it, will you?"

"What about my cat?" said Clay. "My cat climbs all over me sometimes. She likes to climb up and ride on my shoulder," he said through barely open lips.

"No way. No cat on your shoulders, young man. That is just too risky." Kuldeep looked at Clay's parents and said, "Cat scratches on new skin would be a very bad idea, Mr. and Mrs. Davis. You'll have to watch your boy to ensure that this doesn't happen." He paused, as if thinking, and then added, "And watch that cat, too!" They laughed again. "If the skin is itchy and bothering Clay, apply a cool, damp cloth to the area for a while. That is helpful. And, of course, as you said, perhaps a little aloe vera gel, but only a little. Your pediatrician may have some other suggestions for you, too." Clay's parents nodded.

"Now, you are going to go home today, Clay. I want your mom and dad to take you to a doctor before the end of this week, okay? You need your jaw and your burn looked after for quite a while yet." Kuldeep Singh gently placed the Clay's gown back over the burn and tucked it behind his shoulder. "Now, I'm not going to put gauze on this anymore. That skin needs some fresh air. The nurse will come in soon and bandage it again for you so that you can go home safely." Kuldeep turned toward Clay's parents as he said, "You don't have to wear a bandage over it all the time, Clay. Mom, perhaps you can put a clean one on him if he's going to be very active for a while, just to protect the site from injury, all right?" Mickey nodded. "Very good then. Well, it's been a pleasure to meet you all, and I wish you all the best in your recovery, Clay." Kuldeep shook the boy's hand and then the parents' hands before leaving.

Reflective Questions

Consider what you've just read to answer the following questions.

1. What is Kuldeep Singh's profession? ______________________________

2. How does a burn cause pain? ______________________________

3. What measures can Clay take to avoid any skin contractures as his burn heals?

   ____

4. Initially, the scald burn was covered. Why? ______________________________

Critical Thinking Questions

Think deeply about what you've been learning and what you've read in this latest Patient Update, and then answer the questions.

1. Name three muscles that Clay will need to flex and extend to promote the healing of tissue at the burn site. ____________________
2. Why might Clay Davis experience skin contractures? ____________________

Key terms: burn healing

Key terms from the conversation between PA Kuldeep Singh and the Davis family are italicized in the example and highlighted below with the explanation.

"... he has *donned* gloves ..."

donned: put on.

"... piece of *cotton gauze.*"

cotton gauze: a type of dressing or material that is used in wound care (see Figure 13-17). A cotton gauze is also called a *cotton sponge.* Sterile cotton gauzes are highly effective for the promotion of skin healing. They allow for some free flow of air to the wound bed while at the same time protecting the raw or damaged skin from microorganisms in the environment. These are used in the healing stages of various types of burn recovery. Before the healing stages begin, gauze may be used, but it will be applied in combination with an antibiotic cream or gel.

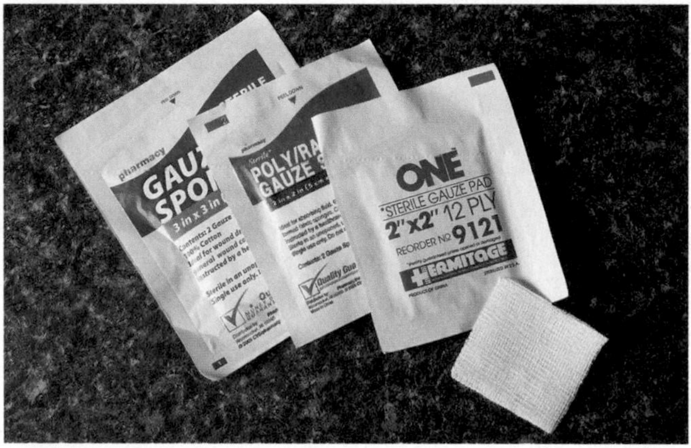

Figure 13.17: Cotton gauzes (From Eagle S, Brassington C, Dailey CS, Goretti C: *The Professional Medical Assistant: An Integrative, Teamwork-Based Approach.* Philadelphia: FA Davis, 2009, p. 405. With permission.)

"... when *baring the wound* ..."

baring the wound: common medical language that means *uncovering a wound.* Another common way to say this is to use the term *exposing the wound.*

"... healing and *pigmentation would recover* ..."

pigmentation would recover: Melanin- and carotene-producing cells will recover to secrete pigment once more (optimally this will pigment that is the natural skin tone of the person).

"... to promote tissue regeneration and *pliability.*"

pliability: flexibility or suppleness. This is a natural characteristic of healthy skin.

"Cat scratches on new skin ..."

cat scratches: The significance of this example is that cat scratch disease is common among children (see "Focus Point: Cat Scratch Disease"). In addition to putting the child at risk for this infection, scratches to the surface of damaged or recovering skin can produce scars and delay healing.

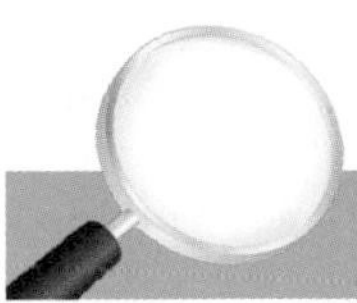

FOCUS POINT: Cat Scratch Disease

Cat scratch disease, which is also known as *cat scratch fever,* is a condition that is caused by the *Bartonella henselae* bacteria. This condition adversely affects the lymph nodes near the infection site, thereby causing lymphadenopathy. It is contracted as a result of contact with an infected cat through the cat's saliva, bites, and scratches. Symptoms include fever, lymphedema near the contact site, headache, and fatigue. When the skin is penetrated, a first sign of the disease might be a papule (bump) or an infected pustule. Cat scratch disease is a common cause of lymph node swelling in children.

Eponyms: *Rochalimaea* and *Bartonella henselae*

Bartonella is a genus (classification) of bacteria in the biological order of *Rickettsiales.* Originally, the *Bartonella* genus was known as *Rochalimaea,* in honor of the Brazilian microbiologist Henrique da Rocha Lima. It was later renamed *Bartonella* in honor of Antonio Bartonella, a Peruvian physician and scientist. *Bartonella* bacteria are found in animals such as cats, fleas, and ticks.

Diane Hensel is a contemporary American laboratory technologist who works in the field of microbiology. During the late 1980s and the early 1990s, she discovered and isolated bacteria of the genus *Rochalimaea.* This new bacteria was originally named *Rochalimaea henselae,* but, during subsequent years, it was renamed *Bartonella henselae* for its more direct similarities to Dr. Bartonella's findings. *Bartonella henselae* is the medical name for cat scratch disease or cat scratch fever.

Figure 13-18 clarifies the sequence of names by which *Bartonella henselae* bacteria are classified.

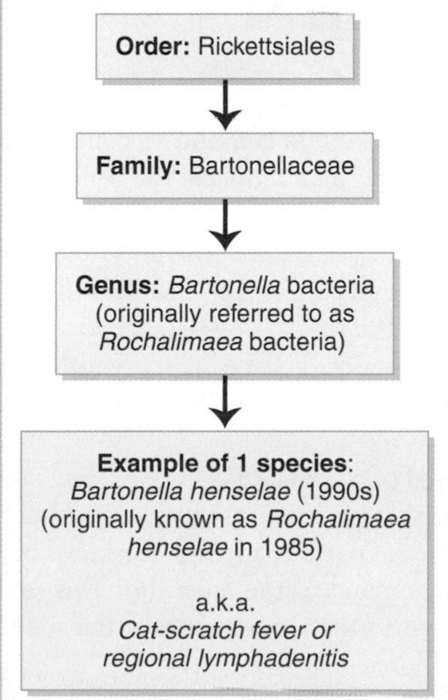

Figure 13.18: Classification of *Bartonella henselae* bacteria

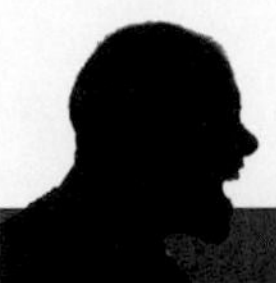

PRONOUNCIATION PRACTICE

Say these words aloud to a friend or classmate, if you can. Here you are given the phonetic pronunciation. Your instructor can help you with pronunciation,

or you can visit **http://www.MedicalLanguageLab.com.**

bacteriology	băk-tēr″ē-**ŏl**′ō-jē	genus	**jē**′nŭs
Bartonella	băr″tō-**nĕl**′ă	*Rickettsia*	rĭ-**kĕt**′sē-ă
carotene	**kăr**′ă-tēn	*Rochalimaea*	rō″chă-lī-**mē**′ă
gauze	gawz		

Skin tissue: regeneration and repair

When skin tissue is damaged, it goes through four stages of recovery:

Stage 1: *Collagenation* begins at the end of and overlaps with the inflammatory response process. Macrophages clear damaged tissue, and fibroblasts appear to construct a collagen matrix, which is the framework on which new skin cells will grow.

Macrophages develop at the end stage of the life of a monocyte, when it settles into tissue. Macrophages are part of the immune system. They can ingest foreign antigens (i.e., agents that stimulate growth of antibodies) and clean the blood of old or abnormal cells and debris (see chapter 14).

Stage 2: *Angiogenesis* is the development of blood vessels at the wound or injury site. During this stage, which is also known as *revascularization,* capillaries grow anew and bring needed circulation and nutrients to the area.

Stage 3: *Proliferation* is the rapid and repeated production of new tissues. This proliferation is the result of **mitosis**, which is the process of cell division. The period of proliferation can be as short as 4 weeks in duration.

Stage 4 = *Remodeling* involves new cells molding into the shape of the tissue that surrounds them and taking on the same functions. A gentle stretching of this new tissue is important to prevent contractures.

More about collagen

Collagen is a major protein in the body. It is found in connective tissue, cartilage, tendons, and bone. In essence, collagen is like glue that connects the cells of the body. Collagen dressings for wounds are commonly used in medical facilities.

The root *colla* means *glue;* the root *gen* means *generation or growth.*

Collagen keeps the skin smooth and supple (i.e., pliable or flexible). As a person ages, the supply of collagen in the skin is depleted. The result is a dryness and wrinkling of the skin because it is no longer able to retain moisture naturally. To maintain a youthful appearance, some middle-aged people may opt for cosmetic surgery in which collagen injections are used to plump up aging or sagging skin, including the lips.

The dermis is densely composed of collagen (95%). However, a severe burn destroys this collagen. To promote healing, treatments that involve a collagen substitute being applied topically can help with skin reconstruction. For cases of partial- and full-thickness burns, artificial or natural collagen (i.e., from cattle or pigs) can be applied to the burn site. This topically applied collagen protects the wound and works together with natural fibroblasts at the site to stimulate and support natural collagen production again.

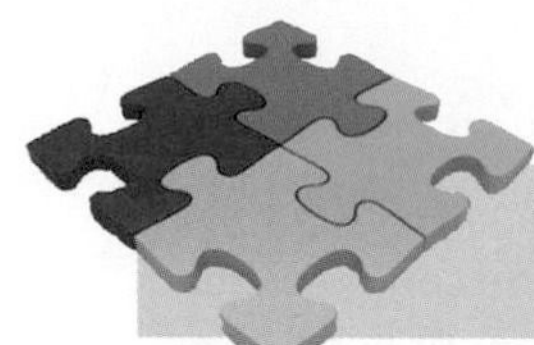

WORD BUILDING: Formula for Creating Words with the Root Word *Colla*

colla = *glue,* from the original Greek *kolla*

colla + gen + ase = *collagenase*

Definition: a type of enzyme that breaks down collagen. (The suffix *-ase* means *enzyme.*) *noun*

Example: For burn victims, a *collagenase* ointment may be used to break down and remove necrotic (dead) tissue.

colla + gen/o + blast = *collagenoblast*

Definition: a type of fibroblast cell that eventually produces collagen. (The suffix *-blast* refers to an embryonic state of development.) *noun*

Example: *Collagenoblasts* are found at the site of inflammation.

pro + colla + gen = *procollagen*

Definition: the stage before something becomes collagen. *noun*

Example: *Procollagen* creams and nutritional supplements are now on the market. The producers of these creams claim that they improve skin health, defend against hair loss, and combat other signs of aging.

colla + gen + o + lysis = *collagenolysis*

Definition: the degradation or destruction of collagen. (The suffix *-lysis* means *dissolution.*) *noun*

Example: *Collagenolysis* may be indicated as part of the disease process of rheumatoid arthritis and the destruction of joints.

tropo + colla + gen = *tropocollagen*

Definition: the molecular unit of collagen. (The combining form *tropo* derives from *trope,* meaning *turn or turning.*) *noun*

Example: The collagen molecule is more properly referred to as the *tropocollagen* molecule.

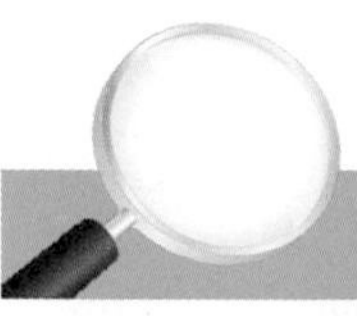

FOCUS POINT: The Suffix *-ase*

The suffix *-ase* identifies a word as an enzyme. The preceding word part is the name of the substance upon which the enzyme works. The work of enzymes is to break substances down into their chemical components.

Build a Word

Use the word parts that you've just been working with and others that are given here to create medical terms. You will recognize the other word parts from previous chapters. Define each full term.

1. trope myo -ic Term: ________________ Meaning: ________________
2. trope dermat -ic Term: ________________ Meaning: ________________
3. -ase creatine Term: ________________ Meaning: ________________
4. mono -cyte pro- Term: ________________ Meaning: ________________
5. cephal pro- -ic Term: ________________ Meaning: ________________

Fill in the Blanks

Complete the following sentences by filling in the blanks with the proper medical term or expression.

1. The potential for skin infection after a burn is always high. To help prevent infection, health care professionals will ______________________ gloves during the initial stages of burn treatment.
2. ______________________ is a common type of dry, fabric dressing that permits air to flow through it.
3. Because skin cells can ______________________, healing can occur.
4. Supple skin is ______________________, which means that it can move easily.
5. The dermis is made up largely of ______________________.
6. ______________________ is a term that refers to the coloration or discoloration of the skin.
7. After a burn or another serious injury, muscles and ______________________ can both ______________________.
8. The enzyme that decomposes collagen is ______________________.

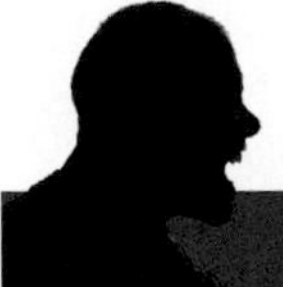

PRONOUNCIATION PRACTICE

Say these words aloud to a friend or classmate, if you can. Here you are given the phonetic pronunciation. Your instructor can help you with pronunciation,

or you can visit **http://www.MedicalLanguageLab.com.** 

angiogenesis	ăn″jē-ō-**jĕn**′ĕ-sĭs	fibroblast	**fī**′brō-blăst
collagen	**kŏl**′ă-jĕn	macrophage	**măk**′rō-fāj
collagenase	kŏl-**lăj**′ĕ-nās	procephalic	prō″sē-**făl**′ĭk
collagenoblast	kŏl-**lăj**′ĕ-nō-blăst	proliferation	prō-lĭf″ĕr-ā′shŭn
collagenolysis	kŏl″ă-jĕn-**ŏl**′ĭ-sĭs	tropocollagen	trō″pō-**kŏl**′a-jĕn
dermatotropic	dĕr″mă-tō-**trŏp**′ĭk		

Tissue regeneration after a burn injury

Clay Davis has a scald burn; in his case, it is a partial-thickness burn of the left side of his upper thorax. He has suffered tissue damage, blistering, tissue loss, and pain as a result. Physician assistant Kuldeep Singh has confirmed that the patient's skin is healing well.

During the initial stages of burn care, medical and nursing staff will take extreme care to protect the burn site. For example, when Clay Davis was transported to the hospital, he was covered with a **sterile burn sheet**. This is simply a light, non-woven sheet of synthetic material that can be used either wet or dry to cover burns. It provides a sterile environment for the tissue, it is not abrasive, and it does not contain any harsh detergents or other chemicals that may aggravate the wound (see Figure 13-19).

Recall that, in the emergency department, the priority of care for Clay Davis was his fracture. The trauma doctors deemed his scald burn to not be life threatening. Therefore, in the ER, Clay had his wound covered with a fresh burn sheet until the treatment team had the opportunity to thoroughly cleanse the wound and apply a silver sulfadiazine cream (i.e., Flamazine 1% cream). This topical antibiotic was applied liberally to the affected area, which was then covered lightly with a cotton gauze dressing. (This dressing would need to be changed immediately after the craniofacial surgery to avoid contamination and infection.)

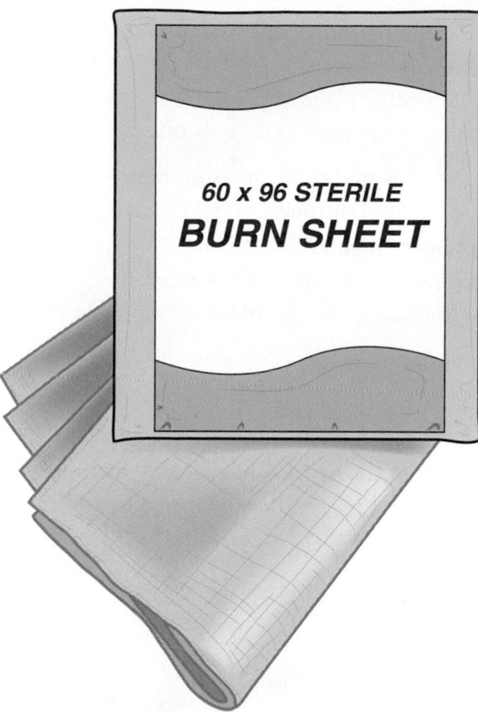

Figure 13.19: Sterile burn sheet

The team may also have applied a paraffin gauze dressing, such as Jelonet (see Figure 13-20). This is a loose-weave cotton gauze that is impregnated with soft paraffin (wax) to prevent adherence (sticking) to the wound. It is often used as the primary or first layer of a dressing that is to be applied to raw skin or wounds. It provides a barrier between the wound bed and the dressing that goes on above it.

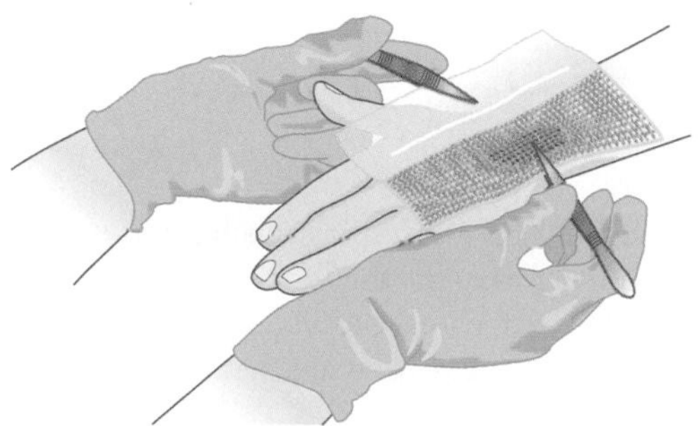

Figure 13.20: Paraffin gauze dressing

After Clay Davis's surgery, he was admitted to the Pediatric Unit for further care and treatment. During Clay's week there, the nursing staff and the PA treated the burn site with a variety of dressings, and they changed the type of dressing as the skin began to heal. These different dressings probably included gauze dressings, with or without a layer of antibiotic or petroleum-based cream, to keep the skin hydrated (but not wet) and clear of infection and to prevent the sticking of the dressing to the healing tissue and the associated blisters.

Enhanced terminology for pigmentation

Recall that melanin and carotene pigments lie in the epidermis layer of the skin. When this layer is burned away, so are these pigments. This loss of pigments may lead to a discoloration of the skin, which can be temporary or permanent.

Discoloration is described as generalized, focal, or segmental:

- *Generalized discoloration:* widespread.
- *Focal discoloration:* only in a specific place or places.
- *Segmental discoloration:* affecting or appearing on only one part of the body (i.e., only on one side).

When skin becomes lighter, it is said to be **hypopigmented** or **depigmented** (i.e., no color). When skin becomes darker than it normally should be, it is said to be **hyperpigmented**.

Enhanced terminology for burn blisters

Recall from Chapter 11 that blisters or *bulla* are not uncommon among patients with burns. Key terms related to the status and healing process of blisters include the following:

- **flaccid:** loose, limp, drooping, or not firm.
- **rupture:** burst.
- **degrade:** diminish, reduce or corrupt.

When Clay was first brought to the hospital, he already had burn blisters on his skin that were similar to the ones shown in Figure 13-21. After the initial treatment of his burn, the hospital staff followed a clinical pathway (i.e., a treatment algorithm) like the one shown in Figure 13-22 while allowing the blisters to heal.

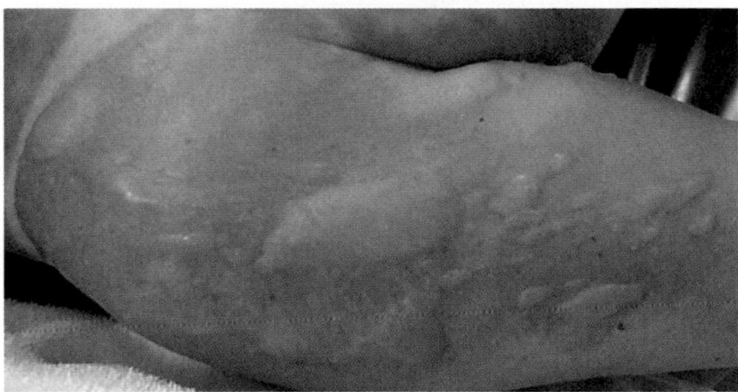

Figure 13.21: Burn blisters (From McCulloch J, and Kloth, L: Wound Healing: Evidence-Based Management, ed. 4. FA Davis, Philadelphia, 2010, p 361, with permission.)

Peeling skin

Skin peeling is a natural process. During the healing of a burn, the function of peeling is to **slough off** (i.e., cast off) dead skin to make way for the new skin that is developing underneath it. The epidermis will also peel if it is irritated, damaged, diseased, infected, or exposed to an allergen.

Among the conditions that may cause peeling are the following:

- *Contact dermatitis:* a localized skin reaction at the site where an allergen or irritant comes in contact with the skin.
- *Psoriasis:* a medical condition in which the skin cells grow too quickly and the body is unable to shed old ones quickly enough to make way for these. The result is the buildup of skin cells on the surface of the body, where lesions form (see "Focus Point: Lesions").
- *Athlete's foot* (see Chapter 5)
- *Staphylococcal infection:* an infection caused by staphylococcal bacteria. *Staph,* as it is commonly known, is naturally found on the skin and in the nose. Usually, it causes no harm. However, when a person has a weakened immune system (see Chapter 17), staph bacteria can invade the bloodstream and become life threatening. Although there are at least 20 types of staphylococci, only two are particularly relevant to humans: *Staphylococcus aureus* and *Staphylococcus epidermis. Staphylococcus aureus* is the most common cause of staph infections. (See "Focus Point: MRSA.")

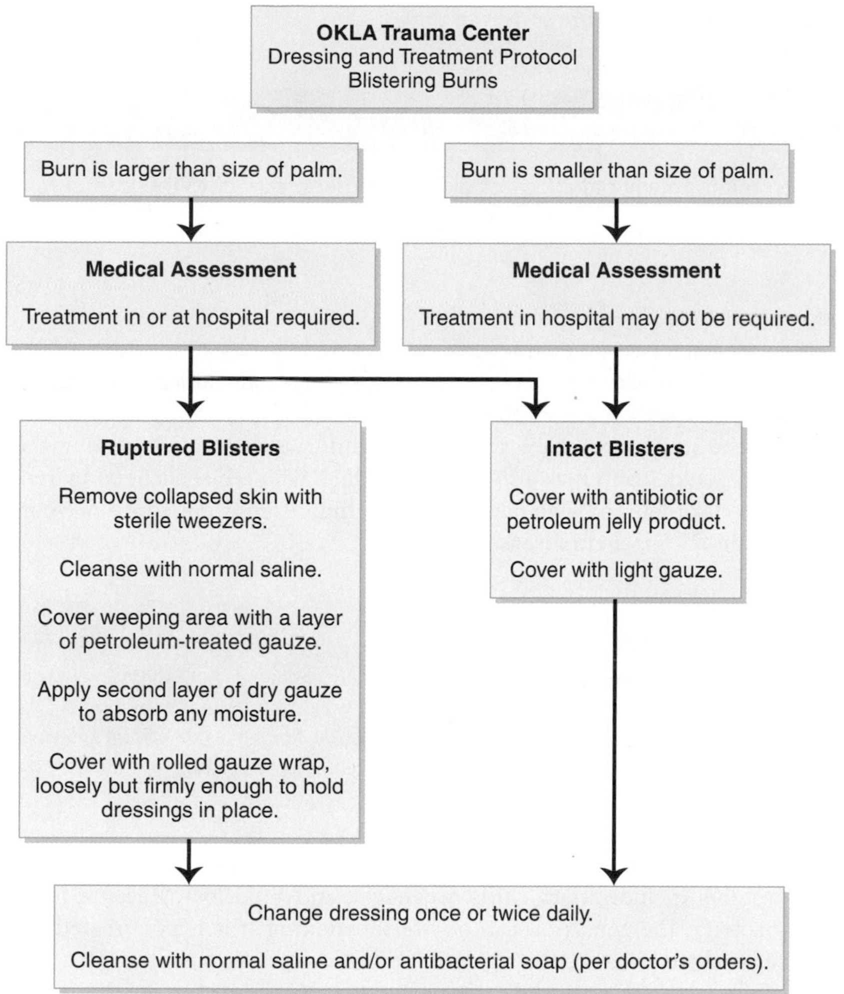

Figure 13.22: Clinical pathway for burn blisters

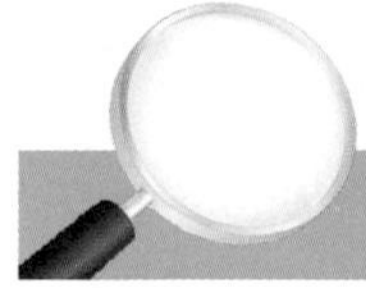

FOCUS POINT: MRSA

MRSA is the abbreviation for *methicillin-resistant Staphylococcus aureus,* a very common and extremely hard-to-treat infection that is caused by *Staphylococcus aureus* bacteria (*Staph A* or *S aureus*). It has earned its name as a result of its resistance to the antibiotic methicillin.

MRSA strains are also resistant to other antibiotics, particularly those of the penicillin family (i.e., penicillin, amoxicillin). MRSA is spread by contact with people or objects that have become contaminated with it, and it has the potential to become life threatening. Patients are often screened for its presence upon admission to a hospital or a health care facility, and a clinical pathway is followed for positive or negative results. If the screening determines that MRSA is present, the patient may be put into isolation during treatment. MRSA is one of the so-called "super bugs," a new group of antibiotic-resistant pathogens increasingly present today.

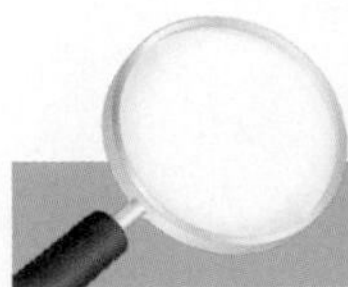

FOCUS POINT: Lesion

The word *lesion* refers to any pathology or disruption of the skin or to the loss of function of a body part.

Scalded skin syndrome

Although we have been focused on a true scald burn, there is an infection with a similar name and symptoms: **scalded skin syndrome**, also known as **staphylococcal scalded skin syndrome (SSSS)**. The etiology of this disorder is very different from that of a burn. It is a type of staphylococcal infection that is seen in newborn babies and young children, particularly among those who are younger than 6 years old. SSSS may also appear in adults who are challenged by renal failure or immune deficiency disorders and who have become immunocompromised. In newborns, it is also known as **Ritter von Ritterschein disease**.

Eponyms: Ritter von Ritterschein Disease

Baron Gottfried Ritter von Ritterschein was a German physician working with newborn Czechoslovakian children in 1878 when he discovered the disease that would subsequently be named for him. The official name given to the disease was *dermatitis exfoliativa neonatorum,* but it has come to be known as *Ritter von Ritterschein disease of newborns.* (*Ritterschein* is sometimes spelled *Rittershain* in older texts.)

SSSS has the appearance of a severe burn. The skin is reddened, and it peels. As with all infections, symptoms include fever, chills, weakness, and fluid loss. Because its origin is the *Staphylococcus* bacteria, the condition can be life threatening if it is not treated promptly and effectively. The condition is treated with antibiotics and intravenous fluids in a hospital, often in a burn unit, where the skin can be expertly treated. With treatment, the infection should resolve within 7 to 10 days.

SSSS is sometimes missed during an initial diagnosis. Because it occurs predominantly among pediatric patients and appears to be a severe burn, erroneous assumptions can be made about its cause. This misdiagnosis can temporarily delay the necessary rigorous treatment of the infection. The diagnosis of SSSS is made through a skin biopsy and a bacterial culture.

biopsy: a tissue sample removed from the body and examined microscopically.

culture: the result of reproduction (propagation) of microorganisms or cells in an environmental medium such as a Petri dish. This procedure occurs in a laboratory.

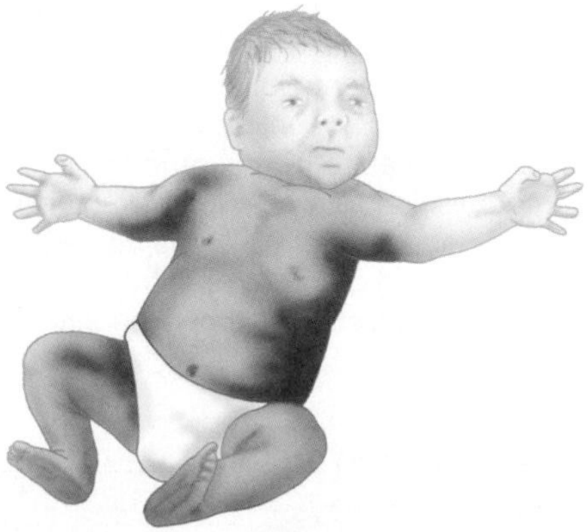

Figure 13.23: Patient with scalded skin syndrome

Eponym: Petri Dish

The name for this piece of laboratory equipment was given by Julius Richard Petri, a German physician and bacteriologist in the late 1800s. *Petri dishes* are shallow, covered plastic or glass dishes that contain a growth medium (usually *agar,* a gel made of algae and nutrients). Bacteria and other microorganisms or tissues are grown in this medium. Some Petri dishes are used for dissection purposes.

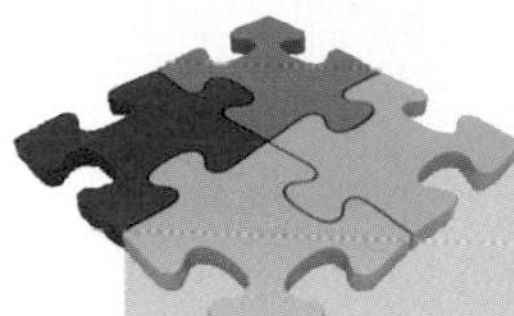

WORD BUILDING: Formula for Creating Words with the Combining Form *Staphylo-*

Staphyle = Greek root meaning *a bunch of grapes.* In microbiology, this root word describes how bacteria clump together in irregularly shaped masses. The combining form is *staphylo-*.

staphylo + cocci = *staphylococci*

Definition: the plural form for a certain genus of bacteria. *noun*

Example: When cultured in the lab, some strains of *staphylococci* produce white, yellow, or orange colonies of bacteria.

staphylo + cocc + al = *staphylococcal*

Definition: pertaining to or caused by *Staphylococcus* bacteria. (The second root is *coccus,* meaning *berry.* It is used in its combining form.) *adjective*

Example: Clay Davis's burn site and his surgical wound have been kept under medical asepsis to prevent a *staphylococcal* infection.

Critical Thinking

On the basis of what you've read, answer the following question.

What is the main reason for covering a burn site? ______________________________

Build a Word

Use your word skills and knowledge to build medical terms from the word parts that are given.

1. -emia cocco staphylo- Term: ________________ Meaning: ________________
2. dermat/a staphylo -itis Term: ________________ Meaning: ________________

Let's Practice

Write the correct medical term for each definition or description.

1. a bacteria that lives on your skin and in your nose and that is usually harmless ______________________________
2. another way to say "weakened immune system" ______________________________
3. abbreviated as *SSSS* ______________________________
4. commonly called *blisters* ______________________________
5. a synthetic covering that is used for patients who have been burned ______________
6. describes a blister that has not burst and that is still intact ______________
7. the shedding of dead skin cells ______________________________
8. a burn dressing that is coated with a waxy substance ______________
9. a topical antibiotic that is often used for burns ______________
10. a condition in which pigmentation is lighter than normal ______________

Mix and Match

Match the term on the left with one that means the same thing on the right.

1. supple	everywhere
2. deplete	bulla
3. gauze	pliant
4. sloughing off	cotton dressing
5. blister	casting off
6. generalized	diminish

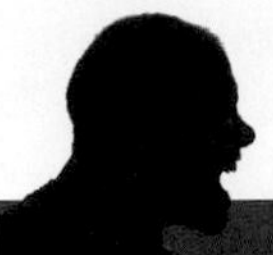

PRONOUNCIATION PRACTICE

Say these words aloud to a friend or classmate, if you can. Here you are given the phonetic pronunciation. Your instructor can help you with pronunciation,

or you can visit **http://www.MedicalLanguageLab.com.**

flaccid	**flăk**´sĭd or **flă**´sĭd	mitosis	mī-**tō**´sĭs
lymphadenopathy	lĭm-făd″ĕ-**nŏp**´ă-thē	revascularization	rē-văs″kū-lăr-ī-**zā**´shŭn
lymphedema	lĭmf-ĕ-**dē**´mă	staphylococcus	stăf″ĭl-ō-**kŏk**´ŭs

The language of discharge

Patient Update

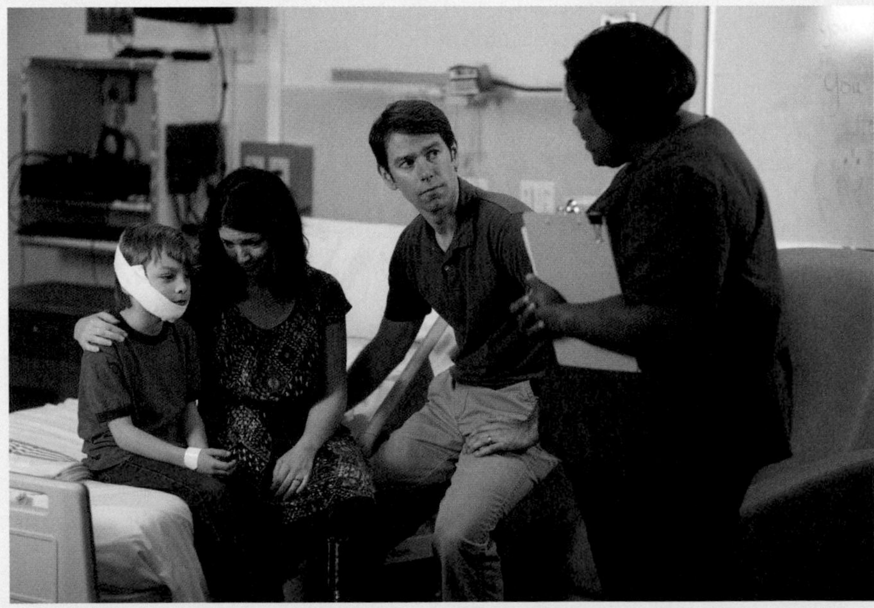

Mickey and Steve Davis are preparing for their son's discharge from the hospital. They've met with Marvane, the nurse on duty, and they have discussed Clay's follow-up care and discharge plans with her. During Clay's recovery, the nurse has told his parents, they must pay careful attention to Clay's nutrition, exercise, and hygiene, in addition to providing wound care for his mouth, jaw, and burn. She has also reinforced with them which appointments will need to be made and kept to ensure optimal patient outcomes from treatment. She instructed Clay and his parents that he should keep his jaw wrap on for the trip home and only take it off intermittently as per the doctor's earlier instructions. Key elements of the discharge plans are explained below.

Infection

Marvane talked to Clay's parents about risks for infection and reinforced the importance of keeping both wound sites and the surrounding tissue clean, as well as the need for all family members to wash their hands frequently with soap and water. She strongly advised that, if Clay should have a temperature of 101°F or higher, the family should report the fever to a health-care provider immediately or go to the nearest Emergency Department. They agreed that they would.

Nutrition

Recall that, after surgery, Clay was seen by a speech pathologist to assess his ability to move fluids and semisolid foods through his oral cavity for swallowing. He began the week on a liquid, full-fluid diet, and he has now progressed to soft foods (see Chapter 11). Marvane explained to Mr. and Mrs. Davis that Clay could continue to add a variety of solids and liquids to his diet as his jaw and his reluctance to move it both improved. Clay's ability to overcome his reluctance to use the recovering muscles would require his parents' encouragement, and Marvane suggested using foods that he particularly likes for inspiration. She cautioned Clay to chew slowly and thoroughly before swallowing to avoid choking. Marvane pretended to choke to show the child not only how dangerous this was for him but also how her jaw moved and her tongue protruded as she gasped for air. Clay quickly understood that choking would cause him pain in addition to creating a frightening situation for him.

Exercise and activity

The nurse reinforced with the family that exercise promotes health and healing, and she encouraged them to be sure that Clay did some physical stretching and that he was up and about during the day. This activity would promote circulation and prevent respiratory infections or other complications that could result from immobility. However, she also cautioned the family that Clay should not involve himself in strenuous activity or play for the next week or two to avoid the risk of his suddenly looking downward, perhaps causing pain, loss of balance, and a fall that could reinjure his jaw.

They all talked about the need for movement to avoid contractures of the skin and muscles. Mrs. Davis shared what she had learned about preventing contractures from the physician assistant, Kuldeep Singh. Marvane gave the family a brochure that illustrated some simple stretching exercises and suggested a scheduled routine for these to which the parents agreed.

Hygiene and bathing

Although it would be safe for Clay to have a shower if one of his parents assisted him, Marvane explained, it would be wiser to give Clay a sponge bath every day until his burn wound is fully healed. The nurse explained that his new, healing skin was going to be particularly tender to the touch for a few more weeks and that the sensation of a shower may feel like pins and needles for him. Even so, a shower would be a healthier option than a tub bath because a tub bath would expose the injured skin to water that may contain contaminants from the perianal area, thus exposing the skin to potential pathogens and infection. Marvane also cautioned the family about the temperature of the water in a bath or shower. New skin is extremely sensitive to hot and cold, and it can be injured by extreme temperatures. She suggested a warm temperature for the water and a soft towel to be used afterward. She stressed the importance of patting (rather than rubbing) the new skin dry.

Clay mentioned that he probably wouldn't be able to brush his teeth for "a long time now," but the nurse and his parents disagreed with him. Marvane reinforced the idea that Clay could use mouthwash to clean his mouth and that a very gentle toothbrush or tooth swab, such as the ones that they were using in the hospital, would be adequate for the job (see Figure 13-24). She also reinforced the importance of gum health to avoid further dental problems.

Skin care

Next, Marvane discussed skin care with the Davises. She spoke to them about the potential for Clay developing dry skin and itching at the burn site. They knew that dryness might occur as a result of lack of fluid in the tissues. Marvane explained that as healing progressed, dryness may also be caused by damage that had occurred to the sebaceous glands in the area. She clearly and assertively told Clay that he must not scratch the new skin for fear of damaging, scarring, or infecting it. He quickly told her that he already knew this because Mr. Singh had told him about it. Mrs. Davis said that she'd also learned that, to combat the dryness and itch, she could apply a damp cloth momentarily or perhaps a little aloe vera gel. The nurse suggested a light application of mineral oil to the skin as a better remedy.

Sun exposure

Finally, the family talked about the fact it was the beginning of summer and that Clay would likely want to be outside a good deal of the time. He put both thumbs up to indicate that he would indeed like this. Marvane taught the family about the negative effects of the sun on new skin. She advised them to keep Clay's burn covered whenever he was out in the sunlight. She explained that, even when the burn appeared to be completely healed, the new tissue remained vulnerable to the sun for at least a year. For that reason, she advised them to use sunscreen diligently.

Referrals and follow-up care

In closing, the nurse presented the family with a short list of referrals and reminders for follow-up care with their own pediatrician or family doctor. Clay's parents said that they had already set up an appointment with their doctor for the following Monday morning. Marvane told them that the unit clerk in Pediatrics would also book them an outpatient appointment with Dr. Reka Sandor to follow up on the craniofacial surgery that the surgeon had performed on Clay. The nurse explained that, 2 weeks from now, Dr. Sandor would want to assess the state of Clay's fracture and make some plans with the family regarding having the titanium plate removed.

Finally, Mr. and Mrs. Davis thanked the nurse for her help and her kindness toward their son. They helped Clay off of his bed and picked up his little bag of clothes, books, and personal items. Marvane explained to Clay that he must ride in a wheelchair out to their car, but he didn't want to that. She encouraged him by saying how far the walk was, and she told him that it was quite a privilege to be escorted out of the hospital in a chair like this. He smiled a bit and said okay. He sat in the chair, and Marvane pushed it. Together, they all went into the hall. As they passed the nursing station, the nurses, care aides, and the unit clerk all came to say their goodbyes. At the front door of the hospital, Marvane transferred the care of the child to his father. Mr. and Mrs. Davis took their son home.

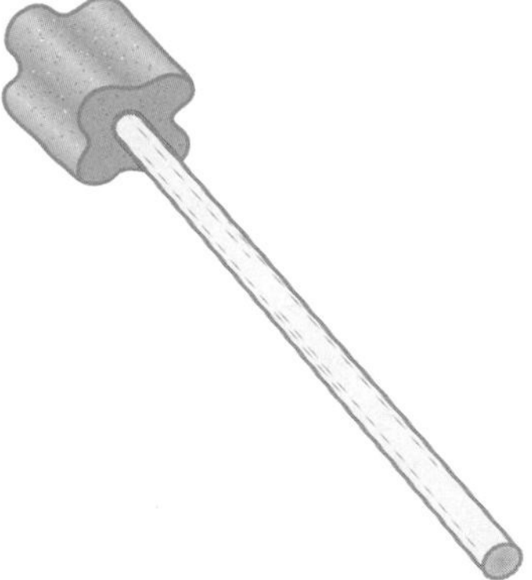

Figure 13.24: Tooth Swab for Oral Hygiene

Critical Thinking

According to this chapter and the introduction to Unit 4, what are the "3 Rs" of patient treatment (i.e., the three desired patient outcomes)?

____________________ ____________________ ____________________

CHAPTER SUMMARY

Chapter 13 provided an opportunity for you to learn and use medical and anatomical terminology related to the healing of bones, muscles, and skin tissues. Enhanced vocabulary for the muscles and the language of pathology was presented in the context of Clay's treatment, ongoing recovery, and discharge from hospital care. New terms for movement and direction were introduced. Examples of the pathology of the integumentary system were explained, and the career of the physician assistant was introduced. Formal and informal medical language was used in discussions between health-care providers, the patient, and his family to further expand the vocabulary that is necessary for health and allied-health careers. Throughout the chapter, exercises afforded numerous opportunities for you to practice new language to reinforce what you have learned and to facilitate deeper understanding.

See How Much You've Learned

For audio exercises, visit **http://www.MedicalLanguageLab.com.** 

Chapter 13 has introduced you to some medical abbreviations. These have been organized into a study table here for quick reference. Some of them you will recognize immediately, and some will reappear throughout the following chapters with more explanation and application.

TABLE 13-6: Abbreviations in Chapter 13

Abbreviation	Meaning	Abbreviation	Meaning
HMO	health maintenance organization	PA	physician assistant
LPM	lateral pterygoid muscle	PPA	pediatric physician assistant
MTS	musculotendinous stiffness	SSSS	staphylococcal scalded skin syndrome
MRSA	methicillin-resistant *Staphylococcus aureus*	SCMs	sternocleidomastoid muscles
OCI	occipitocervical injury		

Key Terms

accompanied by
ambulate
baresthesia
bathroom privileges
biopsy
bone healing
buccinators
calcification
cartilage
collagen
cotton gauze
crown
culture
deep muscles
degrade
depigmented
distorted
excruciating pain
extracellular matrix
fibroblasts
flaccid
hard callus
healing process
HMO
hyoid
hyoid bone
hyperpigmented
hypopigmented
incremental steps
intraoral space
jaw wrap
mammillary line
mandibular alignment
mastication
mesenchyme cells
mitosis
muscle
musculature
nipple line
normal dental occlusion
ossa
ossification
osteoblasts
physical therapy
plate
pliability
proliferate
pursed lips
residual
Ritter von Ritterschein disease
rupture
scalded skin syndrome
semispinalis capitis
skin discoloration
slough off
soft callus
staphylococcal scalded skin syndrome (SSSS)
sterile burn sheet
sternoclavicular joint
stiff
superficial muscles
tender to the touch
united fracture

CHAPTER REVIEW

Critical Thinking

Consider all that you've learned in this chapter to answer the following questions.

1. What steps did the treatment team at Okla Trauma Center take to prevent Clay Davis from acquiring an infection while he was there? ______________________
2. Why must the titanium plate in Clay Davis's jaw be removed in the near future?

____

Right Word or Wrong Word: *Physician's Assistant* or *Physician Assistant*?

Which of these titles is correct? Are they both correct?

Label the Diagram

This is a bone that is found in the neck. Name it. ______________________

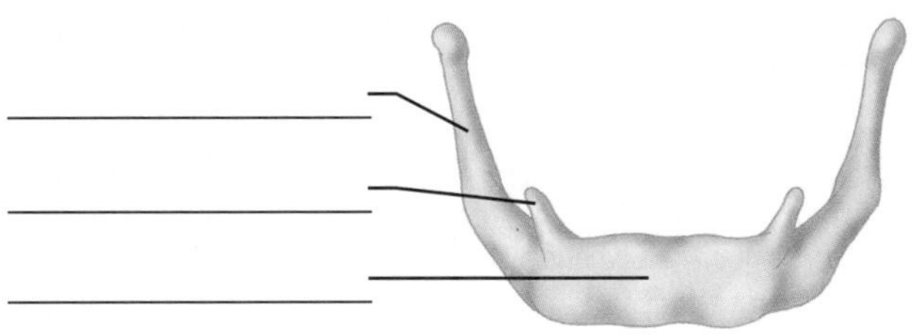

Prefixes and Suffixes

Write the meaning of each prefix or suffix.

1. -ase Meaning: ______________________
2. pro- Meaning: ______________________
3. -cyte Meaning: ______________________
4. -lysis Meaning: ______________________
5. antero- Meaning: ______________________
6. re- Meaning: ______________________
7. di- Meaning: ______________________
8. supra- Meaning: ______________________

What Do You Know?

Use medical terminology to answer the following questions.

1. Name the type of cell that develops from a monocyte and that can ingest foreign matter as a way of cleansing the blood. ______________________
2. Identify the three stages of bone healing.

   ____
3. Name two types of ossification.

   ____
4. Identify the four stages of skin tissue healing.

   ____

Mix and Match

Match the synonyms by drawing a line between the correct answers.

1. ossification	morphosis
2. mammitis	injury
3. stress response	unbearable
4. insult	mammary
5. morphogenesis	osteogenesis
6. excruciating	sternalgia
7. masticate	mastitis
8. mamillary	lower
9. depress	fight or flight response
10. sternodynia	chew

Define the Terms

Write the meaning of each descriptive term.

1. generalized Meaning: ______________________
2. focal Meaning: ______________________
3. segmental Meaning: ______________________
4. sternal Meaning: ______________________
5. mandibular Meaning: ______________________
6. hyperpigmented Meaning: ______________________

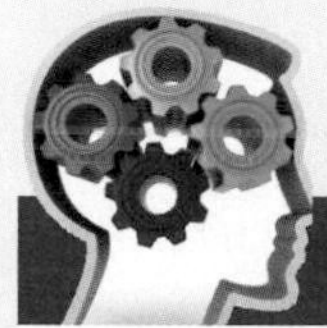

MEMORY MAGIC

1. Mnemonic

Lateral and Medial Pterygoid Muscles

Notice the placement of your jaw when saying the first part of the words *lateral* or *medial.*

LA: The jaw is open. *Lateral* muscles open the mouth.

ME: The jaw is closed. *Medial* muscles close the mouth.

2. Study Skills

The **ASPIRE** Approach

A = Approach, Attitude, and Arrange

- Approach your studies with a positive attitude.
- Arrange your study schedule to eliminate distractions.

S = Select, Survey, and Study

- Select a reasonable amount of material to study.
- Survey the headings, graphics, and any introductory or review questions. This survey will provide an overview of the material.
- Study! Mark any information that you don't understand so that it can be clarified later with a teacher, colleague, or the Internet.

Continued

P = Put aside and Piece together

- Put aside all books and notes after you've studied them.
- Piece together what you have learned: discuss it with other students, peers, or friends; write a summary.

I = Inspect, Investigate, and Inquire

- Inspect things that you didn't understand (i.e., that you marked earlier), and try to find meaning.
- Investigate alternative sources of information to make this material more clear.
- Inquire: ask questions of support professionals such as teachers, librarians, and other experts; seek their assistance.

R = Reconsider, Reflect, and Relay

- Reconsider the content of the material. For example, if you could speak to the author, what questions would you ask or what comments would you make?
- Reflect on the material, and consider how it might apply to the things in which you are interested.
- Relay understanding: teach the material to a friend or another student to reinforce your own learning.

E = Evaluate, Examine, and Explore

- Evaluate the grades you have achieved, and look for a pattern.
- Examine your learning process, and think about ideas for improving.
- Explore options and alternatives for studying, learning with teachers, and so on.

Oncology and Cancer Care

Focus: Lymphatic and Respiratory Systems

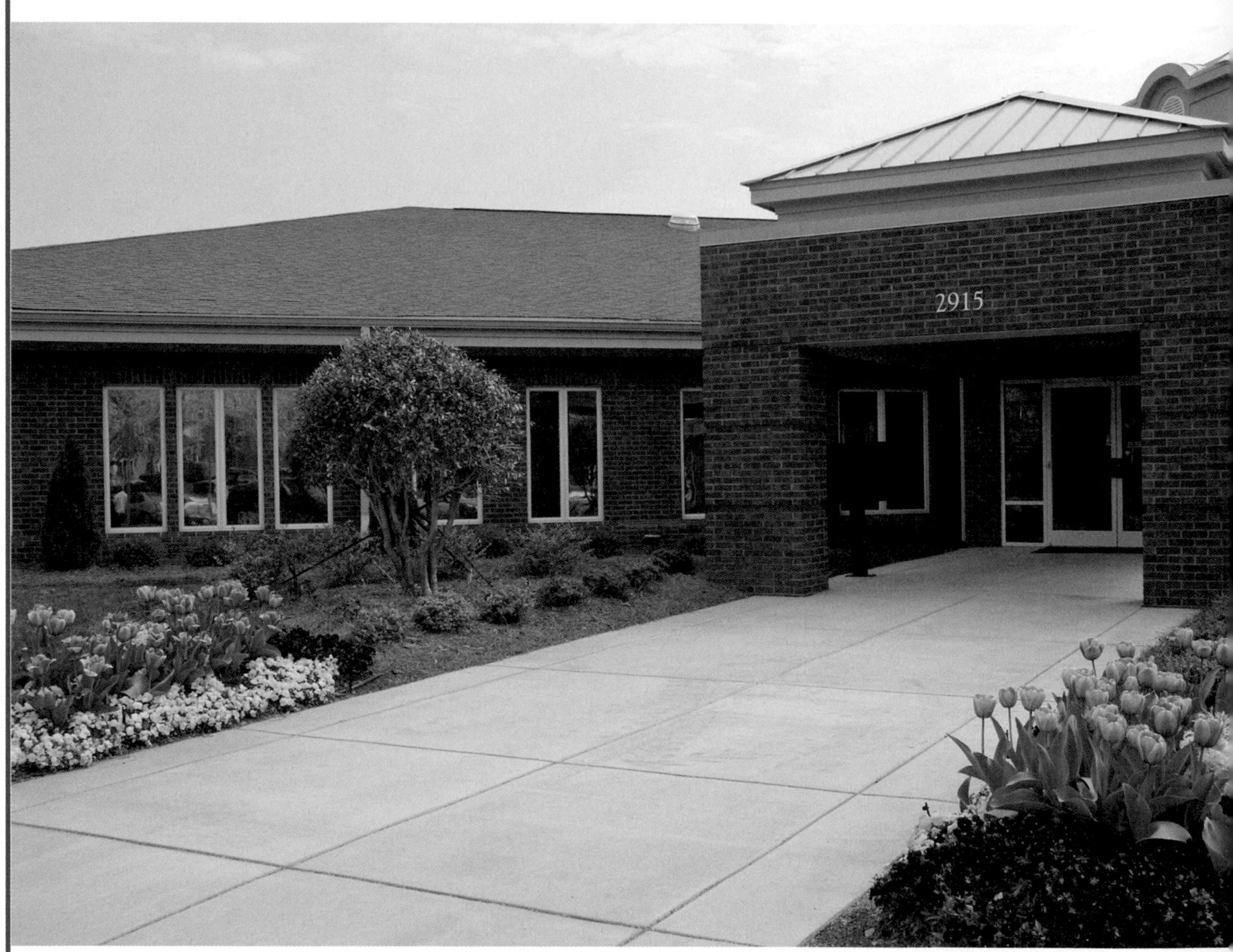

It's been 2 weeks since the motor vehicle accident at the intersection of Shawnee and Sheridan. Seventy-four-year-old Zane Davis, a victim in that incident, was taken from the site to Okla Trauma Center under the suspicion that he may have been experiencing a cardiac or cerebrovascular event. A complete assessment was performed, and these diagnoses were ruled out. However, because of the comprehensiveness of the diagnostic assessments that he underwent, physicians at Okla Trauma found shadows on Zane's lungs. They have referred him to Kootenay Cancer Care Center for follow-up. He has his first appointment today, and he is attending in the company of his wife, Stevie-Rose Davis.

Patient Update

"Hello, I'm Jacob Sweetgrass. I'm an oncologist, a specialist in diagnosing and treating cancer. Thank you for coming. Please, sit down," said a man in his early 40s who was neatly dressed in slacks, a shirt, and a tie. He was accompanied by a woman wearing a lab coat, blouse, and slacks. He moved behind his desk, speaking as he did so.

"Before we begin, let me introduce Reilly-Jo Jackson. She's a medical e-scribe working with me this summer. As you can see, she has a laptop computer in hand. She will take my notes and ensure documentation of our interactions. She won't be commenting or participating in your care other than that," he explained. Reilly-Jo moved off to a nearby chair, where she could work while still observing and listening to the doctor and the patient. The Davises introduced themselves and asked to be called by their first names.

"Oh, I see. Electronic medical records, but Reilly-Jo here writes them as you work rather than listening to dictation after the fact," reflected Zane. "That's interesting." He smiled at Reilly-Jo and she smiled back, nodding in agreement.

"Yes, that's it," said Dr. Sweetgrass. "We've had medical e-scribes here for a while at the care center, and they are just invaluable to us. We have many on staff permanently, but Reilly-Jo is actually working on her master's degree in nursing and working here as a part-time job." Dr. Sweetgrass took a seat at his desk near Zane, where he could access his computer. He then pulled up Zane's patient file.

"Sir, I would like to ask a number of health history questions today. Please bear with me. Some of these you will have answered before with your own physician or over at Okla Trauma Center, but it's important that I confirm these answers so that we know where we are headed with your care, okay?"

Zane spoke up. "Your nurse... um ...Carmelle was her name? Well, she called me the other day, and we had a good, long interview by phone. We're not going to go through all of that again, are we?" The patient looked annoyed, worrying that valuable time would be wasted repeating himself. The oncologist assured Zane that he had studied that data, Zane's past family and social history (PFSH), and the review of systems (ROS). Dr. Sweetgrass added that it was all recorded in the medical record in front of him; and that he would simply be confirming the information that he found salient to the case. He proceeded.

The interview continued for close to 30 minutes, stopping once when the patient went into a short coughing spasm. Dr. Sweetgrass began by asking Zane how he was feeling and if he was aware of any symptoms of shortness of breath, pain in his chest, or dizziness since his release from the hospital. The client commented that these symptoms were not atypical for him and confirmed that he had, indeed, experienced them recently. They talked about Zane's history of smoking. Zane and Stevie-Rose were surprised to hear the doctor call it a smoking addiction, and they commented on this.

"Research and treatment have now shown that smoking cigarettes is indeed an addiction," Dr. Sweetgrass said. "By clearly identifying it as an addiction, the medical profession is now in a much better position to both treat it as such and also to try to prevent it." The Davises nodded in agreement. Zane said he understood his own challenges over a lifetime of trying to stop smoking and having failed repeatedly. He thought that his shortness of breath was a result of smoking. This admission led them to the actual reason for this appointment.

"Mr. Davis—I mean Zane—I have a referral for you from Okla Trauma Center. I understand that you were in a car accident a couple of weeks ago that led to your care there. During the comprehensive assessment that was performed at that time, some shadows were discovered on your lungs. That's what has brought you here." Zane nodded. "I see here, too, in the consult, that your blood tests seem to rule out cancer, but the team at Okla wanted you to have a more comprehensive workup to understand those shadows, as well as the respiratory symptoms that you're experiencing." Dr. Sweetgrass paused for the couple. They said nothing, but they were listening carefully to him. "I see, too, that you were in the Navy, sir."

"Yes, yes, that's right," said Zane. "I was a communications officer in the U.S. Navy for... oh ...many years. Dr. Jackson over at Okla told me that I might have been exposed to asbestos. I spent a lot of time aboard ship during the '60s and '70s." Dr. Sweetgrass nodded and confirmed that this may indeed have exposed Zane to asbestos, but at this point there was no definitive proof of that. The oncologist then shared some of his medical knowledge about exposure to asbestos.

"I'm not sure if you are aware of this, but up to 90% of cancers have some connection to our genetic makeup, our own physiology, our lifestyle, and our environment. Working in an environment where you were surrounded by asbestos may have contributed to those shadows on your lungs and could be a source of celiothelioma for you, but we cannot be sure." The doctor stopped then, noticing a look of dread coming across the client's face. Stevie-Rose gasped. "Zane, let me rephrase that," continued Dr. Sweetgrass. "I am not saying that you have mesothelioma. Please, I didn't mean to imply that. At this point, it would be premature to offer a diagnosis. We are not sure exactly what you have or even if you have anything at all, other than what might be scar tissue of some sort. That's what you're here to find out."

This statement had a slight calming effect on the patient and his wife, but their nervousness and concern remained clear in their body language and facial expressions. Dr. Sweetgrass noticed this, and he went on in a lighter—yet still professional—tone. "So, here's what I'd like to do," said the doctor. "I'd like to do a toxicology screen for asbestos. It's just a blood test. In addition, I'd like to redo some basic blood work, particularly to look for evidence of any cancer anywhere in your body." Zane and Stevie-Rose looked at each other apprehensively.

"I had a PSA at Okla," interjected Zane. "It should be there in my file." Dr. Sweetgrass confirmed that he had those results, but he wondered if Zane wanted to have the test again because he would be undergoing a battery of tests. The doctor pointed out that one of the physicians at Okla Trauma Center had suggested a visit with a urologist and that there were oncologists at Kootenay Cancer Care Center who specialized in urology as well.

"Oh, I see, well, okay," said Zane. "I guess you know too, that I had a urinary tract infection of some sort recently. It should be there in that report." Dr. Sweetgrass confirmed that he knew about the UTI. "Well, maybe I should come clean and tell you that I have had some trouble going to the bathroom. I told the nurse at Okla that this didn't happen often—well, not much anyway—but I do have some trouble starting a ... a ...flow? Is that what you call it?" Dr. Sweetgrass nodded. "And I get up in the night fairly frequently." Zane paused a moment, thinking. "I just figured that was part of growing older." He looked inquiringly at the doctor. "So, I guess having this test done again here would be a good idea, just to be sure about what's really going on. And it would get around me having to set up a separate appointment somewhere else." Dr. Sweetgrass agreed.

"These are all very necessary diagnostic steps, I assure you," the doctor continued. "I'd also like to assure you both that here at Kootenay Cancer Care Center we are firmly committed to excellence in diagnostics and care. We, just like you, want to know exactly what your health status is and if you are facing any health challenges that we can help you with." The doctor paused for the Davises to digest this information. "So, we'll get some blood work done STAT, right while you are here today. And I'd like to get another chest CT as well, if that's all right with you." He paused, and Zane nodded. "Good. We'll do all of that today, too. That's why you were given an early morning appointment—so that we can get as much information as possible about your health today and save you multiple trips in and out of the center." The Davises nodded and thanked him for this. "When those results come back, we can talk about next steps, okay?" The couple nodded and Dr. Sweetgrass stood up. "Zane, what I'd like to do now is my own physical exam. My nursing assistant is going to escort you to an examining room to get you set up. I'll be in to see you in just a few moments."

Dr. Sweetgrass smiled and picked up the office phone to summon a CNA to his office. The certified nursing assistant arrived within minutes.

"Corey, this is Mr. Zane Davis. Please escort him to the examining room for a physical assessment. Give the lab a ring and ask them to come for some blood work, okay? And book a CT scan for this morning, too. I'll write orders." Corey smiled and nodded. "Stevie-Rose, perhaps you would like to sit in the waiting room? I think you'll find some coffee or tea available there for you, if you'd like," said the physician, graciously.

"We have a lovely coffee shop in the lobby, too," said Corey, "and a bright and sunny cafeteria on the third floor as well."

Stevie-Rose stood and put her hand on her husband's shoulder. Smiling at him. "Honey," she said softly, "I'll be right here in the waiting room, waiting for you."

Reflective Questions

Reflect on the story that you've just read.

1. What does the abbreviation *CNA* stand for? ____________________
2. What is the reason for Zane Davis's appointment at Kootenay Cancer Care Center?

____

Critical Thinking

Think back on all you've learned about Zane Davis in this Patient Update and in the previous chapters, and then answer this question.

What is the etiology of mesothelioma? ____________________

For audio exercises, **visit http://www.MedicalLanguageLab.com.** 

Learning Objectives

After reading Chapter 14, you will be able to do the following:

- Differentiate between cancer and oncology.
- Recognize and use the language of oncology.
- Recognize and use the language of cancer.
- Recognize and use medical terminology that identifies the etiology, pathophysiology, and diagnostics related to oncology.
- Recognize and use medical terminology related to cancer care and treatment.
- Differentiate among the stages, grades, and classifications of cancer.
- Appreciate the education and training of an oncology technician and an oncology surgery technician.
- Achieve an introductory awareness of the types of cancer treatment medications.
- Recognize, interpret, and use medical and anatomical terminology for the lymphatic system.
- Enhance your understanding of medical and anatomical terminology related to respiratory diagnostics.
- Recognize, interpret, and use terminology related to the care and treatment of asbestosis and similar pulmonary diseases.
- Develop an awareness of respiratory therapy.
- Appreciate the education and training of a medical e-scribe.
- Appreciate the education and training of a respiratory therapist and technician.

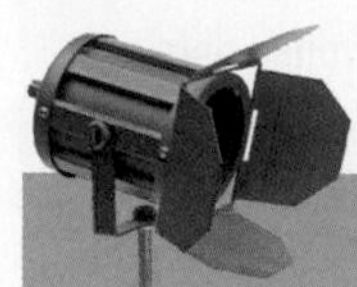

CAREER SPOTLIGHT: Medical E-scribe

The word *scribe* means *writer.* A *medical e-scribe* is a paraprofessional: he or she is someone who assists a professional with the performance of that professional's job. Medical e-scribes assist professionals by documenting the interactions that occur among the physician, the patient or client, and the treatment team as it occurs. In addition, the e-scribe may process the orders for laboratory diagnostics, referrals, and so on. All of these notes and documents become part of the patient's electronic medical record. Medical e-scribes are sworn to patient and client confidentiality, and they work silently in the background. They do not participate in any other way than as a recorder of the physician's words and actions and the patient's story. The physician is ultimately responsible for this documentation and must verify its accuracy.

Medical e-scribes are usually undergraduate students in health care and allied health fields. This background allows them to see, understand, and interpret the interactions in which the physician is involved. Medical interns and nurse practitioners may also work as medical e-scribes; if they do so, they must not have any other clinical responsibility for or involvement with the patient or client, and they may not count this work as their own billable service. Documentation is taken by hand, on a laptop computer, or on a workstation on wheels (WOW), which is a computer on a cart that can be taken where needed. Additional training in medical documentation is expected.

The term *e-scribe* is sometimes written without the hyphen as *escribe.* Emergency medical e-scribes may also use the acronym *EMS* to identify themselves. Note that medical e-scribes are not found in every hospital, clinic, and care facility; this is a newer occupation.

Cancer Care Centers

Zane Davis has come to Kootenay Cancer Care Center on a referral from Okla Trauma Center for further assessment of his lungs and respiratory system. A *cancer care center* or *cancer treatment center* is a highly specialized facility that includes inpatient and outpatient care. Their mandate is the diagnosis, treatment, recovery, restoration, rehabilitation, and maintenance of health, and they specialize in different types of cancer. Cancer care centers offer advanced diagnostic and treatment options that may not be available in general hospitals.

Patients come to a cancer center via referral, or they may have self-selected this avenue of health care. As outpatients, they may be referred to as *clients.* After they have been admitted, they may be referred to as *patients.* Should they be admitted to a palliative care unit, they may be referred to as *patients, clients,* or even *residents.* Family members are welcomed and encouraged to attend appointments and programs at cancer centers. Support programs are also offered for patients and family members as they cope with the experience of cancer.

Cancer care centers are staffed by a variety of health and allied health professionals, all of whom have specific expertise in their own fields, as well as in how those fields relate to cancer. All staff members work within an *integrated care* model, and they work together to achieve optimal patient outcomes. Staff members may include—but are not limited to—the following: oncologists, physician assistants, oncology nurses, oncology technicians, gastroenterologists, immunologists, radiologists and radiology technicians, laboratory technicians, nutritionists, psychologists, psychiatric nurses, and medical office assistants.

Reflective Questions

Medical e-scribes and cancer care centers may be new concepts for you. Consider what you've just learned about them, and then answer these questions.

1. What is the function of a medical e-scribe? ______________________
2. What qualifications are necessary to become a medical e-scribe? ______________________

____

3. Our patient, Zane Davis, has not been diagnosed with cancer. At this time, cancer is only a possible diagnosis. So why is he at a cancer care center? ______________________________

Key terms and concepts

Key terms from the Patient Update and the passage about cancer care centers are explained below.

"... includes both *inpatient* and *outpatient* care."

inpatient: a label given to patients who are admitted to and staying in a hospital.

outpatient: a label given to patients who do not require full admission to a hospital but who still need medical treatment or follow-up care. These patients are ambulatory. They come and go to outpatient appointments on their own.

"... listening to *dictation* after the fact ..."

dictation: the transcription of spoken words into a print document.

"... *review of systems* (ROS) ..."

review of systems (ROS): a series of questions that relate to each of the patient's body systems to provide a comprehensive overview of the patient's health history.

"... that he found *salient* to the case."

salient: significant, relevant, or noteworthy.

"... these symptoms were not *atypical* for him ..."

atypical: unusual.

"... a smoking *addiction* ..."

addiction: physical or emotional dependence on a harmful or toxic drug, substance, person, or behavior (see "Focus Point: Addiction" and Chapter 7 for more information)

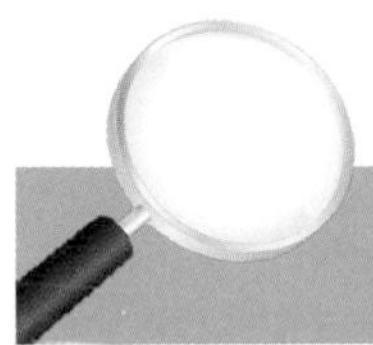

FOCUS POINT: Addiction and Criteria for Diagnosing an Addiction

An addiction is a severe, persistent, uncontrollable, and compulsive physical or psychological need to do or have something, regardless of the fact that the desired object or activity is harmful to the addict. An addiction leads a person to behave in a multitude of ways to obtain the desired substance or activity. Addictions are habit forming, and attempts to halt the addiction can cause uncomfortable physiological or psychological effects to the degree that many people who suffer from addiction cannot tolerate the symptoms of withdrawal itself. Addictions can be to foods, substances, activities, and even people.

Criteria for the diagnosis of an addiction include but are not limited to the following:

- developing an increasing tolerance to the desired object or substance, thereby causing a need to have more of it to achieve the desired effects;
- increasing the amount of time spent in pursuit of attaining the object or substance;
- increasing the distance from others in one's social sphere (i.e., at work or at home);
- developing an awareness of the addiction and a desire or a history of unsuccessful attempts to quit; and
- having a history of unsuccessful attempts to cut down consumption.

For more information about addiction, see Chapter 7.

"... a source of *celiothelioma* ..."

celiothelioma: a synonym for mesothelioma (see Chapter 9).

"... it would be *premature* to offer a diagnosis."

premature: too early or ahead of time.

"I had a *PSA* ..."

PSA: prostate-specific antigen test (see Chapters 5 and 9).

"Give the lab *a ring* ..."

a ring: slang term for *call them by telephone.*

"... *advanced diagnostic and treatment options* ..."

advanced diagnostic and treatment options: access to and the provision of the most up-to-date equipment, laboratories, tools, treatments (i.e., medical, psychological, pharmaceutical, radiological, naturopathic, palliative, support), and care staff. This phrase is often used in reference to highly specialized facilities such as trauma centers, wound care centers, addiction centers, and cancer care centers.

"... admitted to a *palliative care unit* ..."

palliative care unit: a highly specialized unit that provides comfort and quality of life for patients with serious, often (but not always) terminal, life-ending medical challenges.

"*Support programs* are also offered ..."

support programs: any type of program that is designed to offer encouragement, education, comfort, and help to people with illnesses, injuries, addictions, and psychological or psychiatric needs. There are also many support programs for the family members of patients. Examples include support groups for patients with cancer, Alzheimer's disease, alcoholism, or post-traumatic stress disorder.

"... *optimal patient outcomes.*"

optimal patient outcomes: the best possible results of care and treatment.

Free Writing

Use the new terminology that you have learned to write sentences. You are given some clue words to help you. Use these words in your sentence, although you might have to change them slightly. Of course, you will also need to add a number of your own words to make a logical sentence.

Example: welcomed family attend encouraged to members appointments

Sentence: Family members are welcomed and encouraged to attend a patient's appointments.

1. programs clients optimal promotes offering outcomes

___

2. period mesothelioma exposure long can asbestos

___

3. addiction atypical to smokers not cigarettes

___

4. source be environment asbestos in lung disease can

___

5. diagnostic premature without offer would full a to workup diagnosis

___

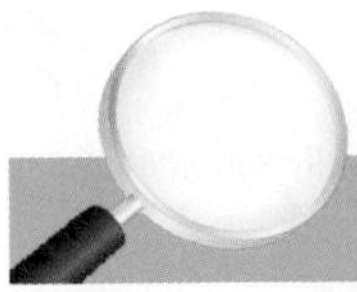

FOCUS POINT: The History of Scribes

Scribes have been in existence since mankind learned to draw and write in an effort to record thoughts, observations, and experiences. In ancient civilizations, scribes were also scholars, and theirs was a position of esteem. They were generally chosen for the position by a monarch or another member of the ruling elite for their intelligence and ability to learn. They became the keepers of knowledge and of private information, particularly in times when the great masses of people could not read or write.

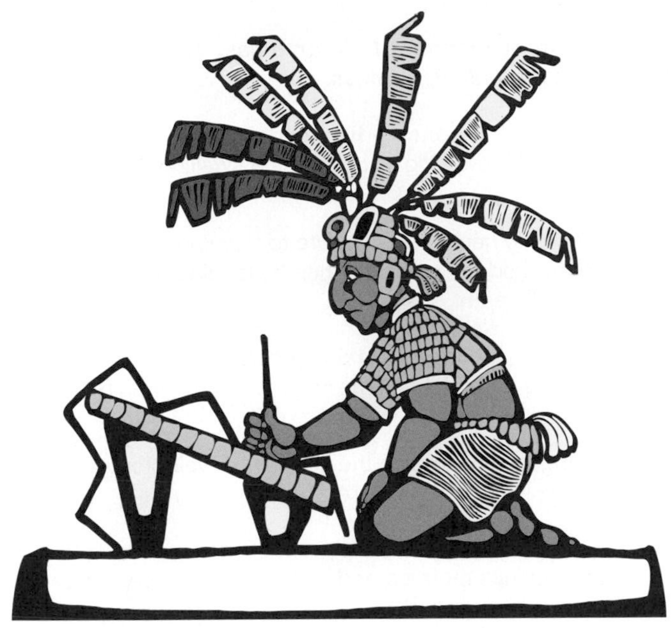

Figure 14.1: Mayan scribe (© Thinkstock)

Cancer and Oncology

Cancer is one of the most prevalent diseases of the 21st century to date. It is not unlikely that each reader of this book will know someone who has experienced it. The likelihood of acquiring some form of cancer among people who live in the United States and Canada is estimated to be approximately 33% over a lifetime.

Cancer (CA) is the growth of abnormal cells that eventually overtake and destroy healthy, normal cells. It is caused by *carcinogens* (see Chapter 9). **Oncology** is the branch of medicine that deals with swollen tissue, tumors, and masses, as well as with cancer research, care, and treatment.

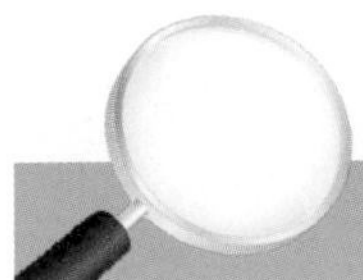

FOCUS POINT: The Abbreviations *Ca* and *CA*

The accepted medical abbreviations for cancer are *Ca* and *CA*. Remember that the context of an abbreviation is extremely important when you are trying to decipher it. These two letters can also mean many other things; consider the following examples:

Ca: calcium

CA: cardiac arrest, chronological age, cancer antigen, or cytosine arabinoside (an antimetabolite that is used to treat neoplasms)

Right Word or Wrong Word: *Oncology* or *Cancer*?

Do these two terms refer to the same thing? They are often used synonymously, but are they really synonyms?

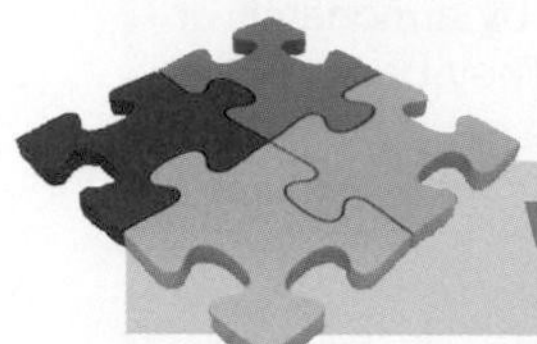

WORD BUILDING: Formulas for Creating Words From the Combining Form *Onco-*

onkos = an early Greek root meaning *bulk or mass.* The modern combining form is *onco-*, which means *tumor, swelling, or mass.*

onco + tic = *oncotic*

Definition: caused or marked by swelling or concerning swelling. (The suffix *-tic* means *pertaining to.*) *adjective*

Example: In the case of *oncotic* necrosis, exposure to toxins or injury can cause some molecules within the cells to produce cytokine, thereby leading to cell swelling, the leakage of the cell's contents, and cell death.

onco + fetal = *oncofetal*

Definition: concerning tumors in the fetus. (The second word part is *fetal,* which refers to a fetus.) *adjective*

Example: An *oncofetal* antigen is present in the normally developing gastrointestinal tissues of an embryo, but it is also specific to colon cancer.

onco + gene = *oncogene*

Definition: a type of gene that has mutated and that now makes cells grow and divide more quickly. *noun*

Example: Cancer cells contain *oncogenes.*

onco + cyto + oma = *oncocytoma*

Definition: an epithelial tumor cell in which the cytoplasm and the mitochondria of a cell are involved (see Chapter 2). *noun*

Example: An *oncocytoma* is usually benign and found in the kidneys or the glands.

onco + tomy = *oncotomy*

Definition: the incision of a tumor, abscess, or boil. *noun*

Example: An *oncotomy* of an abscess or boil on the skin may be performed to relieve pressure.

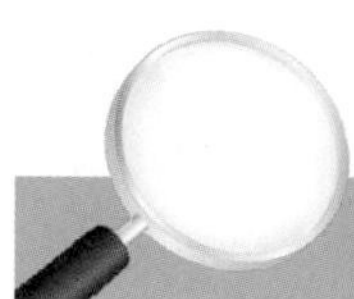

FOCUS POINT: Mitosis

Mitosis is a process of cell division in which the nucleus divides, thereby creating two identical chromosomes. Chromosomes are the structures within cells that carry genes.

Build a Word

Combine the word parts to create a medical term, and then define each term.

1. logy onco Term: ________________ Meaning: ________________
2. -genesis onco Term: ________________ Meaning: ________________
3. virus onco Term: ________________ Meaning: ________________
4. -lysis onco Term: ________________ Meaning: ________________
5. therapy onco Term: ________________ Meaning: ________________
6. logist onco Term: ________________ Meaning: ________________

Key oncology and cancer suffixes

The recognition of suffixes is a key tool used to decipher medical terminology. The more often you see and use medical suffixes, the more likely you will be to recognize and remember them in the future, even if you do not understand the root of the word right away. Table 14-1 highlights a number of suffixes that are common to oncology and cancer.

Build a Word

Build medical terms with the use of the suffixes listed in Table 14-1. Use the prefixes, roots, or combining forms that are given. Remember, you may have to change a word part slightly to get it to combine correctly. For example:

Laryng/o + suffix____________ = ____________

Possible answer:

Laryng + itis = laryngitis

Skeleton + suffix ____________ = ____________

Possible answer:

Skelet + al = skeletal

(If you need help with suffixes, please refer to Chapter 2)

1. psycho + suffix ________________ = Word: ________________
2. endo + suffix ________________ = Word: ________________
3. hypo + suffix ________________ = Word: ________________
4. endotheli/o + suffix ________________ = Word: ________________
5. aller + suffix ________________ = Word: ________________
6. melan + suffix ________________ = Word: ________________
7. hallucin/o + suffix ________________ = Word: ________________
8. non+ carcin/o + suffix ________________ = Word: ________________
9. cyto + suffix ________________ = Word: ________________
10. proto + suffix ________________ = Word: ________________

TABLE 14-1: Key Oncology and Cancer Suffixes

Suffix	Meaning	Examples
-gen	producing	carcinogen
-oma	tumor or mass	sarcoma
-plasia	growth or formation	aplasia (the failure of a tissue or an organ to develop normally)
-plasm	form or mold; growth or formation	neoplasm
-therapy	treatment	chemotherapy

Break It Down

Study the following terms that contain the root word *cancer*. Break down each term into its component parts, and then define the term.

1. cancercidal ______________________ Meaning: ______________________
2. cancerophobia ______________________ Meaning: ______________________
3. precancerous ______________________ Meaning: ______________________

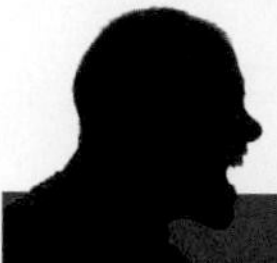

PRONUNCIATION PRACTICE

Say these words aloud to a friend or classmate, if you can. Here you are given the phonetic pronunciation. Your instructor can help you with pronunciation, or you can visit **http://www.MedicalLanguageLab.com.**

atypical	ā-**tĭp**´ĭ-kăl	mitosis	mī-**tō**´sĭs
carcinogen	kăr-**sĭn**´ō-jĕn	oncocytoma	ŏng″kō-sī-**tō**´mă
celiothelioma	sē″lē-ō-thē-lē-ō´mă	oncofetal	ŏng″kō-**fē**´tăl
endoplasm	**ĕn**´dō-plăzm	oncolysis	ŏng-**kŏl**´ĭ-sĭs
endothelioma	ĕn″dŏ-thē-lē-**ō**´mă	oncotic	ŏng-**kŏt**´ĭk
lymph	**lĭmf**	oncotomy	ŏng-**kŏt**´ō-mē
lymphatic	lĭm-**făt**´ĭk	protoplasm	**prō**´tō-plăzm
melanoma	mĕl″ă-**nō**´mă		

Etiology of cancer: carcinogens

In the Patient Update, Dr. Sweetgrass explained to Zane Davis that cancers have many causes. Carcinogens can be found in a person's genetic makeup. In addition, influential factors in a person's lifestyle and environment can play a significant role in increasing that person's risk of acquiring cancer. Pathogens (i.e., bacteria, viruses) can also be carcinogenic if they are harmful enough to injure or damage DNA (see Figure 14-2). The following sections explain some of the factors that may affect a person's chances of getting cancer and of surviving a cancer diagnosis.

Genetics

Genetics is the study of heredity. Medical histories include questions about the health of a patient's relatives because many health challenges are hereditary, the result of a genetic predisposition. Table 14-2 highlights a few of these hereditary conditions. However, simply having genes identified as markers of a health challenge do not guarantee that the condition will occur. Environment, prenatal care, nutrition, and many other factors play into the outcome.

Genes

Genes molecules are contained within every living cell. They function as a set of instructions for the physical structure and function of organisms. Genes string together to create **deoxyribonucleic acid (DNA)**, a material found in every cell of the body. It contains genetic or hereditary information. Strings of DNA make up **chromosomes** (see Figure 14-2). Simply put, chromosomes are the structures that carry genes and that determine the characteristics and sex of an organism. Every cell in the human body contains 23 pairs of chromosomes.

Each strand of DNA contains four bases or chemical compounds: adenine (A), cytosine (C), guanine (G), and thymine (T). These bases are called **nucleotides**. (Note: A simple awareness of these terms is all that is required at this level of medical terminology. Anatomy, physiology, and microbiology texts can provide more detail, if needed.)

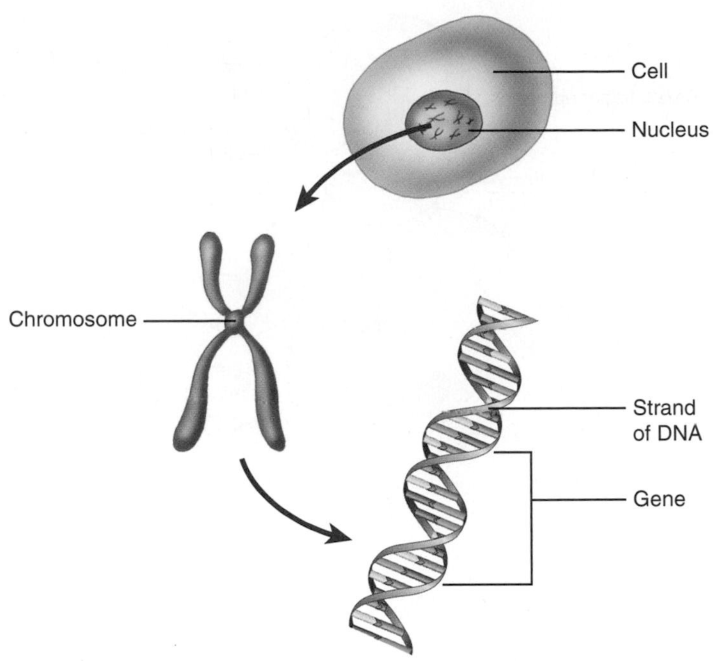

Figure 14.2: Genes on a strand of DNA

TABLE 14-2: Health Challenges with Genetic Predispositions
diabetes mellitus (see Chapter 12)
multiple sclerosis: a progressive and chronic condition of the central nervous system
spina bifida (see Chapter 8)
Alzheimer's disease (see Chapters 7 and 12)
congenital hip displacement: an abnormal formation of the hip joint
cleft lip or palate
hypertension (see Chapters 5 and 13)
manic depression (see Chapter 7)
schizophrenia (see Chapter 7)
alcoholism (see Chapter 7)
addiction (see Chapters 7 and 14)
certain cancers (i.e., breast, prostate, cervical, stomach, and lung)
heart disease (see Chapters 5 and 9)
hemophilia: a rare bleeding disorder
arthritis (see Chapters 7 and 16)

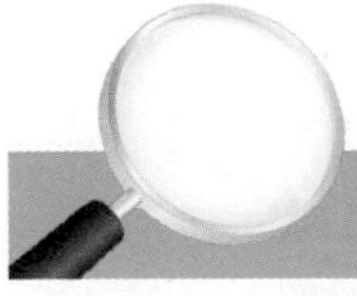

FOCUS POINT: Aneuploidy

Aneuploidy refers to genomic change (i.e., an alteration in a gene or genes) that is not a mutation but rather a loss or gain of at least one chromosome through an error in mitosis. In simple terms, the result of aneuploidy is a birth defect. An example of an aneuploidy disorder is trisomy 21 (Down syndrome).

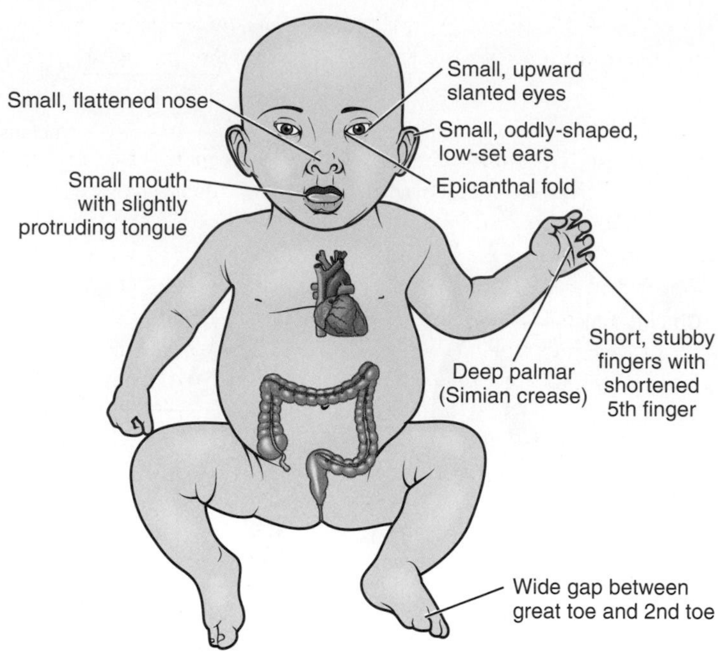

Figure 14.3: A child with Down syndrome (From Eagle S: *Diseases in a Flash!: An Interactive, Flash-Card Approach.* Philadelphia: FA Davis, 2012, p 579. With permission.)

Hardiness and resiliency

A person's hardiness and resiliency are determined by the genes that are passed on by that person's biological parents, as well as by his or her lifestyle choices, belief systems, and environmental influences. **Hardiness** refers to the vitality of a person; it can also be thought of his or her strength, energy, and drive. A person's degree of hardiness is influenced by his or her own health-promoting behaviors in life (i.e., eating healthy foods, exercising), but it also includes a person's philosophical, spiritual, psychological, and emotional approach to life. A person who is hardy will be able to cope more effectively with physical or mental hardship than someone who is not. In other words, he or she will be capable of surviving under unfavorable conditions.

Resiliency refers to a person's ability to bounce back or to recover quickly from an unfavorable circumstance or situation. A resilient person is one who is able to withstand physical or mental stressors. Resiliency is also referred to as *stamina,* which means *strength, endurance, and resistance.*

Right Word or Wrong Word: *Hardiness* or *Heartiness?*

If you were not listening carefully to a conversation, you might not be able to distinguish between the words *hardiness* and *heartiness.* Would that matter? Are these words the same? Is one spelled differently simply because it is written in American English rather than British or Canadian English?

Lifestyle

The term **lifestyle** refers to a way of life that reflects a person's life choices, circumstances, and behaviors. It includes a person's attitudes and beliefs about life, as well as that person's attitudes and beliefs about health and illness. Exploring a patient or client's lifestyle is a routine part of health assessment. This exploration can provide important information related to the etiology and onset of illness, the potential for recovery, the access to or likelihood of using health services (including the patient's own physical and mental health resources), and the patient's daily routines. The exploration of the patient's lifestyle may provide important information about his or her exposure to risks for cancer. An example is Zane Davis's history of smoking, which has increased his risk for lung cancer.

Environment

In health care, the term **environment** refers to environmental factors that may influence a patient's health. Although these factors are often thought of as elements in the physical environment, they can also include psychological environmental factors. For example, living in dire poverty without adequate housing and nutrition involves a risky physical environment, whereas living in a household in which drug addiction is present involves risks in one's psychological environment.

Environmental toxins are chemicals that adversely affect physical well-being and that may be disease producing. Environmental toxins that produce cancer are called **carcinogens**. For example, working in agriculture—where pesticides are frequently used—exposes farm workers to high degrees of carcinogens. Our patient, Zane Davis, spent many years in a work environment in which asbestos insulation lined the walls, ceilings, floors, and water pipes. Exposure to environmental toxins over time increases the risk of acquiring cancer.

Name the Term

Write the term that fits each description.

1. agents or toxins that cause cancer ______________________________
2. a structure that is formed when genes combine into string-like shapes ______________
3. two environmental toxins that can lead to cancer ______________________________
4. structures that carry genes and determine the characteristics and sex of an organism ____
5. found in pairs and made of DNA ______________________________
6. the ability to bounce back from illness or trauma ______________________________

Critical Thinking

Recall all that you know about the patients whom we are following in this book: Zane Davis, Stevie-Rose Davis, Clay Davis, Gil Loeppky, and Glory Loeppky. Answer these questions about possible hereditary links to disease among these patients.

1. Which patient may have a genetic predisposition to arthritis? ____________________
2. Which patient may have a genetic predisposition to heart disease? ________________
3. Which patient may have a genetic predisposition to cancer? ____________________

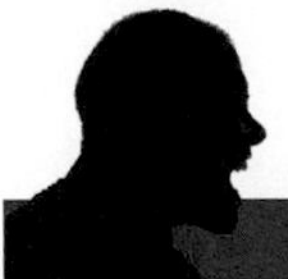

PRONUNCIATION PRACTICE

Say these words aloud to a friend or classmate, if you can. Here you are given the phonetic pronunciation. Your instructor can help you with pronunciation,

or you can visit **http://www.MedicalLanguageLab.com.** mll

chromosome	**kr**ō´mō-sōm	hardiness	**här´**dē-nĕs
deoxyribonucleic	dē-**ŏx**´ē-rī-bō-nū-**klē**´ĭk	heartiness	**här´**tē-nĕs
etiology	ē″tē-**ŏl**´ō-jē	trisomy	**trī**´sō-mē
genetics	jĕ-**nĕt**´ĭks	vitality	vī-**tăl**´ĭ-tē

Pathophysiology of cancer

Cancer is a disease that involves the regulation of tissue growth. It occurs when the genes that regulate tissue growth and **cell differentiation**, which is the process of creating cells that are different in function, are somehow altered.

Cancer cells and neoplasms

Expand your vocabulary of cell physiology as you explore the pathophysiology of cancer cells and cancerous genes.

A cancer cell is part of a **neoplasm**, an abnormal formation of tissues that may be malignant or benign. A neoplasm serves no function, and it takes over space where healthy, normal tissues should exist at the expense of those healthy tissues. The adjective form of this word is *neoplastic* (see Tables 14-3 and 14-4).

A cancer cell differs from a normal cell because of its irregular shape, the changes in the size of its nucleus and cytoplasm, and because *mitosis* or cell division is much more frequent (see Figure 14–4). Cancer cells have the ability to *metastasize* (spread) throughout surrounding tissue or the entire body. Cancer cells can also be **anaplastic**, which means that their structures can revert to a state of being undifferentiated rather than differentiated by function and size. Anaplastic cells divide rapidly and have little resemblance to normal cells.

Anaplastic is the adjective form of *anaplasia,* which is derived from the prefix *ana-,* meaning *backward,* and the suffix *-plasia,* meaning *growing or developing.*

Although neoplasms can develop into tumors, not all cancer cells become tumors. For example, leukemia cancer cells are found in the blood and the bone marrow.

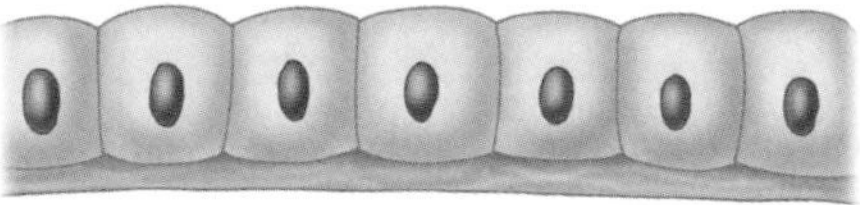

Normal cell

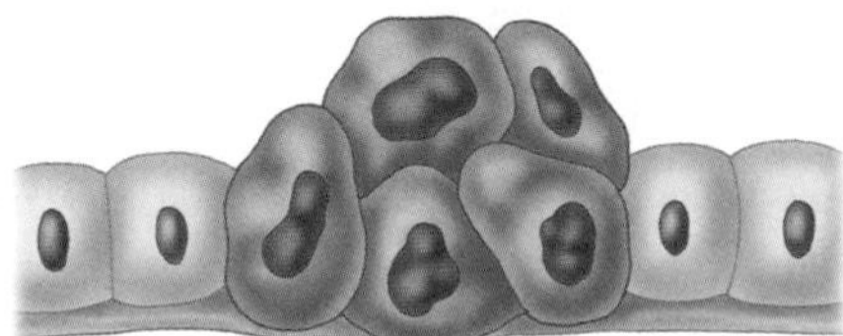

Cancer cell

Figure 14.4: Normal cells vs. cancer cells

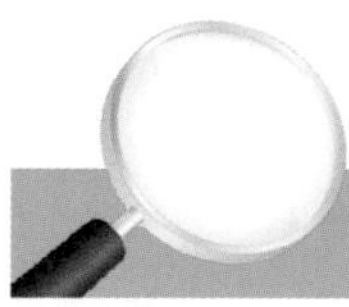

FOCUS POINT: *Benign vs. Malignant*

These two words are medical antonyms.

Benign means *not progressive* or *not likely to recur.* Some neoplasms, such as moles, are benign. Benign tumors grow slowly. (See Table 14-3.)

Malignant means *severe, harmful, progressively worsening, and capable of invading.* In a medical context, it means *cancerous.* Malignant tumors grow quickly. *Malignant* is an adjective, whereas *malignancy* is a noun. The words derive from the Latin root *malignare,* which means *to plot against or to be malicious.*

TABLE 14-3: Examples of Benign Neoplasms

Neoplasm	Description
Histoid	Resembles the structures that surround it; consists of only one type of connective tissue Example: histoid leprosy (skin lesions or tumors caused by a variant and more rare form of leprosy)
Noninvasive	Does not spread Example: a birthmark or mole (nevus)
Desmoid	Scar-like connective tissue that forms a benign tumor, often (but not only) in the abdominal muscles of women who have borne children Example: Gardner syndrome (a condition in which there are colorectal polyps and soft- and hard-tissue neoplasms)
Lymphocele	A cyst that contains lymph, which can occur after surgery Example: a pelvic lymphocele (this is caused by leakage when a lymph node is injured during surgery of the pelvic region)

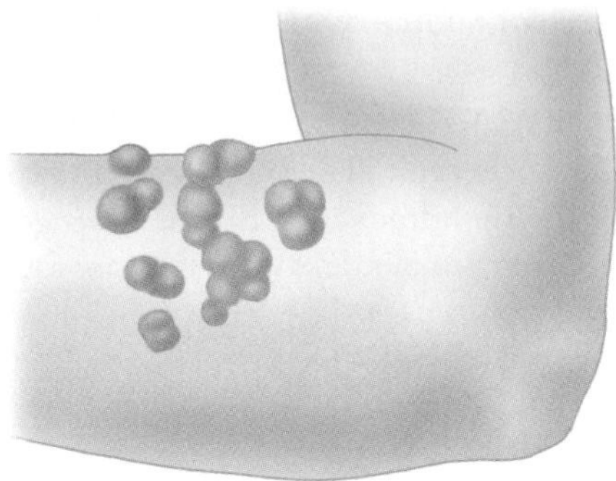

Figure 14.5: Patient with histoid leprosy

The term **neoplasia** refers to an uncontrolled proliferation of cells. These tumors may be benign or malignant. *Neoplasia* is generally used to refer to the spread of malignancies and the invasion of the lymphatic system by cancer cells. An example of neoplasia is a condition called *multiple endocrine neoplasia* (MEN), which has types 1, 2, and 3. This condition is a syndrome of symptoms that involve more than one endocrine gland. A specific example of a neoplastic disorder is Wermer's syndrome.

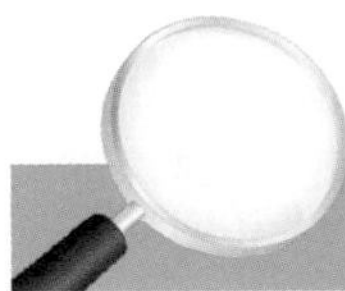

FOCUS POINT: Hyperplasia

Hyperplasia is an abnormal condition in which there is an increase in the production of normal cells.

physiologic hyperplasia: when cells remain normal, even though they are in excess; however, this condition may eventually be determined to be precancerous
pathologic hyperplasia: when hyperplasic cells are determined to be precancerous

Eponyms: Wermer's Syndrome or Multiple Endocrine Neoplasia Type 1

Dr. Paul Wermer was a 20th-century American medical internist and scientist. Around the middle of the century, he became the first to describe the group of symptoms that would later be named *Wermer's syndrome.* Wermer's syndrome is also known as *multiple endocrine neoplasia type 1.* The syndrome is determined by the presence of a number of tumors occurring at approximately the same time or consecutively. Tumors that are associated with this syndrome primarily affect the islets of Langerhans and the thyroid, parathyroid, and pituitary glands, but other locations may also be involved. A diagnosis of Wermer's syndrome signifies a diminished life span. Some examples of conditions that are associated with this syndrome include the following:

parathyroid hyperplasia: increased growth of the parathyroid cells
medullary thyroid cancer: cancer of the thyroid gland (the term *medullary* refers to *the center or the innermost portion)*

Cancerous genes

Cancer cells have genes that are different from those of healthy cells.

Proto-oncogenes produce proteins for normal cellular activities, particularly cell growth and division. If a proto-oncogene mutates or is adversely affected by a virus or an environmental toxin, it may be transformed into an oncogene.

Oncogenes are the precursors of cancer cells. They are genes with proteins that have been altered, thus transforming normal cells into tumor cells. Because oncogenes activate growth and cell division, cancer cells begin to proliferate. When they are found at high levels, they can facilitate the growth of malignant tumors.

Tumor suppressor genes are situated in healthy DNA. Their normal function is to prevent cancer by inhibiting cancer cell growth and division. However, after oncogenes have been activated, the tumor suppressor genes become inactive.

The term **mutation** describes any change or alteration of the genetic material. When mutation occurs on a large scale, chromosomes are affected. The shape or function of a complete organism could be affected.

The term **translocation** describes an abnormal fusion or merging of two separate regions of chromosomes on the DNA strand. Translocation has the potential to lead to a type of cancer called *chronic myelogenous leukemia.*

Chronic myelogenous leukemia (CML) is a slow, progressive, malignant disease of bone marrow and the blood stem cells (immature blood cells) that is the result of translocation. With this condition, the production of white blood cells (granulocytes) is excessive, and these cells are all abnormal. It is caused when two pieces of different chromosomes break off and attach to each other (see Figure 14-6). This disease usually occurs during middle age. CML is also known as *chronic myeloid leukemia (CML)* and *chronic granulocytic leukemia.*

Acute myelogenous leukemia (AML) is a fast-acting, progressive, and terminal disease of the bone marrow and the blood stem cells. When these stem cells differentiate (a natural process), they can become blood stem cells: *myeloid stem cells* (red, white, or platelet cells) or *lymphoid stem cells.* In patients with AML, all white blood cells are abnormal, whereas red cells and platelets may or may not be so. The result is a type of leukemia that strikes across the life span. Other names for this cancer are *acute myeloid leukemia (AML), acute granulocytic leukemia,* and *acute non-lymphocytic leukemia.*

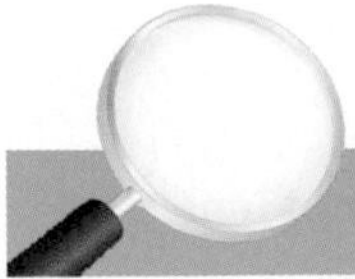

FOCUS POINT: The Philadelphia Chromosome (Ph+)

In patients with chronic myeloid leukemia (CML), two separate chromosomes break and a piece of each one detaches. Subsequently, these different pieces migrate to each other and attach themselves, thereby creating a new chromosome known as the *Philadelphia chromosome* or the *Philadelphia-positive chromosome.* This new structure contains or is positive for an abnormal gene called *bcr-abl.* Next, bcr-abl produces something called a *BCR-ABL protein,* which stimulates the rapid production of abnormal white blood cells. (See Figure 14-6.)

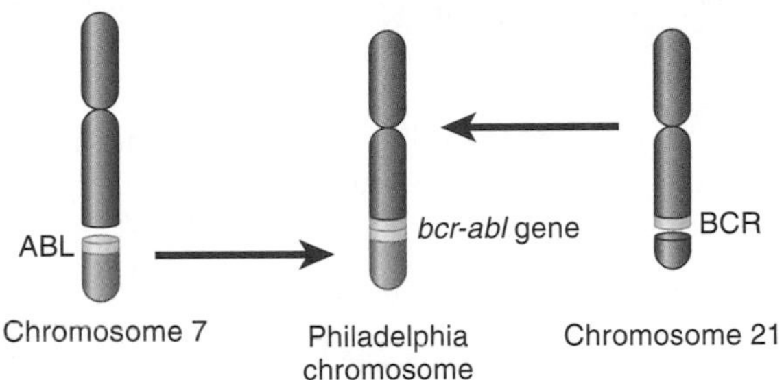

Figure 14.6: The Philadelphia chromosome

Metastasis

The term **metastasis** refers to the spread of cancer cells through a process of invasion, which involves the moving into and taking over of other cells (see Figure 14-7). The plural form of this word is *metastases.* When referring to metastasis, the abbreviated term *mets* is frequently used. The word *metastasis* is derived from two word parts:

meta: a prefix meaning *after, beyond, over or subsequent to*

stasis: a root word meaning *standing, staying in one place, or remaining static*

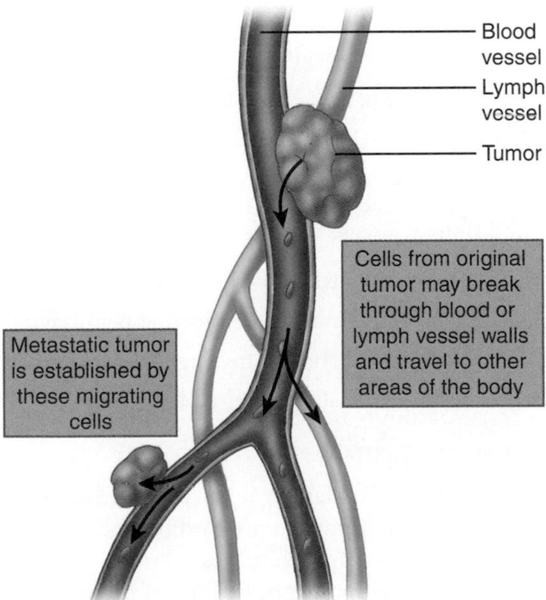

Figure 14.7: The process of metastasis

Let's Practice

Write the term that fits each description below.

1. a change in many chromosomes that affects, for example, the shape or number of limbs that an organism may have ______________
2. there are 23 of these in each human cell ______________
3. the increased production of normal cells that are considered precancerous ______________
4. a cancer of the white blood cells ______________
5. a more formal way of saying "come together" or "collect in one spot" ______________
6. the abnormal fusion of unrelated pieces of different chromosomes ______________
7. referring to cells that evolve for a unique purpose or function ______________

Build a Word

Combine each set of word parts to form a medical term. Remember to add or drop a combining vowel or consonant, if needed. Think critically about the meaning of the word parts when writing a definition of each new term.

1. -tion trans- loc- Term: ______________ Meaning: ______________
2. -emia leuk/o Term: ______________ Meaning: ______________
3. -plasia meta- Term: ______________ Meaning: ______________
4. -oid hist/o Term: ______________ Meaning: ______________
5. -plasm cyto- Term: ______________ Meaning: ______________
6. infect meta- -ive Term: ______________ Meaning: ______________
7. -plasia hypo- Term: ______________ Meaning: ______________
8. -cyte leuk/o Term: ______________ Meaning: ______________

What Do You Know?

Answer each question on the basis of what you have learned in this chapter and earlier chapters.

1. What is a synonym for *mole*? ______________
2. What is the prefix that means *normal*? ______________
3. What does the suffix *-cyte* mean? ______________
4. What does the combining form *leuk/o* mean? ______________
5. What is a chromosome? ______________
6. What is the function of genes? ______________

Mix and Match

Match the name of the condition or disease with its synonym.

1. acute non-lymphocytic leukemia	trisomy 21
2. chronic granulocytic leukemia	multiple endocrine neoplasia, type 1
3. Wermer's syndrome	chronic myelogenous leukemia
4. Down syndrome	acute myeloid leukemia

Pathophysiology of malignancy

If something is malignant, it has the potential to get worse, to cause harm or suffering. *Malignant tumors* are those that are composed of abnormal or poorly differentiated cells that proliferate rapidly and in a disorganized manner. This rapid growth makes cell nutrition problematic, and it leads to the *necrosis* (death) and *ulceration* (development of lesions) of the cells; these are the two cardinal signs of a malignant tumor. Malignant tumors are metastatic, initially invading localized tissue and quickly forming similar tumors in distant organs. There are three main types of malignant tumors: *carcinomas, sarcomas,* and *teratomas.* Table 14-4 provides examples to illustrate each type.

TABLE 14-4: Examples of Malignant Tumors

Malignancy	Description
glioma	• a primary tumor of the brain
hepatoma (also known as *hepatocellular carcinoma)*	• a tumor of the liver
brainstem glioma	• a secondary tumor of the brain that is situated at the brain's base • surgical intervention is not possible
exocrine pancreatic cancer (also known as *pancreatic cancer*)	• a tumor of the pancreas • adversely effects the production of the pancreatic juices that flow into the intestines (see Chapter 12) • poor survival rate
malignant rhabdoid tumor (also known as *rhabdoid tumor of the kidney [and brain]*)	• a pediatric cancer of the kidney • rapid metastasis throughout the body, including the central nervous system • poor survival rate

Carcinomas

Carcinomas are cancerous tumors of the epithelium (see Chapter 2). From there, they either infiltrate local tissues or metastasize via their own extensions, annexing or taking over nearby cells of the bloodstream or the lymphatic system. Carcinomas can be divided into three types: *squamous cell carcinomas, transitional cell carcinomas,* and *adenocarcinomas.*

Squamous cell carcinoma: a cancer of the squamous epithelium; the most common type of skin cancer.

squamous: a term meaning *covered with or resembling thin or flat scales; consisting of one or more layers of scales*

squamous epithelium: the surface-layer epithelium, which is composed of squamous cells

mesenchymal epithelium: a squamous epithelium lining in the subarachnoid and subdural spaces of the cranium (see Chapter 10), the paralymphatic spaces around the ears, and the cavities of the eyes

Transitional cell carcinoma: a specific type of cancer that occurs in the lining of the bladder, the renal pelvis, and the ureters (see Chapter 5).

Adenocarcinoma (glandular cancer): a cancer of the glands or the epithelium of the glands (see Chapter 7).

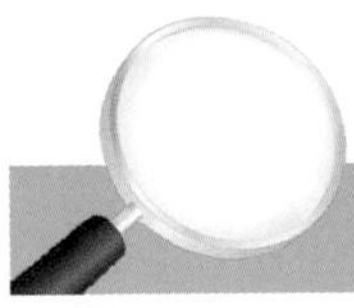

FOCUS POINT: Organoid

The term *organoid* refers to any structure that is glandular in nature and that is similar to another body organ. An organoid can be benign or malignant.

A type of benign organoid is the *organoid nevus* or birthmark that occurs as a result of hyperplasia of a blood vessel.

An organoid that can be either benign or malignant is the *carcinoid tumor* or argentaffinoma, which is generally found in the gastrointestinal tract. The tumor has an affinity for the appendix, and it may metastasize from there into the liver, thereby causing the liver to secrete large amounts of serotonin into the bloodstream. If this occurs, the carcinoid tumor is malignant.

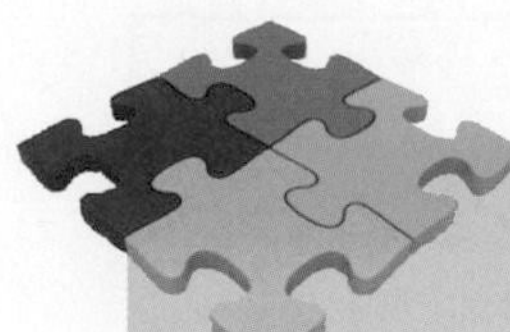

WORD BUILDING: Formulas for Creating Words from the Combining Form *Carcin/o-*

karkinos = an early Greek root meaning *cancer.* The modern combining form is *carcin/o-*.

carcin + oma = *carcinoma*

Definition: a new growth or malignant tumor that occurs in epithelial tissue and that may infiltrate of other local tissues and then metastasize. *noun*

Example: *Carcinoma in situ* is a term used to describe the localized presence of cancer cells at a very early stage, when no other tissues are affected.

carcin + osis = *carcinosis*

Definition: widespread carcinoma throughout the body. (The suffix *-osis* means *condition.* A synonym is *carcinomatosis.*) *noun*

Example: Peritoneal *carcinosis* refers to an advanced stage of cancer and the spread of cancer tumors within the peritoneum.

carcino + sarc + oma = *carcinosarcoma*

Definition: a malignant tumor that contains elements of both carcinoma and sarcoma. (The second root is *sarco,* meaning *flesh.*) *noun*

Example: Uterine *carcinosarcoma* is a rare type of cancer that is both aggressive and life ending.

Sarcomas

Sarcomas are cancers of the soft tissues (connective tissues) of the body. They most notably arise from the mesenchymal tissues of the bones and muscles (see Chapter 11) and the glial cells of the brain. They negatively affect the kidneys, spleen, liver, lungs, and other organs.

Mesenchymal tissue is also known as *embryonic mesenchyme.*

Soft-tissue sarcomas (STSs) can be found anywhere in the body; however, they are more frequently identified in the arms and legs. Examples of soft-tissue sarcomas include the following:

- angiosarcoma: cancer of the blood and lymph vessels
- liposarcoma: cancer of the fatty tissues
- leiomyosarcoma: cancer of the smooth muscles
- osteosarcoma: cancer of the bones
- rhabdomysarcoma: cancer of the striated muscles

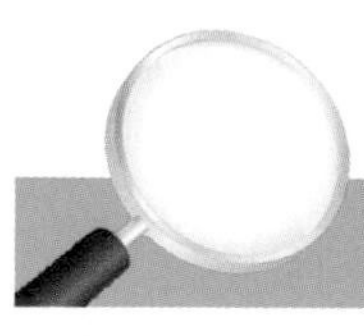

FOCUS POINT: Kaposi's Sarcoma

Kaposi's sarcoma (KS) is a soft-tissue sarcoma that is a multifocal vascular neoplastic malignancy. It affects both the lymphatic system and the endothelium (the lining of blood vessels). It is the most common cancer related to acquired immunodeficiency syndrome (AIDS). It is visible as lesions on the skin or mucous membranes, but it can also involve the internal organs. This sarcoma grows rapidly and metastasizes. KS is believed to be the result of sexual or blood contact with someone who is infected with human herpesvirus 8 (HHV-8), which is also known as *herpes 8 virus.*

Eponyms: Kaposi's Disease and Kaposi's Sarcoma

Moritz K. Kaposi was a Hungarian physician and dermatologist during the 19th century. He completed medical school at the University of Vienna, Austria, which was one of the most prominent and prestigious medical schools in Europe at that time. He was the head of the Vienna School of Dermatology and a professor of medicine. In addition to Kaposi's sarcoma, Moritz Kaposi lent his name to a number of dermatological conditions and diseases:

Kaposi's disease (xeroderma pigmentosum): a degenerative disease of the skin in which dry patches with a rash-like, pigmented appearance occur and the skin is highly photosensitive (i.e., the patient needs to stay out of the light); the onset of this disease occurs during the first year of life

Kaposi's varicelliform eruption (eczema herpeticum): a reaction that occurs when herpes simplex virus is present in the body; large patches of skin develop vesicles (bumps) that are filled with pus; this may occur in infants who already suffer from eczema (a particular itchy, weeping type of rash), which is usually hereditary

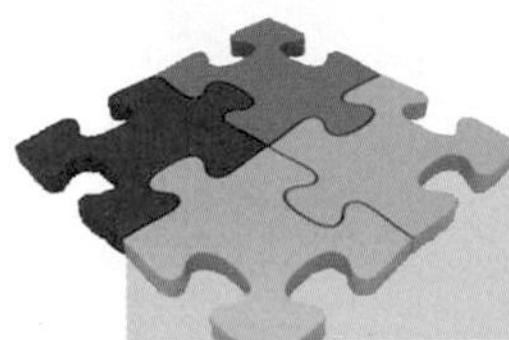

WORD BUILDING: Formulas for Creating Words from the Combining Form *Sarco-*

sarx = an early Greek root meaning *flesh* or *muscle.* The modern combining form is *sarco-*.

sarc + osis = *sarcosis*

Definition: an abnormal formation of flesh. *noun*

Example: A state of *sarcosis* exists when fleshy or flesh-like tumors appear.

sarco + adeno + oma = *sarcoadenoma*

Definition: a fleshy tumor of a gland. (The root *adeno* means *gland.* A synonym is *adenosarcoma.*) *noun*

Example: *Sarcoadenoma* of the lungs is a serious, complicated cancer that is very difficult to treat because it metastasizes across the entire pulmonary region.

sarco + cele = *sarcocele*

Definition: a fleshy tumor of the testicles. *noun*

Example: *Sarcocele* of the epididymis is usually benign.

sarco + logy = *sarcology*

Definition: the science and field of medicine that deals with the soft tissues of the body. *noun*

Example: *Sarcology* includes the study and treatment of soft-tissue sarcomas.

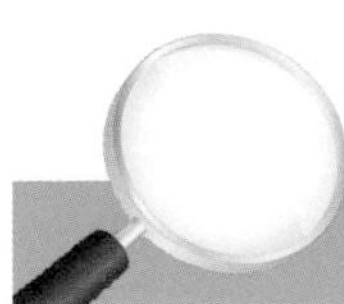

FOCUS POINT: *Sarco-*

The combining form *sarco-* is used in other contexts in addition to involving cancer. The root means *flesh,* and it is also used to refer to muscles. Consider the following examples:

sarcopenia: a loss of muscular mass and strength (as occurs with aging)
sarcolemmopathy: any form of muscular dystrophy
sarcoplasm: cytoplasm of the muscle cells (particularly the striated muscle cells)

Teratomas

A **teratogen** is anything that can adversely affect the normal cell development of an embryo or fetus. Teratogens include certain types of chemicals, medications, illicit drugs, radiation, and viral infections of the uterus. A synonym for teratogen is *mutagen.*

A **teratoma** is a cancerous tumor in an embryo or a tumor that has extraembryonic features (i.e., it may lie just outside of the embryo, perhaps in the amnion or the amniotic sac). A teratoma is congenital (inborn), and it consists of embryonic material that does not resemble the normal epithelium of an embryo. A synonym for teratoma is *terablastoma.* The suffix *-blastoma* means *germ,* and it refers to genetic cell material that is capable of becoming an organ or organism. In general, a **blastoma** is an immature tumor. It develops or arises in tissue that forms part or all of an organ. The root *blast* means *to sprout.*

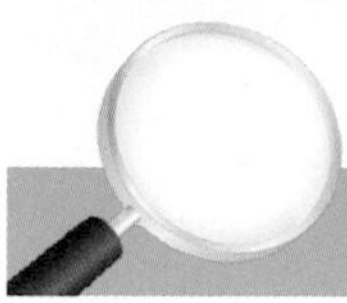

FOCUS POINT: Germ

The word *germ* has two different—and confusing—meanings:

In everyday English and many medical contexts, we often use the word *germ* as a general term to refer to any pathological microorganism.

In the context of genetics and microbiology, however, the term *germ* refers to a mass of genetic material (i.e., protoplasm and cells) that has a reproductive function. It can produce a new organ, parts of an organism, or an entire organism.

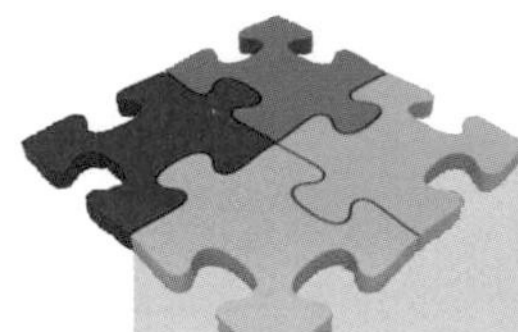

WORD BUILDING: Formulas for Creating Words from the Combining Form *Terat/o*

teras = a Greek root meaning *a severely deformed fetus.* The plural form is *terata.* The combining form is terat/-.

terat + ism = *teratism*

Definition: a structural abnormality or anomaly that is either inherited or acquired; a deformity. *noun*

Example: Spina bifida is an example of a *teratism.*

terat/o + logy = *teratology*

Definition: the study of congenital deformations and abnormal development. *noun*

Example: In medicine, *teratology* concerns itself with abnormalities of development that occur before birth and during life.

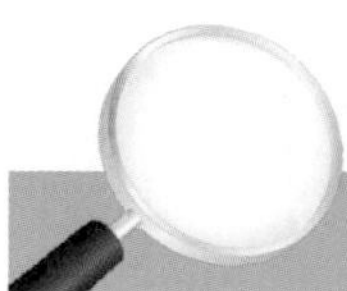

FOCUS POINT: *Gen, Carcin/o, Sarc/o, Terat/o,* and *Onco*

The combining forms *gen, carcin/o, sarc/o, terat/o,* and *onco* are derived from various root words, and they are often used as either suffixes or prefixes. Identifying which type of word part they are in any given term is often less important than simply understanding their meaning, although it can be good practice to try to determine which role a combining form is playing in a certain word's construction.

Build a Word

Use your word-building skills to create medical terms, and then define each term.

1. -lysis sarco Term: ______________ Meaning: ______________
2. -gen carcin/o Term: ______________ Meaning: ______________
3. carcin/o terat/o -oma Term: ______________ Meaning: ______________
4. carcin/o sarco -oma Term: ______________ Meaning: ______________
5. -tomy onco- Term: ______________ Meaning: ______________
6. -lysis carcin/o Term: ______________ Meaning: ______________
7. gene terat/o -tic Term: ______________ Meaning: ______________
8. -cidal onco- Term: ______________ Meaning: ______________

Break It Down

Break down each term into its component parts of prefix, root, and suffix, as applicable. Each part has been taught in this chapter or in previous chapters. You do not need to define the terms in this exercise. However, as you build each word, its meaning should become clear to you. Follow this example:

oncotomy = onco (combining form) + tomy (combining form)

1. carcinogen = ______________________________
2. sarcoplasmatic = ______________________________
3. adenoangiosarcoma ______________________________
4. adenocarcinoma = ______________________________
5. hepatocarcinogen = ______________________________
6. teratocarcinoma = ______________________________
7. teratophobia = ______________________________
8. osteocarcinoma = ______________________________

Mix and Match

Match the name of each condition or disease with its description.

1. blastoma	squamous
2. development of a lesion of the skin or a mucous membrane	Kaposi's disease
3. resembling normal tissue	teratism
4. genetic material able to become organs	germ
5. covered with or formed by scales	histoid
6. cancer of the bone	osteocarcinoma
7. congenital structural abnormality	germs
8. xeroderma pigmentosum	ulceration

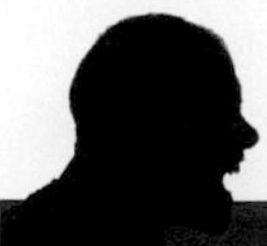

PRONUNCIATION PRACTICE

Say these words aloud to a friend or classmate, if you can. Here you are given the phonetic pronunciation. Your instructor can help you with pronunciation, or you can visit **http://www.MedicalLanguageLab.com.**

anaplasia	ăn″ă-**plā**′zē-ă	myelogenous	mī-ĕ-lō-**lŏj**′ĕn-ŭs
benign	bē-**nīn**′	myeloid	**mī**′ĕ-loyd
hyperplasia	hī″pĕr-**plā**′zē-ă	neoplasm	**nē**′ō-plăzm
leprosy	**lĕp**′rō-sē	neoplasia	nē′ō-**plā**′zē-ă
leukemia	loo-**kē**′mē-ă	nucleotide	**nū**′klē-ō-tīd
malignant	mă-**lĭg**′nănt	pheochromocytoma	fē-ō-krō″mō-sī-**tō**′mă

The Language of Tumors

Patient Update

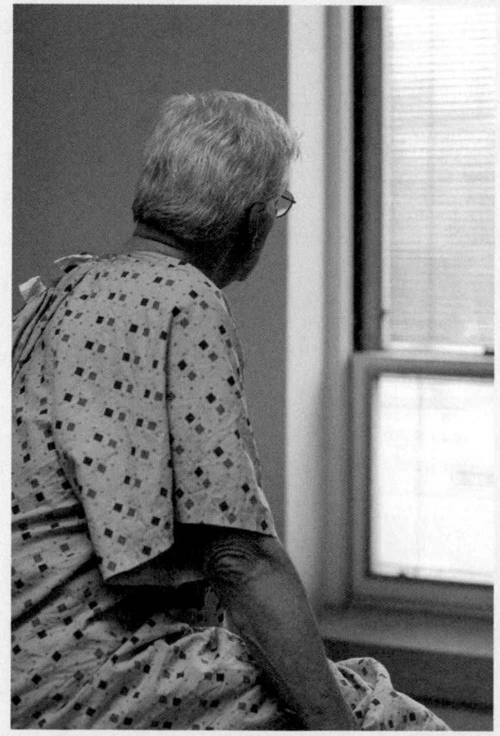

While he was in the examining room waiting for Dr. Sweetgrass, Zane Davis was worried about what might happen to him today. He was coming to accept that he had breathing problems, including shortness of breath (especially on exertion), and that he had become more susceptible to colds and respiratory infections over the last year or two. He had thought that these symptoms were just normal signs of aging and partially due to the fact that he was a chronic smoker. Now, sitting in the room at Kootenay Cancer Care Center, he wasn't so sure. Zane understood what cancer meant; it was a frightening and unwelcome disease. He dreaded the assessment and was afraid of the outcome, yet he was hoping for the best. His wife was right, he supposed, when she said that it would be better if he knew for sure whether he had cancer. If it was bad news, he would be able to make some plans with Stevie-Rose to enjoy his remaining years and get treatment. He struggled to accept either possibility: it could be good news, and he hoped it was a false alarm. Still, what if it was cancer? What if he had a malignant tumor that had metastasized?

Identifying tumors

In medical terminology, the names of tumors can often be recognized by the use of suffixes such as *-blastoma, -carcinoma,* and *-sarcoma.* Tumors are also identified by their location. The term **primary site** indicates the original location of the cancer cells, where the primary tumor first appears.

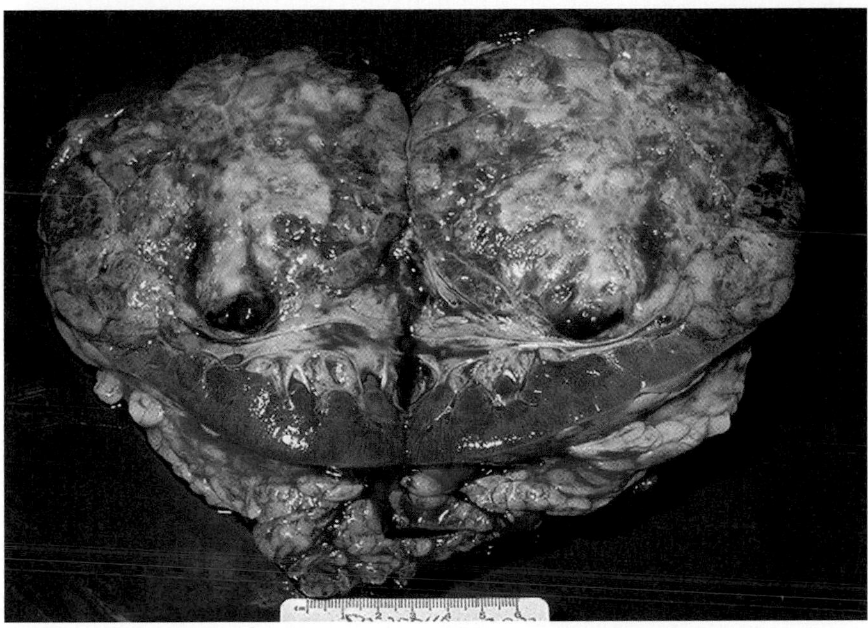

Figure 14.8: Bisected kidney showing large renal cell carcinoma (Courtesy of the Centers for Disease Control and Prevention and Dr. Edwin P. Ewing, Jr., 1972.)

Metastatic tumors

A *metastatic tumor* is one that has formed away from or separate from the primary site as a result of spreading cancer cells. Abbreviations that are relevant to naming and describing metastatic tumors are included in Table 14-5. Note that these abbreviations should be used only in the context of cancer and that they are not generally accepted medical abbreviations. Although it is important to be aware of these abbreviations, they may not be useful to professionals who are not working in oncology or with patients who have cancer.

TABLE 14-5: Abbreviations: Naming and Describing Metastatic Tumors

Abbreviation	Full Term	Abbreviation	Full Term
ADR	adrenal(s)	PLE	pleura
BRA	brain	PUL	pulmonary
HEP	hepatic	OSS	osseous
LYM	lymph nodes	OTH	other
MAR	bone marrow	SKI	skin
PER	peritoneum		

Critical Thinking

To answer these questions, you will need to think back to previous chapters and to consider what you have learned in this one.

1. The abbreviation *MAR* can mean two very different things. Name them. ______________________________
2. What is the antonym of *invasive*? ______________________________
3. Define *osseous*. ______________________________
4. In Chapter 13, the suffix *-static* was introduced with the term *orthostatic*. Provide an example of a new term from this chapter that uses the same suffix. ______________
5. Are metastatic tumors neoplasms? Explain. ______________________________

Fill in the Blanks

Complete the following sentences by filling in the blanks with the proper medical term.

1. A ______________ is a tumor that has not yet fully matured.
2. ______________ ______________ is a term that describes where a tumor originated.

Classification of tumors

Tumors can also be classified after a microscopic analysis of the cancerous tissues. The main classifications are carcinomas, sarcomas, and mixed-tissue tumors.

Histogenesis is a microscopic process that is capable of identifying cells that produce tumors.

Mixed-tissue tumors are those with cells that are capable of differentiating into either epithelial or connective tissue. This type of tumor is quite uncommon.

Staging of tumors

Cancers are staged from I to IV to reflect how far and how much the cancer has spread or the stage of progression. Staging allows the care team to provide appropriate treatment and to determine a prognosis for the patient. Cancer stages can be written in ordinary numbers or in Roman numerals. When referring to a stage of cancer, medical personnel will say the word "stage," but they may use an abbreviation for it when writing, as seen in the following example:

Oncologist speaking to radiologist: "I see that the patient has stage 4 melanoma."

Oncologist writing in medical record or chart: "St. IV melanoma" or "St. 4 melanoma"

Refer to Table 14-6 to learn more about the stages of cancer.

TABLE 14-6: Stages of Cancer

Stage of Cancer	Stage by Roman Numeral	Description
0	0	Cancer in situ (CIS): abnormal cells are identified, but only in the top layer of cells within a region of the body; stage 0 means that the abnormal cells are found only in a particular region and that there is only a trace amount (few) of them present
1	I	Precancerous or cancer cells are present at one site (i.e., the organ of origin) in a very small amount
2	II	Cancerous cells have now congregated in an organ to create a tumor
3	III	Lymph nodes and organs near the primary tumor may have been invaded by cancer cells
4	IV	Full metastases: the cancer has spread to other organ(s); also known as *metastatic cancer* or *secondary cancer*

The TNM staging system

The **TNM staging system** is widely used to identify the presence or absence of tumors. This system classifies cancers by assessing the tumor, the lymph node involvement, and the degree of metastasis. Table 14-7 provides a simple overview of this system.

The TNM staging system is actually quite complex. Each element in Table 14-7 is broken down further as the patient is more comprehensively assessed. The data that result from such an assessment are scored appropriately. The final score leads the medical team to the most appropriate avenues of treatment. Tables 14-8, 14-9, and 14-10 describe how tumors, nodes, and metastasis are graded to obtain the final score with the TNM staging system.

TABLE 14-7: Brief Overview of the TNM Staging System for Cancer

TNM Staging System	Description
tumor	classifies by the size of the primary tumor
nodes	classifies by the number of regional lymph nodes that are affected
metastasis	classifies by the presence or absence of metastasis to the rest of the body

TABLE 14-8: Comprehensive Classification of a Tumor: The TNM Staging System

Primary Tumor (T)	Description
TX	tumor cannot be evaluated
T0	no evidence of tumor
Tis	tumor in situ or carcinoma in situ; it is not invasive disease at this point
T1, T2, T3, T4	gradually increasing size and extent of tumor; T4 is the worst

TABLE 14-9: Comprehensive Classification of the Lymph Nodes: The TNM Staging System

Regional Lymph Nodes (N)	Description
Nx	node(s) cannot be evaluated
N0	no evidence of involvement
N1, N2, N3	regional lymph node involvement; measured in increasing stages of the number of lymph nodes involved or the extent of the disease's spread

TABLE 14-10: Comprehensive Classification of Metastasis: The TNM Staging System

Distant Metastasis (M)	Description
Mx	metastasis cannot be evaluated
M0	no evidence of metastasis
M1	presence of distant metastasis (i.e., disease that is distant from the primary tumor)

Although TNM staging is common, there are a number of other systems in use across North America. If your career takes you into the field of oncology, you may eventually become familiar with systems such as the Ann Arbor Staging system for lymphoma and the FIGO staging system for ovarian cancer.

Grading of tumors

Tumor grading systems classify tumors by evaluating how abnormal they appear under microscopic examination and by predicting how fast they will grow and spread. Each type of cancer is assessed and graded with the use of very specific criteria and grading systems.

Nuclear grading focuses on the nucleus of a tumor cell to assess its size and shape. It then estimates the percentage of tumor cells in the body that are dividing.

Histologic grading evaluates how closely the tumor cells resemble normal cells of the same kind. In other words, it evaluates the degree of cell differentiation.

To grade cancerous tumors, tissue samples must be taken through a procedure called a *biopsy*. You will learn more about biopsies in the diagnostics sections of this chapter.

The grading system for cancer is a progressive numerical system that evaluates the severity of a tumor. Table 14-11 provides an overview of the tumor grading system.

TABLE 14-11: Grading System for Cancer

Grade	Description	Grade	Description
Gx	undetermined grade; cannot be assessed	G3	high grade; poorly differentiated
G1	low grade; well differentiated	G4	high grade; undifferentiated
G2	intermediate grade; moderately differentiated		

Reflective Questions

Answer the following questions on the basis of the information and terminology related to tumors and how they are classified and staged.

1. What type of cells form tumors? ____________________
2. What is the most common system that is used to stage tumors and the spread of cancer?
____
3. What is a primary tumor? ____________________
4. What is the abbreviation and stage for a tumor in situ? ____________________
5. For optimal patient outcomes, at which stage is it best to catch cancer?
____
6. What is the most severe grade of cancer and the one that suggests a loss of life?
____

Critical Thinking

1. What does the term *distant* refer to in the context of the phrase *distant metastasis*?
____
2. Are all abnormal cells cancerous? Explain. ____________________

Fill in the Blanks

Complete the following sentences by filling in the blanks with the proper medical term.

1. The pathologist is looking at the size and shape of some tumor tissue because he wants to ____________________ it.
2. ____________________ ____________________ is full metastatic cancer that is terminal.
3. The most common type of ____________________ system for cancer in North America is the TNM.

Right Word or Wrong Word: *Staging* or *Grading?*

Do these two words mean the same thing? Don't they both measure or indicate the same thing? Surely there is no difference, is there?

Patient Update

Zane Davis has changed into a hospital gown and is waiting for Dr. Sweetgrass to perform a physical assessment.

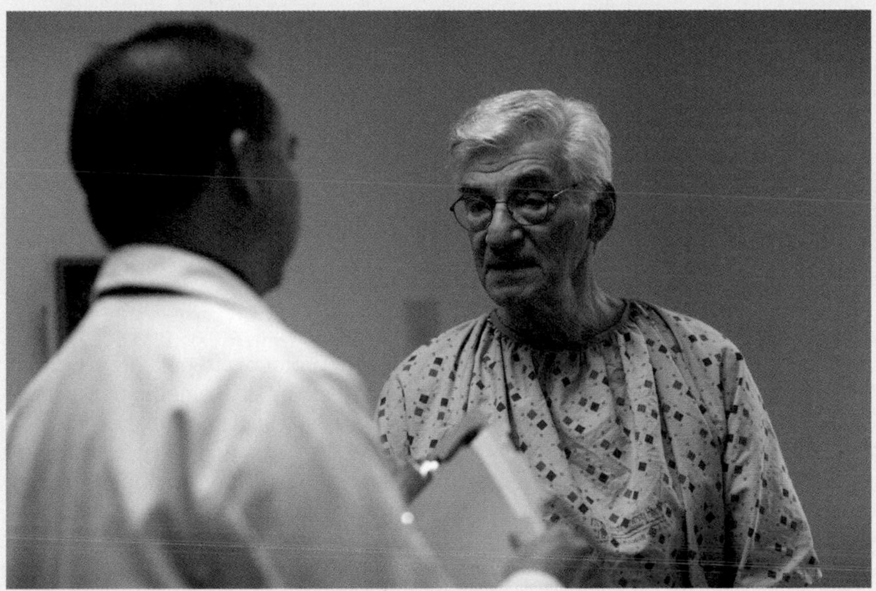

"Ah, I see you're ready for me, Mr. Davis," said Dr. Sweetgrass, as he entered the examining room with his medical e-scribe, Reilly-Jo. Zane noticed the doctor was now wearing his lab coat and looked very official. "Has the lab been in to take a blood specimen?" Zane nodded. "Good. So, I'd like to start the physical exam now." Dr. Sweetgrass moved closer to Zane, who was sitting on the edge of the examining table wearing a light cotton hospital gown that opened at the back. "I'm going to start with a full chest exam. I'm going to observe for symmetry, measure for diameter, and then auscultate—or listen to—the thorax and the abdomen. I'll check for peripheral pulses, skin color, and so on. I'll do a thorough assessment of your lymphatic system today, too." At this point, Zane interrupted the doctor.

"Lymphatic system. I know what that means. You're looking for metastases," the patient said gloomily.

"You sound worried," the physician said, pausing to look a little more directly at the patient to assess his mood. Zane nodded. "Let's not go there yet, Mr. Davis. As I've said before, the jury is still out on what your health condition really is. We've got a lot of work to do before we arrive at anything near that conclusion. We'll be performing a whole battery of tests. For example, when we're done here, Radiology will be ready to see you, and we'll get some radiographs of your thorax as well, and then they'll take you right next door for a CT scan. I'm sure you'd like to get that done soon, so you can have something to eat this morning," the doctor said. Zane nodded and commented that not eating since last evening was difficult for him. "I can appreciate that, Zane, but it won't be much longer now," the doctor responded. "It's going to be a very busy day for you here, sir, and you'll need to have something to eat and drink to get you through it." Dr. Sweetgrass smiled reassuringly. "To help you through all of those tests and procedures, one of our oncology technicians will be with you through every step."

"That's okay, I'm up to it," said Zane. "I want to get as much done here today as possible. I can't stand not knowing what's going on with my own body. But I have to tell you, I'm afraid to hear the answer today.

I don't want to hear bad news, but I've been preparing myself, just in case. My wife was a nurse in the armed forces, you know. She's been researching asbestosis and mesothelioma on the Internet for a week now. Everything we've learned is pretty awful. We both know what it means if you find mesothelioma," Zane said, with a tone of resignation in his voice. "Malignancy; metastases. I'll be terminal." He choked up slightly on this last word. Dr. Sweetgrass jumped in quickly.

"We don't know that, Mr. Davis, but I'm glad that you and your wife have done some research. If you have any questions at all about what is going to occur here today, ask any one of us at any time. No question is considered foolish or unreasonable. All of us here at Kootenay Cancer Care Center are here to help you get through this." Reilly-Jo looked up and smiled at Zane in confirmation. Dr. Sweetgrass began the physical examination.

Reflective Questions

Answer these two questions on the basis of the Patient Update.

1. What is Zane Davis afraid of? ______________________________

2. In addition to his wife, who will be accompanying Zane through his diagnostic tests today?

   ____

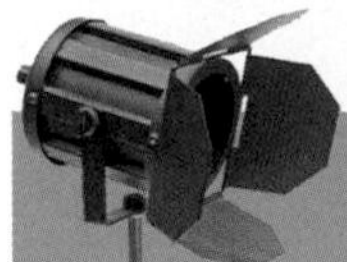

CAREER SPOTLIGHT: Oncology Technician and Oncology Surgery Technician

Oncology technicians provide direct care and support to cancer patients as part of their treatment and palliative care. They are well trained to explain treatment protocols to patients. They work subordinately and collegially with oncologists, nursing staff, and other members of the multidisciplinary team. They are also able to give medications that are associated with cancer treatment.

Oncology technicians have a minimum of a high school diploma, and most have been certified as nursing assistants; others may have been trained as medical assistants. After receiving their general training, they take additional courses to specialize in oncology and cancer care. Requirements for registration or certification as an oncology technician vary from state to state.

An *oncology surgery technician* trains to work in the operating room, the surgical day-care clinic, or a similar facility. This position requires the same educational background needed for an oncology technician; however, the oncology surgery technician will undertake a special course of training (which ranges in length from 9 months to 2 years) to qualify to assist with surgical procedures.

Critical Thinking

Think about everything that you know about our patient, Zane Davis, to answer the following questions.

1. There is evidence in the Patient Update that Zane and Stevie-Rose Davis are informed consumers of health care services. What does this term mean, and what evidence supports this idea?

   ____

   ____

   ____

2. Fill in the following table to identify Zane Davis's health strengths and weaknesses as he is about to proceed through an assessment for cancer. These strengths and weaknesses will be important factors in how well he is able to tolerate the day's procedures and the diagnosis that he will hear at the end of the day. Think holistically, and consider all that you have learned about Zane Davis to date. You may have to review previous chapters about him to refresh your memory, particularly Chapter 9.

TABLE 14-12: Zane Davis's Health Strengths and Weaknesses

Health Strengths	Health Weaknesses

3. On the basis of the data in your table, how hardy or resilient do you think Zane is at the moment? Provide your rationale.

____

____

Key terms in the patient update

"... *to observe for symmetry* ..."

observe for symmetry: As part of the physical assessment protocol, the thorax is examined visually from a number of angles to evaluate its evenness and proportion. For example, if a barrel chest is observed, this may be a result of chronic hyperinflation of the lungs and a sign of emphysema. In addition, if the sternum does not appear to be midline to the chest, if it does not seem to be straight, if it is retracted (sunken inward), or if it is protruding somehow, then the physician will be able to see this and subsequently hear that the patient's breathing is impaired as a result.

"... *measure for diameter* ..."

measure for diameter: This measure will be taken when the chest muscles are at rest and when the patient is expanding the chest by breathing in. Unequal chest expansion can be the result of chronic obstructive pulmonary disease, chest trauma, or other conditions.

"... then *auscultate*—or listen to—the thorax ..."

auscultate: To listen to with a stethoscope. In this context, auscultation of the thorax allows the physician to assess for the symmetry of airflow bilaterally in the lungs. It also lets Dr. Sweetgrass hear whether Zane has normal or abnormal breath sounds. (It is likely that he will have some abnormal breath sounds because he seems to have a persistent cough.)

"I'll be *terminal*."

terminal: Incurable; dying.

Fill in the Blanks

Complete the following sentences by filling in the blanks with the proper medical term.

1. Synonyms for the term ____________________ are *evenness, equilibrium,* and *balance.*
2. Another way to say "____________________" is to say "span" or "breadth."
3. A patient on a palliative care unit quite possibly has a ____________________ illness.
4. When the care provider ____________________ the chest and abdomen, he or she is listening to them.

Right Word or Wrong Word: *Metastasis, Metastases,* or *Metastasize?*

Say these words aloud. Do they sound exactly the same? If not, would you be able to distinguish which one was being said? Would it be important for you to do so? Explain.

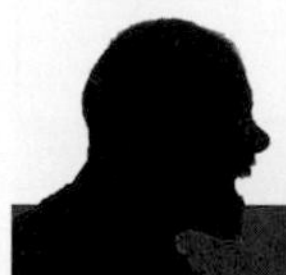

PRONUNCIATION PRACTICE

Say these words aloud to a friend or classmate, if you can. Here you are given the phonetic pronunciation. Your instructor can help you with pronunciation, or you can visit **http://www.MedicalLanguageLab.com.**

auscultate	**aws´**kŭl-tāt	metastasis	mĕ-**tăs´**tă-sis
blastema	blăs-**tē´**mă	metastasize	mĕ-**tăs´**tă-sīz
blastoma	blăs-**tō´**mă	symmetry	**sĭm´**ĕt-rē
metastases	mĕ-**tăs´**tă-sēs		

The Lymphatic System

The lymphatic system is frequently studied as part of the circulatory system or as part of the immune system. It is more akin to the latter. The lymphatic system and the immune system are very closely related: they both protect the body from invasion or infection. The lymphatic system is actually an integral part of the *immune system,* which will be introduced and explored in more detail in Chapters 16 and 17.

The primary function of the lymphatic system is maintaining the fluid and protein balance of the body. The system transports fluids called *lymph* (an interstitial fluid) and *chyle* (a fluid product of the intestines). Lymph carries some red bloods cells back into the circulatory system. It accomplishes these functions through its own network of lymphatic vessels (see Figure 14-9). Larger lymph vessels resemble veins, and lymphatic capillaries are scattered throughout the body just as blood capillaries are. Lymph capillaries connect to small lymph vessels, which connect to larger ones, which eventually flow into the thoracic and right lymphatic ducts. These branching lymphatic vessels that are present throughout the body are referred to as *lymphatic channels*.

The lymphatic system also plays a central role in providing immunity by attempting to halt the spread of infection or invasion by disease. In addition, it facilitates the absorption of fats from foods in the gastrointestinal tract.

Anatomy and physiology

Sometimes referred to as the *lymphatic drainage system* or the *lymph system,* the lymphatic system consists of lymph, lymphatic vessels, lymph organs, lymph nodes, and lymph ducts.

Lymph

During the process of blood circulation, fluid seeps into the body's tissues through the walls of capillaries. The fluid contains oxygen and nutrients that nourish body tissue. Although some of this fluid may return back through the capillary walls and into the bloodstream, some of it is diffused into the lymphatic vessels. This fluid becomes **lymph**, which is a clear fluid that is able to transport and remove any perceived harmful or unwanted matter within it. Examples of these include cancer cells, bacteria, and dead or damaged cells. The movement of materials through this system is accomplished by the contraction of skeletal muscles, which causes lymph to move through lymph valves and vessels.

Lymphocytes

Lymphocytes are lymph cells, and they are produced in bone marrow. They are a type of leukocyte (white blood cell). They include B-lymphocytes (B-cells) and T-stem cells. Lymphocytes are formed by the process of mitosis in the bone marrow itself. Their function is to respond to antigens by producing antibodies (B-cells) and lymphokines (T- and B-cells) to fight them (see "Focus Point: A Review of Antibodies and Antigens").

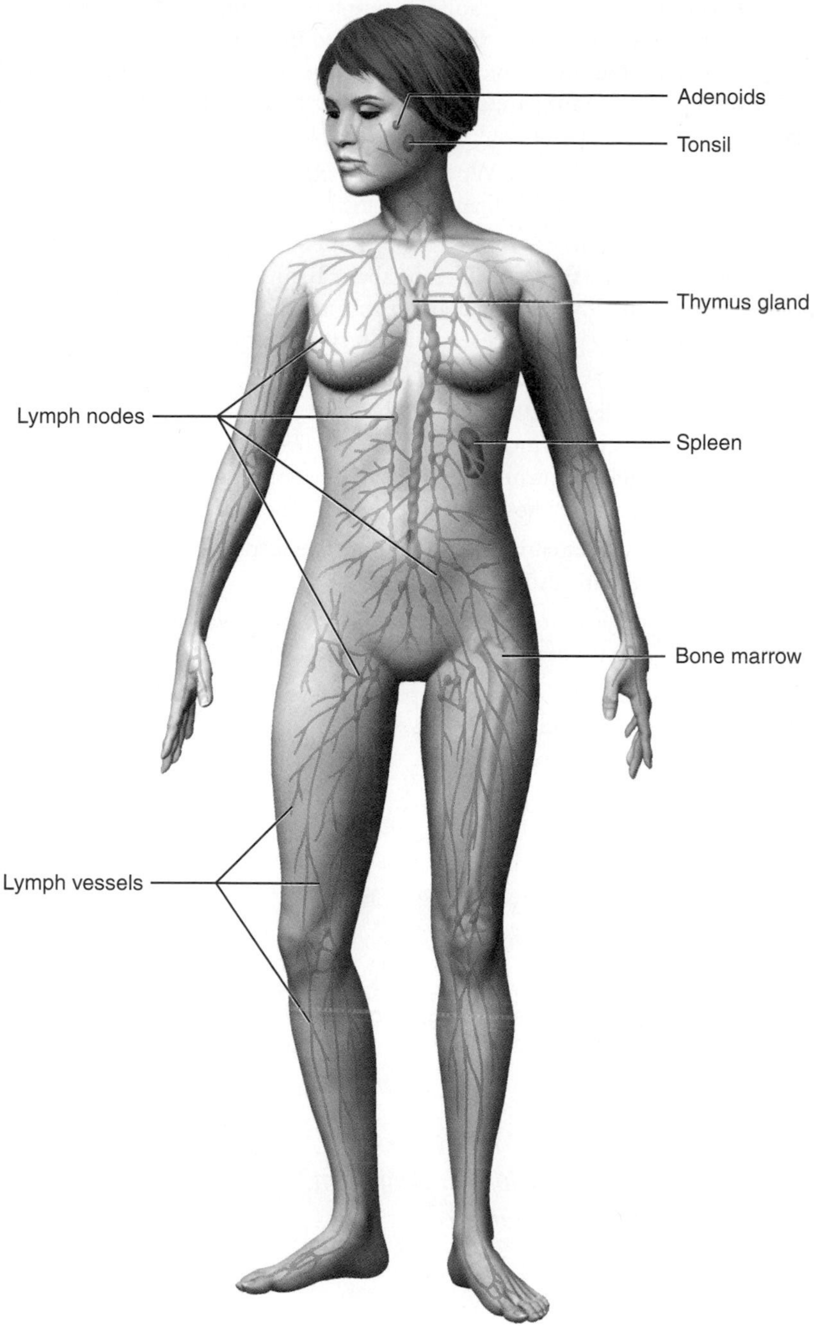

Figure 14.9: The lymphatic system and its channels

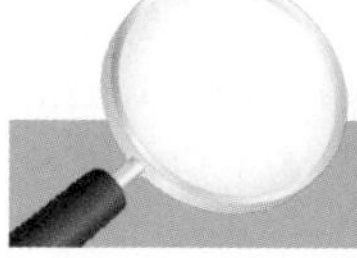

FOCUS POINT: A Review of Antibodies and Antigens

Although antibodies and antigens were introduced in Chapter 8, a brief reminder of their definitions may be helpful for this chapter.

Antibodies are protein particles that bind with unwanted foreign matter in the lymphatic and circulatory systems to contain and destroy that matter. The singular form of *antibodies* is *antibody.*

Antigens are molecules that stimulate the production of antibodies.

B-lymphocytes (B-cells) are antibodies, and they are fundamental to the immune system. They form in the bone marrow; from there, they are released into blood and lymph circulation. Each individual B-cell can uniquely recognize and target a specific foreign antigen. When a B-cell recognizes a particular antigen, it rapidly divides and differentiates into plasma cells or B-memory cells to combat that antigen.

Plasma cells are the factories of B-cells. When they are triggered by the presence of an antigen, they produce multitudes of antibodies that are specific to the fighting of that one specific antigen.

B-memory cells are also antigen-specific cells: they remember a particular type of antigen after they have been exposed to it. What is different about B-memory cells is that they do not react to the antigen the first time that they encounter it. Instead, they hold back in case there is a second attack, and then they provide a secondary response or a line of defense should that antigen appear again. They are also known as *memory B-cells.*

T-stem cells (immature T-cells) are produced in the bone marrow. They are the precursors of T-cells. T-cells mature in the thymus gland. (The *T* in *T-cells* refers to the thymus.) T-cells regulate the immune system by turning the immune response on or off. More importantly, these cells directly attack and destroy infectious agents. There are three main types of T-cells:

Suppressor T-cells are those that curb or limit an immune response by B-cells or T-cells when an antigen is present. They are also referred to as *T-8 cells* or *CD8 cells.*

Cytotoxic T-cells destroy cells that are infected with bacteria or viruses. Sometimes referred to as "killer cells," they can at times successfully kill cancer cells.

Memory T-cells are found in lymphoid organs, peripheral tissue sites, and all sites of inflammation. Like memory B-cells, they are antigen-specific cells and they function in the same manner.

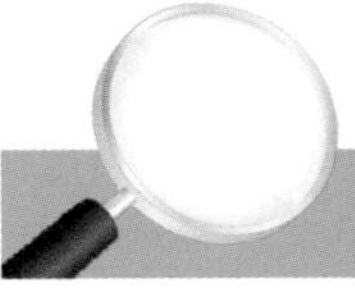

FOCUS POINT: Helper T-cells

Helper T-cells are *macrophages,* which are another type of white blood cell. They digest harmful antigens, viruses, and other microbes by engulfing and destroying them. Helper T-cells also activate B-cells to produce antibodies.

Right Word or Wrong Word: *Bacteria* or *Bacterium?*

Which of these two terms is plural? Can you recall?

Diagnostics: lymphocyte count

A **lymphocyte count** is a diagnostic measure; it is a blood test that measures or estimates the number of white blood cells in the body. It is also known as a *white blood cell differential test* or a **WBC-diff.**

Because lymphocytes are activated in response to the presence of a foreign invader within the body, the number of lymphocytes found in a single blood sample will indicate the degree of protective immune response that has been activated. For example, the normal value of lymphocytes ranges from 20% to 40% of a total leukocyte count (i.e., 10,000 to 40,000/mm3). This level will be elevated when an immune response is occurring.

The term **lymphocytosis** refers to an increase in the number of lymphocytes. This is particularly seen in cases of viral infection, including measles and chicken pox. This condition is also present in patients with tuberculosis, bone marrow cancer, and leukemia and in those who have undergone radiation therapy.

The term **lymphocytopenia** refers to a decrease in the number of lymphocytes. This can occur in cases of starvation, malnutrition, lupus (a chronic autoimmune disease), and acquired immunodeficiency syndrome.

A lymphocyte count is able to do the following:

- assess the body's ability to respond to or eliminate infection
- detect allergy and drug reactions
- detect the presence of parasites
- detect the presence of infections
- identify stages of leukemia
- measure the effectiveness of chemotherapy (for cancer)

Right Word or Wrong Word: *Lymphocyte* or *Leukocyte?*

It seems that these two terms may be synonymous, but are they?

Lymphoid or lymphatic tissue

Lymphoid tissue refers to any group of lymph cells that work together to perform a particular function. It is composed of lymphocytes, which assist in the formation of antibodies to fend off and fight infection. Examples of lymphoid tissues are the spleen, tonsils, adenoids, and the thymus.

Spleen: a lymphoid organ located on the left of the abdominal cavity, just below the diaphragm and posterior to the stomach. It is a reservoir for blood that makes blood available when it is needed. The spleen contains lymphocytes and macrophages that trap and destroy foreign bodies that enter it.

Tonsils: two masses of lymphoid tissues that sit bilaterally on the pharynx and that are embedded at the side of the palate and adjacent to the posterior portion of the tongue in the oral cavity (see Chapters 6 and 11).

Adenoids: a mass of lymphoid tissue that sits at the nasopharynx, near the uvula at the back of the oral cavity.

Thymus: a lymphoid organ that is also a gland. It sits near the lower posterior portion of the neck, behind the sternum. The thymus contains lymphocytes and epithelial cells. Its main function is the production of T-lymphocytes (T-cells), which it secretes into the body to mature and circulate when stimulated by a hormone. During the early years of life, the thymus is instrumental to the development of the body's immune system. The thymus becomes inactive after childhood.

Lymph nodes

Lymph nodes are clusters of lymphatic tissue. Within each node are lymphocytes (B-cells and T-cells), macrophages, and dendritic cells. These dendritic cells come in contact with the external environment, where they first encounter antigens and notify the immune system of these antigens via lymphoid tissue.

Each lymph node is surrounded by a capsule of connective tissue and contains entry and exit ducts (see Figure 14-10). Lymph enters a lymph node through *afferent* lymph vessels found at one end and exits through the other end into *efferent* lymph vessels.

Lymph nodes serve as filters. Their mesh-like structure removes harmful substances from the lymph before it is returned to the bloodstream. All substances that travel through the lymphatic system pass through and are filtered by the lymph nodes. Lymph nodes are found along the branches of lymphatic vessels, particularly in (but not limited to) the neck, groin, and armpits (axillaries). They are small oval or bean-shaped structures.

Swollen lymph nodes can be a sign of infection, and it is important to note that lymph nodes are one of the first hosts of cancer cells. For this reason, physicians, nurse practitioners, and other health professionals who complete physical assessments are inclined to palpate the lymph nodes (where possible) to assess for swelling.

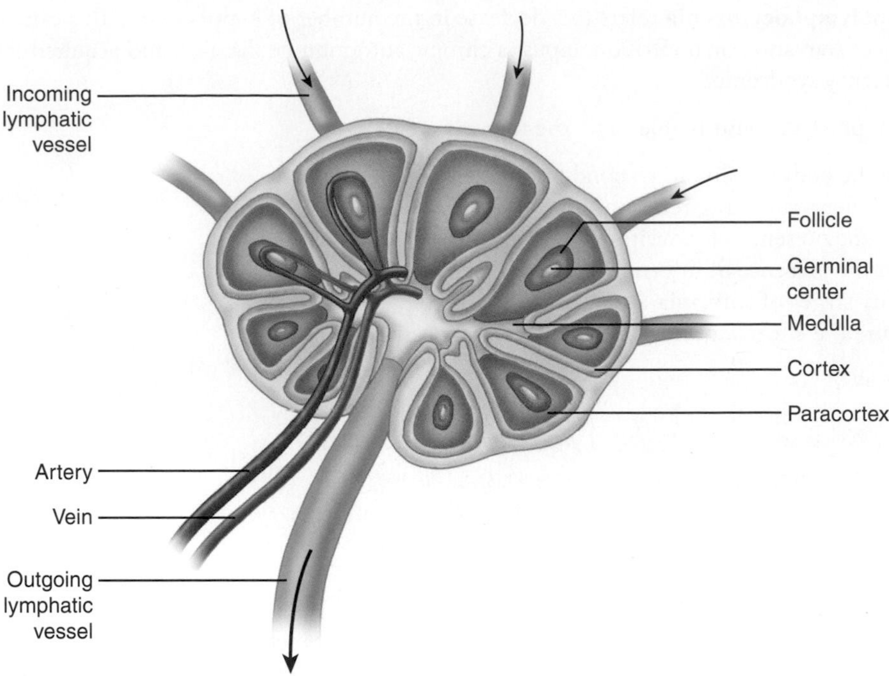

Figure 14.10: Anatomy of a lymph node

Lymph ducts

Lymph flows through lymphatic capillaries to lymphatic veins and into lymph vessels. These eventually empty into two very large lymphatic ducts: the thoracic duct and the right lymphatic duct. These ducts drain into the subclavian veins (under the clavicle) before they enter the heart (see Figure 14-11).

The *thoracic duct* is the largest of the lymph ducts. All lymph vessels of the internal organs, the lower limbs, the left side of the thorax, the left side of the head and neck, and the left arm drain into this duct. By connecting with the subclavian veins, this duct facilitates the entry of lymph into the bloodstream.

The *right lymphatic duct* receives drainage from the lymph vessels of the right side of the body: the right side of the thorax, the right side of the head and neck, and the right arm. It opens into the right subclavian vein only.

Remember that the lymphatic system also has a function related to the gastrointestinal tract. *Lacteal ducts* are very small ducts that are found in the lining of the small intestines. They receive absorbed fat from the digestive system for eventual transport into the bloodstream via the thoracic duct. This fatty substance is called **chyle**.

Right Word or Wrong Word: *Lymph Nodes* or *Lymph Glands?*

Are these two terms interchangeable? Are they synonymous?

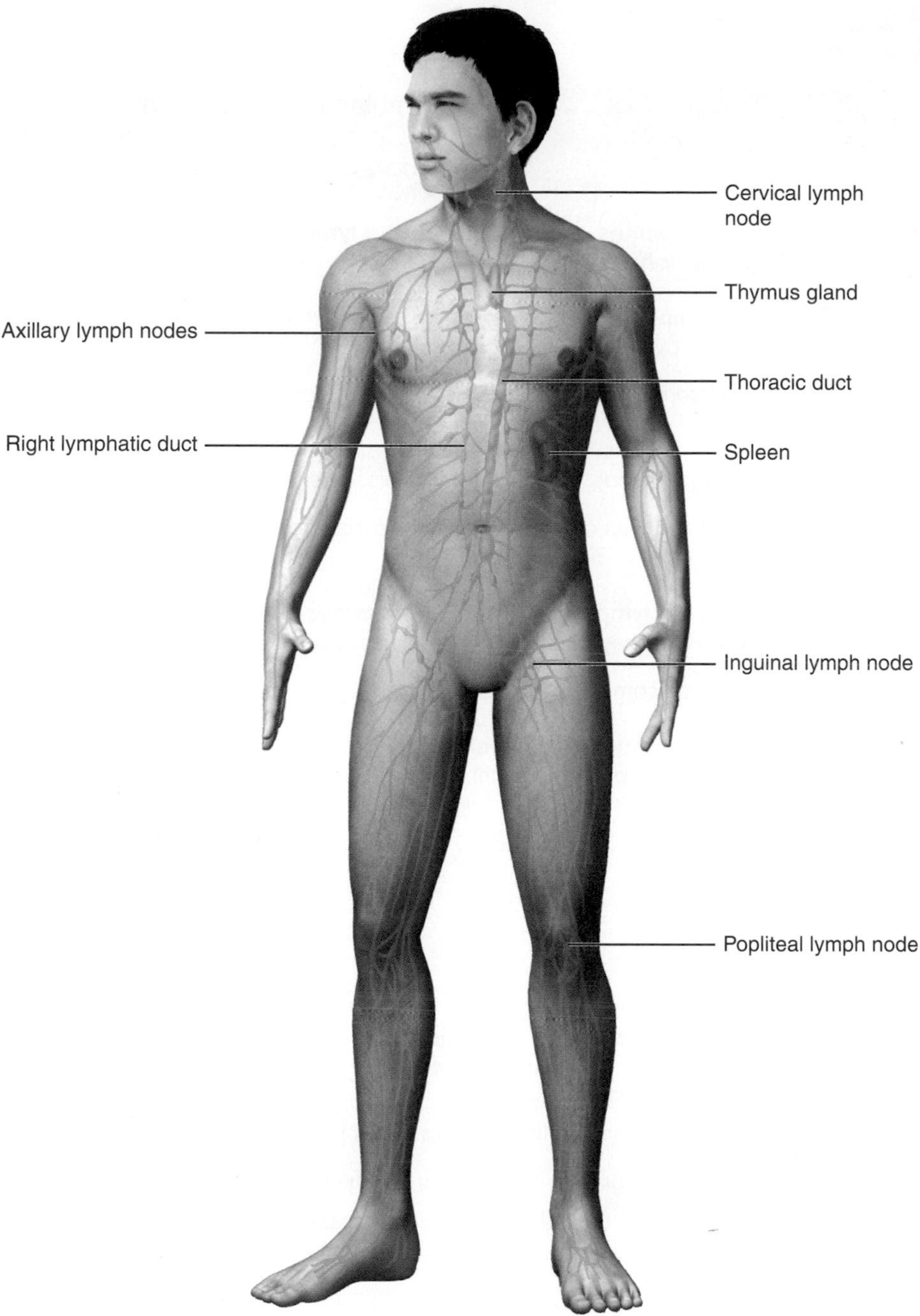

Figure 14.11: Lymphatic system: nodes and ducts

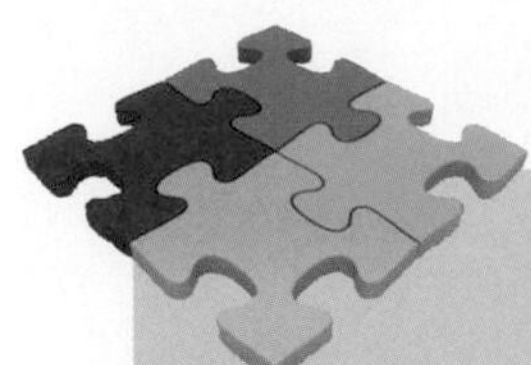

WORD BUILDING: Formulas for Creating Words from the Combining Forms *Lymph/o-* and *Lymphat/o*

lymph = a root word that names a tissue fluid in the lymphatic system. The combining forms are *lymph/o* and *lymphat/o.*

lymph + aden + ectomy = *lymphadenectomy*

Definition: the surgical removal of a lymph node. *noun*

Example: A *lymphadenectomy* may be necessary in the case of testicular cancer.

lymph/o + angi + al = *lymphangial*

Definition: concerning or pertaining to the lymph vessels. *adjective*

Example: The treatment team was concerned that there may be new *lymphangial* involvement as part of the patient's cancer.

lymphat/o + lysis = *lymphatolysis*

Definition: the destruction or dissolution of lymphatic tissue or vessels. *noun*

Example: *Lymphatolysis* can sometimes be used to destroy lymphatic vessels within tumors.

lymph/o + kinesis = *lymphokinesis*

Definition: the circulation of lymph in the lymphatic system. (The root *kinesis* means *movement.*) *noun*

Example: *Lymphokinesis* may provide a pathway through which carcinogens can access the entire body.

Cancer, lymphoma, and lymphangiogenesis

Zane Davis is at Kootenay Cancer Care Center today for a comprehensive physical assessment to determine if he does or does not have any form of cancer. To this end, a diagnostic study of his lymphatic system will be essential because cancer cells often migrate to this system. Dr. Sweetgrass will want to rule out any lymphatic involvement as soon as possible.

A **lymphoma** is a malignant tumor that is a cancer of the lymphatic system.

Lymphangiogenesis is a medical term that describes how cancer cells influence the development of any new lymphatic vessels or channels by influencing where, how, and by which route cancer cells are able to metastasize.

TABLE 14-13: Disorders of the Lymphatic System

Disorder	Definition or Description
primary lymphedema	• a condition that involves the swelling of tissues, usually in the extremities, as a result of the poor drainage of fluid from them; the lymphatic system is unable to drain • congenital (hereditary)
secondary lymphedema (also known as *acquired regional lymphatic insufficiency*)	• a condition that involves the swelling of tissues, usually in the extremities, as a result of trauma or the blockage of the lymphatic system • acquired (not inherited)

TABLE 14-13: Disorders of the Lymphatic System—cont'd

Disorder	Definition or Description
filariasis	• a tropical disease caused by infestation of filarial nematodes (small worms) in the body; these are transmitted through the bite of an infected mosquito • the last stage of this disease is elephantiasis (i.e., the painful and disfiguring swelling of the arms, legs, and genitalia)
lymphoma	• tumors of the lymphatic cells
lymphadenopathy	• swelling of the lymph nodes of the axilla, groin, neck, chest, and abdomen • caused by lymph node infection or lymphoma • a classic symptom of human immunodeficiency virus (HIV) infection
primary pulmonary lymphangiectasia (PPL) (also known as *congenital pulmonary lymphangiectasia [CPL]*)	• widespread dilation of the lymphatic vessels of the lungs • cause is unknown • cases are rare • seen in infants (in whom it can be fatal) and in children
scleroderma (sclera [meaning *hard*] + derma [meaning *skin*])	• a group of autoimmune diseases of the connective tissues (i.e., skin, tendons, cartilage, blood vessels) • includes a loss of the lymphatic capillaries, which leads to a tightening or hardening of the tissue

FOCUS POINT: Hodgkin's Lymphoma and Non-Hodgkin's Lymphoma

Hodgkin's lymphoma (HL) is the name of a group of malignant cancers that originate in the lymph nodes and that metastasize from there. It is a B-cell lymphoma. Abnormal cells called *Reed-Sternberg cells* cause the disease. Symptoms of HL include swelling in the lymph nodes around the armpits, groin, or neck; fever; unintended weight loss; and an enlarged spleen. These symptoms persist over time. HL is treated with radiation therapy, chemotherapy, and stem cell transplantation, particularly if it is caught early. However, it can be terminal. HL occurs in patients of all age groups. The life expectancy of individuals with HL may be 5 years or more if the disease is caught and treated early. HL was originally named *Hodgkin's disease,* and this term can still be heard in medical circles.

Non-Hodgkin's lymphoma (NHL) is another group of malignant cancers of the lymphatic system. NHL can be either a B-cell lymphoma or a T-cell lymphoma. In either case, the affected cells divide and proliferate uncontrollably, and they eventually form tumors. The type of NHL is identifiable only through the microscopic analysis of cells. The symptoms of NHL are often the same as those of HL, and the disease is treated in the same manner as well. NHL is seen more often among people who are more than 60 years old. Life expectancy rates for patients with NHL range from 7 to 10 years if the disease is caught and treated early.

Reflective Questions

Answer these questions on the basis of the anatomy and physiology of the lymphatic system.

1. Which of these produces antibodies: T-cells or B-cells? ______________________
2. What is the name of the fluid that is moved through the lymphatic system by contractions of the smooth muscles? ______________________
3. What is a lymphoma? ______________________

Let's Practice

Write the medical term that fits each description.

1. a type of B-cell that produces and releases antibody molecules into the blood ____________________
2. where both lymphocytes and leukocytes are found ____________________
3. a mass of lymphoid tissue found in the oral cavity ____________________
4. lymphoid organ that produces T-cells, particularly during the early years of life ____________________

Fill in the Blanks

Fill in the blanks with the missing word.

1. Lymph nodes are ____________________ of lymphatic tissue.
2. Lymphocytes assist in the formation of ____________________ to defend against invasion by antigens.
3. ____________________ turn off the production of B-cells and T-cells.
4. ____________________ protect, whereas ____________________ invade and harm.

Build a Word

Use the word parts given to build a word, and then define it.

1. -it is lymph/o	Term: ____________	Meaning: ____________
2. adeno- lymph/o gram	Term: ____________	Meaning: ____________
3. toxin cyto lymph/o	Term: ____________	Meaning: ____________

PRONUNCIATION PRACTICE

Say these words aloud to a friend or classmate, if you can. Here you are given the phonetic pronunciation. Your instructor can help you with pronunciation,

or you can visit **http://www.MedicalLanguageLab.com.**

afferent	**ăf**´ĕr-ĕnt
chyle	**kīl**
efferent	**ĕf**´ĕr-ĕnt
elephantiasis	ĕl″ĕ-făn-**tī**´ă-sĭs
lymphadenectomy	lĭm-făd″ĕ-**nĕk**´tō-mē
lymphangial	lĭm-**făn**´jē-ăl
lymphatolysis	lĭm″fă-**tŏl**´ĭ-sĭs
lymphocytopenia	lĭm″fō-sīt″ō-**pē**´nē-ă
lymphocytosis	lĭm″fō-sī-**tō**´sĭs
lymphogenesis	lĭm″fō-**jĕn**´ĕ-sĭs
lymphoid	**lĭm**´foyd
lymphoma	lĭm-**fō**´mă
macrophage	**măk**´rō-fāj
thymus	**thī**´mŭs

Cancer Center Diagnostics

Patient Update

It's been a long morning of tests for Zane Davis. He and his wife, Stevie-Rose, are enjoying a break now and talking over lunch in the cafeteria. Zane has an hour before he goes for his next set of assessments. He was booked at Kootenay Cancer Care Center for the entire day.

"Gosh, honey, I feel like a pincushion," said Zane. "I've had so many needles in me and so many vials of blood taken, and then an intravenous line of something while I had that CT scan and then the PET scan. Sheesh, I can't recall when I have ever been poked and prodded so much." Zane and Stevie-Rose sat down to begin their lunch. He had chosen a clear soup, a whole-wheat bun, and a cup of French vanilla yogurt; she was having a cucumber and cheese sandwich. He smiled then and said, "Well, maybe that's not true. Maybe I can remember a time when I had a similar—but really very different—experience." He laughed. "Remember when I got this crazy dragon tattoo on my upper arm? That was when we were on rest and relaxation in Shanghai in '65." They both laughed. They started to eat, but they were both picking slowly at their meals. "I don't feel very hungry, Stevie-Rose," Zane commented quietly. She nodded.

"No, I don't, either. It's a long, tough day, isn't it," Stevie-Rose stated rather than inquired. They looked across the table at each other. Zane took her hand in his.

Zane said, "If it's bad news. ..." But Stevie-Rose cut him off nervously.

"Let's talk about something else right now, okay?" she said, trying to distract him. "You've got a big afternoon ahead of you yet. Why don't we talk about that," she suggested. "Please, eat some soup. You need it. You've got to eat something, Zane." Zane nodded, and the two of them started to eat again.

"Yeah, okay," he said. "Well, I'm going to the respiratory department shortly. I have to have some tests done there for my lungs."

"Yes, pulmonary assessment. That's really why we're here: your lungs," Stevie-Rose observed. They talked a bit about that. Zane would be having a forced vital capacity (FVC) assessment (an exercise test to assess his oxygen consumption), among other things.

"How many tests do you think I had this morning, honey?" asked Zane. "I know I had about six vials of blood taken by the lab. Then I gave a urine specimen. And I had to cough into a cup to give them a sputum sample."

"Well, you had a CT scan of your entire body. That took a bit of time," said Zane's wife. "And that's why you couldn't have any breakfast or coffee this morning before you got here. You had to be NPO for that test." Her husband nodded his understanding.

"Oh yeah, I know, but my whole body? I thought they were only going to do my chest or my torso. How come they did the whole body?" Stevie-Rose explained that this full scan would provide information about Zane's lymphatic system and assess his prostate. Zane nodded and frowned, commenting that he didn't like the sound of that. Stevie-Rose smiled, aware that they both understood the relationship of the lymphatic system to cancer.

"I had a number of x-rays, too," Zane added, steering away from any discussion of the lymphatic system. "The team here hasn't said they want to do a biopsy or anything like that. Nobody's said anything about taking that type of specimen."

"No, honey, they won't do a biopsy today," said Stevie-Rose. "Dr. Sweetgrass didn't mention that he found any lumps or masses when he did your physical exam, so they'll wait to see what they find on the radiographs and scans. If they do find anything—and I'm sure they won't, dear—then I suspect they'll book another appointment for you to come into surgical or ambulatory day care to get that done." They sat in silence for a moment then. Stevie-Rose took a bite of her sandwich, and Zane managed a few spoonfuls of soup. They continued like that for a while.

"It's almost time to go, Zane. You've got to see the respiratory technician on the fourth floor in about 15 minutes. Would you like to go outside in the courtyard and get a breath of fresh air till then? It would do you good," suggested Stevie-Rose.

"No, not really. What I'd really, really like is a cigarette! Let's go out the front door so that I can do both: get some sunshine and have a smoke," said Zane. "We'll have to walk back over to the parking lot. You can't smoke right outside the hospital, I guess."

Stevie-Rose frowned but agreed, knowing full well this was not the time or the place to push him to quit smoking. Zane always smoked under stress. However, Stevie-Rose also knew that, by the end of the day, Dr. Sweetgrass would likely be telling him he must stop at all costs. Stevie-Rose bit her lip, worried, but she kept her silence as they went outside.

Reflective Questions

Answer the following questions on the basis of the Patient Update.

1. Zane had two diagnostic exams that required an intravenous line concurrently and for which he had to be NPO. Which exams were these? ______
2. During the afternoon, Zane's testing will be focused in a specific department. Name it, and explain why he will be there. ______
3. How soon will Zane be able to get the results of most—if not all—of his diagnostic assessments? ______

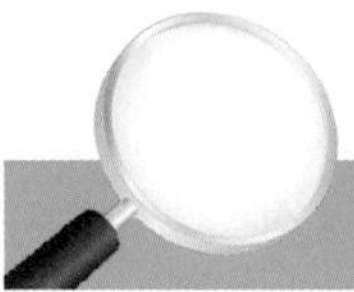

FOCUS POINT: CT/PET Scans

A physician can order a joint test—a CT/PET scan—to reduce the patient's exposure to radioactive substances in the body. Diagnostically, the benefits of the CT/PET scan include the ability to see the two images together, thereby illuminating areas of high metabolic activity and precisely locating them.

Critical Thinking

Consider what you've learned about coping, addiction, and the stress response to answer this question.

Why does Stevie-Rose choose not to bring up the subject of stopping smoking at this point in time? Wouldn't it be a good opportunity to drive this message home for Zane?

______

______

______

______

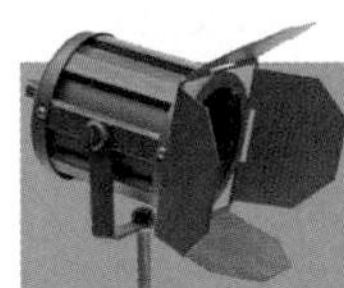

CAREER SPOTLIGHT: Registered Respiratory Therapist (RT) and Respiratory Technician (RT)

A *respiratory therapist* is a health professional with a minimum of a bachelor's degree in science or the health sciences. This professional's responsibilities focus on the assessment, care, and treatment of patients with pulmonary and cardiopulmonary disease, which are conditions in which breathing and gas exchanges are impaired or have the potential to become impaired. Respiratory therapists are skilled in the use of complex technology; they use diagnostic tools and equipment that have been specifically designed for the assessment and treatment of respiratory conditions. They work under the direction of a physician or a nurse practitioner, yet they also take responsibility for setting the modes of assessment, intervention, and treatment in consultation with the treatment team. They are an integral part of the recovery, rehabilitation, and maintenance of health of patients with breathing disorders. Respiratory therapists are able to treat patients with oxygen and aerosol preparations, and they can connect and monitor patients on ventilators. These therapists can also perform chest physical therapy. In almost all states, respiratory therapists require licensing, which is dependent on the candidate's ability to pass a national examination. The credential of *registered respiratory therapist (RRT)* is granted by the National Board of Respiratory Care (NBRC). Respiratory therapists are also known as *respiratory care practitioners.*

A *respiratory technician* is quite similar to a respiratory therapist, although he or she does not work autonomously with regard to clinical decision making for patient care. This type of technician is subordinate to respiratory therapists and physicians and carries out the directions of those professionals. Even so, as a member of a care team, the respiratory technician fully collaborates in all aspects of patient assessment and care. Respiratory technicians may administer oxygen, oxygen mixes, and aerosols. They may teach clients how to use inhalers and nebulizers. In addition, they may also participate in chest physical therapy. Respiratory technicians may also work in obstetrics to assist with the breathing functions of mothers and newborn infants. An associate's degree in one of the health sciences and focused education in respiratory technology are required for entry into practice, and certification may be required. Credentials for these individuals include *RT* and *certified respiratory technician (CRT),* and they are granted after the successful completion of a licensing examination. These credentials are conferred by the National Board of Respiratory Care.

Respiratory diagnostics

Chapter 9 introduced the respiratory system, asbestosis, and mesothelioma. As you know, signs that our patient Zane Davis may have asbestosis or mesothelioma were the main reasons that he was referred to Kootenay Cancer Care Center for additional diagnostic assessment. This afternoon, Zane can expect to undergo pulmonary function tests—including lung capacity studies that will use exercise, a plethysmograph, and a spirometer—in addition to all of the blood work and radiographs he's already had. Table 14-14 describes a number of these diagnostics.

Pulmonology is the branch of science and medicine that is concerned with pathologies of the lungs, the bronchioles, and the upper respiratory tract (see Chapter 9) particularly, although cardiopulmonary involvement is also important. A **pulmonologist** is a medical internist (a doctor of internal medicine) with advanced training in pulmonology.

Table 14-15 identifies a battery of tests for respiratory system and pulmonary (lung) status assessment. Note that pulmonary function tests are included. You may notice from Table 14-15 that some of these diagnostics are invasive rather than noninvasive. Those tests that require the taking of tissue (i.e., biopsies), involve the injection of radiopaque dyes or contrast mediums, or that necessitate the use of an anesthetic or sedative may require a patient to remain in bed and in the hospital for a longer period of time than is scheduled for our patient, Zane Davis. For that reason, if Dr. Sweetgrass determines that these tests are needed, he will reschedule the patient to return to Kootenay Cancer Care Center in the near future, with the possibility of admitting him to a unit, at least for overnight.

Spirometry

Spirometry is a pulmonary function test or a series of breathing tests that ascertain and monitor lung capacity and function. It is accomplished with the use of a device called a **spirometer** (see Figure 14-12), which measures flow rates and the amount of air that is moving through the lungs. Depending on the style of the device, the user either blows into a mouthpiece that is attached to a tube that flows into a meter, or else he or she blows into a small device that sends measurements to a nearby computer or other monitoring device.

The term spirometer is deconstructed as follows:

spiro: to breathe

meter: measure

Incentive spirometry is a procedure that is used to encourage patients to breathe deeply, in and out. Although it is a diagnostic test, it also demonstrates to the patient how deep or shallow his or her breathing is at any given time.

TABLE 14-14: Pulmonary Function Tests

Test	Description
Forced expiratory volume (FEV)	• After the patient takes a deep breath, air is forced out of the lungs purposely, into a spirometer. The measurement is taken during the first second of expiration. It measures the functional ability of the bronchus and the trachea in the respiratory tract. • Values: FEV, 80% to 100% • Percentages that are lower than these indicate increasing severity of lung disease. Values for patients with severe lung disease can be < 35%.
Forced expiratory flow 25-75 (FEF 25-75)	• During the forced expiration of a deep breath, this measure is taken midway. It assesses how smaller airways (i.e., the bronchioles) are functioning.
Forced vital capacity (FVC)	• After the patient takes the deepest breath possible, this test measures the total amount of air that can be blown out forcefully into a spirometer. • It is indicative of how much air the lungs can actually hold.
Progressive exercise test	• This test evaluates the functional capacity of the lungs and the circulatory system during progressive efforts that are made when the patient is riding a stationary bike, including oxygen consumption levels. Oxygen levels may be measured by the use of a mask device or a pulse oximeter.
Respiratory inductance plethysmography	• This test involves the use of a specific instrument to measure total lung capacity and the residual volume of air in the lungs after it has been forced out.
Pulmonary plethysmography	• This is a measure of how much air can be held in the lungs when they are at rest.

TABLE 14-15: Respiratory and Pulmonary Assessment Status Examination

Test	Description and Purpose
chest x-ray	• detects fluids, tumors, or foreign bodies in the thorax
bronchoscopy	• insertion of a fiberoptic tube into the trachea and bronchi to allow for the assessment of the airways through observation • requires NPO status and mild sedation to decrease muscle spasms, the gag reflex, and the anxiety response created by the passing of the bronchoscope
thoracoscopy	• surgical insertion of a fiberoptic tube into the chest wall to visualize the pleural space and the intrathoracic structures (see Chapter 9) to assess for pleural disorders (i.e., in the membranes surrounding the lungs); a tissue biopsy may also be taken by this route • requires NPO status and a mild or general anesthetic • assesses for metastatic cancer, mesothelioma, tuberculosis, mediastinal lymph nodes (i.e., between the spine and the sternum), and other conditions
thoracentesis	• insertion of a needle or thin tube into the chest wall • determines the cause of pleural effusion (i.e., excess fluid in the pleural space of the thorax caused by heart failure, infection, or tumors); removes fluid for diagnostic and treatment purposes (Note: Excessive fluid in the pleural space puts pressure on the lungs and makes breathing challenging.)
sputum specimen	• a sample of mucus and other secretions expelled from the lungs; these samples are analyzed in the laboratory for pathogens (bacteriological analysis) or malignancy (cytological analysis)
pulse oximetry	• a non-invasive method of measuring the saturation of oxygen in the hemoglobin of the circulating blood
fluoroscopy	• a continuous x-ray of movement in an area of the body; for example, fluoroscopy can detect movement of the diaphragm or veins • requires the insertion of an intravenous line plus the use of a dye or contrast medium that can be visually observed and followed through the body on an adjacent video monitor; before the use of any such dyes or contrast mediums, an allergy assessment is completed and, if necessary, an alert is placed in the patient's file and on his or her arm bracelet • can be used to track tumors

TABLE 14-15: Respiratory and Pulmonary Assessment Status Examination—cont'd

Test	Description and Purpose
PET scan (positron emission tomography)	• a type of nuclear imaging that makes use of a small amount of radioactive dye (radiotracer) that is introduced into the body intravenously or that is inhaled or swallowed; this material can be visually observed and followed through the body on an adjacent computer monitor • in addition to assessing for the presence and metastases of cancerous tumors and masses, a PET scan is able to confirm adequate blood supply to targeted areas of the body, to assess for heart disease, and to measure glucose metabolism (Note: Only diabetics who are dependent on insulin or medication are candidates for a PET scan).
CT scan (computed tomography)	• completed with or without a contrast medium, which is given intravenously (see Chapter 4)
angiography (pulmonary)	• another type of continuous x-ray procedure to assess how blood flows through a body part or region • requires a mild sedative and then the insertion of a dye or contrast medium through the femoral vein that can be visually observed and followed through the pulmonary arteries on an adjacent video monitor • requires the patient to be NPO before the procedure and to lay flat for up to 8 hours after the procedure • assesses for pulmonary emboli, pulmonary hypertension, tumors, narrowed blood vessels, and blood clots in the lungs • other types of angiograms include cerebral, cardiac, and retinal

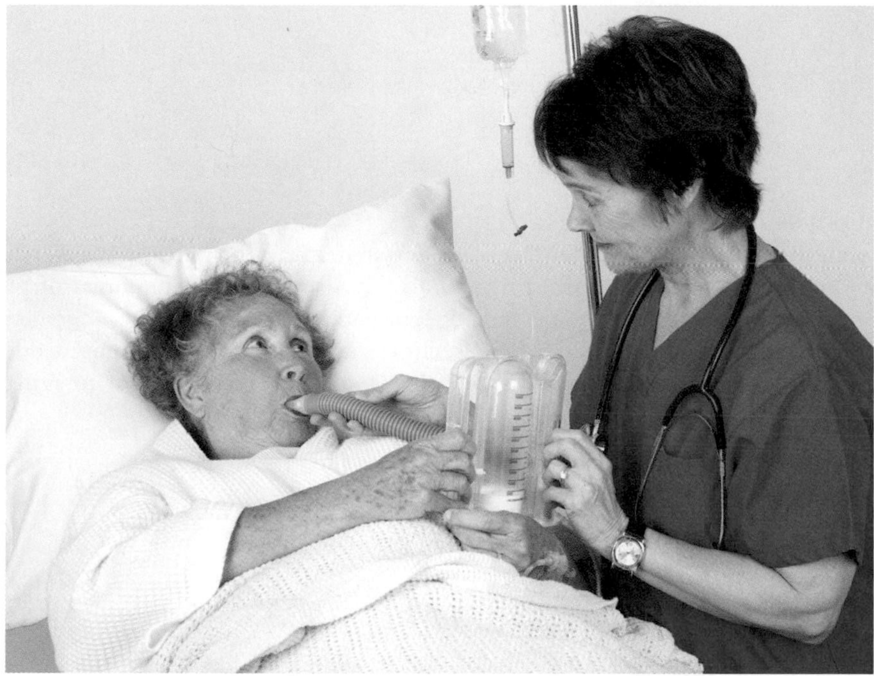

Figure 14.12: Spirometer (© Thinkstock)

Pulmonary plethysmography

Pulmonary plethysmography is the measure of how much air can be held in the lungs (i.e., lung volume) during times of rest. It can help to determine if there is structural damage to the lungs or if they have lost the ability to expand properly as the patient inhales.

Pulmonary plethysmography requires the use of a **plethysmograph**. This device is a small chamber in which the client sits for the test. The client's nose will be plugged, and he or she will breathe into a mouthpiece (see Figure 14-13).

The term *plethysmograph* is deconstructed as follows:

plethysmo: to increase
graph: to write or record

Pulmonary plethysmography is also known as *static lung volume determination.*

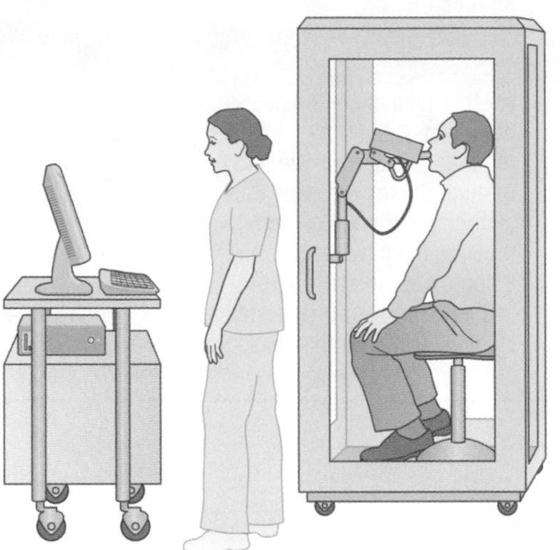

Figure 14.13: Plethysmograph

Positron emission tomography (PET)

A **PET scan** machine is an extremely sensitive device that can pick up and measure even the tiniest amounts of radioactive matter in the body. It also uses trace amounts of glucose—the cells of which begin to metabolize quickly—to detect tumors. PET scanners are part of the Nuclear Medicine department in hospitals, clinics, and laboratories. A combined PET/CT scanner is a newer and more modern device that combines both types of imaging in one machine (see Figure 14-14).

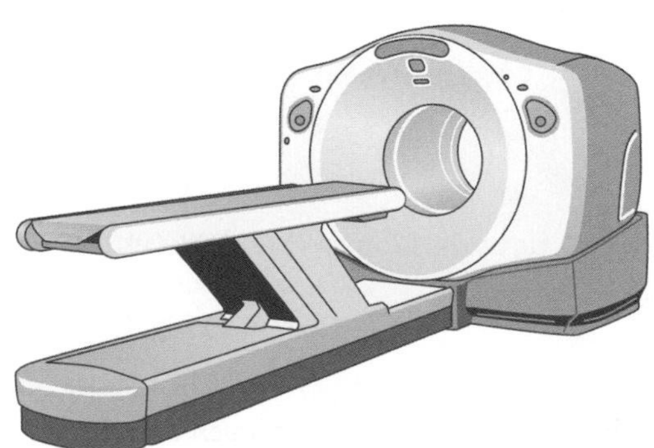

Figure 14.14: Combination CT/PET scanner

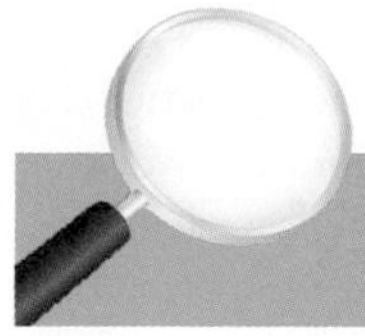

FOCUS POINT: The Basic Difference Between a CT Scan and PET Scan

Here is a quick and easy way to remember the difference between a CT scan and a PET scan:

A *CT scan* shows detailed anatomical locations.

A *PET scan* shows areas of increased metabolic activity.

Reflective Question

Refer to Tables 14-14 and 14-15 to answer the following question.

Identify all of the tests that you are certain Zane Davis has had already today at Kootenay Cancer Care Center. ______________________________

Critical Thinking

To answer these questions, study the section about respiratory diagnostics. Recall the five patients in this textbook and their own assessments. For some of the questions, you will need to practice the skill of research to do so. (In other words, you will have to go back through some of the chapters to search for the answers.)

1. Name the patients who have had a CT scan. ______________________________
2. Name the patients who have been clearly identified as having been assessed via pulse oximetry. ______________________________
3. Which of our patients has had a change in one of his or her health challenges that may lead him or her to become a candidate for a PET scan in the future? ______________________________
4. Which respiratory or pulmonary diagnostic tests is Zane Davis likely to undergo this afternoon at Kootenay Cancer Care Center? ______________________________

Free Writing

In your own words, answer the following question.

What is the basic difference in procedure among an FEV, an FEF, and an FVC test?

____

____

____

____

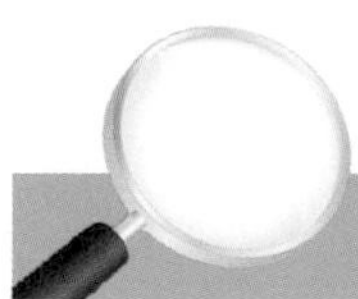

FOCUS POINT: RT

Once again, it is important to stop and think about the context in which a word or abbreviation is heard before interpreting it. For example, be very careful when you hear the initials *RT* after someone's name or used in a sentence.

RT is the credential of a respiratory technician, but it is sometimes used as a simple abbreviation to refer to respiratory therapy or the respiratory therapist.

RT is also the credential of a *recreational therapist,* which is an entirely different health-care career.

Cancer diagnostics

Patients who are undergoing assessment for cancer may undergo some or all of the diagnostic tests and procedures identified in Table 14-16 in addition to a complete physical and laboratory workup. Note that this list is only a sample. As with all health care careers, should your career lead you to the specialty of oncology and cancer care, the special and complex language of that branch of medicine will be essential to learn at the time. These are merely examples.

Our patient, Zane Davis, will have a protein marker test done at Kootenay Cancer Care Center today because this test can detect prostate-specific antigen and the acid phosphatase in the blood, both of which are indicators of the presence of prostate cancer. This test can also detect such cancers as breast, ovarian, and testicular cancer, among others.

TABLE 14-16: Diagnostic Tests and Procedures for Cancer

Test or Diagnostic Procedure	Description
cytogenic analysis	• the cellular analysis of blood or bone marrow for chromosomes and genetic makeup
immunohistochemistry (ICH)	• a very specific laboratory test that is performed to assess for disease and most specifically for lymphomas; the procedure involves a tissue sample and the use of antibodies (referred to here as *matching molecules*) to seek out and attach to antigens by their identifying characteristics • the tissue sample may be collected with a biopsy if it is internal or with a skin scraping if it is external
protein marker test	• a blood test that measures circulating proteins and tumor cells; cancers often produce a specific protein in the blood that is known as a *marker;* circulating tumor cells are those that have broken off of the tumor and are circulating in the bloodstream • high circulating tumor cell counts may indicate that a cancer is growing • this test is often used as an early indicator of the presence of cancer or to look for evidence of metastasis
core needle biopsy	• the removal of a small sample of tissue via a nonsurgical medical procedure; this is performed with the use of a long, thin needle being inserted into the targeted location and a sample of tissue being cut out; the specimen is then sent to a laboratory for analysis
fine-needle aspiration (FNA) or fine-needle aspiration biopsy (FNAB)	• a procedure for extracting a small tissue or cell sample from an identified mass or tumor for analysis in a laboratory; a very fine needle is used (it is smaller than the core needle biopsy needle)
incisional biopsy	• a surgical procedure that is performed to extract a sample from a specific tissue by cutting into it and retrieving it
excisional biopsy	• a surgical procedure that is performed to extract or remove an entire mass or a targeted area of tissue

Let's Practice

Use the new terminology that you have learned. You are given a description; write the medical term to which it refers.

1. a biopsy that removes an entire mass ______________________
2. a test that does not involve a large needle but that still involves aspiration ______________
3. the removal of a sample of tissue for microscopic analysis ______________________
4. a person who scrutinizes for genes and chromosomes ______________________
5. a test that employs antigens during the laboratory analysis of tissue ______________
6. testing looks for tumors and cells with this characteristic ______________________

Critical Thinking

1. What is a biopsy? ____________________
2. What is the difference between an excisional biopsy and an incisional biopsy? ____________________

PRONUNCIATION PRACTICE

Say these words aloud to a friend or classmate, if you can. Here you are given the phonetic pronunciation. Your instructor can help you with pronunciation,

or you can visit **http://www.MedicalLanguageLab.com.**

angiograph	**ăn**´jē-ō-grăf˝
biopsy	**bī**´ŏp-sē
bronchoscopy	brŏng-**kŏs**´kō-pē
cytogenic	sī-tō-**jĕn**´ĭk
excision	ĕk-**sĭ**´zhŭn
fluoroscopy	floo-or˝**ŏs**´kō-pē
incision	ĭn-**sĭzh**´ŭn
plethysmograph	plē-**thĭz**´mō-grăf
positron	**pŏz**´ĭ-trŏn
spirometer	spī-**rŏm**´ĕt-ĕr
thoracentesis	thō˝ră-sĕn-**tē**´sĭs
thoracoscopy	thō˝ră-**kŏs**´kō-pē

The Language of Cancer Care

Zane Davis has been accompanied to a number of his assessments today by an oncology technician named Ethan. Zane has found the young man to be both knowledgeable and very helpful when answering questions regarding his concerns about his health. Zane has also asked Ethan what he knows about chronic obstructive pulmonary disease (COPD), and the technician told him. They talked about the services available at Kootenay Cancer Care Center, and Ethan informed Zane that there were many ways to treat cancer, should he turn out to have it. Ethan explained that these treatments have been very successful for either eradicating the disease from the body, putting it into remission, or simply providing a high degree of comfort and quality of life to those with the more difficult-to-treat forms of the disease. Realizing that Zane was here for assessment, particularly of his lungs, Ethan described a program called *interventional pulmonology* with which symptoms such as shortness of breath, coughing, and some chest pain can be treated without surgery. At one point, Zane and Ethan even talked about the motor vehicle accident that was the beginning of Zane's journey to Kootenay Cancer Care Center for assessment.

Radiation therapy

Radiation therapy is a common intervention for cancer. It uses the energy of radiation to kill cancer cells and to shrink tumors. It can also provide some relief for certain types of symptoms related to cancer, which may occur in patients who are receiving palliative care.

Radiation therapy can be used before, during, or after surgery, depending on the type of cancer in question and its stage. The goal of radiation therapy is to eliminate the cancer or at least to halt its progression and to prevent it from recurring.

external radiation: therapeutic doses of radiation that are given from outside the body

internal radiation: radioactive material is injected into the bloodstream or placed into the body near a tumor site

Bone marrow transplantation (BMT)

This therapeutic procedure delivers healthy bone marrow to patients with cancer, particularly those with lymphoma or leukemia. The marrow may be infused by an intravenous route or injected directly into the breastbone or a hip bone. The route of delivery is dependent on how the bone marrow was collected.

Hyperthermia

This cancer treatment exposes the patient to high temperatures to kill or damage cancer cells. It is not a stand-alone treatment; rather, it is performed concurrently with either chemotherapy or radiation therapy.

Surgical oncology

Surgical intervention is not uncommon as part of cancer treatment. The goal of surgery is to remove a tumor to prevent the further spread of the disease. Oncology surgery may include the reconstruction of a part of the body. It is also used to relieve symptoms of pain when no other remedy will suffice.

Chemotherapy

Chemotherapy is the systemic treatment of cancer with use of chemical compounds (i.e., drugs, anticancer agents) that target pathogens. The goal is to destroy the cancer cells or to prevent their proliferation. Table 14-17 provides just a few examples of the many anticancer agents that are used in this large and complicated field. The field of chemotherapy is constantly changing, with new medications being developed and used all the time. If you are working in this field, it is critically important to keep abreast of new medications and their manner of administration.

Chemotherapy is a difficult form of intervention for patients. For all of the good outcomes that it can produce, there are many possible adverse effects that can make the person feel very uncomfortable and ill. These can include—but are not limited to—hair loss, nausea, vomiting, weight loss, and fatigue.

TABLE 14-17: Anti-Cancer Agents

Type of Medication	Examples	Functions
alkylating agents: genotoxic drugs	cyclophosphamide cisplatin	• modifying the bases of DNA and interfering with its reproduction
biological response modifiers (BMTs)	cytokines (i.e., interferon and interleukin-2) antibodies (i.e., monoclonal) vaccines gene therapy	• making use of the immune system directly or indirectly, thereby strengthening it • destroying cancer cells, minimizing the adverse side effects of other treatments, or both
nitrosourea	carmustine	• interfering with enzymes that facilitate the repair of DNA
enzyme inhibitors	topoisomerase aromatase	• binding to enzymes to decrease their activity to a degree that pathogens are destroyed
antimetabolites	mitomycin C methotrexate	• inhibiting the function of metabolites • acting as decoys for cell metabolism and preventing normal cell growth and function

TABLE 14-17: Anti-Cancer Agents—cont'd

Type of Medication	Examples	Functions
antitumor antibiotics	bleomycin	• preventing cell division by preventing the division of DNA or preventing enzyme synthesis in RNA
plant alkaloids (derived from natural substances in plants)	vinblastine	• blocking cell division
hormonal agents: corticosteroids	prednisone	• decreasing the amount of circulating lymphocytes • inducing cell differentiation • producing anti-inflammatory effects
hormonal agents: steroid (sex) hormones	tamoxifen	• reducing swelling around tumors of the brain and spinal cord • blocking the effect of a steroid on the cells
antifungals	itraconazole	• possibly blocking angiogenesis
antiemetics	prochlorperazine	• relieving chemotherapy-induced nausea and vomiting
antidiarrheals	calcium aluminosilicate	• relieving diarrhea caused by cancer treatments
anti-infectives	penicillin and other antibiotics	• interfering with cancer cell metabolism and reproduction

Let's Practice

Answer the following questions on the basis of what you have learned about cancer care.

1. Name an invasive treatment that is used to remove or repair. ____________________
2. Write out the full term for the abbreviation *BMT.* ____________________
3. Identify the type of treatment that may cause hair loss. ____________________
4. Which type of cancer treatment can be done both internally and externally? ____________
5. Which kind of treatment can cause emesis (vomiting) as a side effect? ______________

Fill in the Blanks

Use new terminology that you have learned. Fill in the blanks with the missing word.

1. An ____________________ agent is one that does not promote the growth of a neoplasm.
2. Should chemotherapy or cancer cause frequent or abnormal bowel movements, an ____________________ might be in order.
3. The opposite of ____________________ is *depress* or *slow.*
4. The infusion of healthy bone marrow into the body is known as ____________________.
5. A genotoxic agent is also an ____________________ agent.
6. The purpose of ____________________ is to expose cancer cells to high temperatures.

PRONUNCIATION PRACTICE

Say these words aloud to a friend or classmate, if you can. Here you are given the phonetic pronunciation. Your instructor can help you with pronunciation,

or you can visit **http://www.MedicalLanguageLab.com.** 

alkylating	**ăl**´kĭ-lā-tĭng	chemotherapy	kē˝mō-**thĕr**´ă-pē
antiemetic	ăn˝tĭ-ē-**mĕt**´ĭk	hyperthermia	hī˝pĕr-**thĕr**´mē-ă
antimetabolite	ăn˝tĭ-mĕ-**tăb**´ō-līt	radiation	rā-dē-**ā**´shŭn

Diagnosis, Prognosis, and Health Maintenance

Read aloud

Read the following Patient Update aloud to practice using new medical terms and medical language. As you do so, notice how familiar you now are with most—if not all—of the medical terminology contained within it. These terms have come from this and previous chapters. Congratulate yourself on your progress!

Patient Update

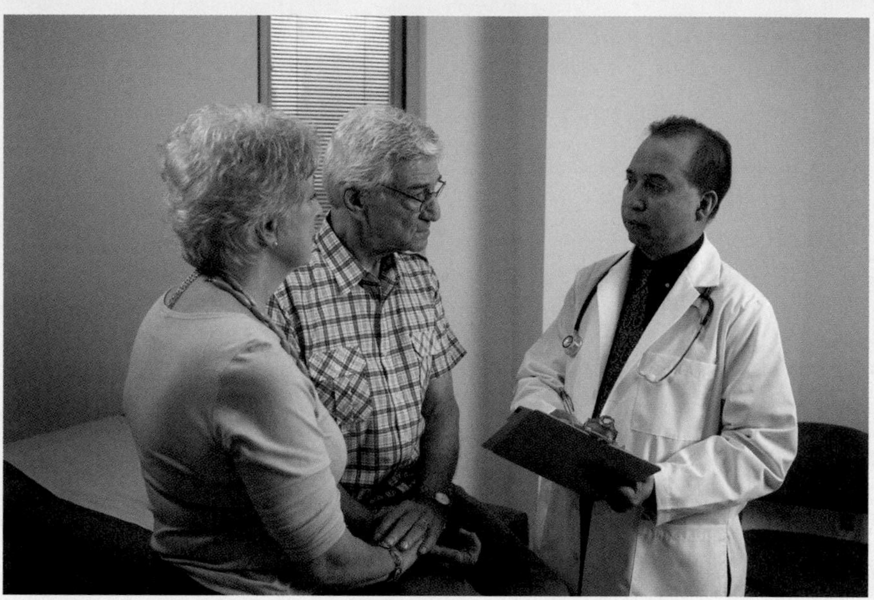

It is now late in the day, and Zane Davis has returned to Dr. Sweetgrass's office to learn the results of his many tests. His wife Stevie-Rose is with him. They are both nervous and tired. Dr. Sweetgrass enters the room with his medical e-scribe. He is not smiling, and the Davises notice this immediately.

"Oh, you don't look happy," observed Stevie-Rose. "I hope that doesn't mean we're about to hear bad news," she said with a tone of inquiry in her voice. She squeezed Zane's hand, and Zane squeezed hers back.

"Oh, I'm sorry, please forgive me," said Dr. Sweetgrass. "My facial expression was one of deep thought, and I was actually thinking about something else when I walked in," reassured the doctor. He moved to take a seat at his desk, facing the Davises. Reilly-Jo moved to a chair nearby and sat down. "You've had an extremely busy day, Zane. How are you feeling?"

"I've got to tell you, I'm really tired now. I don't know why. Maybe it's all the running around I did today or simply the stress of not knowing what will happen," Zane replied.

"And you've barely had anything to eat, either, dear," added Stevie-Rose, while looking at her husband with concern. Zane coughed then, and they all waited for this short burst to subside before continuing the conversation.

"I have good news and bad news," began Dr. Sweetgrass. "First, there is no evidence of prostate cancer, but it does appear that you have some degree of benign prostatic hyperplasia. Your family doctor will be able to follow that with you." The Davises smiled. Dr. Sweetgrass continued: "And I am happy to tell you that we don't believe that you have mesothelioma." The Davises sighed in relief. "Having said that, though," the doctor said, "there is one more test I'd like to order to be absolutely sure. That would require you coming back to us one more time for a thoracoscopy. You'd need to be NPO again for that procedure, and we'd want to give you a general anesthetic. A thoracoscopy would give us a chance to look internally at the tissues of your lungs and to take just a small sample of tissue, a biopsy for further analysis."

"But you said that I don't have mesothelioma," Zane stated. "Why would you need to do that if I don't have it?" He sounded worried. Dr. Sweetgrass explained the importance of using whatever means necessary to completely rule out the disease.

"Sir, you do have asbestosis," the doctor then said, and he waited a moment for this to sink in. "A thoracoscopy would confirm that as well. So, it would be a good idea to do the exam. But that is entirely up to you. You can think about this and just let us know if you're interested at a later date." He paused again, waiting for their reaction or thoughts.

"Okay, so let's see," began Stevie-Rose. "You're saying that Zane doesn't have cancer, but he does have asbestosis." Dr. Sweetgrass agreed.

"Let me explain," said the doctor. "I'd like to go over what's been done here today and some of the results of your tests, all right?" He went on to summarize that the patient had had a physical exam, imaging studies, and laboratory tests. He noted that, during the physical examination, he was able to hear abnormal breath sounds and that this was to be expected with chronic smoking, as well as with scarring on the lungs from asbestos exposure in the past. Blood tests revealed that Zane's hemoglobin and hematocrit values were somewhat elevated, but this too was to be expected under these circumstances. Zane's WBC-diff (lymphocyte count) was normal, and the physician pointed out that this meant that Zane was not currently fighting a viral or bacterial infection that could have caused his coughing or shortness of breath. He added that this test also helped to rule out leukemia.

He went on then to discuss Zane's pulmonary function test results, noting a slightly elevated $PaCO_2$ level. This was explained as an indicator of hypercapnia or impaired gas exchange. Zane also had an FEV of 40% to 59%, which is moderately indicative of lung disease. Finally, Dr. Sweetgrass reported that the PET/CT scan and the chest x-ray still showed some scarring in the lungs, but they revealed no evidence of cancer. He went through these results slowly, stopping from time to time to explain any abbreviations that he may have used that the Davises were not familiar with and to answer any questions that they had about the tests.

"So, Zane, you do have asbestosis," said the doctor. "You are a chronic smoker. You have a history of chronic bronchitis and pneumonia. All of these symptoms mean that you have chronic obstructive pulmonary disease." He paused. The Davises looked at each other as the diagnosis set in for them.

"I want to suggest that you begin a regimen of respiratory therapy to keep your lungs as healthy as possible. I'm sure that you are well aware that smoking is harmful and that it is even destructive and disease producing. I have to say to you today that you should, at all costs, quit smoking now. We can help you with that," said Dr. Sweetgrass firmly. "You have tar deposits in your lungs that block the passage of air. You are unable to get a full, clean breath; the plethysmograph study that you underwent today showed us that. You cough often as well. This is the body trying to expel the toxins of the tobacco tar. On top of this, you have a mild case of asbestosis. This, too, impairs your ability to take in fresh air and to achieve the necessary gas exchange that your body needs." As he spoke, Dr. Sweetgrass looked directly at his patient. "Quitting smoking can help to restore some of that lung function." He waited for Zane to comment.

"I know, I know, but I've tried and tried to quit. I just can't," said Zane. "I hear what you're saying, but I don't know if I can do it." Dr. Sweetgrass advised Zane that Kootenay Cancer Care Center offered a smoking cessation program on an outpatient basis and that perhaps Zane may want to join it. The doctor described the program and then added that he could order some nicotine patches or medications to help Zane through the withdrawal process, if needed. Zane agreed to consider the program and wanted some time to do so, and he did agree to take a prescription for the nicotine patches.

"I'd like to talk about your diagnosis of asbestosis now," said Dr. Sweetgrass. "From what you've told me, your exposure to this toxin seems to have been minimal, and the tests bear this out. You have a minor form of the disease, but that in itself is serious, because it is confounded or complicated by the presence of your other respiratory problems." He explained that, when he listened to Zane's lungs, he heard late respiratory crackles over the lung fields (see Chapter 9), and he observed and heard shortness of breath, particularly on exertion. The doctor stated that the radiographs taken today confirmed those taken at Okla Trauma Center in that they showed lower- and middle-zone shadowing with small opaque spots on the lobes of the lungs. He pointed out that these spots were what they were referring to as "scarring"; there was pleural thickening or calcification of the tissue at those sites.

"I know that the two of you have done some research on asbestosis, but I want you to clearly hear that this is a progressive pulmonary disease," said Dr. Sweetgrass. "It can lead to a shortened life expectancy if it is not treated and monitored regularly. Luckily, you were in a car accident that led you to a hospital, where your lungs were assessed. We have found this disease early. We don't want it to progress to anything cancerous." Dr. Sweetgrass paused to give the Davises time to think about all of the information that they had learned. They looked directly at him, listening intently.

Then the doctor went on. "I am confident that I can treat you for this condition, Zane." The Davises looked at each other then and held each other's gaze for a moment as Dr. Sweetgrass continued. "I want to start you on an anti-inflammatory medication to prevent further damage to your lung tissue. You need to stop smoking immediately. And, finally, respiratory therapy should begin this week to improve or maintain the optimal level of healthy lung function that is possible for you. Will you do all of those things? Take care of yourself like this?" Zane Davis smiled, looked at his wife, and said softly yet firmly, "I will."

Reflective Questions

1. During the auscultation of the chest, what did Dr. Sweetgrass hear?____________________
2. What will be the goal of respiratory therapy for this patient?____________________
3. How many diagnoses were identified for Zane today? Name them.____________________

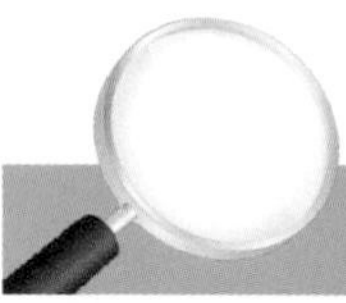

FOCUS POINT: Nicotine Patch

A nicotine patch is a transdermal patch that is applied to the surface of the skin. Over a specific period of time, it releases nicotine into the body to circumvent the craving that the body has for it. In this way, controlled doses that are gradually diminished can be given and thus withdrawal symptoms eased. The use of nicotine patches is referred to as *nicotine replacement therapy (NRT).*

Critical Thinking

Consider the interaction between Zane and Dr. Sweetgrass as Zane's diagnoses are identified.

1. Why does the heading for this section include the words *health maintenance*?

____

____

2. Zane hesitates with one health-promoting initiative that is presented to him. Which one is it? ______________________________
3. In addition to lung cancer, our patient was also assessed for another type of cancer today. Luckily, he does not have it. What was it? ____________________

CHAPTER SUMMARY

Chapter 14 has followed our patient, Zane Davis, through his day-long appointment at Kootenay Cancer Care Center. This context has provided you with the opportunity to discover the language of cancer diagnostics, care, and treatment. The health careers of medical e-scribes, respiratory therapists, respiratory and oncology technicians, and oncology surgical technicians have been introduced. The lymphatic system was introduced, and you were given the opportunity to explore the construction of medical terminology for that body system. A variety of exercises allowed for practice with the use of new terminology in meaningful ways.

See How Much You've Learned

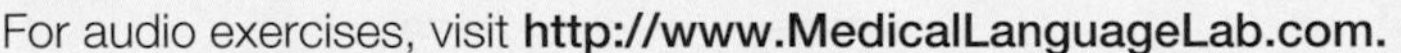

For audio exercises, visit **http://www.MedicalLanguageLab.com.** 

Chapter 14 also introduced new abbreviations. A number of them appear again here in a concise table to promote study.

TABLE 14-18: Abbreviations in Chapter 14

Abbreviation or Acronym	Meaning
AML	acute myelogenous leukemia; acute myeloid leukemia
AIDS	acquired immunodeficiency syndrome
Ca	cancer, calcium
CA	cancer, cardiac arrest, chronological age, cancer antigen, or cytosine arabinoside
CEA	carcinoembryonic antigen
CIS	cancer in situ
CML	chronic myelogenous leukemia; chronic myeloid leukemia
DNA	deoxyribonucleic acid
FNA	fine-needle aspiration
FNAB	fine-needle aspiration biopsy
HHV-8	human herpes virus (herpesvirus) 8
HIV	human immunodeficiency virus
HL	Hodgkin's lymphoma
ICH	immunohistochemistry
KS	Kaposi's sarcoma
mets	metastases
NED	no evidence of disease
NHL	non-Hodgkin's lymphoma
NRT	nicotine replacement therapy
PET	positron emission tomography
St	stage
STS	soft-tissue sarcoma
T and A	tonsils and adenoids
Tis (or TIS)	tumor in situ
WBC-Diff	white blood cell differential test (lymphocyte count)

Key Terms

addiction
adenoids
anaplastic
atypical
auscultate
B-lymphocytes (B-cells)
blastoma
cancer (CA)
carcinogens
carcinomas
celiothelioma
cell differentiation
chemotherapy
chromosomes
chyle
deoxyribonucleic acid (DNA)
dictation
environment
environmental toxins
genes
genetics
hardiness
histogenesis
inpatient
lifestyle
lymph
lymph nodes
lymphangiogenesis
lymphocyte count (WBC-diff)
lymphocytes
lymphocytopenia
lymphocytosis
lymphoma
metastasis (mets)
mutation
neoplasia
neoplasm
nucleotides
oncology
optimal patient outcomes

Continued

outpatient	**pulmonary plethysmography**	**sarcomas**	**terminal**
palliative care unit	**pulmonologist**	**spirometer**	**thymus**
PET scan	**pulmonology**	**spirometry**	**TNM staging system**
plethysmograph	**resiliency**	**spleen**	**tonsils**
premature	**review of systems (ROS)**	**support programs**	**translocation**
primary site	**salient**	**teratogen**	**T-stem cells**
PSA		**teratoma**	

CHAPTER REVIEW

Critical Thinking

Use your new knowledge of medical terms and medical language to answer the following questions.

1. At this point in his journey through the medical system, Zane Davis's condition is no longer acute, and he is not in need of inpatient care. Is he in the recovery, rehabilitation, or maintenance phase of health care now? How do you know?

 ____

2. Which blood test related to the health of his urinary system did our patient have again at Kootenay Cancer Care Center?

 ____

3. A young man named Ethan accompanied Zane throughout the tests and procedures that he underwent today. What position on the care team does Ethan hold?

 ____

4. In the radiology and nuclear medicine department of Kootenay Cancer Care Center, what co-occurring examination did our patient have?

 ____

Antonyms

Provide the antonym for the term given.

1. lymphocytosis ______________________________
2. antigen ______________________________
3. antifungal ______________________________
4. stimulating ______________________________
5. infective ______________________________

Mix and Match

Match the synonyms.

1. teratoma	trisomy 21
2. carcinosarcoma	Wermer's syndrome
3. Down syndrome	oncofetal
4. carcinosis	sarcocarcinoma
5. carcinoembryonic	terablastoma
6. MENS, type 1	carcinomatosis

Translate the Terminology

Use your new skills to decipher medical language. On the line provided, rewrite each statement in your own words using everyday language to convey the meaning of the terminology.

Example: Current research focuses on the gradiation potency of carcinogens present in aromatic amines.

Answer: Scientists are now studying the grades of carcinogens in aromatic amines to see how strong they are.

1. Insulinomas are rare and hold only moderate significance in the realm of pancreatic cell tumors.

   ____

2. Clinical determination of the degree of carcinogenicity in substances falls to the oncologists.

   ____

3. During the transition from hyperplasia to neoplasia, angiogenesis was induced.

   ____

Synonyms

Provide a synonym for each of the following medical terms.

1. suppress ______________________________
2. B-cells ______________________________
3. T-stem cells ______________________________
4. macrophages ______________________________
5. T-lymphocytes ______________________________
6. WBC differential ______________________________
7. adenosarcoma ______________________________
8. mesothelioma ______________________________
9. static lung volume determination ______________________________
10. white blood cell ______________________________

Name the Suffix

Read each definition, and then write the suffix with that meaning.

1. growth and development ______________________________
2. production or birth ______________________________
3. tumor or swelling ______________________________

Right Word or Wrong Word: *Werner Syndrome* or *Wermer's Syndrome?*

Which of these terms refers to multiple endocrine neoplasia, and which refers to a form of adult progeria (i.e., abnormal aging)?

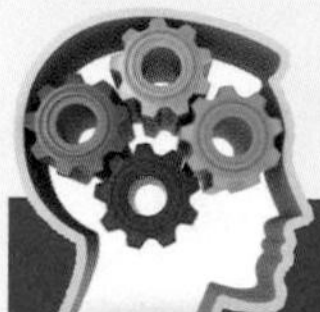

MEMORY MAGIC

Here are two mnemonics to help you remember important information related to cancer.

1. **CAUTION** (early signs and symptoms for cancer screening)

   C: Change in bowel or bladder habits

   A: A sore that doesn't heal

   U: Unusual bleeding or discharge

   T: Thickening or lump

   I: Indigestion or difficulty swallowing

   O: Obvious changes in a wart or mole

   N: Nagging cough or hoarseness

   *This mnemonic is promoted by the American Cancer Society, and it is quite well known in the health sciences.

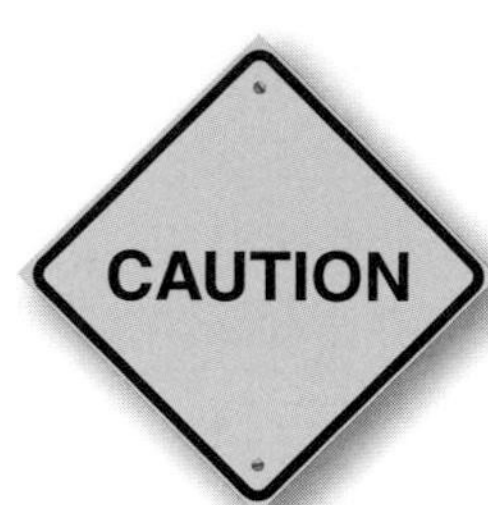

2. **ABCD Rule** (to assess the malignant potential of a mole)

   A: Asymmetry: Does the mole have an irregular shape?

   B: Border: Is the border of the mole irregular, notched, or poorly defined?

   C: Color: Does the color of the mole vary among shades of brown, red, white, blue, or black?

   D: Diameter: Is the diameter more than 6 mm (0.24 inches)?

CHAPTER FIFTEEN

Rehabilitation: Physical and Occupational Therapy

Focus: Muscles and the Brain

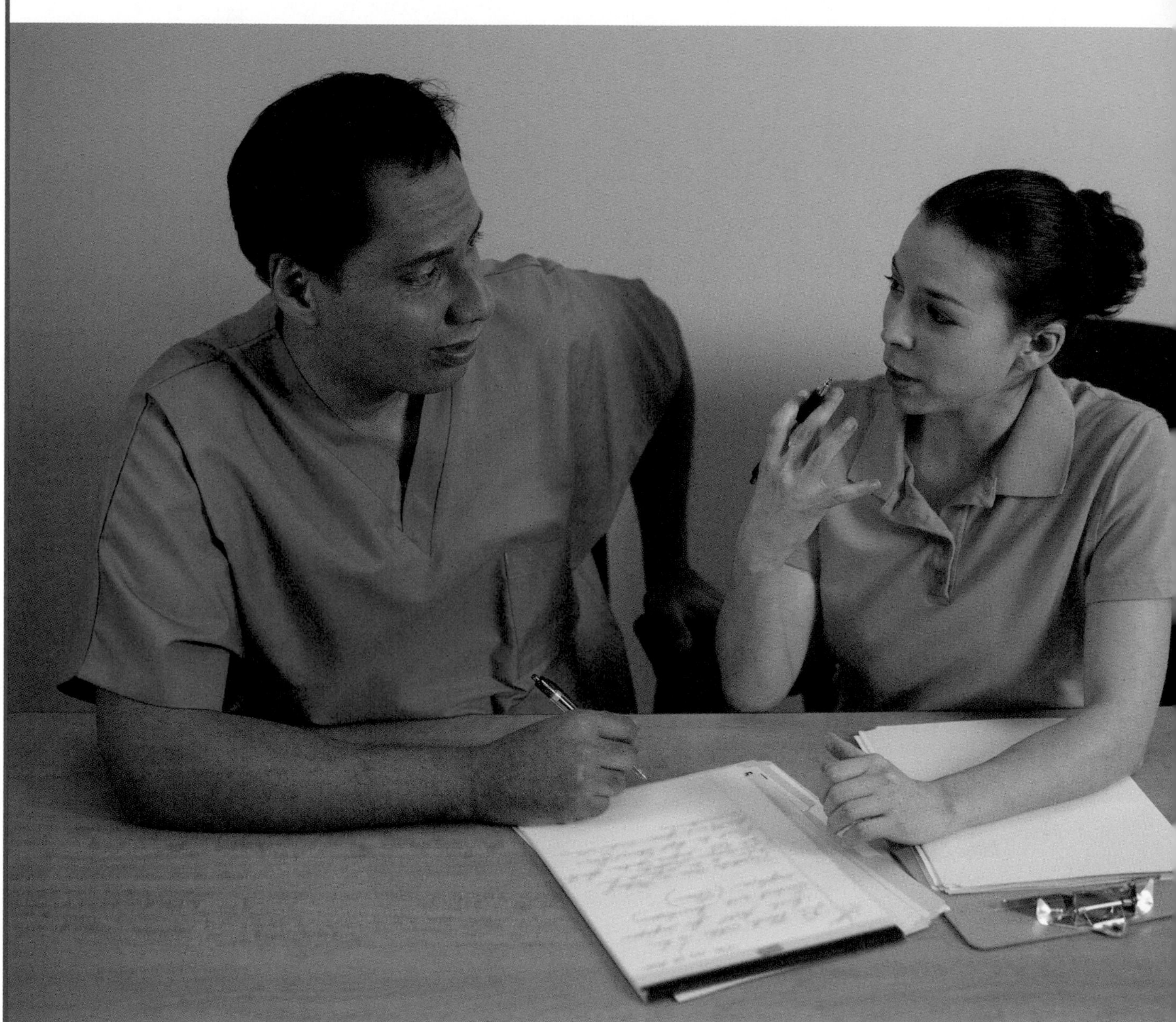

Thirty-six-year old Gilbert Loeppky is the driver of a delivery truck that was involved in a motor vehicle accident 3 full weeks ago. His injuries led him to Okla Trauma Center (see Chapters 4 and 10). He was in the hospital for the injuries that he sustained: a spiral fracture of the right hip, a pilon fracture to the distal portion of his right tibia, an acute patellar injury to the right knee, and a moderate concussion.

During our last encounter with this patient, he was recovering postoperatively from an acute subdural hematoma, the result of a fall from his hospital bed (see Chapter 10). Subsequent to that, he emerged from his medically induced coma with very minimal neurological and motor deficits. This meant that within days, he was able to have the necessary orthopedic surgery to reduce his right hip fracture. In addition, an anteromedial joint arthrotomy was successfully performed, thus reducing and repairing the pilon fracture.

Gil spent a total of 10 days at Okla Trauma Center. After he stabilized, he was transferred to an orthopedic floor at Fayette General Hospital for ongoing care and recovery. He has now been there for 11 days. He continues to recover and has begun physical therapy for his fractures and for the acute patellar injury to his right knee. Gil has now spent a total of 3 weeks in two hospitals.

Patient Update

"Hi, Tamron, how are things going in the physical therapy department today?" greeted Scott Kanesewah, one of the registered nurses on the orthopedic unit. Tamron Epp, a physical therapist, smiled as she walked into the small consulting room behind the unit's nursing station.

"We're very busy, but I like it that way," she replied. Tamron pulled up a chair at the small table where Scott sat with a small writing pad and a pen in hand. They began to talk about their mutual patient, Gil Loeppky. Their meeting was arranged to provide a progress report from both perspectives and to collaborate on the next steps in Gil's recovery and rehabilitation. They were holistic in their approach, understanding the importance that the mind-body connection played in a patient's resiliency.

"He's generally quite friendly, and his mood is good. However, I wonder if he's really as optimistic as he says he is," commented Scott. He then provided an explanation, noting that Gil knew he would not be able to return to work as a delivery truck driver for at least another 6 months. Scott pointed out that although Gil had sufficient medical coverage for his inpatient stay, as well as for some follow-up physical therapy and rehabilitation, he had not been alone in the car accident that brought him to this crisis in his life. They discussed the financial implications of Gil's wife having been hospitalized and the birth of their baby, who remains in neonatal care at Fayette General. Scott shared that he knew that the police had been in earlier during the week to talk to Gil about the circumstances of the accident, and that this visit had upset the patient. Tamron wondered if Gil's presentation of optimism was designed to get himself discharged from the hospital as soon as possible to prevent his medical costs from climbing even higher.

"That's really a lot for him to think about, isn't it?" said Scott.

"Well yes, but even so, I have to make the most of that upbeat mood whenever I have him in my care," commented Tamron. "In my job with orthopedic patients, it's important that they approach their rehabilitation with hope—hope for some degree of recovery or at least for the ability to function as closely to normal again as they can possibly manage." Scott nodded in agreement. The physical therapist went on to talk about her plan of care for Gil, noting that he'd been started on high-frequency PT since his arrival at Fayette General.

She explained that research has shown that patients who received this level of PT in the hospital achieved earlier ambulation than those who did not. Gil had been started on some isometric exercises and some light stretching and bending exercises that he could perform in bed and in a chair.

"When he's in bed, we've been placing him in a supine position while I or one of the other physical therapists on duty support some passive range-of-motion exercises for the quadriceps femoris. You've probably seen us do this." Scott nodded, and Tamron continued. "We spend about 5 to 7 minutes per leg. We gently support the dorsal aspect of the lower leg with one hand, and we place our other hand on the anterior of the knee. Then we gently guide his upper leg into a flexion position, with just a slight amount of pressure, and then push the knee over his abdomen. Still supporting the limb, we then gently extend it back to a normal position. Of course, for his right leg, we are extremely careful with that injured patella. We don't want to stress it in any way, but we need to keep the other leg muscles healthy and strong. Gil seems to be tolerating these exercises quite well. There's not much we can do with the ankle right now. It's just been pinned, and we need to allow that to heal without too much stress on the entire ankle area. That's where some simple isometrics are helpful."

"And are you doing these exercises bilaterally?" asked Scott, nodding in acknowledgement of all that was said.

"Oh, yes. It's important to do this bilaterally to prevent any kind of muscle atrophy in either leg, especially this patient's left leg, since he won't be able to bear any weight on his right leg for some time yet." They talked then about the complication of Gil's broken right ankle and his patellar injury. The physical therapist explained that she had begun getting Gil to stand up at the parallel bars with direct assistance to see how long he could tolerate being upright in this position. Tamron continued: "He seems to be able to tolerate the sit-to-stand procedure, and he can stand with the assistance of the rails for about 4 to 5 full minutes now before his strength begins to diminish. So far, his locomotion is limited to the use of a wheelchair. We've had him fitted for crutches as well, but I'm just not sure his balance is good enough for crutches yet. That may have something to do with his head injury." Tamron also explained her staff's inability to use a lifting device to bring Gil to an upright position because of the complications of his hip and leg surgeries. "We don't want to apply any unnecessary pressure to those fractures," said Tamron.

"Uh-huh," said Scott. "It sounds like Gil is making progress." Tamron nodded, and Scott continued. "Tell me more about his balance and about his motor functioning? Any thoughts or observations on that? You know that he had a concussion and then a fall out of bed at Okla Trauma that led to a subdural hematoma, ICP, and an emergency craniotomy?"

"Yes," said Tamron, "I did know that, and, of course, you can see where his head has been shaved and where the sutures were originally in place." She paused for a moment to think. "Because of the multiple traumas to his right leg, I'm not sure that I can fully comment on his balance and gait just yet. When he tries to perch on one leg, he has a tendency to wobble, and I'm worried that he'll put his injured foot down. We're trying to avoid that at all costs because the doctor has not given him permission to do that yet and because it would be painful as well. We run the risk that, if he steps down on the right foot, he'll immediately retract it and then fall. I am absolutely sure that he doesn't have enough balance to manage that kind of situation yet."

Scott nodded in agreement and then asked, "What about tremors or spastic gait? Have you noticed anything like that?"

"No, Scott," said Tamron, "I haven't seen any evidence of spastic gait. You're thinking of neuro-involvement here, aren't you?" The nurse confirmed this. "No, no evidence. Gil's stiff and hesitant when he moves, but he's not spastic, and I haven't observed any type of muscle spasm, either. Although his muscle tone seems good, I think the hesitancy may be psychological, or it could also be associated with the impairment of muscle innervation along a neuropathway. I've noticed some tremors of the upper limbs when he does our lifting exercises, but only if he does too many repetitions of those. I'm gradually increasing the repetitions, though. We want to ensure that he doesn't lose any muscle function in his arms and that he's able to lift himself up and down off of chairs, the toilet, and so on prior to discharge. Has he had another CT scan since arriving here to check for neuro-involvement?"

Scott shook his head, replying that Gil had not undergone such a scan because his insurance company was not willing to pay for it. Scott advised Tamron that the nursing staff on his unit were continuing to do some Glasgow Coma Scale evaluations to assess the patient's neuro-functioning from time to time (see Chapter 4). He reported that Gil's left pupil sometimes seemed a bit sluggish when tested and that, when he woke in the morning, it took a moment or two for him to clear his slurred speech. Tamron and Scott talked about this for a while and reviewed what they knew about traumatic brain injury and recovery (see Chapters 4 and 10). They then worked through the physical therapy care plan and the nursing care plan as they related to the rehabilitation of the patient's musculoskeletal system.

"Okay," said Scott, planning aloud. "So if someone from physical therapy comes to see Gil in his room in the morning for some gentle stretching to start his day around 0930 hours, we can give him a minor analgesic/anti-inflammatory about half an hour beforehand prepare him for the exercises." Tamron nodded, and Scott continued: "Then, if you've got him scheduled to attend in the PT department at 1400 hours, we can do the same thing before that." The physical therapist agreed that this would be helpful. In turn, she or her colleagues would be sure to report about Gil's ability to tolerate the PT activities and would speak to the nurses about the patient's need for ice for the muscles or pain management after each session.

"The nurses will supplement with the range-of-motion exercises that you've identified for him once during the day shift, once during the afternoon, and once before bed," added Scott. "We'll also continue to get him up into a chair throughout the day, allowing for periods of rest in his bed. We're helping him change position routinely when he's in bed to keep pressure off of the left hip and heel, too." Scott and Tamron agreed about all of the interventions.

Before departing, Tamron said, "Gil told me that he's only seen his little baby in pictures and in a video that his family shot through the glass of the NICU. Is that true? Hasn't he been allowed to go into the unit to hold his baby yet?" Scott explained that the neonatal nurses did not want to put the babies at risk of infection from someone who was also an inpatient at the hospital, pointing out the risks of MRSA and other infections (see Chapter 13). He said they had also told him that the unit was very small and crowded with equipment, so it was not possible for Gil to get near his baby's incubator in his wheelchair.

"That must be hard on Gil. This is his first baby, you know. He's very excited about it. His wife comes in a couple of times every day to see him, and each time she brings him photos of their new baby girl. That seems to cheer him up immensely, but then, after she leaves, he is suddenly quiet and pensive for a while. He certainly has a lot to deal with, doesn't he?" The two health professionals nodded at each other, said their goodbyes, and then went on about their duties.

For audio exercises, visit **http://www.MedicalLanguageLab.com.** 

Reflective Questions

Reflect on the dialogue that you've just read as you answer these questions.

1. How long has Gil Loeppky been at Fayette General?

____

2. In this scenario, which two professions are managing patient care?

____

3. The patient is not allowed to bear weight on his right leg. Why not?

____

4. What type of unit has Gil been admitted to at Fayette General?

____

Learning Objectives

After reading Chapter 15, you will be able to do the following:

- Use enhanced terminology related to the muscles of the lower limbs.
- Understand and use the terminology of rehabilitation.
- Understand and use the language of physical therapy and musculoskeletal rehabilitation.
- Appreciate the education, training, and responsibilities of a physical therapist.
- Understand the role of physical therapy in rehabilitation.
- Appreciate the education, training, and responsibilities of an occupational therapist.
- Understand the role of occupational therapy in rehabilitation.
- Use enhanced terminology related to brain function in the context of rehabilitation.

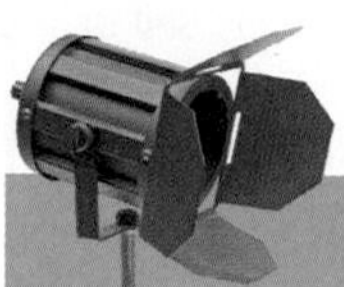

CAREER SPOTLIGHT: Physical Therapist

Physical therapy is the branch of health care that is dedicated to the treatment, restoration, or maintenance of optimal function of the musculoskeletal system.

A *physical therapist (PT)* is a health professional who provides direct patient care to clients who are experiencing disorders, impairments, or limitations of movement. Their work includes working with individuals with developmental impairments. PTs are found in hospitals (inpatient and outpatient services), rehabilitation and care centers, clinics, private practices, and education. They consult with physicians and other members of the health-care or workplace team about patient care. They promote the ability to move, they prevent or minimize disability, and they restore function and reduce pain.

To become a PT, a person must achieve a master's degree in physical therapy from a program accredited by the Commission on Accreditation of Physical Therapy Education (CAPTE). This organization is a branch of the American Physical Therapy Association. A license to practice is required in all states, and there is a National Physical Therapy Examination (NPTE). Doctoral programs are also available.

Physical therapy assistants work under the direction and supervision of physical therapists. The content of their work includes hands-on assistance provided to patients as they participate in their therapy. This assistance can include using hot and cold compresses, as well as certain devices and equipment that are relevant to physical therapy. These individuals participate with physical therapists and their patients in the creation of care plans that are designed for optimal patient outcomes (i.e., recovery, rehabilitation, or maintenance of health).

Licensure as a PT assistant requires graduation from a program that has been accredited by the American Physical Therapy Association. In addition, most states require an associate's degree for entrance into practice. These allied health professionals can go on to earn specialty certificates in fields such as gerontology. They may also rise to positions in administration.

Physical therapy aides do not require special education or training, and they are more often than not taught on the job. They facilitate the running of a physical therapy department. They do not perform any hands-on care. Physical therapy aides ensure that the treatment area is clean and ready to receive patients. They may also be involved in other support services, such as ensuring that supplies are available and assisting with clerical and reception work. Physical therapy aides do not require licensing.

Enhanced Vocabulary: Musculoskeletal System

Terminology for the muscles and the skeleton has been presented in a number of chapters in this book, most specifically Chapters 3, 4, 6, and 10. This terminology will now be enhanced in the context of Gil Loeppky's physical rehabilitation.

Key terms: physical therapy/musculoskeletal system

In the opening scenario, the nurse and the physical therapist used both medical terminology and medical jargon as they discussed their plans for Gil Loeppky's rehabilitation. Key terms and phrases from their dialogue are italicized in the example and highlighted below with the explanation.

"... the *mind-body connection* ..."

mind-body connection: a term derived from holistic health care that reflects an understanding of how the mind influences the body in all aspects of functioning and vice versa. From this perspective, Gil Loeppky's optimistic outlook will positively influence his ability to heal and recover on both a psychological and a physical level. Conversely, if Gil were to be pessimistic, the mind-body connection would suggest a negative impact (i.e., one that is slower or less effective) on his body's ability to heal from its injuries.

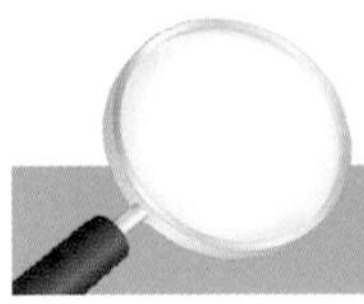

FOCUS POINT: Holistic Health Care

Holistic health care is an approach that believes that each patient is the sum of all of the domains of his or her existence and that one aspect (i.e., a broken limb) cannot be treated without consideration of the entire person and his or her situation in life. The term *holistic* is derived from the early Greek root *holos*, meaning *whole*. The term first appeared in a medical context during the 1960s.

The philosophy that underpins holistic care is *holism*; this is the belief that an entity such as an individual or a family is not simply a single unit but rather a collection of parts that all work together toward optimal or healthy functioning. When one or more of the parts is impaired, disturbed, or diseased, the unit ceases to function as well as it should or could. In other words, a unit is really a complex system of parts. In health care, those parts are referred to as *domains*. A person's domains of health include the biological, psychological, social, spiritual, occupational/economic, and environmental health domains. Each domain contributes to the general overall health of the individual.

hol + ism = holism

↓ ↓

root: *whole* + suffix: *belief*

Right Word or Wrong Word: *Holism* or *-holism*?

Do you think that the word *holism* can be used as a suffix? Does the suffix *-holism* have the same meaning as the term *holism*? Explain your answer.

"... started on *high-frequency PT* ..."

high-frequency PT: jargon meaning *numerous visits from and interactions with physical therapists.*

"... achieved *earlier ambulation* ..."

earlier ambulation: recovering the ability to walk more quickly than would have occurred without early intervention via physical therapy.

"... some *isometric exercises ...*"

isometric: a specific type of strength-training exercise that is common for muscle rehabilitation. The muscle is required to push against something (i.e., the physical therapist's hand) for short intervals of time. At no time does the muscle lengthen or do any joints move. The goal is to maintain muscle strength while a patient is bedridden or chair bound.

"... some *passive range-of-motion exercises ...*"

passive range-of-motion exercises: moving parts of the body without causing the muscles to contract or relax.

"... the *quadriceps femoris.*"

quadriceps femoris: a group of muscles in the upper leg.

"... any kind of muscle *atrophy ...*"

atrophy: wasting, weakening, or degenerating.

"... at the *parallel bars ...*"

parallel bars: an apparatus that consists of two bars that are side by side between which a person can walk while holding onto one bar with each hand. In physical therapy and rehabilitation programs, parallel bars are used for gait training (walking). Gil is not yet able to walk with the parallel bars because he cannot put his weight down on his right ankle (see Figure 15-1).

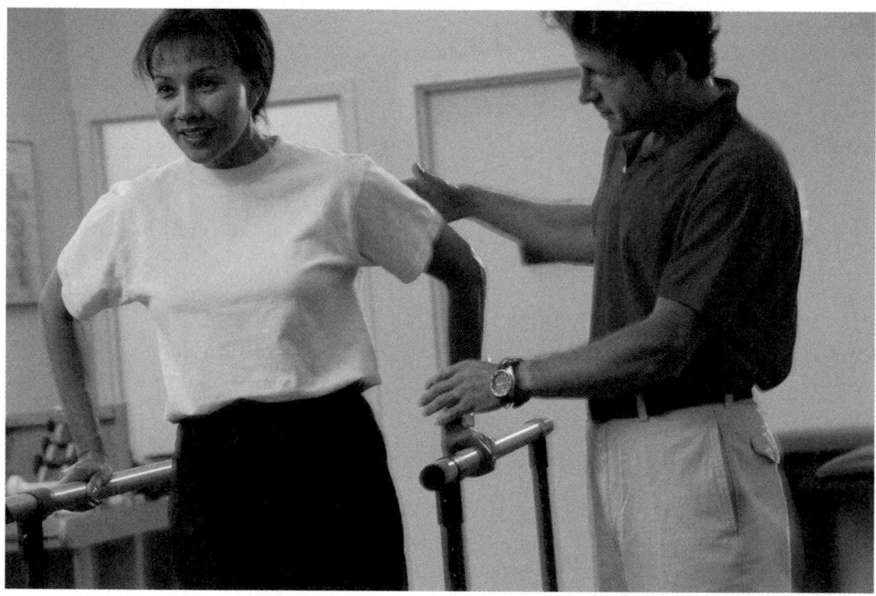

Figure 15.1: Physical therapy patient using parallel bars (© Thinkstock / Comstock)

"... with *direct assistance ...*"

direct assistance: a term from physical therapy and nursing that describes how a client or patient is not allowed to stand, move, or sit up independently but rather must rely on trained staff at his or her side.

"... able *to tolerate the sit-to-stand procedure...*"

tolerate: endure or withstand.

sit-to-stand procedure: an approved procedure for moving a patient from a sitting position to a standing position. Each care facility (and some States) will have its own policy and procedures for this. During the early stages of postoperative care or rehabilitation for a patient, the nursing staff, care aides, physical therapists, or rehabilitation technicians must be within arm's reach of the patient as he or she arises (see Figure 15-2). To understand this in the context of our patient, Gil, study the picture of the sit-to-stand device. Notice that the support pad on the device is placed directly on the tibia. In this position, it will slowly push against the legs, exert pressure on the hip to move, and cause an upward, standing motion. As this occurs, the patient will hold onto the support bars, and the support around his back and under his arms will pull him up and forward, toward the machine. It would be impossible to use this device with our patient, Gil, because he has an orthopedic support on his right knee, and he has had recent surgery and pins placed in the distal end of his right tibia (see Figure 15-2). The pain that this would cause the patient and the chance of reinjury would be intolerable.

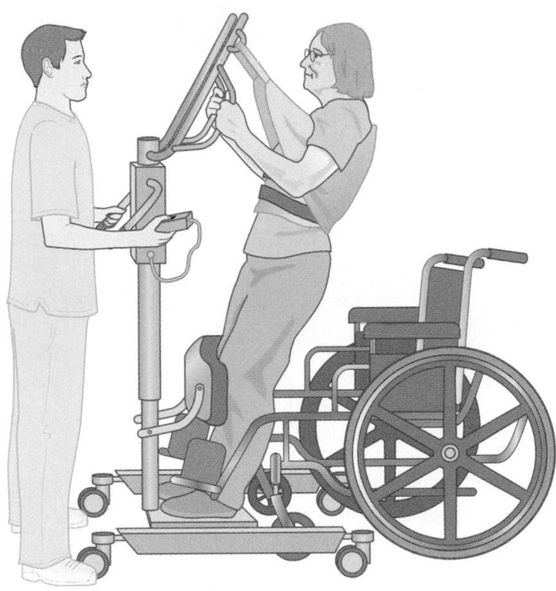

Figure 15.2: Patient using a sit-to-stand device

"... his *locomotion* is limited to the use of a wheelchair."

locomotion: the ability to move oneself from one place to another. Walking is a form of locomotion, and so is using a wheelchair, driving, or even riding a bus or train.

"... to use a *lifting device* to bring Gil to an upright position ..."

lifting device: also known as a *patient lift*, a *medical lifting device,* or a *mobile lifting device*; a mechanical apparatus that is designed to prevent back injury among health-care providers and to protect patients from falls. These devices are used to assist the patient from a bed or chair to a standing position, and they can also swing about to transfer the patient to a bed, a toilet or commode, or a chair. Lifting devices can be activated by hydraulic action (pumping), or they may be run by an electric motor. In many care facilities, electronic or mechanical lifting devices are attached to tracks on the ceiling around the patient's bed, as well as in the shower or bathroom (see Figure 15-3).

"... his *motor functioning?*"

motor functioning: the ability to use and control muscles to achieve movement.

"... balance and *gait* ..."

gait: a person's style or manner of walking (see Table 15-1).

"... thinking of *neuro-involvement* here ..."

neuro-involvement: medical jargon that refers to the involvement of the neurological system, particularly the brain, but including all aspects of the neuropathway through the spinal cord (see Chapter 4).

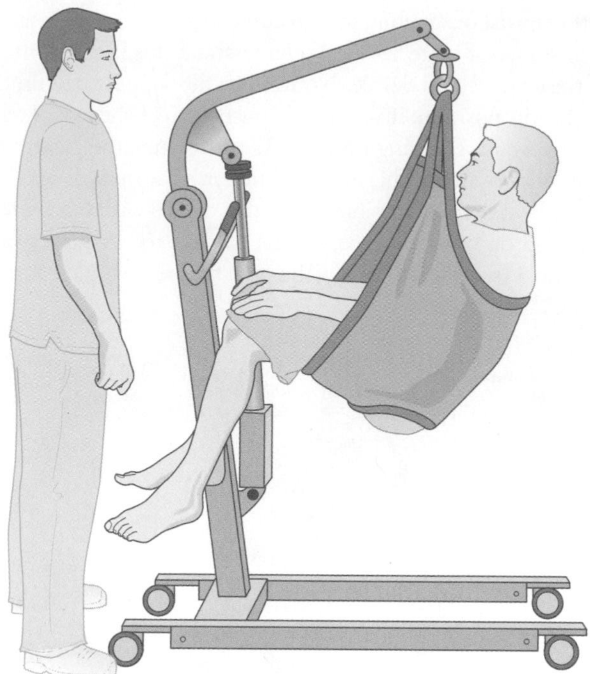

Figure 15.3: Sling lift device

"... the *hesitancy may be* psychological ..."

hesitancy: an involuntary delay in action, the cause of which may be physiological or psychological. The term is frequently used to refer to urination and the inability to initiate a urine stream, but it can be used in a musculoskeletal context as well.

"... noticed some *tremors ...*"

tremors: a type of continuous, involuntary muscle activity that causes the movement of a limb. Muscle fatigue from overuse may be one cause of tremors, but there are many others. For example, neurological impairments that result from injury or disease can lead to tremors. In the case of injury, the tremors may or may not eventually subside. With a disease state, there is always the possibility that the tremors will worsen.

"... too many *repetitions ...*"

repetitions: tasks (in this case, exercises or movements) that are repeated for a set number of times.

"... to assess the patient's *neuro-functioning ...*"

neuro-functioning: medical jargon for what is more properly referred to as *neurological functioning*. The term refers to the ability of the neurological system to detect and respond to stimuli and to function at a normal capacity with regard to cognition, learning ability, and coordination.

"... a bit *sluggish ...*"

sluggish: slow. In this context, the pupil is reacting to light more slowly than normal.

"... for him *to clear his slurred speech. ...*"

to clear: a common medical expression that means that a situation or condition has resolved. In this context, within a short time after waking, Gil no longer slurs his words.

"... about the patient's *need for ice ...*"

need for ice: a reference to using ice or an ice pack on an injury to reduce pain and swelling. This treatment is commonly used for muscle and joint injuries.

"... through *the glass of the NICU ....*"

the glass: slang for the window that surrounds a unit or ward.

NICU: the neonatal intensive care unit.

TABLE 15-1: Types of Gait

Type of Gait	Description
Antalgic gait	• The patient limps when walking to avoid any chance of pain that might occur from bearing weight on the affected foot or limb. • Steps are noticeably shorter or quicker on the affected side.
Spastic gait (also known as *circumduction gait*)	• Steps are taken without flexing the knee or ankle. The legs are held stiffly when walking. • With each step, the leg is swung out in a semicircle, with the feet touching or near to the ground. The foot goes down when the process is completed.
Stuttering gait	• There is an obvious hesitancy before completing a step.
Quadriceps gait	• When stepping down on the affected leg, the knee hyperextends, thereby causing the trunk of the body to lurch forward.
Ataxic gait	• The patient has an unsteady and uncoordinated manner of walking. • The feet and legs are far apart (i.e., the patient has a wide base). • When stepping, the feet appear to be thrown forward and away from the body.
Festinating gait	• The legs are stiff and inflexible, and the trunk is flexed forward, thus affecting balance. • Very short steps are taken, and these are at risk for involuntary hastening (i.e., they can rapidly speed up, without control). • Shuffling occurs; the feet do not come off of the ground as they should.

Critical Thinking

These questions require the application of new knowledge and vocabulary from Table 15-1.

1. A neurological impairment or pathology, such as Parkinson's disease, can lead to a type of gait that involves shuffling, stiffness in the legs, and the potential for taking rapid, short steps. What is this gait called?

___

2. In a normal stance, the feet should normally be no more than 12 inches apart. What is the term that describes a stance that is greater than that?

___

3. What is the formal term for a process in which something speeds up and cannot be slowed voluntarily?

___

4. Eventually, Gil Loeppky might experience one of the types of gaits identified in Table 15-1. Which one? Why?

___

Fill in the Blanks

Fill in the blanks with the proper medical term or expression. These terms were first used in the Patient Update. Now, use them in other health-care contexts to show that you understand them. You are given the first letter of each word as a hint.

1. Zane Davis, who is 74 years old, advised one of his physicians that he has some difficulty urinating. At times, he experiences **h** ____________, even though he knows that he needs to urinate.
2. The optimal **p** ____________ for a fetus before birth is head down in the birth canal.
3. When people who are not used to exercising engage in vigorous activity and then stop, they may temporarily feel or see some **t** ____________ in their hands or limbs.
4. In Chapter 4, you learned that a test for pupillary response will identify if both pupils are equal and reactive to light or whether the response is normal or **s** ____________ .
5. In Chapter 2, Stevie-Rose Davis exhibited an unsteady **g** ____________ when she was walking with the EMT.
6. In Chapter 3, the emergency treatment team tended to a deep laceration involving Glory Loeppky's **q** ____________ **f** ____________ muscles.

Enhanced terminology: muscles of the upper leg

The muscles of the upper leg are identified in Table 15-2 and can be seen in Figure 15-4. Study the descriptions and locations of these muscles. Notice the language of direction and the composition of words as you prepare for upcoming exercises related to these terms. Referring back to Tables 2-8 and 2-10 in Chapter 2 for a quick review of terms related to direction and movement may be helpful.

TABLE 15-2: Muscles of the Upper Leg

Muscles of the Upper Leg: Posterior Thigh	Function
biceps femoris (part of the group known as *the hamstrings*)	extends the hip rotates the femur laterally (out to the side) tilts the pelvis in the posterior direction flexes the knee
semimembranosus (part of the group known as *the hamstrings*)	extends the hip rotates a flexed knee medially tilts the pelvis in the posterior direction flexes the knee
semitendinosus (part of the group known as *the hamstrings*)	extends the hip rotates a flexed knee medially tilts the pelvis in the posterior direction flexes the knee
Muscles of the Upper Leg: Medial Thigh	**Function**
adductor brevis	adduction of the hip assists with hip flexion assists with the rotation of the hip medially
adductor magnus	adduction of the hip assists with hip flexion assists with the extension of the hip
adductor longus	adduction of the hip assists with hip flexion assists with the rotation of the hip medially
pectineus	adduction of the hip flexes the hip rotates the hip medially
gracilis	adduction of the hip flexes the knee rotates a flexed knee medially

TABLE 15-2: Muscles of the Upper Leg—cont'd

Muscles of the Upper Leg: Anterior Thigh	Function
sartorius (see Chapter 3)	assists with the flexion of the knee assists with the medial rotation of the knee assists with the abduction of the hip assists with the rotation of the hip laterally
quadriceps femoris (see Chapter 3)	the basic function of this group of muscles is to extend and straighten the leg
vastus lateralis	extends the knee
vastus medialis	extends the knee
vastus intermedius	extends the knee
rectus femoris	extends the knee helps to flex the hip

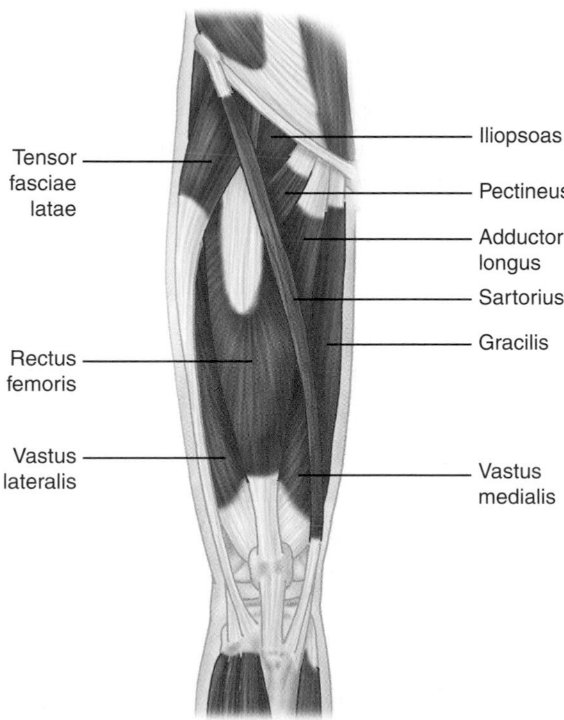

Figure 15.4: Muscles of the upper leg

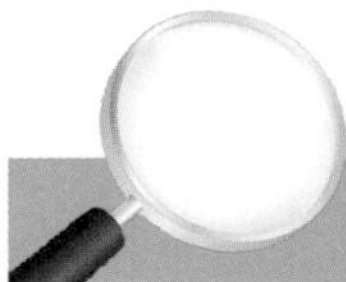

FOCUS POINT: Hamstrings

The *hamstrings* are a group of muscles that work together to flex the knee. These are located on the back of the upper leg, and they include the biceps femoris, as well as the semimembranosus and semitendinosus muscles.

Right Word or Wrong Word: ***Hip*** **or** ***Thigh?***

Are these two terms interchangeable? Are they technically physiologically the same?

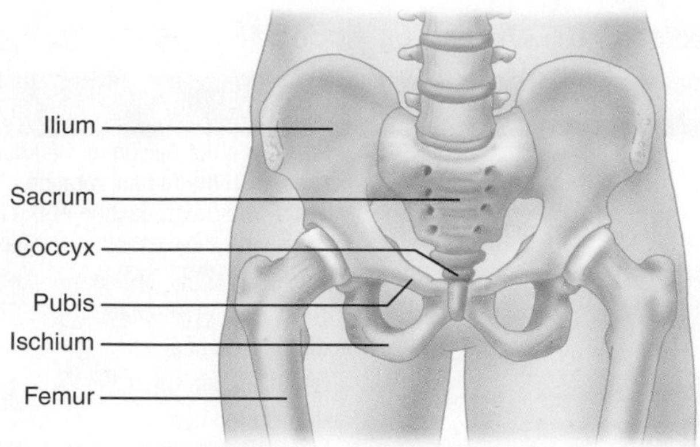

Figure 15.5: Anatomy of the hip and pelvis

Enhanced terminology: muscles of the lower leg and foot

Explore the muscles of the lower leg and foot in more detail in Table 15-3 and Figure 15-6. Once again, pay attention to the language of direction and the composition of words as you prepare for upcoming exercises related to these terms.

TABLE 15-3: Muscles of the Lower Leg, the Ankle, and the Foot

Muscles of the Lower Leg and Foot: Anterior	Function
extensor digitorum longus	extends the of toes (except for the great toe) dorsiflexes the ankle everts the foot
extensor hallucis longus	extends the great toe (the big toe) dorsiflexes the ankle inverts the foot
tibialis anterior	dorsiflexes the foot inverts the foot supports the arch of the foot
Muscles of the Lower Leg and Foot: Medial and Lateral	**Function**
peroneus brevis (also known as the *fibularis peroneus brevis*)	plantarflexes the foot (weakly and minimally)
peroneus longus (also known as the *fibularis peroneus longus*)	plantarflexes the foot (weakly) adducts the foot everts the foot
peroneus tertius (also known as the *fibularis peroneus tertius*)	dorsiflexes the foot everts the foot
Muscles of the Lower Leg and Foot: Posterior	**Function**
flexor digitorum longus	flexes the toes (except for the great toe) plantarflexes the foot inverts the foot
flexor hallucis longus	flexes the great toe plantarflexes the ankle (minimally) inverts the foot
popliteus	flexes the knee releases the knee from a position of extension rotates the femur laterally

TABLE 15-3: Muscles of the Lower Leg, the Ankle, and the Foot—cont'd

Muscles of the Lower Leg and Foot: Posterior	Function
gastrocnemius	flexes the knee plantarflexes the ankle
tibialis posterior	plantarflexes the ankle inverts the foot
plantaris	plantarflexes the ankle
soleus	plantarflexes the foot

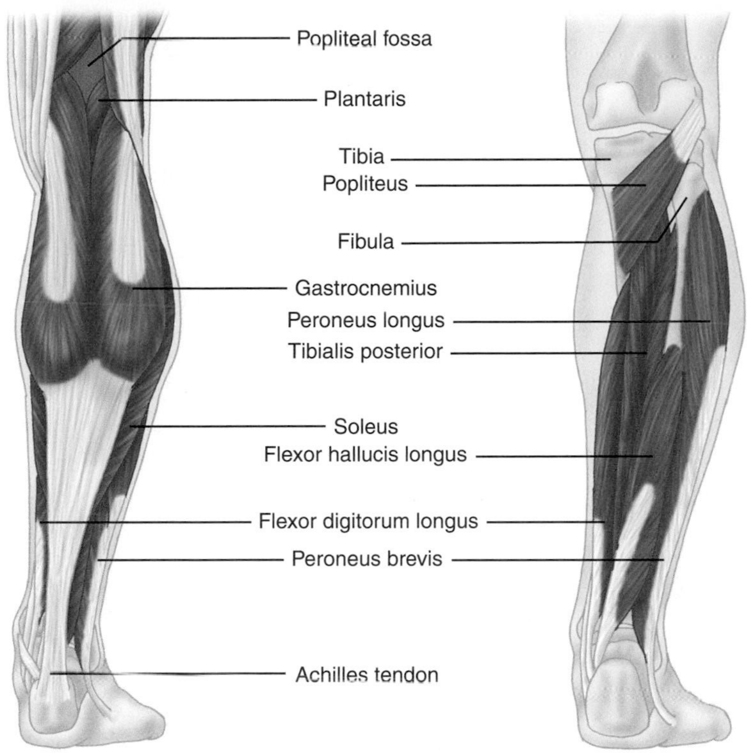

Figure 15.6: Muscles of the lower leg

Right Word or Wrong Word: *Dorsal, Posterior,* or *Caudal?*

Do these three words have anything in common? Are they synonyms, or do they mean almost—but not quite—the same thing?

Define the Term

Define each medical term that refers to an anatomical term of location. These terms were first introduced in Chapter 2, and you have also seen them in other chapters throughout this book.

1. plantar ____________________
2. dorsal ____________________
3. anterior ____________________
4. lateral ____________________
5. medial ____________________

Let's Practice

Identify each muscle or group of muscles described below. The answer will include the muscles that are directly responsible, as well as any helper muscles.

1. extends the great toe ______________________
2. flexes the great toe ______________________
3. extends the hip ______________________
4. everts the foot ______________________
5. flexes the knee ______________________
6. rotates the femur into a lateral position ______________________
7. flexes the hip ______________________
8. achieve(s) plantar flexion of the ankle ______________________

Fill in the Blanks

Answer the following questions by filling in the blanks.

1. One thing a(n) ______________ muscle *cannot* do but that a(n) ______________ muscle *can* do is to extend the great toe.
2. Two adductor muscles of the upper leg—the ______________ and the ______________ can rotate the hip, but only one adductor of the upper leg—the ______________ can extend it.
3. The ______________, ______________, and ______________ muscles can tilt the pelvis in a posterior direction.
4. The root of the word *digitorum* is ______________, meaning *finger or toe.*
5. The first few letters of the muscle name ______________ tell you that the muscle is related to the knee.

Label the Diagram

Label the muscles of the upper leg.

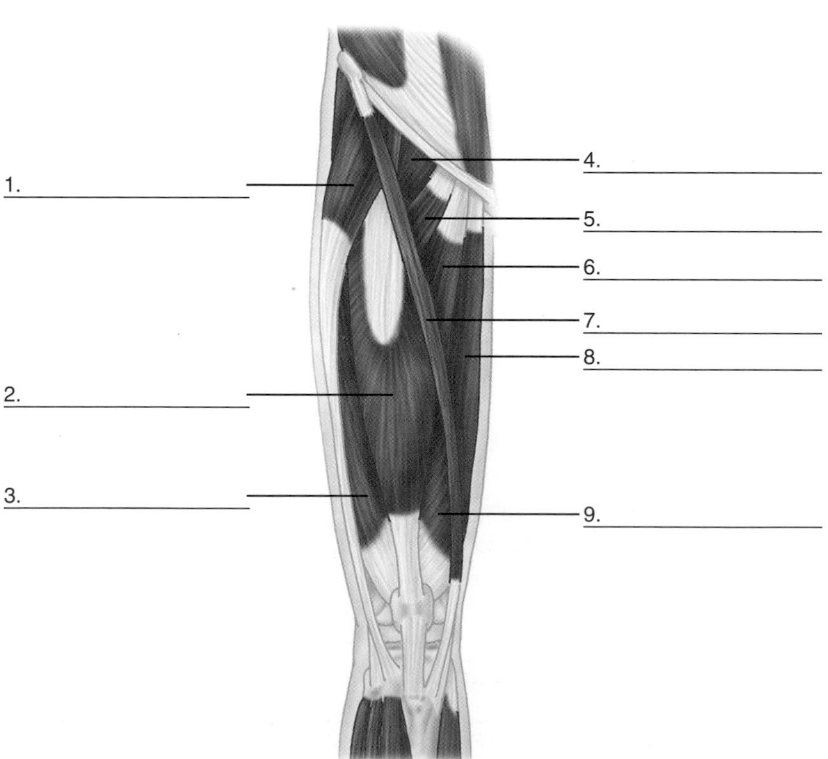

PRONUNCIATION PRACTICE

Say these words aloud to a friend or classmate, if you can. Here you are given the phonetic pronunciation. Your instructor can help you with pronunciation, or you can visit **http://www.MedicalLanguageLab.com.**

ataxia	ă-**tăk**′sē-ă
ataxic	ă-**tăk**′tĭk or ă-**tăk**′sĭk
atrophy	**ăt**′rō-fē
circumduction	sĕr″kŭm-**dŭk**′shŭn
festinating	**fĕs**″tĭ-nā′tĭng
gastrocnemius	găs″trŏk-**nē**′mē-ŭs
gracilis	**grăs**′ĭ-lĭs
isometric	ī″sō-**mĕ**′trĭk
pectineus	pĕk-tĭn-**ē**′ŭs
peroneus	pĕr″ō-**nē**′ŭs
plantaris	plăn-**tăr**′ĭs
popliteus	pŏp-**lĭt**′-ē′ŭs or pŏp-lĭt-**ē**′ŭs
quadriceps	**kwŏd**′rĭ-sĕps
sartorius	săr-**tō**′rē-ŭs
spastic	**spăs**′tĭk
tibialis	tĭb″ē-ā′lĭs

More about muscles

As you know, muscles flex, extend, contract, and release (see Chapter 3). They work in groups and pairs. Muscles are composed of muscle fibers, and these are under *tension*, which keeps them firm and able to maintain the body's posture and position. Muscles also work against *resistance* (an outside force). A working muscle may resist the force of gravity or the force of weights, exercise bands, and so on. There are a number of types of muscles:

Synergist muscles help a primary muscle to accomplish its task. The quadriceps femoris group is a good example.

Stabilizer muscles are those that contract with no significant body movement. Their function is to maintain a posture or to fixate a joint.

When muscles are stimulated or *innervated*, they react by agonistic or antagonistic responses. Through this interplay of opposites, one muscle or group of muscles can flex while the others extend. This combination permits movement.

Agonist muscles are those that respond directly to produce an action or movement. For example, when you wish to take a step, the anterior muscles of the upper leg are agonists when they flex.

Antagonist muscles respond to the stimulation of the agonists by performing the opposite action. In the context of taking a step, the posterior muscles of the upper leg will be the antagonists when they extend.

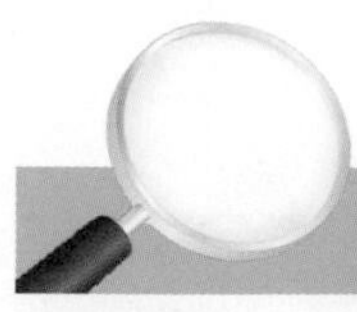

FOCUS POINT: Agonist and Antagonist

Context is always key to understanding medical terminology. You have been studying the words *agonist* and *antagonist* in the context of the muscular system. However, *agonist* and *antagonist* have different meanings in the realm of pharmacology:

An *agonist medication* is one that mimics some types of body functions or processes. An agonist medication binds to a receptor site and then causes it to respond in a desired therapeutic manner. For example, a *dopamine agonist* can help to reduce muscle spasms when there is an insufficient supply of natural dopamine (a neurotransmitter) in the brain. (For more about neurotransmitters, see Chapter 10.)

An *antagonist medication* is one that does the opposite of an agonist. Although it, too, will bind to a receptor site, it will inhibit the receptor's ability to respond to stimuli or to function. Again, dopamine can be used as an example. A *dopamine antagonist* will stop the overproduction of this neurotransmitter; this is a condition that occurs in patients with schizophrenia (see Chapter 7).

Innervation

Muscle fiber is stimulated by electrical impulses that are processed by the neurological system. Segments of the spinal cord conduct these impulses to specific motor and sensory regions of the body. This is the process of **innervation**. When the innervation of an agonist muscle occurs, a **reciprocal innervation** occurs at the same time. The reciprocal innervation stimulates the antagonist muscle response. For example, when a skeletal muscle is innervated to contract, the antagonist muscle simultaneously relaxes.

Muscle contractions

The anatomy and physiology of muscle contractions were previously introduced in Chapters 3 and 8. Table 15-4 now enhances your vocabulary and understanding by adding a number of terms that describe the different types of muscle contractions.

TABLE 15-4: Types of Muscle Contractions

Type of Contraction	Description and Result
concentric	muscle shortens
eccentric	muscle lengthens
dynamic	muscle contraction that results in movement; concentric and eccentric contractions are both types of dynamic contractions
isokinetic	muscle contraction that takes place against a co-occurring force of resistance or speed; the type of contraction that occurs, for example, when using an exercise bicycle
isometric (also known as *static tension*)	muscle contracts without any lengthening of a muscle or movement of the accompanying joint or angle of that joint
isotonic (also known as *same tension*)	muscle contraction that manipulates a joint through a range of motion working against a fixed force of resistance; the type of contraction that occurs, for example, when raising your hand to your shoulder while holding a book

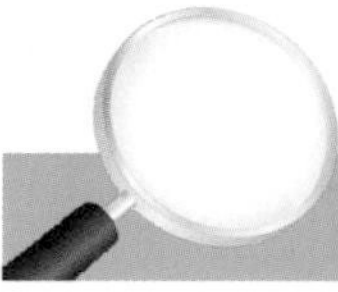

FOCUS POINT: The Prefix *iso-*

The prefix *iso-* means *equal*. A few more words that make use of this prefix include the following:

isoenergetic: demonstrating equal forces or equal activity

isochromatic: having the same color

Spasms and cramps

Spasms are brief involuntary muscle contractions that can happen anywhere in the body. They may occur with or without pain. Etiologically, muscle spasms can arise from irritated, pinched nerves or from trauma. They can also occur in response to pain. *Tonic* and *clonic spasms* can both be evident during an epileptic seizure.

Tonic spasms are sustained over period of time.

Clonic spasms are those that occur at intervals of contraction and relaxation.

Cramps are contractions that last much longer than muscle spasms, and the contraction is painful. They may be the result of decreased electrolyte levels in the blood (i.e., potassium, calcium, magnesium); the ingestion of toxins, poisons, or other pathogens; excessive muscle strain; certain medications; vigorous activity; or dehydration.

Muscle tone

The term **muscle tone** refers to the natural or normal firmness of a muscle and its functionality. Muscles are frequently assessed for tone by reviewing their ability to respond to a stretch (extension) and then, afterward, to automatically contract to their normal resting position. At rest, muscles are in a state of slight or partial contraction. This condition helps the body to retain its form while at the same time facilitating posture and coordination. Healthy tone means that the muscles have the innate capacity to contract quickly when they are stimulated (rather than having to start from the point of being fully relaxed).

The term **tone** is derived from the Latin root *tonus,* which means *tension* (the partial contraction of a muscle). The opposite of tonus is *clonus.*

The term *tonicity* refers to the *firmness* of a muscle or its *tension.*

Amyotony, which is also referred to as *amyotonia*, is a condition in which a person lacks or is deficient in normal muscle tone (tonus). This state could be the result of a disease, but it can also stem from a severe brain or spinal cord injury.

Alternatively, **myotonia** refers to *tonic spasm* or a state of temporary rigidity after a muscle contraction.

Amyotony and myotonia are often present with the same disease or muscle disorder, and sometimes the terms are used interchangeably to name these conditions. Muscular dystrophy is a clear example of a disorder in which both amyotony and myotonia are present.

Eponyms: Steinert's Disease and Myotonia Dystrophica

Dr. Hans Steinert was a German physician who spent the first part of his career in the field of cardiology and infectious diseases. Near the end of the 19th century, he turned his interest to neurology; in this field, he discovered specific signs and symptoms of a muscle disorder. During the early 20th century, this pathology would be named in his honor.

Steinert's disease is also known as *myotonia dystrophica* or *dystrophia myotonica;* it is a rare disorder of muscular dystrophy. The condition is genetic in origin, and it is caused when a section of DNA repeats itself on either chromosome 3 or 19. Symptoms worsen over the course of the patient's lifetime, thus making this a chronic disease of muscle wasting (atrophy) related to muscle dysfunction. Onset is typically diagnosed during adolescence. Learning disabilities may accompany this disease.

Eponyms: Thomsen's Disease and Myotonia Congenita

Asmus Julius Thomsen was a Danish physician of the 19th century. Thomsen was a medical doctor for most of his career, but he eventually gave up his practice and became a medical advisor for his district in Denmark, likely as a result of his chronic muscle pain and impairment. Dr. Thomsen suffered from a muscle disorder, and he was able to track similar symptoms back through five generations through his family. The disorder that he suffered from and identified became known as *Thomsen's disease.* Most of its symptoms are identical to those of the broader disease myotonia congenita, whereas some are unique to the disorder.

Continued

Myotonia congenita (or congenital myotonia) is a disease that affects muscle contraction. The muscles are hyperexcitable; they will react to sudden noises or light touch, and they will rapidly go into spasm or contraction. After the muscles contract, they are difficult to relax. Myotonia congenita is non-progressive: it does not worsen after onset, but it is chronic and difficult to treat.

Alternatively, Thomsen's disease is progressive: it worsens over the life span. Onset can occur later in life, but the disease is genetic in origin. This disease adds the symptom of painful muscle stiffness, which is not always present with other congenital myotonia disorders. An observable sign of Thomsen's disease can be seen in the patient's grasp. When the hand grasps something, it cannot let go on cue, and it will take several seconds to do so. Even then, the hand may not fully relax.

Right Word or Wrong Word: *Myotonia* or *Myotomy*?

Say these two words aloud. Do they sound somewhat similar? Would you be able to differentiate them if you heard colleagues using these terms in a conversation? Are you sure? Explain your answer.

The term **dystonia** means *disordered tonicity of the muscles*. The term is also used to identify a group of neurological disorders of movement. A diagnosis of dystonia is made by a neurologist. Dystonia disorders include the diagnostic criteria of involuntary muscle activity such as sustained or prolonged muscle contraction that results in abnormal posturing, repetitive twisting movements, and pain. These symptoms may be preceded by tremors, cramps, and muscle spasms. Dystonia disorders are classified by the parts or regions of the body that are affected (see Table 15-5) or by the age at which they occur.

Primary (idiopathic) dystonia disorders may occur across the life span. Their cause is generally unknown, but there is some evidence of genetic predisposition. *Idiopathic* means that the cause is not clearly known or has yet to be determined.

Secondary (symptomatic) dystonias are conditions that include the above-noted signs and symptoms but that are caused by head injury, cerebrovascular accident, birth injuries, medications, exposure to toxins or poisons, or the secondary effects of disease.

TABLE 15-5: Classification of Dystonia by Affected Area

Classification of Dystonia	Involvement
focal	affects one area of the body
generalized	affects the entire body
hemidystonia	affects the arm and leg of the same side of the body
multifocal	affects two or more unrelated body parts or areas
segmental	affects two or more areas that are near each other

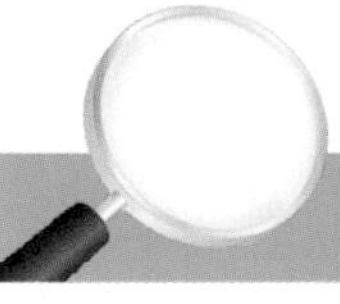

FOCUS POINT: Writer's Cramp and Dystonia

Perhaps the best way to remember *dystonia* (disordered tonicity of muscles) is to remember that it includes the involuntary movement of muscles. Associating this term with something that almost all of us have experienced will help you to remember this. For example, a transient form of a *focal dystonia* that you may have personally experienced is *writer's cramp*. Symptoms of this condition include cramps in the hand with which you write and sometimes the adjoining forearm. The ability to continuing writing is impeded. Writer's cramp may be preceded or followed by fine tremors (dystonic tremors) and the inability to write at all for a short period.

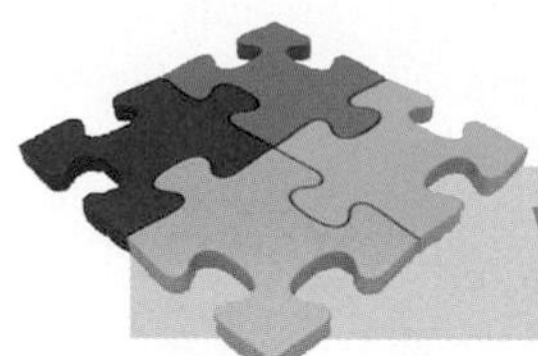

WORD BUILDING: Formulas for Creating Words from the Root *Tonos* and the Suffix *-tonia*

tonus = tension. The combining form is *ton/o.* The suffix form is *-tonia*, meaning *the degree or state of muscle tension (tonicity).*

tono + graph = *tonograph*

Definition: an instrument used to record and measure pressure or tension. *noun*

Example: A *tonograph* can be used to diagnose intraocular pressure related to glaucoma.

acro + myo + tonia = *acromyotonia*

Definition: myotonia of the extremities. (The combining form *acro-* means *extremities or top.*) *noun*

Example: *Acromyotonia* can cause spastic deformities in the body, such as those seen in some cases of cerebral palsy.

neuro + myo + tonia = *neuromyotonia*

Definition: a rare neuromuscular disorder that involves continuous peripheral nerve stimulation of the muscles. *noun*

Example: Stiffness, pain, and dysarthria result from *neuromyotonia*.

hypo + tonia = *hypotonia*

Definition: severely diminished or low muscle tone. *noun*

Example: Floppy infant syndrome is a form of *hypotonia* in which the muscles are loose and do not naturally flex; the body is unable to maintain its posture.

Classifying muscles

Muscles can be classified as either *tonic muscles* or *phasic muscles.* These terms differentiate the time that a muscle needs to respond to a stimulus. Tonic muscles are also classified as *postural*, which means that they function to maintain or stabilize the body's posture and position.

Tonic muscles are postural and designed to hold the body upright for long periods of time. They work against the force of gravity. Tonic muscles contain something called *slow-twitch muscle fibers.* These muscles work slowly but steadily, expending small but continual amounts of energy over prolonged periods. Under stress or exertion or as the result of trauma, they can tighten or knot, thereby becoming shorter and *hypertonic*. Muscle relaxation and stretching exercises promote the healthy functioning of these muscles. An example of a tonic muscle is the soleus.

Phasic muscles provide movement for the skeleton. They conduct impulses rapidly, and they are referred to as *fast-twitch muscles.* This means that they are helpful for situations in which a quick response or a strength response is required (i.e., the sudden need to run or to protect the face with an arm). They contract and relax rapidly. Powerful bursts of energy lead quite quickly to energy depletion in these muscles, and they fatigue easily. Phasic muscles tend to elongate and weaken when they are not used over time. Phasic muscles can be inhibited or weakened in response to pathology or trauma. Treatment for phasic muscle dysfunction could include the use of a transcutaneous electrical neve stimulation (TENS) device. These muscles are treated only after the tonic muscles are stretched and relaxed.

Muscle strength

The term *muscle strength* refers to the maximum amount of force that a muscle or muscle group can generate with a single effort. It is not the same as tone. A person can have lower tone but still exhibit some strength. Muscle strength is key to healthy functioning, and it plays a major role in the body's ability to physically endure periods of extended activity. Our patient, Gilbert Loeppky, will be undergoing muscle strengthening exercises as part of his physical therapy.

Key terms related to muscle strength and strengthening include the following:

muscle endurance: a term that describes a muscle's ability to contract and release repeatedly over a period of time.

muscle fatigue: a term that refers to a situation in which a muscle has been worked to its maximum point of endurance, beyond which its performance declines. Our patient, Gil, faces this potential if his exercise program focuses too long on certain muscles or muscle groups when he may be too weak to continue.

muscle failure: a state of muscle exhaustion in which a muscle simply cannot function one more time. This state has been known to occur after strenuous exercise in which specific muscles are repeatedly involved. Physical therapists are quite attuned to this potential when working with clients who are trying to gain muscle strength through exercise. For example, when muscles in the leg fail, a person can collapse.

muscle overload: a core concept in physical therapy, kinesiology, rehabilitation, weight training, and exercise training. It refers to the principle that, to strengthen a muscle, that muscle must be worked above its current capacity. In other words, muscle strength increases when the muscle is forced to work against increasing resistance. This principle can be seen when body builders are in a weight-training program.

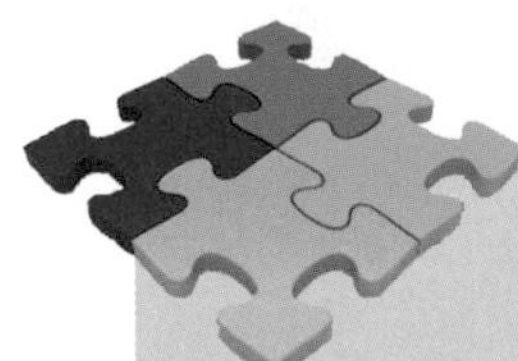

WORD BUILDING: Formulas for Creating Words from the Roots *Sthenos*, *Sthenia,* and *Asthenia*

1. sthenos = Greek root meaning strength. The combining form is sthen/o.

2. sthenia = a root word meaning *strength or unusual strength*. The term refers to a person's overall bodily strength and vitality. It is not exclusive to the musculoskeletal system. The combining form is *sthen/i/ia*

3. asthenia = a root word meaning *lack of strength*. It is the antonym for *sthenia*. (Note: This term is not exclusive to the musculoskeletal system. For example, it can refer to fatigue, a lack of strength when breathing, or the weakness that can accompany anxiety.)

hyper + sthenia = *hypersthenia*

Definition: abnormal strength or a state of excessive tension of a part or all of the muscles. *noun*

Example: *Hypersthenia* of the uterine wall can lead to miscarriage of the fetus.

cali + sthen + ics = *calisthenics*

Definition: a type of exercise that is designed to improve range of motion, tone, suppleness, and gracefulness. (The prefix *cali-* means *beautiful*. The suffix *-ics* means *pertaining to.*) *noun*

Example: *Calisthenics* are generally light exercises of stretching that are not intended to build muscle but rather to tone and shape the muscles.

my/o + asthenia = *myasthenia*

Definition: muscle weakness that is accompanied by abnormal muscle fatigue. *noun*

Example: *Myasthenia gravis* is an autoimmune disorder that includes increasing weakness and fatigue of the muscles.

Right Word or Wrong Word: *Asthenia* or *Anesthesia*?

Is there a spelling error in the first or second word here, or are both words spelled correctly? What do these words mean? Are they the same (except that one is spelled incorrectly)? Finally, are they pronounced the same? Explain your answers.

TABLE 15-6: Assessment of Muscle Strength

Assessment of Muscle Strength	Criteria
0	no muscle movement whatsoever
1	only the barest flicker of muscle movement; this is not enough to move the attached structure (i.e., a leg or an arm)
2	some weak voluntary movement of the muscle but not enough to overcome the force of gravity
3	voluntary movement of the muscle with the ability to overcome the force of gravity; unable to push against any applied resistance (i.e., the therapist's hand)
4	voluntary muscle movement is present and able to overcome the force of gravity, as well as some amount of resistance
5	normal muscle strength and function that is able to overcome gravity and multiple degrees of applied resistance

Let's Practice

Name the term that fits each definition or description.

1. muscle tension ______
2. a muscle's normal firmness and functionality ______
3. the cause is yet to be determined ______
4. the muscles of limbs on the same side of the body are affected ______
5. can *both* be evident during an epileptic seizure ______
   ______ and ______
6. the muscle that responds by doing the opposite ______
7. the type of muscle that provides movement for the skeleton ______
8. a root word that means *strength* ______
9. when one skeletal muscle contracts, this process makes another muscle extend ______
   ______
10. Another name for *floppy infant syndrome* ______

Build a Word

Use each word part to build a word that describes or names an action or a condition of the muscles. You may need to change the form or spelling of the word part that you are given.

1. neuro ______________________________
2. nerve ______________________________
3. calo ______________________________
4. hyper ______________________________
5. meter ______________________________

PRONUNCIATION PRACTICE

Say these words aloud to a friend or classmate, if you can. Here you are given the phonetic pronunciation. Your instructor can help you with pronunciation, or you can visit **http://www.MedicalLanguageLab.com.** mll

acromyotonia	ăk″rō-mī-ō-**tō**´nē-ă
agonist	**ăg**´ŏn-ĭst
antagonist	ăn-**tăg**´ă-nĭst
asthenia	ăs-**thē**´nē-ă
calisthenics	kăl″ĭs-**thĕn**´ĭks
clonic	**klŏn**´ĭk
concentric	kŏn-**sĕn**´trĭk
dystonia	dĭs-**tō**´nē-ă
eccentric	ĕk-**sĕn**´trĭk
hypotonia	hī″pō-**tō**´nē-ă
idiopathic	ĭd″ē-ō-**păth**´ĭk
isotonic	ī″sō-**tŏn**´ĭk
myasthenia	mī-ăs-**thē**´nē-ă
myotomy	mī-**ŏt**´ō-mē
myotonia	mī″ă-**tō**´nē-ă
neuromyotonia	nū″rō-mī″ō-**tō**´nē-ă
phasic	**fā**´sĭk
sthenia	**sthē**´nē-ă
tonic	**tŏn**´ĭk
tonicity	tō-**nĭs**´ĭ-tē
tonograph	**tō**´nō-grăf
tonus	**tō**´n̆us

Rehabilitation

Rehabilitation is a key element of any treatment plan. It is included in all aspects of recovery and health maintenance. **Rehabilitation (rehab)** is the process of recovering function—and as much self-sufficiency and independence as possible—after a physical or psychological trauma, injury, or disease. Rehabilitation also plays an important role in assisting people with chronic disabilities to maintain optimal functioning. Some rehabilitation programs help patients to overcome deficits by teaching them how to use compensatory devices such as *prosthetics* (artificial body parts) when a limb has been amputated; walking or mobility aids such as electric wheelchairs or leg braces; and speech and communication aids such as highly individualized keyboards and picture boards.

The term *rehabilitation* is derived from the Latin root *rehabilitare*, which means *to become fit again.*

Rehabilitation is commonly referred to as "rehab" by the medical community.

The rehabilitation professional is a therapist who also makes suggestions for modifying the individual's environment so that he or she is able to function more efficiently. Rehab therapists work under the supervision of a physician. In the broad field of rehabilitation, professionals include—but are not limited to—the following:

- prosthestists: makers of **prostheses,** which are artificial limbs or organs;
- counselors and psychotherapists;
- occupational therapists (see "Career Spotlight: Occupational Therapist");
- physical therapists (also known as *physiotherapists* in some jurisdictions; see "Career Spotlight: Physical Therapist");
- physical therapy assistants;
- speech therapists (see Chapter 11); and
- physiatrists: physicians who specialize in rehabilitation, as well as pain assessment and treatment.

Rehabilitation technicians are also found in this field. These allied health professionals work under the supervision of a rehabilitation professional. Qualifications include a high school diploma or its equivalent plus some training and experience in a health career (i.e., a certificate in addiction care, in long-term care, or in working with patients with disabilities).

Rehabilitation services are provided in hospitals, care homes, medical and health clinics, therapists' offices, sports medicine centers, and a wide variety of rehabilitation clinics. Services may also occur in the client's home.

Recall the terminology for muscle movements from Chapters 2 and 3 as you now apply that terminology to rehabilitation, specifically to the physical therapy of Gil Loeppky's right leg, as well as the support of his uninjured left leg.

Physical Therapy

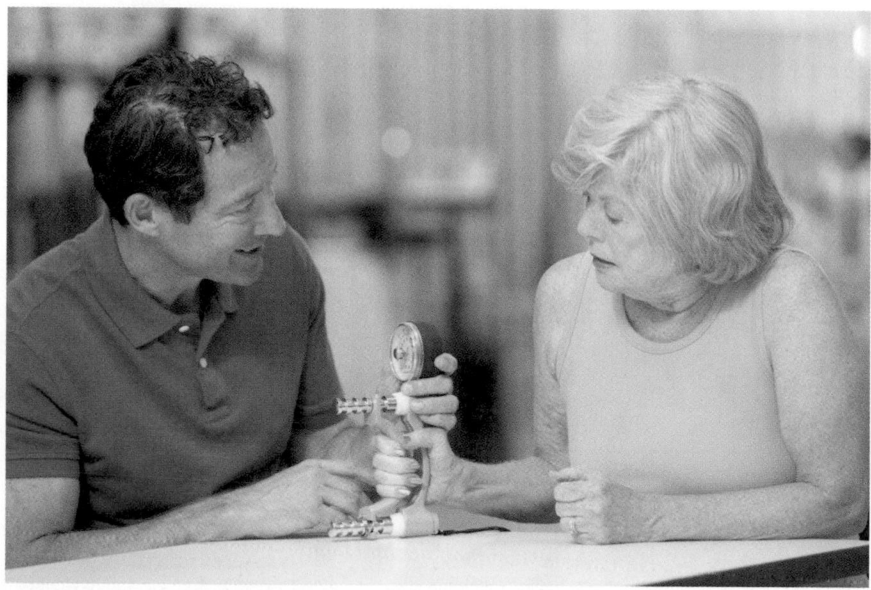

Figure 15.7: Physical therapist at work (© Thinkstock)

Physical therapy is a health-care discipline that is concerned with the care, treatment, maintenance, and rehabilitation of injuries and pathologies that affect the musculoskeletal system. Physical therapists work with patients who have enormous variability with regard to the reasons that they have come for treatment. What they all have in common, however, is an impaired ability to function related to the musculoskeletal system: their motor functioning has somehow been adversely affected.

Physical therapy includes the assessment of a patient's general motor functioning and his or her current range of motion and strength. Physical therapists also evaluate a person's posture, balance, and coordination. They are concerned with overall functional outcomes, and they plan care with this goal in mind. To achieve this goal, collaboration with other health disciplines is essential so that the physical therapy staff can have an accurate picture of what is or is not possible for the client. In the opening scene of this chapter, you saw PT Tamron Epp involved in a collaborative discussion with nurse Scott Kanesewah related to therapy goals for their shared patient, Gil Loeppky.

Physical therapy works to restore motor functioning through the treatment of muscles and bones and of the nervous system because the nervous system is responsible for stimulating muscles into action.

Assessment techniques

Physical therapists employ a wide range of assessments to determine a client's current level of functioning. Some of these are listed in Table 15-7.

TABLE 15-7: Physical Therapy Assessment Techniques

Assessment Technique	Description
Myotonometer	An electronic device is placed topically and used to assess muscle tone, stiffness, and strength. It also assesses muscle compliance (i.e., the muscle's ability to alter its size and shape in response to weight or force applied). The myotonometer functions like a small handheld computer. It can generate charts and graphs of changes in the status of the muscle over a number of separate assessments.
Functional Balance Grades	A series of measures that assess the balance of a person who is standing and shifting his or her weight, picking up something from the floor, turning around, and so on, all with or without support, as needed.
Goniometer	A measuring device that is used to assess angles and degrees of range of motion of the knees, elbows, and other joints (see Figure 15-8).
Gait Assessment Rating Score (GARS)	The client is observed while walking, and an assessment is made against 16 criteria for abnormal aspects of gait. The main purpose is to assess the patient for his or her risk of falling.
The Walk Test	A series of tests that assess the patient's walking performance by the distance walked within a specific time frame. The goal is the measurement of function, which includes the musculoskeletal, respiratory, cardiovascular, and neurological systems working together on the walking task.
Functional Independence Measure* for Locomotion (also known as *the FIM Locomotion Scale and Score*)	A scale that measures mobility and the ability to walk from dependence to independence on an interval-level scale and that scores each interval to measure progress. The scale is progressive, with one step leading to the next. Criteria include the following: walking with total assistance → walking with direct assistance → walking with supervision → modified independence (using a walking device) → complete independence: walking independently and using stairs independently

*Note: Functional Independence Measures are also available for cognition, communication, activities of daily living, and so on.

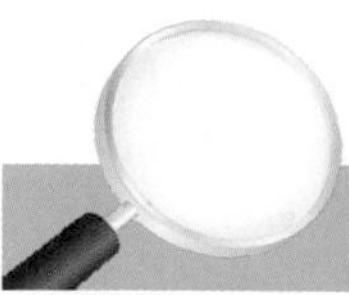

FOCUS POINT: Abasia and Astasia

Abasia is the inability to walk or impaired motor coordination when walking. The term is derived from the early Greek word for *basis* (base) and the prefix *a*-, which means *without or none*.

Astasia refers to unsteadiness when standing or the inability to stand or hold a standing position. This term is derived from the early Greek as well. *Statos* is the Greek root for *standing*.

The causes of abasia and astasia are thought to be both neurological and psychological.

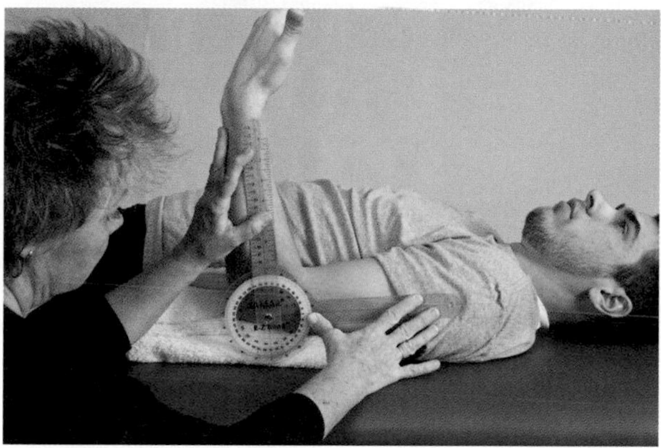

Figure 15.8: Patient assessment with the use of a goniometer (From Houglum PA, Bertotit DB: *Brunnstrom's Clinical Kinesiology*, ed. 6. Philadelphia: FA Davis, 2012, p. 14. With permission.)

Treatment modalities

Treatment during physical therapy can include the following:

- *application of heat or cold:* the use of cold compresses to decrease inflammation or the use of heat to relax the muscles. The application of heat also warms the blood, thereby causing dilation in the blood vessels. (Note that Gil Loeppky would not have been treated with heat or hot compresses as long as he was medically unstable because this would have put him at risk for the dilation of blood vessels and possible hemorrhage.)
- *massage:* the manipulation of the muscles to reduce muscle tension, to improve flexibility of movement, and to decrease pain.
- *hydrotherapy* or *aquatherapy:* the use of whirlpool baths, exercises in a pool, and so on to reduce muscle tension and to provide an environment for exercise that provides resistance to muscle but that does not put additional stress on the joints.
- *various types of exercises:* exercises that are performed with and without resistance to target specific muscles. These are designed to improve the patient's range of motion and to assist with his or her stretching and flexibility (see Figure 15-9). They may also involve the use of a wide variety of exercise equipment. Exercise has the added benefit of improving circulation, respiration, and general mental health and cognition.
- *endurance and strength-building exercises:* these types of exercises can be enhanced with the use of specialized equipment such as stationary bikes, stair climbers, treadmills, pulleys, and lifting devices.
- **electrical stimulation of muscles (E-stim, EMS)**: electricity is used to elicit contractions and to force muscles to function until they can do so on their own again. This stimulation is accomplished with special equipment. Small cloth pads that contain electrodes are placed strategically over muscles and connected to a small control device, which sends an electrical current that causes the muscles to contract. The goals of E-stim are to strengthen the affected muscles and to prevent

atrophy. This treatment can also help to alleviate muscle spasms by working the muscles isometrically until they are spent (i.e., energy is drained and the muscles are weakened or fatigued.) For our patient, Gil Loeppky, therapy with an E-stim device may be helpful for his upper leg and knee while he is recovering in the hospital, as well as after discharge (see Figure 15-10).

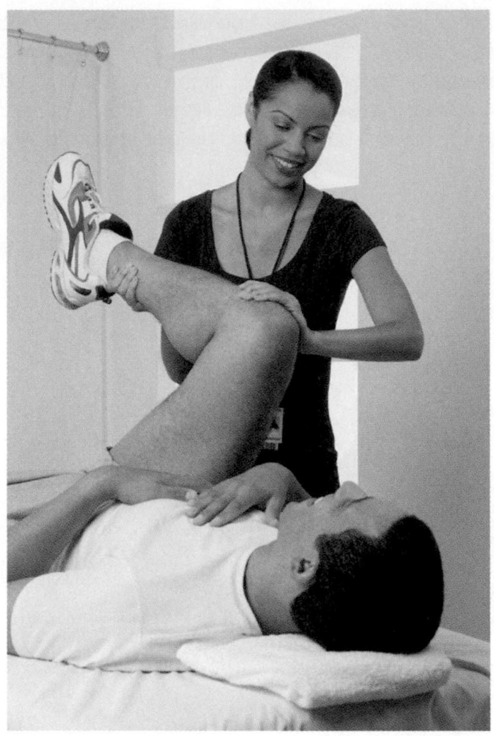

Figure 15.9: A supported stretch. (© Getty Images / Jupiterimages)

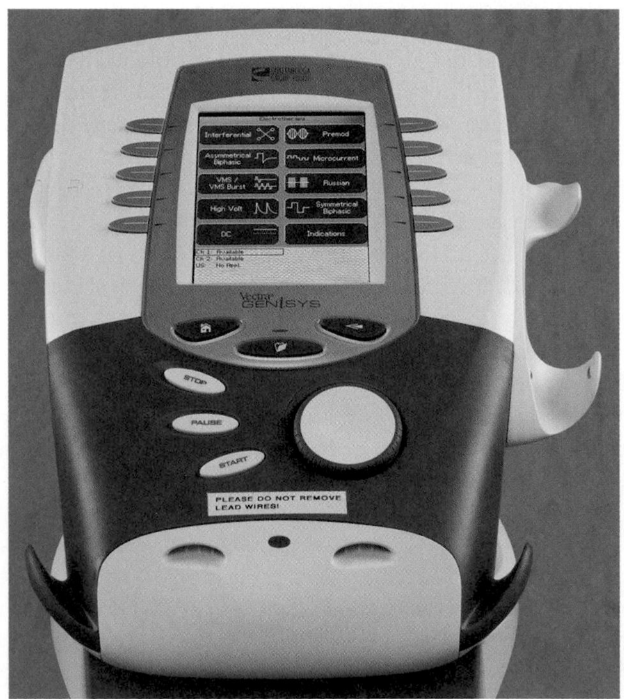

Figure 15.10: An electrical stimulation of muscles (E-stim or EMS) device. (From Michlovitz SL, Bellew JW, and Nolan TP Jr: *Modalities for Therapeutic Intervention*, ed 5. Philadelphia: FA Davis, 2012, p. 288. With permission.)

- **transcutaneous electrical nerve stimulation (TENS)**: an electrical technique that targets pain and the peripheral nerves rather than the muscles. In other words, a TENS unit treats localized neuropathic pain that is the result of disease, inflammation, or trauma to the peripheral nerves caused by injury or surgery. Gil may at some point require TENS therapy if the surgery to his hip or tibia incised nerves and if these injured nerves continue to cause him pain months after his discharge from the hospital.

Pain relief is accomplished by placing electrode pads on the skin over targeted peripheral nerves. An electrical impulse is sent from a small battery through the skin to the affected nerves and nerve receptor sites (see Figure 15-11). When this electrical impulse is received, the pain response is temporarily blocked, thus providing some relief for the patient.

There are two theories regarding how the TENS technique relieves pain. One is the **gate theory**, which asserts that only one message can be carried along a nerve at a time. If that message is incoming from the TENS unit, then the pain that was previously occurring in the nerve cannot travel along the nerve at the same time. The second theory is the **endorphin theory**. According to this theory, when the nerves are stimulated by certain frequencies, endorphins (natural morphine-like substances) are released by the brain, thereby providing analgesia.

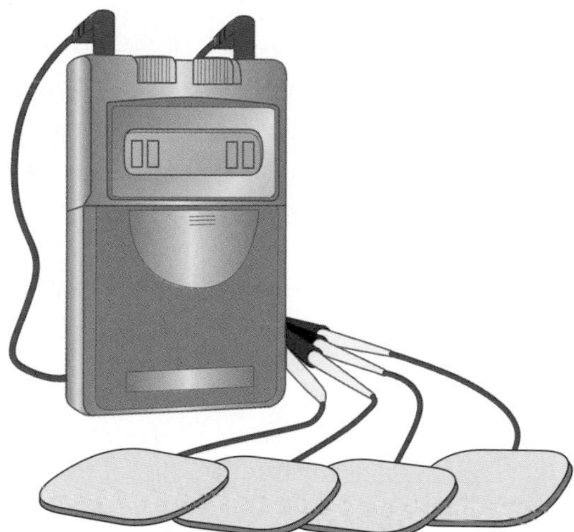

Figure 15.11: A transcutaneous electrical nerve stimulation (TENS) unit. (From Eagle S, Brassington C, Dailey C, Goretti C: *The Professional Medical Assistant: An Integrative, Teamwork-Based Approach.* Philadelphia: FA Davis, 2009, p. 742. With permission.)

Reflective Questions

Consider what you have learned about physical therapy treatments to answer the following questions.

1. What is the key difference between the purpose of a TENS unit and the purpose of an E-stim device? ______________________________
2. Is resistance necessary for all types of exercise? Explain. ______________________________
3. What is an endorphin? ______________________________
4. What is the medical term for *pain relief* or *pain control*? ______________________________
5. What effect does the application of something cold have on muscles? ______________________________

Mix and Match

Match each description with the name of the test that is used to assess it.

1. ambulation or ability to move	The Balance Test
2. angle of the knee	GARS
3. muscle stiffness	A myotonometer
4. distance walked at defined intervals	A goniometer
5. watching a person walk	The Walk Test
6. standing, turning, bending, and shifting	The FIM Locomotion Scale

Fill in the Blanks

Apply your understanding of new physical therapy terminology that you have learned by filling in the blanks.

1. Mrs. Vegreville, who is 82 years old, suffers from neuralgia. Today, the physical therapist has decided to start her on ____________ treatment to help alleviate this condition.
2. Electronic muscle stimulation devices provide the client with a form of ____________ exercise.
3. Treadmill exercises help to build the strength and ____________ of muscles.
4. When the nurse or physical therapist helps a patient to gently rotate a stiff or injured wrist, he or she is performing ____________ - ____________ - ____________ exercises.
5. Mr. Kleinschmidt, who is 87 years old, is afraid of taking the stairs now and does not feel safe on them unless he can hold onto both handrails or to someone's arm. He needs a ____________ ____________ test.
6. Mrs. Samson is 64 years old and has arthritis in her knees. Her physician has suggested that she participate in ____________, where she can get some exercise without putting undue stress on her joints.
7. After her car accident, Shaka finds her neck to be very, very stiff on occasion. This condition is painful. She is diagnosed with a whiplash injury (i.e., soft-tissue damage), and her doctor has suggested that ____________ may release the muscle tension, relieve some pain, and promote the overall relaxation of her muscles, mind, and body.
8. Madge is a paraplegic (paralyzed from the waist down). To prevent muscle atrophy, she does daily exercises with assistance of a care attendant, but she also sees a physical therapist twice weekly, who attaches a device that provides ____________ ____________ of her leg muscles.
9. Monique has a diagnosis of fibromyalgia; the main features of this disorder are pain and tiredness. She wonders if treatment with a ____________ unit might help to relieve this pain.
10. A ____________ scale will assess a patient's ability to move from one place to another.

Critical Thinking

To answer the following question, you will need to recall something that you learned much earlier in this textbook.

Provide two meanings for the acronym *EMS.*

1. ____
2. ____

Recovery and rehabilitation: leg injuries

Another day has passed at Fayette General Hospital for our patient, Gil Loeppky. His recovery continues to be good, and he is nearing discharge.

Patient Update

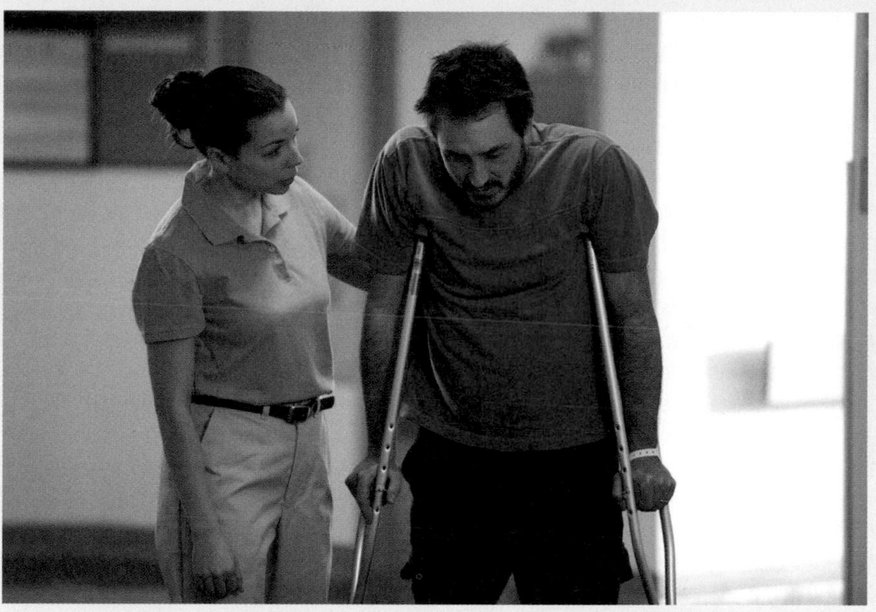

Tamron Epp greeted her patient in the physical therapy department. "Hi, Gil. I see that it's that time again." Gil smiled. "How was the ride here in that chair?" Tamron asked, observing that Gil was in a wheelchair. "Did you manage to wheel yourself here, or did someone bring you and drop you off?" Gil explained proudly that he had managed the journey on his own, propelling the wheelchair with his own upper body strength. Tamron smiled and congratulated him. "You certainly are determined to get better fast, aren't you?" Gil agreed.

"Have you spoken to your doctor today, Gil?" Tamron asked.

"Yes, and he says that I can go home in 24 to 48 hours," Gil said, pausing to let this news sink in. "Can you imagine? Finally going home! Sleeping in my own bed, being home with my wife. It's great news!"

"Well, I had heard that from the doctor, so I prepared some discharge plans for you that I'd like to go over today," said Tamron. "I'd also like to work through a complete review of your physical therapy needs, and then we can get into some activities for today. How does that sound?" she asked. Gil responded positively and was eager to begin.

They began by discussing Gil's hip fracture, what progress had been made toward full recovery, and what rehabilitative measures were still remaining. Tamron spent some extra time on this aspect of Gil's rehabilitation. "As you know," she said, "you had a complex spiral hip fracture at the distal end of your right femur, right where it impacted the acetabulum." Gil nodded and mentioned that he'd learned quite a lot about what that meant when he was at Okla Trauma Center.

Tamron continued: "That fracture was surgically reduced, and the wound site was covered with a padded dressing that not only protected the incision and the suture line but also the hip area itself, thus preventing skin breakdown and pain along the bony prominences of the hip." Gil reported that the stitches along his hip, as well as those on both sides of his lower leg, had been removed by the nurse earlier today and that fresh padded dressings had been applied. The physical therapist nodded her acknowledgement.

Tamron reviewed the progress of Gil's physical therapy: "We've had you sitting up and standing quite frequently throughout the time that you've been with us here at Fayette. You and I have been working on some very gentle range-of-motion exercises for your right ankle over the past week. These have helped to keep the muscles and tendons from stiffening, to promote muscle strength, and to ensure that healthy circulation was maintained."

"So when will I finally be able to walk?" asked Gil. "When will I be able to get back on both feet?"

"Generally, when an internal fixation of a fracture like this occurs, you can expect to start walking on the affected side within 2 to 3 months," answered Tamron. Gil grimaced in disappointment. "In the interim," Tamron went on, offering some hopeful information, "once you've been able to tolerate those range-of-motion exercises for a bit—as you have—you can be fitted for a short removable brace or a cast to protect and support the healing tibia and the adjacent ankle. I'm not sure if the doctor plans to arrange that for you before your discharge. If not, your physician will be able to plan this transition with you." Tamron paused, giving the patient time to think about this information. "In the interim," she repeated, "you will be able to use crutches in addition to using a wheelchair." Gil commented that at least that would be some progress, although not as much as he'd hoped.

"Gil, we haven't been able to progress to crutches as quickly as we'd hoped to because of the complications of your knee and shinbone injuries," said Tamron. Gil nodded, following her train of thought, and then she continued. "You're wearing a knee support, and, although that does not weigh a great deal, it still exerts pressure on your quadriceps and on the ball-and-socket joint of your hip. The distal end of your fractured right tibia is only minimally supported by the dressing and the tensor bandage that cover it now. It's absolutely impossible for you to bear weight on that foot and ankle under these circumstances. Even so, you are strong enough now to start walking more independently. Today, I have permission from the physician to try you out on crutches." The patient smiled at this; he was glad to hear the news and eager to continue with his recovery and rehabilitation.

"Gil, when you're released from the hospital, you'll need to rent or buy a wheelchair," said Tamron. "You'll need to use that for at least the next 3 or 4 weeks. That being said, you will be able to ambulate with crutches intermittently throughout your day, as long as you're at home, where it's safe. As you continue as an outpatient while receiving rehabilitation services, your therapist and physician will notify you when you can use the crutches more often and where. It won't be long until you are weaned off of the chair," she said.

"All right," sighed Gil. He summarized. "What you're telling me is that I've got a long way to go yet before I can walk without support. I can see that I've got the same amount of time—or even more—to wait until I can drive again, too, right?" he said, in a tone that was partly resigned and partly hopeful. Tamron nodded in confirmation that he had understood her correctly: he wouldn't be able to drive for some time. She knew what this meant to him. He drove a delivery truck for a living.

"Today, and after your discharge, you'll need to continue those bilateral leg exercises so that, when you're standing erect, you will be able to maintain your balance and gradually begin to distribute your weight equally on both feet when standing," said Tamron. "So, we'll do a couple of warm-up exercises first, to prepare your hip, knee, and ankle for standing. After a few repetitions for each muscle and muscle group, we'll move over to the parallel bars so that I can watch you stand up by yourself, as you've already done now a couple of times. When we get there, you'll be in control. When you're ready to stand, just let me know." Gil nodded.

The PT went on: "When you're in that standing position, I'll make an assessment of your current postural alignment. Next, Conrad—one of our rehab technicians—and I are going to measure you for crutches. Then, with us standing near at hand, we'll wait for you get your balance and take your first steps with them." Tamron then paused, waiting as Gil confirmed his readiness for this. She then continued. "Afterward, depending on how well you tolerate the activities, we may have you lie down on one of the beds here while we apply some ice to those muscles that have been working so hard." Tamron smiled.

"Let's do it!" came Gil's enthusiastic reply.

"One more thing, Gil," said the physical therapist. "I have a surprise for you." Gil looked up at her from his wheelchair with curiosity. She smiled and said, "I've invited your wife to join us today." Gil broke into a great grin. "She's sitting in the waiting room right now. I wanted to bring her in so that I can teach her how to help you with your exercises, applying ice, using the crutches, and so on. I hope you don't mind."

"Mind?" said Gil. "No, no. This is great!" Tamron turned to the rehabilitation technician nearby and asked him to escort Mrs. Loeppky into the department. Gil quickly turned his chair around to face the doors in happy anticipation of seeing his wife. "Does she know I'm going home soon?" he asked the PT.

"No, I haven't told her. I thought maybe you'd be the one who'd like to tell her," Tamron said softly, smiling.

Key terms: recovery and rehabilitation

Did you notice the kinds of language that the physical therapist used as she discussed Gil's recovery and rehabilitation with him? She used a mixture of medical terminology and common speech. By doing so, she was rightly acknowledging to him that he now had some knowledge of medical terms and that he had become informed about his own health challenges. She treated him respectfully, as an informed consumer of her services, while still appreciating that he did not have the same level of technical medical vocabulary that she did. She adapted her way of communicating to a level at which mutual understanding could and did occur. Key terms from the dialogue are explained below.

"... *propelling the wheelchair* ..."

propelling the wheelchair: moving the wheelchair forward. The root word *propel* mans *to drive, push, or force.*

"... that fresh *padded dressings* had been applied."

padded dressings: coverings for a wound that provides some form of cushioning to protect it from further injury. The cushioning may be cotton, a cotton-like fabric, or foam (see Figure 15-12).

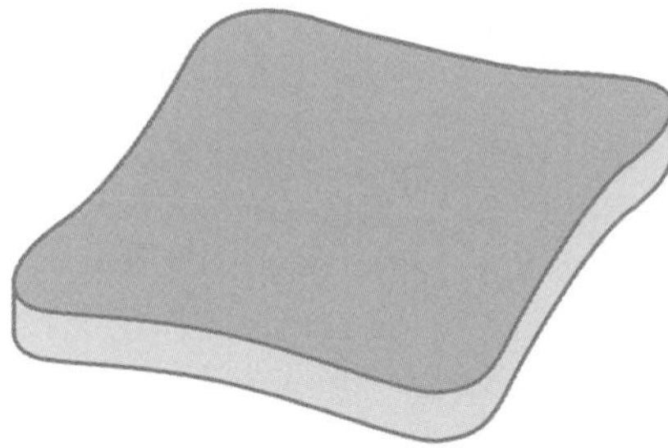

Figure 15.12: Foam dressing

"... and the *suture line* ..."

suture line: an incision creates a break in the skin called an *incision line*; the *suture line* is the row of stitches (sutures) over the incision line (see Figure 15-13).

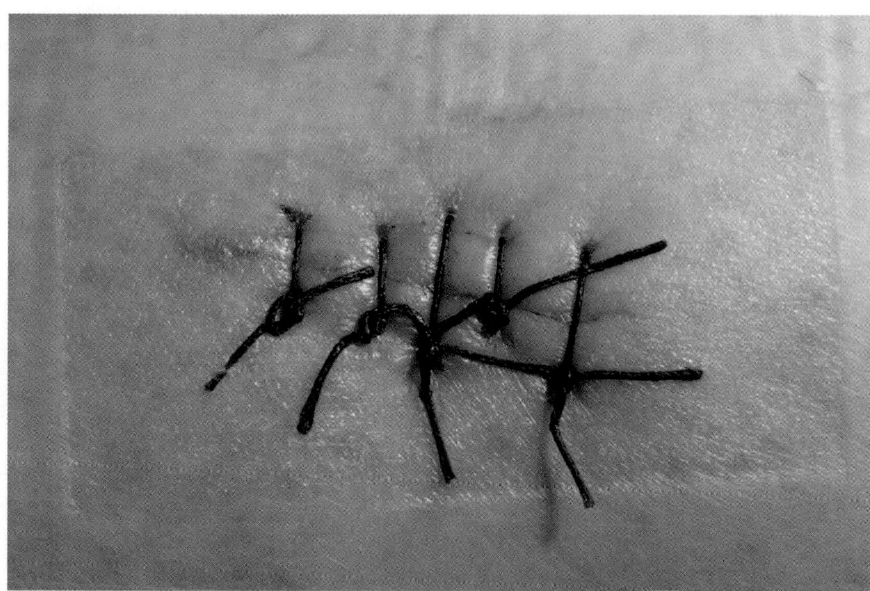

Figure 15.13: Suture line (© Thinkstock)

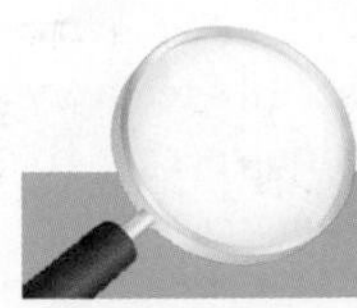

FOCUS POINT: Suture Lines

In wound care, a *suture line* is a line of sutures or stitches that are placed to hold two sides of a wound together so that they may heal. The word *suture* can also refer to the anatomical lines of the cranium where various bony plates come together. In this context, the term *suture line* can have a different meaning. For example, newborn infants are born with soft skulls. During the pressure of birth, the bones of their skulls may be pressed together and overlap. This condition is usually temporary; however, if the condition does not resolve, ridges and altered shapes in the skull may occur. Examples include the following:

- A *sagittal suture line* extends along the length of the skull where the parietal bones meet; this condition will result in a head shape that is long and narrow.
- A *coronal suture line* develops across the skull where the frontal and parietal bones meet; this condition will result in a head shape that is short and wide.

"... thus preventing *skin breakdown* and pain along the *bony prominences of the hip.*"

skin breakdown: a process during which the integrity of the surface of the skin is broken and the underlying tissue is exposed to the air. This situation can result from long periods of immobility, allergies, exposure to the sun, wounds, and other causes (see "Focus Point: Skin Integrity and Skin Breakdown").

bony prominences: places on the body where a bone is near the surface of the skin, such as the hip, the elbow, or the ankle.

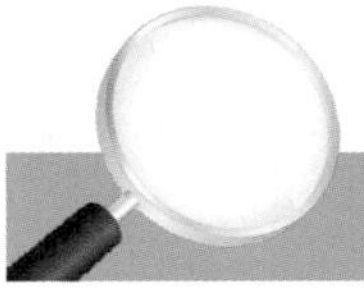

FOCUS POINT: Skin Integrity and Skin Breakdown

In a medical context, the word *integrity* means *wholeness or without impairment*. The maintenance of *skin integrity* is a priority in health care because the skin is the first line of defense against trauma and invading microorganisms.

Skin breakdown is also referred to as *skin impairment*. Among patients who spend long periods of time in bed or sitting in wheelchairs, the skin will begin to break down over the bony prominences as a result of pressure being placed on the area in addition to heat being generated there. Multiple other causative factors may also apply, such as poor nutrition, dehydration, and a lack of adipose tissue.

"... an *internal fixation* of a fracture like this ..."

internal fixation: the use of pins and screws to fixate or hold bone segments together (see Chapter 11).

"... a short *removable brace* or a cast ..."

removable brace: an orthotic device made of lightweight plastics or polymers that protects and stabilizes fractures and joints after injury. These braces are often held in place by Velcro strips or straps and can be removed at night for some relief and to protect the skin from breakdown (see Figure 15-14).

"... knee and *shinbone* injuries ..."

shinbone: an everyday word for the tibia.

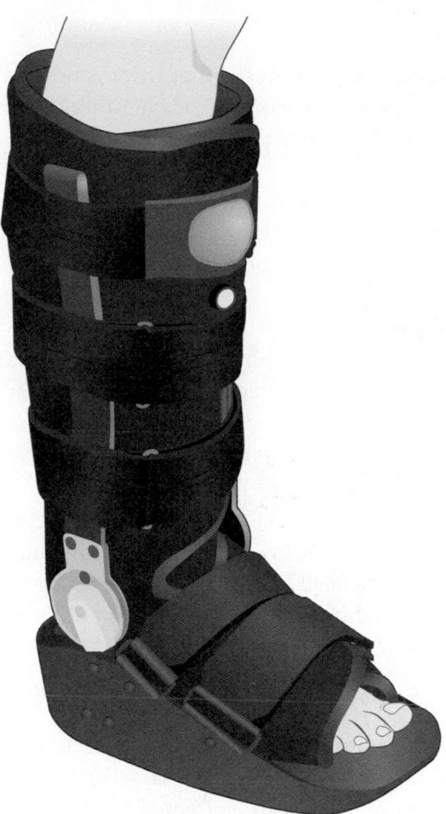

Figure 15.14: Removable leg brace

"... wearing a *knee support* ..."

support: any type of brace, wrap, or other device that provides stabilization and that may also enhance circulation surrounding a joint or a moveable body part.

knee support: a pull-on or wraparound orthotic device designed to provide medial and lateral stabilization of the knee. Some include bilateral hinges to help support movement. All prevent hyperextension of the knee. Our patient, Gil Loeppky, will likely be using either a lightweight stabilizing knee brace made of a synthetic material called *neoprene* or a practical hinged knee support (see Figure 15-15).

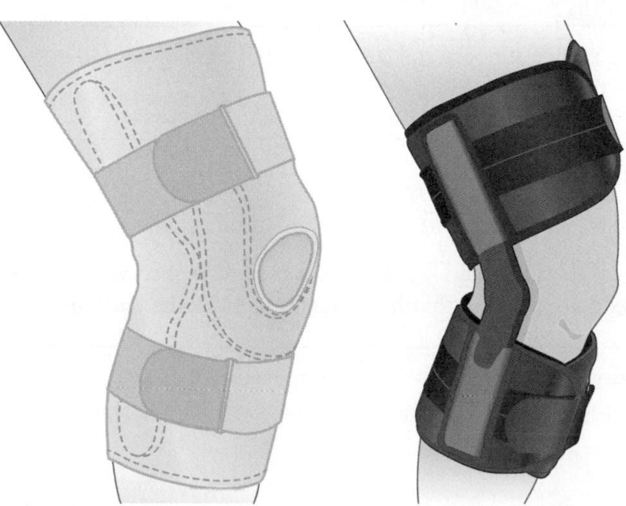

Figure 15.15: *A*, Lightweight stabilizing knee brace; *B*, Practical hinged knee support

"... to *try you out on crutches.*"

try you out on crutches: medical jargon that means that there is no guarantee that the patient will actually be able to use the crutches successfully today; rather, he or she will be fitted for a pair his or her size and then assisted to use them to the best of his or her ability.

"... are *weaned off of* the chair ..."

weaned off of: adjusted to the gradual withdrawal from something. In this case, Gil will gradually withdraw from the use of the wheelchair until it is no longer used at all.

"... *you'll be in control.*"

you'll be in control: a common expression that is used in health care to allay the patient's fears of loss of control and of being pushed into something that he or she does not feel ready to do.

"... your current *postural alignment.*"

postural alignment: the proper placement of the bones of the skeleton related to the posture. Ideal postural alignment involves standing up straight. Individuals who limp, use crutches, or have other health challenges may need assistance or therapeutic interventions (i.e., physical therapy, chiropractic care) to maintain postural alignment. There are many exercises that promote correct postural alignment.

"... to *measure you for crutches.*"

measure you for crutches: a procedure that involves the lengthening or shortening of crutches to promote good postural alignment while at the same time supporting the patient enough to avoid the risk of a fall or a reinjury of the affected lower limb. Crutches should sit 2 inches below the axilla (armpit) along the ribs to achieve proper posture. At no time should the individual lean forward to support himself or herself on crutches. Leaning forward throws off the person's center of gravity and balance, thereby greatly increasing the risk of falls and back strain.

Critical Thinking

Consider what you've just learned about rehabilitation and physical therapy as you answer the following questions.

1. Is it likely that Gil will receive a TENS treatment today? Explain your answer.

   ____

2. Why was it a good idea to invite Gil's wife, Glory, to this particular physical therapy session?

   ____

3. How does having a knee support and cast on his right leg affect Gil's ability to stand and walk?

   ____

Reflective Questions

Answer the following questions on the basis of the Patient Update.

1. When the physical therapist said "sutures," the patient replied with a more common word for sutures, thus demonstrating that he understood what she had said. What word did he use? ______________________________
2. From which wound sites were Gil's sutures removed today? ______________________________
3. What is the job title for the person who is assisting Tamron today? ______________________________

Translate the Terms

Translate the following terms into everyday English.

1. acetabulum ______
2. reduced ______
3. tibia ______
4. rehabilitation ______
5. prominence ______
6. erect ______
7. dressing ______
8. propel ______
9. distal ______
10. bear ______

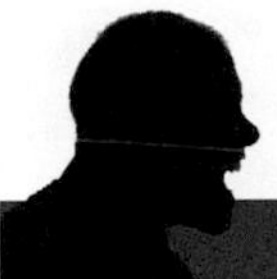

PRONUNCIATION PRACTICE

Say these words aloud to a friend or classmate, if you can. Here you are given the phonetic pronunciation. Your instructor can help you with pronunciation, or you can visit **http://www.MedicalLanguageLab.com.**

abasia	ă-**bā**´zē-ă
astasia	ă-**stā**´zē-ă
goniometer	gō″nē-**ŏm**´ĕ-ter
rehabilitation	rē″hă-bĭl″ĭ-**tā**´shŭn
transcutaneous	trăns″kū-**tā**´nē-ŭs

Occupational Therapy and Brain Injury Rehabilitation

Thirty-four-year-old Gilbert Loeppky recently suffered two brain injuries and underwent brain surgery. His path to recovery will be unique to him: how each individual patient responds to and recovers from brain injury varies greatly. Although Gil seems to be doing exceptionally well, he will need to be monitored for at least 6 months or even a year post-injury.

The rehabilitation of patients with neurological disorders falls within a specialized branch of medicine called *physical medicine and rehabilitation.* The physicians involved are called *physiatrists.* Luckily, Gil has not required the skills of these practitioners. There has been no evidence to date that he has sustained serious nerve damage or significant impairment of his neuropathways. Our patient's brain traumas have led to minimal physical, cognitive, and emotional deficits. As a result, he can be assessed and cared for neurologically by his own physician, as well as occupational and physical therapists. Gil is expected to make a full neurological recovery.

Occupational therapy (OT) is a branch of health care that focuses on self-care activities and the promotion of independent functioning. It is concerned with the maintenance and restoration of fine-motor functioning and coordination, particularly those of the upper limbs. OT also concerns itself with an individual's ability to perform an occupation at home or at work. In this context, the term *occupation* refers to any goal-directed activity; it does not refer strictly to employment or a job. We are "occupied" each time we are busy completing a task such as reading, brushing our teeth, taking a walk, or even watching television.

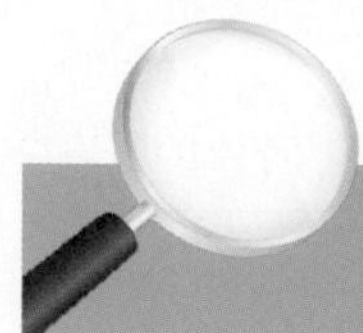

FOCUS POINT: Fine Motor Functioning vs. Gross Motor Functioning

Fine motor functioning refers to the actions of small (fine) muscles, such as those in the fingers, which are used to complete precise or delicate movements, such as picking up a pin, typing, or writing.

Gross motor functioning refers to the use of larger muscles or muscle groups to move and to maintain balance and posture.

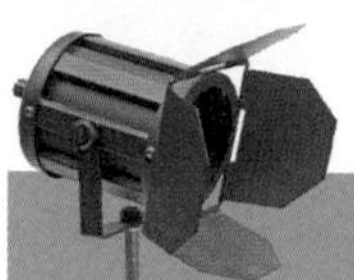

CAREER SPOTLIGHT: Occupational Therapist

An *occupational therapist (OT)* has specialty training at the graduate (master's degree) level, and all states require licensure for these health professionals. OTs work at a variety of sites, both inside and outside of health-care facilities. They can be found in schools, businesses, and industrial settings.

Many occupational therapists follow a *person-environment-occupation-performance (PEOP) approach* to their work. This theory asserts that the ability to perform an activity is based on an individual's capacity to do so, the characteristics or demands of that activity, and the resources and task requirements in the environment in which the activity is to occur. Simply put, these therapists assess a person's ability to do a task, assess whether the task is possible in a particular environment, and assess all the elements of the task. This information leads to the development of strategies to intervene with or to help the client proceed. OTs are able to make recommendations for changes or adaptations to the client's environment to support the successful completion of the task.

OTs work with clients who have a wide array of limitations, including cognitive, psychosocial, sensory, and motor function impairments. These professionals understand that the ability to function as independently as possible improves self-esteem and confidence. With that in mind, they develop interventions that will restore or enhance patient success through task accomplishment. These interventions include teaching the client to relearn skills that may have been temporarily lost or to learn new adaptive skills in the face of a new disability.

To become an occupational therapist, a person must obtain a master's degree in occupational therapy from a program that has been accredited by the Accreditation Council for Occupational Therapy Education (ACOTE), which is an arm of the American Occupational Therapy Association (AOTA). The successful completion of national examinations facilitates licensing and credentialing. OTs may go on to complete doctoral programs.

Right Word or Wrong Word: *Occupational Therapist* or *Physical Therapist*?

According to what you've learned in this chapter, are these two careers the same? Is an OT the same as a PT but with a slightly different background education? Explain your answer.

Read aloud

Read the following patient history aloud to practice talking about patients and their care. While you do so, you might want to imagine that you have just admitted or received this patient into your care. After introducing yourself to him, you would review his medical record in depth and then share your findings in a review like this with your colleagues. Could you summarize this material for them?

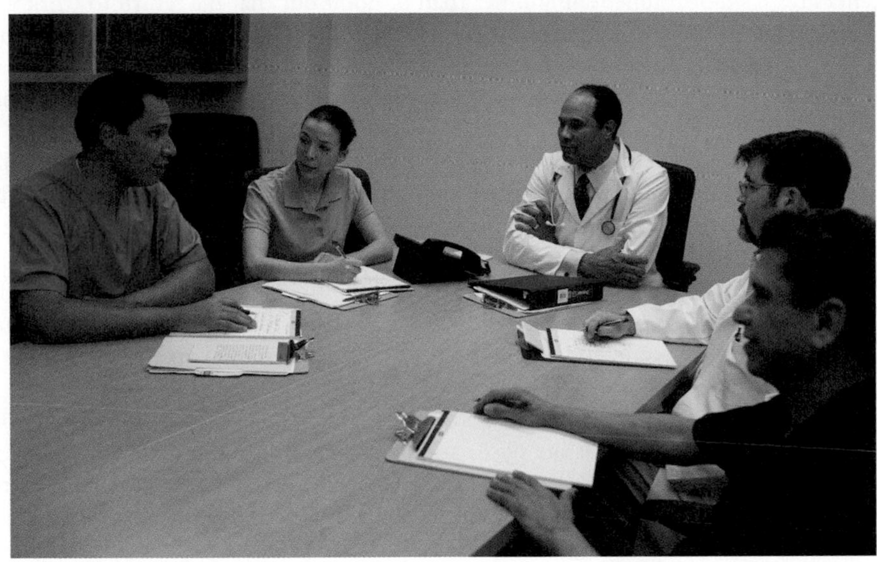

Patient history: Gil Loeppky

When he arrived at Okla Trauma Center, Gil Loeppky was diagnosed with a mild concussion, the result of a blunt force trauma to the head that he received during a motor vehicle accident. Subsequent to that, he fell out of bed while in the hospital and acquired a secondary impact concussion with a subdural hematoma. That was treated immediately; intracranial pressure in the brain was relieved, and the patient has demonstrated little to no adverse effects of either trauma. Even so, the medical team at Fayette General Hospital has been monitoring Gil's neurological signs routinely to ensure that no changes in his status occur.

Gil was started on anticonvulsant medications at Okla Trauma Center as well. Convulsions (seizures) are not uncommon with brain injury, and starting the patient on this medication is an important prophylactic measure so that, should any signs of seizure activity occur, the patient does not reinjure his body or brain. Gil did not exhibit any seizure activity, and this medication was discontinued by the physician at Okla 7 days after commencement. The admitting physician at Fayette General Hospital was aware of the continuing possibility of seizure risk and understood that the patient should continue to be monitored for seizure activity for 6 months or more. He did not choose to restart the anticonvulsants, which showed that he appreciated how Gil's overall recovery contraindicated the need for such medications. He did instruct the nurses to continue to monitor the patient for seizures, and he recently ordered an electroencephalogram (EEG) to assess the electrical activity in Gil's brain. The EEG was normal.

Gil Loeppky was seen by a speech and language pathologist (SLP) at Okla Trauma Center as well. This is standard procedure for patients with brain injuries to ensure that these patients have recovered their ability to masticate (chew), drink, and swallow correctly; these functions are controlled by the brain (see Chapter 10 and 11). Although Gil did not have any difficulties with these functions, he did have some initial slurring of speech and drooling post-operatively. The SLP worked with Gil on muscle exercises of the lips, tongue, and jaw to improve his articulation of speech and his ability to keep his lips closed in a natural position. These exercises worked to stave off the drooling. Gil's speaking improved, particularly when he was not tired. At Fayette General, the staff noted that the patient is still prone to some slurring when he is fatigued. The team believes that this will resolve as the patient's overall recovery continues.

Shortly after Gil's admission to Fayette General Hospital, his physician asked that he be seen by an occupational therapist to assess his neurological functioning. The OT identified the patient as right-hand dominant. She found that Gil had a slower grasp response in his left hand than normally expected, and she was working with him on holding a fork to cut food while eating and other activities that required the use of this hand. She was able to send an OT assistant to Gil's room to help rehabilitate function in that hand. He no longer requires this type of intervention. The OT was optimistic that this challenge would also resolve itself in time. She noted no other impairments in Gil's motor functioning other than to point out that his return to work would be difficult because his occupation as a truck driver required further assessment of his reaction times while driving a vehicle. The treatment team was aware that Gil's health insurance provider would follow through with his case and determine his ability to safely return to work through their own assessment processes and occupational therapists.

Impairments in memory, concentration, judgment, decision making, and mood can all be the result of head injuries. The treatment team at Fayette General is monitoring Gil's cognitive and emotional functioning to assess for these impairments. He was seen for a comprehensive neurological assessment after his arrival at this facility. At that time, some impairments in short-term memory and concentration were noted. In addition, during those first few days at the facility, Gil had a number of spontaneous outbursts of anger. These have subsided, and the team has considered that they may have been caused by the residual effects of intracranial pressure on the impulse control center of his brain.

To improve his short-term memory and his ability to concentrate, Gil has been attending half-hour rehabilitation sessions in the occupational therapy department once per day for just over a week. His plan of care includes support for his self-efficacy and self-esteem as he recovers from his traumas. The team is also very mindful to not overtax the patient with occupational therapy and physical therapy appointments that are scheduled too closely together. They understand that patients with head injuries require time to rest between sessions. Both OT and PT have identified that Gil becomes increasingly distracted and then irritable when he is fatigued or when his pain reappears (most notably the pain that he feels around the pins and screws in his tibia).

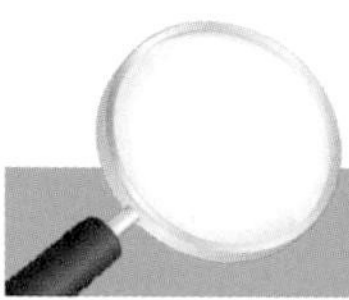

FOCUS POINT: Prophylactic

Prophylactic is an important term in health care that means *preventative*. The word is used in many different contexts, such as the following:

- Vaccines are prophylactic for diseases.
- Bike helmets are prophylactic for head injuries.
- Condoms are prophylactic for sexually transmitted diseases.
- A small dose of acetylsalicylic acid (aspirin) every day is prophylactic for cerebrovascular accidents.

Reflective Questions

Answer these questions related to Gil Loeppky's patient history.

1. Which hand does Gil Loeppky use for most activities? ______________________
2. Where is the impulse control center located in the body? ______________________
3. Who has worked with Gil for the rehabilitation of his grasp? ______________________
4. What kind of comprehensive assessment did Gil receive when he first arrived at Fayette General Hospital? ______________________

Key terms: patient history

Gil Loeppky's patient history provided a summary or overview of his care since he was in a motor vehicle accident just over 3 weeks ago. Key terms from the patient history are explained below.

"... Gil's overall recovery *contraindicated* the need for such medications."

contraindicated: indicated that they were not advisable, not warranted, or not necessary.

"... continue to *monitor* the patient ..."

to monitor: jargon for *to observe or to watch for.*

"... ordered an *electroencephalogram (EEG)* ..."

electroencephalogram (EEG): a recording of the electrical activity of the brain. This is achieved by placing electrodes on the surface of the skull and recording brain-wave patterns on a computer-like monitoring device called an **electroencephalograph**. This procedure may be performed by an EEG technician.

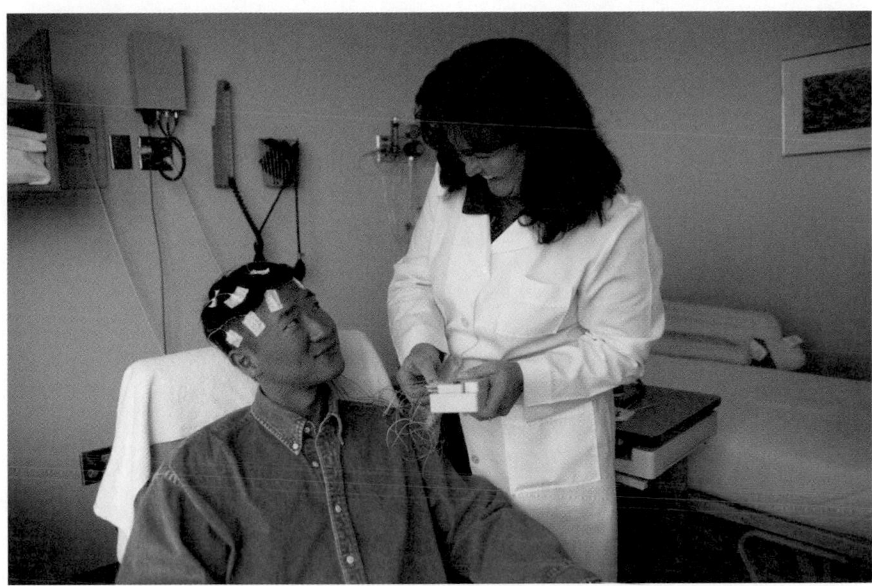

Figure 15.16: Patient receiving an electroencephalogram (EEG) (© Thinkstock)

"... *electrical activity in Gil's brain* ..."

electrical activity in Gil's brain: The operation of the nervous system is electrochemical in nature: in the axon of a neuron, an impulse (signal) is transformed into a chemical (a neurotransmitter) that is then released into the space between neurons (the synapse). The next neuron is triggered, and the activity repeats. The process continues as the signal is transmitted through the neurological system. During this process, each axon generates a small electrical charge (see Chapter 4 for more detail). The brain continuously generates electrical impulses, even during sleep. Seizure occurs when there is a misfiring of neuronal impulses and the brain is suddenly bombarded with excessive and random bursts of electrical activity. An electroencephalogram (EEG) can be used to measure the electrical activity of the brain.

"... to *stave off* the drooling."

stave off: to ward off or prevent the occurrence of.

"... *right-hand dominant.*"

right-hand dominant: medical term for being right-handed.

"... had a slower *grasp response*..."

grasp response: a reflexive action that occurs when the fingers or interior surface of the hand (the palm) are stimulated and they immediately begin to close around the stimulus.

"... his *reaction times*..."

reaction times: the amount of time that elapses (the interval) between a stimulus occurring and a response to it. In the context of Gil's safety at work, appropriate reaction times to any hazards on the road, changes in the traffic lights, and so on are critically important.

"... the *residual effects* of intracranial pressure..."

residual effects: aftereffects. In this context, the swelling of the tissues in the brain from the surgical intervention to decrease ICP may be a residual effect. The swelling may put pressure on certain functional centers of the brain, thereby impeding their ability to perform as they should.

"... *impulse control center* of his brain."

impulse control center: located in the frontal lobe of the brian, the impulse control center affects how reactions occur (i.e., whether with thought and judgment or impulsively). Impulse control can be a challenge for patients who have experienced frontal head injuries. It is also a factor in decision making during adolescence, as this part of the brain is not fully developed until the early 20s.

"... to not *overtax* the patient..."

overtax: overwhelm or exhaust.

Right Word or Wrong Word: *Response Time* or *Reaction Time*?

Are these two terms synonymous? Do they mean the same thing? Explain.

Fill in the Blanks

Use terminology from the patient history to fill in the blanks.

1. Continuing on anticonvulsant medications is not indicated; it is ____________________ at this time.
2. A sudden burst of anger or risky behavior may be indicative of immature development of the ____________________ of the brain.
3. The driver of the car saw the broken bottle in the road, but his ____________________ was too slow to avoid it. He got a flat tire.
4. When you touch a small baby, it will reach out to take hold of you. This is an example of the ____________________.
5. To apply sutures to a wound, the physician or nurse practitioner must have good ____________________ functioning.
6. A career that focuses on helping a patient to achieve optimal functioning in his or her activities of work and daily living is ____________________.

Free Writing

Practice the skill of summarizing what you've read or heard. In a short paragraph and with the use of complete sentences, summarize what you've just learned about Gil Loeppky's cognitive and emotional deficits. Include rationales for your answers. In other words, explain why you are writing what you are writing or what evidence you have to support what you've said. Refer to Gil as "the patient."

____

____

____

____

Occupational therapy: assessment techniques

After an operation or a trauma, the goal of any treatment team is to return the patient to a *premorbid* level of functioning. To ascertain this level, various formal and informal interviews are held with the patient and his or her support persons or family. Next, more formal measures in the form of written tests or activities are used.

The term **pre-morbid** means *occurring before the medical incident, trauma, or disease.*

Morbid is a root word that means *diseased or sick*. In health care, the term is used widely to describe many conditions or situations that require intervention or treatment.

For patients with head or brain injuries, it is crucial to explore their pre-morbid functioning to prepare care plans that will include goals that are appropriate for their personalities, interests, needs, activities, and capabilities.

The global assessment of functioning (GAF) scale

The **Global Assessment of Functioning (GAF) Scale** is by far the most commonly used test of overall (global) functioning. It may be administered by nurses, physicians, psychiatrists, occupational and physical therapists, medical social workers, and other health professionals. This test evaluates the occupational, social, and psychological functioning of adults. It also assesses how well an individual is coping with or adapting to the challenges that they meet during their lives. The patient is given a score from 1 to 100 to evaluate his or her overall level of occupational, social, and psychological functioning. The GAF (or a version of it) is also used to collect data for health benefits.

In addition to the GAF, occupational therapists employ a wide range of other assessments to determine a person's level of functioning. Some of these are described in Table 15-8.

TABLE 15-8: Occupational Therapy Assessment Techniques

Assessment Technique	Description
Bay Area Functional Performance Evaluation (BaFPE)	• developed for use with patients in psychiatric care and psychiatric occupational therapy • evaluates two sets of functions: social interaction and task orientation (attention or focus on task) • results show cognitive, affective (emotional), and performance levels
Cognitive Assessment of Minnesota (CAM)	• assesses a broad range of cognitive skills using a variety of subtests for memory, arithmetic, following directions, and attention
Chessington Occupational Therapy Neurological Assessment Battery (COTNAB)	• developed for patients with brain injuries or strokes (i.e., neurological patients) • measures visual perception, ability to follow directions, ability to construct things, and sensory-motor ability on a variety of subtests
Loewenstein Occupational Therapy Assessment (LOTCA)	• for use with patients who have mental health challenges or neurological deficits • through multiple subtests, assesses visual-spatial perception, orientation, cognition, and praxis (i.e., ability to perform a skill)
Rivermead Behavioural Memory Test, Third Edition (RBMT-3)	• designed for people with an acquired brain injury • assesses memory deficits and impairments
Kinetic Self-Image Test	• a psychological test that is helpful for the assessment of children and adolescents but that can also be used across the life span • evaluates self-image and self-esteem

Continued

TABLE 15-8: Occupational Therapy Assessment Techniques—cont'd

Assessment Technique	Description
Canadian Occupational Performance Measure	• designed for adults to detect any changes that they themselves perceive in their occupational performance over time • assesses perceived quality of function, as well as performance and satisfaction with same
Rancho Los Amigos Level of Cognitive Functioning Scale (LCFS)	• designed to be used with patients with severe head trauma • measures response levels to stimuli or requests • evaluates level and evidence of self-awareness, as well as purposeful and appropriate response to stimuli and requests • assesses levels of confusion and agitation
Psychosocial Adjustment to Illness Scale (PAIS) (also known as *the Derogatis tests*)	• designed for adults with medical issues • assesses coping and adjustment to health challenges on multiple dimensions: past experience with illness, patterns of coping, psychosocial adjustment to current situation, and so on
Psychosocial Adjustment to Illness Scale—Self-Report (PAIS-SR)	• designed for adults with medical issues • a subjective, self-reporting scale performed by the patient that measures how he or she is coping with and adjusting to his or her medical issue

Daily living assessments

A priority for the OT assessment of a client's functional status is an *activities of daily living (ADLs)* assessment. A number of evaluative tools are used to measure the client's strengths and limitations. Each tool scores the person on the following scale:

- able to do independently;
- needs assistance to do; and
- cannot do.

ADL assessment may include the following:

basic ADLs (BADLs) assessment: a means of evaluating the patient's ability to carry out a series of self-care tasks, including dressing oneself, brushing the teeth, combing the hair, using the toilet, and so on.

instrumental ADLs (IADLs) assessment: an advanced form of the BADLs that is used to assess the patient's ability to carry out a series of tasks that require more complex cognitive functioning. These may include talking on the phone or making a phone call, managing finances and budgets, setting up and following a daily medication regimen, using the bus, doing one's laundry, cooking meals, and so on. The occupational therapist may also assess a patient's driving skills if the ability to drive is important to the client. This assessment can be accomplished with the use of technology in a safe setting rather than in a vehicle.

Eponyms: The Katz Index of Independence in Activities of Daily Living

Dr. Sydney Katz is an American physician, professor, researcher, and author. He has written extensively on issues that face the elderly, particularly issues related to their physical functioning. During the 1960s, Katz created the Index of Activities of Daily Living with the elderly in mind. The index has since been adapted into similar assessment tools that are used across the life span and across disciplines in health care. Dr. Katz is currently Professor Emeritus in Geriatric Medicine and Public Health at Columbia University.

Eponyms: The Lawton Instrumental Activities of Daily Living Scale

Until his death in 2001, M. Powell Lawton, PhD, was an American research scientist and Director Emeritus of the Polisher Research Institute of Philadelphia Geriatric Center (PGC). His long and distinguished career in psychology and education began at Columbia University. He was also a professor of psychiatry at Temple University School of Medicine. He is well known for his work in human development, particularly with regard to the elderly. In 1969, he developed the Lawton Instrumental Activities of Daily Living Scale (IADL) for this target population. This tool is in common use across the United States and Canada. In addition, his interest in how the environment affects older adults led the PGC to open the first American nursing home that was specifically designed for persons with Alzheimer's disease. The Lawton IADL scale is also referred to as the *Lawton-Brody IADL scale*. This was named after Dr. Lawton and Elaine M. Brody, MSW, a long-time colleague of Dr. Lawton who works as a senior research consultant for PGC.

Cognitive treatment modalities

Gil's treatment in occupational therapy includes the paying of attention to his short-term memory deficit, his distractibility, and his difficulty with staying focused on a task or conversation. The OT will want to discover the length of time that Gil can remember information and how well he can pay attention. The OT will then design a plan of treatment to assist with the rehabilitation of these cognitive skills.

Types of memory

Memory is a complex phenomenon with many different aspects. Two basic types of memory are differentiated below:

Retrospective memory allows us to remember *how* to do things. It forms the content of our actions. In cases of severe brain injury or pathology (i.e., dementia), people can forget how to do things and what steps are needed and in which order. This type of memory is involved in all kinds of everyday tasks, including those as simple as knowing what to do with a fork when you see it sitting on the table next to a plate.

Prospective memory allows us to remember *what* we need to do and *when*. Although posting notes and using calendars facilitate this ability, our own memories are able to perform this function unaided for the most part. Prospective memory can be affected by cerebrovascular accidents, alcoholism, and brain trauma.

Memory strategies

People use two different kinds of strategies to help them to remember:

External strategies are those that rely on cues in our environment to remind us to do something.

Internal strategies are mental techniques that we have trained ourselves to use to remember things. These might include repeating a word, phrase, or name over and over in our heads until we are sure that it's committed to long-term memory. Another internal strategy involves the use of mnemonics, such as those found at the end of many chapters in this textbook.

Memory rehabilitation

Gil's occupational therapy will include external compensatory strategies that have been designed to teach him the importance of labeling and posting notes in his hospital room or home to alert him to things that he should remember. He will also practice identifying cues that are important reminders. For example, a cue of a growling stomach might mean that he forgot to eat, a cue of the phone ringing might mean that he should answer it, and a cue of the sound of the doorbell may mean that he needs to answer the door.

The OT will start with simple memory tasks and gradually move to more complex ones. The use of memory books (journals), calendars, and alert devices (i.e., cell phones, pagers, alarm clocks) will also be part of Gil's memory rehabilitation plan. Memory practice activities in OT can include table games, card games, and even seek-and-find games such as treasure hunts. However, the treatment team must be careful that these are age appropriate and not demeaning to an adult if they wish the patient to participate.

Gil Loeppky will also need internal compensatory strategies to help restore his memory. Teaching mnemonics may help; the use of verbal and visual cues such as laying out a particular shirt for the next day or setting towels on the sink or bed to remind the patient to shower may also be useful. When Gil sees these reminders, his memory will be activated.

Learning to draw associations is another internal memory strategy. We associate many sights, sounds, and smells with our thoughts and memories. For example, the smell of fresh coffee can stimulate the memory of coffee and perhaps the desire to find the source of the smell. Another strategy in Gil's rehabilitation may be to teach him to use rhymes to help him remember because these can also be a form of association. However, if rhyming is not something that is familiar or interesting to the patient, this technique will not be helpful.

Rehabilitation of concentration and attention

Occupational therapists will work with Gil to help him stay on task for longer and longer periods. This training will occur over time so that it does not to overwhelm him. OTs will observe and discover how and when Gil is distracted. Discovering the reasons for his distraction will help them to plan how to intervene successfully and to build a treatment plan to rehabilitate his ability to concentrate longer. The occupational therapists will also pay attention to how many tasks, stimuli, or interruptions in the environment are occurring at the same time so that they may decrease these to a level that is manageable for the patient.

Psychosocial treatment modalities

Patients who have suffered brain injuries may find that their ability to cope has been adversely affected. Sometimes this loss of coping skills is related to actual damage to the brain or residual swelling in the cranium. Often, however, it is related to the patient's own frustration with his or her situation, a sense of helplessness, and a loss of the patient's self-concept as a person who is capable and in control of his or her own life. Another goal of Gil Loeppky's occupational therapy will be to help restore his self-concept and his internal locus of control.

Locus of control

The term **locus of control** is taken from psychology to describe how a person perceives the events of his or her life. It reflects personal attitudes and beliefs about one's own power to influence life events. *Locus* means location.

People with an *internal locus of control* believe that they have control of and responsibility for their own situation in life.

People with an *external locus of control* believe that they do *not* have control of or responsibility for their situation. They believe that other people are in control of their lives, and they rely on other people to take responsibility for them.

Possessing an *internal* locus of control is important for patients during recovery or rehabilitation. These patients believe and accept that they have some control and responsibility for their own treatment and recovery. Research has shown that people who accept responsibility for their health challenges are more active participants in their treatment. They work more collaboratively during care planning with multidisciplinary team members. They don't simply hope for recovery, rehabilitation, or the restoration of functioning; they actively work toward these things. Through their observations and interactions with Gil Loeppky, the nursing, occupational therapy, and physical therapy staff members of Fayette General Hospital have found Gil to have this important ingredient for successful rehabilitation.

Alternatively, patients with an *external* locus of control tend to rely on others to make them feel better. They believe that any control over their health is beyond them and thus located in their external world. These patients are more likely to have longer stays in the hospital and in rehabilitation programs, and they are more likely to become depressed.

The patient's sense of self

There are a number of concepts related to the self that are relevant to recovery and rehabilitation, and they are all related. These include the following:

self-concept: a person's internal self-image and beliefs about himself or herself. A person's self-concept includes all that you know about yourself and what meaning you draw from this knowledge.

self-image: one's view of oneself. For example, you might believe that you are good-looking and strong, that you have the look of a professional, or that you exude confidence or charm. A self-image is often projected onto others. However, a person's self-image can be quite different from how others actually see him or her. For example, a person may believe that he is fun to be with and has a good sense of humor, but other people may not see him that way at all.

self-esteem: an appraisal that a person makes of his or her own value or worth. It consists of beliefs about one's own strengths, weaknesses, talents, capabilities, likability, and so on. Our self-esteem differs from our self-concept and self-image in that it is full of positive or negative value judgments that can help or hinder psychosocial functioning. Occupational therapists understand how important the maintenance of healthy self-esteem can be; they engage patients in activities at which the patients can succeed and which are personally meaningful for those patients so that the patients can feel proud. Self-esteem and self-efficacy are closely linked.

self-efficacy: the belief that one is capable of performing tasks that will lead to the attainment of goals. An example is the process of food shopping, preparing a meal, and then eating it. At each stage of this process, self-efficacy is shown. A more complex example is going to college, graduating from college, being interviewed for a job, and getting the job. Occupational therapists who are working with clients in return-to-work programs or with clients who are preparing to re-enter the home or community after a hospitalization will work with these clients on self-efficacy tasks related to the client's personal goals. For example, an OT may help Gil prepare to return to his job of driving a delivery truck by assessing and planning with Gil how to get up into the cab or how to apply pressure to the gas and brakes with a healing yet still somewhat fragile leg.

Frustration tolerance or frustration intolerance

Sudden changes in our health can be very frustrating. Health problems add physical, psychosocial, financial, and even spiritual stress to our lives. During a period of recovery and rehabilitation, even the tiniest setbacks or mistakes (i.e., dropping a toothbrush) can lead to sudden manifestations of frustration, including irritability, impatience, and even angry outbursts. Although stress, mood lability (changes), and frustration tolerance or intolerance often fall into the purview (scope) of mental health professionals, these emotional factors are also key elements in the assessment and care that are provided by occupational therapists. To combat problems with frustration intolerance, OTs will design activities and tasks that minimize the patient's chance of failure. By doing so, the patient stays engaged in the activity and feels a better sense of control and accomplishment.

Critical Thinking

Consider what you've just learned about the work of occupational therapists with regard to assessment, treatment, and rehabilitation. Apply your learning to the following real-world situations.

1. Martha is 92 years old. She is participating in her ADLs with a care aide this morning. She is handed a comb. She holds it and stares at it, seemingly at a loss for what to do with it. What type of memory deficit is this woman showing? ________________________
2. Ibrahim uses his mobile device to log every appointment and reminder that he can think of for what he needs to do each day. It often rings or buzzes during his time at work, and this aggravates the person who sits at the desk next to him. What memory strategy is Ibrahim using? ________________________
3. Grant finds that using an alarm clock in the morning does not work for him. Instead, he sets his coffeemaker to the appropriate time so that it will brew a pot of coffee for him. The smell is his memory trigger. It always awakens him on time. What memory strategy is this man using? ________________________
4. Which assessment tests from Table 15-8 do you think may be appropriate to use with our patient, Gil? Explain your answer. ________________________

Let's Practice

Name each assessment test or evaluation tool described below. Use the full name, not the acronym (initials).

1. evaluates self-image and self-esteem ______________________
2. commonly used to assess how individuals are coping with or adapting to the challenges that they meet in their lives ______________________
3. in gerontology, used to evaluate activities of daily living ______________________
4. targeted assessment for patients who have suffered severe head or brain injury __________
5. evaluates coping and adjustment to current illness and more ______________________

PRONUNCIATION PRACTICE

Say these words aloud to a friend or classmate, if you can. Here you are given the phonetic pronunciation. Your instructor can help you with pronunciation, or you can visit **http://www.MedicalLanguageLab.com.**

electroencephalogram	ē-lĕk″trō-ĕn-**sĕf**′ă-lō-grăm
kinetic	kĭ-**nĕt**′ ĭk
locus	**lō**′ kŭs
morbid	**mor**′ bĭd
pre-morbid	prē-**mor**′ bĭd
prophylactic	prō-fī-**lăk**′ tĭk
retrospective	rĕt-rō-**spĕk**′ tĭv

Recovery and rehabilitation: emotional health

Recall the conversation between two members of Gil's treatment team at the beginning of this chapter. At one point, they discussed this patient's optimistic approach to rehabilitation and recovery. This is another example of the mind-body connection at work. There is now a good deal of scientific evidence that shows that the pace of and success of recovery from trauma or surgery may depend on the patient's personality, as well as his or her psychological health and philosophical and spiritual beliefs before these medical events.

The recovery of our patient, Gil, has been going well. He has been tolerating the tasks of occupational therapy. He's mentioned that he's found them quite helpful and that they have kept him from feeling bored or ruminating about his difficult situation. He has learned a few memory assistance skills to help with his short-term memory challenges. His mood is less labile now that some of the initial swelling in his brain has subsided, and his pain levels have decreased significantly, although he continues to suffer from headaches from time to time. He has just arrived in the OT department for his last session before discharge.

Patient Update

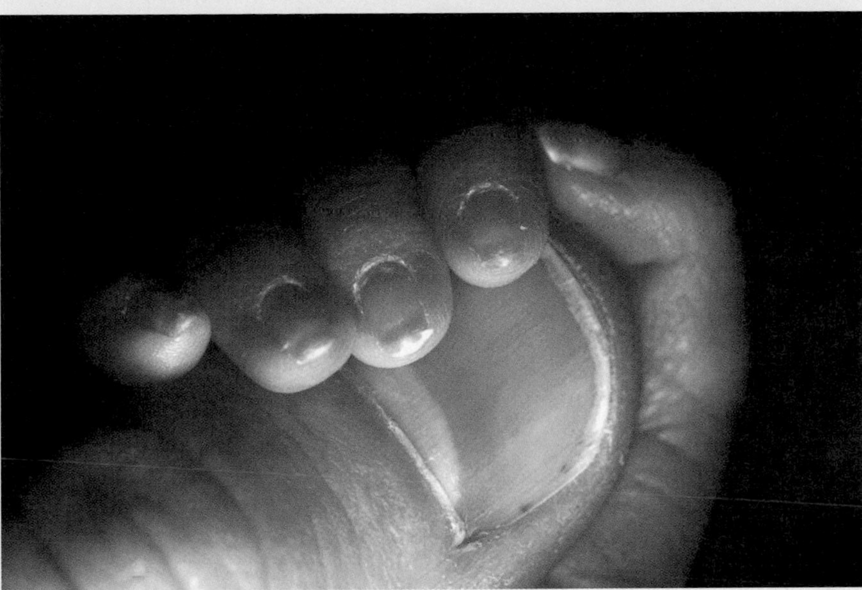

"Hello, Gil," said an OT as the patient entered the department. Maryanne rose from the chair where she had been waiting for Gil and advanced toward him. "I have a big surprise for you for your last session," she said enthusiastically. He wheeled up to her in his chair.

"A surprise? What kind of a surprise, Maryanne?" Gil found himself smiling back, caught by her infectious smile. "What are you up to?" he asked amiably.

Maryanne stooped down beside Gil so that she could speak to him face to face. She touched his arm and spoke. "Gil, I know that you're going to be discharged tomorrow and we ...," she said, waving her hand around the occupational therapy department, "well, we were talking about you and how well you've done and how many complications you've faced. We wanted to make this last day here with us not just a good one, but a healthy, healing, and inspiring one." She paused for a moment. Gil watched her, sensing her sincerity, waiting for her to go on. "Gil, I'm taking you to see your baby! To touch your baby!"

"What?" Gil said incredulously. He was speechless for a moment. Maryanne waited. "What do you mean? I can't go there. They won't let me in with this wheelchair and all my casts and things. They said I can't visit her like that. I've only been able to see her on Glory's cell phone pictures and videos and only twice have I been able to make it over there to see her through the glass window."

Maryanne explained that, because his status was pre-discharge, his treatment team (the nurses, physical therapists, and occupational therapists) had all agreed that it would be very good for him emotionally to see and touch his little girl in person. Maryanne volunteered to advocate on his behalf with the neonatal intensive care unit to arrange this visit. She added that the NICU had taken a bit of convincing but that they were quite agreeable in the end.

"We've worked this out with your wife, too, Gil," said Maryanne. Gil raised his eyebrows, amazed by all that was transpiring. "She's over there now with the baby. They're waiting for you, Gil," Maryanne said with compassion. "They're waiting for you," she almost whispered. "Let's go." Maryanne stood up, stepped behind Gil, and began to push him through the long corridors to the pediatric and obstetrics wing of Fayette General Hospital. He was quiet the whole time, lost in thought and anticipating what was to come. They arrived, and his wife, Glory, was there. She met Gil at the door to the unit and held the door open for him to enter. A nurse approached.

"Let me help you, Mr. Loeppky," the nurse said gently. She covered him lightly with a simple long-sleeved isolation gown and tied it behind his neck. She smiled. "You'll want to wear this to keep your daughter safe from any microorganisms on your clothes." Gil looked up at her and thanked her. The nurse stepped behind Gil's wheelchair and took over from Maryanne, and Glory took Gil's hand. The nurse stopped a moment and asked both parents to wash their hands with an antimicrobial preparation that she gave them. They did so, and then they maneuvered past just a few incubators before stopping in front of one.

"This is our Emily Grace, Gil," said Glory softly but proudly, squeezing Gil's hand again.

"Emily Grace," whispered Gil as the nurse wheeled him as close as possible and showed him how to reach into the incubator. Gil moved forward in the chair and reached out to touch his daughter's forehead. "She's so little," he commented to no one in particular. "Emily," he called to her softly. "Emily, it's Daddy." He had tears in his eyes as he touched his baby girl for the very first time. She opened her eyes, and then she reached out to grasp her Daddy's finger with her tiny hand.

Critical Thinking

Answer the following questions on the basis of the Patient Update.

1. Why would the treatment team think that it is health promoting to arrange this face-to-face visit for Gil and his new baby?

   ____

   ____

   ____

2. Why did the nurse put a gown over the top of Gil's clothing in the NICU?

   ____

3. Gil's daughter responded in a specific way to her father's touch. Use medical terminology to identify her response. ______________________________

CHAPTER SUMMARY

This is the end of Chapter 15, and Gil Loeppky will soon be discharged from the hospital to continue his recovery at home. In this chapter, medical terminology related to rehabilitation and recovery was introduced in the context of the patient's treatment with physical and occupational therapy. A number of PT and OT assessment tests and techniques were described to familiarize you with some of the ones that you may encounter during your health-care career. Terminology for the musculoskeletal system was enhanced as well. Many opportunities were provided to use new language in meaningful ways through critical thinking, reflection, and application to real-world scenarios.

See How Much You've Learned

For audio exercises, visit **http://www.MedicalLanguageLab.com.** 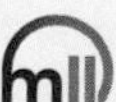

Chapter 15 has introduced you to some medical abbreviations. These have been organized into a study table here for quick reference.

TABLE 15-9: Abbreviations in Chapter 15

Abbreviation or Acronym	Meaning
BaFPE	Bay Area Functional Performance Evaluation
CAM	Cognitive Assessment of Minnesota
COTNAB	Chessington Occupational Therapy Neurological Assessment Battery

TABLE 15-9: Abbreviations in Chapter 15—cont'd

Abbreviation or Acronym	Meaning
EEG	electroencephalogram
FIM	Functional Independence Measure
GAF	Global Assessment of Functioning
GARS	Gait Assessment Rating Score
LOTCA	Loewenstein Occupational Therapy Assessment
MG	myasthenia gravis
OT	occupational therapist or occupational therapy
PEOP	people-environment-occupational-performance
PT	physical therapist or physical therapy
PAIS	Psychosocial Adjustment to Illness Scale
RBMT-3	Rivermead Behavioural Memory Test, Third Edition
TENS	transcutaneous electrical nerve stimulator

Key Terms

amyotony
atrophy
bony prominences
contraindicated
cramps
dystonia
electrical stimulation of muscles (E-stim, EMS)
electroencephalogram (EEG)
electroencephalograph
endorphin theory
gait
gate theory
Global Assessment of Functioning (GAF) Scale
grasp response
hesitancy
impulse control center
innervation
internal fixation
isometric
knee support
locomotion
locus of control
memory
mind-body connection
morbid
motor functioning
muscle tone
myotonia
Neo-natal intensive care unit (NICU)
occupational therapy (OT)
overtax
padded dressings
parallel bars
passive range-of-motion exercises
physical therapy
postural alignment
pre-morbid
prostheses
quadriceps femoris
reaction times
reciprocal innervation
rehabilitation (rehab)
removable brace
repetitions
residual effects
right-hand dominant
skin breakdown
sluggish
spasms
stave off
support
suture line
tolerate
tone
transcutaneous electrical nerve stimulation (TENS)
tremors

CHAPTER REVIEW

Critical Thinking

Use your new knowledge of medical terms and medical language to answer the following questions.

1. In anatomy and medicine, what is a *digit*?

____

2. In mathematics and medication administration, what is a *digit*?

____

3. Gil Loeppky is experiencing two cognitive deficits that occupational therapy is helping to rehabilitate. What are these cognitive deficits?

____

Agonists and Antagonists

Name the opposing muscle(s) for each muscle or muscle group listed.

1. extensor digitorum longus ________________________
2. quadriceps ________________________
3. extensor hallucis longus ________________________
4. peroneus tertius ________________________

Break It Down

Deconstruct the following medical terms into their component parts. Follow this example: musculoskeletal = muscul/o + skelet/o + al

1. myotonometer ________________________
2. locomotion ________________________
3. dystrophy ________________________
4. antagonist ________________________
5. electroencephalogram ________________________
6. anticonvulsant ________________________

Right Word or Wrong Word: *Self-Esteem* or *Self-Image?*

Do these two words have the same meaning? If not, what is the difference between them?

Label the Muscles

Label the three muscles that are identified in this diagram.

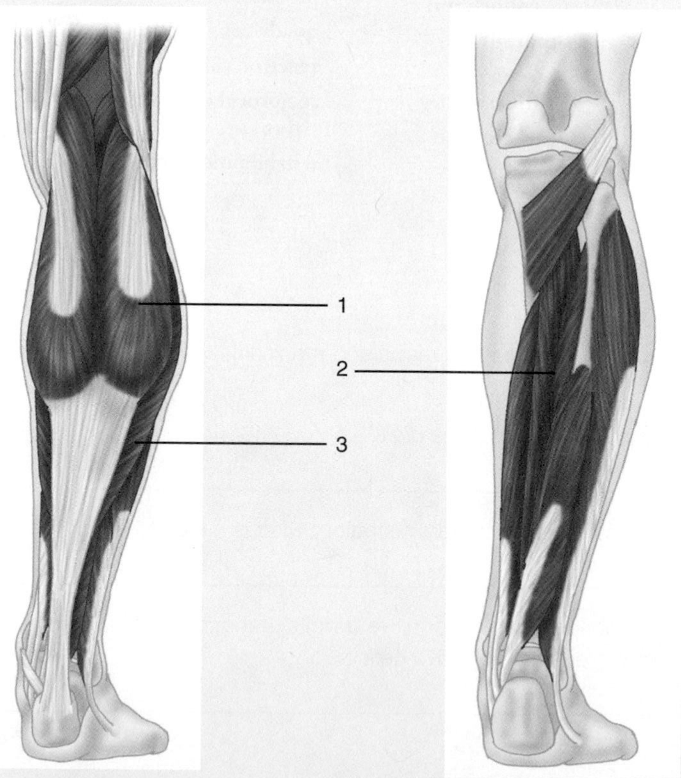

1. ____________________

2. ____________________

3. ____________________

Word Accuracy

Demonstrate that you are reading and interpreting accurately. Differentiate the following three medical terms by defining each one.

1. myotonia ____________________
2. amyotony ____________________
3. dystonia ____________________

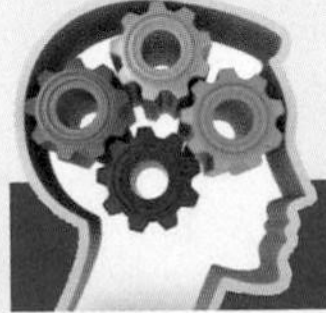

MEMORY MAGIC

Use the following mnemonics to remember which bone is which in the lower leg:

T-I-B
The tibia is the ...

Thicker
Inner
Bone

Fibula: *Little* fib (little white lie)
Tibia: *Big fat* tib (big fat lie)

The *F*ibula is thin like a *F*lute.
The *T*ibia is thick like a *T*uba.

CHAPTER SIXTEEN

The Mind–Body Connection

Focus: Mental Health, the Limbic and Immune Systems

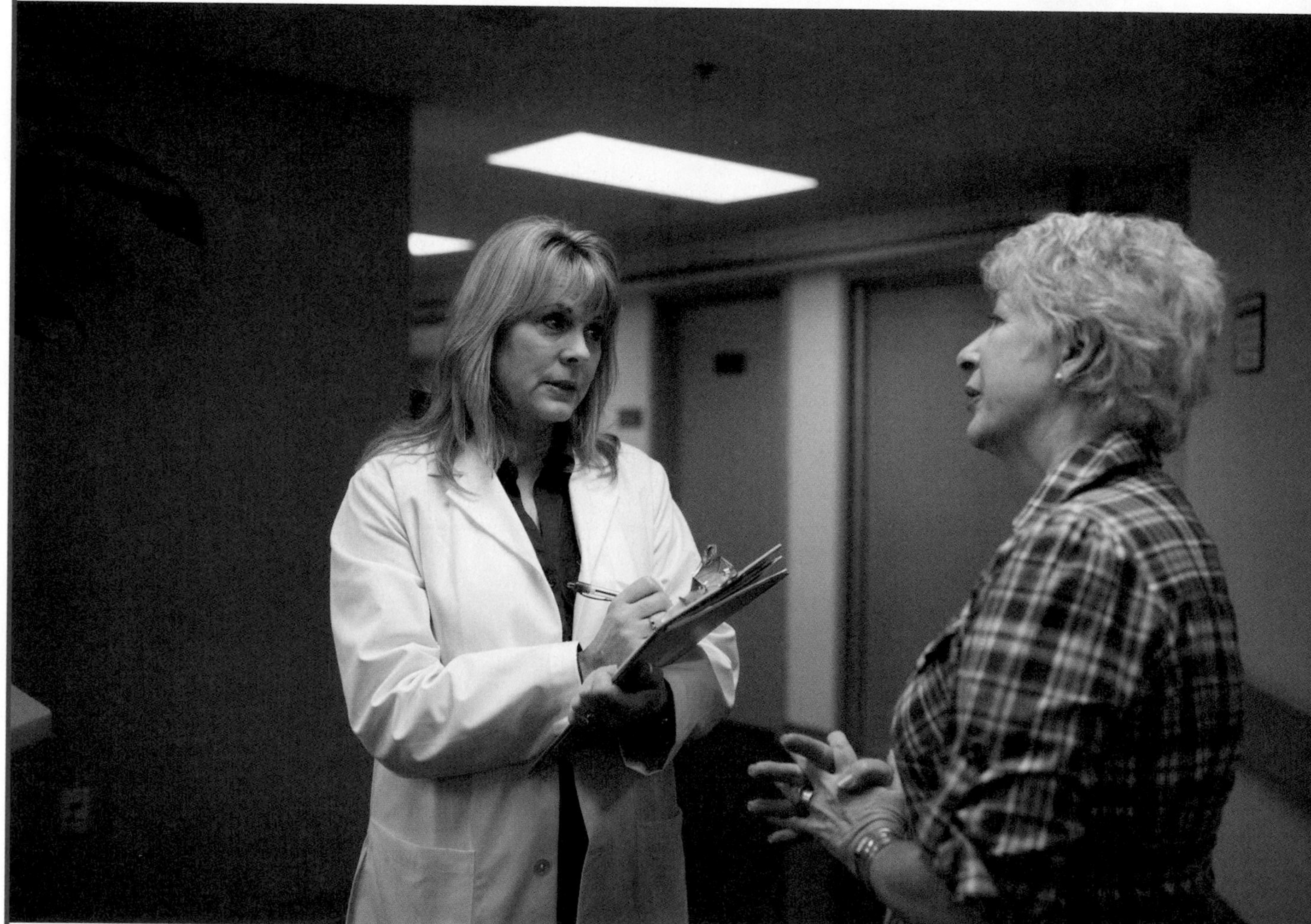

Four weeks ago, Stevie-Rose Davis, 72 years old, was in a motor vehicle accident with her husband, Zane, and her grandson, Clay. She did not incur any serious injuries during the accident, and after an overnight stay in the hospital for observation, she was quickly discharged home. Since that time, she has been taking an antidepressant to help keep her calm and to help her to sleep at night (see Chapter 12). Stevie-Rose has a number of chronic medical conditions as well. She lives with arthritis, diabetes, and thyroid challenges, which affect her everyday quality of life. While she was in the hospital, some evidence surfaced to suggest that she also suffers from post-traumatic stress disorder. However, she denies this possibility. Adding to her stress level, her husband of more than 40 years has recently been diagnosed with asbestosis and he may also be facing criminal or traffic charges arising from the motor vehicle accident.

Stevie-Rose Davis is at Sumac Veterans Medical Center (Sumac Center) today. She has asked for an appointment with a nurse practitioner in the ambulatory care clinic there—the A.L. Murphy Clinic—to discuss some of her ongoing health concerns and to get a physical exam.

Patient Update

Stevie-Rose Davis arrived precisely on time at the Sumac Center for her 10 a.m. appointment. She skirted by the medical center's main doors and headed to the southeast door and the entrance to the "Audie Murphy Clinic," as she liked to call it. She checked in with the busy MOA at the reception desk and took a seat in the waiting room. After a short time, a tall, middle-aged woman who was professionally dressed in street clothes under an open lab coat appeared at the entrance to a nearby hallway. She called Stevie-Rose's name, and Stevie-Rose followed the woman to her office.

"Good morning," said the woman, as the two of them sat down in a small, windowless office full of books and health promotion posters. She looked up then and said, "I'm Ophelia Lambert, a nurse practitioner here at Murphy Clinic. I do the intake interviews and physical examinations." She smiled warmly. "And you're Stevie-Rose Davis?" The client smiled. The nurse opened Stevie-Rose's medical record on the computer at hand. "Yes, here you are. Good. And I see that you are a retired army lieutenant? And a nurse?" Ophelia looked back at Stevie-Rose inquisitively, and Stevie-Rose confirmed this information. The women talked very briefly about Stevie-Rose's years in the service. Then, to break the ice, the nurse said, "And how can I help you today?"

"I'm not really sure," answered Stevie-Rose. "I'm feeling run down. I've got no energy to speak of, I seem to have lost my sense of humor, and ... well ... I don't know. I just seem to be dragging myself through each day. I'd like to get some blood work done to check my thyroid and diabetes, although I'm pretty sure they're okay. Maybe I've got low B_{12} or something. I'm on some medication for sleep, too, and I wonder if maybe that's too strong of a drug for me. Can we check that?" Ophelia nodded and asked Stevie-Rose a few questions about her medications. Ophelia then entered the requests on a laboratory requisition on her desktop computer.

"Please go on, Stevie-Rose. I have a sense there's more you'd like to share," said Ophelia.

"Yes, well, I've got a number of things on my mind ... a number of things," Stevie-Rose began. "I haven't been in to the clinic for a couple of years, and I thought maybe I'd start back. My life seems to have gotten complicated lately, and, well ..." She paused for a moment, looking down at her hands, thinking. The nurse encouraged her to continue and then waited patiently.

Stevie-Rose explained that she was under a lot of stress lately and wondered if it was related to physical or emotional health problems. "In the past, when I was under a lot of stress, I used to meditate and do yoga. They really helped me clear my head. I practiced them at home and sometimes with a women's group in my neighborhood." She paused a second before going on. "I learned meditation when I was posted overseas years ago, but I learned yoga here at the VA. I don't know why I gave those things up, but life happens, and I just let them slide, I guess. No discipline, I'm sorry to say." Stevie-Rose looked at the nurse as she spoke to try to gauge her reaction. Ophelia remained open in her posture and her manner as an encouragement for Stevie-Rose to continue. "My husband's sick now, and we were recently in an accident, and my grandson got injured and that was all my fault," she blurted out. "My hands hurt, and I seem to be rubbing them all the time, but maybe I'm wringing them out of nervousness instead. I just don't know." Stevie-Rose spoke more rapidly now.

"You sound anxious, and it sounds like you have a lot going on in your life right now, Stevie-Rose," Ophelia responded. "Let's slow things down a bit so that I can get some more information about each of these challenges. Then you and I can work together to try to find you some help or guidance or whatever else you may need today." The two women began to examine Stevie-Rosie's current situation and her concerns, and they talked for more than half an hour. Intermittently throughout, Ophelia made notes on Stevie-Rose's electronic medical record.

"If I may summarize, Stevie-Rose, here's what I've heard and what health matters I think need to be addressed." Ophelia stopped typing and turned to speak directly to her. The client confirmed that this was a good and timely idea. "Based on what you've been saying about your hands in particular but also about your knees, it seems that your arthritis is giving you grief. You haven't seen a rheumatologist for many years, and I would suggest that you do so now. Arthritis is a chronic and progressive disease that can cause considerable pain and discomfort. Some of your perceived inability to deal with stressors in everyday life may be related to problems with pain management."

"I don't even notice the pain in my joints. I think I'm used to that," interjected Stevie-Rose. The nurse nodded.

"While it is sometimes possible to ignore pain or to force yourself to ignore or endure pain, pain continues in the body," said Ophelia. "It is a sympathetic nervous system response to your disease of arthritis. In this case, it won't simply go away without treatment. As you know, underlying pain can affect a person's ability to concentrate, to solve problems, to experience humor, to rest comfortably, and so on. All in all, underlying chronic pain can diminish functioning and quality of life." Stevie-Rose nodded that she understood, and Ophelia continued: "I'd like to set you up with an appointment with one of our rheumatologists here at the Murphy Clinic." When she received permission from the client to do so, Ophelia typed a referral into the medical record and explained that someone from that office would contact Stevie-Rose later today or tomorrow to set up an appointment. Then she went on.

"I have also learned from you today that you have some emotional challenges right now. You are quite, quite concerned for your husband's health, and you want to be there for him as both his wife and his nurse." Ophelia smiled. "While I applaud that and would probably want to do the same thing if it were my husband, I have to caution you that your own age and health may prevent you from being that full-time nurse. I wonder if you're aware that, here at Veteran's Affairs, we offer support groups for family members and care providers. We can offer some home-care services, too, to help you care for your husband, if needed."

"Oh, no, no thanks. No home care for us. I'll take care of Zane. I know him best," said Stevie-Rose adamantly. "But ... well ... ," she hesitated, "I might be interested in a support group if you have one for spouses of ... well, he doesn't have cancer, but he does have COPD. Asbestosis, to be exact. Are there support groups for that kind of thing?" The nurse practitioner said she wasn't sure if there were groups specific to chronic illnesses such as lung disorders, but she was very pleased to hear that the client was open to the possibility of attending a group like this. Stevie-Rose mentioned that she was very familiar with support groups. She related that, when she was on active duty many years ago, she had actually run some support groups for wounded patients.

The nurse practitioner told Stevie-Rose where the counseling department was and suggested that she pop in there before leaving today to see what they had to offer in this regard. Ophelia reinforced what the client had said: that support groups could help people work through stress, doubt, fear, disease, and distress. They helped people to maintain a healthy balance in life and enhanced the ability to cope.

The nurse practitioner continued. "I'd like to talk just a bit more about your own mental health, if I may." She paused, waiting for permission. "You've told me today that you're experiencing a number of stressors above and beyond your husband's illness. You've suggested that you aren't handling these very well, am I right?" Stevie-Rose agreed. "I heard the emotion in your voice when you said that Zane might be charged with a criminal offense or a motor vehicle violation because of an accident some weeks ago."

"Yes, yes, but we spoke with our lawyer," Stevie-Rose interrupted. "He says everything's going to be okay. He says the accident was just an accident. Zane wasn't to blame. The lawyer says a charge of driving without due care and concern or whatever ..." She broke off, her voice began to rise, and her words came more quickly again, which was clear evidence of her anxiety about this situation. She was wringing her hands again as she spoke. Ophelia intervened; she had Stevie-Rose take a couple of deep breaths to calm herself before proceeding. Stevie-Rose explained that an investigation was still ongoing and that the driver of the other vehicle was still being investigated as well. The nurse practitioner validated her client's efforts to follow through with a lawyer and suggested that they move on to the rest of the summary.

"We've been talking about your stressors, and clearly we've just identified two major psychological stressors in your life right now. However, I also heard the distress and anxiety in your voice when you told me about the accident and the injuries incurred by your grandson. Correct me if I'm wrong, but I think that is your third major stressor." Ophelia paused while Stevie-Rose confirmed this. "I'd like to talk to you about how you're coping in more detail. For example, you told me about your sleep pattern. You explained that you have been prone to insomnia of late but that, since the motor vehicle accident, you have been sleeping better. You believe that is due to the effects of an antidepressant medication that a physician prescribed for your insomnia and restlessness. However, you're also worried that the med is too strong for you. Am I right so far?" Stevie-Rose nodded. She mentioned her surprise that this type of drug would be able to improve her sleeping, and she hoped that she wouldn't have to stop taking it right now. Ophelia acknowledged what Stevie-Rose had said and then went on.

"You've mentioned that you're having some difficulties concentrating, too. You feel distracted or disconnected sometimes," the nurse practitioner said.

"It's as if my mind goes vacant and I just seem to drift away," said Stevie-Rose. "Funny, it's not like a daydream, because there don't seem to be any thoughts or images. I just go blank." Ophelia made a sound of acknowledgment and then entered this information into the client's medical record.

"Have there been any changes in your diet?" asked Ophelia. Stevie-Rose confirmed that she seemed to have lost her appetite, and she noted that this was typical for her when she was under a lot of pressure.

Ophelia Lambert, RN, NP, then went on to share her clinical thoughts. "All right. You're certainly dealing with three major psychological stressors, as well as a possible physical stressor of some exacerbation or progression of your arthritis." Stevie-Rose concurred, and Ophelia continued. "I've referred you to someone for the physical aspect of your health, but we need to address your emotional health." Ophelia went on to explain that Stevie-Rose was exhibiting some symptoms of anxiety but also of depression and that Stevie-Rose had given some historical evidence of having had struggles with her emotional or psychological health before. Stevie-Rose nodded. They talked a bit more about that, exploring what the contributing factors might be, including any unresolved issues that may cause these symptoms to recur from time to time. Ophelia was about to broach the subject of post-traumatic stress disorder when suddenly the client spoke up.

"I was in Vietnam in a MASH unit for a year and a half. I have nightmares about it. Things in my day suddenly remind me of it. It plagues me ... it haunts me," Stevie-Rose said, glancing upward and around the room as she began wringing her hands. She then looked directly at the nurse. "I've got it," she said firmly. "I don't want to have it, but I've got it." Stevie-Rose paused for a split second. "I've got PTSD, and I don't know what to do about it." Ophelia Lambert picked up the phone and called the PTSD counselor on duty.

Reflective Questions

Reflect on the dialogue that you've just read as you answer the following questions.

1. Why has Stevie-Rose Davis made an appointment to speak with a nurse practitioner today?

   ____

2. Which physical symptom might be causing some of Stevie-Rose's psychological or emotional difficulties? Name those difficulties.

   ____

Critical Thinking

Consider all that you've learned about Stevie-Rose Davis—during this interaction and others—to answer the following questions.

1. What is PTSD? ______________________________
2. Why is Stevie-Rose referred to as a "client" in this most recent scenario?
____

For audio exercises, visit **http://www.MedicalLanguageLab.com.** 

Learning Objectives

After reading Chapter 16, you will be able to do the following:

- Enhance your vocabulary and knowledge related to mental health concepts.
- Understand the concept of the mind-body connection and its relationship to health and healing.
- Enhance your vocabulary and knowledge related to the anatomy and physiology of the brain.
- Gain an appreciation of the different functions of the right brain as compared with the left brain.
- Understand and use terminology that applies to the limbic system.
- Appreciate the relationship between the limbic system and emotional health.
- Appreciate the education, training, and work of counselors.
- Enhance your knowledge of terminology related to the immune system.
- Understand and acquire terminology that applies to the concept of autoimmunity.
- Acquire language and knowledge related to allergies.
- Understand the education, training, and work of a rheumatologist.
- Enhance vocabulary and use terminology related to the joints.
- Understand and use medical terms for the disease of arthritis.
- Acquire and use terminology related to aging.
- Acquire and use terminology related to chronicity.
- Identify and explain common treatment modalities for health maintenance and for the promotion of the health of the mind and the body.

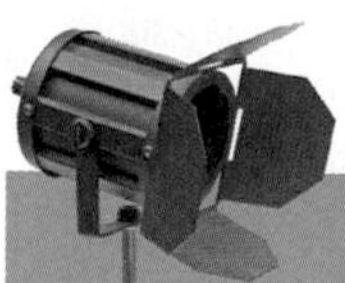

CAREER SPOTLIGHT: Counselor

Counselors are not health professionals per se, although their education certainly includes core coursework in the broad field of mental health: psychology, group and individual counseling, growth and development, and counseling techniques. This background facilitates their work in the area of mental health and wellness, which are core components of their profession. Counselors often function as guides, facilitators, or problem solvers in the realm of interpersonal relationships and behavioral challenges. They work with people who are facing everyday challenges of coping and role functioning. This work may occur in one-to-one counseling sessions, in groups, or with families.

Unless counselors have specialized (i.e., in mental health or illness, addictions, or rehabilitation), it is not likely that they have had education and training in biology, anatomy, physiology, medical terminology, pharmacology, or other core subjects that are part of a standard health sciences curriculum. Even so, counselors are key members of multidisciplinary health care teams. They hold positions in outpatient and private clinics, schools, vocational centers, rehabilitation and substance abuse centers, and a variety of other support centers in the community. They work with people across the life span to help them cope with issues in the here and now. They do not provide psychotherapy, which deals with a person's past and with his or her issues in the present, unless they have specific advanced training.

Education and training for counselors varies by state and by the counselor's specialty. A graduate degree (i.e., a master's degree) is required to become a *licensed professional counselor* (LPC). Educational counselors may require certification before they can practice. Professional counselors are those with graduate degrees from accredited university programs. A counselor who attains a doctoral degree may apply to become a licensed psychologist.

Note that there are many people who work in the capacity of counselors; however, they may or may not be professionally qualified to do so. Some counselors are *paraprofessionals* and may have received training through an employer, a self-help group, or a diploma program at a lesser level of education than that required to be considered fully professional. These counselors should be working under the supervision of an LPC, an advanced practice psychiatric nurse, a psychologist, a psychiatrist, a physician, or another fully qualified professional.

Right Word or Wrong Word: *Counselor, Therapist,* or *Psychologist*?

Are these three terms interchangeable? Is the work of a counselor the same as the work of a therapist or a psychologist? Are their qualifications the same? Explain.

The Mind-Body Connection: Enhanced Vocabulary

The concept of the mind-body connection was first introduced in Chapter 15. This concept involves the belief that how people think about themselves and their situations can positively or negatively affect the ways that they are able to deal with those situations. Simply put, the mind-body connection implies that negative thoughts and energy lead to negative outcomes. For example, if you do not believe that you will recover from an illness, your recovery will involve a much more difficult and lengthy process. This philosophical stance is not uncommon in health care. In the opening scenario of this chapter, the mind-body connection is suggested in the interaction between the client and the nurse practitioner. Notice the links that are made between the client's thoughts and emotions (i.e., her psychological health) and her physical symptoms and conditions (i.e., her physical health).

The mind-body connection is linked through the autonomic nervous system and particularly via the limbic system, which is described in more detail later in this chapter.

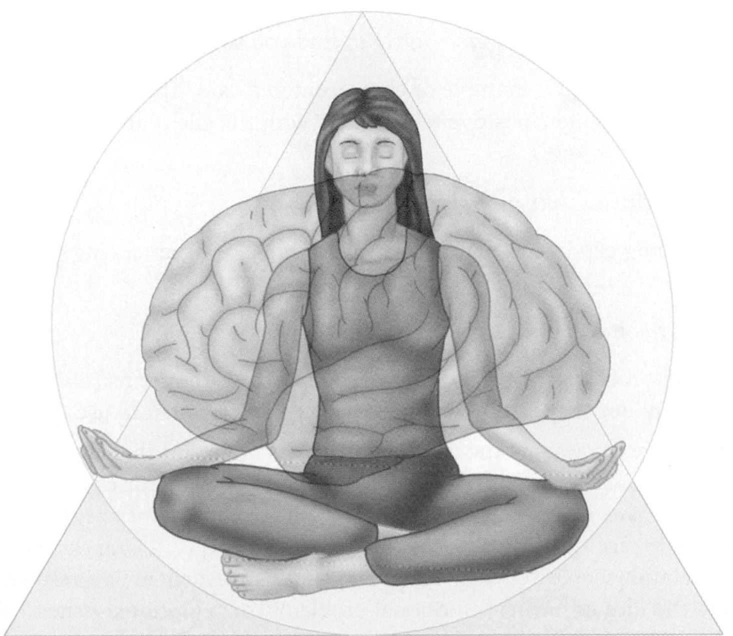

Figure 16.1: The mind-body connection

Key terms: mind-body connection

In the Patient Update at the beginning of this chapter, our client, Stevie-Rose Davis, was speaking with a nurse practitioner named Ophelia Lambert. They used a combination of colloquialisms and medical language in their conversation. The context of the interaction was the client's sense that she was not functioning as well as she should be, either physically or mentally. To that end, Stevie-Rose is looking for an assessment of her physical and mental health, as well as for suggestions regarding health and healing initiatives that encompass the mind-body philosophy. Terms and phrases from this interaction are italicized in the example and highlighted below with the explanation.

"I do the *intake interviews* ..."

intake interviews: medical jargon that refers to the admission interviews that are used to assess the patient's needs and wants.

"I'm *feeling run down.*"

feeling run down: an expression that describes a sense of low energy or not feeling well. The medical term for a nondescript sense of not feeling well is *malaise.* Stevie-Rose Davis has a general sense of malaise.

"I've *got no energy to speak of* ..."

got no energy to speak of: a colloquialism that describes a sense of low energy. A more formal way to say this is "I don't seem to have any energy" or "I haven't got any energy."

"Maybe I've got low B_{12} or something."

B_{12}: a vitamin that assists with the maintenance of the central nervous system and that facilitates metabolism and the formation of red blood cells. A person's B_{12} level can be measured with a simple blood test. Physical symptoms of having a low level of B_{12} can include low levels of energy, fatigue, numbness in the hands and feet, difficulty concentrating, and mood lability.

"... *open in her posture and her manner* ..."

open in her posture and manner: professional behavior on the part of the health-care professional that helps to build a relationship in which the client will feel at ease and thus able to speak freely. This is an interpersonal communication skill that is used in the health professions. It is a form of nonverbal body language that communicates a nonjudgmental, warm, open, patient, and willing attitude.

"Then *you and I can work together* to try to find you some help or guidance ..."

you and I can work together: an example of client-centered care. This phrase is commonly used in health care to build a positive relationship with the client and to create a sense of partnership.

"... your arthritis is *giving you grief.*"

giving you grief: a slang expression that means that a person is experiencing pain, aggravation, or discomfort.

"... you have some *emotional challenges* right now."

emotional challenges: medical jargon. Although you may hear the terms *issues* or *problems* in your own work, try not to use these words. It is more professional to use the term *challenges.*

The word **challenge** suggests to the client that there is hope and that something can be overcome. The word *problem* is rarely used in health care today because it carries a negative connotation or association that may subtly encourage patients or clients to think that they won't be able to face the difficulties of treatment or recovery. Using the word *challenges* is especially helpful when discussing emotional issues with a client as a result of the stigma attached to the idea of having "emotional problems" or "emotional issues." These phrases seem to suggest that the patient has a mental illness, and there is still a great stigma attached to mental illness in our society.

Stigma refers to the shame attached to negative labels. This may be shame felt for oneself or demonstrated by others who feel shamed or ashamed. It is usually caused by misunderstanding or a lack of knowledge about a condition.

"... we offer *support groups* for family members and care providers."

support groups: groups of patients, family members, friends, significant others, or coworkers who come together voluntarily to seek emotional support and information about specific issues. No matter where you work in health care, you will become acquainted with a wide variety of support groups that help clients and patients to transition through physical or mental health challenges or to deal with the everyday challenges of chronic physical or mental illness. Table 16-1 provides some examples of organizations that offer support groups that appreciate the mind-body connection. In other words, they employ a holistic approach (see Chapter 15).

"... she had actually *run* some support groups ..."

run: medical jargon for having facilitated or led something.

TABLE 16-1: Support Groups with a Holistic Approach

Support Group	Description
Irritable Bowel Syndrome Self-Help and Support Group	• provides an online support group for persons with this diagnosis, including forums, blogs, pen pals, and meeting opportunities
Al-Anon/Alateen	• offers self-help groups to strengthen and facilitate hope for friends and families of alcoholics, including providing an understanding of the disease process
Mothers Against Drunk Driving (MADD)	• offers psychological support groups for the families and friends of victims of drunk drivers
National Breast Cancer Foundation: Support Network	• provides support for women with breast cancer and their supporters (i.e., friends, family members, significant others) through an online community, including providing an understanding of the disease process
Us TOO International: Prostate Cancer Education and Support Network	• offers links to regional support meetings and groups for men who have been diagnosed with prostate cancer • offers support groups for significant others, family members, and friends; health professionals are also invited • includes discourse and dialogue to help provide an understanding of the disease process
Depression and Bipolar Support Alliance (DBSA)	• offers online and in-person support groups for individuals with either or both of these diagnoses, as well as for their families, friends, and significant others • includes discourse and dialogue to help provide an understanding of the disease process
Brain Injury Association of America	• provides links to regional support groups that focus on teaching affected individuals about brain injury, that offer information about available services, and that provide opportunities to meet with others who are facing or who have faced similar challenges
The Wounded Warrior Project	• offers support for military personnel who have been wounded during service • focuses on the well-being of family members and care providers; offers caregiver retreats (therapeutic getaways) with support groups and peers to assist with coping, hardiness, and resiliency
Operation Home Front: Wounded Warriors' Wives	• offers support groups and assistance for wives of military personnel who have been wounded during service • focuses on developing and supporting knowledge and skills, including interpersonal skills, coping, hardiness, and resiliency in preparation for caring for a person with a lifelong disability • offers support for transition and coping while the person with the disability and his or her spouse come to terms with the changes taking place in their lives

"... worried that the *med is too strong* for you ..."

med is too strong: a medical phrase that suggests that the amount or dosage of a medication is stronger than necessary to achieve a therapeutic effect and that this same amount is causing a number of adverse side effects.

"... or *disconnected* sometimes ..."

disconnected: a medical descriptor for a client's sense of being apart from his or her external world or surroundings. Some people describe this as feeling like they are watching the events occur around them as if they are in some sort of waking dream and not really participating. This feeling can be brought about by some types of medications, certain mental health issues, and hypnosis or psychological shock. Another medical term for this feeling is *depersonalized.*

"... when she was *under a lot of pressure.*"

under a lot of pressure: a colloquialism to describe what in medical language this would be translated as *was experiencing numerous stressors.*

"... to share her *clinical thoughts.*"

clinical thoughts: medical jargon that refers to well-informed, well-thought-out, and medically based thoughts, ideas, conclusions, and so on. Clinical thoughts do not include personal (as compared with professional) opinions or judgments about the client's situation or health.

"... was *exhibiting* some symptoms ..."

exhibiting: demonstrating, showing, or expressing.

Chronicity

Ophelia, the nurse practitioner, used the word *chronic* with our client several times. A **chronic** illness or medical condition is one that lasts for a very long time. It is not easily cured, if it even ever is. Synonyms for the word *chronic* are *constant, unremitting, continual, unrelieved,* and *persistent.*

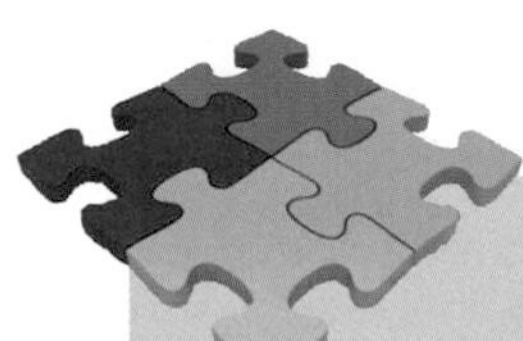

WORD BUILDING: Formulas for Creating Words from the Combining Form *chron/o*

chronos **= a Greek root word meaning *time*. In modern English, the root word is *chronic*, which means *persisting over a long period of time.* The combining form is *chron/o*.**

chrono + ology = *chronology*

Definition: the science of determining the dates of events in sequential order of time. *noun*

Example: Patient records are an example of a written *chronology*.

chrono + onc + ology = *chrono-oncology*

Definition: a type of anticancer treatment. *noun*

Example: The practice of *chrono-oncology* focuses on the timing of the administration of a drug to a patient.

chrono + tropic = *chronotropic*

Definition: affecting the rate of movements that are rhythmic. The suffix *-tropic* means *having the ability to influence. adjective*

Example: *Chronotropic* drugs can affect the heart rate and heart rhythm and thus must be used with care.

algesi + chrono + meter = *algesichronometer*

Definition: an assessment instrument that records how long it takes for pain to be perceived. (*Algesi* is a combining form that is derived from *algesia*, meaning *pain*.) *noun*

Example: An *algesichronometer* may be used to assess pain perception and tolerance in patients with neuromuscular diseases or paralysis.

chrono + pharmac + ology = *chronopharmacology*

Definition: the study of the effects of medications on the timing of certain biological events and rhythms. *noun*

Example: The birth control pill is an example of how the principles of *chronopharmacology* are applied to contraception.

Right Word or Wrong Word: *Chronic* or *Chorionic*?

Are these two medical terms the same? Is one spelled differently because it is the more formal, technical version of the word?

Critical Thinking

You have encountered the career of nurse practitioner a number of times in this textbook. You'll need that knowledge to answer this question.

What is a nurse practitioner? ____

____

Fill In the Blanks

Use terminology from the Patient Update at the beginning of this chapter to complete the following sentences.

1. Excessive worrying is an example of an _________ health challenge.
2. In our earlier encounters with Stevie-Rose Davis, she was _________ some confusion, but she is completely alert and oriented today.
3. When Stevie-Rose accompanied her husband for assessment in Chapter 14, Dr. Jacob Sweetgrass met with the couple at the end of the day to share his _________ thoughts.
4. When you arrive at a health-care facility, at least two people speak to you to complete an _________ form about why you've come.
5. Stress and certain medications can cause a sensation of being depersonalized or _________ from your body and your environment.
6. The way that a health professional sits or stands during one-to-one time with a patient or client is referred to as professional _________.
7. Body language that invites another person to continue to speak is referred to as _________.

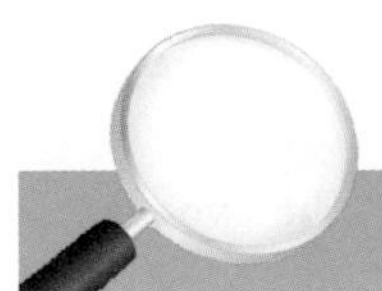

FOCUS POINT: A Veterans' Medical Center

A *veterans' medical center* is a hospital that provides full in-patient clinical and medical services for veterans and members of their immediate families. Such a center will also include a pharmacy, dietary services, physical and occupational therapy, prosthetics and auditory services, and psychiatry and psychology services.

A *veterans' medical clinic* provides ambulatory care services just as any other medical clinic might. The clients at these clinics are outpatients. Such clinics also provide a wide range of mental health and addiction services, rehabilitation programs, and family support programs.

Principles of the mind-body connection

All illnesses and traumas elicit emotional and psychological responses, in addition to the physical response of the body's immune system. For example, the physical sense of pain affects the mind when a person starts to think about or anticipate the pain. When cognition or thinking about the pain is combined with an emotion such as dread or fear, the degree of pain experienced when it does physically occur can be greater.

Just as physical symptoms can elicit emotional responses, emotions can also elicit physical symptoms. When an emotion is triggered by a stimulus, the emotional stimulus-response center of the brain, the hypothalamus, is activated, and a physical response occurs. An example of this is the loss of a loved one. The emotion of grief originates in the mind (the psyche), but it is also experienced quite physically through crying, sobbing, nervous or restless behavior, changes in appetite (even stomach pain or diarrhea), headaches, and so on.

According to the mind-body connection, the right side of the brain is an important source of health and healing. Shifting from the logical, workaday left side of the brain, where we often spend most of our psychic energy, to the right side—which is more creative, visual, and holistic—can help to restore a balance in the flow of energy in the brain. Although humans are naturally prone to do this, the circumstances of life can upset this delicate balance.

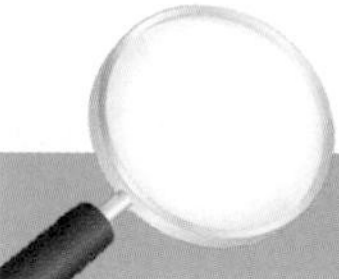

FOCUS POINT: Psychic Energy

In the context of medicine, *psychic energy* is a term that arises from the field of psychology. It refers to the physiology behind the thoughts, the emotions, and their accompanying behaviors, as well as the biochemical production of energy in the brain that facilitates its function. Energy patterns in the brain can be detected by PET, MRI, and other scans. For example, some brain scans can observe where energy flows in the brain when you are suddenly asked to sing while you are being scanned. A PET scan is particularly helpful for assessing energy flow and consumption by the brain. It can even detect simple psychological changes when they occur (see Figure 16-2). Psychic energy is also referred to as *mental energy*.

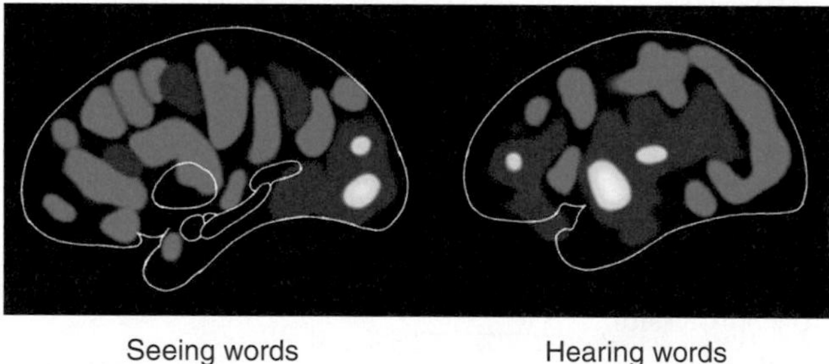

Figure 16.2: Positron emission tomography scan showing a map of psychic energy

Enhanced brain anatomy: centers of function

Chapter 7 differentiated the concept of the mind from that of the physical brain. The two are inextricably linked. **Inextricably** means that two or more things are so intricately enmeshed or combined that one of them cannot be separated from the other. To fully understand the mind, it is essential to understand more about how the brain functions.

In Chapter 10, you studied the anatomy and physiology of the brain and the central nervous system. Now, explore the sites of many more activities that are part of the brain by studying Figure 16-3. Notice the locations or centers of various brain functions. As you do so, consider how a trauma to a particular lobe of the brain may disrupt a person's cognitive or emotional functioning. For example, in Chapter 15, the treatment team was concerned that there may be damage to Gil Loeppky's occipital lobe. They were worried that, if he had suffered such damage, he could have some impairment of muscle coordination. Luckily, this was not the case.

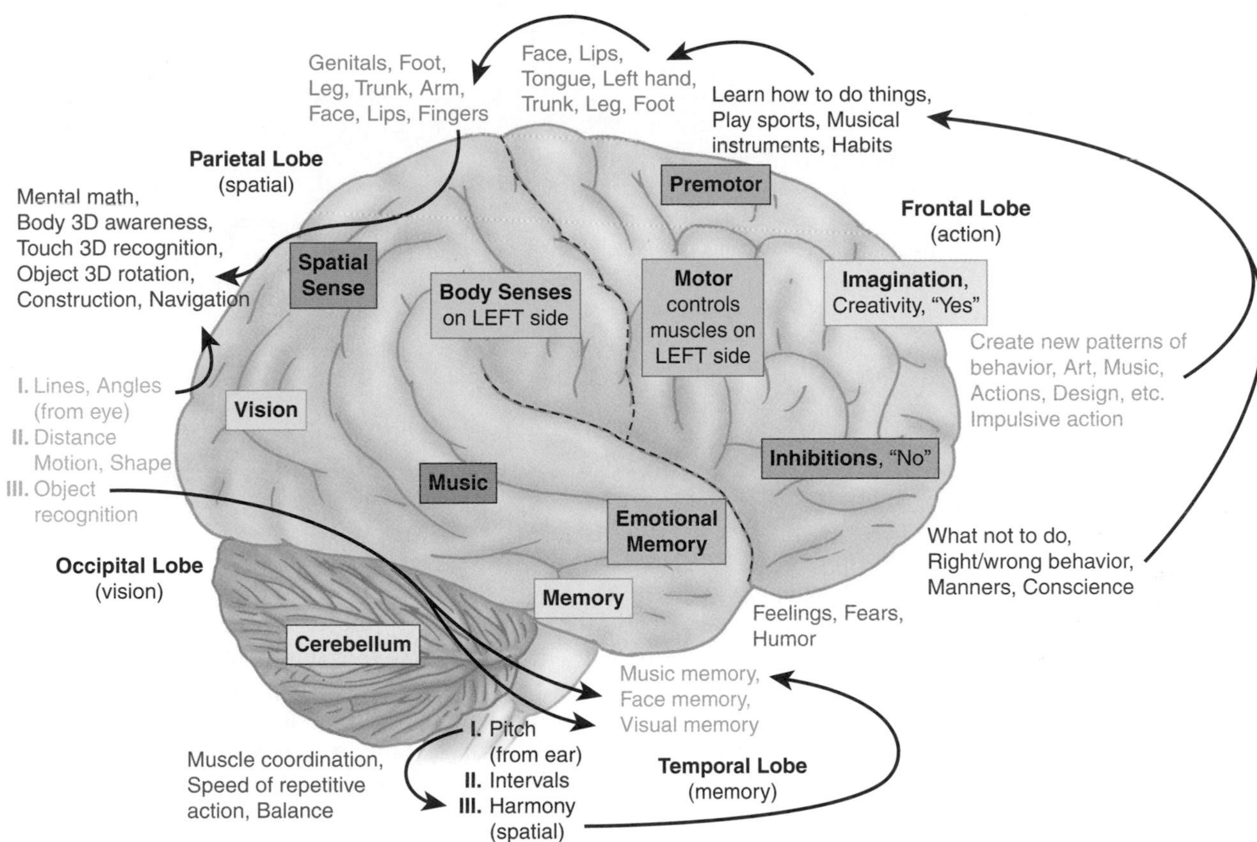

Figure 16.3: Map of the brain showing centers of function

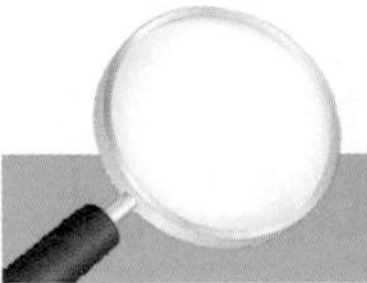

FOCUS POINT: Mapping the Mind vs. Mind Map

Mapping the mind is a medical and diagnostic term that is used to refer to exploring the brain's function and finding the functional centers of the brain. An example can be seen in Figure 16-3. Mapping the mind or mapping the brain is the purview of the field of neurology.

Alternatively, a *mind map* is a cognitive tool that is used to enhance a person's clarity of thought and to help a person sort through the relationships among his or her ideas and to come to a clear understanding of them. Mind maps show branches of ideas that stem from a central core thought or concept. Figure 16-4 shows an example of a mind map that Stevie-Rose Davis might make about concepts related to her husband's illness.

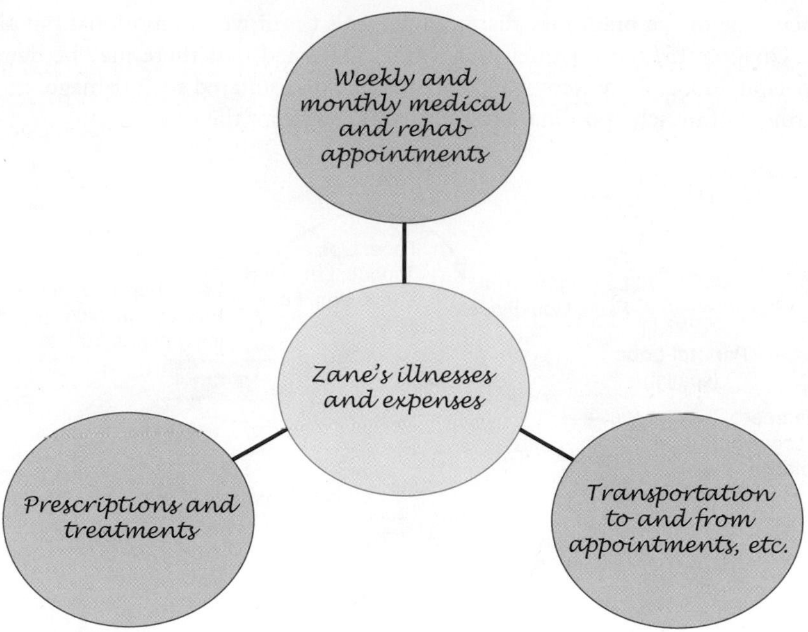

Figure 16.4: Sample mind map written by Stevie-Rose Davis

Left brain function and right brain function

The brain can be divided into two *hemispheres*—the left hemisphere and the right hemisphere—that run midline from the frontal lobe to the occipital lobe. Research into the functions of the brain has mapped these hemispheres for their functions. Figure 16-5 further identifies which functions lay on which side of the brain. Notice that these functions are singular: they are not paired with a partner on the other side of the brain. The importance of this fact is that injury to a particular center may mean impaired functioning or the full loss of that specific function. The brain can only sometimes compensate for the loss of a center of function. The brain and the mind have the ability to learn to compensate for a loss but not necessarily replace it. **Compensate** is a common term in medicine that means to counterbalance, to offset, or to oppose or mitigate (lessen) the effects of something.

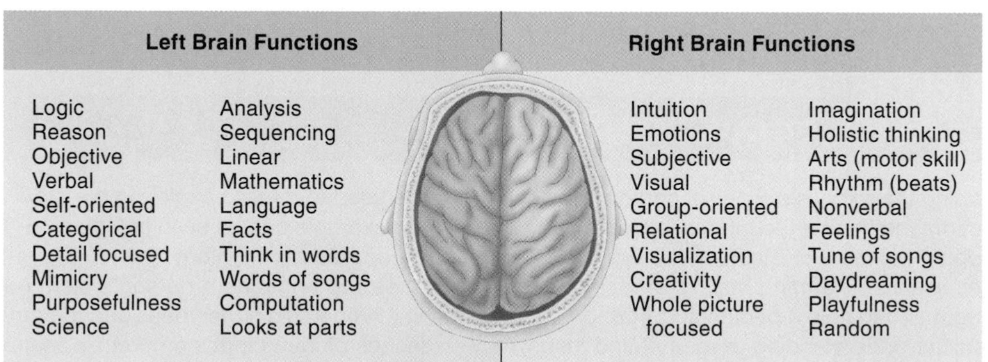

Figure 16.5: Left brain functions vs. right brain functions

Right Word or Wrong Word: *Compensate* or *Complement*?

These two words seem similar, but are they? Can they be used interchangeably? Explain.

Critical Thinking

Consider what you know about Stevie-Rose Davis's mental health. In Chapter 7, you observed her having a flashback related to her experiences years ago when she was serving in Vietnam. Apply that knowledge and the new information from Figure 16-5 as you answer this question.

From where in the physical brain do flashbacks arise? ______________________

Let's Practice

Answer the following questions on the basis of Figures 16-3 and 16-5.

1. What is the term for the ability to add and subtract in your head without the use of a pen, paper, or calculator? ______________________
2. If you're busy and preoccupied or if you've suffered a brain injury, you may see someone whom you are sure that you know, but you just can't place the person's identity. You can't remember their name or from exactly where you know them. What center of the brain is not functioning clearly at this moment, and where is it located? ______________________
3. The last portion of the brain to fully develop is the occipital lobe. For that reason, teens and some young adults are not good at making decisions. How do they often react or respond? ______________________
4. A very busy and growing part of the brain during the preschool and primary (elementary) school days is the ______________________.
5. One of the first signs of the onset of a dementia such as Alzheimer's disease is the inability to do basic arithmetic. Where is this center located in the brain? ______________________
6. Sometimes you hear a song on the radio or the television and that song sticks with you all day long. What part of the brain has been engaged? ______________________

Supporting the mind-body connection

Health care providers are increasingly focusing on the mind-body connection by incorporating health promotion and healing activities into care planning with and for patients and clients. Table 16-2 provides some examples of how this new awareness is put into action and describes some techniques and their possible benefits. You may or may not believe in the efficacy of some of these techniques, but it is important to recognize that they exist and are used by many Americans. As a health-care provider in any field, you may have opportunities to hear or use these terms in your work.

Endorphins

Endorphins play a significant role in the mind-body connection. An **endorphin** is a substance that is produced in the brain. It is a neurotransmitter that has an *opioid* or analgesic effect. There are many types of endorphins.

Opioid refers to synthetic narcotics or opium-like substances. The term breaks down as follows:

opium (Latin) + eidos (Greek) = opioid
↓ ↓
opium + shape

Opium is a narcotic substance that is obtained from certain types of poppy flowers. It has analgesic properties, it is addictive, and it alters the user's level of consciousness.

An **opiate** is a drug that contains opium.

Endorphins respond to stimuli such as pain and stress, whether physical or psychological. They are natural painkillers (analgesics) that lower the heart rate, decrease blood pressure, improve airflow to the lungs, and promote a healthy immune system. At certain high levels, endorphins can induce a sense of happiness, joy, and euphoria. Certain foods, drugs, and beverages can also stimulate the release of endorphins.

TABLE 16-2: Health Initiatives That Support the Mind-Body Connection

Initiative	Definition or Description	Mind-Body Connection: Benefits
Physical exercise	• includes all types of exercise, especially those that promote healthy circulation (i.e., aerobics) and that enhance blood flow to the brain	*Mind:* decreases anxiety; improves concentration and academic performance *Body:* enhances circulation; improves physical strength and endurance; promotes physical growth and development; staves off diminishing physical and functional effects of aging; maintains optimal body weight; releases endorphins
Nutrition	• provides energy sources for physical and mental activities	*Mind:* improves attentiveness and concentration; improves alertness *Body:* assists with weight loss or the maintenance of a healthy weight; enhances immunity
Visualization (creative imagery performed by oneself or guided imagery facilitated by a therapist)	• involves envisioning positive images in the mind and focusing on them • images may be related to psychosocial stressors or physical health challenges; positive thoughts may also accompany these	*Mind:* promotes relaxation and relief from stress or anxiety; enhances ability to focus (Envisioning oneself as healthy or free of pain provides a goal and a state of being for which the mind and body can strive.) *Body:* allows the body to physically relax so that healing may occur and pain can be managed; increases the release of endorphins (Focusing on a positive or healthy image alters the brain waves in a manner that has a calming and healing effect.)
Meditation	• a technique of focusing inward while ignoring the external world and its stressors	*Mind:* calms the mind; promotes a sense of well-being; decreases depression, anxiety, moodiness, and irritability *Body:* potentially positively alters brain waves and flow of energy, thus increasing the release of endorphins
Mindfulness	• a conscious state of being fully aware of your existence in the immediate, present time • a technique of focusing inward • a type of meditation • provides a technique for reaching a relaxed state of mind and body	*Mind:* improves mood and self-awareness; promotes relaxation; enhances observation of one's physical and emotional surroundings, as well as coping and problem-solving *Body:* enhances immune system function
Therapeutic touch	• a noncontact technique during which the practitioner's hands are moved over energy fields of the client's body to restore balance (i.e., the hands skim the body)	*Mind:* reduces anxiety; promotes relaxation; improves ability to think and cope with stress *Body:* reduces pain and high blood pressure; enhances the immune system
Deep breathing	• a conscious state of tuning into one's breathing and changing its rhythm and rate	*Mind:* provides stress release (calming effect) and clarity of thinking *Body:* improves oxygenation of the brain (which leads to the ability to think more clearly); enhances the immune function that is present in the respiratory tract; decreases high blood pressure; releases endorphins; relaxes muscles
Yoga	• a discipline of mastering one's own thoughts and bodily processes that includes specific practices of meditation, diet, and exercise	*Mind:* leads to a state of tranquility and insight *Body:* improves ability to control own blood pressure, body temperature, and brain waves (i.e., calming or slowing them); improves ventilation and respiration; positively affects metabolism

Sleep and the Mind-Body Connection

The human body cannot function at its optimal level without adequate sleep. For example, most adults need 7.5 to 8 hours of sleep per night to function at their best.

Sleep lowers the metabolism and allows the body to slow down and function less vigorously. During this rest period, cells, tissues, and organs are able to grow, regenerate, or heal. The immune system is able to work more efficiently when less stress (whether physical or mental) is coming its way. This is the situation during sleep. For these reasons, sleep has a physical healing effect. However, sleep also affects the mind. Lack of sleep leads to irritability, low frustration tolerance, heightened distractibility, some degree of clumsiness, and other symptoms of impaired mental functioning.

Let's Practice

Write the term that fits each definition.

1. a neurochemical that is an analgesic substance ______________________
2. a natural state that is characterized by a full loss of consciousness ______________________
3. a narcotic that is produced by a specific type of poppy ______________________
4. a type of drug that alleviates pain but that also alters consciousness ______________________
5. a technique of focusing inward to clear the mind ______________________
6. a health-promoting or healing technique that simulates touch without involving actual touching ______________________

Critical Thinking

In your own words, explain how sleep and the mind-body connection are related.

1. How does a lack of sleep influence physical health, which then influences mental health?

____

____

____

2. How does a lack of sleep influence mental health, which then influences physical health?

____

____

PRONUNCIATION PRACTICE

Say these words aloud to a friend or classmate, if you can. Here you are given the phonetic pronunciation. Your instructor can help you with pronunciation,

or you can visit **http://www.MedicalLanguageLab.com.** mll

chronic	**krŏn**´ĭk
chronotropic	krŏn˝ō-**trŏp**´ĭk
chorionic	kō´rē-**ŏn**´ĭk
endorphin	ĕn-**dor**´fĭn
neurochemical	nū˝rō-**kĕm**´ĭkl
opioid	**ō**´pē-oyd
opiate	**ō**´pē-ăt
psychic	**sī**´kĭk

Mental Health: Enhanced Terminology

Detailed definitions and explanations of mental health and mental illness appear in Chapter 7. Recall that **mental health** is a state of mental well-being that allows a person to cope with life, to function effectively to take care of himself or herself, and to achieve a sense of wellness, satisfaction, or contentment.

Mental wellness is achieved when a person is able to maintain a positive attitude and an appropriate physical and psychological balance in his or her personal life. This balance can be assessed though a number of domains or dimensions including a positive attitude and an appropriate balance of aspects of one's personal life and interpersonal relationships that enhance and maintain that attitude (see Chapter 7). These domains can be used for assessment purposes to determine a client's strengths, weaknesses, resiliency, and hardiness. For example, in the domain of psychological wellness, an assessment of a person's coping strategies, personal characteristics, past experiences with the stressor, and so on can produce baseline data from which a health-care provider can begin working with the client to restore balance and thus to restore a state of mental health.

Right Word or Wrong Word: *Domains* or *Dimensions* of Health?

Are these two words interchangeable? Do they both refer to the multiple aspects of a person's life that contribute to his or her state of health?

Our client, Stevie-Rose Davis is not mentally ill, but she is also not completely mentally well. She acknowledges this fact. She is experiencing and exhibiting certain signs and symptoms that confirm the fact that she may not be coping well with current stressors. Stevie-Rose's mental health situation includes the following:

- *stressors:* numerous family issues and possible pain management issues related to her arthritis. The fact that her husband is ill may also prevent her from enjoying some of the social activities in which they are involved, such as square dancing.
- *signs, symptoms, and behaviors:* a recent history of insomnia, the use of a psychotropic medication (in this case, an antidepressant), restless behaviors (i.e., wringing of the hands), rapid speech when discussing certain topics, a sense of feeling fatigued or rundown, some difficulty with concentration, and her acceptance of the fact that she has post-traumatic stress disorder.

Stress and stressors

Recall from Chapter 13 that, although stress and stressors can be physiological, there is also psychological stress. In psychology, **stress** is a descriptive term that explains a myriad of experiences during which demands are placed on the individual to cope or act. These demands are called **stressors**.

Some amount of stress is healthy and normal; in fact, it can act as a motivator. However, recurrent episodes or prolonged periods of stress deplete the body's natural energy resources and its strength. This energy depletion adversely affects a person's ability to cope with and resolve any stressful issues.

An internal state of stress leads to feelings of tension, anxiety, and worry, as well as the restlessness of the mind. Rumination or preoccupation with thoughts can occur.

rumination: repeatedly and deeply going over and over a subject of concern or an anxiety-producing subject to the point that normal daily functioning is impaired. It is very difficult for someone who ruminates to stop doing so without some therapy or medication.

preoccupation: a state of being fully absorbed in one's own thoughts to the exclusion of the external world. In other words, a preoccupied individual may not be not fully aware of when he or she is being spoken to or able to give his or her full attention to a task at hand. A preoccupied person may not make good decisions because he or she cannot give enough attention to the decision-making process. Preoccupation is less disruptive than rumination, however, and the preoccupied person can be brought back into a conversation or activity.

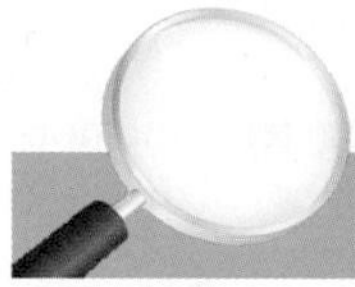

FOCUS POINT: *Rumination* in Context

Be very alert to the context in which you hear the term *rumination*.

In psychiatry and mental health, the term *rumination* refers to an obsessional preoccupation with a thought or thoughts that an individual is unable to dismiss.

In neonatology and pediatrics, *rumination* refers to a disorder of infancy in which the child repeatedly regurgitates food (i.e., throws it up). The result is often a failure to thrive that can result in death.

Disturbed thought processes

In a medical or psychiatric context, the word **disturbed** means *showing signs of mental illness or disorder.* **Disturbed thought process** is a broad term. It refers to alterations in cognition or thinking. These can be minor or major, depending on the wellness or illness of the patient. Disturbed thought processes include confusion, disorientation, altered mood states, inappropriate social behaviors, and hallucinations. Rumination and preoccupation are also examples of disturbed thought processes. The etiology (cause) of these symptoms may be pathological, or it may be related to emotionally challenging circumstances and life events. Illicit drugs and some medications can also lead to disturbed thought processes.

Our client, Stevie-Rose, notices that she has trouble concentrating lately. She feels distracted or loses her train of thought (i.e., her mind goes blank). She notices some shifts in her mood, and she has commented particularly on what she perceives to be a loss of her sense of humor. She may be preoccupied with her husband's health, worrying in particular about his new diagnosis of asbestosis and what this will mean to both of them. She is experiencing symptoms of disturbed thought processes.

The limbic system and emotional health

The limbic system sits deep within the brain. It is responsible for learning, emotions, and emotional behaviors and expressions. The limbic system also motivates us to survive. It is a core component of the physiology of mental health and wellness. It includes a number of structures that regulate emotional responses and that maintain emotional health. The limbic system also exerts influence over two other systems: the autonomic nervous system, through the hypothalamus, and the endocrine system, where it triggers the release of hormones.

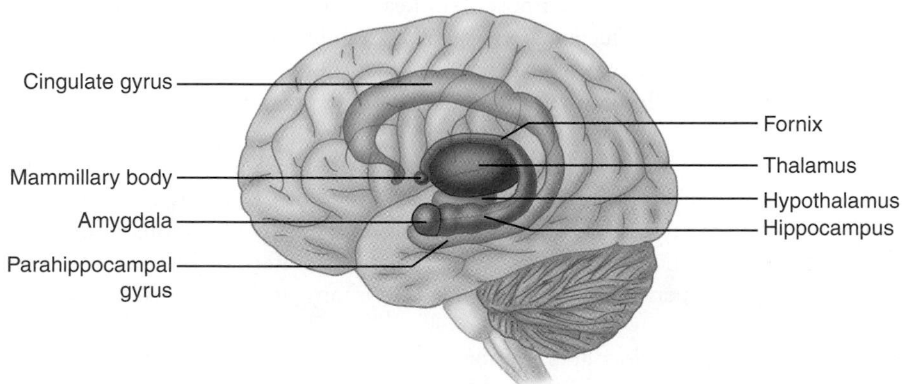

Figure 16.6: The limbic system

Structures of the limbic system

Hippocampus

The hippocampus plays a role in memory by transferring our experiences into the long-term memory and then recovering them as needed. It also assists with spatial navigation (i.e., recognizing and understanding distances). There are two hippocampi: one is in the left hemisphere, and one is in the right hemisphere. Pathology in the hippocampus is seen in patients with Alzheimer's disease.

Cingulate gyrus

The cingulate gyrus regulates aggression and receives sensory input. It also processes emotional experiences, and it is involved in memory. This structure is actually a fold in the brain itself.

Parahippocampal gyrus

The parahippocampal gyrus connects the structures of the limbic system.

Fornix

The fornix is a communication pathway within the limbic system. It consists of a band of neural fibers. This structure is also known as the *fimbria*.

Thalamus

The thalamus receives sensory stimuli and transmits them to the cerebral cortex of the brain. It is involved in alertness and short-term memory. It also plays a role in initiating or inhibiting movement, as well as the planning and coordination of movement. It plays an important part in the learning process as well. Anatomically, the thalamus consists of two lobes.

Hypothalamus

The hypothalamus controls the autonomic nervous system and regulates the hormones that are secreted by the adrenal and pituitary glands, as well as the hormones that regulate sex drive, hunger, and thirst. It is located at the base of the brain, posterior to the thalamus (see Chapter 7).

Mammillary bodies

There are two small mammillary bodies located near the fornix. They function as message relay centers between the hippocampus, the thalamus, and the amygdala.

The amygdala

The amygdala is a structure that is found deep within the brain and that influences our emotions and triggers automatic responses to them. It also plays a role in both hormone secretion and memory. The amygdala decides which of our memories will be stored and where they will be stored in the brain (i.e., an olfactory or smell memory may be stored separately from one that is visual). This structure plays an important role in the recognition of and response to fear and anxiety. Functional changes in the amygdala are seen in individuals who are diagnosed with depression, autism, and borderline personality disorder (see Chapter 12). The amygdala and the hippocampus together are thought to be responsible for our ability to laugh.

Humor: functional and health promoting

Humor is functional (i.e., it serves a purpose) and health promoting. It plays an important role in mental health by positively influencing an individual's ability to cope both psychologically and physically. Stevie-Rose Davis mentions that she fears that she has lost her sense of humor. This is often a symptom of stress, anxiety, and depression. The subject of humor may very well be one that a counselor will address with her.

An appreciation of how humor influences health (or illness) is another example of the mind-body connection. Research has increasingly shown that humor is not only a normal and natural function of the brain but that it is also health promoting. The positive emotions generated through humor benefit both the sender and the receiver of humorous material. Humor leads to a sense of cohesiveness and shared experience between people, and it mitigates any stress that may be present in a situation.

Anatomically, humor detection, appreciation, and response are located in the frontal and temporal lobes and more specifically in the amygdala, which is a structure that is highly involved in all emotional response and memory. When the brain perceives humor, it releases endorphins. Laughter, which is a response to perceived humor, is believed to lower blood pressure and to reduce levels of stress hormones that circulate in the body. Laughter is also thought to enhance immune system function by stimulating the production of T-cells, B-cells, and interferon (see Chapter 14).

Humor therapy and laughter therapy are becoming more common in health care. Across the life span, a wide variety of laughter-invoking and humorous interventions are now being included in patient and residential care. An example of this trend is the presence of clowns on pediatric units, where they distract from negative stressors that the children are experiencing while at the same time stimulating the play and imagination areas of the children's brains. Clowns are also sometimes used to help alleviate the anxiety that a child experiences before a surgical procedure.

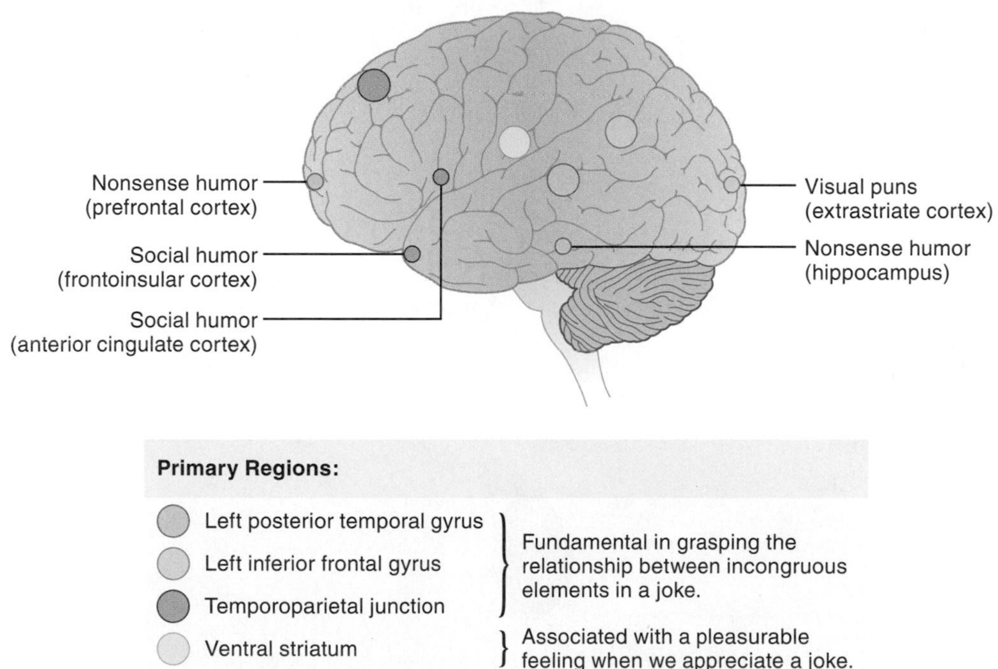

Figure 16.7: An anatomy of humor

Stress and the limbic system

Stress is a phenomenon of both the mind and the body. When a stressor is perceived, the limbic system is activated. The amygdala triggers a response in the hypothalamus, which triggers the pituitary gland, which in turn triggers the adrenal glands to release adrenaline and cortisol. This process is referred to as the **hypothalamic-pituitary-adrenal (HPA) pathway**. Figure 16-8 illustrates this process.

Cortisol and adrenaline are *stress hormones*. This means that they contribute to the body's overall response to stress with a goal of homeostasis and self-preservation.

Cortisol or *corticosteroid* has a number of functions. Its normal physiological tasks are to remove toxins from the body and to reduce inflammation. It also plays a role in short-term memory acquisition. Psychologically, cortisol influences the expression of moods (including fear) and an individual's motivation. When a stress response is initiated, cortisol is produced in greater amounts to help the body to physically deal with the stressor.

Adrenaline (epinephrine) boosts the energy levels of both the body and the mind when it is produced; it also elevates blood pressure and heart rate. The production of adrenaline is initiated by the limbic system's perception of a threat. It too is part of the stress response.

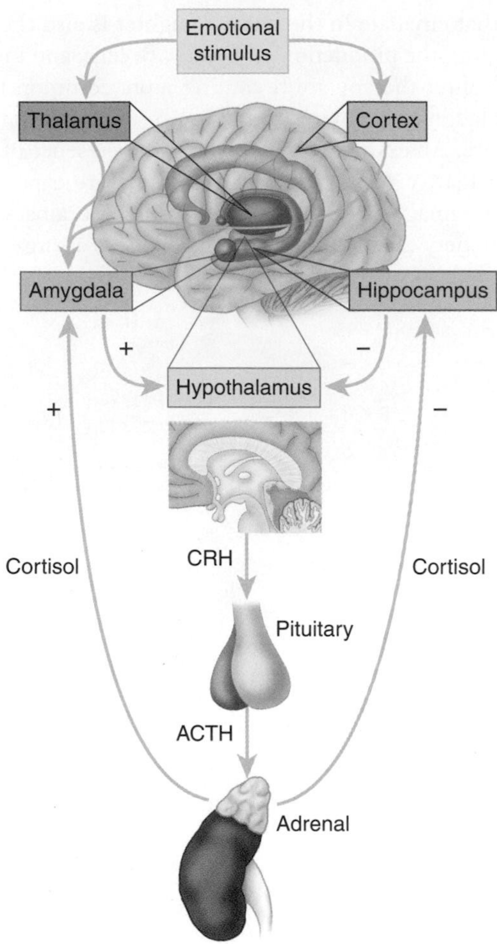

Figure 16.8: The stress response and the hypothalamic-pituitary-adrenal pathway

Critical Thinking

Review the structures of the limbic system to answer the following question.

Which aspects of the limbic system might be influencing or influenced by Stevie-Rose Davis' current situation in life? Explain your answer.

____

____

____

____

Mix and Match

Match the description of each limbic system structure with its name. You will need to think carefully about anatomy and physiology to complete some of the matches.

1. indicated with a diagnosis of Alzheimer's disease	amygdala
2. sits centrally in the limbic system	thalamus
3. not involved in memory	ingulate gyrus
4. involved in the regulation and expression of aggression	hypothalamus
5. implicated in depression	hippocampus

Fill in the Blanks

Use medical terminology in a meaningful way to finish the following sentences.

1. When you have a job, go to night school, and also have young children in the home, you could be said to have multiple ____.
2. Stress can lead to and is part of ____.
3. If a student has a job to go to after class and the instructor seems to be dragging out the lecture, it is likely the student will be thinking excessively about leaving. The term for this type of thinking is ____.
4. A way of thinking that signals that a person is not thinking clearly or rationally is called ____.
5. A small system that is located in the brain and that is responsible for our emotions, how we express them, and how we react to the emotions of others is called the ____.
6. The saying "Laughter is the best medicine" recognizes a philosophical approach to wellness called the ____.
7. Recall that the autonomic nervous system, which was introduced in Chapter 10 and which has been referred to many times since, is controlled by the ____________________.
8. The sudden loss of a job can cause a person to be preoccupied with thoughts of that loss. When an unemployed person repeatedly goes over and over what happened that led to his or her job loss, the person is said to be ____.

Label the Health Assessment Diagram

Complete this health assessment diagram. Within each domain of health, identify Stevie-Rose's strengths and weaknesses. In other words, which aspects of Stevie-Rose's current situation have the potential to influence her health in a positive or negative way? For each of the circles in the diagram, list positive or negative points in Stevie-Rose's life. Follow the example given in Figure 16-9; this figure provides an evaluation of Stevie-Rose's situation in the economic domain, which is also sometimes included in these types of assessment diagrams.

Economic
• Retired
• VA pension with medical coverage
• Owns a car
• No complaints voiced for financial

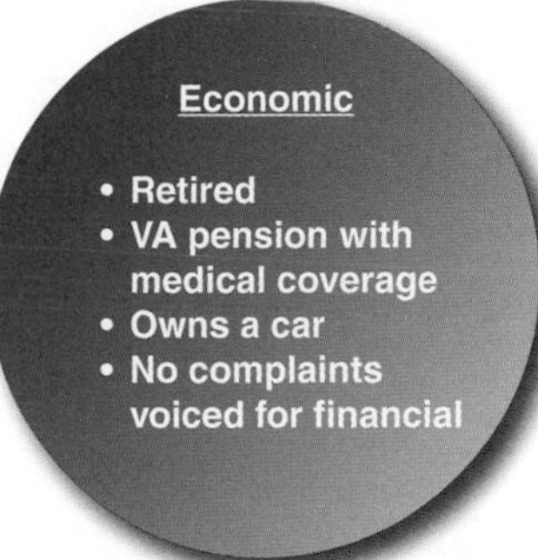

Figure 16.9: Sample health assessment diagram: economic domain

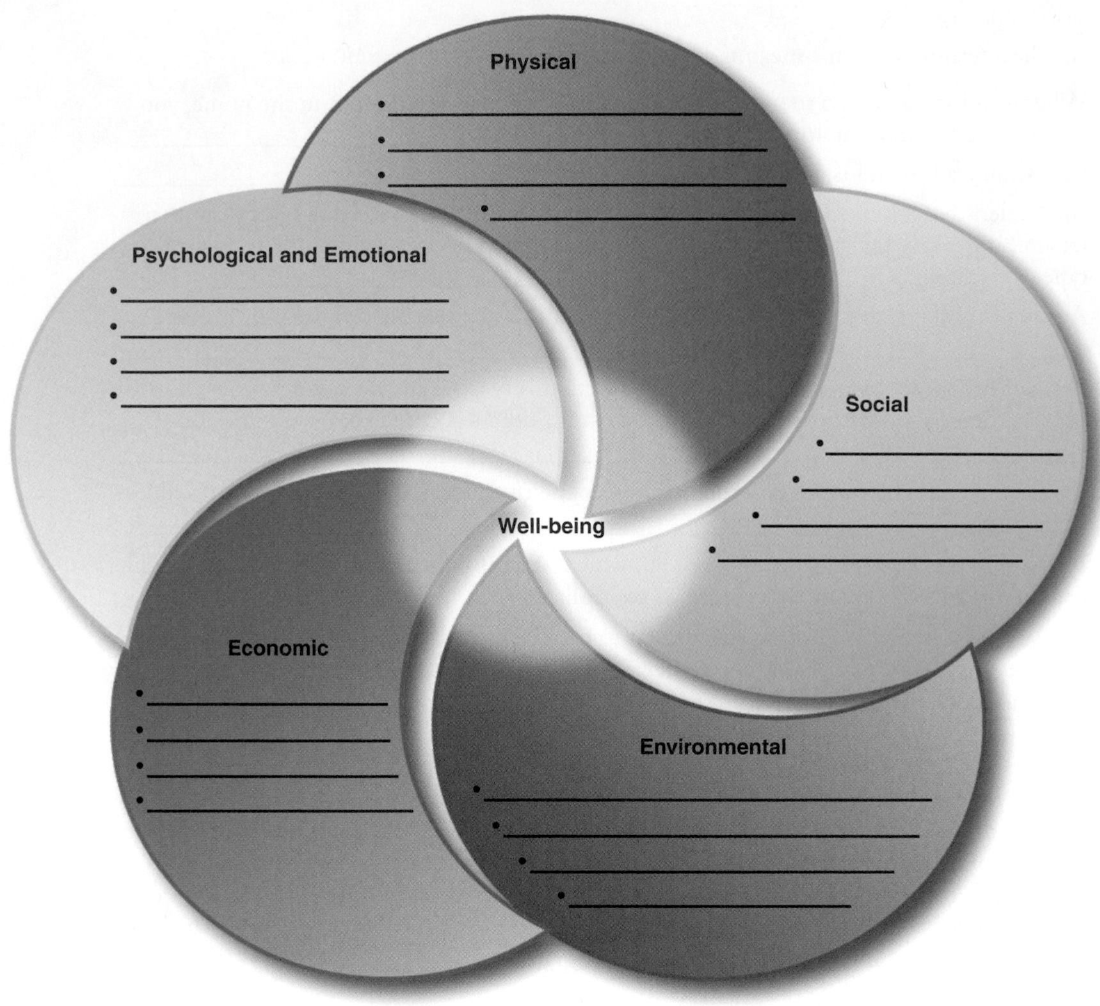

Critical Thinking

On the basis of the health assessment diagram, decide whether our patient is in an optimal state of physical or mental health. What is her state of wellness from a holistic perspective?

___

PRONUNCIATION PRACTICE

Say these words aloud to a friend or classmate, if you can. Here you are given the phonetic pronunciation. Your instructor can help you with pronunciation,

or you can visit **http://www.MedicalLanguageLab.com.** 

adrenaline	ă-**drĕn**´ă-lēn *or* ă-**drĕn**´ă-lĭn	hippocampus	hĭp″ō-**kăm**´pŭs
amygdala	ă-**mĭg**´dă-lă	hypothalamus	hī″pō-**thăl**´ă-mŭs
cortisol	**kor**´tĭ-sŏl	limbic	**lĭm**´bĭk
gyrus	**jī**´rŭs	thalamus	**thăl**´ă-mŭs

Mental health maintenance

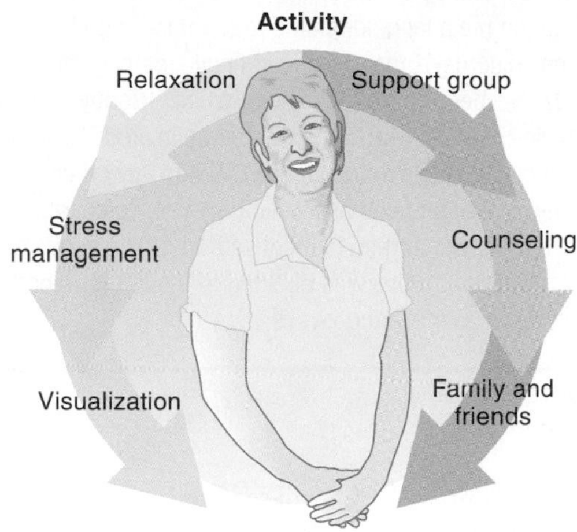

Figure 16.10: Maintaining mental health: the importance of balance

Patient Update

Stevie-Rose wants to maintain or improve her mental health. She senses that she has somehow lost balance in her life, and she made a number of comments to the nurse practicioner (NP) about this. In response, Ophelia contacted the clinic's counseling center to refer the client for help with managing stress and anxiety, as well as with addressing her post-traumatic stress disorder. Stevie-Rose is going to meet with a counselor in Ophelia's office briefly this morning to set up a counseling plan; that will occur after the nurse completes a physical examination of the client. As a health-care professional, Ophelia is very aware that a physical assessment must first be made to rule in or out any physiological disturbances that may be contributing to the client's expressed symptoms.

During the physical, Stevie-Rose Davis had her blood pressure, TPR, weight, and height assessed. Ophelia also assessed her client's skin turgor (elasticity) to see if Stevie-Rose was hydrated. She checked Stevie-Rose's vision and examined the ear canals. In addition, the NP learned that, in most regards, the client was quite physically fit for her age. She also learned that Stevie-Rose had received a very minor concussion during an MVA that occurred 4 weeks ago and that the client had also bruised her knee at that time. The client wondered if the pain and stiffness that she was experiencing in her right knee were related to that accident, to her chronic arthritis, or simply to aging. Ophelia examined all of the client's reflexes, as well as her range of motion. She recorded the information in the e-medical record, and she advised the client that the information would be forwarded to the rheumatologist. She also asked the client if there were any residual effects from the concussion, such as headache or blurred vision. There were not.

Just as the exam ended, a knock came at the outer door to the office. "Hi," a male voice said, "it's Bobby Pontiac from Counseling. Are you in there, Ophelia?" The man poked his head into the office just as Ophelia entered it through the door from the examining room.

"Glad you could make it, Bobby." Ophelia smiled. "I have a client here whom I'd like you to see. She'll be right out." Ophelia pointed at a chair and invited Bobby to sit down. "When I heard her blurt out 'PTSD,' I called you immediately. I know how tenuous these cases can be. The client can be hesitant or afraid to admit that he or she has the disorder or to pursue help. I didn't want her to change her mind." Stevie-Rose entered the room and took a seat near the counselor. Ophelia introduced them and left them to chat.

"Lieutenant Davis," the man began, with a voice that was warm, friendly, and respectful, "I'm Bobby Pontiac, a counselor here at Murphy Clinic. I understand that you may want to talk to me about something." Stevie-Rose smiled and nodded, looking away. Bobby waited. Stevie-Rose looked him over, assessing whether or not she should speak. She noticed his casual Western way of dressing, the long salt-and-pepper ponytail that was neatly tied at the back of his neck, a turquoise ring on one of his fingers, and cowboy boots. She could relate to these things, and so she began.

"I ... uh ... I ... well, it's taken me a long, long time to say this—and I never thought I would—but I think I've got post-traumatic stress disorder," the client said finally, before she quickly added, "And please, call me Stevie-Rose, won't you? I've been retired for a long while." Bobby smiled and said that he would. He then began to talk with Stevie-Rose about PTSD a bit. Bobby invited her to meet with him again later that day, around 2 p.m., so that they could talk more about PTSD and any other concerns that she may have. She looked at him carefully as he spoke, and she assessed his eyes, voice, and mannerisms for sincerity. She decided that she liked him, and so she agreed to meet with him. The appointment was set, and Bobby said goodbye. Ophelia returned, and Stevie-Rose was directed to the lab for blood work and urinalysis and then to the radiology department for knee and hand x-rays.

Counseling

At the Murphy Center, Bobby Pontiac, LPC, will see Stevie-Rose Davis for an intake assessment into the counseling department. He will speak with her later today about her activities, her level of social engagement, her present and past methods of coping, and any issues that she wishes to talk about that reflect her mental and emotional health. With Stevie-Rose's help, Bobby will ascertain her counseling needs and develop a plan of action for and with her. Most importantly, though, Bobby will speak with the client today about post-traumatic stress disorder (see Chapter 12) and how she has begun to come to terms with having this condition. He will get a personal history from Stevie-Rose. Finally, he will speak with her about her current life stressors and discover how she would like to proceed to get help managing them. Treatment modalities that are open to Stevie-Rose will include support groups for veterans with PTSD, as well as one-to-one or group counseling for coping with stress. Bobby will make it clear that, if Stevie-Rose would like more in-depth psychotherapy for her PTSD on an individual or group basis, he will need to refer her to the clinic's psychologist.

Stevie-Rose Davis may also be a candidate for **rehabilitation counseling**. This service helps people to deal with disabilities of a personal, social, or vocational nature. It can include assistance with recovery from accidents, dealing with diseases, and living with congenital or acquired disabilities (i.e., amputation). Stevie-Rose may benefit from rehabilitation counseling to deal with her chronic arthritis, which may worsen over time. In this regard, her self-image and sense of self-efficacy will play a prominent role in her counseling sessions.

If the counselor determines that his client has some other mental health issues, such as depression or an anxiety disorder, he will refer her to an advanced-practice psychiatric nurse (an NP), a psychologist, or a psychiatrist for diagnosis. After that, Stevie-Rose may become part of Bobby's own caseload. He is a mental health counselor who is qualified to work with individuals, families, and groups who are living with the challenges of mental illness.

Reflective Questions

Demonstrate your cumulative knowledge by answering the following questions.

1. What is an MVA? ______________________________
2. What is an NP? ______________________________
3. What does *TPR* stand for? ______________________________
4. Why did the nurse practitioner complete a physical examination for this client?

   ____

Let's Practice

Answer the following questions by choosing "T" or "F."

1. Bobby Pontiac is fully qualified to engage Stevie-Rose in psychotherapy for PTSD. T ___ F ___
2. Mental health counselors are able to work only with individuals. T ___ F ___

3. Rehabilitation counseling is performed by occupational therapists who work in the counseling department. T ___ F ___
4. A licensed professional counselor is able to make a diagnosis. T ___ F ___
5. In addition to counseling for PTSD, Stevie-Rose Davis may also receive rehabilitation counseling. T ___ F ___

Critical Thinking

Think carefully and critically about what you have learned over time about Stevie-Rose's response to the possibility of having post-traumatic distress disorder. Consider what has occurred today as you answer this question.

Why did the nurse practitioner call Counseling immediately when Stevie-Rose blurted out that she had PTSD?

____

____

The Immune System: Enhanced Terminology

The immune system was briefly introduced in Chapter 2. References to it have appeared throughout this textbook, particularly in Chapters 13 and 14. Your accumulated knowledge and vocabulary will now be enriched by an overview of the elements of the immune system and its function. Your knowledge and terminology will be enhanced as you move through the system to its subsystem: the autoimmune system. The autoimmune system as it is relevant to our patient, Stevie-Rose Davis, will be presented in depth as a basis for her visit to a rheumatologist.

Recall that the immune system is not an organ system like the other body systems that have been studied in this book. It is a type of circulatory system. It circulates lymph and antibodies that protect the body from attack by pathogens. (See Figure 16-11)

The immune system revolves around antibodies and antigens:

Antigens provoke an immune response. They are foreign invaders in the body such as pathogens or toxins.

Antibodies are proteins found in the body. They respond to being provoked by antigens. They detect, trap, and neutralize foreign invaders. **Lymphocytes** are cells that produce antibodies.

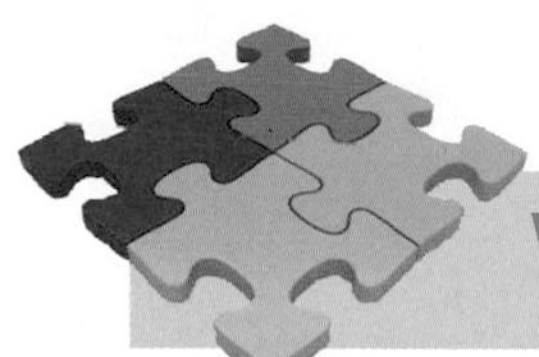

WORD BUILDING: Formulas for Creating Words from the Root Word *immune*

immune* = protected from or resistant to disease or infection from a pathogen. The combining form is *immun/o.

immun/o + deficienc + y = *immunodeficiency*
Definition: the condition of having a decreased or compromised ability to respond to antigens. (The second word part is derived from the root *deficere*, meaning *to want or to need.*) *noun*

Example: Cancer patients who are undergoing chemotherapy can acquire *immunodeficiency*.

immun/o + gen/e+ tics = *immunogenetics*
Definition: the study of how genes influence susceptibility to infectious or autoimmune diseases. *noun*

Example: *Immunogenetics* is involved when ascertaining whether a recipient is physically able to accept an organ transplant.

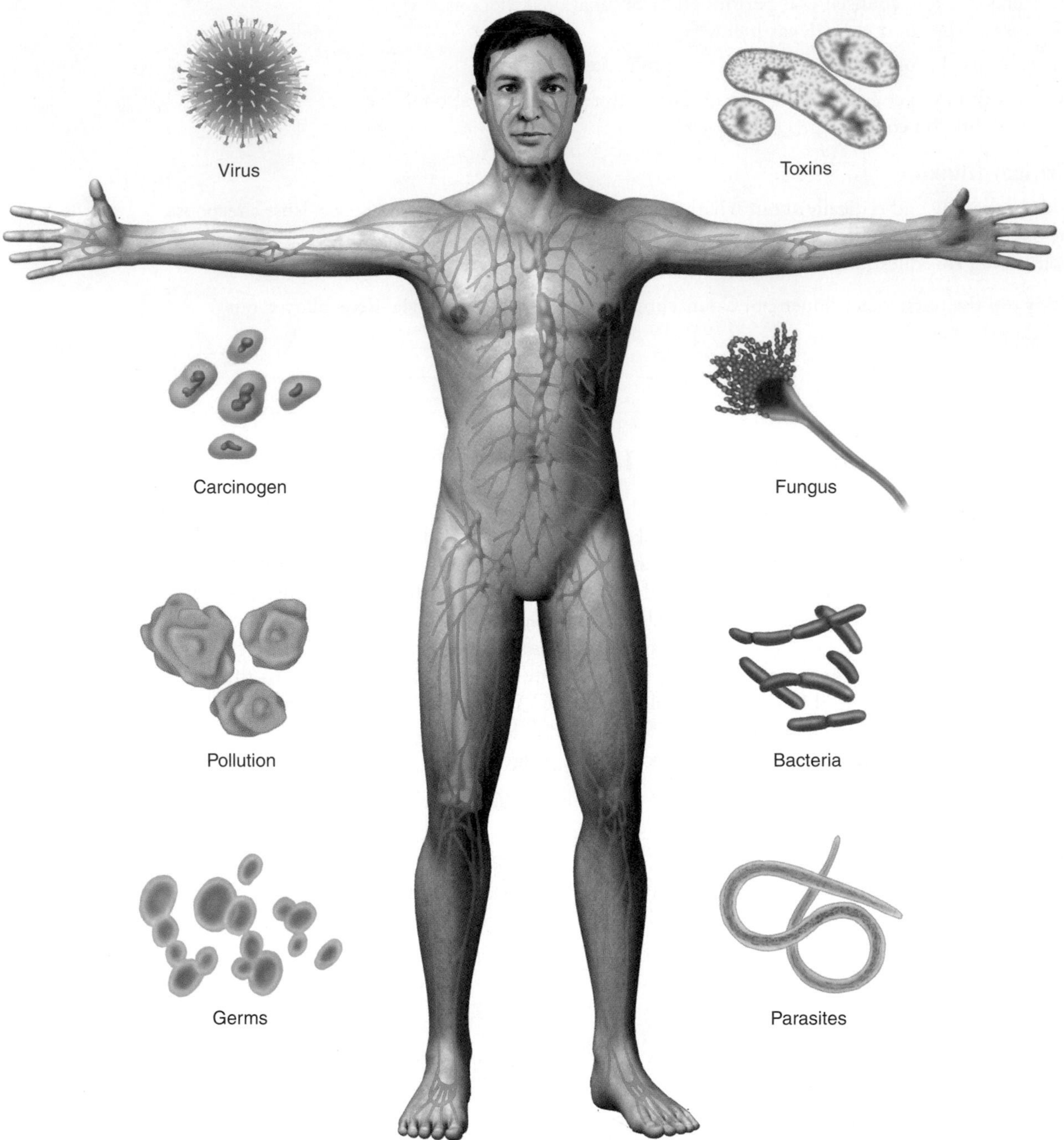

Figure 16.11: Immune system protection

The immune response

The **immune response** is a series of steps that occur when the body perceives a threat from pathogens. These include germs, parasites, bacteria, pollution, viruses, fungi, toxins, or carcinogens. It may take as many as 2 or 3 weeks to produce sufficient numbers of antibodies to fight the infection or disease. A successful immune response is one in which the foreign pathogens are eradicated or depleted to the extent that they are no longer viable and thus can no longer harm the body. The term **pathogen** means disease producing.

Lysis is the medical term for the process of dissolving, destroying, or disintegrating cells. An enzyme called *lysozyme* is generally responsible for this process.

Pathogens and toxins make contact with their hosts (i.e., the people that they infect or invade) by various modes of transmission, which are explained in Table 16-3.

TABLE 16-3: Modes of Transmission: Pathogens and Toxins

Mode of Transmission	How Transmission Occurs
Contact: direct or indirect	direct contact = person to person or body to body indirect contact = between a person and a contaminated object
Droplets	spread through respiratory secretions via coughing, sneezing, talking, or the use of contaminated equipment (i.e., a bronchoscope)
Airborne	carried by dust particles or other small particles that can be suspended in the air and inhaled
Fecal-oral route	infection occurs generally through the ingestion of foods, the licking of hands, or poor hand hygiene
Vector-borne route	infection occurs through contact with an animal or an insect that is carrying a pathogen (i.e., mosquito bites that transmit malaria)

There are two types of immune responses: the specific response and the nonspecific response. During the *nonspecific immune response,* pathogens are blocked from entry into the body and thereby prevented from spreading. During the *specific immune response,* antibody-mediated and cell-mediated responses attack specific antigens:

Antibody-mediated immunity is the first line of defense against invading pathogens. It is regulated by B-cells and by the antibodies that are produced by B-cells (see chapter 14). Antibody-mediated immunity is also known as *humoral immunity.*

Cell-mediated immunity is the second line of defense that is initiated by the immune system. Here, cells that have been infected are targeted by T-cells for destruction (see Chapter 14).

Sensing invasion and an upset in the homeostasis of the body, the immune system produces and releases antibodies and lymphocytes to combat the invaders. This process occurs in two stages.

The *primary immune response* begins immediately upon contact with or the detection of an antigen. This leads to the production and circulation of immunoglobulin M within the first 48 to 72 hours (see Table 16-4).

The *secondary immune response* begins within 24 to 48 hours and produces immunoglobulin G. This response is prolonged, and the battle continues until all antigens have been addressed (see Table 16-4).

Immunoglobulins

Immunoglobulins (Ig) are glycoprotein molecules. They are antibodies that have a distinct "Y" shape (see Figure 16-12). The function of immunoglobulins is to identify foreign invaders in the body. Once they do so, they attach to each invading cell, thereby creating an *immune complex,* which is a cell made up of an antibody and an antigen that are bound together. Immunoglobulins do not destroy cells on their own. They trap antigens, and they then require the assistance of T-cells to help them to destroy invaders (see Chapter 14).

The roles of immunoglobulins include the following functions:

- neutralization: preventing antigens from binding to cells where they could cause harm or spread.
- agglutination: the gathering together of like antigens so that they may be engulfed by macrophages; this is discussed in more detail later in this chapter.
- activation of a complement: the act of a pathogen binding with an antigen, as well as with a complementary protein to create a membrane that will contain the pathogen. This will cut it off from nutrients and inhibit its ability to reproduce.
- activation of effector cells: the activation of specific sites on lymphocytes (F-receptors), platelets, and phagocytes that can recognize specific types of antigens.These sites are only activated in the presence of the specific antigens that they are designed to respond to and destroy.

There are five different types or *isotopes* of immunoglobulin. Each isotope responds to a specific type of antigen. For example, if the measles virus presents itself, then only the antibody that is programmed to attack measles will be triggered during an immune response. Table 16-4 provides the names, locations, and descriptions of these different isotopes.

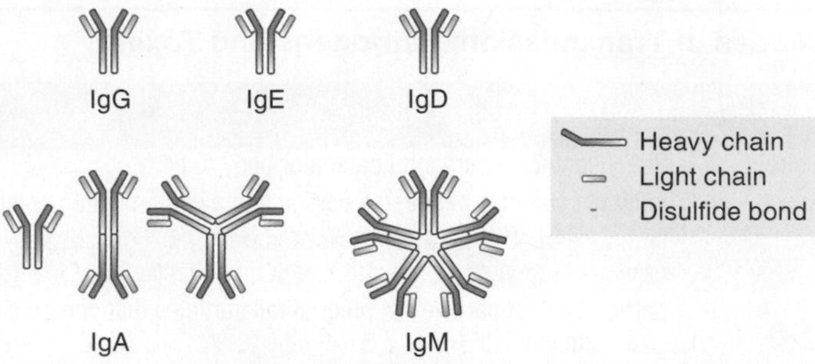

Figure 16.12: Type of immunoglobulin molecules

TABLE 16-4: Types of Immunoglobulin

Type	Location	Function
Immunoglobulin A	• located in the nose, saliva, airways, digestive tract, ears, eyes, and vagina	• protects the body's surface
Immunoglobulin D	• found in the tissues that line the abdominal and chest cavities	• may play a role in response to allergies, including those to dairy products
Immunoglobulin E	• located in the lungs, the mucous membranes, and the skin; provides mucosal immunity	• induces a bodily response to allergens such as fungus, animal dander, parasites, dust, and pollen
Immunoglobulin G (the most abundant of all of the antibodies but also the tiniest)	• present in all body fluids; can cross the placenta	• fights bacterial and viral infections
Immunoglobulin M (the largest in size of the antibodies)	• located in the bloodstream and the lymph	• first responder to infection • stimulates macrophages (a type of immune cell)

Interleukins (ILs)

Interleukins are also part of the immune response. They are proteins that are naturally secreted when the presence of a foreign invader is detected. Interleukins trigger the immune response by alerting lymphocytes and antibodies and then stimulating them into action. They are thought to play a significant role in the fight against fever, inflammation, and pain. They are also involved in the allergy response and cell regeneration. There are many interleukins, and they are numbered from 1 through 15: IL1 through IL15.

Phagocytes

Phagocytes are leukocytes (white blood cells) that attract and engulf harmful foreign bodies (i.e., viruses, bacteria) and dead or dying cells. They kill them by ingestion via a process called **phagocytosis**. Phagocytes play a significant role in fighting infection and providing immunity.

The term *phagocyte* is derived from the Greek verb *phagein*, which means *to eat or devour.*

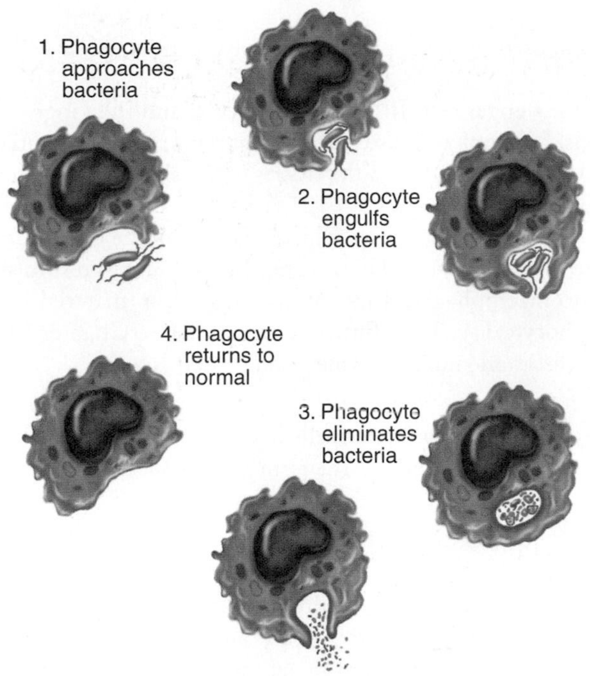

Figure 16.13: Phagocytosis: microscopic view (From Eagle S, Brassington C, Dailey CS, Goretti C: *The Professional Medical Assistant: An Integrative, Teamwork-Based Approach.* Philadelphia: FA Davis, 2009, p. 295. With permission.)

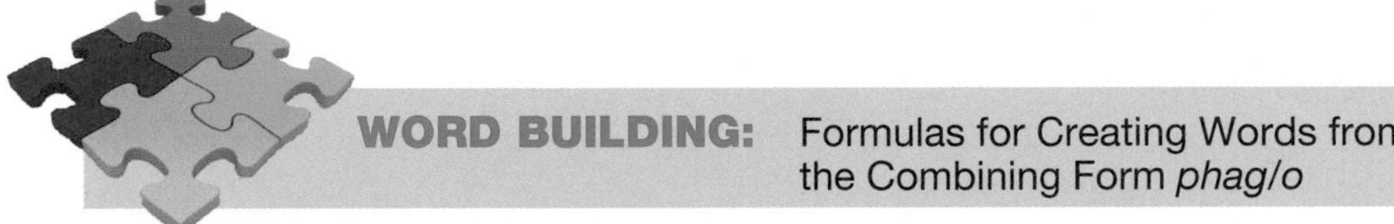

WORD BUILDING: Formulas for Creating Words from the Combining Form *phag/o*

phagein **= Greek root meaning *to eat*. The modern combining form is *phag/o*, which means *eating, ingesting, or devouring.***

phag/o + cyt/o + blast = *phagocytoblast*

Definition: a cell that develops into a phagocyte. *noun*

Example: The generation of *phagocytoblasts* occurs in the lymphatic system.

phag/o + cyt/o + lysis = *phagocytolysis*

Definition: the destruction of phagocytes. (The suffix *-lysis* means *dissolution*.) *noun*

Example: There is some evidence that acupuncture may be able to facilitate the action of *phagocytolysis*.

phag/o + some = *phagosome*

Definition: a membranous structure of a phagocyte in which foreign matter or other material is waiting to be digested. *noun*

Example: *Phagosomes* are essential to the function of macrophages.

Right Word or Wrong Word: *Phagocyte* or *Phacocyst*?

Are these two terms the same? Do they have the same pronunciation? Do they have the same meaning?

Macrophages

Phagocyte cells are composed of macrophages and polymorphonuclear cells, which are central to phagocytosis.

A **macrophage** is a scavenger cell. It hunts for, detects, and then ingests foreign matter, dead cells, or other cell debris. Macrophages also play an important role in the initiation of some immune responses. They are found in abundance in the tissues of the skin, the digestive tract, the lungs, the spleen, and some blood vessels.

Blood macrophages develop from *monocytes,* which originate in the bone marrow. Monocytes enter the blood and circulate for a short period of time until they come to rest in specific types of tissue. There, they mature into macrophages. These macrophages trap material in sufficient quantity to then transfer it to lymphocyte T-cells for further destruction (see Chapter 14). Blood macrophages secrete substances such as interleukins, enzymes, and proteins.

Polymorphonuclear cells

There are three types of polymorphonuclear cells that also provide protection to the body. These are neutrophils, basophils, and eosinophils. The term *polymorphonuclear* refers to the unusual shape of the nuclei of these cells.

Neutrophils have the following characteristics:

- They are found in the blood.
- They are the major cells involved in the anti-inflammatory response.
- Abnormally low levels of neutrophils in the blood can increase the risk of infection.
- Increased levels of neutrophils in the blood signal the presence of infection, inflammation, malignancies, or the use of corticosteroid drugs.

The root word is *neuter,* meaning *neither.*

The combining form is *neutr/o.*

Basophils have the following characteristics:

- They are found in the blood and in the mast cells of the skin; **mast cells** are a type of immune cell found in connective tissue.
- They play a role in atopic allergy responses (i.e., in the skin) and the anaphylaxis response, which is initiated by extreme sensitivity.
- They contain some amounts of serotonin, heparin, histamine, and enzymes.
- They contribute to a basic, nonspecific immune response to inflammation.

The root word for *basophils* is *basis,* meaning *base.*

The combining form is basi/io.

Eosinophils have the following characteristics:

- They are found in tissues.
- They play a role in parasitic infection, inflammation, and allergic reactions.

The root word is *eos*, meaning *rose colored.*

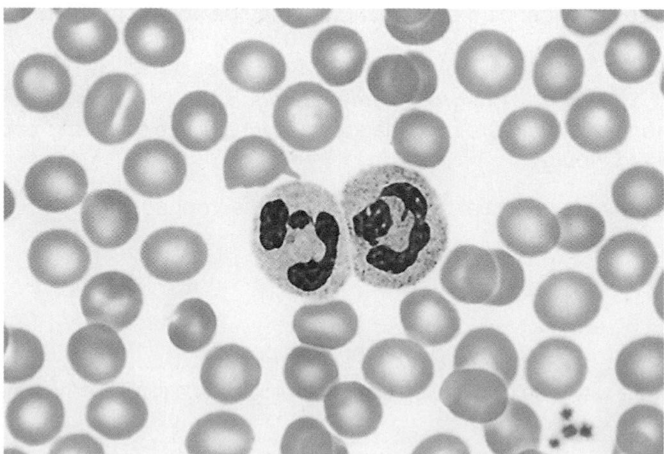

Figure 16.14: Neutrophil: microscopic view (From Harmening DM: *Clinical Hematology and Fundamentals of Hemostasis,* ed 5. Philadelphia: FA Davis, 2009, p. 4. With permission.)

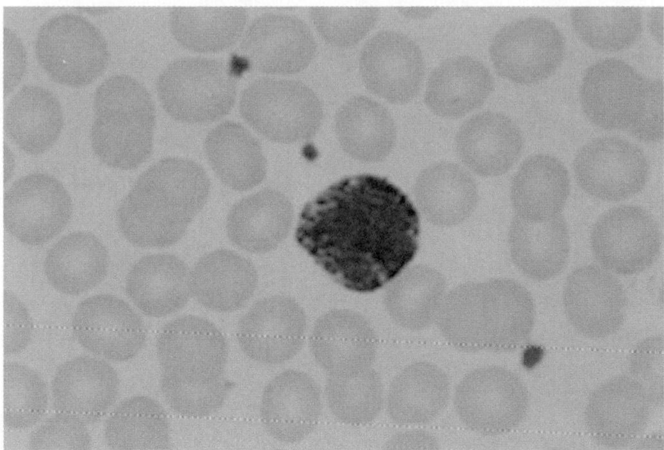

Figure 16.15: Basophil: microscopic view (From Harmening DM: *Clinical Hematology and Fundamentals of Hemostasis*, ed 5. Philadelphia: FA Davis, 2009, p. 5. With permission.)

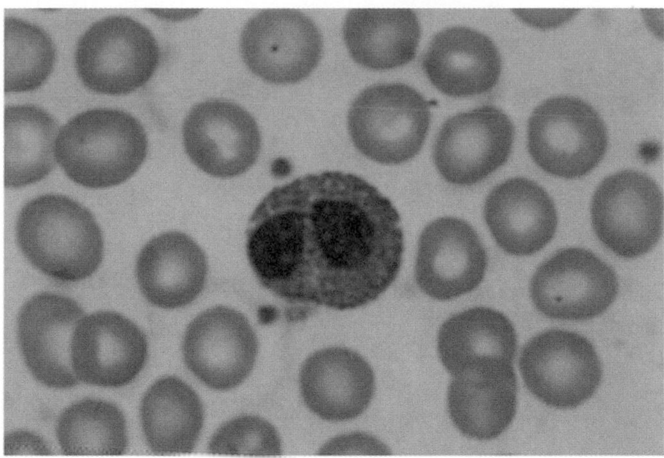

Figure 16.16: Eosinophil: microscopic view (From Harmening DM: *Clinical Hematology and Fundamentals of Hemostasis*, ed 5. Philadelphia: FA Davis, 2009, p. 5. With permission.)

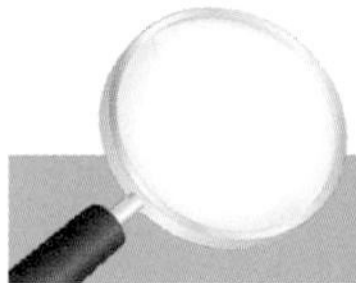

FOCUS POINT: The Suffixes *-philia* and *-phobia*

The suffix *-phil* or *-philia* means *to love or have a preference for.* The opposite of *-philia is -phobia*, which indicates a fear or hatred of something. The use of these suffixes in medical terms is understood to mean an excessive or obsessive love or fear of something, respectively.

Critical Reflection Questions

Consider what you have learned about the immune system to answer the following questions.

1. If a pathogen is spread when someone sneezes, what is the mode of transmission?

   ____

2. If you are bitten by a tick and get Lyme disease, what is the mode of transmission?

   ____

3. Which type of phagocytes in particular ingest pathogens? ______________
4. Name the type of antibody that is instrumental to the allergic response. ______________

5. Which antibody is involved in the inflammatory response to a pathogen? ____________
6. Which microorganisms in the body trigger lymphocytes and antibodies and are involved in the allergy response? ____________

Critical Thinking

Apply your new knowledge and the new terms that you have learned to the following question.

You have just returned from a 4-hour airplane flight. During that time, you heard the man behind you cough incessantly. Now you are afraid that you might catch whatever illness he had. What would be the mode of transmission for this illness?

____

Break It Down

Use the word construction and deconstruction skills that you have learned over the course of many chapters to break down the following medical terms.

1. phagolysis ____________
   Meaning: ____________
2. eosinopenia ____________
   Meaning: ____________
3. basophilia ____________
   Meaning: ____________
4. neutropenia ____________
   Meaning: ____________

Let's Practice

Practice with suffixes. Change the medical term that you are given into its opposite. Take the root word or combining form, and then change the suffix.

Example: arachnophobia (fear of spiders) *Antonym:* arachnophilia

1. affinity for dead things or dead people: necrophilia
   Antonym: ____________
2. love of being alone or in solitude: autophilia
   Antonym: ____________
3. affinity for writing blogs: blogophilia
   Antonym: ____________
4. affinity for a person of same gender: homophilia
   Antonym: ____________
5. fear of clowns: coulrophobia
   Antonym: ____________
6. excessive fear of pain: agliophobia
   Antonym: ____________
7. excessive fear of growing old: gerascophobia (gerontophobia)
   Antonym: ____________
8. fear of going bald: phalacophobia
   Antonym: ____________

PRONUNCIATION PRACTICE

Say these words aloud to a friend or classmate, if you can. Here you are given the phonetic pronunciation. Your instructor can help you with pronunciation,

or you can visit **http://www.MedicalLanguageLab.com.**

agglutination	ă-gloot″ĭn-**ā**′shŭn	lysis	**lī**′sĭs
autophobia	aw″tō-**fō**′bē-ă	lysozyme	**lī**′sō-zīm
basophil	**bā**′sō fĭl	macrophage	**măk**′rō-fāj
basophilia	bĕ-sō-**fĭl**′ē-ă	neutropenia	nū-trō-**pē**′nē ă
eosinopenia	ē″ō-sĭn-ō-**pē**′nē-ă	neutrophil	**nū**′trō-fĭl
eosinophil	ē″ŏ-**sĭn**′ō-fĭl	phagocyte	**făg**′ō-sīt
gerontophobia	jĕ-rŏn″tŏ-**fō**′bē-ă	phagocytolysis	făg″ō-sī-**tŏl**′ĭ-sĭs
immunifacient	ĭ-mū″nĭ-**fā**′shĕnt	phagolysis	făg-**ŏl**′ĭ-sĭs
immunodeficiency	ĭm″ū-nō-dĕ-**fĭsh**′ĕn-sē	phagosome	**făg**′ō-sōm
interleukin	ĭn″tĕr-**loo**′kĭn	polymorphonuclear	pŏl″ē-mor″fō-**nū**′klē-ăr

Immunity

In a medical sense, **immunity** means protection from disease and infection. It is the body's mechanism for defending itself as well as the body's capability or capacity to do so successfully. Immunity is also a process: it is the result of the activities of antibodies that are specific to certain types of antigens binding to those antigens to destroy or inactivate them. Immunity can be acquired or innate (inborn). The term *immunity* is derived from the Latin word *immunitas,* meaning *exempt from.*

Immunology is the field of science and medicine that is concerned with how immunity is established.

Humoral immunity refers to a type of acquired immunity in which there is an abundance of antibodies in circulation.

Types of immunity

There are three main types of immunity: innate, active (acquired), and passive. Figure 16-17 helps to clarify the differences between these types.

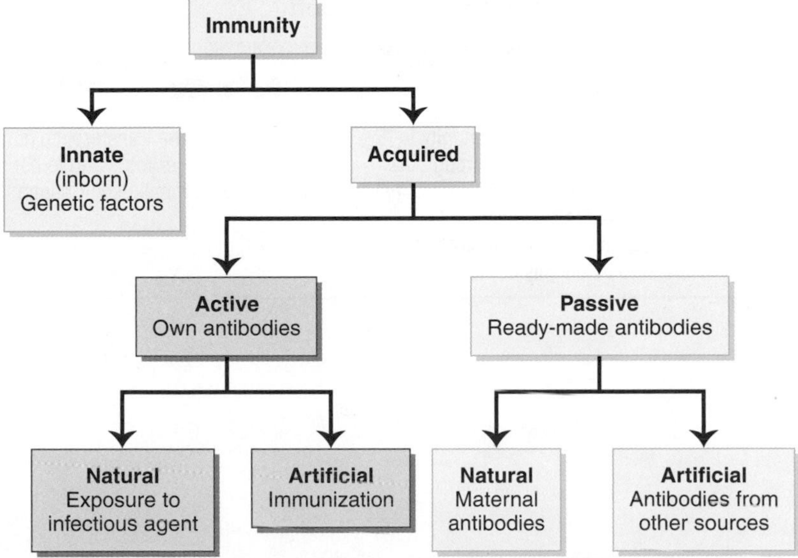

Figure 16.17: Types of immunity

Innate immunity is that with which we are born; it is a state of natural immunity to some pathogens. Physiologically, innate immunity is found in the body's external barriers of the skin and the mucous membranes.

Innate immunity is assessed by the way in which the body is able to mount or initiate the immune response and whether or not it is successful in doing so.

An example of innate immunity is the protection that humans have from illnesses that are present in other species, such as cats or dogs. For example, even when they are exposed to the pathogen of the dog disease canine parvovirus, humans do not contract it.

Active immunity is a state of immunity that is achieved. In other words, it does not come naturally. Active immunity is also known as acquired or adaptive immunity. This type of immunity develops in two response stages:

The *primary response* stage triggers lymphocytes to produce antibodies that will lock onto specific antigens and code for them (memorize them) for future reference and use.

The *secondary response* stage is the ongoing state of immunity that occurs as a result of memorization of the antigen and preparation to combat it when it is next encountered.

Active immunity is dependent on exposure to an antigen and the ability of the lymphocytes involved in the immune response to remember it (see the information about memory cells Chapter 14):

The *humoral response* of active immunity involves the activation of B-cells (lymphocytes), which in turn activate antibody production (i.e., the production of immunoglobulin).

The *cellular response* of active immunity involves the activation of T-cells (lymphocytes), which destroy antigens.

Passive immunity is the result of exposure to antibodies that are produced in one person's body and then acquired by another.

Tables 16-5, 16-6, and 16-7 provide more information about active and passive immunity.

TABLE 16-5: Active Immunity vs. Passive Immunity

Active Immunity	Passive Immunity
achieved *naturally* through exposure to infection	achieved *naturally* through the receipt of maternal antibodies
achieved *artificially* through immunization	achieved *artificially* through antibodies obtained from other sources

TABLE 16-6: Active and Passive Natural Immunity

Active Natural Immunity	Passive Natural Immunity
Active naturally acquired immunity entails being exposed to a pathogen or an infection and building immunity to it. An example of acquired immunity achieved through the active natural process is seen with rubeola (the measles). After a person has been exposed to the measles, it is extremely unlikely that he or she will ever contract it again, even when exposed to this highly contagious virus.	*Passive naturally acquired immunity* comes about as a result of the transference of a mother's antibodies to her fetus and to her newborn through breast milk (see Chapter 17).

TABLE 16-7: Active and Passive *Artificial* Immunity

Active Artificial immunity	Passive Artificial immunity
Active artificially acquired immunity requires immunization to prevent an individual from contracting a disease. A vaccine contains trace amounts of a pathogen (i.e., a virus). By exposing the body to the pathogen, the immune system is able to remember that pathogen and to build an immunity to it should that pathogen be encountered again. Low exposure builds immunity without causing the symptoms of the disease.	*Passive artificially acquired immunity* results from the injection of antiserum or antibodies from another host. The person's tissues play absolutely no role in the provision of the immune response. The inoculation (i.e., the injection or vaccination) provides protection immediately. This route is used when an individual is known to have been exposed to a pathogen and when it is dangerous to wait to see how the body will respond (or if it will). Hepatitis immunoglobulin (HBIG) is an example of a passive artificial immunizing agent. Immunization against rubella (German measles) will also be given when a pregnant woman finds herself exposed to the disease.

Right Word or Wrong Word: *Rubeola* or *Rubella*?

Which one of these words is the correct one for measles? Or is one spelled in its Latin form and the other in American English?

Eponyms: German Measles and Rubella

The disease *rubella* is well known by its second name, *German measles.* The name *German measles* originated during the late 18th century in Europe. It is thought to derive from the work of German scientists who first differentiated the rubella virus from others that were similar to it; they named the virus *rotheln.*

There is also a theory that the word *German* has been applied to this disease for another reason. This belief is based on the use of the medical term *germinaus,* which is from the Latin and means *germane or closely related to.* After all, the rubella virus is related to and similar to other measles viruses.

The name *rubella* is thought to have originated with the 19th-century Scottish physician Dr. Henry Veale. He wrote extensively about this disease, and he treated many cases of it.

Immunization

Immunization is the process of converting an individual who is not immune to a pathogen(s) or toxin(s) to a state of immunity against that pathogen or toxin. Artificial immunization is achieved through vaccinations.

Vaccinations or **inoculations** are injections that contain small doses of an antigen. They stimulate the primary response to the antigen without causing the illness. Memory cells (B-cells working with T-cells) develop the ability to detect and intervene in cases of future exposure to the pathogen. This process provides active, ongoing immunity.

In most cases, **vaccines** are used to prevent disease. A vaccine is a biological substance; a biological preparation used to promote immunization. The names of many vaccines include the name of the disease or infection that they are targeting. Examples of some of the more common vaccines are presented in Table 16-8. An example of a vaccine that prevents infection is the rabies vaccine, which prevents rabies, a viral infection that is transmitted by animals and that causes encephalitis (inflammation of the brain).

TABLE 16-8: Common Vaccines

Name of Vaccine	Target and Details
Gardasil HPV4	• It protects against human papillomavirus (HPV). HPV can lead to cervical cancer and genital warts. • Recent evidence shows that HPV is also a contributor to the development of mouth cancer. • HPV is spread through sexual conduct.
Hep A Havrix VAQTA	• It protects against a specific type of liver infection, hepatitis A (infectious hepatitis). The illness persists some months and requires treatment. Symptoms include jaundice, fever, vomiting, and loss of appetite. • Hepatitis A is spread via the ingestion of the virus. It is found in water, food, beverages, or ice cubes that have been contaminated with fecal material. This is called the *fecal-oral route of transmission.*
Hep B HPV Engerix Heptavax	• It protects against a specific type of liver disease, hepatitis B (serum hepatitis). This disease can become chronic and enduring. Symptoms include jaundice, fatigue, loss of appetite, and diarrhea. • Hepatitis B is spread through contact with the blood or other body fluids of an infected person, including through contaminated blood transfusions, shared needle use, or the infection of a fetus when the disease is passed on through the placenta.
Varicella VAR Varivax VZV ZOS	• It protects against the highly contagious varicella-zoster virus. The varicella virus causes chickenpox, whereas the zoster virus causes a painful condition called *shingles.* These two diseases are innately connected; symptoms of both include a rash and blister-like sores. • This virus is spread through direct person-to-person contact (touch) and through the air by droplets that are expressed during sneezing or coughing.
TIV Afluria Agriflu Fluarix Fluvirin Fluzone FluLaval	• This is the most common of the influenza vaccinations. • It protects against several types of influenza. Flu vaccines are updated continuously to protect against new strains of the illness. • Influenza is spread through airborne droplets (i.e., droplets of contaminated moisture that travel through the air) via sneezes, coughs, and so on.
Bacille Calmette-Guérin BCG	• It protects against tuberculosis (*Mycobacterium tuberculosis*). A carrier of tuberculosis can be asymptomatic, or he or she may exhibit symptoms of respiratory infection, including coughing, chest pain, fever, chill, pallor, and fatigue. Symptoms can also include the expression of bloody sputum. • The tuberculosis virus is spread through droplets.
Tetanus toxoid TT	• It protects against the infection tetanus, which causes uncontrolled muscle spasms and rigidity as it attacks the brain and the central nervous system. • Tetanus is spread through direct contact with *Clostridium tetani* bacteria spores, which are found in soil that has been contaminated by animal feces. These bacterial spores enter the body through open wounds.

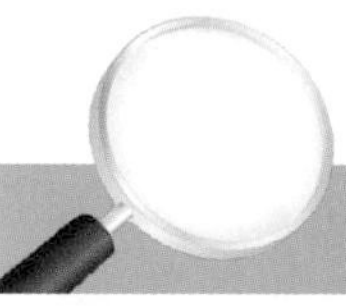

FOCUS POINT: The Smallpox Vaccine

Smallpox is a highly contagious and potentially deadly disease. In earlier times, it was quite common. It was introduced to North America by early immigrants and settlers. This devastating disease almost annihilated the Native American population of North, Central, and South America. Smallpox has now been eradicated in many countries, including the United States and Canada.

Vaccinations were given for smallpox until sometime around the 1970s, but the vaccine is no longer routinely given. However, because the vaccine is only effective for 10 years and there is now increasing consideration of the possibility of biological warfare, some countries are considering bringing it back. The vaccine contains the vaccinia virus.

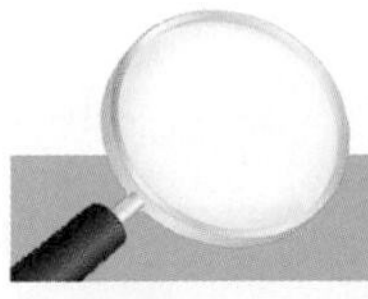

FOCUS POINT: Combination Vaccines

Some vaccines can be combined with others to provide protection from disease. Here are a few:

TwinRx (protects against both hepatitis A and hepatitis B)
TwinRx Jr (provides pediatric protection against both hepatitis A and hepatitis B)
MMR vaccine (protects against measles, mumps, and rubella)
MMRV vaccine (provides protection from measles, mumps, rubella, and varicella)

Eponyms: Bacille Calmette-Guérin (BCG)

The BCG vaccine for tuberculosis was discovered by A. Calmette and C. Guérin in 1905 in Paris, France. These scientists worked at the famous Institut Pasteur, which was named after Louis Pasteur (Pasteur discovered the process for pasteurizing milk). The BCG vaccine was first used with humans for immunization against tuberculosis in France in 1921.

Reflective Questions

Answer the following questions on the basis of what you've just learned about immunity.

1. What does the root word *immune* mean? ______
2. What does the combining form *phago-* mean? ______
3. What does the suffix *-lysis* mean? ______
4. What modern English term is derived from the root *deficere,* and what does it mean?
______
5. Which stage of the immune response occurs when you touch a tissue that someone has used to blow his or her nose? ______
6. When a person is diagnosed as having ongoing immunity to a disease, he or she does not require any further immunization at that time. Use medical terminology to describe what type of immunity this person has. ______
7. Although some people are allergic to cat dander, others seem to have a type of immunity to this allergen. What is this type of immunity called? ______
8. Which disease has the potential to return with effects so devastating that health officials in the United States are considering restarting a vaccine program for it?
______
9. Provide a synonym for the word *vaccination.* ______

Let's Practice

In this exercise, you will be given the formal medical name of a disease or infection. Provide the less formal—but equally appropriate—name for it.

1. infectious hepatitis ______
2. *Clostridium tetani* bacteria ______
3. *Mycobacterium tuberculosis* ______
4. rubella ______
5. serum hepatitis ______
6. rubeola ______

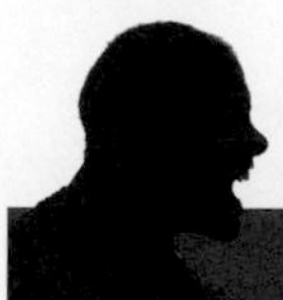

PRONUNCIATION PRACTICE

Say these words aloud to a friend or classmate, if you can. Here you are given the phonetic pronunciation. Your instructor can help you with pronunciation,

or you can visit **http://www.MedicalLanguageLab.com.**

hepatitis	hĕp″ă-**tī**′tĭs	rubeola	roo-bē-**ō**′-lă
influenza	ĭn″floo-**ĕn**′ză	tetanus	**tĕt**′ă-nŭs
inoculation	ĭn-ŏk″ū-**lā**′shŭn	tuberculosis	tū-bĕr″kū-**lō**′sĭs
rubella	roo-**bĕl**′lă		

Pathology of the immune system

When the immune system is not functioning or not functioning well, investigation is necessary to ensure that protection from invading pathogens or toxins is maintained in some manner. The source of the dysfunction must be identified and remedied. Immunosuppression, immunodeficiency, or allergies may be at the root of the problem.

The study of the pathology of the immune system falls to chemical pathologists. These professionals focus on the immune system and the function of antibodies, the pharmacological function of drugs in the body, and the role and function of hormones. Chemical pathology is a subspecialty of clinical pathology. Although it is not necessary to be a physician to hold these jobs, degrees in the health or biological sciences are requisite.

Immunosuppression

The term **immunosuppression** indicates that the immune response has been diminished or turned off altogether. When this happens, the patient is said to be in a state of immunosuppression. This condition can be the result of exposure to disease, certain types of drugs, or radiation. Immunosuppression can also be the result of the deterioration of the immune system over long periods of illness, such as that which occurs among patients with HIV/AIDS, alcoholism, or diabetes.

The word *suppression* is derived from the Latin word *suppressio,* which means *pressing under.*

Immunodeficiency disorders

When a person is diagnosed as *immune deficient,* a co-occurring state of disease is not only possible but probable. For whatever reason, the immune system is dysfunctional, and the individual is highly susceptible to infections and diseases that would not normally do him or her serious harm. In simple terms, the immune response is not functioning as it should. Patients who are immune deficient suffer from multiple incidents of infection, mostly respiratory and mucosal.

Congenital immunodeficiency disorders are caused by genetic abnormalities and are quite rare. They involve defects in B-lymphocytes, T-lymphocytes, or both. The individual will face a lifetime of dealing with infections. An example of one of these disorders is DiGeorge syndrome (see the Eponyms box that discusses this condition).

People with congenital immunodeficiency disorders are said to have *primary immunodeficiency.* These individuals are highly susceptible to infection and generally die when they are quite young.

Eponyms: DiGeorge and the DiGeorge Syndrome

DiGeorge syndrome is a collection of symptoms and birth abnormalities that can be detected prenatally through amniocentesis (i.e., a test of the amniotic fluid that surrounds the fetus). It can be inherited, or it may occur as a spontaneous mutation of chromosome 22. With this rare disorder, there is a defect in the genes of this chromosome, and many of the genes are missing. Core physical abnormalities, proneness to infection, and behavioral challenges result (see Figure 16-18). Prompt recognition and treatment prenatally or during infancy can lead to a normal life expectancy.

DiGeorge syndrome is also known as *CATCH-22.* This acronym identifies the faulty chromosome and the core features of the disease:

*C*ardiac defects
*A*bnormal facial features
*T*hymus underdeveloped or absent, which leads to T-cell deficiency or absence
*C*left palate
*H*ypocalcemia

A.M. DiGeorge was a 20th-century American pediatrician, professor of pediatric medicine, and geneticist who, during the 1960s, made the link to the chromosome involved in the disorder that came to have his name. However, the group of symptoms and abnormalities associated with the disease was first identified in Sweden by W. Wernstedt and E. Bottinger decades earlier, during the 1920s.

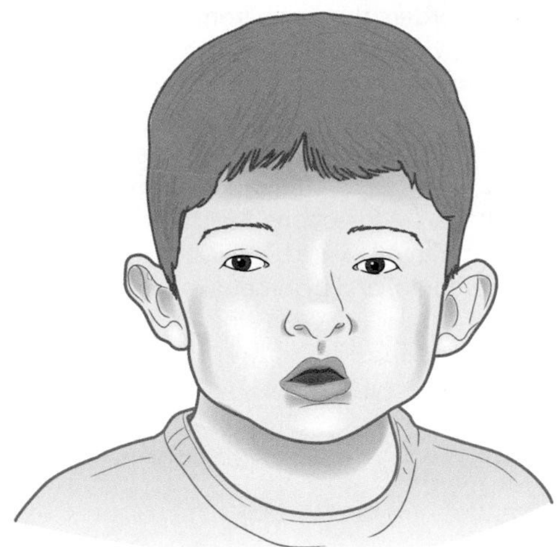

Figure 16.18: Child with DiGeorge syndrome

Combined immunodeficiency disorders or severe combined immunodeficiency disorders (SCIDs) are the result of the complete absence of both cell-mediated and antibody-mediated immune responses. SCIDs can be genetic (congenital). These conditions are difficult to treat; if they are untreated, they lead to the death of the affected children within the first year or two of their lives. An example is adenosine deaminase deficiency, which predisposes an infant to viral and fungal infections. Stem cell transplantation may be the most effective treatment for some types of SCIDs.

Acquired immunodeficiency disorders usually develop as a result of a disease or disorder such as the following:

- specific types of infectious diseases, such as varicella, rubella, tuberculosis, and hepatitis
- diabetes mellitus
- Down syndrome
- cancer
- human immunodeficiency virus (HIV)
- hepatitis

Other possible causes include the following:

- burns
- malnutrition
- alcoholism
- radiation therapy

- medications that are immunosuppressant:
  - anti-rejection drugs used after organ transplantation
  - chemotherapy agents used for cancer treatments
  - corticosteroids used to treat inflammation

A patient with a disorder of this type is said to have *secondary immunodeficiency*. The best known of the acquired immunodeficiency disorders is AIDS (see Focus Point: Acquired Immunodeficiency Syndrome)

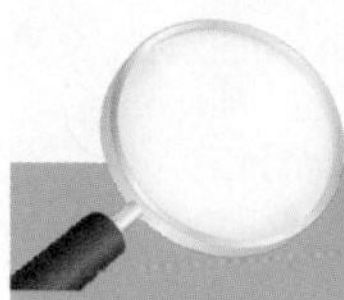

FOCUS POINT: Acquired Immunodeficiency Syndrome (AIDS)

AIDS is a group or syndrome of disorders that arise from the destruction of T-cells by the *human immunodeficiency virus (HIV).* This virus also attacks T-helper cells (see Chapter 14). AIDS develops from prolonged exposure to the HIV antibodies that are produced by the immune system to combat the virus. AIDS-related symptoms include severe weight loss and even brain tumors. Treatment is offered via antiretroviral therapy, which slows the progression of HIV. Because the body is hosting a virus that attacks the immune system, it becomes more susceptible to other *opportunistic infections;* these are infections that take advantage of a weakened immune system when they attack. Persons with AIDS are highly vulnerable to these infections, particularly pneumonia, *Candida,* Kaposi's sarcoma, and cytomegalovirus (an eye infection). There is no cure for AIDS, and it is life threatening.

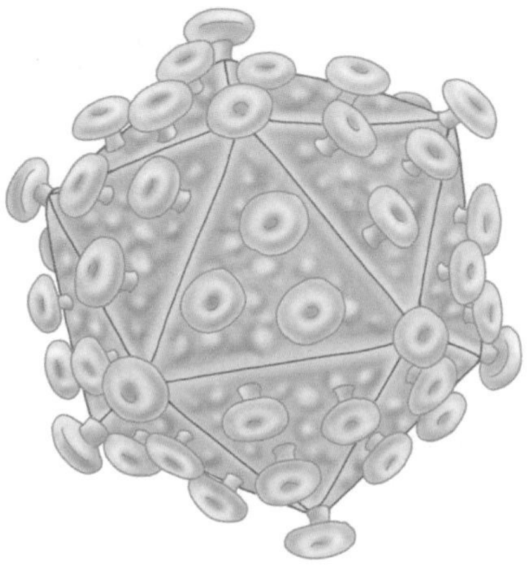

Figure 16.19: Human immunodeficiency virus: microscopic view

Allergies

An **allergy** is an immune response to a foreign antigen that leads to inflammation, organ dysfunction, or both. It is a hypersensitivity or an inability to tolerate exposure to an allergen, which is the foreign antigen. Exposure causes the body to overreact. This reaction is often respiratory in nature, but the response can also be topical. Although it may seem that what a person is allergic to can change over time, this is not actually true. If a person has an allergy, he or she can expect to have it for life. What does change is the amount of exposure that a person has to the allergen. Exposure is the key to whether or not the patient is symptomatic (i.e., showing symptoms). The exception to this may be an egg allergy; children have been known to outgrow this as they grow up.

The term *allergy* is derives from two Greek roots: *allos* and *ergon.*

all + ergon = allergy
↓ ↓
other + *work* = working against the other (i.e.: the pathogen or antigen)

Allergens

The term **allergen** refers to any substance that triggers an allergy response, which is a hypersensitive reaction or an abnormal immune response. Allergens can include substances such as pet hair and dander, shellfish, bee stings, dust, mold, and pollens. Some people are allergic to certain medications. Table 16-9 offers more examples. Although allergies are specific to individuals, most people will experience at least one allergic reaction to something during their lifetime.

Allergy responses

Contact with allergens is made physically through touch, ingestion, inhalation, and the olfactory sense (smell). This contact is referred to as *exposure* to the allergen. When exposure occurs, the immune response is initiated. An **allergy response** can include symptoms of sneezing, watery eyes, inflammation, and rash. An allergy response is also known as an *allergic response,* or *allergic reaction,* or a *hypersensitivity response.* An allergic response can range from mild to life threatening.

Some types of allergy responses are explained here; others appear in Table 16-9.

TABLE 16-9: Common Allergies, Symptoms, and Treatments

Scientific Name	Common Name	Class of Allergen	Primary/Cardinal Symptoms	Treatment
Apis mellifera	allergy to bee stings or honeybee venom	insect venom allergen	anaphylaxis	epinephrine avoidance; (carry an epinephrine injector [EpiPen])
Penaeus spp.	allergy to shrimp	food allergen (shellfish)	hives, nasal congestion, wheezing, dizziness, anaphylaxis	avoidance; epinephrine for anaphylaxis
Felis domesticus (Fel)	allergy to cats (to their dander, saliva, or sebaceous gland excretions)	pet allergen	rhinoconjunctivitis, hives	avoidance; medications; allergy shots
Beta-lactam (Pcn)	allergy to penicillin	drug allergen	anaphylaxis	avoidance; medication for mild symptoms; epinephrine for anaphylaxis
Hevea brasilensis (Hev b)	allergy to latex (rubber) or to the chemicals that are used to manufacture latex	occupational exposure allergen	contact dermatitis, rhinitis, bronchospasms	avoidance
Arachis hypogaea (Ara h)	allergy to peanuts	food allergen	rashes, cardiac arrhythmia, anaphylaxis	epinephrine avoidance; (carry an epinephrine injector [EpiPen®])
Apovitellin; ovalbumin; ovomucoid (Gad d Gal) or *Gallus gallus domesticus*	allergy to eggs, egg whites, or egg yolks	food allergen	hives, conjunctivitis, wheezing, rhinitis, anaphylaxis	avoidance; epinephrine for anaphylaxis (carry an epinephrine injector [EpiPen®])

Urticaria is a form of dermatitis, which involves inflammation of the skin that is characterized by small bumps on the skin that are raised, red, and itchy. The common term for urticaria is *hives*. Hives are a type of rash, but not all rashes are allergy responses.

The term *urticaria* is derived from the Latin word *urtica,* meaning *nettle*. The medical term for *itchiness* is **pruritus**.

Contact dermatitis is a localized skin reaction where the skin has come into contact with either an irritant or an allergen.

Allergic contact dermatitis occurs from external contact with an allergen such as poison ivy, latex, or certain soaps.

Irritant contact dermatitis occurs as a result of exposure to an irritant that does some damage to the skin (i.e., breaks it down). Examples of irritants include detergents and other cleaning products.

Rhinoconjunctivitis is an allergy response that is characterized by itchy, watery eyes and a runny nose that may also itch.

Anaphylaxis is an acute and potentially life-threatening allergy response. It results from an extreme sensitivity to an allergen. Symptoms may appear within seconds, although food allergy symptoms may not express themselves for up to 2 hours after ingestion. *Anaphylaxis is an emergency situation.* Symptoms can include urticaria, pruritus (itchiness), bronchospasms, dyspnea, laryngeal edema, angioedema (i.e., swelling of the lips, tongue, and face), vertigo, tachycardia, and loss of consciousness. Respiratory distress may ensue when the airways close as they swell. When the airways are completely blocked, death may result.

Right Word or Wrong Word: *Hives* or *Rash*?

Are these two terms always interchangeable? Are they true synonyms? Explain.

Allergy treatments

Allergies are most often diagnosed and treated by allergists. These medical specialists are able to pinpoint the causes of allergy responses. After the cause is identified, clients are taught how to adapt to and manage their allergies autonomously (i.e., on their own). In other words, the client is taught to avoid allergens by reducing or eliminating his or her exposure to them. When exposure cannot be avoided or controlled to limit its negative effects, medications may be prescribed. These may include antihistamines and corticosteroids. Immunotherapy (allergy shots) may also be recommended to help desensitize an individual to an allergen. This process is known as *antigen desensitization*. Immunotherapy of this type is done mostly with children.

Histamines are naturally occurring substances that are released by the immune system. They play a role in triggering the allergic responses of rhinitis, conjunctivitis, urticaria, breathing irregularities, and nausea. To combat these reactions, *antihistamine* medication is given orally, intravenously, or intramuscularly. An example of a very commonly used antihistamine is diphenhydramine (Benadryl).

Anaphylaxis is treated with epinephrine (adrenaline) administered via intramuscular or intravenous injection. Epinephrine has the ability to counteract allergic reactions. It also serves as an effective bronchodilator by keeping the airways open. Many people with severe allergies carry a syringe or a syringe-like device filled with epinephrine in case of a sudden exposure to an allergen that may be life threatening in a very short time frame. This epinephrine delivery device (trade name: EpiPen®) can relieve symptoms immediately. Transport to a hospital is expected after its use to ensure that the individual is safe and that the allergy response has subsided.

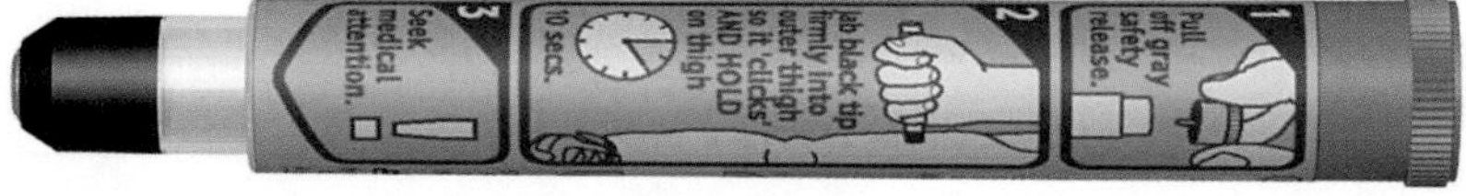

Figure 16.20: Epinephrine delivery system (EpiPen®) (From Eagle S, Brassington C, Dailey CS, Goretti C: *The Professional Medical Assistant: An Integrative, Teamwork-Based Approach.* Philadelphia: FA Davis, 2009, p. 654. With permission.)

Right Word or Wrong Word: *Food Allergy* or *Food Intolerance*?

Are these two terms synonymous? Are food allergies and food intolerances the same thing?

Autoimmune diseases

The immune system has a built-in mechanism for identifying the body's own natural cells and substances (i.e., hormones, lymph). It can distinguish *own* from *foreign* or *self* from *non-self*. However, it is possible for this recognition system to fail. When this type of failure occurs, autoimmune diseases result. There are many possible causes of an autoimmune reaction. For example, if the immune system should overreact or overrespond to a pathogen or toxin, it can alter elements of the immune response to a point at which phagocytes and lymphocytes can no longer discern foreign from familiar. When this happens, the immune system attacks and destroys the body's own cells and tissues. It becomes autoimmune.

A state of **autoimmunity** occurs when the immune system produces antibodies that are directed against the self. These are called *autoantibodies*. As they bind with self-antigens, they create *immune complexes*. When these immune complexes build up in tissues, they cause inflammation, pain, and injury to tissue. A very common autoimmune disease that illustrates this process is arthritis.

In this textbook, you have been introduced to a number of autoimmune diseases in the context of body systems and physical illnesses, including the following:

- diabetes (Chapter 12)
- Graves' disease (Chapter 7)
- multiple sclerosis (Chapter 14)

Table 16-10 provides details about more autoimmune diseases. The Rheumatology section of this chapter will explore the group of autoimmune diseases referred to as "arthritis" in detail.

Autoimmune diseases are not curable. However, they are treatable. Treatment modalities can include anti-inflammatory medications (including corticosteroids), analgesic medications, the use of hot and cold compresses, physical therapy, occupational therapy, relaxation, mindfulness, meditation, and changes in diet.

Stress and the immune system

When the immune system is forced to work for extended periods of time as a result of disease or exposure to stressors, it eventually becomes fatigued and less capable of defending the body. A prolonged stress response can lead to headaches, hypertension, and a lack of physical and mental energy.

Adrenal fatigue or *hypoadrenia* is a syndrome that is just gaining recognition in the medical world. Its symptoms include fluid and electrolyte imbalances, alterations in mood and motivation, the inability to think as clearly as normal, fatigue or exhaustion, sleep difficulties, food cravings, and weak muscles. Adrenal fatigue is often misdiagnosed as other disorders, including depression. A buccal swab (a swab of the inside of the cheek) is used to diagnose this syndrome.

Vitamin B_{12} and the autoimmune system

When she first arrived at A.L. Murphy Clinic, Stevie-Rose Davis suggested to the nurse-practitioner that she may have "low B_{12}." She will be tested for that deficiency via the blood work that was ordered. A deficiency in the level of vitamin B_{12} in the body can frequently be seen in patients with autoimmune diseases such as diabetes, hypothyroidism, and rheumatoid arthritis. Our client has two of these conditions. Other contributors to low B_{12} that may or may not influence or be influenced by the autoimmune system are an individual's history of smoking, high alcohol consumption, inadequate nutrition, and coping with significant stress. Stevie-Rose certainly meets two of these criteria.

TABLE 16-10: Autoimmune Diseases

Disease	Description
Lupus (systemic lupus)	• a chronic autoimmune disease • symptoms include joint inflammation, pain, and damage to the tissues of the joints, heart, lungs, kidneys, and skin
Scleroderma	• a rare, chronic, rheumatic, autoimmune disease of the connective tissues • symptoms include the thickening and hardening of the connective tissues
Ankylosing spondylitis (AS)	• a form of chronic arthritis • symptoms include the chronic inflammation of the joints of the spine and the sacroiliac joint (i.e., the joint where the sacrum and the ilium meet in the lower back)
Juvenile dermatomyositis (JDM)	• a rare autoimmune disease in children • symptoms include skin rash and weak muscles caused by the inflammation of the blood vessels under the skin and in the muscles (vasculitis)

Let's Practice

You are given a term or description. Provide the medical term.

1. itchiness ______________________________
2. adrenaline ______________________________
3. hives ______________________________
4. swelling of the lips, tongue, or face ______________________________
5. difficulty breathing ______________________________
6. olfactory ______________________________
7. swelling of the throat ______________________________
8. desensitize to an allergen ______________________________
9. showing symptoms ______________________________
10. free of or lacking any symptoms ______________________________

Mix and Match

Match the scientific name of the allergy with its more common name. Be careful: there is one here that you may have not seen before, but you should be able to discover it through the process of elimination.

1. *Gallus gallus domesticus*	milk allergy
2. *Felis domesticus*	penicillin allergy
3. *Arachis hypogaea*	egg allergy
4. Beta-lactam	cat allergy
5. *Bos taurus*	peanut allergy

Build a Word

Add the prefix *auto-* to each term or set of word parts below to create a new term, and then define each new term that you create.

1. vaccine	Term: ______________	Meaning: ______________
2. hypnosis	Term: ______________	Meaning: ______________
3. toxin anti-	Term: ______________	Meaning: ______________
4. genesis	Term: ______________	Meaning: ______________
5. lysin hemo	Term: ______________	Meaning: ______________
6. phagia	Term: ______________	Meaning: ______________

Critical Thinking

Consider all that you know about our client, Stevie-Rose Davis, to answer the following questions.

1. Although no one has ever mentioned that she may be immunosuppressed, Stevie-Rose is a potential candidate for this condition. What condition does she have that may contribute to immunosuppression?

   ____

2. What evidence is there that Stevie-Rose may have a vitamin B_{12} deficiency?

   ____

   ____

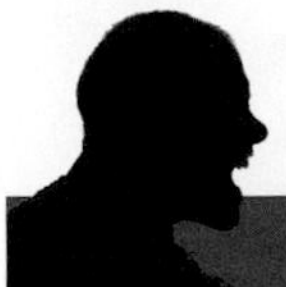

PRONUNCIATION PRACTICE

Say these words aloud to a friend or classmate, if you can. Here you are given the phonetic pronunciation. Your instructor can help you with pronunciation,

or you can visit **http://www.MedicalLanguageLab.com.**

anaphylaxis	ăn″ă-fĭ-**lăk′**sĭs	epinephrine	ĕp″ĭ-**nĕf′**rĭn
angioedema	ăn″jē-ō-ĕ-**dē′**mă	lupus	**lū′**pŭs
autoantitoxin	aw″tō-ăn″tī-**tŏk′**sĭn	pruritis	proo-**rī′**tŭs
autophagia	aw″tō-**fā′**jē-ă	scleroderma	sklĕr″ă-**dĕr′**mă
conjunctivitis	kŏn-jŭnk″tĭ-**vī′**tĭs	urticaria	ŭr-tĭ-**kā′**rē-ă
dermatomyositis	dĕr″mă-tō-mī″ō-**sī′**tĭs		

Rheumatology and Arthritis

Rheumatology is the field of medicine that specializes in disorders of the joints, muscles, and bones, as well as the diagnosis and treatment of arthritis, which is really a group of autoimmune diseases. Stevie-Rose Davis is going to be seen by a rheumatologist, who will evaluate the severity of her arthritis. She has been noticing some uncomfortable changes in the joints of her hands and knees. Rheumatic diseases are assessed and classified by a system created by the American College of Rheumatology, which sets out criteria that are based on a client's functional ability (see Table 16-11).

TABLE 16-11: Functional Classes of Rheumatic Diseases

Class	Functional Assessment Criteria
I	completely and wholly functional; no handicaps present as the result of rheumatic disease
II	adequate functional capacity for normal activities; some handicap or discomfort present; limited mobility of one or more joints
III	functional capacity is limited to doing only a few or none of the activities of daily living; limited self-care
IV	wholly incapacitated by a rheumatic disease; likely bedridden or confined to a wheelchair

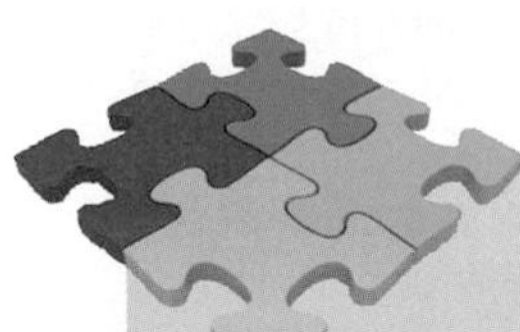

WORD BUILDING: Formulas for Creating Words fom the Root *rheum* or *rheuma*

rheum **or** ***rheuma*** **= Greek roots meaning** ***flowing, watery, or running (as in water running).*** **The combining forms are** ***rheum/a*** **and** ***rheumat/a*****.**

rheumat + ism = *rheumatism*

Definition: an older medical term (that is less used today) that refers to acute and chronic conditions of inflammation, muscle soreness, and stiffness; pain and stiffness in the joints. *noun*

Example: The term *rheumatism* used to be applied to all types of arthritis and other joint diseases.

Continued

rheumat + oid = *rheumatoid*

Definition: resembling or similar in nature to rheumatism (or to illnesses previously defined as rheumatism). *adjective*

Example: *Rheumatoid* arthritis can be the result of having had rheumatic fever.

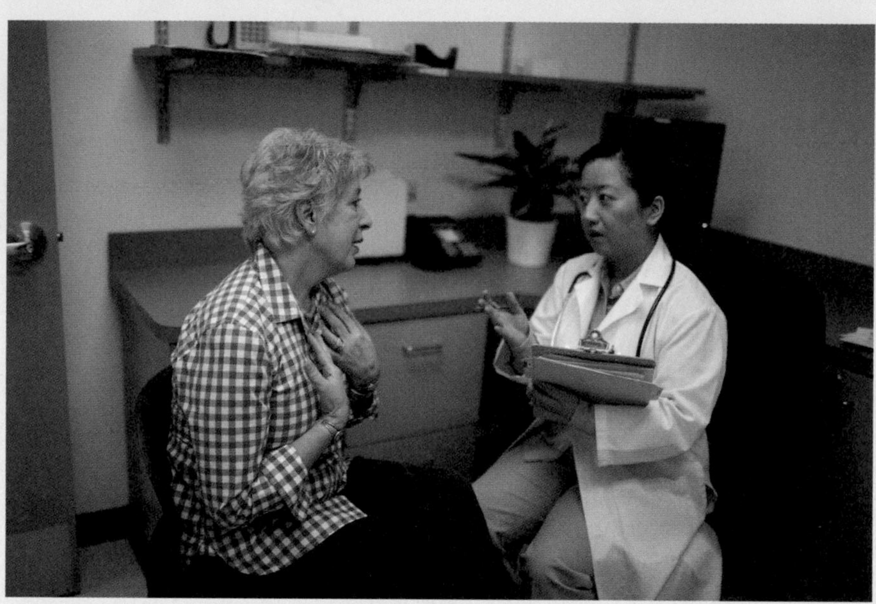

Patient Update

Stevie-Rose Davis was not able to see a rheumatologist at the A.L. Murphy Center until the next day. She met with Dr. Maggie Chan, a pleasant woman with a very professional demeanor. As they began, the physician pulled up the client's medical records on her computer and perused the information from the radiographs of the client's hands and knees, taken the day before. She then began the client interview.

"Mrs. Davis, I see here that you have a history of arthritis. I believe that's osteoarthritis, correct?" Stevie-Rose did not take the opportunity to ask Dr. Chan to call her by her first name; she sensed a more formal and professional manner in the doctor, which was not conducive to the use of first names.

"Yes, that's correct," said Stevie-Rose. "I've had it for about 10 years or so now. For a long time, it just gave me some minor aches and pains in my joints, but lately, my finger joints are beginning to swell and stiffen." She showed the doctor. "I don't really notice any changes in my knees, other than some stiffness in the morning when I get up or if I have been sitting for too long, but I chalk that up to old age. Unfortunately, I'm not as young as I used to be, and I know full well that aging affects the joints, as well as every other part of the body." Dr. Chan nodded, listening carefully as she took the client's hands into her own to examine them more carefully.

"While I agree that aging plays a role in how our joints function and that mobility overall does change with age, I am not certain that all of the symptoms you have been describing to me today are simply the result of aging," Dr. Chan commented. "As a geriatric patient yourself, you can appreciate that your age does play a significant role in the changes that you are experiencing in your body, but there are other pathological processes at work here—namely osteoarthritis—that are responsible for your symptoms. Osteoarthritis is not old-age specific." Stevie-Rose sat there and listened, aghast at the terminology that the physician was using.

"I beg your pardon," Stevie-Rose interjected. "Please do not call me a 'geriatric patient'! I take great offense at that. I may be growing old, but I do not under any circumstances consider myself to be a geriatric patient," she asserted. "Nor do I appreciate your term *old-age specific.*" She sat then in silence, awaiting a reply.

"Forgive me," said the doctor. "I had not meant to offend. I was simply using proper medical terminology when I was speaking. Perhaps I should not have ..." Stevie-Rose interrupted Dr. Chan and was somewhat calmer after having heard an apology, but she was still assertive.

"I'm not sure that it's even proper medical terminology these days for people who are aging," said Stevie-Rose. "You know, more and more people are living to be 100 years old—and I very well may be one of them—so 50 is now the beginning of middle age. I believe middle age is usually a span of 20 years. I'm 72, so I've just recently become a senior citizen in my mind. You may refer to me as a 'senior,' but I do *not* consider myself to be one of the elderly. Not yet. I reserve that term for people who are 80 years old and older. I am an older adult, and, quite frankly, I am generally in very good health. I am physically active; I have all of my memory and intellect intact; and I am very involved with my family, my friends, and my community. I take good care of myself." Stevie-Rose paused again to let this information sink in.

"Very well," replied Dr. Chan, "I stand corrected. Once again, I hadn't meant to offend. What you say is very true today. People are living longer, and this necessitates a change of terminology when speaking about older adults versus, say, the elderly or the frail elderly. Even so," she pointed out, "the field of gerontology is the discipline and science of aging during the later years of life." Stevie-Rose conceded this point. They then agreed to continue talking about Stevie-Rose's arthritis.

"When I look at your x-rays," said Dr. Chan, "I can see that you certainly have inflammation in the joints of your hands. I see some pathological changes in the synovial fluid of a number of your finger joints and perhaps even in your left wrist. I think I can help you with this. We could take some further studies, if you'd like. Perhaps a CT scan or an MRI." The client said that she would think about it. Dr. Chan then continued: "I think it's important that you've come for assessment and treatment now. It's always better to treat or intervene with a disease before the symptoms become unmanageable." They went on to talk about Stevie-Rose's knees and her other joints in more detail. The doctor then asked Stevie-Rose to step into the exam room so that she could more thoroughly assess Stevie-Rose's range of motion, her reflexes, and the functional capacity of her joints.

As the interview and assessment progressed, Dr. Chan also said that she'd like to prescribe an anti-inflammatory medication specifically for arthritis. She spent some time discussing pain management, and she inquired as to how the client was coping with her arthritic pain and what methods of coping the client used. Stevie-Rose informed Dr. Chan that she tried to take daily walks and that she was involved in a square-dancing group to keep herself physically fit and her joints mobile. She noted that warm baths helped to ease the pain and stiffness that she felt in her knees and hands and that she always carried a pair of light cotton gloves with her. She found these very helpful to reduce the pain in her fingers that occurred if she found herself in a very cold air-conditioned room. Dr. Chan wondered if Stevie-Rose may be interested in attending either physical therapy or occupational therapy for a short while to help improve her range of motion and her joint stamina. The client was interested, but she noted that Veterans Affairs may not fund both types of treatment. They talked about available options, and Stevie-Rose decided that she'd like a referral to physical therapy.

As the appointment was about to end, Dr. Chan said, "I see here on your chart that you have been referred to our Counseling Department." She waited for a response.

"Yes, yes ..." Stevie-Rose responded, not wanting to go into details about her mental health with a rheumatologist. "I'm under quite a lot of stress lately. My husband's ill, and ...." She chose to let the sentence fall uncompleted. Dr. Chan nodded. Sensing the client's unease with the topic, the physician did not press her to continue. Instead, she spoke with Stevie-Rose about the implications of having a chronic illness, such as osteoarthritis in addition to other stressors in a person's life. She talked about the mind-body connection with arthritis and how pain, inflammation, stiffness, and other symptoms can lead to frustration, disappointment, and even depression. The client had not previously thought about this idea, and she agreed that the effects of her arthritis may be a subject to discuss during her counseling sessions at some point.

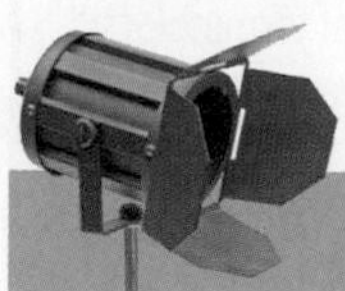

CAREER SPOTLIGHT: Rheumatologist

A *rheumatologist* is a physician who specializes in the musculoskeletal system: the joints, some autoimmune diseases (i.e., arthritis), and disorders of the soft and connective tissues. Rheumatologists complete undergraduate education, medical school, and a medical residency, and they then specialize in rheumatology. To practice, they need to be certified by the American Board of Internal Medicine.

Key terms: rheumatology and aging

During the conversation between Dr. Chan and Stevie-Rose Davis, a number of terms related to the client's physical health and her age were used. Key terms from the dialogue are italicized in the example and highlighted below with the explanation.

"... I *chalk that up* ..."

chalk that up: an idiom that means *attribute that to* or *explain the cause of that.*

"... there are other *pathological processes* at work here ..."

pathological processes: the progression and effects of a disease or illness.

"... not *old-age specific.*"

old-age specific: occurring only during old age.

"... *aghast* at the terminology ..."

aghast: horrified or shocked by.

"... or the *frail elderly.*"

frail elderly: a classification of older adults who are unable to manage or care for themselves.

"... take some further *studies* ..."

studies: diagnostic tests.

"... her reflexes, and the *functional capacity* of her joints."

functional capacity: the ability or potential ability to function.

"... improve her range of motion and her *joint stamina.*"

joint stamina: the resiliency or strength of a joint.

Critical Thinking

Stevie-Rose Davis had not made the mind-body connection between her arthritis and her mood or her concentration levels of late. Think about that connection as you answer these questions. Be careful; these two questions may seem similar, but they are not the same.

1. How is mood affected by pain or increasing disability?

   ____

2. How is mood affected by a progressive disability, such as that which occurs in patients with severe cases of arthritis throughout the body?

   ____

Anatomy and physiology of joints: enhanced terminology

Stevie-Rose Davis suffers from osteoarthritis. Before terminology can be introduced for that autoimmune disorder, terminology for the anatomy and physiology of the joints must be acquired.

Recall from Chapter 3 that a **joint** is a point of connection or articulation between two or more bones. As you know, without fully functional joints, movement is impaired. There are 360 joints in the body (as compared with 206 bones).

To work, joints need the presence, support, and assistance of the bones, ligaments, cartilage, synovial fluid, and synovium. Joints can be classified according to the degree and type of movement that they allow. Table 16-12 explains these classifications, and Figure 16-21 illustrates the movement of different types of joints.

TABLE 16-12: Classification of Joints: Structures and Types of Movement

Name of Joint and Structure	Type of Movement
Ball-and-socket joint (a joint that consists of a bone with a rounded head that fits into a cup-shaped bone socket)	Facilitates swinging and rotating movements Examples: hips and shoulder joints
Condyloid or ellipsoidal joint (a joint at the site of two or more bones; a *condyle* is an oval-shaped tip on a bone that fits into the hollow shape of a nearby ellipsoid bone to form a knuckle)	Facilitates moving from side to side, bending, and extending Examples: jaws and fingers
Fibrous or immovable joint (a joint that is held firmly together by connective tissue)	No movement occurs Examples: sutures of the skull
Gliding joint (a joint between the surfaces of two flat bones that are held together by ligaments)	Permits movement between the flat surfaces of bones, mostly in a sideways direction; the bones are able to glide past each other Examples: wrists
Hinge joint (bones come together at the joint and fit into each other while being supported by very strong ligaments that keep the joint in place)	Facilitates movement in one anatomical plane only; extends and flexes; opens and closes only Examples: fingers, elbows, and knees
Pivot joint (a joint at end of one bone that rotates around another bone)	Facilitates rotation Examples: the radius and ulna at the wrist; the neck's ability to turn from side to side
Saddle joint (a joint that sits between a *concave* [curved inward] bone and a *convex* [curved outward] bone)	Allows movement in two different directions; enables grasping, as well as rocking back and forth or side to side Examples: thumbs

Physiology of joints

Cartilage is a type of dense, strong connective tissue that can withstand physical pressure, exertion, and tension. *Cartilaginous joints* are those in which the bones are attached to each other by cartilaginous discs and ligaments. These joints provide only a limited degree of movement.

Examples: the vertebrae of the spine and the symphysis pubis in the pelvis.

Compound joints consist of several joints between several bones that provide a wider range of movement.

Examples: the joints of the cervical spine

Synovial joints are the most common type. Each of these joints is encapsulated by a ligament that is lined with a synovial membrane. This synovial membrane secretes synovial fluid between the bones, which lubricates the joint. Ligaments hold the joint in place, thus preventing dislocation. The *articulating bones,* which are the ones that communicate with or work with each other, are covered by protective cartilage (see Figure 16-22).

Examples: ball-and-socket, hinge, saddle, ellipsoidal/condyloid, gliding, and pivotal joints. With many types of arthritis, the synovial joints are pathologically affected.

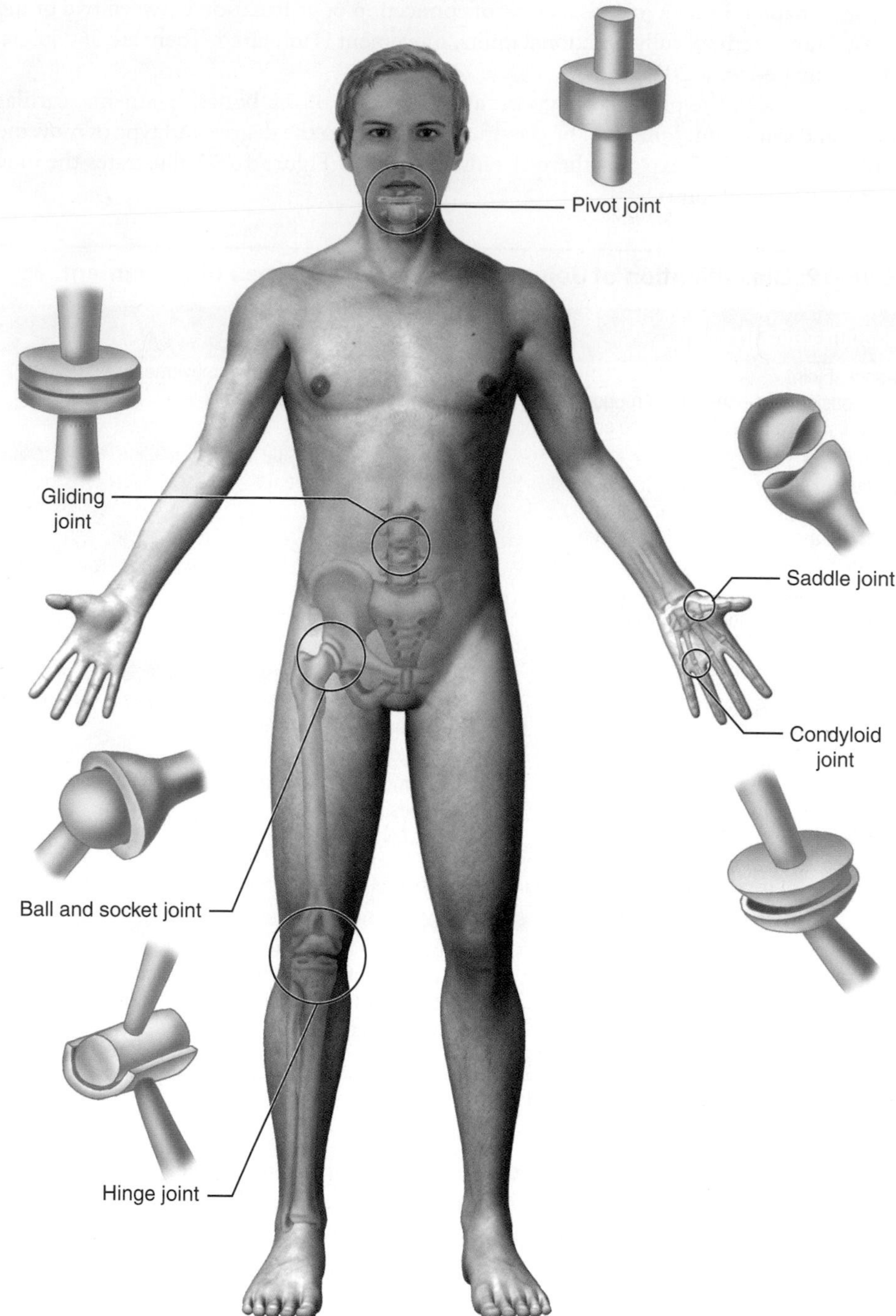

Figure 16.21: Types of joints: classified by movement

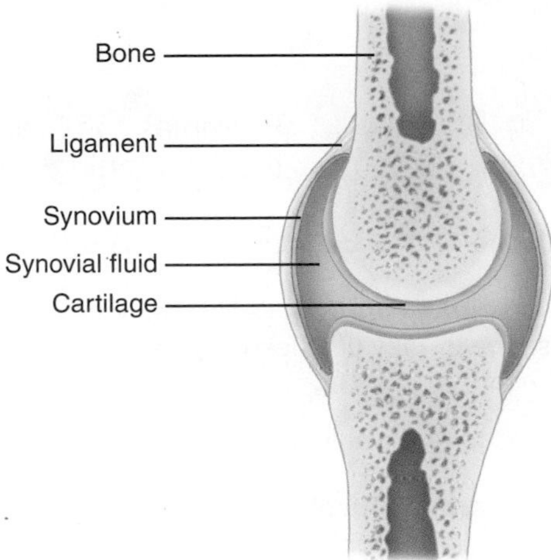

Figure 16.22: Detailed anatomy of a synovial joint

Arthritis and the joints

Arthritis is a term that applies to a number of autoimmune diseases that affect the joints and movement. These include the following:

- rheumatoid arthritis
- osteoarthritis
- gouty arthritis (gout)

Medically, arthritis is situated in the context of rheumatology because a core feature of this group of diseases is pathology of the fluid or **rheuma** in the joint spaces. In particular, there may be pathological changes in the synovial fluid; this is called *synovial membrane hypertrophy.* A comparison of a normal, healthy joint with an arthritic joint can be seen in Figure 16-23.

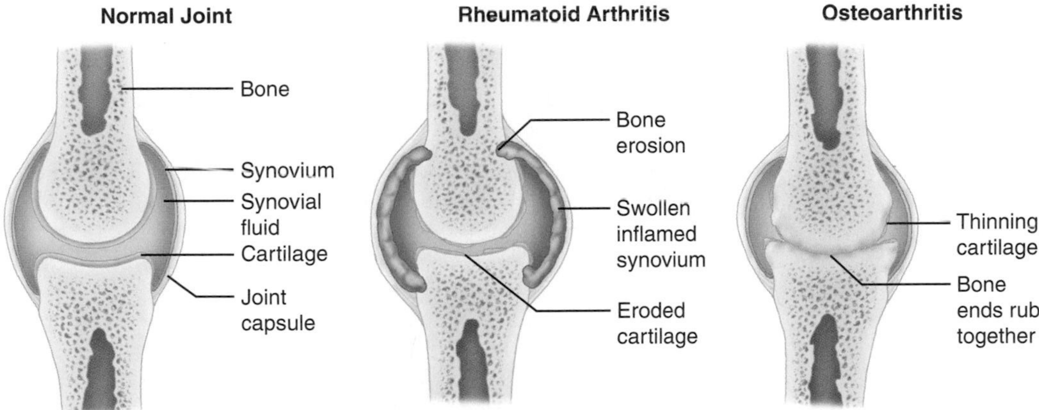

Figure 16.23: Normal joint vs. joints with osteoarthritis and rheumatoid arthritis

Deconstructing the word parts of *arthritis* reveals the word's meaning:
arthr/o + itis = arthritis
↓ ↓
joint inflammation = inflammation of the joint(s)

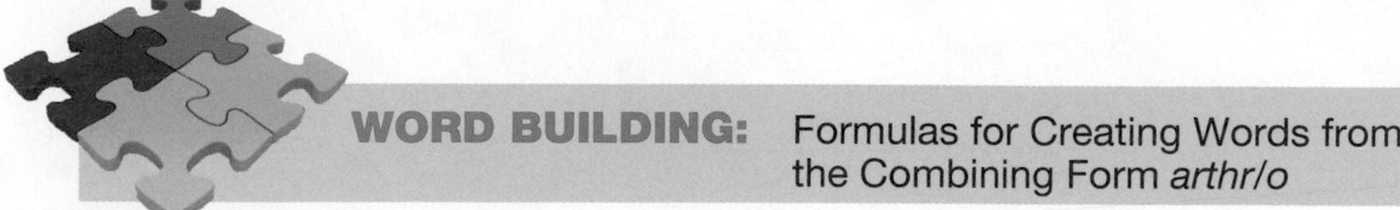

WORD BUILDING: Formulas for Creating Words from the Combining Form *arthr/o*

***arthron* = Greek root meaning *joint*. The combining form is *arthr/o*.**

arthro + centesis = *arthrocentesis*

Definition: entry into a joint space by way of a needle. (The second root word is derived from *kentesis,* meaning *puncture.*) *noun*

Example: *Arthrocentesis* is used to remove fluid from a joint for laboratory analysis.

arthro + desis = *arthrodesis*

Definition: the fusion of two bones. (The root *desis* means *binding*.) *noun*

Example: Ankle *arthrodesis* may be necessary when a fracture at the site does not heal correctly or promote weight bearing.

arthro + graph + y = *arthrography*

Definition: a radiograph taken after the injection of contrast dye into a joint. *noun*

Example: *Arthrography* of the knee is very common; it is often performed for people who have persistent pain.

Rheumatoid arthritis (RA)

Rheumatoid arthritis is a chronic inflammatory autoimmune disorder that attacks the synovial joints and causes inflammation of the soft tissues that surround them. The cause is unknown. Symptoms include pain, stiffness, limited movement, and the thickening of the soft tissues, which can be seen on an x-ray (see Figure 16-23).

Osteoarthritis (OA)

Stevie-Rose Davis has *osteoarthritis*, which is a very common form of the disease. There are two types. With each type, the shape of the joints may change over time (Figure 16-24).

Primary osteoarthritis runs in the family and involves the hands, the hips, and the finger joints. Bunions on the great toe of the foot may also appear.

Secondary osteoarthritis is a degenerative joint disease that progresses over a lifetime. It is influenced by wear and tear on the joints or the spine. It involves the hands (including the thumb), the hips, and the knees.

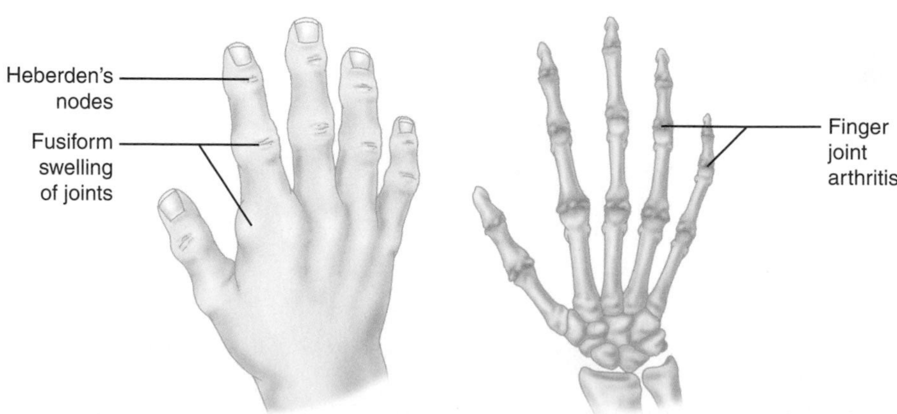

Figure 16.24: Osteoarthritic hand: external view and internal view

Gout (gouty arthritis)

Gout is a type of arthritis that is caused by a buildup of crystals of uric acid in the joint capsules. It often affects only one joint, and that is usually a great toe. This disease is chronic, but it offers periods of remission (i.e., no symptoms) that help the individual to endure it. Gout can be very painful. The affected joint becomes red and inflamed during the acute phase.

Symptoms of arthritis

General symptoms of arthritis can include swelling, pain, stiffness, limited movement, muscle weakness, and fatigue. Disfigurement of the knuckles may also occur. Consider the following examples:

Inflammatory arthritis leads to the swelling of the joint, which is caused by synovial membrane hypertrophy.

Non-inflammatory arthritis leads to the development of **osteophytes**. These are swellings on the bone that are eventually seen as knobby, gnarled, or disfigured joints.

Treatments for arthritis

Arthritis is not curable. However, there are many types of treatment available to help relieve the symptoms. These include medications, hydrotherapy, physical and occupational therapy, decreasing the amount of stress in one's life, making changes in one's dietary habits, and performing daily exercise. Surgical treatment may also be an option.

Arthroplasty is a surgical procedure to remove bone or to replace tissue to facilitate the function and stability of a joint. There are three types:

- *Resection arthroplasty* removes a small portion of bone to repair a joint.
- *Interposition arthroplasty* takes new tissue from somewhere else in the body and places it between the damaged surfaces of an elbow joint.
- *Revision arthroplasty* is a surgical procedure that is performed to replace a failing joint. An example of this is a hip replacement.

Prefixes related to arthritis

The prefixes *mono-*, *oligo-*, and *poly-* are used to identify how many of the patient's joints are involved in the arthritic disease process. You should be familiar with these prefixes at this point.

monoarthritis: 1 joint

oligoarthritis: 2 to 4 joints

polyarthritis: 5 or more joints

The prefixes *amphi-*, *syn-*, and *di-* are used to classify arthritis by functional ability. These prefixes may be unfamiliar to you. Their definitions are provided.

syn: without or none
- synarthrosis: limited or no mobility, particularly in the fibrous joints; an immovable joint

amphi: on both sides, all around, or double
- amphiarthrosis: some mobility, although it is limited, particularly in the cartilaginous joints

di: twice, two, or double
- diarthrosis: a wide variety of movements are possible. This term refers to the synovial joints.

Right Word or Wrong Word: *Athero-* or *Artho-*?

You have had an opportunity to work with each of these combining forms. Do they have the same meaning? In which body system will you find each word part used? Give an example for each.

Pain Management

Dr. Chan also spoke with Stevie-Rose about **pain management**. This is a broad medical term that pertains to how individuals perceive and cope with pain when they experience it. In a hospital or clinical setting, nurses and doctors help patients to manage their pain. During outpatient or home care, patients and clients manage their pain independently, with the guidance of a care provider. Whether they are in or out of a care facility, all patients and clients are taught how to identify, evaluate, and intervene with pain so that they may take care of themselves or ask a health professional for assistance.

In Chapter 11, Clay Davis was taught to use a pain scale that had been adapted for pediatric care. Pain assessment was also described in Chapters 11 and 13. Stevie-Rose Davis will be familiar with pain scales for adults because she is a retired nurse who has worked with adult patients. Adult pain scales are similar to those that are used in pediatric care, but they lack the cartoonish or childlike features in the images that are used. More generally, health professionals will explore and assess pain with patients or clients with the use of the following *rubric* or set of established steps:

The PQRST assessment:

P: palliative or provocative factors for the pain (i.e., what is causing or contributing to it)

Q: quality of pain (i.e., burning, stabbing, aching)

R: region of body affected (i.e., the location or site of the pain)

S: severity of pain

T: timing of pain (i.e., does it occur after meals? in the morning?)

Pain management includes the use of medication, hot and cold compresses, increasing periods of rest and sleep, ensuring a well-balanced diet (so that the body has all of the nutrients it needs to respond fully to the pain), and referrals to physical and occupational therapists, chiropractors, and massage therapists. It can also include acupuncture, meditation, and yoga.

Mix and Match

Match each type of joint with a corresponding body part.

1. saddle	wrist
2. pivot	hip
3. gliding	thumb
4. hinge	knee
5. immovable	neck
6. ball and socket	skull sutures

Let's Practice

Answer the following questions by identifying what is being described.

1. a surgical procedure that is performed to replace a failing joint ____________________

2. limited mobility in the cartilaginous joints ____________________

3. identified by a buildup of crystals of uric acid in the joint capsules ____________________

4. a type of pain assessment for all aspects of the pain, not just its severity ____________________

Build a Word

You are given parts of a medical term. Combine the parts to build a term, and then define the term.

1. scopy arthr/o Term: ____________________ Meaning: ____________________

2. emia olig Term: ____________________ Meaning: ____________________

3. dynia arthr/o Term: ____________________ Meaning: ____________________

Reflective Questions

Consider what you've learned about joints, arthritis, and pain management to answer the following questions.

1. What is a rubric? ____________________

2. What does the "Q" in *PQRST* stand for? ____________________

3. What is a PCA? ______________________________
4. How many joints are involved in the diagnosis of polyarthritis? ______________
5. What is the name of the procedure that is used to replace a hip joint? ____________
6. What is the difference between *convex* and *concave* (see Table 16-12)? ____________
____

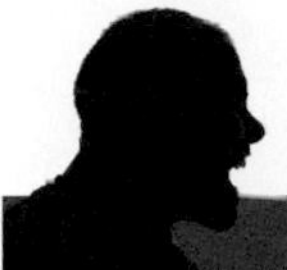

PRONUNCIATION PRACTICE

Say these words aloud to a friend or classmate, if you can. Here you are given the phonetic pronunciation. Your instructor can help you with pronunciation,

or you can visit **http://www.MedicalLanguageLab.com.**

amphiarthrosis	ăm″fē-ăr-**thrō**′sĭs	diarthrosis	dī″ăr-**thrō**′sĭs
arthrocentesis	ăr″thrō-sĕn-**tē**′sĭs	ellipsoid	ē-**lĭp**′soyd
arthrodesis	ăr-thrō-**dē**′sĭs	gout	gowt
arthrodynia	ăr″thrō-**dĭn**′ē-ă	rheumatoid	**roo**′mă-toyd
arthroscopy	ăr-**thrŏs**′kō-pē	rheumatology	roo″mă-**tŏl**′ō-jē
cartilaginous	kăr″tĭ-**lăj**′ĭ-nŭs	synarthrosis	sĭn″ăr-**thrō**′sĭs
condyloid	**kŏn**′dĭ-loyd	synovial	sĭn-**ō**′vē-ăl

The Language of Aging

Aging refers to the natural process of growing older. However, it is used as a broader concept when it is applied to older adults. It becomes a category for identifying people as old, older, or elderly. It is important to recognize which medical terminology is appropriate to use with which clients or patients.

For example, Stevie-Rose Davis took exception to Dr. Chan referring to her as a "geriatric patient," and she brought forward a number of key points to support her argument. Even so, being referred to as "geriatric" has bothered her ever since. Before leaving the A.L. Murphy Clinic, Stevie-Rose phoned her husband, Zane, to tell him about this issue. As you proceed through that conversation now, pay attention to Zane and Stevie-Rose's attitudes toward aging, and take note of their health-promoting activities. Reflect on what you have learned in this chapter. Can you evaluate this aging couple's domains of health and wellness?

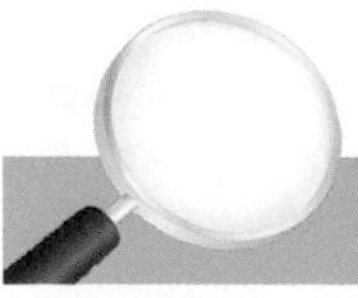

FOCUS POINT: Geriatric and Gerontology

Geriatric stems from the Greek root *geras,* which means *old age*. *Gero* and *geront/o* are the combining forms.

Geriatrics is the medical specialty that is concerned with pathophysiological changes during later life.

The field of research and medicine that deals only with the adults during later life is called *gerontology.*

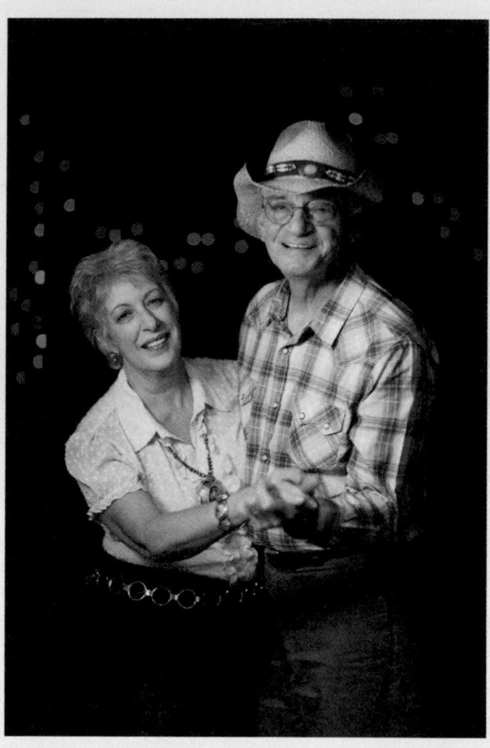

Patient Update

"Hi, Zane, I'm just finishing up here at the clinic now," Stevie-Rose said into her cell phone. "I thought I'd call and let you know I should be home in about an hour."

"How'd it go, honey?" Zane asked. Stevie-Rose told him about her meeting with the rheumatologist and that she had made an appointment to begin physical therapy for her arthritis later in the week. She didn't tell him about her pending appointment with the counselor; she didn't want to burden him with what she thought was unnecessary information at this time. Instead, Stevie-Rose told her husband about something that had been bothering her all day.

"Zane, that woman ... that doctor ... oh, I just have to get this off my chest," she began. "That doctor called me a 'geriatric patient'!" Stevie-Rose's voice rose in pitch and became louder. When no response came, she said, "Zane, Zane, love ... did you hear me? Zane, are you listening to me?" She shook the cell phone in her hand, as if it wasn't working.Then she heard him begin to laugh.

"Honey, I don't know what you're getting all worked up about. We aren't young anymore, you know. That doctor might be right," he said gently.

"Right? Right???" Stevie-Rose said incredulously. "I am just barely out of middle age, and you think I'm a geriatric? No siree, Bob! Not me. I'm still young and spry and smart as a whip. I have my own cell phone, for crying out loud!" She paused a moment. "And you're not doing so badly yourself, Zane," she pointed out. She heard him say "Uh-huh," and then she continued with her story. "I told her—that doctor—that she should choose her words more carefully, you know. I offered her a few suggestions about how she might refer to people of our age without making us feel really old and helpless, for heaven's sakes." Zane chuckled in the background. Stevie-Rose listened and finally started laughing, too. "Oh, Zane, you're right. I've gotta face it sometime. I'm getting up there in years. Darn it, anyway."

"That's all right, honey," said Zane. "As long as you and I are 'up there' together, it doesn't matter what anyone else calls us or how they see us. We know who we are and how we are, and we know we aren't what most people think of as 'old people.' We're a new breed, my love: the young-old!" They laughed. "Now come on home," Zane said. "Quincy will be here soon for supper." Stevie-Rose reminded her husband gently that she had not forgotten about their dinner plans. Then Zane added, "Oh, by the way, Mickey called. She and Steven want to know if we want to join them for supper on Saturday night and get in a little Texas line dancing."

"Oh, honey, I'd love that!" Stevie-Rose replied, and then she muttered just loud enough for Zane to hear as she hung up, "Old, my foot!"

Key terminology: aging

Political correctness, respect, and an appreciation for whom clients are as human beings are all important aspects of the day-to-day work that health and allied health professionals do with clients, patients, and their families. Therefore, it is important to keep abreast of new terminology and trends in health care that address not just science and medicine but that consider the human experience as well. Aging is a good example of this. It is important for all health professionals to avoid any signs of **ageism**, discrimination against, stereotyping of, or stigmatization of older adults.

Whether you work directly with clients or in medical research, population health, or a similar field, familiarity with the terms of reference for aging will be necessary. Table 16-13 provides a number of these, including some euphemisms. A *euphemism* is a descriptive term or phrase that is considered milder than others; it is less offensive or painful to hear or to have applied to oneself. It is very important to avoid any signs of ageism in your interactions with clients and patients.

Table 16-14 provides information about how older adults are divided statistically into age groups and what these categories are called. As the human life span is extended to 100 years or more, the terms of reference for adult age groups will change to reflect healthier and more productive populations of older adults. As Stevie-Rose has said, she still considers herself to be young at the age of 72 years. For now, the most appropriate and currently acceptable term to use when working with someone who is more than 65 years old is *older adult.*

TABLE 16-13: Using Appropriate Language for the Aging Population

Euphemism	Definition or Description	Polite or Politically Correct?
(the) aged (pronounced ā′jĕd)	• people who have grown old	Yes
elder	• a person who is more than 65 years old • connotes respect for maturity	Yes
elderly	• a person who is more than 65 years old • a word that some older people dislike because they believe it signifies frailty and perhaps being of less value to society	Yes, in a medical and professional context Use caution when using this term with an older patient or client.
frail elderly	• an older adult (usually more than 75 old) who has multiple health challenges and who is at risk for more	Yes, in a medical and professional context and with family members and support persons of this client, patient, or resident of a care facility. The person would not be called a *frail elder* but simply *frail.*
geriatric	• synonymous with *aged,* as discussed previously • has a connotation for many people of being unable to care for oneself or of being mentally and physically less capable	Yes, in a medical and professional context No, with clients or patients who do not perceive themselves to be this
old age	• a very broad and commonly used term that is used to identify anyone who is perceived to be older than middle aged and who is in their later years of life	Some individuals may take offense when this term is used in reference to them.
old-timer	• an archaic, colloquial term	No, not professional This is considered impolite and rude to use unless the person is someone whom you know and who allows this term to be used.
baby boomers *or* boomers	• people who were born between 1946 and 1960, during the post–World War II population boom	Yes
senior	• a mature adult who is generally more than 60 or 65 years old • term may also be recognized by governments and agencies to identify eligibility for benefits and discounts	Yes However, do not call clients *seniors* until they have identified themselves as such. Remember, a person may look older than he or she really is.
senior citizen	• a term much like *senior* that engenders some respect	Yes

TABLE 16-14: Current Terms for Adult Age Groups

Term	Age
middle age	approximately 45 to 66 years old
young-old	66 to 75 years old
old	76 to 84 years old
old-old, oldest-old, or very old	85 years old or older

CHAPTER SUMMARY

Chapter 16 has come to an end and Stevie-Rose Davis is on the road to improving her mental and physical health with the help of the A.L. Murphy Clinic at the Sumac Veterans Medical Center. In the context of her assessment and treatment there, terminology for the limbic and immune systems was introduced and used. The language of anatomy, physiology, pathology, and treatment provided the anchors from which to complete vocabulary and knowledge-building exercises. The concept of the mind-body connection was enhanced with new terminology and opportunities to apply it were provided. Critical thinking exercises afforded us opportunities to assess our client and to apply concepts and terms to her care and to the care of others, as shown for the examples that addressed immune and autoimmune disorders. The language of aging illustrated the importance of word choices when engaging clients (in this case, the older adult).

See How Much You've Learned

For audio exercises, visit **http://www.MedicalLanguageLab.com.** 

Chapter 16 also introduced new abbreviations. A number of them appear again here in a concise table to promote study.

TABLE 16-15: Abbreviations in Chapter 16

Abbreviation or Acronym	What It Means
AIDS	acquired immunodeficiency syndrome
BCG	bacille Calmette-Guérin; a tuberculosis vaccine
Ig	immunoglobulin
ILs	interleukins
HPV	human papillomavirus
HBV	hepatitis B virus
TB	tuberculosis
MMR	measles, mumps, and rubella (vaccine)
MMRV	measles, mumps, rubella, and varicella (vaccine)
TT	tetanus toxin
HIV	human immunodeficiency virus
AS	ankylosing spondylitis
JDM	juvenile dermatomyositis
ACTH	adrenocorticotropic hormone

KEY TERMS

active immunity
ageism
aging
allergen
allergy
allergy response
anaphylaxis
antibodies
antigens
arthritis
arthroplasty
autoimmunity
B_{12}
cartilage
challenge
chronic
compensate
disturbed
disturbed thought process
endorphin
frail elderly
functional capacity
hypothalamic-pituitary-adrenal (HPA) pathway
immune response
immunity
immunization
immunoglobulins (Ig)
immunosuppression
inextricably
innate immunity
inoculations
interleukins
joint
joint stamina
lymphocytes
lysis
macrophage
mast cells
mental health
opiate
opioid
osteophytes
pain management
passive immunity
pathogen
pathological processes
phagocytes
phagocytosis
preoccupation
pruritus
rehabilitation counseling
rheuma
rheumatology
rumination
stigma
stress
stressors
support groups
vaccine
vaccination

CHAPTER REVIEW

Critical Thinking

1. Define the term *syndrome* in the context of health care.
___
2. Why doesn't Stevie-Rose want to be referred to as *elderly*?
___
3. Why is arthritis treated by a rheumatologist rather than an orthopedic physician?
___

Reflective Questions

Use your new knowledge of medical terms and medical language to answer the following questions.

1. What is the plural form of the term *hippocampus*? ___
2. Antibodies alone cannot kill cells. What else do they need to carry out or complete this process? ___
3. What is the difference between an antigen and an antibody? ___
4. Define *acquired immunity*. ___
5. Can a counselor provide psychotherapy to clients? ___
6. Which type of arthritis produces disfigurement of the joints (i.e., gnarled fingers)?
___

Translate the Terminology

Here is an opportunity to apply your knowledge of medical terminology in a new way and to generalize your learning to a more complex passage. Translate the following passage into your own words.

Within the depths of the cerebrum lie a number of sizeable aggregates of limbic neurons. In the forebrain, limbic structures and the hypothalamus are essential to survival as they initiate food-seeking behaviors, self-protection mechanisms, and adaptation to environmental factors. In addition, there is a functional interface between the limbic system and the motor neurons that support it. During the first 3 years of life, the amygdala and the cingulate are implicated in the acquisition of synaptic interconnections that result in sociability, emotional attachments, and the development of appropriate emotionality. Conversely, when these structures are deprived of sufficient stimulation during the same time period, inappropriate or explosive emotionality may occur, as may pathological shyness or diminished sociability.

____

____

____

____

Fill in the Blanks

Answer the following questions by filling in the blanks.

1. A synonym for the *fornix* of the limbic system is ________________.
2. Psychologists and psychotherapists provide long-term treatment for their clients; however, counselors provide ________________ treatment.
3. The type of arthritis that most often affects only the big toe is ________________ arthritis.
4. ________________ is a type of arthritis that is thought to be inherited or familial.
5. Stress can influence or be influenced by the ________________ and ________________ systems.
6. ________________ is a belief system that stereotypes the older adult as frail or less valuable to society.

Break It Down

Deconstruct the following medical terms into their component parts. Follow this example.

Example: Musculoskeletal = muscul/o + skelet/o + al

1. geropsychiatry ______________________________
2. rheumatic ______________________________
3. arthroscopy ______________________________
4. immunodeficiency ______________________________
5. phagocytolysis ______________________________

Right Word or Wrong Word: *Osteo-* or *Artho-*?

Do these two roots have the same meaning? If not, what is the difference between them?

Right Word or Wrong Word: *HPV* or *HBV*?

Do these two acronyms have the same meaning? Write out the words for which each set of letters stands, and then explain any difference in meaning.

Word Accuracy

Demonstrate that you are reading and interpreting accurately. Differentiate between the medical terms in each set by defining each term.

1. counselor, therapist

____

____

2. active immunity, passive immunity

____

____

3. senior, elderly

____

____

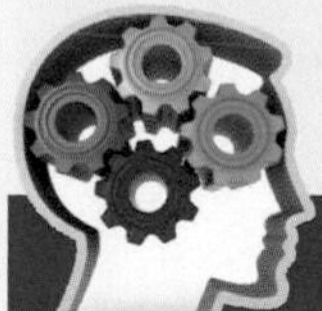

MEMORY MAGIC

Here are a couple of mnemonics that can be used to remember key elements that apply to the assessment and care of the older adult.

1. **OVAH**

This mnemonic can be used when admitting an older adult to the hospital and beginning his or her medical record or chart.

O = outpatient and over-the-counter medications reviewed

V = vision assessment

A = advance directives (do-not-resuscitate orders, power of attorney, and so on)

H = hearing assessment

2. **PULSE PROFILE**

This mnemonic can be used to remind you how to perform a cursory assessment of the functional ability of an older adult. It looks at activities of daily living, mobility, medical conditions, and psychosocial involvement.*

P = physical condition

U = upper limb function

L = lower limb function

S = sensory components

E = excretory functions

S = support factors

*Granger, C.V., Albrecht, G.L., Hamilton, B.B. Outcome of Comprehensive Medical Rehabilitation: Measurement by PULSES profile and the Barthel Index. *Arch Phys Med Rehabil.* 1979 April; 60(4): 145-154.

CHAPTER SEVENTEEN

Reproductive and Family Health

Focus: Reproductive Systems, Infant/Child/Family Growth and Development

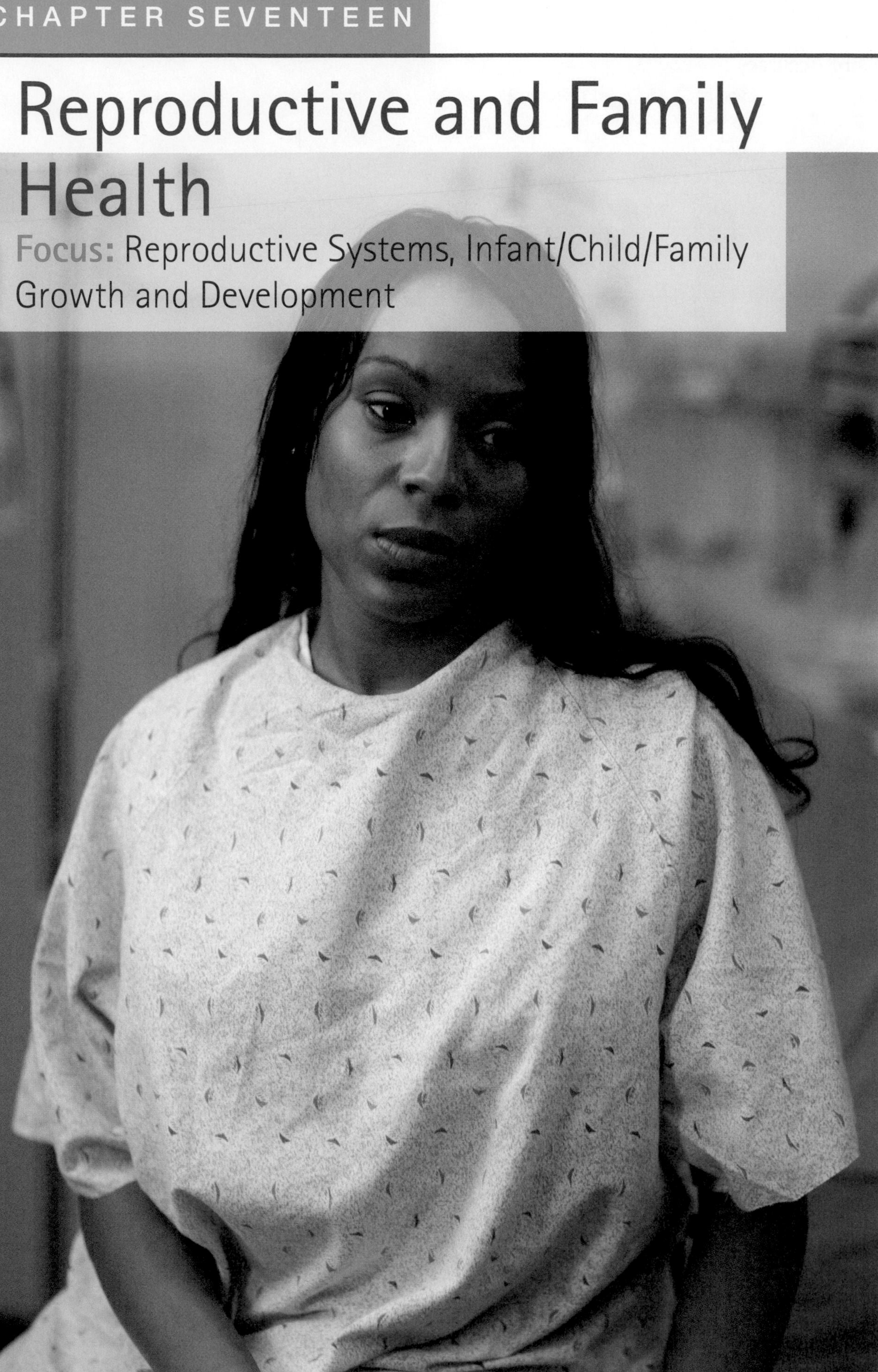

Glory Loeppky, a 32-year-old married mother of a premature infant, has an appointment with her family practice physician this morning, for a postpartum checkup. Although she has already been seen by the obstetrician who delivered her baby by Cesarean section, a checkup with a family physician is also routinely scheduled from 4 to 6 weeks postpartum. Glory was a passenger in the vehicle with her husband when a motor vehicle accident occurred 5 weeks ago. This led to the premature birth of her daughter, Emily Grace, who remains in neonatal care at Fayette General Hospital. Glory also sustained a deep laceration wound to her thigh and an injury to her thumb, which were treated in the ER upon her arrival there.

Patient Update

"Hello, there," said Dr. Antoine in a friendly tone as he entered one of his examination rooms at Mary Ezra Mahoney Clinic. Glory was sitting on the examining table, wearing a paper gown, waiting for him. She smiled back at him. He took a seat at his desk and logged in on his computer to pull up her medical record.

"It's good to see you again, Dr. Antoine."

"So, how's that new baby of yours?" he inquired cheerfully. "Doing well? Still in NICU?" Glory explained that the staff at Fayette General Hospital had told her that Emily Grace was doing "remarkably well" given the circumstances of her very early premature birth. The baby had been moved to a step-down unit, the neonatal nursery. Dr. Antoine nodded and expressed his pleasure at hearing this, understanding what it meant to Glory.

"I have to get another pediatrician," Glory continued. "My HMO says I have to take the baby to one of the doctors in its network once she's discharged from the hospital. Dr. Jasper was there at Fayette General when Emily Grace was born, so they're going to allow him to continue her care as long as she's there."

"All right then, Glory, let's talk about you and your health now." Dr. Antoine stood up and walked over to take her TPR and BP. He talked as he worked. "I see my medical assistant weighed you today and that you've lost some of that baby weight already."

Glory smiled and told him she had lost nearly 10 pounds in 5 weeks; she wondered if that was normal, or a combination of normal and her running back and forth to the hospital and helping her husband to get moving around the home. He agreed with the latter.

"Are you getting any sleep? Eating regularly?" Dr. Antoine asked. Glory confirmed that these issues were not posing a problem for her, but she expected her sleep to be reduced once the baby came home. Again, Dr. Antoine nodded his agreement. Then he asked about the status of her bowel movements and her ability to void. She confirmed that the frequency and consistency of her bowel movements had returned to what she perceived to be normal for herself and that she was not experiencing any abnormal changes in frequency of urination, nor had she noticed any unusual color in the urine. "I'm going to order a urinalysis and a couple of blood tests today just the same," said Dr. Antoine. "This is strictly routine postpartum, Glory. I just want to be sure that you're not fighting off any infections or having any other difficulties." She agreed that this was a good idea.

"I'd like to begin your physical exam now, Glory. Would you like the nurse to join us so that there is another female present in the room?" Glory considered this question for a moment and then declined the offer, saying that she felt comfortable with her doctor. "All right, but if you decide you'd like to have the nurse here at any time, please just let me know, and we'll stop for that." She nodded her agreement.

"Okay, let's begin. I'm going to check your abdomen now, so if you'll please lie down here on the examining table. I'm just going to palpate here and here. Let me know if there is any tenderness. I won't press directly on your incision line." She smiled and thanked him for that consideration, commenting that the site was still somewhat tender. Then she lay down.

The doctor began by examining her breasts, looking for tenderness there, as well as any redness, discharge, or abnormal changes to the nipples. Other than the typical postpartum tenderness and swelling, Dr. Antoine did not find anything that concerned him. He inquired if she was breastfeeding the baby yet.

"Yes, yes," she said happily, "I was able to start breastfeeding 3 weeks ago when the baby reached 33 weeks gestation. Oh, it's wonderful to hold my baby!" She paused, as if remembering. "But, as you know, I've also been pumping my breast milk so that the nurses can give her some by bottle. I really think this is important for Emily Grace." Dr. Antoine confirmed the importance of not just bonding with the baby through the act of breastfeeding whenever that was possible. He also spoke about the importance to the infant's immune system of receiving antibodies by way of breast milk. She nodded.

"Now, I'm going to use a speculum to do an internal exam, to look at your vagina and cervix." Glory positioned herself on the table, feet in stirrups. Dr. Antoine continued speaking as he prepared. "I know you had a cesarean birth. This procedure will let me feel your uterus, too, to see if it has reduced in size appropriately for 5 weeks postpartum." He proceeded and then asked her to sit up. He took off his gloves and washed his hands. "Everything's looking good, Glory. You're recovering well, and I can't find anything to be concerned about."

"You mean you're giving me a clean bill of health, Dr. Antoine?" She smiled. "Oh, I almost forgot. Please take a look at that big scar that's forming on my left thigh. I know you've seen it before, but I was just wondering if it's okay, or if it's going to always look so big and red and ugly." He took a look at her request, inspecting for color, depth, and tenderness.

"You're healing well. That wound was quite deep, as I recall, and you had internal and subcuticular sutures that dissolved over time. I don't see any real marking from the sutures, just the mark where the edges of the skin have approximated. The coloring and size of this wound will certainly diminish over time, but you might want to consider keeping it out of the sunlight for awhile to avoid any further tissue damage." She asked about applying Vitamin E cream, and he agreed that many people have found positive results with this treatment of newly formed scar tissue.

"And what about your thumb ... the left one? I see you're wearing a brace on it still. How's that going?" Glory said that she had regained most of her range of motion and function in her thumb following the ulnar collateral injury, and that she was following the instructions of the physical therapist, who had seen her in the hospital, to promote healing. She reported that she continued to wear the brace to protect the thumb. She said this was important when she was helping Gil get dressed or helping him with some of his other ADLs. She also mentioned she wore the brace when driving and while performing various activities around the house. He validated her need to protect the thumb and its saddle joint.

"So, all in all, Glory, I am happy to say you are doing very well, physically. Why don't you get dressed now and come in to my office so that we can talk." Dr. Antoine smiled and left the room to give her some privacy.

For audio exercises, visit **http://www.MedicalLanguageLab.com.** 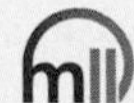

Reflective Questions

Reflect on the dialogue you have just read as you answer these questions.

1. How long has it been since Glory was in the motor vehicle accident?

   ____

2. What is the status of her leg wound from the MVA?

   ____

3. What is the status of the ulnar collateral injury to her thumb?

   ____

Learning Objectives

After reading Chapter 17, you will be able to:

- Understand concepts and use medical terminology related to postpartum health.
- Understand and use the language of sexual and reproductive health.
- Appreciate the education, training, and work of family practice physicians.
- Appreciate the education, training, and work of reproductive health clinicians, biologists, and technicians.
- Acquire terminology and knowledge related to the pathology of sexually transmitted infections and diseases.
- Enhance vocabulary related to the anatomy, physiology, and pathology of the male reproductive system.
- Enhance vocabulary related to the anatomy, physiology, and pathology of the female reproductive system.
- Recognize key terminology related to family practice medicine.
- Appreciate the education, training, and work of public health nurses.
- Acquire and use vocabulary related to family health, lifecycles, and family practice medicine.
- Develop vocabulary for and knowledge of childhood growth and development, illness, and wellness.
- Understand and use medical terms for pathologies of childhood.
- Enhance terminology for immunity to include newborns, infants, and children.
- Understand terms and concepts pertaining to breastfeeding and immunology.

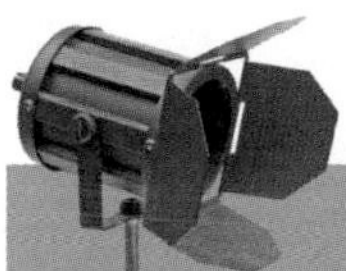

CAREER SPOTLIGHT: Family Physician

A *family physician* is a medical professional who treats families as a unit, as well as caring for each individual in that unit. The family and its individual members are this physician's clients or patients. Family physicians study *family practice medicine.* This includes health care across the life span, including not only medicine but also the behavioral, social, and psychological aspects of health. Family physicians are educated in the same manner as all doctors, but with a specialty in family care.

Postpartum Health

Postpartum health, or *maternal health,* includes attention to all the changes that occur following giving birth. A physical and psychosocial assessment of postpartum health is important for all new mothers. Depending on the woman's circumstances, this checkup may include environmental and financial assessments as well. If necessary, referrals to agencies that can help and that support the mother and infant will be made at the time of the appointment. Typically, an initial assessment occurs within the first 2 weeks and then 4 to 6 weeks after delivery of the baby. For example, Glory was first seen by the obstetrician who delivered her child and now has been seen by her family practice physician, who will manage all of her care again.

Postpartum health checkups also include assessment and discussion of breastfeeding, if the mother has decided to nurse her baby. However, counseling about breastfeeding itself is most often managed by nurses, nurse practitioners, and other specialists who work directly with the new mother to assist her.

The term *breastfeeding* can be written in the following ways, and all are quite acceptable:

breast feeding–two distinct words
breastfeeding–one word
breast-feeding–hyphenated

The term *breastfeeding* is synonymous with *nursing*. For example, a woman who is breastfeeding her infant is nursing her infant. A mother who breastfeeds her infant is referred to as a *nursing mother*.

Right Word or Wrong Word: *After birth* or *Afterbirth*?

Are these two different ways of writing the same term? Or does writing the term as one word change the meaning? Explain.

Right Word or Wrong Word: *Postpartum* or *Postnatal*?

Are these two words synonyms? They certainly look like they might be. What do you think? Explain.

Key terms: postpartum health

Dr. Antoine completed a postpartum physical assessment of Glory Loeppky, including an external and internal exam. Key terms from his dialogue with the patient are italicized in the text and highlighted below with the explanation.

. . . wearing a *paper gown* . . .

paper gown: disposable paper garment worn by patients during a physical exam.

. . . moved to a *step-down unit*, the *neonatal nursery* . . .

step-down unit: medical jargon meaning a unit for those who now need less continuous monitoring or care but still have medical needs.

neonatal nursery: a step-down unit from neonatal intensive care. It is much like any other infant nursery in a hospital, but it makes provisions for the special needs of premature and other at-risk infants. These might include special precautions for infection control, direct access to the NICU in case the baby's condition suddenly changes, and so on.

The neonatal nursery is sometimes referred to as the *special care nursery*, *intermediate care nursery*, or less professionally, the *preemie unit.*

. . . *bowel movements* . . .

bowel movements: acts of defecation, widely referred to as *BMs* by health care providers.

. . . the *frequency and consistency of her bowel movements* . . .

frequency . . . of her bowel movements: how often defecation occurs.

consistency . . . of her bowel movements: the firmness, density, viscosity, and uniformity of the patient's stool (feces).

. . . directly on your *incision line* . . .

incision line: the line on the skin where two sides of an incision (a surgical cut) have now come together.

. . . I've been *pumping my breast milk* so . . .

pumping breast milk: extracting, or *expressing*, milk from the breast; this is accomplished with a device called a *breast pump*.

...going to use a *speculum* to do an internal exam...

speculum: a device used for internal exams for women to dilate (open) the vaginal canal for examination. A speculum can be either plastic or metal.

...on the table, feet in *stirrups*...

stirrups: an apparatus attached to an examining table in which the heels of the feet are placed; the knees are bent.

...*subcuticular sutures* that dissolved over time...

subcuticular sutures: sutures below the epidermis, below the surface of the skin.

...don't see any *real marking* from the sutures...

real marking: reference to a specific type of cross-hatch scarring from the sutures themselves, as opposed to the incision line. Suture scars can initially be more predominant when staples are used to close a wound/incision; however, all suture scars are likely to fade over time (see Figure 17-1).

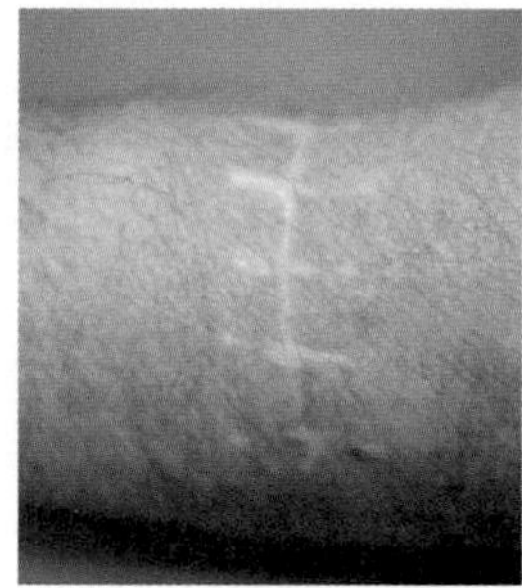

Figure 17.1: Surgical suture scar (From Barankin, B, and Freiman, A: *Derm Notes: Clinical Dermatology Pocket Guide*, FA Davis, Philadelphia, 2006, p 145, with permission.)

...edges of the skin have *approximated*...

approximated: come together in close proximity, in a manner that closes the wound or incision. Figure 17-1 shows an approximated incision line that has begun to heal.

...asked about applying *Vitamin E cream*...

Vitamin E cream: an antioxidant topical cream that enhances production of collagen (see Chapter13). Vitamin E is more formally known as *tocopherol.*

Reflective Questions

Demonstrate cumulative knowledge.

1. What caused the two opposing sides of Glory's incision to come together, to heal?

____

2. What term could be applied to describe the activities of a patient who has several bowel movements in a day?

____

3. What type of sutures did Glory have to close her leg wound?

____

Critical Thinking

Use new terminology in other contexts. Consider what you have previously learned about another patient in this book to answer this question.

Zane Davis was originally admitted to the ICU, but he was soon transferred. What new terminology have you just learned that could describe where he went?

____

Fill in the Blanks

Fill in the blanks with the correct terms.

1. Some sutures need to be removed, whereas others ____________.
2. Women who are unable to be present when their baby needs feeding may opt to ____________ breast milk and store it for these occasions.
3. A ____________ is a device used for internal exams for women to open the vagina and cervix for inspection.

Postpartum mental health

A rollercoaster of emotions occur during and after pregnancy for every member of the family, friends, or support group involved in the birth of a child. However, these emotional changes are much more significant for the woman who has given birth. As you have learned previously, there is a fundamental interplay of hormones, the limbic system, and the reproductive system that can contribute to mood swings, both prenatal and postnatal. Although all pregnant women can expect these mood swings, which usually dissipate gradually after birth, some new mothers may develop mental illnesses, such as postpartum depression and, possibly, even postpartum psychosis.

Patient Update

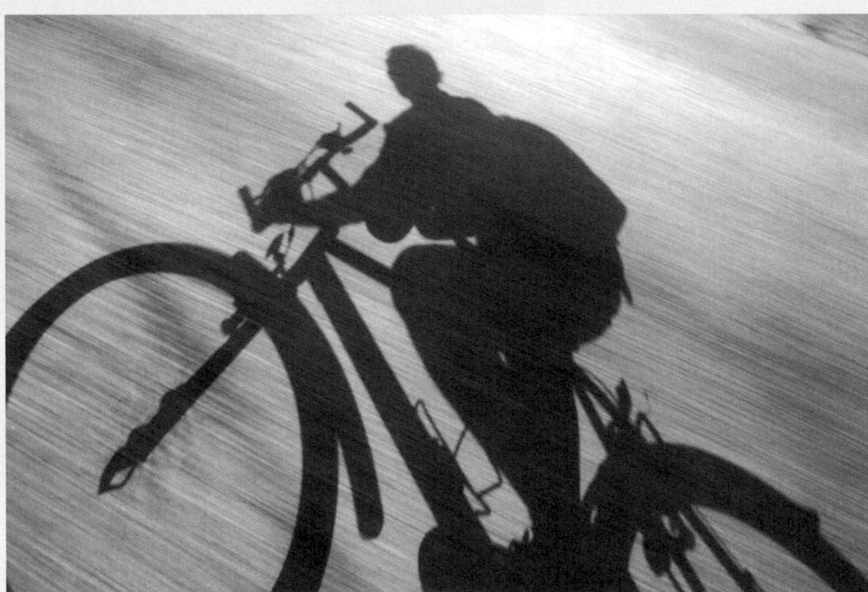

Glory got dressed and stepped into Dr. Antoine's office next door. He was standing by the window, lost in thought. She joined him there for a moment before they took their seats.

"I'd like to talk more about how you're doing, Glory. You've been through a stressful time that I suspect has been both happy and troublesome for you. Am I correct?" She nodded.

"Let's talk for a minute about your husband, Gil, and how you and he are both managing," said Dr. Antoine. He paused, waiting for her to signal that he should go on. She did. "When you were here a couple of weeks ago, you said he was about to be discharged from the hospital. How did that go?" Glory explained that Gil was indeed home, but that his mobility was limited. She was helping him move about the house. She reported that he was still in recovery and receiving physical therapy for his leg, as well as his brain injury. Dr. Antoine explored how her husband's condition was affecting her—emotionally and physically—knowing that she was also attending to her baby at the hospital for most of the day and into the evening. He also inquired about how she helped her husband get around, worrying about undue stress on her abdomen post-Cesarean section. She reported this had not been an issue, and she had been very careful about this possibility.

"I've been very lucky that way, you know. Thankfully, Gil is in recovery and, although he seems impulsive and moody sometimes, that doesn't happen a lot. And I don't want to leave him alone too long during the day because I worry that he might fall or—and this is a big fear of mine—he might pass out or bump his head or something ..." Her voice trailed off. The physician talked with her about her fears.

Then Glory added, "Well, Gil's mom and dad live nearby. They both work but are able to check up on him when I'm at the hospital with Emily Grace. And my mom and dad help out, too. They don't live that far away, and they take turns coming in to stay with him sometimes. Of course, he wants his independence back, so he won't allow any of the family to stay too long. He says it makes him think he's being babysat!" She laughed and went on to express her empathy for his position. She paused for a moment or two before going on. Dr. Antoine waited patiently, knowing she would.

"Dr. Antoine, you know we were in a car accident," she said, looking at him for confirmation. He gave it. "Well, that's put another big amount of stress on us." She paused again, thinking. She bit her lip nervously. "Well," she said, "the police came to investigate the crash. First, they asked me all kinds of questions when I was in the hospital about who was driving, what I was doing at the time of the crash, what color the traffic lights were, that kind of thing."

She drew a breath. "It was very uncomfortable. It sounded like they wanted to blame Gil for the accident. I knew it wasn't Gil's fault ... but he was unconscious and couldn't defend himself." She sounded increasingly distressed as she told this story. "I think they wanted to blame me, too," she said anxiously, averting her eyes from the doctor. "And then ... well, they told me that the people in the other car were also injured, particularly a little boy," she said with a tone of distress. "Oh, Dr. Antoine ... a little boy. That was just awful to hear!" Tears gathered in her eyes.

Glory went on to say that their motor vehicle insurance company had provided a lawyer for them. When Gil was able to, the three of them had sat together in the hospital at his bedside and gone over all the events of the day. She noted how difficult this was, since Gil had some short-term memory loss, and how stressful this was for her, on top of worrying about the baby and Gil's health. However, they did piece it together.

"You know what happened, doctor?" she asked. "We were coming up to the intersection to cross it and turn left. The light had been red as we approached, so Gil slowed to a stop. As he was doing this, the baby kicked a couple of times. I was so excited to be with Gil for the day, and when this happened, I had to put his hand on my belly. I called out to him just as we were braking at the red light, grabbed his hand, and pulled it over to my belly. He was half-looking at me and half-looking at the light. It changed at that very moment, and just as he started into the intersection, a guy on a bicycle suddenly appeared! He darted right out in front of our truck from my side. He crossed right in our path! Gil slammed on the brakes and we went skidding through the intersection!" She stopped abruptly. Her eyes were locked on her doctor, expecting comment or judgment. The animated recounting of events was done.

Dr. Antoine spoke. "So, the accident wasn't Gil's fault, Glory? Is that what you're saying?" She nodded vigorously. She said that it took almost a month for the police and insurance companies to figure this out. They had taken measurements of the skid marks, recorded eyewitness accounts, and so on. Then she explained that the people in the other vehicle had also had something going on at the moment of the crash, but the police had determined that they too had been proceeding properly into the intersection when the driver saw Gil's truck skidding as he tried to avoid hitting the cyclist. The other vehicle was unable to avoid hitting them.

"So the other driver tried to avoid both us and that guy on the bicycle. But in the end, we skidded into each other. What a mess!" said Glory, still upset. "But we've all been absolved of any responsibility, including me. I know I shouldn't have taken Gil's hand off the wheel, but that's not what caused the accident. Thank heavens, Dr. Antoine. I don't know what I would have done if things had turned out differently. What if our injuries had been worse or ... the baby ..." She let the sentence hang in the air. "We couldn't take the financial or emotional blow, you know." Dr. Antoine consoled her, saying he empathized with her and recognized the fear and stress this event had put on her. They talked for awhile about the emotional impact of a motor vehicle accident in general, and then for Gil and Glory, specifically.

"Glory, I want you to know that if you are having any emotional or psychological difficulties now or in the next few months, I'd like you to feel free to tell me. You are facing a number of unusual stressors right now, in addition to those involved with having a new baby. And giving birth itself can bring on mood changes: self-doubt, joy, and anxiety. If your mood swings become problematic, or if you're feeling overwhelmed in any way, please, please let me know." She smiled and promised she would.

Reflective Questions

Reflect on the dialogue you have just read as you answer these questions.

1. Dr. Antoine completed a psychosocial assessment with Glory Loeppky in his office. He assessed her current situation by framing questions within the domains of health (see Chapter 16). Which domains did he address?

____

2. Why is Dr. Antoine concerned about his patient's mental health?

____

Critical Thinking

To answer these questions, consider all that you have just learned about the motor vehicle accident that Glory was in recently.

1. Do you think that Glory feels some sort of guilt or blame for what occurred in the accident? Explain your answer. _______________
2. What unspoken outcome did Glory fear the most from this accident?

   ____
3. Why would Glory's husband, Gil, take exception to having his relatives look after him all the time? _______________
4. Why did Dr. Antoine bother with this interview in his office? Why did he not just send his patient home after the physical?

   ____

   ____

   ____

Postpartum depression

Postpartum depression is a serious type of major clinical depression that can occur within the first six months after delivery. Symptoms of the illness include persistent anxiety and fatigue. The new mother becomes preoccupied with thoughts of worthlessness, inadequacy to the tasks of motherhood, and lack of self-confidence in her ability to care for and protect her baby. **Despondency** (feeling discouraged and sad) and tearfulness are present, and the new mother may experience feelings of guilt that she is unable to cope. Physiologically, this illness brings symptoms of headaches, chest pain, and possibly hyperventilation (tachypnea). A general sense of numbness—both emotionally and physically—may occur.

Additionally, the woman experiencing postpartum depression may be **ambivalent** (unsure, undecided, or hesitant) toward the baby, and this ambivalence can have an adverse effect on the ability of mother and child to bond. **Bonding** is a term often used in maternal and child health care. It is also very common in psychiatry, psychology, and social work. It derives from the full term *human bonding*, which refers to the innate, natural proclivity (tendency) to attach ourselves to others to meet biological, psychosocial, and even spiritual needs.

An overwhelming sense of sadness is consistent with a diagnosis of postpartum depression and differentiates it from a very minor form of the disorder that is experienced by a majority of new mothers, *postpartum blues* (see "Focus Point").

Etiology

Current medical research suggests that the cause of postpartum depression may be hormonal; however, environmental and psychosocial stressors cannot be ruled out as contributors above and beyond that.

Treatment

Postpartum depression requires treatment. If left untreated it can last several months to a year. Timely and accurate diagnosis of the symptoms is crucial to early intervention, because the depression will affect both the mother and the child. Individual or group therapy, support groups, or counseling have all been shown to be effective treatments for this disorder. Use of antidepressant medications is also helpful but not always recommended if the mother is breastfeeding.

Right Word or Wrong Word: *Bonding* or *Attachment*?

Do these two words have exactly the same meaning? Explain.

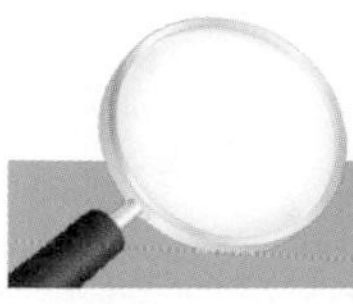

FOCUS POINT: The Baby Blues

The *baby blues,* or *postpartum blues,* are not the same thing as postpartum depression. They can be transient, occurring for a few minutes off and on throughout the day. Baby blues are also short-lived, occurring over a period of only 7 to 10 days.

The onset of symptoms occurs within the first 1 to 3 days postpartum. Symptoms include lack of sleep, tearfulness or weeping, mood lability (including irritability), and an overriding sense of feeling vulnerable and not in control or able to care for oneself. These symptoms resolve themselves.

The cause of this condition is scientifically unknown, but causality is suspected to be linked to sudden hormone changes upon birth and a sudden change in the woman's reality: the baby has arrived and is fully present in her life. For many new mothers, the arrival of the baby is a dream coming true but also very emotionally overwhelming. Emotions tied to the circumstances of the delivery may also have an effect here.

Postpartum psychosis

Recall the symptoms of psychosis and mania from Chapter 7 to help you understand **postpartum psychosis**, a rare mental illness that almost always requires hospitalization. Symptoms include extreme states of erratic or disorganized behavior, confusion, agitation, and lability of mood. These symptoms may be accompanied by rapid speech, manic behaviors, fatigue, and feelings of hopelessness and possibly shame. The woman experiencing postpartum psychosis may also become frantic (panicky, hysterical, or desperate) and paranoid (distrustful, fearful, and suspicious of the intent of others). The most serious of the symptoms often warrant hospitalization, because they can lead to suicide and infanticide (murder of an infant). These severe symptoms include the following:

- auditory hallucinations that may instruct the mother to harm herself or the baby.
- delusions (fixed false beliefs) held by the woman regarding herself or the baby; these may include beliefs that the baby would be better off dead.

Postpartum psychosis is thought to be a type of rapidly occurring mania—an episode of bipolar disorder. The onset is within the first 3 months postpartum, with early warning signs usually seen within the first 2 to 3 weeks. Once symptoms begin, full-blown psychosis occurs rapidly.

> Postpartum psychosis is sometimes referred to as *puerperal psychosis.*
>
> **Puerperal** means *"occurring during or immediately after childbirth."*
>
> Other medical terms that include the adjective *puerperal* are *puerperal depression* (postpartum depression), *puerperal fever*, and *puerperal sepsis.*

Etiology

To date, there are no clearly determined causes of postpartum psychosis. Again, it may be triggered by abrupt hormonal changes during childbirth. A family history of bipolar disorder or postpartum psychosis may lead to a predisposition for its occurrence.

Treatment

Postpartum psychosis is considered a medical, psychiatric emergency. Treatment is essential to protect the lives of both mother and child. The diagnosis is determined only after a full physical assessment is completed, with blood work that includes a CBC, thyroid function, Vitamin B_{12} levels, and folate levels because abnormalities in these may induce some symptoms of confusion and agitation.

Treatment involves administration of antipsychotic medications. Anti-anxiety drugs will also be prescribed to stabilize mood. The patient may or may not be started on antidepressants at this time. In cases in which the psychosis is difficult to treat with medications and in which there are concerns for the patient's safety, electroconvulsive therapy (ECT) may be used to stabilize the mother. There is a good deal of evidence for the efficacy of this medical approach.

Mix and Match

Match each word to its synonym or definition.

1. despondency	distrustful, fearful, and suspicious
2. hyperventilation	panicky, hysterical, or desperate
3. ambivalent	passing, fleeting, temporary
4. proclivity	tendency
5. transient	unsure, undecided, or hesitant
6. frantic	tachypnea
7. paranoid	sadness

Let's Practice

Write the definition of each term.

1. puerperal ____________________

2. delusions ____________________

3. infanticide ____________________

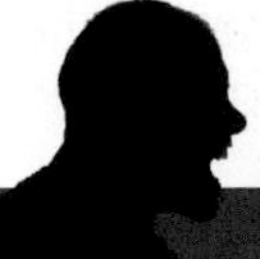

PRONUNCIATION PRACTICE

Say these words aloud to a friend or classmate. You are given the phonetic pronunciation. Your instructor can help you with pronunciation,

or visit **http://www.MedicalLanguageLab.com.**

ambivalent	ăm-**bĭv**´ă-lĕnt
approximated	ă-**prŏk**´sĭ-māt'd
infanticide	ĭn-**făn**´tĭ-sīd
speculum	**spĕk**´ū-lŭm
subcuticular	sŭb˝kū-**tĭk**´ū-lăr

Reproductive Health (Sexual Health)

Reproductive, or sexual, health is a major part of health care for both men and women. The topic will come up in most health careers, so it is important to know the concepts and terminology related to it. Tables 17-1 to 17-3 provide a number of key terms used in this field. The *Career Spotlight* in this section describes the education, training, and expertise of reproductive clinicians, biologists, and technicians.

Human reproductive science supports research and treatment focused on alleviating infertility, developing contraception, and investigating all aspects of human reproduction. A distinguishing feature of this field is its holistic approach to the ability to reproduce, understanding the interplay of the individual with his or her world. There is a fundamental appreciation of and focus on wellness, rather than illness.

Patient Update

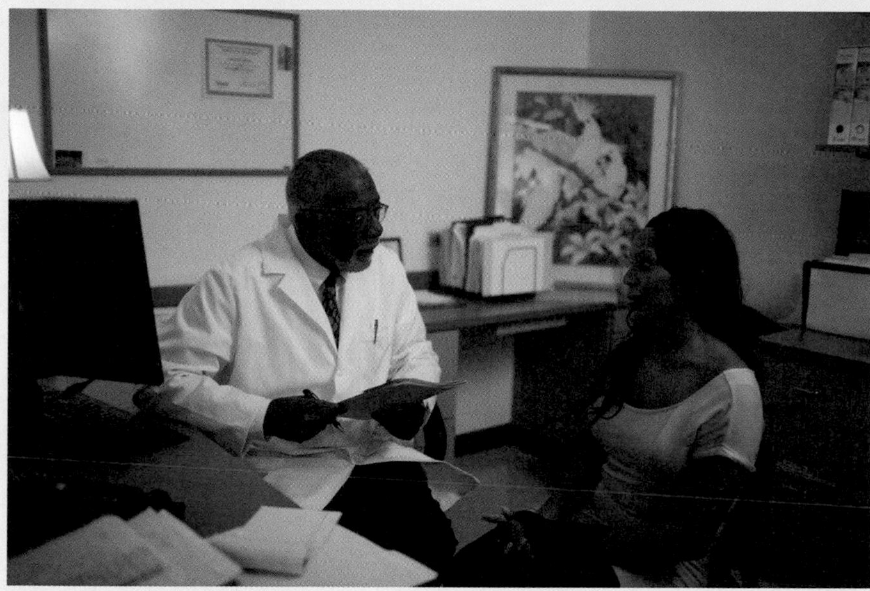

Glory's postpartum checkup with her family practice physician, Dr. Antoine, is coming to an end. He has talked to her about her mental health and examined her physically. He has one more subject to broach with her: her sexual, reproductive health.

"There's just one more thing I'd like to talk with you about today, Glory. And that is about a return to sexual activity and the risks of pregnancy. Have you thought about your sexual health yet, Glory?" he asked. She looked at him inquisitively, not sure which direction he was going with this new topic.

"Sexual health? I'm not sure what you mean, Doctor. Do you mean have I thought about having sex with my husband yet?" She paused and then added, "Well, I've thought it was much too early for that, but then again, Gil's not really in any position to engage in that kind of thing. You know, he has all kinds of apparatuses around his knee, pins in his ankle, and ..."

"Well, let's approach this one topic at a time. Number one, you can begin to have intimate relations—sexual intercourse with your husband—any time now, if you like. I see from the exam that you're no longer bleeding post-delivery, so I think it would be safe for you. And, of course, you did not have a vaginal birth. Secondly, I was asking about family planning, birth control, and so on." He let that sink in for a moment.

"Well, Gil and I do want one more child," she said. "We have always wanted two. I will be able to have another, won't I?" she asked nervously and quickly added, "Dr. Bedard, the OB, said I could have more children. You're saying that, too aren't you?" She sounded nervous.

"Yes, yes, I am, Glory. But now that you might become sexually active again soon, it's not too early to start thinking about contraception again. I'm wondering if you know about the relationship between breastfeeding and conception?" He paused to let her respond. She raised her eyebrows in inquiry and he continued. "Well, it's not likely that you'll conceive again while you're breastfeeding—as long as you feed your baby often and feed her breast milk exclusively. And it is up to you to decide when you'd like to stop nursing. However, you may wish to think ahead about family planning and any contraception needs you might have. I know that I used to prescribe birth control pills for you, and I wonder if you'd like to start them again." She talked about this with him and took a new prescription. They said goodbye then, and Glory left, eager to go to the hospital to see her little girl.

Reflective Question

Reflect on the dialogue you have just read as you answer this question.

How many children would Glory and her husband like to have eventually? ______________________

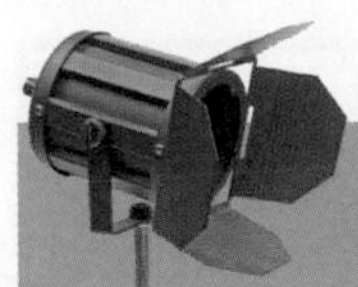

CAREER SPOTLIGHT: Reproductive Clinicians, Biologists, and Technicians

Reproductive clinicians are medical professionals with advanced education and training in reproduction and health or life sciences (biology, microbiology, embryology, medicine, and so on). They are often gynecologists but also obstetricians as well. A focus of the work is sexual health, contraception, and public health (public reproductive health). Reproductive clinicians work in acute and community care settings, in fertility clinics, and in public and global health organizations.

Reproductive biologists and technologists are scientists concerned with human and/or animal embryology in particular, but they may also be involved in the study of genetics. Education and training are at the graduate level. These professionals work in research and laboratories, including field labs out in the community, where they gather data.

To become an embryologist, a minimum of an undergraduate, baccalaureate degree is required, although advanced education that includes laboratory sciences is preferred. Embryologists work in laboratories and fertility clinics and with sufficient training may assist or take responsibility for all aspects of in vitro fertilization.

Reproductive clinicians, biologists, and technologists may be associated or affiliated with organizations such as the Society of Reproductive Biologists and Technologists or the American Society for Reproductive Medicine.

Critical Thinking

Think carefully about what Dr. Antoine has said to his patient. Then answer this question.

Dr. Antoine says it might now be safe for Glory to resume sexual activity with her husband. What does he mean by "safe"?

____

____

Reproduction

Human reproduction refers to the product of the joining of gametes: an **ovum** (egg) from a female with a reproductive cell from a male, which is called a **sperm** (see Figure 17-2). A **gamete** is a reproductive cell that fuses with one of the opposite sex to form a **zygote**, or fertilized egg. Each gamete contains half the genes, or the **haploid** number of chromosomes, of each parent. When a male gamete fuses with a female one, the product is a **diploid** zygote: It contains a full set of chromosomes, half of them from each donor.

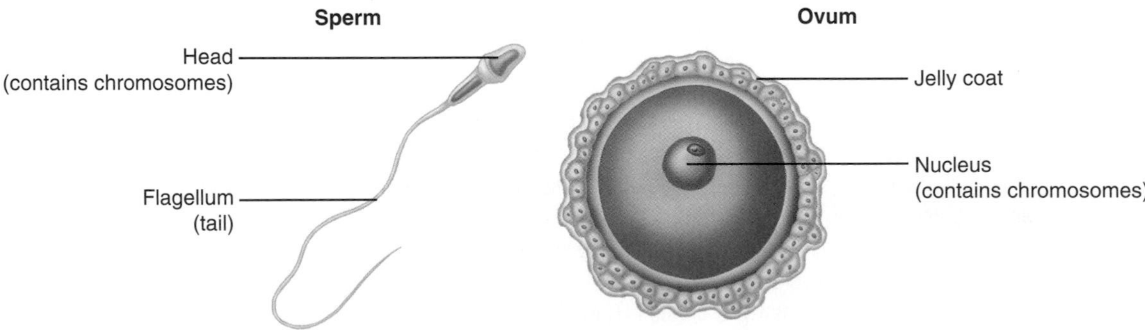

Figure 17.2: Male and Female Gametes

The word *reproduction* literally means "forming again" or "the act of forming again." The term deconstructs as follows:

re	+	produc/e	+	tion	= reproduction
↓		↓		↓	
again	+	make a copy of	+	state of; condition; act of	

The most appropriate term to use for sexual intercourse is coitus, although *pareunia*, *sexual intercourse*, *intercourse*, and *copulation* might also be used.

coitus: penetration of a vagina by a penis. The Latin root is *coire*, meaning "coming together."

pareunia: synonym for *coitus.*

dyspareunia: painful intercourse; pain during intercourse.

copulation: synonym for *coitus.* The root word, *copulate,* means "to link or join together."

intercourse: a term literally meaning "to run between." When used in the context of sexuality it means *coitus.*

Key terms: reproductive/sexual health

It is important to use proper terminology at all times when working with people regarding their reproductive or sexual health. Tables 17-1 and 17-2 introduce important terms related to conception and fertility.

Other key terms related to reproductive and sexual health are introduced and deconstructed in Table 17-3.

TABLE 17-1: Conception and Contraception

Term	Definition
conception	the result of sperm successfully fertilizing an egg; the beginning of pregnancy
contraception contra- prefix meaning *against*	a term that generally refers to a pharmaceutical preparation or a technique that prevents pregnancy; however, people use natural forms of contraception as well (see *Family Planning* section)

TABLE 17-2: Fertile and Infertile

Term	Definition
fertile root word meaning *fruitful, productive, bearing in abundance*	capable of reproduction
infertile in- prefix meaning *not*	not capable of reproduction

TABLE 17-3: Reproductive Health: Key Terms and Word Parts

Term and Definition	Word Parts
impregnation The process of becoming pregnant	*im-* prefix meaning *within* *pregn-* combining form of *praegnans*, meaning *before giving birth* *-ation* suffix meaning "the act or process of; the end result of an action; the resulting state of"

Continued

TABLE 17-3: Reproductive Health: Key Terms and Word Parts—cont'd

Term and Definition	Word Parts
miscarriage The end result of miscarrying an embryo or fetus	*mis-* prefix meaning *bad* or *erroneous* *miscarry* to be unable to carry through; to perish; to die; to come to harm; to be lost or destroyed *-age* suffix that changes a verb to a noun
abortion A spontaneous, naturally occurring, sudden and abrupt end to a pregnancy **or** the end result of a medically induced miscarriage or termination of pregnancy	*abort, aborto* root word and combining form meaning to *miscarry* -tion suffix meaning "the act of/process of/state of"

Puberty

Puberty is the period of growth and development in which a person reaches biological, reproductive maturity. In other words, gamete production occurs, and fertility and impregnation become possible: The reproductive system of both males and females becomes functional.

The word *puberty* derives from the Latin root *pubertas*, meaning *adult* or "age of maturity." The meaning of the English word *puberty* has evolved to mean "capable of sexual reproduction," which signals the onset of biological adulthood. The root of this word may also originate in the Latin *pubescere*, meaning "to grow hair,“ since the appearance of body hair is most certainly a sign of the onset of sexual/reproductive maturity. Modern derivatives of the word *puberty* include the following:

pubertal or *puberal:* of/pertaining to puberty

puberulent: covered with fine, minute hairs

pubescence: the period in which a person reaches puberty

Right Word or Wrong Word: *Puberty* or *Adolescence*?

Do these two words describe the same thing? If so, what is that?

Fertility and infertility

Fertility is the medical term for the ability to conceive children: the ability to become pregnant naturally.

Infertility is the medical term for just the opposite: the inability to conceive children or become pregnant through sexual activity. In medicine, this determination is made only after a year of unprotected sexual intercourse that has not produced a pregnancy. A number of investigative tests and diagnostics can also help make this determination. Causes of infertility can be physiological (including genetic and traumatic), pathological, and/or psychological for both males and females.

Fecundity is another term that refers to the ability to produce offspring, but it more specifically refers to the ability to produce many offspring and to do so frequently.

Fecund is the root word of *fecundity*. It means *fruitfulness* or *fertility*.

Fecundability refers to the likelihood that conception will occur within a determined time period.

Cycle fecundability refers to the likelihood that conception will occur within a single menstrual cycle (see *Female Reproductive Cycle*).

Assisted reproduction

Assisted reproduction refers to a variety of techniques now available to aid in fertilization through intrauterine insemination (IUI). Table 17-4 provides some examples.

TABLE 17-4: Types of Assisted Reproduction

Types of Assisted Reproduction	Explanation of Procedure
Follicle Aspiration, Sperm Injection, and Assisted Follicular Rupture (FASIAR)	• Ova are removed from follicles and then mixed with sperm inside a syringe. Next, they are injected back into the female. There is a risk in this procedure of multiple pregnancies/multiple births.
Gamete Intrafallopian Transfer (GIFT)	• Ova are extracted through the vagina, where they are combined with sperm. Immediately thereafter, the combination of eggs and sperm is placed into one of the fallopian tubes by laparoscopy (insertion of a thin instrument through the abdomen). Fertilization occurs within the fallopian tubes.
Intracytoplasmic Sperm Insertion (ICSI)	• Injection/insertion of sperm directly into an ovum in the lab. *This is the second most common procedure in assisted reproduction. It is used for conditions of male infertility or low sperm count.
In Vitro Fertilization (IVF)	• Ova are harvested (collected; gathered) from the vagina. They are then combined with sperm in the laboratory. Fertilization occurs in the lab. Should a zygote result (2 to 5 days later), it is transferred to the uterus. Usually, between two and four zygotes are implanted, in hopes that at least one will produce a pregnancy. It is possible to have multiple births this way. *This is the most common procedure in assisted reproduction.
Zygote Intrafallopian Transfer (ZIFT)	• Ova are harvested in a similar manner to that of IVF and GIFT, introduced to sperm in the laboratory setting, and then reintroduced to the female body. However, these zygotes are transferred to a fallopian tube, not the uterus.

Pathology: sexually transmitted infections and diseases

Any discussion of the reproductive system requires discussion of sexually transmitted infections and diseases. However, because this is primarily a language book, only key terms will be presented, those that will help you become familiar with sexually transmitted health challenges.

The term **sexually transmitted** identifies the mode of infection (the route taken) by pathogens from one carrier to another. In this case, the mode of infection is person-to-person, skin-to-skin sexual contact: intimate sexual relations of intercourse and/or oral sex.

The symptoms of a sexually transmitted infection or a disease may vary, but core symptoms are present in the genitalia. These include the following: soreness, pain and/or tenderness; itchiness or burning; pain or burning during urination; and unusual discharge from the penis or vagina that often also has an unpleasant odor.

Although the terms *sexually transmitted infection* and *sexually transmitted disease* are often used interchangeably as synonyms, the terms are not really synonymous. Infections are not the sole cause of disease, nor do they always lead to disease.

Sexually transmitted infections (STIs)

Sexually transmitted infections (**STIs**) are just that: infections transmitted through sexual contact with an infected person. They can be treated by various anti-infective medications and antibiotics. Not all infections are diseases. Types of sexually transmitted infection affecting both males and females include the following:

chlamydia: a bacterial infection of the urethra and reproductive system (see Chapter 8). It is treated and resolved with the use of antibiotics. However, if it is left undiagnosed or untreated, chlamydia can lead to problems with fertility for women over time. It might also be a contributor or causative factor in cervical cancer.

gonorrhea: a bacterial infection of the urethra, cervix, rectum, anus, and/or throat. It is well-treated (successfully) with antibiotics. Untreated, it can lead to pelvic inflammatory disease in women and epididymitis in men (see Chapter 9).

trichomoniasis (trich) = a common parasitic infection of the urethra and vagina by the protozoa *Trichomonas vaginalis.* Treatment is by a type of antibiotic suited specifically for this type of parasitic infection. If the infection is left untreated, men may suffer prostate and bladder damage. For women, the risk of inflammation and damage to the fallopian tubes and cervix is present. If undetected or untreated during pregnancy, miscarriage or premature birth is possible. Research also shows a higher possibility for both males and females with undiagnosed or untreated trichomoniasis for contracting HIV.

Sexually transmitted diseases (STDs)

Sexually transmitted diseases (**STDs**) are more enduring (can last longer) and are often much harder to treat than infections. They can cause damage to organs and systems; they can even be life threatening. If the cause of the sexually transmitted disease is viral, then the disease is untreatable and will stay in the body forever, sometimes dormant and sometimes active, producing acute symptoms and/or injury to organs and cells (see Chapter 16). A core example of a sexually transmitted disease is HIV (see Chapter 16). Other types of sexually transmitted diseases affecting both males and females include the following:

syphilis: a bacterial infection that is a disease. It proceeds through a number of worsening stages and takes a great toll on body systems, organs, and the mind. Long-term effects can include blindness, sores on the genitals and other body parts, deafness, heart disease, and insanity. If syphilis is transmitted to an unborn child, it can physically disable the child.

Syphilis can be contracted only by person-to-person contact with a syphilitic sore. Treatment is simple: penicillin by intramuscular injection is warranted. This antibiotic will destroy the pathogen if it is caught in its earliest stages. Even so, it is possible to contract the disease again if in contact with an infected person.

Syphilis was almost eradicated in North America and other parts of the world by the late 20th century. However, it has begun to make a comeback, and it is possible to encounter a patient with syphilis in your career.

genital herpes (Herpes genitalis; herpes simplex II): a very common viral STD. It is transmitted through direct, person-to-person contact only through body fluids (blood, saliva), vaginal, oral, and anal sex and contact with the blisters.

Symptoms of small blisters appear on the genitals and anus. These eventually degrade to become open sores (ulcers). The outbreak of symptoms is sporadic and can last for 1 to 4 weeks at a time.

Although no significant long-term effects have been identified to date, genital herpes does have significant risk during pregnancy. Infection with this virus can be fatal for newborns. If the female with genital herpes is pregnant, a Cesarean section can prevent the spread of the virus to the child during birth.

There is no cure for genital herpes, but antiviral medication can reduce the number of outbreaks that occur. A medication that suppresses symptoms is also available for the carrier of this disease. It helps protect the sexual partner from infection.

human papillomavirus (HPV): a viral infection of the genital tract that cannot be treated, only prevented (see Chapters 9 and 16). It can lead to the development of genital warts and is thought to be causative in cervical and mouth cancer. It is contracted by skin-to-skin, genital contact.

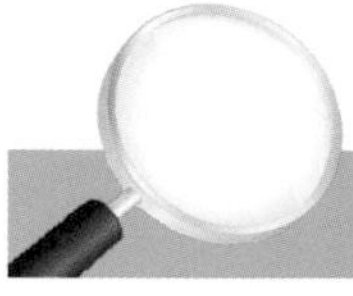

FOCUS POINT: What Is a Venereal Disease?

Venereal disease (VD) is a term for a broad category of sexually transmitted diseases. The term *venereal* means "pertaining to sexual intercourse or sexual desire." It is quite acceptable to use VD interchangeably with STD, although the term VD is less commonly used these days.

Build a Word

Use new terminology. Apply your knowledge of how word parts combine, with consideration as to when to drop or add vowels and consonants. Combine each set of word parts below to create a medical or anatomical term. Then use your knowledge of word parts to define the term you have written.

1. –ive concepti/o ______________________ Meaning ______________________
2. –ity fecund in- ______________________ Meaning ______________________
3. –able pregn im- ______________________ Meaning ______________________
4. concepti/o pre- ______________________ Meaning ______________________
5. –lent puberty ______________________ Meaning ______________________

Let's Practice

Write a word derived from the root word given in each description to identify what is being described. Think carefully. Some of these words may be new to you, but you should have enough medical terminology now to be able to complete this exercise successfully.

1. the period of time just before the onset of *puberty* ______________________
2. the role of sperm in *fertility* ______________________
3. a noun that refers to the act of getting *pregnant* ______________________
4. a synonym of *impregnation* that uses the root *fecund* ______________________
5. a rare type of *fecundity* in which impregnation of two ova on two separate occasions occurs, both within the same menstrual cycle. The term uses the prefix *super*-. ______________

Free Writing

Write sentences using new terminology. Use the words given in the context of reproduction.

1. preceding health timeframe preconception female refers to cycle pregnancy the in the reproductive ______________________
2. years prepubescent age a approximately child 10 to 12 of is ______________________
3. injection syphilis serious a intervention STD intramuscular is that penicillin of early requires an with ______________________

Fill in the Blanks

Use new language and terms in a meaningful way. Complete these sentences by filling in the blanks.

1. Biologically, the ability to ______________ does not occur until puberty.
2. The word ______________ refers to any loss of a pregnancy, not just to one caused by medical intervention.
3. ______________ can occur naturally as the result of intercourse or through the use of in vitro fertilization.
4. A ______________ that is viral in nature cannot be cured.
5. ______________ sexually transmitted infections can be treated with antibiotics.
6. The definition for ______________ is person-to-person, skin-to-skin sexual contact: intimate sexual relations of intercourse and/or oral sex.
7. If pain is experienced during coitus, the symptom is called ______________.

Let's Practice

In the context of reproduction, write the word or word part that fits each definition or description.

1. uses the prefix *im*- and means that conception has occurred ______________________
2. the beginning or origin of a new experience or idea; the formation of something ______________________
3. uses the prefix *in*- and means "not capable of conception" ______________________

Mix and Match

Match the name of each STD or STI to its symptoms. Draw a line to connect them.

1. human papillomavirus	can lead to infertility if not treated
2. syphilis	microscopic parasites infect urethra and vagina
3. chlamydia	can lead to development of genital warts
4. Herpes Simplex Virus II	causes small blisters on the genitals
5. trichomoniasis	can lead to blindness, deafness, heart disease

PRONUNCIATION PRACTICE

Say these words aloud to a friend or classmate. You are given the phonetic pronunciation. Your instructor can help you with pronunciation,

or visit **http://www.MedicalLanguageLab.com.**

chlamydia	klă-**mĭd**´ē-ă	pareunia	păr-ĕ-**ū**´nē-ă
coitus	**kō**´ĭ-tŭs	prepubescent	prē″pū-**bĕ**s´ĕnt
dyspareunia	dĭs″pă-**rū**´nē-ă	syphilis	**sĭf**´ĭ-lĭs
fecundity	fē-**kŭn**´dĭ-tē	trichomoniasis	trĭk″ō-mō-**nī**´ă-sĭs
gamete	**găm**´ēt	venereal	vē-**nē**´rē-ăl
gonorrhea	gŏn″ō-**rē**´ă	zygote	**zī**´gōt
papilloma	păp-ĭ-**lō**´mă		

Male reproductive health

You were introduced to terms relating to the anatomy and physiology of the male reproductive system in Chapter 9, with our patient Zane Davis. Apply that knowledge and terminology now to the context of male reproductive health. Figure 17-3 reviews the major structures of the system.

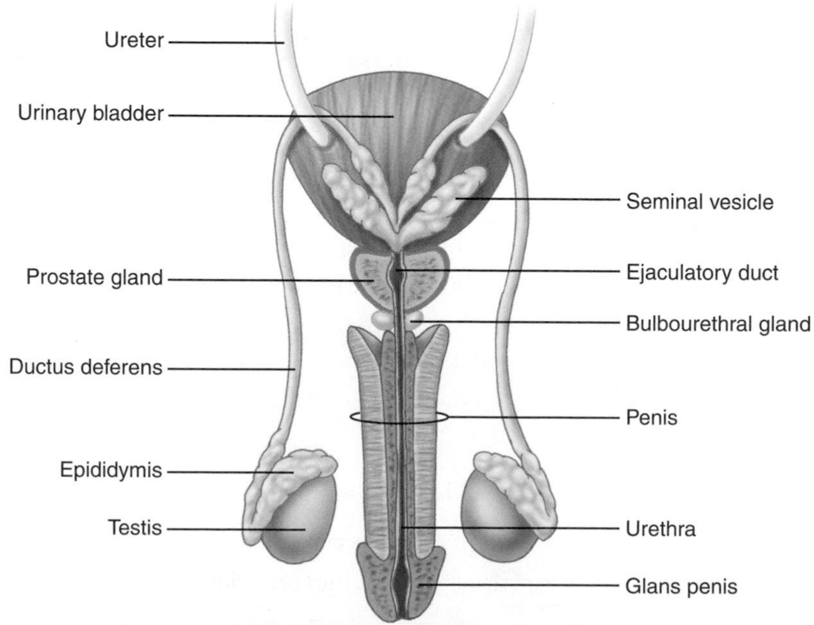

Figure 17.3: Male Reproductive System

The male reproductive system

The function of the male reproductive system is twofold: the production of sperm and the delivery of sperm to the reproductive tract of the female. **Spermatogenesis** is the production of fully mature, functional spermatozoa. This process occurs in the testes, more specifically in the seminiferous tubules of the testes.

Recall from Chapter 9 that spermatozoa are the plural form of *spermatozoon*, a mature male sex cell, or germ cell, also known as sperm. Spermatozoa are the end product of multiple cell divisions in the testes (see Figure 17-4). To review terms built from the combining forms *sperma-* and *spermat/o*, see Chapter 9.

The word *spermatozoon* is deconstructed in this way:

spermato + **zoon** = **spermatozoon**
↓ ↓
seed + life = seed of life

Sperm is a type of *flagellated* cell. This means it has a head, or nucleus, as well as a tail, or *flagellum*. The flagellum provides **motility**, the capacity for movement, which allows sperm cells to travel in a way that is often referred to as *swimming*. Sperm is transported through the penis in viscous (thick) fluid called **semen**.

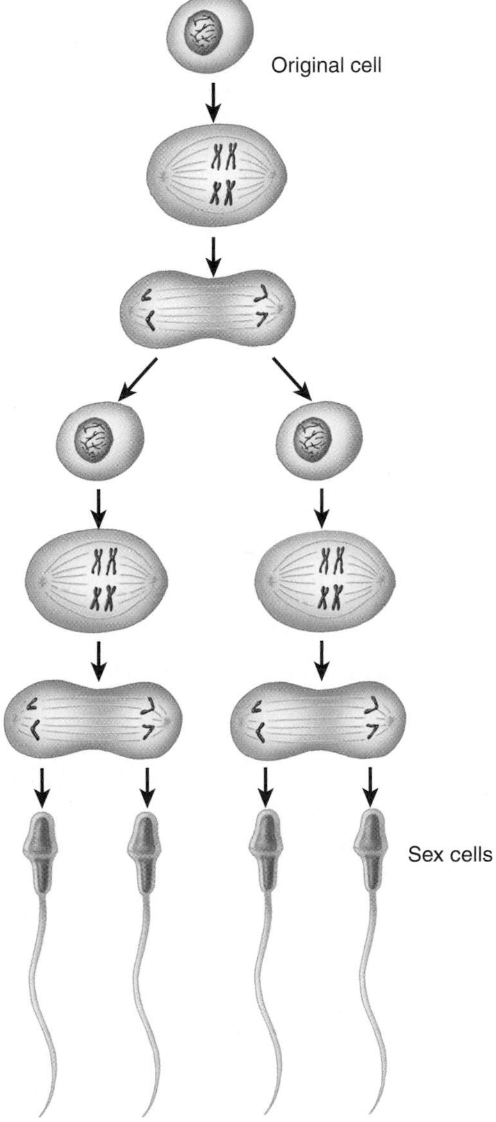

Figure 17.4: Spermatogenesis

The testes

The **testes** are reproductive organs that not only produce sperm but also function as endocrine glands. They produce **testosterone**, a hormone that is important to the development of secondary sex characteristics. Testosterone is produced in the interstitial cells of the testes.

Secondary sex characteristics arise in puberty. They include changes in voice and body shape, as well as the development of internal and external sexual organs. In males, testosterone levels increase during puberty; the result is the growth of body hair on the face, axilla, and genitals. The body shape changes to become more masculine, and the male voice changes to become deeper.

Male pubertal hormones

The onset of puberty is triggered by the release of *growth releasing growth hormone (GRGH)* and *gonadotropin releasing hormone (GRH).* The release of these hormones occurs in the hypothalamus, and their release triggers the anterior pituitary gland to produce *gonadotropins* and growth hormones called *somatotropins* (see Chapter 7). This process is more clearly illustrated in Figure 17-5.

> Gonadotropins include *luteinizing hormone* and *follicle stimulating hormone* (FSH).
> GRGH is also known as *somatocrinin* or *growth hormone releasing factor* (GRF or GHRF).

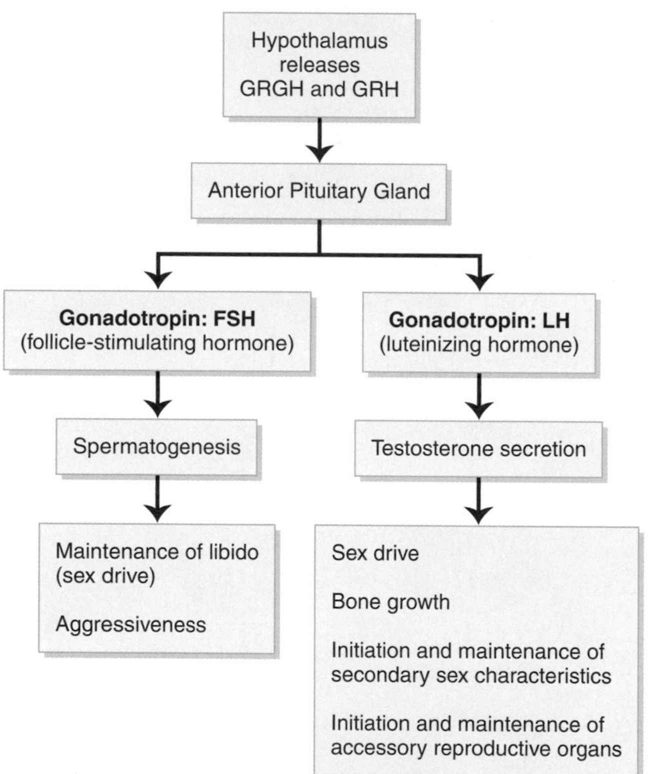

Figure 17.5: Sequential Release of Male Pubertal Hormones

Follicle stimulating hormone

Follicle Stimulating Hormone (FSH) is essential to start the process of spermatogenesis. It also functions to develop and maintain libido. **Libido** is a medical term commonly understood to mean *sex drive. Libido* is also a term from psychology and psychoanalysis. In this context, it refers to the innate psychological and emotional energy involved in striving for sexual activity and sexual intimacy (the sex drive).

Luteinizing hormone

Luteinizing hormone (LH) plays a crucial role in reproduction. It stimulates, or triggers, the release of testosterone by the testes. Without this hormone, or with low levels of it, the physical and emotional characteristics typically associated with being male may not develop or may not develop to their full potential. Note: A low level of testosterone does not necessarily indicate impotency, but it may be a causal factor in infertility.

Male fertility

A male becomes fertile at puberty. Although men continuously produce sperm across the lifespan, reproductive ability decreases with age, particularly after age 25. There is some scientific evidence that says the quality of male sperm is highest during a man's 30s, whereas motility rates begin declining after age 25 and particularly after age 55.

Quality of sperm refers to the genetic makeup and viability of the sperm. A man's age at conception also affects the *viability* of the resulting pregnancy, its likelihood to come to full term, as well as the genetics, growth, and development of the embryo and fetus. Today, there is growing scientific evidence identifying the potential for genetic abnormalities carried in the sperm of older men. These potential abnormalities increase the risk for miscarriages and birth defects. Additionally, a man over the age of 40 faces diminished fertility, a decline in his ability to impregnate.

Assessment of male fertility or infertility is a common task in reproductive health care. Male fertility is measured by *semen analysis (SA)* for sperm concentration, motility, volume, and morphology.

sperm count: assessment of sperm density, or concentration. A semen specimen is collected to determine sperm count. A normal range for fertility is 20 million or more sperm per milliliter of semen, with a total of 80 million or more sperm identified per one ejaculation.

motility: a measure of the percentage of living, moving sperm in a semen sample. The test also evaluates the direction and rate of travel of the sperm.

morphology: a laboratory test that examines the shape, size, and appearance of sperm, looking for any abnormalities that might affect fertility.

Additionally, tests of **sexual function**, the ability to not only produce sperm, but to ejaculate it, may be undertaken. These exams include the following:

white blood cell counts: looking for any interfering pathologies. These can be obtained through urinalysis and/or blood specimens.

sperm agglutination: a microscopic assessment that determines whether or not sperm are agglutinating, or clumping together. If the sperm are agglutinating, they may be unable to swim through the female's cervical mucus.

hypo-osmotic swelling: a sperm specimen is subjected to a salt-sugar solution to assess motility. Under a microscope, the flagellum is observed for its reaction to the solution. If healthy, the flagellum should swell. Results point to whether or not the sperm will be able to penetrate an ovum.

acrosome reaction: a microscopic assessment of the ability of sperm to undergo the chemical changes necessary to dissolve (and thereby penetrate) the outer layer of an ovum.

hemizona assay: another laboratory test to determine if sperm can penetrate the outer layer of an ovum, in this case by exposing the sperm to a dissected, nonviable (nonusable) ovum.

ultrasonography: a sonographic evaluation of the male reproductive tract to locate any damage or blockages (see Chapter 3 for more about sonography).

> A *transrectal ultrasound* (TRUS) can be particularly useful for assessment of the male reproductive tract and its potential involvement in infertility. This sonographic evaluation can determine the status of the seminal vesicles and the ejaculatory duct, assess the prostate gland, and discover cysts and other pathological conditions. The ejaculatory duct (*ductus ejaculatori*) is a canal formed at the meeting point of the vas deferens and the seminal vesicles, passing through the prostate gland.

vasography: a radiograph of the vas deferens to evaluate the patency of the vas deferens and ejaculatory ducts versus vasal obstruction. In other words, this test can determine if there is a blockage in the flow of semen in or damage to the vas deferens. A vasography requires injection of a contrast medium into the vas deferens.

This test is done only when a testes biopsy has indicated: (a) normal spermatogenesis; and (b) low sperm production (low volume ejaculates) with poor motility. These two conditions suggest a blockage may be present.

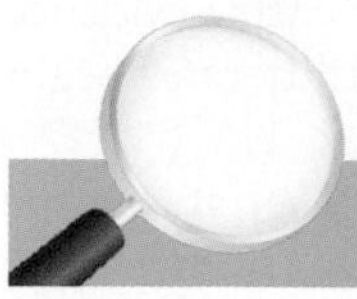

FOCUS POINT: Vasography

Once again, the context in which a medical term is found can alter its meaning. For example, *vasography* refers to radiograph visualization of blood vessels for assessment of blood flow and vasodilation.

vas/o	+	**graph**	+	**y**	=	**vasography**
↓		↓		↓		
vessel	+	write/record	+	process of	=	process of recording a vessel

In the context of male reproductive health, *vasography* refers specifically to the diagnostic test of the blood vessels and tubes of the testes—the male ductal system.

On the other hand, a cardio-vasograph assesses blood flow.

testicular biopsy: an evaluation of testicular tissue surgically removed from the tubules in the testes. The tissue is examined microscopically to determine if normal spermatogenesis is occurring. This test can also determine if the cause of infertility is due to obstructive or nonobstructive reasons. Testicular biopsies are done when two conditions are present: (a) there are no abnormalities in hormone levels or production; and (b) semen lacks sperm (azoospermia).

Testicular biopsies can also be used for in vitro fertilization to collect sperm for intracytoplasmic sperm injection (ICSI—see Table 17-4.)

Note: Testicular biopsies are not used for assessment of cancer.

Right Word or Wrong Word: *Infertility* or *Impotency*?

Are these two terms synonymous? Explain.

Pathology of the male reproductive system

In Chapter 9, you learned about pathology of the male urinary tract. The male reproductive organs were included in the discussion, but only in a limited context. Now expand your knowledge and terminology related to pathology of the male reproductive system. Refer to the Table 17-5 to learn more.

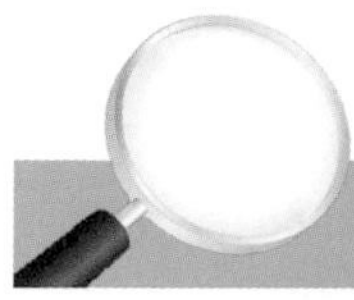

FOCUS POINT: Retractile Testes

The condition of *retractile testes* is quite normal. Occasionally, one testicle (or both) will rise back up into the groin. The condition is temporary, and the testicle will descend again.

TABLE 17-5: Pathology of the Male Reproductive System

Pathology	Definition and/or Description	Treatment
cryptorchidism (crytorchism) * The root word *orchid* appears in Chapter 9	Undescended testicles A condition occurring in up to 40% of all male births. The testicles usually descend naturally within the first 6 months.	Should the testicles not descend, surgical intervention is necessary. Undescended testicles can lead to infertility and other health problems later in life.
erectile dysfunction (ED)	inability to achieve or maintain a penile erection Etiology can be biological, psychosocial, or pharmacological.	Oral medications, medications inserted into the urethra, penile injections; penile pumps (vacuum devices); surgical implants.
testicular torsion	Twisting of the testes around the spermatic cord. This leads to occlusion of the blood supply to the testicle(s) and scrotum. A condition that occurs more often in adolescent males than adults or children. Etiology is physiologic (congenital).	A urologic emergency requiring immediate surgery. Lack of treatment can lead to loss of a testicle.
testicular teratoma *The root, *terato* appears in Chapter 14.	benign tumor of/in the testes in young males may be benign, but it is more often malignant when it occurs in adult males	Early detection through diagnostic screening. Surgery may be indicated (a lumpectomy).
varicocele	A widening of the veins within the scrotum that pass along the ligament that supports the testicle(s) Incidents are more common in adolescence. May be caused by faulty valves within the veins of the spermatic cord.	Associated with azoospermia and/or oligospermia (low concentration of sperm). May cause testicular atrophy. (shrinking of the testicle(s)) A varicocelectomy may be necessary to redirect blood flow.

Reflective Questions

Consider what you have learned about the male reproductive system to answer these questions.

1. What are pubertal hormones?

____

2. Which pathology listed in Table 17-5 can lead to or cause cancer?

____

3. Which pathologies listed in Table 17-5 can lead to infertility problems for males? Why?

____

Mix and Match

Match the description with the medical term. Draw a line to connect them.

1. semen lacks sperm	flagellum
2. ducts for ejaculation	torsion
3. ability to move	libido
4. thick and sticky	agglutinated
5. tail	motility
6. clumped together	viscous
7. sex drive	azoospermia
8. twisting	ductus ejaculatori

Let's Practice

Read each description of a medical condition or assessment. Then write the medical term for what is described.

1. When Zane Davis was being assessed for prostate cancer, he was not concerned about not having any more children, but he was concerned about his ability to function sexually. What two medical terms apply to these two different issues a man might be concerned about? ________________ and ________________
2. Gil Loeppky conceived a child with Glory. What medical term applies to his ability to do so? ________________
3. Rafael is sent for an assessment of the blood vessels and tubes located in his testicles. What is this diagnostic called? ________________
4. Fifty-year-old Sharif wonders why his wife has not gotten pregnant even though they have been trying to conceive for a year. The doctor suggests he should be tested for fertility. What is the name of this test? ________________
5. Roxly mistakenly thinks he cannot father a child because he suffers from an inability to maintain an erection. What is his condition actually called? ________________
6. At birth, male children can have undescended testicles. What is this condition called? ________________

PRONUNCIATION PRACTICE

Say these words aloud to a friend or classmate. You are given the phonetic pronunciation. Your instructor can help you with pronunciation,

or visit **http://www.MedicalLanguageLab.com.**

agglutinized	ă-**gloot**´ĭn-īzd
azoospermia	ă-zō-ō-**spĕr**´mē-ă
cryptorchidism	krĭpt-**or**´kĭd-ĭzm
flagellum	flă-**jĕl**´ŭm
gonadotropin	gŏn″ă-dō-**trō**´pĭn
impotency	**ĭm**´pō-tĕn-sē
libido	lĭ-**bī**´dō or lĭ-**bē**´dō
spermatozoa	spĕr″măt-ō-**zō**´ă
vasography	văs-**ŏg**´ră-fē

Female reproductive health

In the context of Glory Loeppky's pregnancy, a good deal of anatomy and physiology for the female reproductive system was presented in Chapter 8. However, there is still more to learn, particularly about the roles of the menstrual cycle and the female breast in reproduction. Review Figure 17-6 to recall key anatomical terms.

The female reproductive system

The function of the female reproductive system is to generate **ova** (eggs) and to receive sperm. It provides an environment conducive to fertilization. Implantation of the zygote occurs in the uterus, or womb. In addition, this system is designed to house and nourish a developing embryo and fetus prior to birth and to continue nourishing the child after birth.

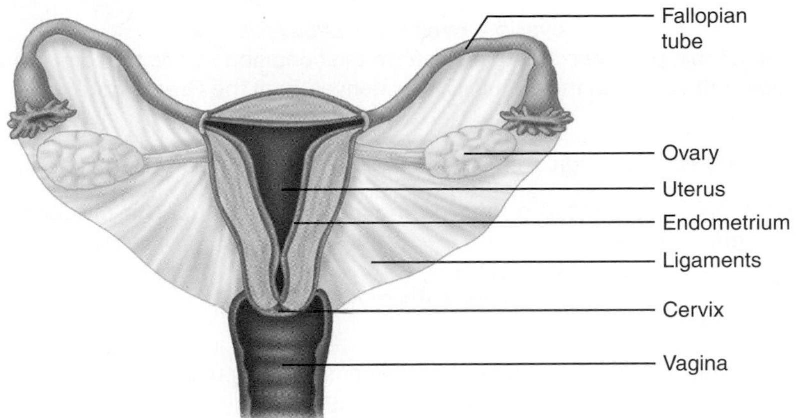

Figure 17.6: The Female Reproductive System

Oogenesis is a process in the female body that eventually produces a mature ovum. This process occurs in the ovaries. It begins soon after conception in the female embryo and continues from puberty to **menopause**, which is the cessation of female reproductive ability.

For the female adolescent and adult, the production of one ovum by oogenesis occurs only once a month, a process that is controlled by the release of hormones. Oogenesis is part of the female reproductive cycle (see below).

Oogenesis is a complex process, the details of which are better studied in anatomy, physiology, and reproductive science courses. However, a few key terms are helpful to know.

The root word of *oogenesis* is *oon*, meaning *egg* or *ovary*.

Oogonia is the plural form of *oogonium,* the cells from which oocytes originate.

Oocytes are types of cells created in the process of oogenesis. They occur between the stages of oogonium and final production of an ovum. In simpler terms, they are immature ova.

Oosperm is a synonym for *zygote*.

Oogenesis is also called *ovigenesis*.

Ovaries

The ovaries are glands that produce ova for reproduction. They also produce the hormones estrogen (oestrogen) and progesterone (see next section). In addition, they produce small amounts of testosterone, an androgen. The ovaries release one ovum per month via oviducts, also known as the fallopian tubes, en route to the uterus and then, if not fertilized, out of the body through the vagina.

There are two ovaries in the female body, sitting bilaterally to the uterus. A condition of *ovarian agenesis* occurs when the body lacks one or both ovaries.

Chapter 8 briefly introduced roots and combining forms related to the ovaries. You can use the Word Building feature that follows to expand your vocabulary of terms that use these roots.

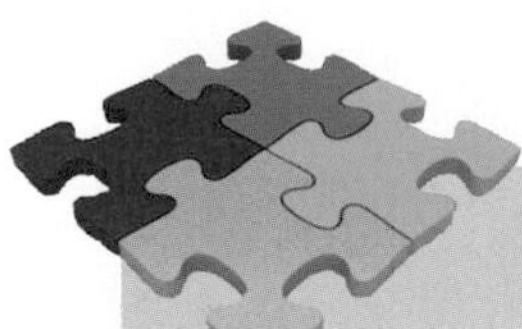

WORD BUILDING: Formulas for creating words from the combining forms *ovari/o* and *oophor/o*

1. The combining forms for *ovary* are *ovari/o* and *oophor/o*.

ovario + centesis = *ovariocentesis*

Definition: surgical puncture and draining of an ovarian cyst; *noun*

Example: An *ovariocentesis* is a minor surgical procedure that can be done in an outpatient setting.

Continued

ovario + cyesis = *ovariocyesis*

Definition: an ectopic pregnancy that results from the condition of a fertilized ovum lodging in a fallopian tube, rather than in the uterus. *Cyesis* derives from the Greek root *kyesis*, meaning *pregnancy*; *noun*

Example: *Ovariocyesis* is a medical emergency, usually requiring surgical intervention.

2. The original Greek root word oophoros means *egg bearing.* The modern combining forms are *oophor/o*.

oophor + itis = *oophoritis*

Definition: inflammation of an ovary; *noun*

Example: The painful condition of *oophoritis* may be caused by unprotected sexual intercourse, having multiple sexual partners, and sometimes by the use of intrauterine devices.

oophoro + cyst + ectomy = *oophorocystectomy*

Definition: surgical removable of an ovarian cyst; *noun*

Example: When an *oophorocystectomy* is performed, tissue samples are sent to the lab to determine if the cyst is benign or malignant.

oophoro = hyster = ectomy = *oophorohysterectomy*

Definition: surgical removal of the ovaries and uterus; *noun*

Example: Not every hysterectomy is as inclusive as an *oophorohysterectomy*.

Eponyms: Fallopio and Fallopian Tubes

Gabriele Fallopio was a 16th century Italian who began his working life as an academic, then went on to become a priest, and finally took up a career as a physician, anatomist, and pharmacist. He is known for his work as a professor of anatomy, particularly in regard to dissection.

Fallopio is credited for identifying, naming, and describing the following structures, conditions, and procedures:

fallopian tubes: structures of the female reproductive system

fallopian pregnancy: an ectopic pregnancy. In an **ectopic pregnancy,** a fertilized egg embeds and begins to develop outside of the uterus (almost always in a fallopian tube). It is not possible for the pregnancy to succeed this way.

fallotomy: a procedure for surgical division of the fallopian tubes

fallopian ligament or *fallopian arch:* an abdominal ligament now called Poupart's ligament

fallopian canal: a facial canal that runs through the temporal bone and through which the facial nerve passes.

Ovarian follicles

Females are born with approximately one million ovarian follicles. These comprise the basic elements of female reproduction: the oocyte. An *ovarian follicle* is a cavity (a pouchlike depression) in the ovary. The **oocyte**, or immature ovum, sits within this follicle, encased in specialized epithelial cells (see Figure 17-7).

Follicle means *sac* or *pouch*.

Folliculogenesis refers to the ripening or maturing of an ovarian follicle.

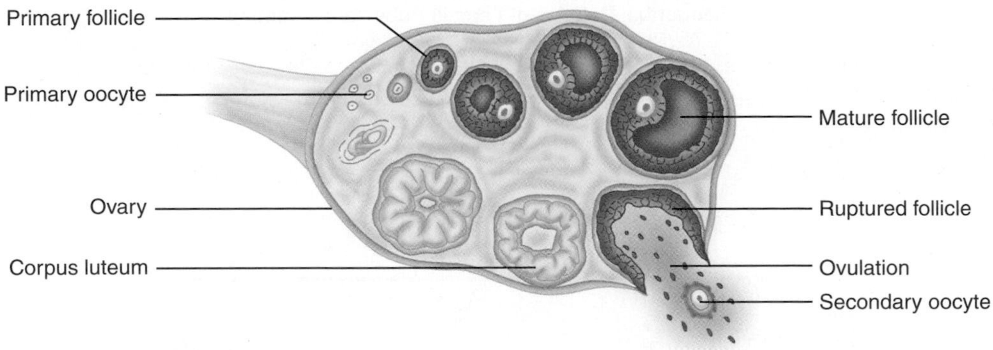

Figure 17.7: An Ovarian Follicle

During childhood, just over half of the ovarian follicles present at birth are absorbed back into the body. By the age of puberty, when the menstrual cycle begins, the remaining ovarian follicles await development into mature eggs. Periodically, the ovarian follicles are stimulated to mature. This process leads to the ovulation of a single mature ovum once per month.

Ovulation refers to the ripening and release of an egg from an ovary. It occurs approximately 2 weeks after the onset of menstruation (see *Female Reproductive Cycle*). At this time, a surge of luteinizing hormone causes the follicle to rupture, releasing the ovum into and down the fallopian tubes.

Ovarian follicles are identified by the following descriptive terms:

primary or *primordial ovarian follicle:* the immature ovum and the cells that encase it.

secondary ovarian follicle: the stage in which there is a maturing, or ripening, of an oocyte in the follicle. As the oocyte grows, it eventually exerts pressure on the follicle that contains it, causing it to rupture. The ovum is then released. Once the ovum leaves the follicle, the empty space is filled by cells called the corpus luteum.

> The *corpus luteum* is a yellow glandular mass that secretes progesterone to prepare and enhance the environment of the uterus in case of pregnancy.
>
> Secondary ovarian follicles are also known as *graafian follicles* and/or *vesicular ovarian follicles.*

atretic ovarian follicles: involuted (upside down; complex) ovarian follicles that are not viable and eventually get reabsorbed into the body.

Female pubertal hormones

The ability to achieve puberty and reproductive status begins in embryo, although the timing of these events is closely regulated by hormone *switches* that do not turn on until approximately 10 years of age (pre-pubescence). From that time onward, the hormones FSH, LH, estrogen, and progesterone play a key role in regulating the female reproductive cycle.

Together, the follicle stimulating hormone (FSH) and the luteinizing hormone (LH) stimulate the ovaries to begin production of the hormone estrogen. These three hormones combined lead to sexual, reproductive maturity and preparation for pregnancy (should conception occur).

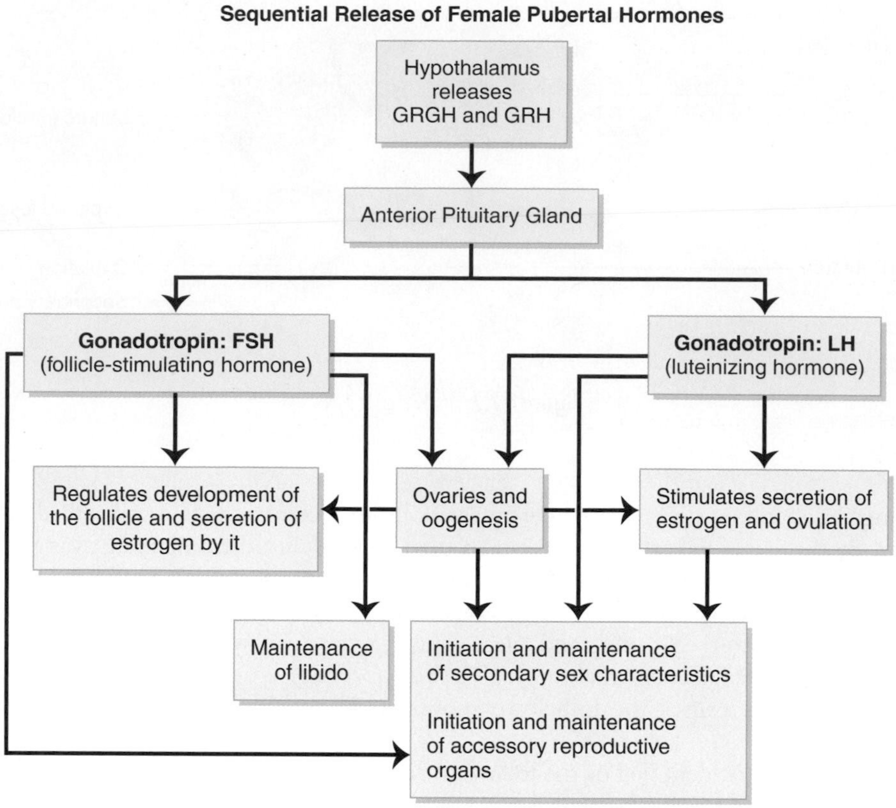

Sequential Release of Female Pubertal Hormones

Hypothalamus releases GRGH and GRH

Anterior Pituitary Gland

Gonadotropin: FSH (follicle-stimulating hormone)

Gonadotropin: LH (luteinizing hormone)

Regulates development of the follicle and secretion of estrogen by it

Ovaries and oogenesis

Stimulates secretion of estrogen and ovulation

Maintenance of libido

Initiation and maintenance of secondary sex characteristics

Initiation and maintenance of accessory reproductive organs

Figure 17.8: Sequential Release of Female Pubertal Hormones

follicle stimulating hormone (FSH): At this point, it should be quite clear how important ovarian follicles are to reproduction, but the entire process of maturation of an ovum and the rupturing of a follicle are dependent on the follicle stimulating hormone (FSH).

Not only is FSH essential to initiating the process of oogenesis, but it also stimulates production of another hormone called *estradiol* (a type of estrogen). In other words, FSH stimulates the secretion of estrogens.

Just as it does in males, FSH serves another reproductive purpose as well, by developing and maintaining the libido.

estrogen: Estrogen is a female steroid hormone. It is produced by both the adrenal cortex and a mature ovarian follicle at the time in the monthly reproductive cycle when the female is most receptive biologically to becoming pregnant.

Estrogen continues to be secreted throughout the reproductive years of women. During this time, it plays an essential role in the monthly menstrual cycle. Increases in estrogen are also associated with an increased sex drive, or libido.

The roots of estrogen are:

estrus + **gen** = **estrogen**
↓ ↓
passion + generate/produce

There is some speculation in the world of linguistics that this term may have arisen to explain how the hormone has the ability to cause sexual excitement and receptivity.

Upon the onset of puberty, estrogen is responsible for the maturing of the female reproductive organs. Additionally, it triggers development of the following *secondary sexual characteristics* in females: development of the breasts, a broadening of the pelvis and hips, the growth of body hair, and the deposit of adipose (fatty) tissues that create the female shape.

Across the life span, estrogen plays a key role in reproductive health and secondary sexual characteristics. It also assists with the maintenance of healthy bones and a healthy heart. With aging, estrogen production ceases. Some menopausal women choose to take estrogen replacement therapy to promote bone health.

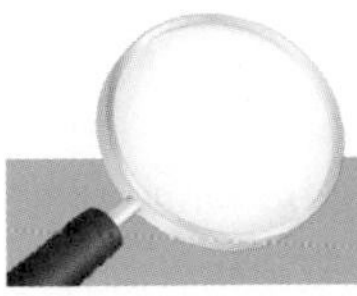

FOCUS POINT: Estrus—A Warning

Although *estrus* is the root word of *estrogen*, it should NEVER be used in relation to human beings. It is highly unprofessional and unacceptable to do so. Today, *estrus* refers only to the period of fertility in female animals, the condition of being in heat.

luteinizing hormone (LH): In puberty, LH triggers ovulation and the production of estrogen in the ovaries. It also stimulates production of the hormone progesterone.

progesterone: Recall that progesterone is produced by the corpus luteum in an empty ovarian follicle, post-ovulation. This hormone plays a critical role in pregnancy:

> Should the released ovum be fertilized, progesterone supports pregnancy by preparing the *endometrium,* the lining of the uterus.
>
> It also suppresses further ova production. It inhibits this cycle by blocking FSH and LH release. It prevents **lactation,** the production of breast milk, from occurring until after birth.
>
> Progesterone is also responsible, in almost all cases, for preventing any early contractions and/or premature birth.

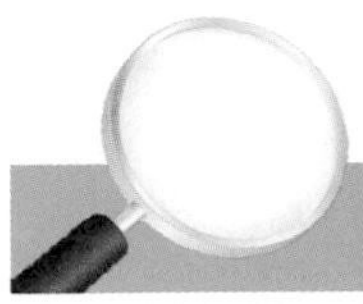

FOCUS POINT: Hormones after Childbirth

Following childbirth, estrogen and progesterone levels fall quite dramatically, which causes the uterus to begin to return to its normal size. Other physiological changes include an improvement in muscle tone in the abdomen (particularly along the pelvic floor) as the body begins its return to normal function and the reproductive cycle reasserts itself.

The female reproductive cycle

The female reproductive ability occurs in a monthly, 28-day *menstrual cycle.* The function of the cycle is to create an ovum and prepare for possible conception.

The root **menses** means *month.* What occurs between days 21 and 28 of the menstrual cycle is referred to as *menses, menstruation,* or the *menstrual period.* The use of proper medical terminology to refer to this cycle is an expected part of professional behavior.

There are three phases in a woman's menstrual cycle: the follicular, the ovulatory, and the luteal phases.

follicular phase: On days 1 to 14, the follicle stimulating hormone (FSH) begins the creation of a single, mature ovum (egg) and the endometrium begins to thicken.

ovulatory phase: As the 14th day approaches, the luteinizing hormone (LH) assists development of the ovum, culminating in ovulation (the release of the ovum) into the fallopian tube.

luteal phase: Days 15 to 28 are the time of ovulation and possible conception. There are two events that can occur here:

- *If the ovum is fertilized*, it continues to travel down the fallopian tube to embed itself in the endometrium by Day 20. At this point, it will become an embryo. Pregnancy begins: the female has been *impregnated.*
- *If the ovum remains unfertilized*, it will pass out of the body by Day 28 (approximately).

Menses

Days 21 to 28 are the period of menstruation. During the reproductive cycle, if an ovum is not fertilized, levels of estrogen and progesterone decrease. This leads to the sloughing off (shedding) of the lining of the uterus, the *endometrium.* It flows out of the body in the form of menstrual blood and tissue. Following menstruation, a new menstrual cycle begins.

Generally, the first menstrual period occurs within 2 to 2½ years of the onset of puberty and the development of the breasts.

A synonym for the *menstrual cycle* is *ovarian cyclicity.*

Table 17-6 explores words formed from the root *menses.* Study the definitions to be sure that you know exactly what you are talking about and can understand what is said or written about regarding this important subject matter. Always remember that the use of professional terminology is essential and expected when dealing with subjects of reproductive or sexual health.

Notice how the words in Table 17-6 break down into prefixes, roots, and suffixes. Identifying these word parts enhances your ability to decipher each word, even if, at first look, you do not think you know the term.

TABLE 17-6: Terms Derived from menses *and menstru/a*

Term	Word Parts	Meaning
menses	a root meaning *month*	the monthly flow of menstrual blood from the endometrium Also known as *menstruation*
menstruation	*menstru-*: derived from the root *menses* + the suffix–*ation* to identify a process	a sloughing off of the lining of the uterus that occurs monthly in women
menstrual	*menstru-:* derived from the root *menses* + the suffix–*al*, meaning "related to"	referring to or related to menstruation
premenstrual	pre- prefix meaning *before* +menstrual	before menstruation; the days immediately preceding menstruation
menarche	men- (combining form of *menses*) +arche root meaning *beginning*	the stage of a woman's life marked by the onset of menstrual activity and the ability to reproduce
menopause	men/o (combining form of *menses*) +pause (derivative of *pausis*, meaning *cessation*)	the stage of a woman's life marked by the cessation (end) of menstrual activity and the ability to reproduce
menorrhalgia	men/o- (combining form of *menses*) -rrh/a (form of suffix, *rrhea* meaning *flow*) +algia meaning pain	pain that accompanies menstrual flow; pelvic pain
dysmenorrhea	dys– prefix meaning *difficult* or *painful* meno– Combining form of *menses* -rrhea suffix meaning *flow* or *discharge*	pain associated with menstruation

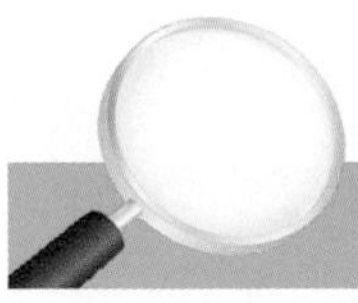

FOCUS POINT: Menarche and Menopause

Menarche is the onset of menstruation. It occurs in puberty.

Menopause is the cessation, or end, of menstruation. It occurs in middle age (50 to 60 years of age). Cessation is determined if the woman has not had a period in a full year.

Female fertility

Female fertility declines over the lifespan, beginning in a woman's 30s. By their mid-to-late 40s, women are unlikely to be fertile, although this is not impossible. In other words, a woman's ability to become pregnant decreases over her lifespan, although conception can occur into the 50s. However, even with the onset of menopause and the cessation of menses, it is still possible for the mature woman to conceive. Medically, contraception is suggested for a period of at least 2 years following the onset of menopause.

Postpartum infertility and *postpartum fertility* are terms used to describe the time period following birth or the end of pregnancy. Generally, women are infertile for approximately 3 weeks postpartum. Then the cycle of ovulation (the menstrual cycle) begins again. To avoid pregnancy too soon, contraception or contraceptive practices are suggested. However for breastfeeding women, the period of infertility lasts until cessation of that activity (since ovulation is biologically inhibited during lactation). Even so, caution may be warranted to avoid an early unwanted pregnancy during this time.

A woman's age at the time she conceives can affect whether or not she can see the pregnancy through to fruition (childbirth), as well as the health of the unborn child. This is not so much about her age itself, but about the quantity and quality of the available oocytes. These also age, and the DNA stored within them can degrade over time or be adversely affected by environmental toxins, disease, and other factors. If there are chromosomal abnormalities in the embryo, women have a higher chance of miscarriage, or loss of the pregnancy.

Infertility in women can have many causes. Besides the natural loss of fertility that occurs in later life, infertility can be caused by the presence or residual effects of diseases such as malaria, tuberculosis, and sexually transmitted diseases, for example. Poor nutrition can also contribute to a state of infertility. Infertility can be the result of natural causes, too. These might include anatomical factors such as insufficient mucosa in the cervix to assist in sperm mobility, poor egg quality that prohibits pregnancy from developing, or atypically shaped organs such as the uterus.

Assessment of female fertility or infertility is a common task in reproductive health care: family practice medicine, obstetrics, and gynecology. Table 17-7 identifies and describes a few of these assessments.

TABLE 17-7: Fertility Tests of Women

Fertility Test	Description
Day 3 FSH Fertility Test of Ovarian Reserve	A blood test to measure for baseline FSH on day 3 of the menstrual cycle. Results indicate the quantity of follicles and ova that are present in the ovaries. Results: A *high* FSH means a *lower* quantity of eggs in the ovaries.
Day 3 Estradiol* testing	A blood test to ascertain decreased egg quantity and quality even with a normal FSH level. Results: Co-occurring low FSH and low estradiol levels are an indication of normal quantity and quality of follicles and ova.
Clomiphene challenge test	Tests the ovarian reserve (how many ova are available). A blood test is taken on day 3 of the menstrual cycle. Then a dose of clomiphene (a fertility drug used to initiate ovulation) is administered on the fifth day. Another blood test is taken on the 10th day of the cycle. Results: Elevated levels of FSH on day 10 indicate problems with follicular development and production of estradiol.

* *Estradiol* is the most potent type of estrogen. It is produced only during the first half of the menstrual cycle.

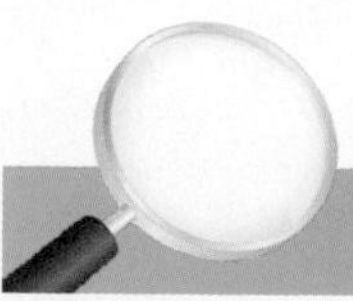

FOCUS POINT: *Barren*

The term *barren* refers to an inability to produce offspring. It can be used to describe an infertile woman or a couple who have been incapable of reproduction. A barren woman can also be one who is able to conceive but unable to carry a pregnancy through to conception, never giving birth to any children. Although this term is used in communication with other health professionals, it should not be used when addressing the infertile couple themselves, who may find the word *barren* hurtful and insensitive in their already painful emotional situation.

Pathology of the female reproductive system

Pathology related to the female reproductive system can be genetic or pathogenic. It can interfere with ovulation, fertilization, and development of an embryo/fetus. Pathology of this system can lead to miscarriages, infertility, or the pregnant female's or her offspring's demise. Table 17-8 provides more information and introduces some of the relevant terminology.

TABLE 17-8: Pathology of the Female Reproductive System

Pathology	Definition/Description	Treatment
chronic anovulation *also known as* hypothalamic chronic anovulation	a condition of chronic dysfunction of the hypothalamus in which it fails to signal the pituitary gland to begin ovulation	administration of gonadotropic releasing hormone
endometriosis	Tissue similar to that of the uterus builds up in other parts of the female body and sheds in response to the cycle of reproductive hormones. causes pains, cramps, and dysmenorrhea *The endometrium is the mucosal membrane that lines the uterine wall. It naturally sheds during menses.	medication (nonsteroidal, anti-inflammatory) surgery
fibroids *also known as* uterine fibroids	ovarian neoplasms; benign	Although often left in place, they can be removed by surgery if they are causing pain or excessive menstrual bleeding.
premenstrual syndrome (PMS)	a group of physical, emotional, and behavioral symptoms occurring prior to the onset of menses (5–11 days prior)	increase fluid intake eat frequent, small meals consider adding supplements of Vitamin B_6, calcium, and magnesium to the diet medication (nonsteroidal, anti-inflammatory)
oophoroma	a rare, malignant ovarian tumor	oophorectomy radiation and chemotherapy
pelvic inflammatory disease (PID)	an infectious, inflammatory disease that begins in the vagina and cervix, but spreads upwards into the uterus, ovaries, and fallopian tubes, as well as the pelvis. produces vaginal discharge, pain and cramping: lower abdominal pain	antibiotics

Ovarian cysts (oophorocystosis)

Ovarian cysts provide an excellent example from which it is possible to see the interrelatedness of hormones to the menstrual cycle and the structures of the female reproductive system.

A **cyst** is a membrane-covered growth consisting of fluid or semi-solid substances, such as pus. A cyst could also simply be filled with air. Although the majority of cysts are harmless, some are not and may need antibiotic therapy and/or surgical removal. All cysts have the potential to become painful.

Ovarian cysts are caused when ovulation does not occur in its normal cyclic and sequential manner (the process is disrupted or disorganized) or when ovulation fails completely.

These cysts can be quite painful. Those cysts that do not resolve on their own and are left untreated can grow to such a size as to exert pressure on other organs of the abdomen, increasing the pain. There are two main types of ovarian cysts:

Follicular cysts are caused when the hormone LH fails to surge (flow) when it should in the reproductive cycle and the follicle is not stimulated to rupture. As a result, the ovum is not released. The follicle then continues to grow unchecked until it forms a cyst.

Follicular cysts are not considered medically dangerous and often resolve themselves within two or three menstrual cycles. They may or may not cause pain.

Corpus luteum cysts: After the follicle has ruptured and the ovum is released, the follicle evolves to house the corpus luteum. Sometimes the ruptured follicle closes off too quickly after the egg's release and other tissues accumulate within it. The corpus luteum itself then expands to accommodate these tissues, and a cyst is formed.

This type of cyst can grow to a good size (3 to 4 inches) but also often dissolves within a week. However, the corpus luteum cyst might also fill with blood, impinging on the rest of the ovary, causing pelvic pain. Should it be blood-filled and rupture, it can cause internal bleeding and sudden pain.

Polycystic ovarian syndrome (**PCOS**) is the term for a number of co-occurring pathological conditions, the primary one of which is multiple cysts on the ovaries. The other conditions might include acne, obesity, anovulation (lack of ovulation), **hirsutism** (growth of facial hair), baldness (male pattern baldness), low bone density, and menstrual irregularities. Insulin resistance and type II diabetes may also be present.

PCOS develops when ovulation fails to occur. Lack of ovulation disrupts a woman's normal reproductive cycle. This disruption, in turn, has an adverse effect on hormone production, brain chemistry, and ovary function. It is a vicious cycle in which hormones continue to be released or not released, causing a build-up of unruptured follicles, which become ovarian cysts. Figure 17-9 illustrates this process.

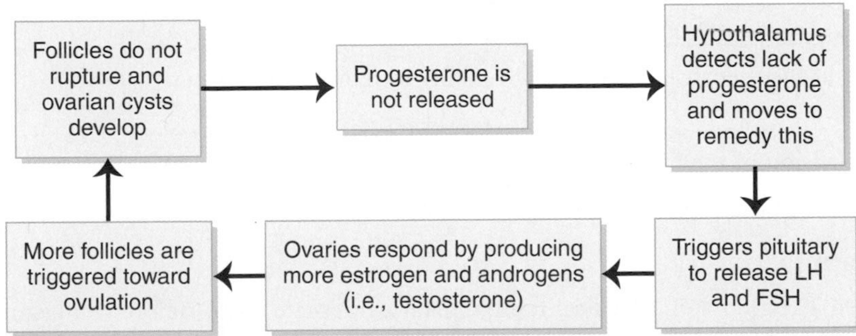

Figure 17.9: Development of Polycystic Ovarian Syndrome

Fill in the Blanks

Use new language and terms in a meaningful way. Complete these sentences by filling in the blanks.

1. Menopause leads to the reproductive change of _____________ in older women.
2. Another way to say *menstrual period* is to simply say _____________.
3. The _____________ phase is when a hormone is released to create and grow an ovum.
4. The term _____________ uses the prefix *im-* to signify that conception has occurred.
5. An _____________ is an immature ovum.
6. _____________ is the main hormone produced in the ovaries.
7. The production of the hormone _____________ is triggered when conception occurs.
8. Heightened levels of _____________ and _____________ fall postpartum.

Mix and Match

Match the medical term with its synonym. Draw a line to connect them.

1. oosperm	ovigenesis
2. uterus	ovaries
3. ova	eggs
4. sloughing	zygote
5. ovum	womb
6. menses	menstrual period
7. oogenesis	egg
8. ovaria	shedding

Break It Down

You are given a description. Identify the medical term for it. Then identify the word part asked for.

1. pain associated with menstruation
   Term: _____________ Word Part – prefix: _____________
2. the stage of life marked by the cessation (end) of the menstrual cycle and the ability to reproduce
   Term: _____________ Word Part – root word: _____________
3. the lining of the uterus
   Term: _____________ Word Part – prefix: _____________
4. the onset of the menstrual cycle and the ability to reproduce
   Term: _____________ Word Part – root word: _____________
5. surgical division of the fallopian tubes
   Term: _____________ Word Part – suffix: _____________

Build a Word

You are given all or parts of a medical term. Create a complete term. Before you begin each task, study the word parts to glean (garner, gather; put together) their meaning. You should recognize all of them. Then define the term in your own words.

1. –ic gen ovari/o _____________ Meaning _____________
2. otomy ovari/o _____________ Meaning _____________
3. rrhexis ovari/o _____________ Meaning _____________
4. ectomy oophor/o _____________ Meaning _____________

The breast

Chapter 8 introduced the basic anatomy and physiology of the breast. Enhance that knowledge and terminology now by exploring the breast in the context of the reproductive system, particularly for the female breast.

Male and female breasts sit bilaterally on the anterior surface of the chest, although they originate within the anterior chest wall itself. Their center point, the *nipple,* is located between invisible midclavicular and midaxillary lines (lines that run vertically down from midcollarbone and midunderarm). Internally, they are positioned anterior to the *pectoralis major* and *serratus anterior* muscles.

The medical field specializing in the breast is **mastology**. This word derives from the Greek root *mast/o,* meaning *breast.* Table 17-9 illustrates how this root can be expanded to form medical terms.

It is also quite correct to identify the medical field specializing in the breast as **mammology**. This word derives from the Latin root *mamm/o,* meaning "the glandular structure found within the breasts of females which secretes milk." Study Table 17-10 to discover how this root can be expanded to create medical terms.

The female breast contains *mammary glands.* To review the structures of the female breast, study Figure 17-10.

Female breast Tissue

Female breasts are composed of three types of tissues: glandular, fibrous, and adipose (fatty).

Glandular tissues are the functional part of the breast, producing milk. Within this tissue are *mammary ducts (lactiferous ducts)* that convey milk to the nipple.

Fibrous tissues provide support for the glandular ones. They do this with the help of bands of ligaments called Cooper's ligaments, which help suspend the breasts (hold them up).

Adipose tissue plays host to the glandular tissue, which is embedded in it. Adipose tissue gives shape, form, and consistency to the breast overall.

TABLE 17-9: Suffixes Used with *mast/o*

Begin with the combining form *mast/o*	Add a suffix	Create Medical Terms
mast	-oid meaning *shape* or *form*	mastoid = shaped like a breast
mast	-algia meaning *pain*	mastalgia = pain in the breast Also known as *mammalgia*
masto	-plasty meaning *to form*	mastoplasty = plastic surgery of the breast
mast	-ectomy meaning *removal*	mastectomy = surgical removal of a breast

TABLE 17-10: Suffixes used with *mamm/a/o*

Begin with the combining form *mamm/a/o*	Add a suffix	Create Medical Terms
mamma	-plasty meaning *to form*	mammaplasty = surgical reconstruction of a breast
mamm	-itis meaning *inflammation* or *swelling*	mammitis = inflammation or infection of the breast that causes swelling to occur Also known as *mastitis*
mammo	-gram	mammogram = a radiograph of the breast/breast tissues

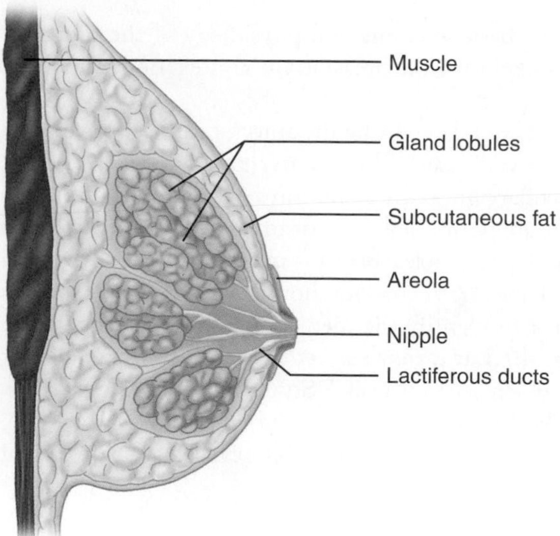

Figure 17.10: Anatomy of the Female Breast

Cooper's ligaments

As you know, ligaments are bands of fibrous tissue that connect bones and/or cartilage. In most cases, their function is to support joints. However, *Cooper's ligaments* are different. These tissues support the breast, creating its structure, shape, and tone. They also hold the breasts in their proper anatomical place. Cooper's ligaments attach anatomically to breast tissue and the chest wall. They extend from the base of the chin distally to the last rib (see Figure 17-11).

When Cooper's ligaments are shorter and tighter, the breasts sit higher on the chest wall and their consistency is firmer. This is quite evident in youth. Conversely, if these same ligaments are stretched (by age or exertion) or if they are longer and laxer for any reason, the breasts will droop (elongate) and their placement on the chest wall may shift. Types of activities that can cause this to occur are repeated high-impact activities (i.e., jogging), breastfeeding, and the loss or gain of weight.

Cooper's ligaments are also known as *fibrocollagenous septa*, *Cooper's suspensory ligaments*, or *suspensory ligaments of Cooper*.

Eponyms: Cooper and Cooper's Ligaments

Sir Astley Paston Cooper was an English surgeon, professor of surgery, and anatomist from the late 1700s through the early 1800s. Along with naming Cooper's ligaments in the breast, he is responsible for identifying, describing, and naming the following:

Cooper's disease: Multiple benign cystic growths in the breast(s), which have a bluish-brown color, occur when a woman is in her early 30s and are the result of pathology in the mammary ducts or the epithelium of these ducts.
Cooper's neuralgia: pain and tissue irritability in the breast
Cooper's testis: recurrent pain in the testis/testes
Cooper's fascia: a fascia (covering) of the spermatic cord

Sir Astley Paston Cooper was also a 1st baronet and Sergeant-Surgeon to royalty. The first royal title was bestowed by King George IV of England, when Cooper successfully removed a sebaceous cyst from the king's scalp. The surgeon was further endowed with the title and position of Sergeant-Surgeon to this king and then to his successor, King William IV.

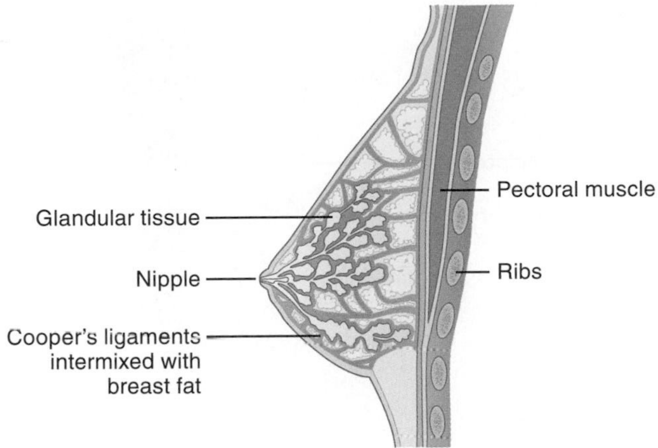

Figure 17.11: Cooper's Ligaments

Mammary glands

Recall that exocrine glands contain ducts. Internally, the female breasts contain **lactiferous ducts**—ducts capable of lactation (generating milk). These are organized into clusters of ducts called *lobules.* There are approximately 15 to 20 lobules in one breast. Lactiferous ducts transport breast milk from the ducts to the nipple (see *Breastfeeding*).

Lactation refers to the yielding or release of milk from the lactiferous ducts. It also refers to the time period in which breast milk is produced. Originally, this term referred to the process of suckling (feeding) an infant at the breast. The Latin root is *lac or lactis*, meaning *milk.* In modern English, the combining form *lac/to* refers to milk and dairy products.

lac/to	+	**a**	+	**tion**	=	**lactation**
↓		↓		↓		↓
milk	+	combining vowel	+	process or state of	=	process or state of producing or giving milk

Lactation is initiated by the hormone prolactin when conception occurs. *Prolactin,* a lactogenic hormone, is released by the pituitary gland at the time of, or immediately after, childbirth. When the newborn is receiving all nourishment from breast milk, he or she is said to be **lactivorous** (living on milk).

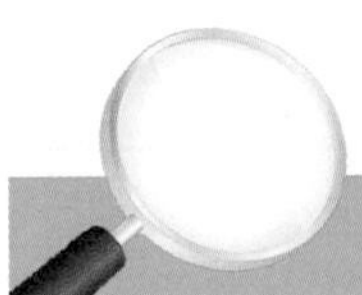

FOCUS POINT: Expressing Milk

The most appropriate and common medical term for the act of yielding or releasing milk through the nipple is *expressing*. For example, a woman *expresses* milk when she breastfeeds.

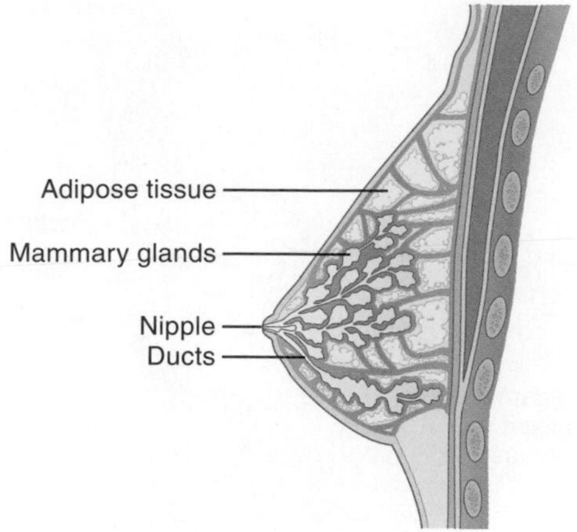

Figure 17.12: Mammary Glands

Breast changes during and after pregnancy

During pregnancy, the hormones estrogen, progesterone, and prolactin cause the breasts to enlarge and prepare to produce milk. Prolactin is the primary hormone of lactation, and its levels increase throughout the entire pregnancy. However, interplay with the hormone estrogen during that time inhibits actual milk production until after childbirth.

Generally, lactation ceases when the female stops breastfeeding, although this may vary by a few months. As lactation ceases, the breasts return to their normal shape and size.

Pathology of the breast

Male and female breasts are susceptible to pathology. Tables 17-11 and 17-12 provide details and terminology related to breast pathology.

Diagnostic assessment of breast health is achieved in a number of ways, including the following:

Histopathology is the microscopic, laboratory testing of tissue and blood. One method for gathering a breast tissue specimen is the *fine-needle aspiration cytology test*. In this test, a long, fine needle is inserted into the breast tissue. A specimen is retrieved by drawing it up through the needle into the body of the syringe. The specimen is then examined by microscope.

Mammograms are a type of radiograph, or x-ray. This test is noninvasive. It can detect cysts, tumors, and other changes in breast tissues. Mammograms are considered an excellent diagnostic tool for the screening of breast cancer.

TABLE 17-11: Pathology of the Female Breast

Pathology	Definition/Description	Symptoms	Treatment
agalactia	• failure to lactate or faulty lactation • Causes might include hormonal imbalances, presence of other diseases, mental or emotional health challenges.	• the inability of the mother to feed the newborn sufficiently or adequately with her own milk	• antibiotics may be indicated • mental health intervention • hormone supplements or other adjustment of hormone levels
ductal carcinoma	• neoplasm and tumors of the lactiferous ducts • may be caused by estrogen, genetic propensity and family history of same, age, exposure to radiation, and various lifestyle and environmental factors	• bone and breast pain • swelling of arm nearest to the cancer site • weight loss	• hormonal therapy • lumpectomy • chemotherapy • radiation therapy • mastectomy

TABLE 17-11: Pathology of the Female Breast—cont'd

Pathology	Definition/Description	Symptoms	Treatment
fibrocystic breast disease (FBD) *also known as* benign fibrocystic disease or fibrocystic breast condition **Note: The name of this condition is slowly changing to reflect the fact that it is not actually a disease, as was first thought.*	• a common condition characterized by a lumpiness or lumpy texture to the breast tissue • can be caused by cyclic release of hormones that affect breast tissue; diabetes or thyroid disease	• symptoms may include breast tenderness and/or pain	• analgesic anti-inflammatory medications for discomfort and inflammation • supplemental Vitamin E • correction of hormonal irregularities by use of anti-estrogen compounds
galactorrhea	• inappropriate, spontaneous lactation that is not associated with/not co-occurring with nursing or childbirth • may be caused by tumors of the pituitary gland, use of oral contraceptives, kidney disease, some prescribed medications and hormone preparations, marijuana or opiates, and some herbal supplements	• Symptoms can include discharge of a milklike substance, acne, headaches, increased facial hair, irregular or absent menses	• medication that inhibits prolactin production • estrogen supplements • If the cause is a prolactin tumor, then surgery or radiation are necessitated.
lobular carcinoma	• neoplasms and tumors of the lobules in the breast • possibly caused by estrogen, genetic tendency, age, exposure to radiation, and various lifestyle and environmental factors	• bone and breast pain • swelling of arm nearest to the cancer site • weight loss	• hormonal therapy • lumpectomy • chemotherapy • radiation therapy • mastectomy

TABLE 17-12: Pathology of the Male Breast

Pathology	Definition/Description	Symptoms	Treatment
phylloid tumors of the breast *also known as* fibroepithelial tumors **may also occur in females*	• a group of smooth, rounded lesions with multiple nodes (lumps; bumps) • generally benign, but can be malignant • may be secondary to gynecomastia	• skin ulceration as a result of the size of the tumor and pressure on the skin	• estrogen administration • hormonal therapy • lumpectomy • chemotherapy • radiation therapy
gynecomastia	• abnormal breast development • lactation may or may not occur • not uncommon during puberty as the result of fluctuations in hormone activity • Possible causes include breast and lung tumors, cirrhosis of the liver (where estrogen cannot be inhibited as it should be), or other diseases • temporary • benign	• enlargement of breasts	• If it does not resolve itself, cosmetic surgery is an option.

Continued

TABLE 17-12: Pathology of the Male Breast—cont'd

Pathology	Definition/Description	Symptoms	Treatment
galactorrhea **also occurs in females*	• the production of breast milk • a pituitary gland disorder • Causes can include reaction to certain medications, very low thyroxin levels, diseases of the hypothalamus.	• Symptoms can include discharge of a milk-like substance, acne, headaches, and increased facial hair.	• adjustments in medications • hormonal therapy • surgery if unresolved: bilateral total duct excision
male breast cancer	• rare, but incidents are increasing • malignant neoplasms of the breast	• presence of a lump • nipple pain • pain or tenderness around the nipple • clear or bloody discharge from nipple • enlarged lymph nodes under arm on affected side	• lymphectomy or dissection • radiation • chemotherapy • hormonal therapy

Critical Thinking

Answer these questions on the basis of what you have learned in this and other chapters.

1. Which reproductive hormone will be dominant for Glory Loeppky now as she cares for her baby? Provide your rationale. ______________________
2. What is the difference between an infection and a disease?
____
____
____

Reflective Questions

Answer these questions based on new terminology relating to the female breast.

1. Name the primary lactogenic hormone. ______________
2. Name the medical condition of abnormal breast development in males. ______________
3. What are clusters of ducts in the breast called? ______________
4. Name two pathologies of the breast that occur in both men and women. ______________ and ______________
5. What do Cooper's ligaments support? ______________
6. Define histopathology. ______________

Build a Word

Unscramble each set of word parts to create a proper medical term. Then define the term.

1. gen lac/to ______________________ Meaning ______________________
2. rrhea lac/to ______________________ Meaning ______________________
3. algia mamm/o ______________________ Meaning ______________________

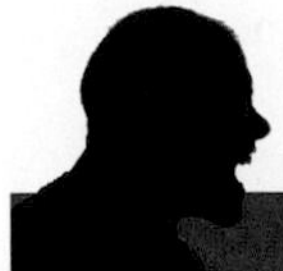

PRONUNCIATION PRACTICE

Say these words aloud to a friend or classmate. You are given the phonetic pronunciation. Your instructor can help you with pronunciation,

or visit **http://www.MedicalLanguageLab.com.**

galactorrhea	gă-lăk″tō-**rē**´ă	lactorrhea	lăk-tō-**rē**´ă
gynecomastia	gī″nĕ-kō-**măs**´tē-ă	mammalgia	măm-**ăl**´jē-ă
lactogen	**lăk**´tō-jĕn	prolactin	prō-**lăk**´tĭn

The Language of Family Practice Medicine

Family practice medicine is concerned with the health, growth, and development of families as a whole and with the individual members making up a family unit. It is a medical specialty providing continuing, comprehensive health care. But it is also more than that. This field of health care integrates a number of other fields, making it more holistic in its approach.

The family practice approach includes the biological, psychological, and behavioral sciences. Careers in this field include physicians, nurses and nurse practitioners, early childhood educators and developmental experts, geneticists, and mental health professionals. Public health nurses (PHNs) also play an important role in family practice medicine (see *Career Spotlight*).

Family practice medicine is also known as *family medicine* or *family practice.*

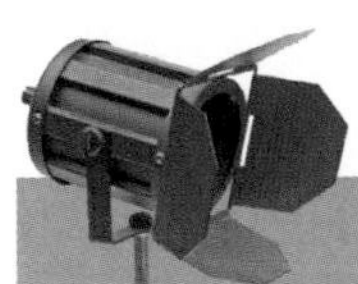

CAREER SPOTLIGHT: Public Health Nurse

A career as a public health nurse (PHN) involves working with individuals, families, and groups across the life span (all ages). Through a public health clinic or agency, PHNs attend to childhood immunizations; offer support and counseling in family planning; facilitate prenatal care and classes; provide postpartum and postnatal follow-up care, education, and home visits; provide parenting classes; and liaise with the local schools regarding matters of health, hygiene, infection control, and some mental health issues. PHNs might also do follow-up home visits for elderly or disabled patients who have just been released from a hospital.

The scope of practice of a PHN also includes working with communities to promote healthy environments. Examples of such community work are holding flu clinics and investigating, documenting, and intervening with outbreaks of communicable diseases.

Public health nurses generally hold a baccalaureate degree in nursing (or in lieu of this, many years in nursing prior to becoming a PHN), and most specialize in public health. However, the work of the PHN is very family-focused, so additional education and training in areas relevant to family medicine are encouraged.

Family can be defined in many ways, and the definition of a family may sometimes become a political, moral, ethical, or religious issue. As a health or allied health professional, you will be required to follow the definition set out by legislation and your regulatory (licensing) body whenever you are on duty. Here are some examples of different ways that the word *family* may be defined:

- a group of people consisting of parent(s) and children
- two or more people sharing a long-term commitment to each other, as well as common goals

- a group with shared values and a sense of identification or belonging with one another
- a couple in a committed relationship with or without children
- all members of one household
- people who share their ancestry or lineage (blood relations)

Families move through **lifecycles**—stages of growth and development. Theoretically, there are a good number of these. They can be described slightly differently by various disciplines: health studies, sociology, anthropology, psychology, and so on. Basically, however, these descriptions of family lifecycles are all based on the same core principles of when and what families do as a unit: how they grow and develop. Figures 17-13 and 17-14 offer a simple overview of the family lifecycle concept. Notice their similarities.

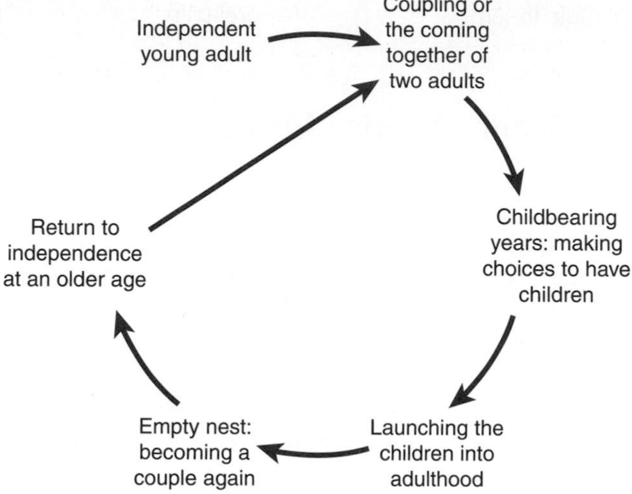

Figure 17.13: The Family Lifecycle with Children

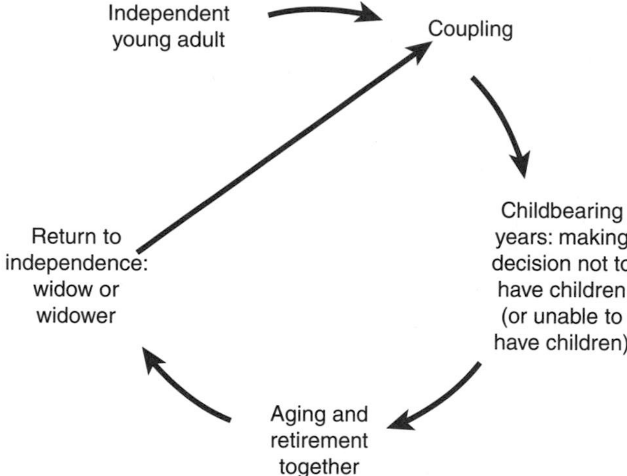

Figure 17.14: The Family Lifecycle without Children

In the world of family practice, **stage theory** is often referenced. This term applies to a number of commonly used theories that group people of certain ages (i.e., children, adults, elderly) and then identify specific physical and psychosocial developmental tasks that each age group should or will complete. Some examples of developmental tasks people complete per age and stage are as follows (although this list is not in any way complete):

- infants: sitting up independently and learning to crawl
- toddlers: learning to walk, feed self, and use the toilet

- school-age children: learning to write, read, spell, do arithmetic
- adolescents: reproductive maturity, finding self-identity (as opposed to seeing self in connection with family)
- adults: coupling; finding and maintaining intimate partnerships/relationships

The childbearing years

This period in the family lifecycle is based on the ages of the parents. As you know, the ability to conceive children occurs with sexual maturity. And although the actual physical ability to bear children is part of female reproduction and women's health, you have learned that the quality and quantity of sperm produced by a male can also affect whether or not a pregnancy can be carried through to birth. Recall that the ability to reproduce ends for women after menopause and declines significantly for men as they reach their later years of life.

Not everyone chooses to bear children, and some people cannot do so. Even so, everyone progresses biologically through the childbearing years. Health care during this period will focus on matters of sexual health (sexual activities that may or may not be related to reproduction) and matters of reproduction (such as fertility, genetics, and contraception). Family planning is an important aspect of health care for clients in their childbearing years.

Glory Loeppky and her husband are in the childbearing years. In that regard, Glory has been speaking with Dr. Antoine, her family physician, about the first addition to their family, baby Emily Grace. She also spoke with him about family planning: the plans that she and Gil have for having at least one more child. In that discussion, they also talked about contraception.

Family planning

Family planning is an ideological approach to childbearing, wherein considerations of the adult's health (including genetics), financial ability, economic stability, environment, mental health (including readiness and ability to cope), and spirituality (philosophical or religious values and beliefs) are all assessed and weighed by that person before conception is attempted. The goal is to find harmony or balance in all the domains of health prior to bringing a child into the world. The belief is that this planning provides the best possible birth and life circumstances for both the parent(s) and the child.

From a professional health care perspective, the decision to start a family or not remains solely with the individual(s) considering it, although the process of making this decision can be facilitated by a wide variety of trained health and allied health professionals. For example, physicians, geneticists, nurse practitioners, psychiatrists, psychologists, and social workers may be involved in helping couples and individuals to make this decision.

Contraception

As part of sexual health and family planning, health and allied health professionals will need to discuss contraception with their clients. Recall that **contraception** is the opposite of conception. In the medical sense, the term refers to multiple pharmaceutical, hormonal, or other interventions that prevent pregnancy. A basic knowledge of the medical terminology for contraception is important for members of the health care team.

Contraception is more commonly known as *birth control.*

There are several main types of contraception:

- barrier methods
- hormonal therapy: oral, topical, or injectable
- sterilization
- behavioral
- chemical

Tables 17-13 through 17-16 provide more details about different forms of contraception.

TABLE 17-13: Behavioral Forms of Contraception

Behavioral Forms of Contraception	Description
abstention	• refraining from sexual intercourse • highly effective
coitus interruptus	• the penis is withdrawn from the vagina before ejaculation occurs • only somewhat effective
rhythm method	• not having sexual intercourse on the days during the reproductive cycle when the female partner is most susceptible to becoming pregnant • somewhat effective

TABLE 17-14: Hormonal Forms of Contraception

Hormonal Forms of Contraception: Oral, Topical, and Injectable	Description
birth control pills, patches, or long-acting injections (*depo* injections: deep muscle injections of time-released hormones)	• pharmaceutical preparations using progesterone at measured doses that release slowly or daily at appropriate levels to prevent pregnancy • highly effective, proven methods of birth control

TABLE 17-15: Barrier Forms of Contraception

Form	Description
condom for males and females	• latex sheath (cover) of two types: male or female. The male condom covers the penis to prevent sperm from entering the vagina. The female condom is inserted into the vagina to prevent sperm from entering. Condoms can only be used once and then need to be safely discarded. • fairly effective in preventing pregnancy. Effectiveness is enhanced with concurrent use of spermicide or other birth control methods.
diaphragm (See Figure 17-15)	• a dome-shaped rubber disk temporarily inserted into the vagina to prevent sperm from traveling to the uterus • quite effective in preventing pregnancy • Use of a spermicide with this device greatly improves its efficacy.
intrauterine device (IUD) (See Figure 17-16)	• T-shaped device inserted into the vagina by a medical professional; it can remain in place for several years but needs to be replaced periodically. • Copper IUDs immobilize sperm and prevent them from traveling up into the uterus. Copper also changes the lining of the uterus to prevent an egg from implanting there. • Hormonal IUDs release progesterone slowly, making the cervix inhospitable and therefore inaccessible to sperm. • highly effective
sponge	• a plastic foam sponge temporarily inserted into the vagina (cervix) to block access to the uterus by sperm • moderately effective

TABLE 17-16: Sterilization as Contraception

Form of Sterilization	Description
tubal ligation	• minor surgical procedure in which the fallopian tubes are severed or cauterized (burned to seal them)
hysterectomy	• surgical removal of the uterus. Sometimes the ovaries are removed as well.
castration	• surgical removal of the testicle(s) This type of contraception does not occur in the United States (although castration for other medical reasons may occur).
vasectomy	• minor surgical procedure in which sperm are prevented from entering the seminal vesicles. This prevents ejaculation. The procedure requires that the vas deferens (both) be surgically severed (cut). • This type of male contraception is becoming increasingly more common, particularly for married men whose wives have already had children.

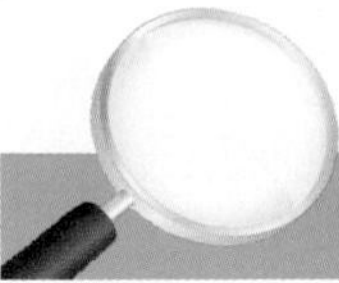

FOCUS POINT: Contragestive

By deconstructing this word, you can glean its meaning:

contra	+	**gest**	+	**ive**	=	**contragestive**
↓		↓		↓		
against	+	gestation	+	quality of/inclined to	=	inclined to prevent gestation

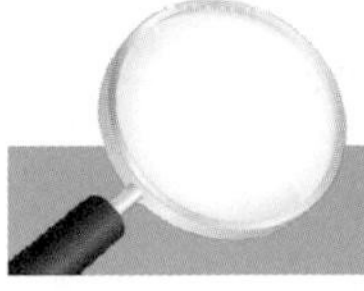

FOCUS POINT: Spermicides

A *spermicide* is a chemical pharmaceutical preparation that kills sperm. It is dispensed in the form of cream, gel, or foam. The preparation is inserted into the vagina at the time of, or just prior to, sexual intercourse. Spermicides are not highly effective in preventing pregnancy, although there is some thought that efficacy is improved (but not perfected) with concurrent use of a condom.

A spermicide is also called *spermatocide*.

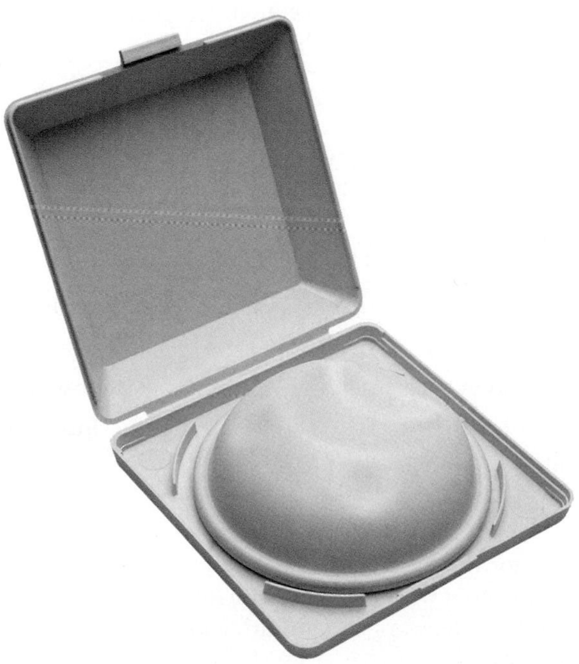

Figure 17.15: A Contraceptive Diaphragm (© Thinkstock / Stockbyte.)

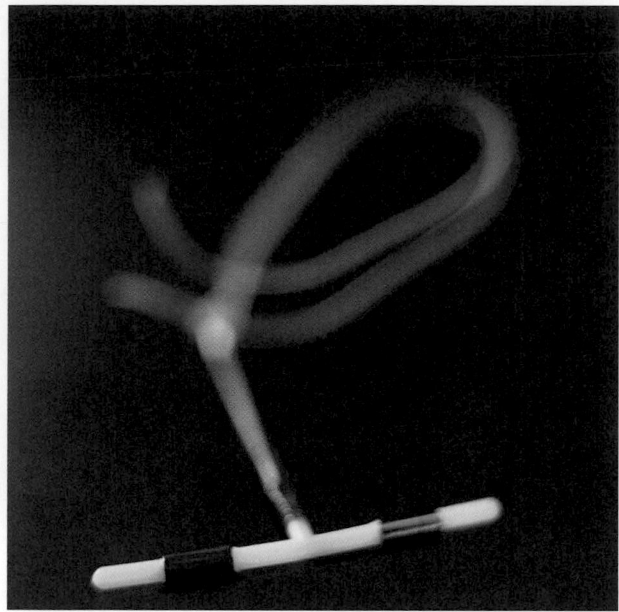

Figure 17.16: An Intrauterine Device (© Thinkstock / Spike Mafford.)

Let's Practice

Answer these questions on the basis of what you have learned about contraception.

1. Give an example of a barrier form of contraception. ______________________
2. What is the opposite of contraception? ______________________
3. In a family planning session with a health professional, who makes the final decision about whether or not to have children? ______________________
4. Which organ is removed in a hysterectomy? ______________________

Mix and Match

Match each description of a contraceptive technique with the medical term for it.

1. chemical pharmaceutical preparation that kills sperm	birth control pills
2. T-shaped device inserted into the vagina	coitus interruptus
3. withdrawal before ejaculation takes place	abstention
4. refraining from sexual intercourse	intrauterine device
5. series of pills containing differing levels of hormone	spermicide

Infancy, childhood, and adolescence

Theories and frameworks for the human lifecycle, growth, and development abound. There is however, general agreement about what ages comprise infancy, childhood, and adolescence. This terminology will be relevant to the work of all health and allied health professionals.

Growth and development

Ongoing growth and development during childhood should be monitored by a family physician or pediatrician. Other health professionals, such as school nurses, public health nurses, dieticians, and mental health counselors, may also play a role in monitoring a child's mental and physical health.

Delayed growth and development may be genetic, pathological, or quite normal. Although there are recognized, predictable trends in growth and development, there is no set rule that says, for example, that a child will grow in height at a certain age. Each child is unique in the way he or she grows.

Growth spurts, sudden onset of periods of physical growth, can lead to physical discomforts of muscle and joint pain, disrupted sleep, changes in appetite, and fatigue. At some point, these might all come to the attention of a health care provider.

Growth and development assessment includes the domains of physical, psychosocial, cognitive, and behavioral evaluation. Assessment is done using standardized protocols and measures. A simple example of this is a growth chart.

Assessment involves screening, a precursor to diagnosis. Screening helps health professionals (and educators) determine if a child is making developmental progress. Examples of these types of tests are found in Table 17-17. Sometimes the same test can serve as both a screening and a diagnostic tool.

Developmental disorders

Developmental disorders require the attention of health and allied health professionals. When present *in utero* or at birth, they are disorders or defects of the genes, the nervous system, the senses, or the brain. Developmental disorders can also be **degenerative**, meaning that the symptoms may not be present at birth but develop over time. Diagnostic screening and assessment are critical throughout childhood to intervene and help these children so that they may lead healthy and productive lives. Examples of developmental disorders include Down syndrome (see Chapter 14), blindness, deafness, and spina bifida (see Chapter 14).

TABLE 17-17: Childhood Development: Diagnostic and Screening Tools

Tool	Description
Denver Developmental Screening Test II (DDST-II)	• for ages 0–6 years • screens for neurological, cognitive, and behavioral disorders via social/personal development, fine and gross motor function, language (and/or the use of sound/voice prior to language)
Developmental Indicators for the Assessment of Learning (DIAL3)	• for ages 3–6 yrs, 11 months • assesses development of motor function, understanding of concepts (i.e., right, wrong; yes, no; big, small), language, self-help and social development
Early Screening Inventory-Revised (ESI-R)	• for ages 3–6 years • assesses sensory and behavioral development, as well as visual, motor, language, and cognitive development • screens for children who may have special needs, particularly in school
Hawaii Early Learning Profile (HELP)	• for ages 0–6 years • assesses cognition, language, gross and fine motor function, self-help behaviors, and social-emotional development
Kaufman Assessment Battery (K-ABC)	• for ages 2.5–12.5 years • assesses achievement and intelligence; verbal and nonverbal abilities; memory and problem-solving ability • diagnoses learning disabilities
Ounce Scale	• for ages 0–3.5 years old • assesses psychomotor and psychosocial development, including cognition and intellect: comprehension, exploration, inquiry, and related problem solving
Peabody Picture Vocabulary Test (4) (PPVT-4)	• for ages 2.5–4 years • measures verbal ability in standard American English vocabulary by asking examinee to point to or say the picture that represents what the examiner says. • can diagnose language disorders, cognitive and intellectual deficits, verbal ability, emotional withdrawal *There are other PPVTs designed for ages across the lifespan.
Social Competence and Behavior Evaluation	• for ages 2.5–6 years • evaluates adaptation and functioning with the child's environment; social competence, affect (emotion and mood), and social adjustment
Wechsler Preschool and Primary Scale of Intelligence III (WPPSI-III)	• for ages 2.6–7.3 years • measures cognitive/intellectual ability through a series of test items that require performance (i.e., object assembly), arithmetic, vocabulary, language competencies

Pervasive developmental disorders (**PDD**) refers to a syndrome of multiple developmental delays occurring together. This syndrome leads to disabilities in function, cognition, social ability, and communication. It may also include the absence of imagination. An example is autism spectrum disorder (see *Focus Point*).

Pervasive means persistent and all-encompassing. In this context, it signifies that the developmental delays encompass all aspects of the person's life: activity, relationships, experiences, and so on.

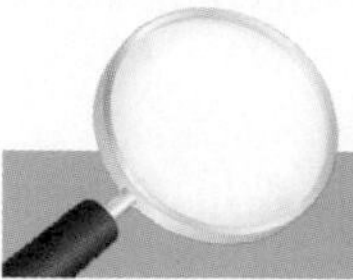

FOCUS POINT: Autism Spectrum Disorder (ASD)

Autism or *autism spectrum disorder* is a syndrome of neurological and mental symptoms, as well as developmental delays, believed to be caused by abnormalities in the brain. The term *spectrum* identifies that no one individual with autism will have exactly the same signs, symptoms, deficits, or behaviors.

The primary characteristics of a person with ASD include the following:

- introspection and isolation (thoughts are involved inward, with limited awareness of or interaction with the world around the individual)
- inability to socialize, to connect with others in meaningful or functional ways
- lack of empathy (inability to understand and/or feel for others)
- avoidance of or reluctance to experience physical contact
- repetitive and routine behaviors that seem to comfort
- hypersensitivity to, and sometimes fear or aversion of, loud sounds, lights, smells
- varying degrees of language competency or incompetency

Infancy

The period of **infancy** extends from birth to the end of the child's first year of life. The term derives from the early Latin word *infantum*, meaning "a young child or babe in arms." The modern version of the word still carries that meaning—that the child is not yet fully ambulant and must often be carried in someone's arms. Some key terms that contain the root word *infant* include the following:

infancy: the period of life prior to walking and feeding self

infantile: pertaining to infancy, infant behaviors, or infant-like behavior(s)

infantilism: a condition of developmental delay in which both the mind and body are slow to attain adult characteristics (i.e., cognitive and psychomotor delays; growth retardation)

post-term infant: a baby born after 42 weeks' gestation

pre-term infant or *premature infant:* a baby born before 37 weeks' gestation (Recall that Glory Loeppky's baby, Emily Grace, was premature, born at 32 weeks' gestation.)

Common illnesses of infancy

There are six very common illnesses that occur in infants and for which many new parents seek medical advice at clinics, pharmacies, and emergency departments at hospitals. These include constipation, diarrhea, ear infections, vomiting, diaper rash, and coughs and colds. These are all quite treatable, especially when attended to early in their onset.

Infection and immunity in infancy

During pregnancy, antibodies pass through the maternal blood into the fetal bloodstream. These antibodies provide a degree of naturally acquired active immunity for the fetus.

To prepare for lactation, the female body produces a liquid substance called **colostrum**. This is the first fluid secreted by the mammary glands after childbirth. The substance contains a large number of antibodies that are able to enter the infant's bloodstream and, by doing so, provide another level of naturally acquired immunity. Colostrum is particularly helpful to ward off the development of asthma and other allergies. It is not produced after the first few days postpartum.

Vaccinations are important for infants. They provide a protective barrier against disease and build immunity (see Chapter16). Some of these vaccines are described below, and others have appeared in previous chapters. Examples of recommended vaccines and their schedule for inoculation are also described in Table 17-18.

Pertussis, or whooping cough, is a highly contagious respiratory disease that is particularly harmful for infants.

Diptheria is a highly contagious disease that causes a thickening and blackening of the back of the throat and can cause breathing problems and heart failure.

Polio has almost been eradicated from the United States, but it is alive and proliferating in other parts of the world. To that end, vaccination of children continues in the United States to prevent the disease. Polio causes disability: muscle weakening, pain, fatigue, and possibly paralysis and death.

Rotavirus is a serious, severe viral infection of the digestive tract. It causes severe diarrhea, vomiting, and dehydration in infants and children and can be life-threatening.

Infant nutrition

Infants require a great deal of sleep and a great deal of nutrition. Infant nutrition in particular is a topic often dealt with in family practice medicine. Physicians, nurses, and dieticians are all knowledgeable resources for new mothers about the nutritional needs of their babies.

TABLE 17-18: Examples of Infant and Childhood Vaccinations

Disease and Vaccine	Frequency and Schedule of Childhood Vaccinations
Measles, mumps, rubella MMR	2 doses: • one dose at 12–15 months of age • second dose at 4–6 years of age
Diphtheria, tetanus, and pertussis DTaP	5 doses: • one dose each at ages 2, 4, and 6 months • fourth dose at 15–18 months • fifth dose at 4–6 years of age
Polio Salk vaccine	4 doses: • one dose each at 2 months and 4 months • third dose at 6–18 months • fourth dose at 4–6 years of age
Rotavirus RotaTeq/RV1 or Rotarix/RV5	3 doses (oral) if using RotaTeq/RVI vaccine at 6–15 weeks of age (but not later) and one dose at 18 months 2 doses (oral) if using Rotarix/RV5 vaccine at 2–4 months of age and one dose at 8 months of age
Varicella (chicken pox) VZV	2 doses: • one at 12–18 months • second dose at 4–6 years of age

Breastfeeding: As you know, breastfeeding is the natural way to nourish a newborn. Not only does breast milk provide antibodies to help the infant build an immune system, but it also provides the insulin, thyroxine, and cortisol necessary for digestion, metabolism, and growth and development. The action of the baby sucking at the breast (suckling) stimulates the production of more prolactin, which in turn stimulates lactation. This is often referred to as the "let down response" (see Figure 17-17).

When it is not possible to breastfeed the infant in person, lactating mothers can use a device called a breast pump to *express* and collect their milk, and then store it for bottle feeding.

When possible, breastfeeding is recommended for the first 6 months of the infant's life. It does not generally continue long after the first year, as the baby gradually moves on to alternative fluids and solids.

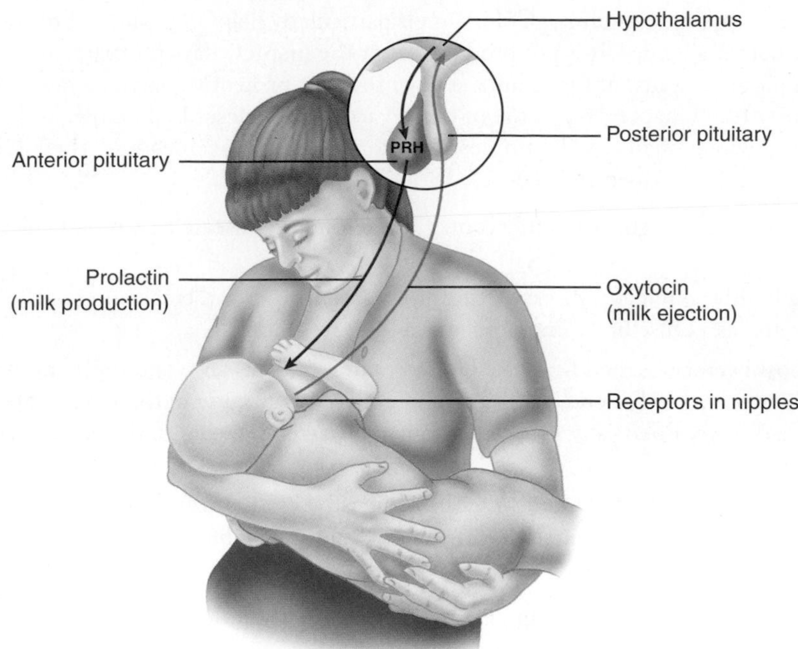

Figure 17.17: The Process of Lactation

Formula and Bottle Feeding: It is not possible in every case to breastfeed an infant. In this situation, the baby will be started on a highly nutritious *formula* that simulates breast milk. The formula will be delivered to the child through a baby bottle (a bottle with a nipple attached to stimulate the sucking reflex in the infant). Formulas come in the following formats:

- powdered form, which needs to be measured and mixed with sterile water
- concentrated liquid form, which needs to be measured and mixed with sterile water
- ready-to-use

Nutritious formulas include the following ingredients that promote the health, growth, and development of the infant:

- oil, which provides a source of fat
- lactose, which provides a source of carbohydrate
- iron, provided through fortified cow's milk
- protein, provided by whey (a by-product of cheese) and casein (a protein in milk)
- vitamins and minerals

Childhood

Children fall into a number of subcategories, or stages, in health and mental health care. These stages help professionals identify developmental tasks and milestones appropriate to certain ages. Identifying such stages of development allows health professionals to assess and intervene, promoting optimal growth and development. The stages of childhood are: toddlers, preschoolers, school-age children, and preadolescents.

toddlers: children ages 1 to 3. The root word *toddle* means "to run or walk with uneasy steps." The term **toddler** is indicative of the developmental task of learning to walk. This child is able to be away for his or her parent or caregiver for longer and longer periods. The toddler is very curious and experiences life by touching, tasting, and asking why.

preschool children: children ages 4 to 6. These children are developing the fine motor skills needed for drawing, coloring, writing, tying shoelaces, and other important skills. By now, the child can skip and ride a bicycle. This child is interested in having and playing with friends, as well as learning.

school-age children: ages 7 to 10. Group play, friendship, and learning are the focus of development. The child can progressively understand arithmetic and mathematics, learn music, problem solve, and think in abstract concepts.

pre-adolescents: ages 11 to 13. Focus increases on comparing self to others, trying on a variety of roles. The child develops opinions about likes and dislikes and offers his or her own opinions about the world.

Adolescence

As you know, *adolescence* is the psychosocial period of growth and development that follows childhood. It coincides with puberty, the biological period of growth in which reproductive maturity ensues.

Developmental tasks in the period of adolescence include developing a self-identity, forming deep and intimate relationships with peers, developing and defending strong opinions and beliefs (which at this point in time may be different from those of the parental figures in his/her life), coming to terms with a new sexuality and sexual desires, and learning socially acceptable behaviors in preparation for young adulthood.

Adolescents are often seen by health care providers for concerns related to reproductive system changes, sexuality (sexual identity and activity), and the challenges that the growth spurt at this time places on young people. These challenges might include disrupted sleep patterns, disrupted appetite (often a large increase), and risk-taking behaviors that can lead to accidents and injuries.

Critical Thinking

Think carefully and critically about what you have learned about the developmental stages of human life.

1. Why should a student of medical terminology be interested in learning about the ages and stages of infancy, childhood, and adolescence?

   ____

   ____

2. Although it is quite common and acceptable to say Glory and Gil Loeppky have a new child, medically and technically speaking they actually have a new

   ____.

3. Accidents and injuries in childhood are not generally the result of risk-taking behavior. On the basis of what you have learned about growth and development, what might be their cause?

   ____

Reflective Questions

Answer these questions on the basis of what you have learned about growth and development.

1. Because adolescence is a time of personal ______________ development, these youth may seek the services of school or community counselors.
2. How can newborn infants acquire some degree of immunization to protect them from the world? ______________
3. Risk-taking behavior in ______________ can lead to accidents and injuries that require medical attention.
4. How is immunity passed to the fetus, and then to the newborn, by the birth mother?

   ____
5. What action stimulates the ongoing production of breast milk, and who performs this action? ______________
6. Identify the stages of childhood. ______________

Mix and Match

Match the vaccination with the description of the illness it prevents.

1. DTaP	pox (blisters; sores on the skin)
2. Rotarix/RV5	respiratory, neuromuscular
3. Salk Vaccine	muscle fatigue and wasting; possible paralysis
4. VZV	severe dehydration and diarrhea

Let's Practice

Provide the full term that each abbreviation stands for.

1. WPPSI-III ____________________
2. DIAL3 ____________________
3. HELP ____________________
4. MMR ____________________
5. DTaP ____________________
6. ESI-R ____________________
7. PDD ____________________
8. DDST-II ____________________
9. PPVT-4 ____________________
10. PHN ____________________

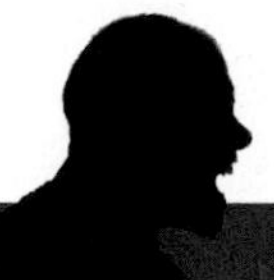

PRONUNCIATION PRACTICE

Say these words aloud to a friend or classmate. You are given the phonetic pronunciation. Your instructor can help you with pronunciation,

or visit **http://www.MedicalLanguageLab.com.** 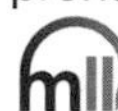

autism	**aw´**tĭzm
colostrum	kō-**lŏs´**trŭm
diphtheria	dĭf-**thē´**rē-ă
intrauterine	ĭn″tră-**ū´**tĕr-ĭn
pertussis	pĕr-**tŭs´**ĭs
rotavirus	**rō´**tă-vī″rŭs
spermicide	**spĕr´**mĭ-sīd

Caring for a Premature Infant

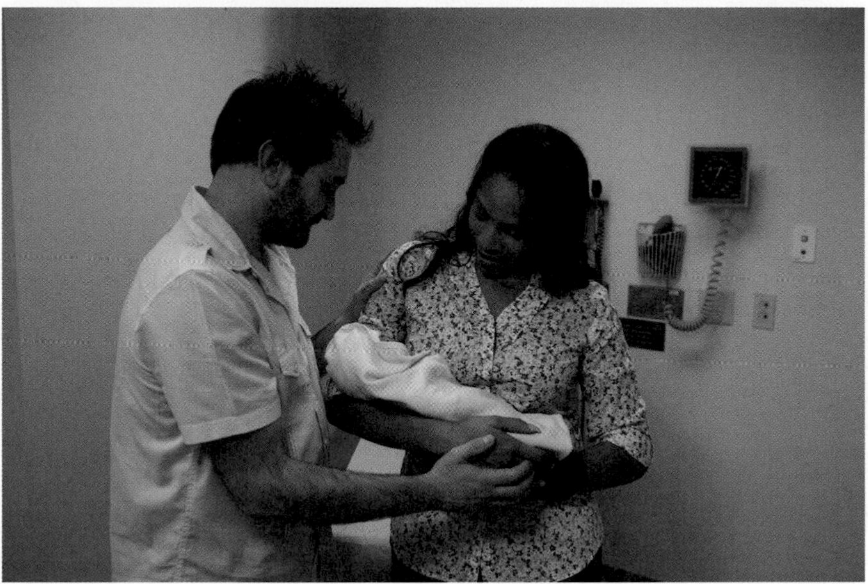

Patient Update

It has been a few days since Glory was at Dr. Antoine's office. She continues to attend to her baby, Emily Grace, in the neonatal nursery daily, sometimes for very long periods each day. She does this to promote bonding and development, and because she is so truly in love with her little girl. She also worries about Emily Grace because the infant was premature. Glory wants to be as close and comforting to the baby as possible under these circumstances.

Gil attends physical therapy as an outpatient at Fayette General Hospital three mornings per week. On those days, he and Glory drive there together. When Gil has completed his treatment, he also goes to be with his daughter. And now that Emily Grace is no longer on a respirator and is doing well, both her mother and father can hold her.

The Loeppkys have been advised that their baby will likely be discharged home to their care in 2 to 3 weeks. They are very excited about this. This morning, Gil will join his wife in the neonatal nursery to meet with the nurse clinician there. They will be discussing Emily Grace's progress, and the parents will be guided in how to care for their premature infant at home.

"Good morning, Glory and Gil," said Roberta, the neonatal nurse clinician. "How are you both doing today?" She took a seat on a chair near them. When the greetings were finished, she began. "Well, as you know, your little girl is doing so well, under the circumstances of her premature birth, that the doctor says it's time to really plan for taking her home." She smiled warmly and looked directly at each parent. They were beaming from ear to ear.

"I've invited you here today to do some pre-discharge planning with you and to answer any questions you may have about caring for Emily Grace." She paused to let them think about this before going on. "As you know, your baby was preterm at 31 weeks gestation, and this is very early for a baby." They nodded that they understood. "She's now 36 weeks old. She has done very well and has gained a good deal of weight."

She looked directly at Glory then and said, "A good deal of the credit goes to you for that, Glory. Your dedication and ability to be here for her has gone a very long way to nurture her physically and emotionally. Babies receive a great deal of comfort from being close to another person, and you have spent long hours holding her, talking to her, and generally caring for her. In addition to that, you have been breastfeeding from the moment this became possible, and I cannot stress enough how important that has been for her physical nutrition and immunity, as well as for helping both of you bond." Glory smiled and nodded her head.

Roberta then turned to her husband. "And you, Gil, have also been terrific. Despite your own injuries and challenges in recovery, you have been here as often as you could. I've seen you holding Emily Grace, rocking her and talking softly to her as well." He smiled in response to her validation of his efforts. "All of that loving, that caring touch, and those soft, gentle words that you share with your baby are extremely important to your little girl's physical and emotional development, Gil. I can just imagine how attached she is becoming to you, too." She offered an affirming smile to him she spoke.

"I love to do it," said Gil. "She is my world—she and Glory—they mean everything to me." He reached out and took his wife's hand lovingly. Roberta nodded her acknowledgement of the bonds this family shared.

"We need to talk a bit about Emily Grace's respiratory system," she continued. Suddenly, the parents looked worried. "No, no ... there is nothing untoward happening in that regard," the nurse clinician reassured them. "I just want to go over some aspects of respiratory health with you. As you know, this is an area of concern with premature babies, and I just want to be sure you understand what that means." She paused to let them think a moment. "As you know, Emily's lung function has improved, and that was why we were able to remove her from the respirator a couple of weeks ago. That's one of the core reasons we were able to move her to the neonatal nursery from NICU. However, because she was so premature, she will be very susceptible to infections for a good while yet, particularly respiratory ones." The parents said they were aware of this, and that it worried them. "I'd like to suggest that you both pop in to your local public health clinic and speak to the nurses there about your situation. Public Health offers a number of services and supports for parents of preemies." She went on to explain these and provided a number of pamphlets about them. They discussed these, and Roberta provided more information and contact details for them.

"You'll also want to ensure that your infant has enough stimulation to encourage the development of neuropathways in the brain and to stimulate her sensory organs. This is important for all newborns, but especially premature ones, who need just a little extra care and attention in that regard." She took a breath before continuing. "By the way," she said, "did either of you know that babies come to know a parent or care provider by that person's scent, rhythm of speech, and tone of voice?" She nodded. "They can even recognize who is touching them! " Both Glory and Gil had felt this was true, but were not sure if their feeling was actually based on fact. Roberta confirmed the accuracy of their feeling and reinforced once again how important skin-to-skin, person-to-person contact with a baby can be.

"What kind of stimulation are we talking about, Roberta?" asked Glory. The nurse clinician offered some suggestions of gently changing the amount of light in the room, exposing the child carefully to different temperatures, allowing her to touch materials of different textures, playing music or a radio softly in the background from time to time, providing interesting visual stimulation such as a mobile above the bed, and so on. Emily Grace's parents loved this. They told Roberta how they had already planned for much of this in the baby's new room.

"I have just one more thing I'd like to talk to you both about, but more specifically, it's something I'd like to go over with you, Gil." He looked up at her inquiringly. "As you know and have now seen, premature infants do very well with bodily contact from a loving, supportive person. They can sense this. It nurtures their mind and body." The parents agreed. "Gil, I'd like to talk to you particularly about kangaroo care." He raised his eyebrows in curiosity, indicating that this concept was new to him. "You may have seen your wife doing this, but I think it's time you thought about it, too. I know your daughter will really benefit from it, and so will you." She smiled warmly and began a mini-teaching session with him. She taught Gil how to wrap his baby (naked or with a diaper on) against his bare chest, covering the infant with a warm blanket. She used a small doll and a blanket in her office to demonstrate. "The practice of kangaroo care has been found to be very soothing, very bonding, and emotional for everyone who does it, and research has shown that it is hugely beneficial to premature infants," she said.

"How often would I do this?" Gil asked with a tone of enthusiasm.

"Just as often as you like, and for long as you like. There are no rules about it, but again the research is showing that the more nurturing contact you provide to an infant like this, the better the outcomes." He smiled happily. Roberta smiled too, watching the new parents. "Between you and Glory both, I think little Emily Grace will be able to spend a good deal of time *snuggled up* to her mom and dad!"

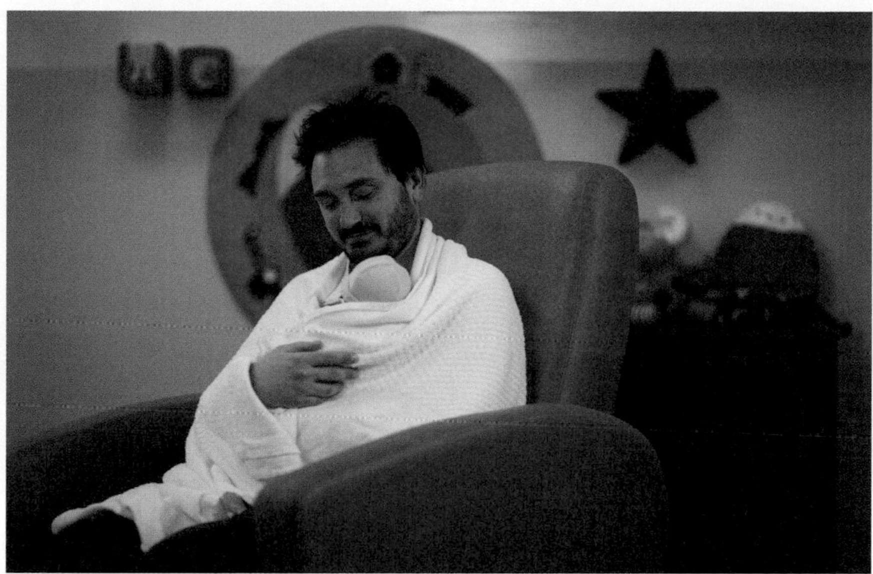

Figure 17.18: Kangaroo Care

Critical Thinking

Consider kangaroo care as you answer this question.

Using the domains of health, what are the biological, psychological, and social benefits of kangaroo care to a newborn?

____

____

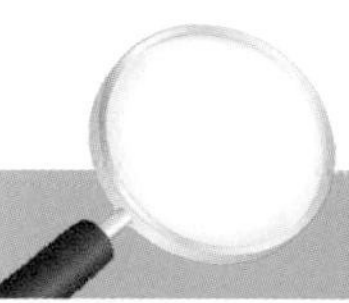

FOCUS POINT: Bonding and Attachment

Research has shown that bonding and attachment are both significant in the growth and development of children physiologically and psychologically. While *bonding* and *attachment* are often used interchangeably, there is a slight difference between the two terms.

In the context of infants and children, *bonding* refers to the feelings that parents or parent figures have for their children. It encompasses the feelings of love, commitment, and an overwhelming desire to cherish and care for the young. The process of bonding begins in infancy, at birth or at the time of adoption. Bonding requires physical contact and presence, nearness and access to the infant or child. It provides the first positive experiences for a child with direct, person-to-person human contact.

Attachment refers to an infant or child's response to the parent or parent figure, the child's developing sense that this person will love and protect him or her. Physical contact with the parent figure provides the child with a deep sense of belonging (attachment) and safety. Attachment is enhanced through physical touch and smell. Even the smallest infants soon learn to recognize their care providers in this way and are able to differentiate them from strangers. Infants are also perceptive to mood, and they will react when the mood of a care provider shifts in such a way that the infant doesn't feel secure.

CHAPTER SUMMARY

In Chapter 17, you have enhanced your vocabulary and knowledge of medical, anatomical, physiological, and psychosocial terminology for family practice medicine. Opportunities were provided for working with new terms and concepts in the context of the care of Glory and Gil Loeppky, new parents to Emily Grace Loeppky. Family practice medicine; family physicians; reproductive clinicians, biologists, and technicians; and public health nurses were introduced. Immunization for infants and children was explored, providing terminology and information, as well as including abbreviations and acronyms. Family lifecycles and human growth and development were presented, including an introduction to stage theory. Exercises provided occasions for practicing with newly acquired terminology and building upon new and previous knowledge and language skills.

TABLE 17-19: Abbreviations in Chapter 17

Abbreviation or Acronym	Meaning
ASD	autism spectrum disorder
DDST-II	Denver Developmental Screening Test II
DIAL3	Developmental Indicators for the Assessment of Learning
ESI-R	Early Screening Inventory-Revised
ED	erectile dysfunction
FASIAR	Follicle Aspiration, Sperm Injection, and Assisted Follicular Rupture
FNAC	fine-needle aspiration cytology
FSH	follicle-stimulating hormone
GIFT	Gamete Intrafallopian Tube Transfer
GHRF	growth hormone-releasing factor
GRGH	growth-releasing growth hormones
GRH	gonadotropin-releasing hormone
HELP	Hawaii Early Learning Profile
ICSI	Intracytoplasmic Sperm Insertion
IUI	intrauterine insemination
IUD	intrauterine device
K-ABC	Kaufman Assessment Battery
IVF	In-vitro fertilization
LH	luteinizing hormone
PID	pelvic inflammatory disease
PCOS	polycystic ovarian syndrome
PPVT-4	Peabody Picture Vocabulary Test (4)
SA	semen analysis
STI	sexually transmitted infection
STD	sexually transmitted disease
TRUS	transrectal ultrasound
VD	venereal disease
WPPSI-III	Wechsler Preschool and Primary Scale of Intelligence III
ZIFT	Zygote Intrafallopian Transfer

KEY TERMS

ambivalent
approximated
assisted reproduction
bonding
chlamydia
coitus
colostrum
contraception
copulation
cyst
degenerative
despondency
diploid
dyspareunia
family practice medicine
fecundity
fertility
gamete(s)
genital herpes
gonorrhea
haploid
hirsutism
histopathology
human papillomavirus (HPV)
incision line
infancy
intercourse
lactiferous ducts
lactivorous
libido
lifecycles
mammograms
mammology
mastology
menopause
menses
motility
oocyte
oogenesis
ova
ovulation
ovum
pareunia
pervasive
pervasive development disorders (PDD)
Polycystic ovarian syndrome (PCOS)
postpartum depression
postpartum psychosis
puberty
puerperal
semen
sexual function
sexually transmitted
sexually transmitted disease (STD)
sexually transmitted infections (STI)
speculum
sperm
spermatogenesis
stage theory
stirrups
subcuticular sutures
syphilis
testes
testosterone
toddler
trichomoniasis (trich)
Vitamin E cream
zygote

CHAPTER REVIEW

Critical Thinking

Consider all that you have learned in this chapter to answer these questions.

1. What is the difference between GRGH and GRH? ____________________

2. What stage of the family lifecycle are Gil and Glory Loeppky in? ____________________

3. What is the difference between a neonatal intensive care unit and a neonatal nursery?
____

4. It is very likely that Gil and Glory Loeppky will visit a public health clinic once their baby is home with them. Why is that? ____________________

Right Word or Wrong Word: ***Oophorectomy or Oophorocystectomy?***

Are these two terms the same? Perhaps one is simply spelled differently. Do you know? Explain your answer.

Reflective Questions

Use your new knowledge of medical terms and medical language to answer these questions.

1. What is the root word of *fecundity,* and what does it mean? ________________
2. What is a zygote? ________________
3. What is the term for a pouchlike or saclike structure that might be filled with air, infected fluids, or substances or even blood? ________________
4. What is colostrum? ________________
5. In vitro fertilization refers to a procedure to ________________ a woman by introducing a fertilized ovum into the uterus.
6. A miscarriage is a form of spontaneous ________________.
7. Which sexually transmitted disease is linked to cervical and mouth cancer? ________________

Mix and Match

Connect the medical term with its synonym or definition. Draw a line between the two.

1. menstrual cycle	pouch
2. sloughing	ovarian cyclicity
3. follicle	ovary
4. ovarium	shedding
5. oosperm	zygote

True or False

Read the following statements and decided if they are true or false. Circle your choice.

1. Impotence is the same as infertility.	T	F
2. The condition of a retractable testicle is called cryptorchidism.	T	F
3. *Contraception* prevents *conception*.	T	F
4. The terms *postpartum* and *postnatal health* both pertain to women.	T	F
5. Aging affects male fertility adversely.	T	F
6. An *STD* and an *STI* are both contagious.	T	F
7. A gamete is a reproductive cell.	T	F
8. All ovarian cysts are cancerous.	T	F
9. Female breasts contain mammary glands.	T	F
10. Female fertility does not continue across the lifespan.	T	F

Translate the Terminology

Here is an opportunity to apply your knowledge of medical terminology to a more complex passage. Translate the following information about possible links between sexually transmitted diseases (STDs) and HIV into your own words.

A possible interrelationship between sexual transmission of HIV infection by those who have or have had a sexually transmitted disease requires investigation. Implications of the resultant scientific data can be significant to prevention, interventions, and treatments. To date, some evidence exists indicating ulcerative and nonulcerative symptoms of STDs may be the determiners of, have a potentiating effect for, or increase susceptibility to HIV infection. Further research is indicated, differentiating the two populations. The question should also be posed regarding bidirectionality of the two key factors to determine sequence: if STDs increase the potential for acquisition of HIV infection or if HIV infection increases the potential for acquisition of STDs.

____

____

____

____

____

Fill in the Blanks

Answer the following questions by filling in the blanks.

1. ________________ is the stage in the lifecycle when the decision to have children is made.
2. The best medical term for *sexual intercourse* is ________________.
3. In the stage of growth and development for ________________, one of the tasks they master is fine motor movements such as holding a pen or pencil to print.
4. ________________ stimulation includes changing the environment in subtle ways to promote neurological growth.
5. ________________ planning is sometimes a collaborative venture between parents and health or allied health professionals.
6. If diseases can be transmitted by sexual contact, then they are ________________.

Label the Diagram

Label the diagram of the male reproductive system.

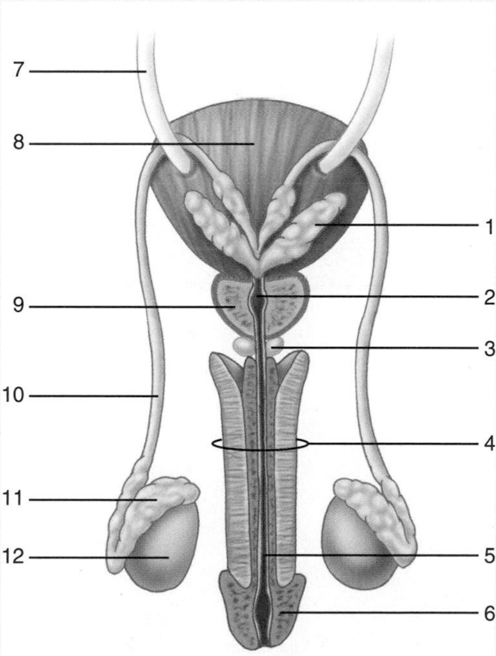

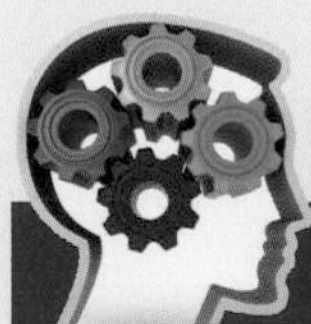

MEMORY MAGIC

The following mnemonics can help you remember important information in this chapter:

1) **Postpartum Assessment = BUBBLE**
   - **B-**reasts
   - **U-**terus
   - **B-**owels
   - **B-**ladder
   - **L-**ochia (discharge from the uterus)
   - **E-**pisiotomy/laceration/C-section incision

2) **Breast Feeding Advantages = PACES**
   - **P** = psychological satisfaction
   - **A** = anti-infective properties/atopic disorders risk
   - **C** = convenient
   - **E** = expenseless (free)
   - **S** = stimulates growth and development

3) **Breast feeding disadvantages = KIDS**
   - **K** = vitamin K deficiency
   - **I** = infection transmission risk (i.e., HIV)
   - **D** = drugs excreted in milk
   - **S** = stressful and tiring for mother

4) **Sperm pathway through male reproductive tract = SEVEN UP:**
   - **S**eminiferous tubules
   - **E**pididymis
   - **V**as deferens
   - **E**jaculatory duct
   - **N**othing left but . . .
   - **U**rethra
   - **P**enis

CHAPTER EIGHTEEN

Putting It All Together

Focus: Forensic Sciences and Documentation

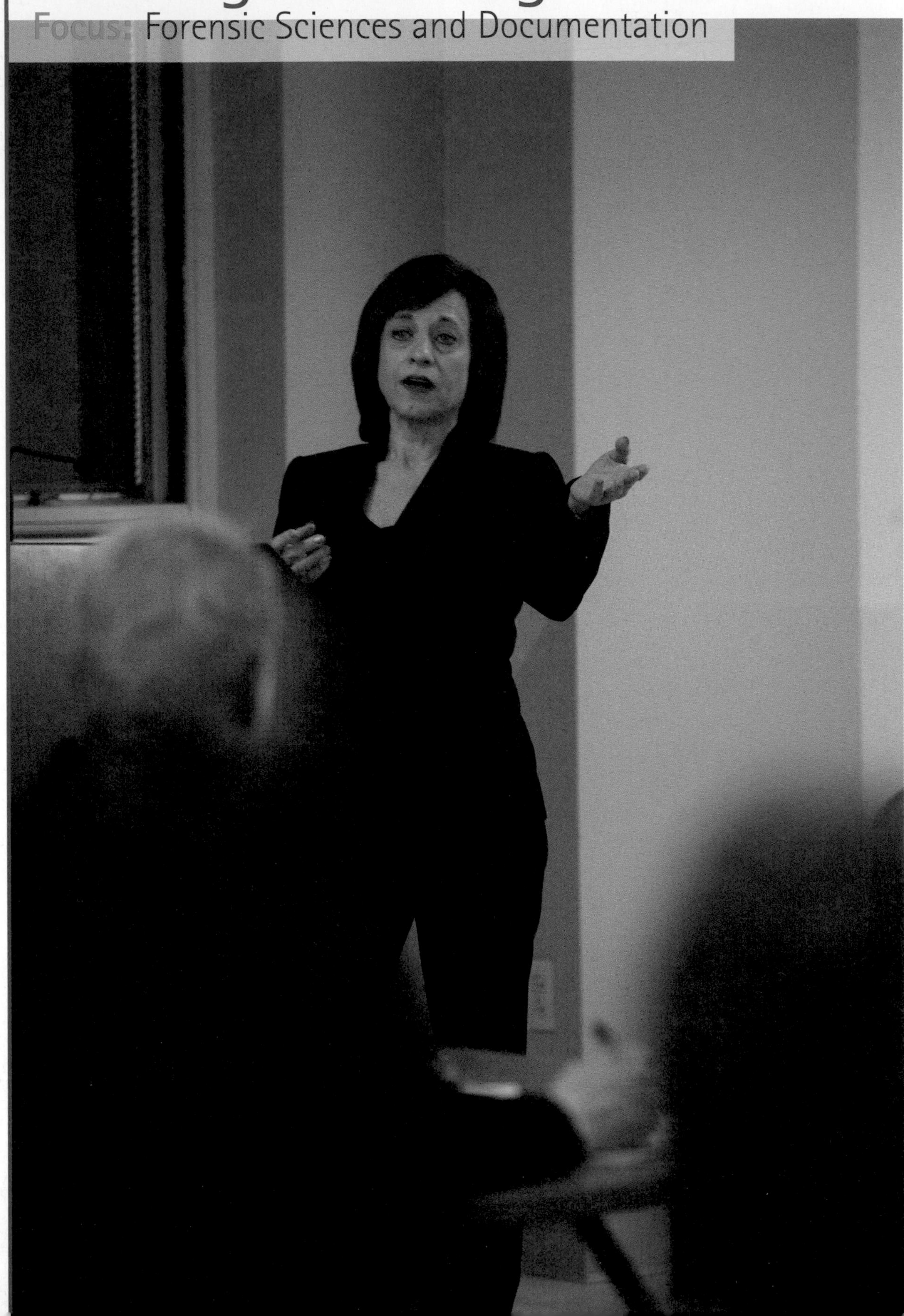

Dr. Robin Haydel, an expert in forensic medicine, has arrived as a guest lecturer at Wyatt College. The health sciences department has invited her to do a presentation on forensic sciences and forensic medicine. When word of her presentation spread around campus, it generated a great deal of interest across multiple disciplines. As a result, the college administration opened up the lecture to everyone. Today Dr. Haydel will be speaking to a group of students majoring in health sciences, criminology, psychology, anthropology, and biological sciences, as well as their faculty.

"Welcome everyone," Dr. Haydel began. "Please take a seat so that we can get started." She waited as the last of the students straggled in to the room, noting a full lecture hall of at least 120 students, all interested in the world of forensics. "I wonder," she thought to herself, "if these students realize that there are many fields of forensics and not just the one they see on TV." She waited another minute, checking her PowerPoint presentation and testing her remote microphone. The room settled and she began by introducing herself, thanking the department of health sciences for the invitation.

"I am aware," she added, "that some of the health sciences courses here at Wyatt College are following a particular case study, that of a motor vehicle accident involving two vehicles and two families. Is that correct?" Voices in the audience confirmed it. "And you are, let me see ..." She checked her notes. "We have medical terminology students, laboratory and radiology students, medical office assistants and medical records students, and first-year nursing students, right?" She looked up from her paper each time she spoke, noting the various cohort groups that had applauded and confirmed her list. She smiled. "Excellent," she said. "I will be tying a good portion of my presentation today to that contextual case study to demonstrate how forensic science and forensic medicine apply to you." She paused before going on. "I want to also thank everyone else for attending, and I hope that this presentation will be inclusive of you and helpful to your own interests and studies here at Wyatt."

Critical Thinking

Why would a health sciences department at a college invite a forensic medical expert to speak to their students?

____

Learning Objectives

After reading Chapter 18, you will be able to do the following:

- Understand the concept of medical terminology as a standard of professional practice.
- Recognize the importance and legal ramifications of accuracy, specificity, and detail in patient/client documentation.
- Internalize and exhibit professional documentation skills in the context of health care.
- Understand the fields of forensic sciences and forensic medicine at an introductory level.
- Appreciate the education, training, and work of forensic scientists and technicians.
- Appreciate the role that medical terminology plays across multiple disciplines.
- Appreciate the education, training, and work of medical transcriptionists.
- Appreciate the education, training, and work of medical coders and billers.
- Develop skills for searching, researching, and locating pertinent information.
- Search for, collect, and use data obtained from various sections and forms in a medical record.
- Understand the elements of a medical record/patient chart.

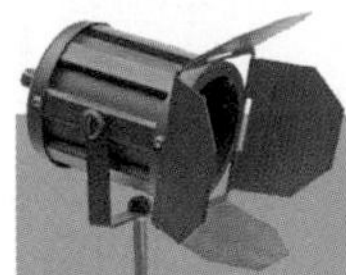

CAREER SPOTLIGHT: Forensic Scientists and Technicians

The field of forensic sciences is vast. Within it, scientific principles and methods are used to determine what has happened and what will happen for civil and/or criminal cases in law. Work in this field requires a strong foundation in biological and life sciences (social sciences, psychology, etc.), as well as criminal justice. Depending on the practitioner's subspecialty, further education and training in fields such as anthropology, criminology or criminalistics, chemistry and toxicology, agriculture, or medicine may be required. For the majority of forensic science professionals, medical terminology is a requisite course.

A *forensic science technician* attains a certificate or diploma in forensic and laboratory sciences, as well as criminal justice. These credentials allow the technician to collect, identify, classify, and analyze physical evidence. Specimens can include tissues, bone fragments, fibers, hair, and so on. They might also include (with special training) weapons and ballistics, information technology, and accounting. The forensic science technician may be called to testify in court.

Forensic scientists are experts with undergraduate, graduate, and doctoral degrees in criminology/criminalistics and/or forensic medicine. Even within these fields, they may specialize as *coroners* (medical examiners) or *criminal profilers*. These experts are often called to testify at cause-of-death inquests and accident inquiries, as well as civil and criminal court cases.

Accuracy, Specificity, and Detail: Key Components of Medical Documentation

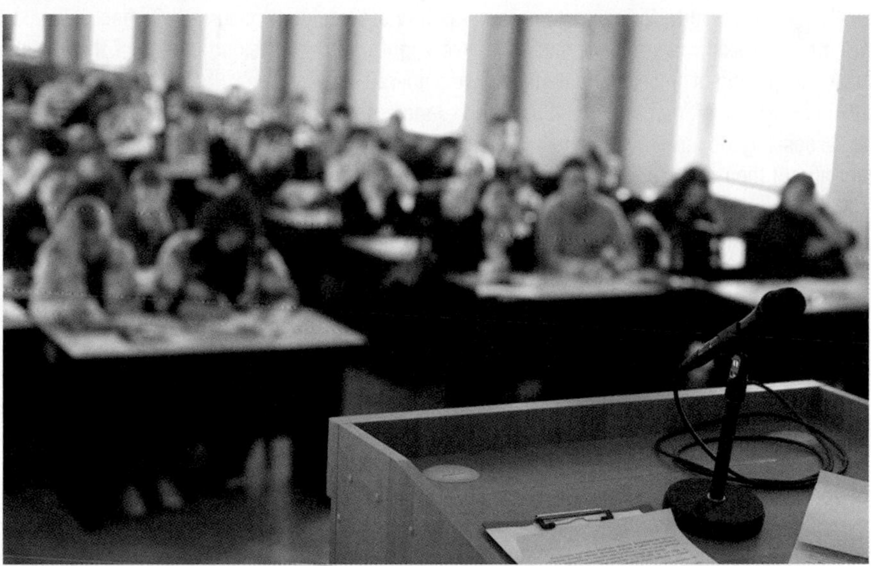

Patient Update

Dr. Robin Haydel continued her lecture by defining the terms *forensic*, *forensic science*, and *forensic medicine*. "The term forensic refers to the application of scientific knowledge, gained through investigation and assessment, to a legal issue or legal proceedings. There are many different specialties in forensic medicine. These include forensic pathology, forensic toxicology, forensic histology, and so on." She paused for a moment to let the audience think about this. "If you look at the handouts I've given you, you will see an expanded list of just some of the careers available in forensic sciences." She waited for them to find the pages and then continued (see Table 18-1).

TABLE 18-1: Careers in Forensic Sciences
forensic pathologist: investigates and determines cause of death
forensic entomologist: studies insects, especially those involved in the decomposition of corpses
forensic special chemist or special drug chemist: performs tests in clinical toxicology, drug analysis, and analyzes specimens to detect evidence of drug use
ballistics expert: analyzes and identifies projectiles such as bullets

"Forensic science deals with skilled observations of situations and circumstances, as well as the collection of evidence. In a criminal case, this can include evidence from both the alleged perpetrator of a crime and the victim. And what might that evidence be?" She stopped and smiled at the roomful of students in front of her. "Well, I'm sure you have a lot of ideas about that," she said warmly. "Anyone who watches crime shows on television will have some idea that evidence can include—but is not limited to—hair and body fluids, tissue samples, various fibers, shards of glass, bullets, and on and on." She showed these and a few other examples on the PowerPoint slides she had prepared. "But evidence is also found in *documentation*: charts, medical records, financial documents, police reports, and a multitude of other paper trails and e-documents." Again she paused to let her words have impact.

"Furthermore," Dr. Haydel continued, "let's not forget that not everything that happens in forensic science happens in the lab. It can happen in the field. A good example of that is your own case study of the motor vehicle accident. Many professionals at the accident scene would have been applying scientific knowledge and techniques specific to forensics to determine how the accident occurred. Someone would be taking measurements of skid marks, while someone else might have been taking photos of the vehicles and the victims and the crowd of onlookers that might have gathered at the scene." She paused to show photographic examples on the PowerPoint screen. "Still others—the emergency medical people—would have been observing, assessing, documenting, and even interviewing the accident victims for the possible causes of the accident and of their injuries. Then, once the accident victims arrived in the emergency room and became patients, the hospital itself became a field of investigation, albeit in a medical, rather than a legal context.

Dr. Haydel explained that every member of the treatment team who observes, assesses, and intervenes with patients is collecting and recording data that in turn will contribute to the team's growing body of evidence. "And this evidence will help inform treatment and other clinical decisions," she said. "For example, the treatment team will determine how an injury was sustained, and if it was recent or not. The physician or nurse, for example, will note the exact trauma site on a body, as well as the angle and depth of a wound. They'll record whether or not wounds were penetrating and how deep they were. And they will take note of the direction or mechanism of injury, such as identifying blunt force trauma to a particular aspect of the skull." She paused and looked around her audience for effect.

"In your own case studies here at Wyatt College, every health and allied health professional involved with the accident victims contributed to the evidence in the case. *And any one of them could have been you.*" For emphasis, she pointed at the audience, sweeping her pointer finger from left to right across the room. She saw understanding dawn across the faces of the audience. She knew she had made her point. Dr. Haydel had begun to bring home the relevance of their studies for them.

"I think we should stop here for a moment to make sure we are clear about some definitions I've been using. I'm sure you can relate to this: the need to know the definition of the key terms for the subject." She laughed lightheartedly. "Let's begin with *evidence*. Please turn your attention to this slide." She turned away from them to look up at the screen. I have a series of about four slides here that help define *evidence* and key terminology related to evidence." She showed them each of the slides, augmenting the information on the slides with her own expertise in the subject (see Figures 18-1 through 18-6).

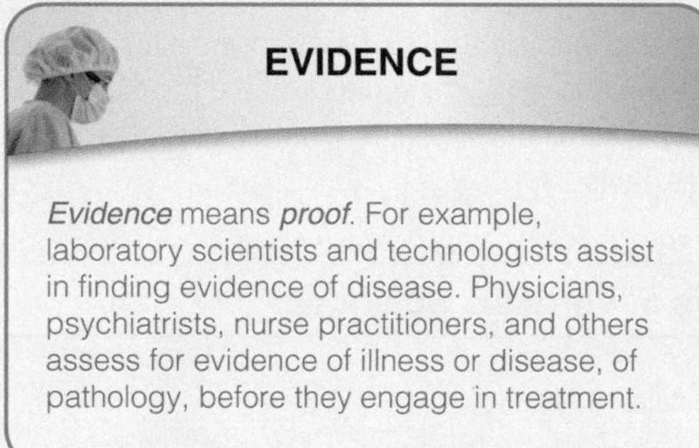

Figure 18.1: *Evidence* PowerPoint slide

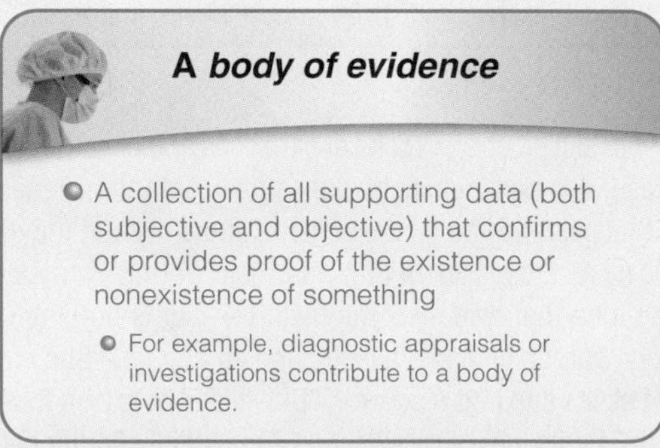

Figure 18.2: *Body of Evidence* PowerPoint slide

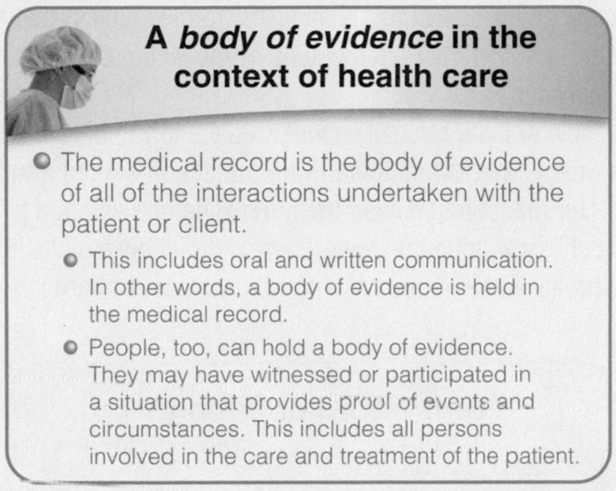

Figure 18.3: *Body of Evidence in the Context of Health Care* PowerPoint slide

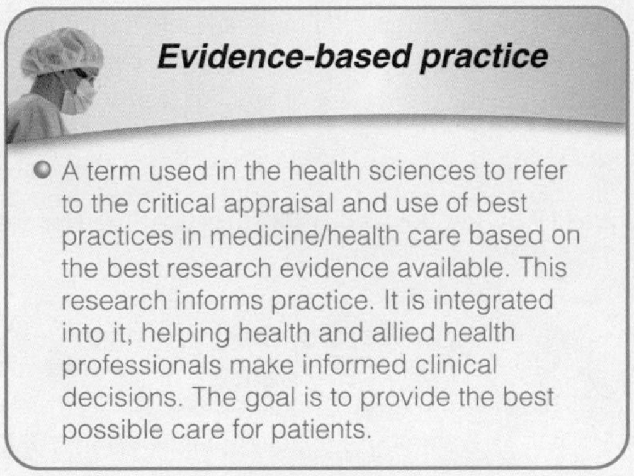

Figure 18.4: *Evidence-Based Practice* PowerPoint slide

"All right," continued Dr. Haydel, turning back to speak directly to her audience. "Let's move on to define forensic medicine. This is a rather broad term as well. I hope I can shed some light on that for you," she said. "Forensic medicine is a specialty in health sciences. Practitioners are medical-legal experts who seek to answer legal questions, based on medical knowledge and practice. The field includes doctors, nurses, coroners (who are actually doctors), and emergency medical personnel. More often than not, though, when we are talking about an expert in forensic medicine, we are almost always talking about a physician who has become an expert in medicine and the law." She turned their attention then to a second table in the handout she had given at the start of the lecture (see Table 18-2).

TABLE 18-2: Careers in Forensic Medicine
coroner/medical examiner
pediatric physical assault nurse, physician, or psychologist
sexual assault nurse (SANE)
emergency room physicians and nurses (with advanced training in forensic assessment and evidence collection) for victims and/or perpetrators of violence
forensic odontology/dentistry
forensic psychiatric nurses, psychiatrists, and psychologists -working with the criminally insane
forensic pharmacist

Subsequently, Dr. Haydel went on to provide an example of someone who practices forensic medicine—the sexual assault nurse examiner (SANE). "In the case of rape or sexual assault," she explained, "a nurse with advanced training in the collection of forensic evidence will attend to the victim in the emergency department.

The sexual assault nurse examiner will collect tissue samples from vaginal swabs and from under the victim's fingernails. She, not the police, will also take photographs of the victim's injuries. This forensic nurse can be called upon to testify in criminal court.

"I'd like to challenge you now to think critically about medical terminology and the titles of health professionals. Take a look at this slide." She turned toward the projection screen and then back to them. "See if you can answer the question for me." She showed them the slide and listened to a number of answers generated by the students. Then she advanced the PowerPoint to the answer slide, emphasizing the importance of paying attention to what appear to be subtle or minor differences, but are in reality quite important.

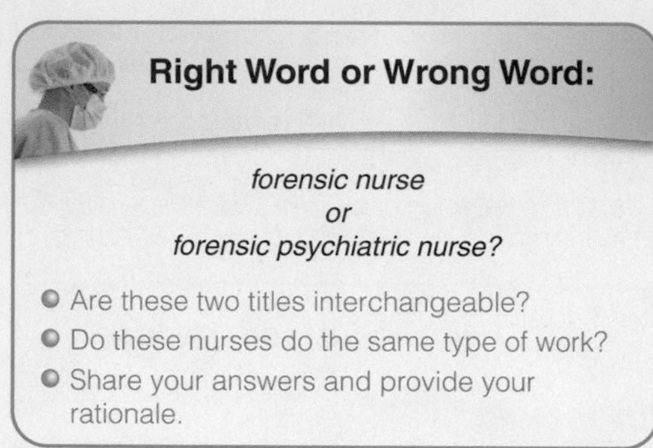

Figure 18.5: *Right Word or Wrong Word* question PowerPoint slide

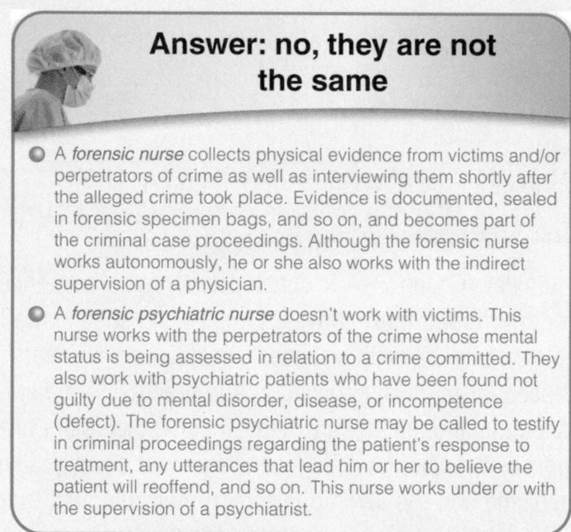

Figure 18.6: *Right Word or Wrong Word* answer PowerPoint slide

Following this, Dr. Hayden drew the audience's attention back to their handouts. She directed them to another table of careers in forensics. "Everyone found it? This table shows you some additional careers in forensics that you may not have ever considered" (see Table 18-3).

TABLE 18-3: Other Careers in Forensics
forensic anthropologist
voice analysts
fingerprint analysts
handwriting analysts
information technology analysts
forensic accountants
forensic photographers
forensic profilers -psychologists, psychiatrists, or criminologists/criminalists with advanced training
forensic social workers
forensic document auditors

Dr. Haydel continued her lecture, making a link that she hoped the student would appreciate. "Although forensic science and medicine are two highly specialized fields, the everyday work of individuals in health care can certainly include an element of forensics. For example, every time you observe and document patient data accurately and specifically, you are contributing to a forensic body of knowledge about that patient's status at any given time—like a snapshot in words. Your entries in a patient's medical record become permanent data in that person's file. Nothing in a medical record can be removed, crossed out, covered up, or deleted. It is permanent. Any action taken to change an entry requires adherence to extremely strict protocols for documentation. Breaches of those protocols can lead to discipline and inquiry actions by employers, regulators, and licensing bodies for your profession and for your workplace."

"I hope that you can see then," she added, "how very important your written communication can be. *A patient's medical record is a legal document.* And forensic medicine is about the law and medicine, combined. Although you may think your documentation might be seen and used only by other members of the patient's health care team, it is possible with or without the patient's consent, that these records will be viewed by others. These might include health insurers, lawyers, and the police." She watched them as she spoke. She saw the look of interest, of learning something new, that crossed the faces of so many in the audience.

"Now, since we want accuracy, specificity, and detail in written documentation, can you all see how absolutely essential it is to have a strong background, not only in biological sciences, but also in medical terminology?" She paused for a moment to let the audience consider this. She saw some people nodding in the affirmative. "I'd like to start with a quick review of word construction before we investigate and analyze your case studies, which will, of course, require you to recognize and use medical language— terminology in context."

"Okay, are you ready?" asked Dr. Haydel, looking up and scanning across the room for a response. "Good. Let's begin with some exercises in medical terminology. Please turn to your handouts. Complete the exercises, and then we'll come back together as a large group to go over the answers."

Medical Terminology: Composition and Decomposition

Throughout this textbook you have worked on word construction and deconstruction through numerous examples and exercises. As you have learned, understanding word composition can help you to make good word choices. It also helps you understand and respond to the words of others.

Composition means *arrangement* or *construction*. In medicine, it can refer to how cells, tissues, and organs are put together. In linguistics (language), *composition* refers to word formation: how words are formed from their pieces or parts.

The root word of *composition* is *compose*, meaning "to put together, arrange or write." The word derives from the French verb *composer*.

Decomposition means *breakdown*. It is the antonym of *composition*. In medicine, it can refer to the decay and putrefaction of living matter such as cells and tissues. In linguistics, the word refers to the deconstruction of words, phrases, paragraphs, and so on. For example, a medical term can be decomposed, or deconstructed, into its various parts: prefixes, roots, and suffixes.

Complete the following exercises to assess your skills of word composition and decomposition.

Critical Thinking

Think carefully about what you have learned about medical terminology and its construction to answer these questions.

1. What is the name of the word part that contains the core meaning of a term?
   ____
2. What is the name of the word part that comes at the beginning of some medical terms and may describe something as *high*, *low*, *big*, or *small*? ______________________________
3. What is the name of the word part that may come at the end of a term and determine whether the word is a noun, verb, adjective, or adverb? ______________________________

Let's Practice

Imagine you are reading a diagnostic report from a laboratory or a diagnostic imaging department. Deconstruct these terms into their parts: prefixes, roots, and suffixes. You do not have to define the term.

1. craniotomy ____________________
2. radiograph ____________________
3. leukocyte ____________________
4. microbiologist ____________________
5. glycemia ____________________
6. sarcoadenoma ____________________
7. ketonuria ____________________
8. sublingual ____________________
9. dentalgia ____________________
10. odontorrhagia ____________________

Free Writing

Many medical terms are composed of prefixes that make them antonyms of their root words. Rewrite the following sentences by changing the highlighted word, replacing it with its antonym, or opposite. Then decide which of the two sentences correctly describes one of the patients you have followed in this book.

Example:

a. When EMS arrived at the scene of the accident, Gilbert Loeppky was *conscious.*

Rewritten with an antonym:

b. When EMS arrived at the scene of the accident, Gilbert Loeppky was *unconscious.*

Which sentence is correct? *Answer:* b.

1. a. Mrs. Davis was increasingly *oriented* the evening after the accident.
   b. ____________________

Which sentence is correct? (Chapter 12) ____________________

2. a. A nurse at Oklahoma Trauma Center noticed that Mr. Davis had *eupnea* and mentioned it Dr. Filmore.
   b. ____________________

Which sentence is correct? (Chapter 9) ____________________

3. a. Despite the effects of Gil Loeppky's accident, he will soon be *ambulant.*
   b. ____________________

Which sentence is correct? (Chapter 15) ____________________

4. a. During the *antepartum* period, Glory Loeppky was able to pump her breast milk and store it for her baby.
   b. ____________________

Which sentence is correct? (Chapter 17) ____________________

5. a. When she was first admitted to the hospital, Stevie-Rose Davis was *hypoglycemic.*
   b. ____________________

Which sentence is correct? (Chapter 7) ____________________

6. a. As Dr. Lincoln prepared to do the *extra-oral* exam on Clay Davis, he noted that the mouth was bloody but the teeth were still in situ.
   b. ____________________

Which sentence is correct? (Chapter 6) ____________________

7. a. Zane Davis has *cancerous* lesions on his lungs.
   b. ____________________

Which sentence is correct? (Chapter 14) ____________________

8. a. Emily Grace Loeppky's respiratory system was *mature* at the time of her birth.
   b. ____________________

Which sentence is correct? (Chapter 8) ____________________

9. a. The paramedic of Ambulance NM421 determined that Glory Loeppky was *bradycardic.*
   b. ____________________

Which sentence is correct? (Chapter 3) ____________________

10. a. The doctors worried that Gil Loeppky might suffer some cognitive *function* when he woke up from his medically induced coma.
    b. ____________________

Which sentence is correct? (Chapter 10) ____________________

Mix and Match

Work with word composition. Match the word part on the left to one on the right to create a medical term.

1. epi-	dontal
2. chemo-	-plasia
3. a-	thermia
4. hyper-	oma
5. ortho-	arachnoid
6. intra-	dermis
7. sub-	therapy
8. blast-	venous

Decoding and Deciphering Terms: Anatomy and Pathology

Health care and forensic science careers both require a comprehensive knowledge of the human body and its pathologies. Acquisition of this knowledge necessitates learning the language of these two subjects and the subsequent use of formal medical terminology. By using this formal language as a standard means of communication, health providers are able to decipher and decode what their peers and others are communicating to them: they are able to interpret words accurately.

Medical codes

Medical terminology and medical language (jargon, etc.) are types of code. A **code** is a system of numbers, letters, or symbols used to hide information so that only those authorized will be able to read it. A code system very popular today is the one used in text messaging. Someone who was unfamiliar with this code would find it difficult to decode, or understand—even the simplest text message, such as LOL (laugh out loud).

A **medical code** is a system of communication known to certain health care agencies, workers compensation organizations, and private insurance companies. Medical codes take a medical description, diagnosis, or procedure and transform it into a standardized code number. One of the most common standardized codes used internationally is the *International Statistical Classification of Diseases and Related Health Problems* (ICD), which is now in its ninth edition (ICD9). Another example is the *Diagnostic and Statistical Manual of Mental Disorders* (DSM), which is now in its fourth edition (DMS-IV). Medical codes can also be used for billing purposes (see Career Spotlight).

An example of *coded language* in health care is the medical jargon used in the health professions. **Jargon** is a set of words and phrases that is recognized and used by only a select group of people.

Another example of a code is a **hospital code**. Recall from Chapter 10, when Gil Loeppky fell out of his bed, that codes are called over the intercom or public address system to communicate specific messages to hospital staff, but not to other people in the hospital. These codes are most often used only for emergency situations.

Medical ciphers

Electronic medical records (**EMRs**) are also known as **electronic health records** (**EHRs**). Documentation within these records can include ciphers. A **cipher** is a type of code that conceals data to prevent access by others. To accomplish this, data is encrypted into something called a **ciphertext**: letters are transformed into systems of numbers (binary codes). Electronic, or digital, health care databases use this process of ciphers and encryption to provide patient identity security in EMRs. This measure also protects patients from unauthorized access to their medical and billing details. To decipher a protected EMR, the person accessing the information must follow a **user authentication protocol**, as well as provide a user-specific password and identification. The access protocol further requires permission of the owner or repository of the records. This permission will be electronically granted by way of an access e-address, to which the user can log in.

Under other circumstances, the abbreviations and acronyms used in health care are also examples of encrypted text. For example, if an EMT says that she has checked an emergency patient's *ABCs*, everyone in the emergency room knows that she is referring to the patient's airway, breathing, and circulation.

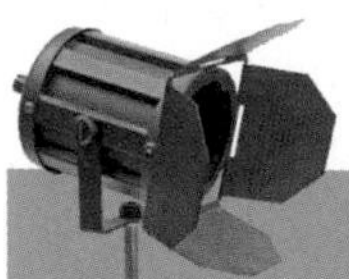

CAREER SPOTLIGHT: Medical Coders and Billers

Medical coders and *medical billers* are health information technologists who work in administration or support services in health care. More specifically, they can be found working in medical records departments, billing and finance departments, clinics, or health insurance companies. These technicians codify medical data: they use computer software to apply codes to diagnoses, procedures, and types of treatment (see Figure 18-7). Although some medical coders also function as medical billers, this is not always the case. For instance, some medical coders participate in research projects in which demographic information about the health of different populations is studied for particular coded diagnoses, for the purpose of prevention and intervention programs.

Education and training for medical coders includes a high school diploma at entry level, or a 2-year associate college degree. A 4-year undergraduate degree is also available. Along with learning medical terminology, courses in various office skills are required and students must learn coding systems and coding terminology. They also study anatomy, physiology, diagnostics, and pathophysiology. Advanced training and certification in specialties such as interventional radiation and cardiovascular coding are possible. Although certification is not a requirement for this allied health professional, it is available through organizations such as the American Academy of Professional Coders (AAPC), and the Professional Association of Health Care Coding Specialists (PAHCS).

Medical billers codify medical information for billing and reimbursement purposes. By assigning standardized, numerical codes to information in the medical record, the medical biller is able to then assign approved fees and costs as set by the employer or agency.

Education and training for medical billers include the same courses as those for medical coding, plus course work in medical documentation and insurance, health insurance billing, medical insurance, and managed care. These students are required to learn to work with medical billing software. Medical billers do not require certification to engage in this work, although certification is available through organizations such as the American Association of Medical Billers (AAMB) and Certified Medical Billing Specialists (CMBS).

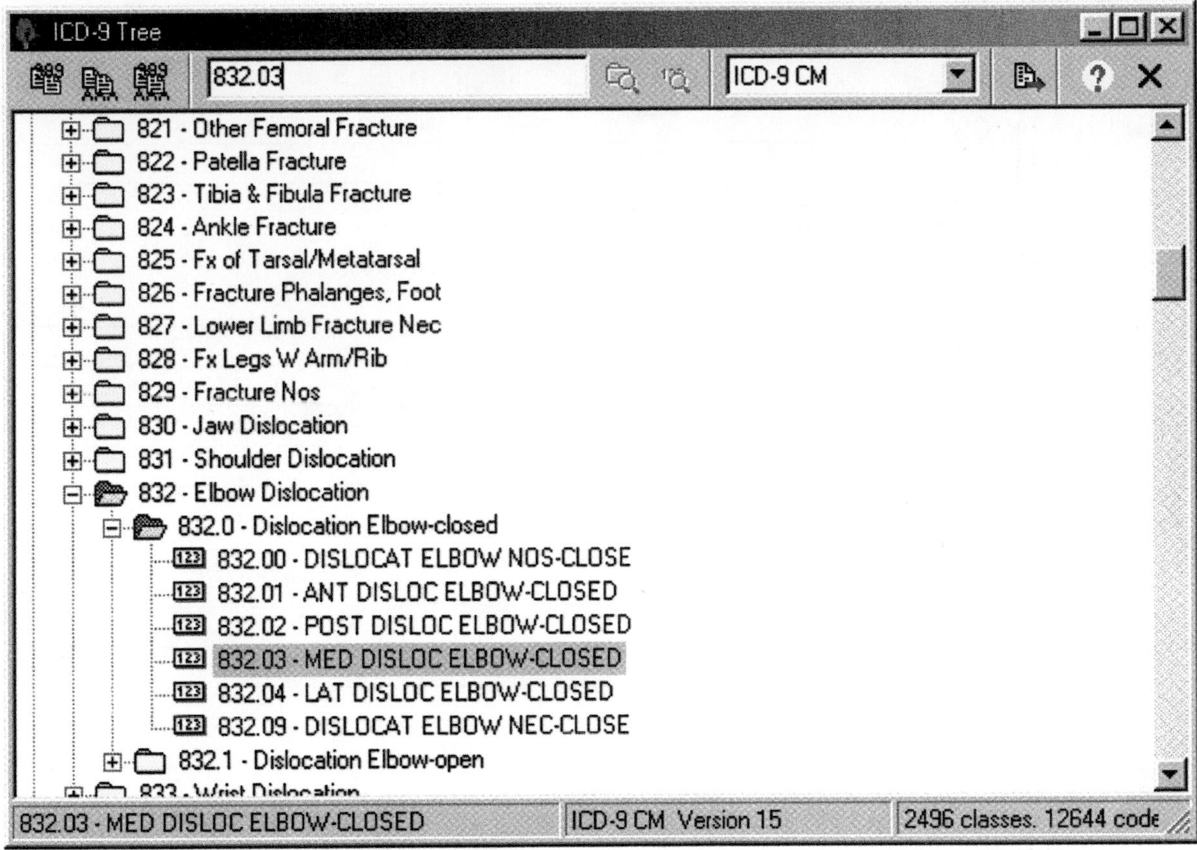

Figure 18.7: Medical codes on an EMR

Decode It: Anatomical Terms

Each term, root, or combining form below refers to a specific structure in human anatomy. Decode each item by explaining, in your own words, what it refers to.

1. ossa ______
2. adren/o- ______
3. placenta ______
4. leukocyte ______
5. mandible and maxilla ______
6. cyte ______
7. hypothalamus ______
8. neuron ______
9. anus ______
10. hemoglobin ______

Decipher It

Decipher the following abbreviations and acronyms by telling what they mean.

1. CSF ______
2. TMJ ______
3. O2 ______
4. DNA ______
5. T and A ______

6. VL ______
7. ROM ______
8. DG ______
9. CN ______
10. ANS ______

Decode It: Pathology Terms

Describe the pathology that each of the following terms refers to.

1. deep vein thrombosis ______
2. abruptio placentae ______
3. diabetes ______
4. neoplasm ______
5. varicella or Varicella zoster ______
6. neuropathy ______
7. hematoma ______
8. lesion ______
9. edema ______
10. osteoporosis ______
11. meningitis ______
12. inflammatory response ______

Decipher It

Decipher the following abbreviations, acronyms, symbols, and jargon used in pathophysiology.

1. COPD ______
2. HIV ______
3. ADHD ______
4. MTBI ______
5. IDDM ______
6. HPV ______
7. UCL ______
8. # ______
9. AML ______
10. mets ______

Decoding and Deciphering Terms: Diagnostics

Searching through medical charts to locate specific information, in order to share it with physicians or other members of the health care team, requires the ability to decode abbreviations and acronyms used by diagnosticians. Use the knowledge acquired in this course to interpret the following examples.

Decipher It

Decipher the following abbreviations and acronyms used in diagnostic assessment.

1. TPR ______
2. ABG ______
3. PT ______
4. BUN ______

5. MRI ______________________________
6. hCG ______________________________
7. FNAB ______________________________
8. PET ______________________________
9. mg ______________________________
10. d/L ______________________________

Identification and Naming

Health and forensic specialists require the skills of identifying and naming all aspects of the body. Again, human anatomy and medical terminology play a critical role in their work.

Identify the Body System

Study the diagrams. Then label each of the body systems, using formal medical terminology.

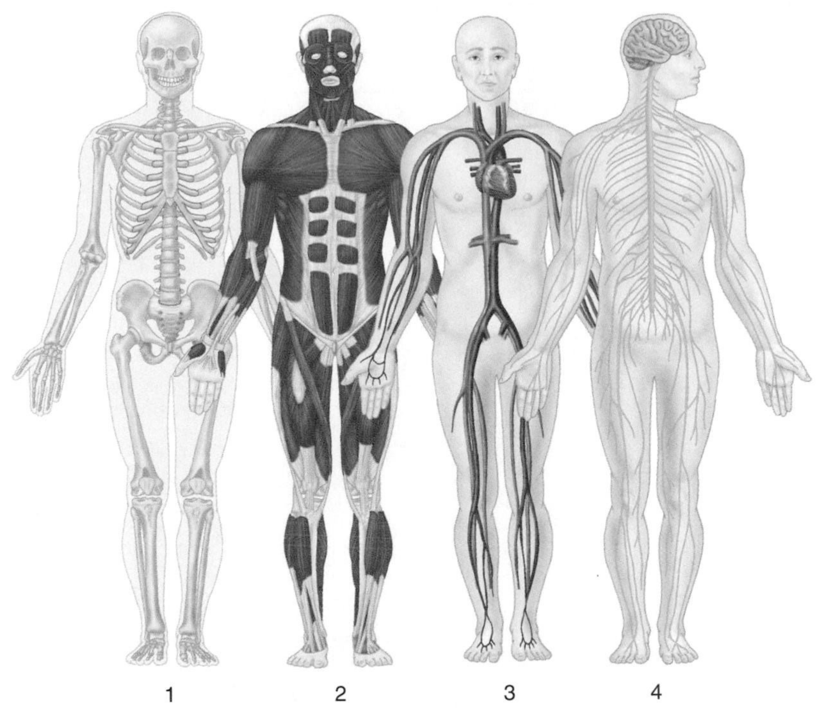

1. ______________________________
2. ______________________________
3. ______________________________
4. ______________________________

Identify the Body Parts

Study the diagrams. Then label the body parts shown, using formal medical terminology.

1. Label the internal organs visible on this diagram.

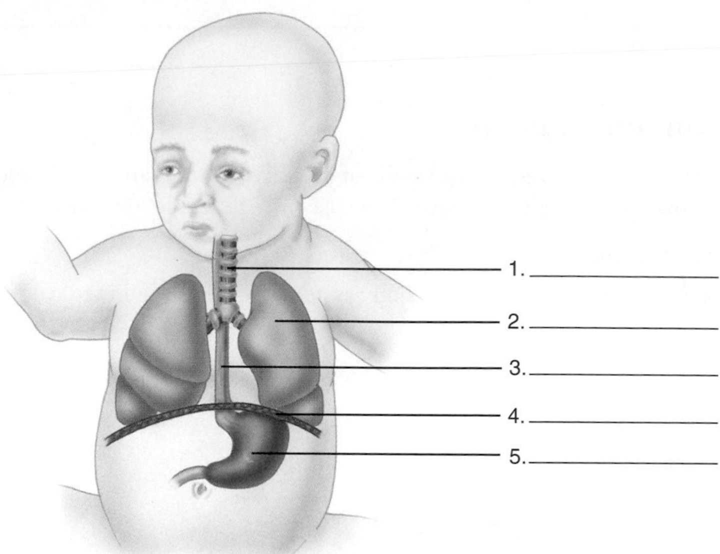

2. Label the craniofacial bones.

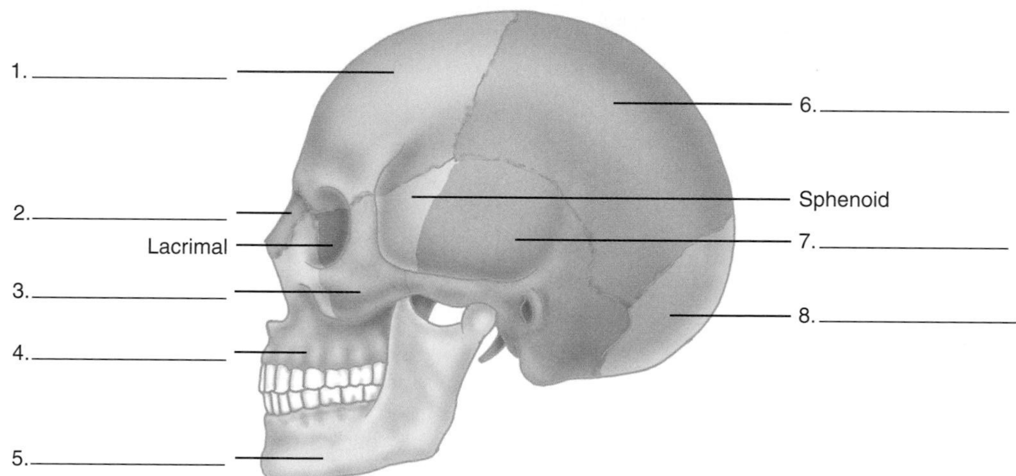

3. Label the organs of the digestive system.

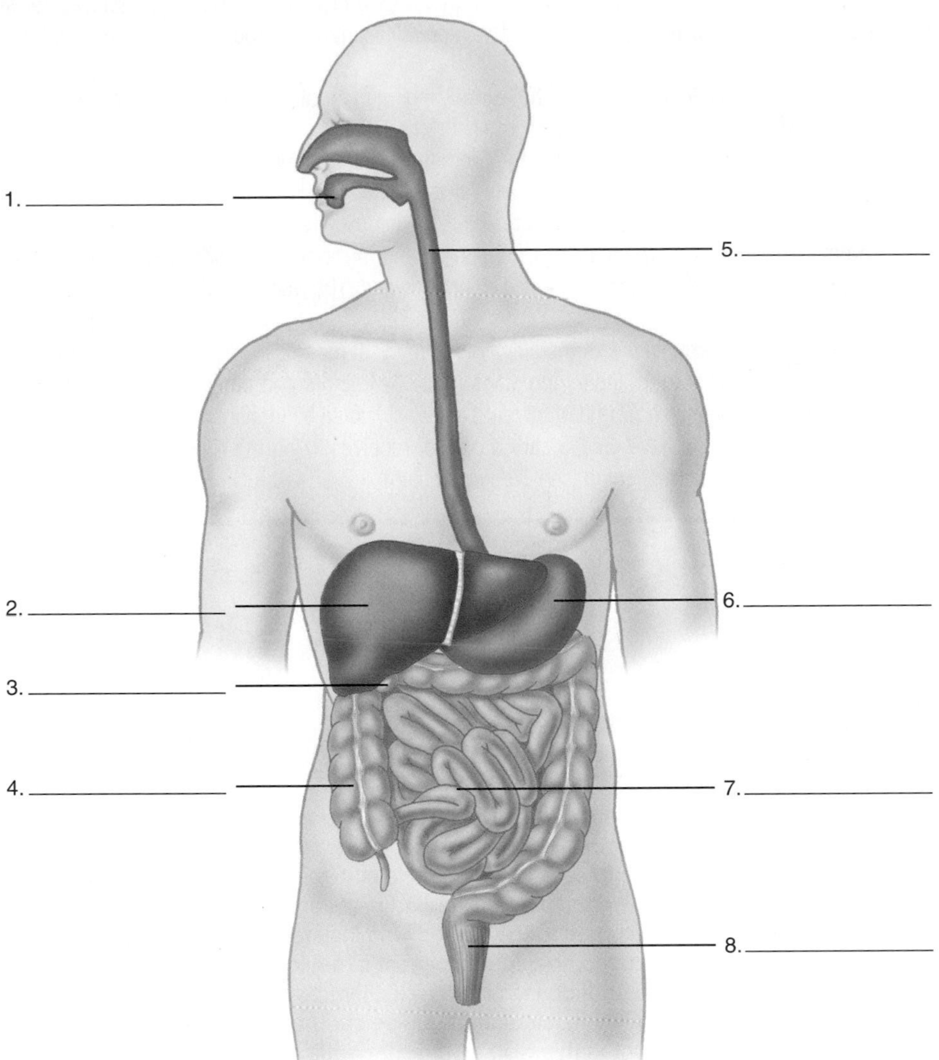

Oral Communication

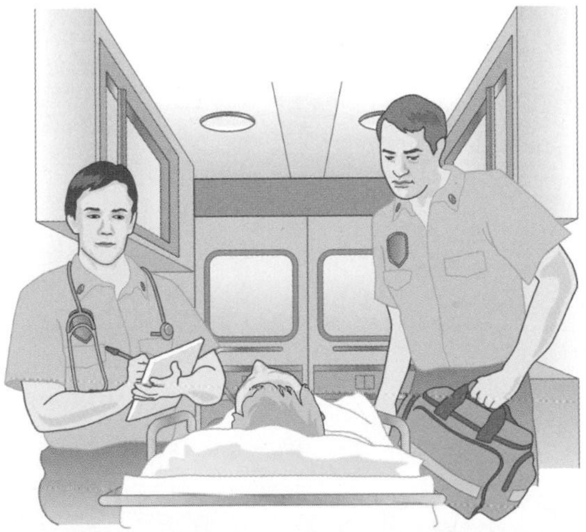

Figure 18.8: EMTs talking to patient and recording data in writing

After going over the answers to the medical terminology questions, Dr. Haydel continued her lecture, explaining that she would now move beyond written messages and focus on the importance of oral communication.

"Oral communication includes all of the verbal and nonverbal messages we send and receive to convey or interpret meaning when we speak to each other. Attention to detail is important in this type of communication, for both speakers and listeners. From time to time, it will be necessary to record in writing some of what you hear. There are many reasons for this requirement. The information someone tells you may be pertinent to the care you are about to provide. For example, if someone accompanied an unconscious patient to emergency and told the staff that the patient had ingested a number of sleeping pills, this oral information would be relevant to the care about to be provided. That fact would need to be documented in the medical record."

Dr. Haydel went on to explain that some elements of medical records have traditionally been transcribed by medical transcriptionists from audio recordings made by doctors and other specialists. She asked the audience to critically reflect on how important word accuracy would be in this type of work and what effects errors in transcription could have on the care a patient receives or on the record of care he or she has received, should it ever be investigated (see Career Spotlight).

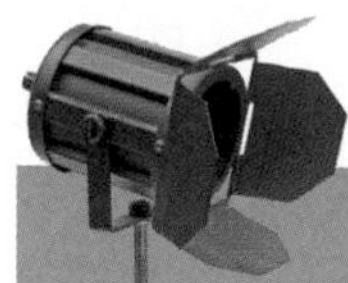

CAREER SPOTLIGHT: Medical Transcriptionists

In Chapter 14, medical e-scribes were introduced. These allied health professionals should not be confused with *medical transcriptionists* or *registered medical transcriptionists (RMTs).*

A medical transcriptionist listens to audio recordings (dictations) made by health practitioners and transcribes what is heard into written medical and administrative documents and letters. Once completed, the material is returned to the person who initiated it for proofreading and signature. These documents then become part of a patient's medical record.

Qualifications for medical transcription include an excellent command of English, including spelling and grammar. The work also requires an attentive ear that can distinguish between homonyms. Accuracy is paramount in this work. A 1-year certificate program or a 2-year associate's degree program will include English grammar courses, medical terminology, and anatomy and physiology, as well as courses in all aspects of medical documentation.

Certification as a medical transcriptionist is voluntary, although employers usually prefer to hire certified transcriptionists. One organization that provides certification is the Association of Health Care Documentation Integrity (AHDI), which can confer an RMT or a certified medical transcriptionist (CMT) designation.

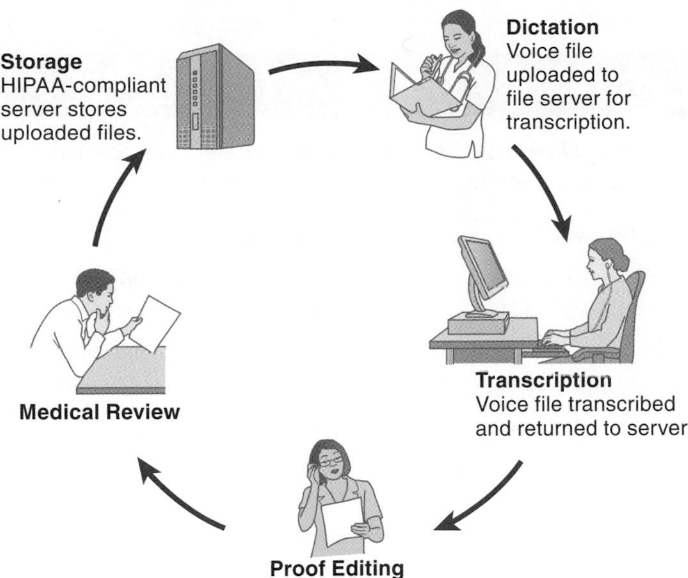

Figure 18.9: The medical transcription process

Following a brief discussion about the importance of word recognition and accuracy, Dr. Haydel added, "Throughout your textbook, a great deal of information was provided in the context of dialogues between health professionals as they discussed the diagnosis, treatment, and recovery of the Loeppkys and the Davises. She directed the students back to their handouts and an exercise in word differentiation. "Let's see how well you *listened* to your case studies. And please note that in these exercises, we are referring to the audio components of your textbook, as well as the written dialogues. You may begin."

Let's Practice

Let's practice accuracy in word usage. Imagine that you are involved in the diagnosis or treatment of patients. Would you be able to use the correct terminology when speaking to a colleague about different kinds of cases? See if you can distinguish the difference in meaning between similar terms.

Explain the difference in meaning between:

1. *-ectomy* versus *-otomy* ______
2. *incise* versus *excise* ______
3. *sonographer* versus *radiographer* ______
4. *EEG* versus *ECG* ______
5. *edema* versus *adrenal* ______
6. *postnatal* versus *postpartum* ______
7. *tachycardia* versus *bradycardia* ______
8. *epithelia* versus *endothelia* ______
9. *rubella* versus *rubeola* ______
10. *HIV* versus *AIDS* ______

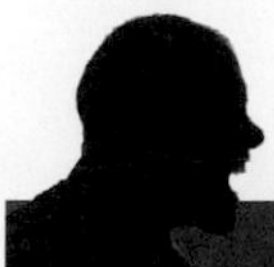

PRONUNCIATION PRACTICE

Say these words aloud to a friend or classmate, if you can. Here you are given the phonetic pronunciation. Your instructor can help you with pronunciation,

or you can visit **http://www.MedicalLanguageLab.com.**

adrenal	ăd-**rē**´năl	natal	**nā**´tăl
bradycardia	brăd″ē-**kăr**´dē-ă	-otomy	**ŏt**-ō-mē
-ectomy	**ĕk**´tō-mē	partum	**păr**´tŭm
edema	ĕ-**dē**´mă	radiographer	rā″dē-**ŏg**´ră-fĕr
endothelia	ĕn″dŏ-**thē**´lē-ă	rubella	roo-**bĕl**´lă
epithelia	ĕp″ĭ-**thē**´lē-ă	rubeola	roo-**bē**´ō-lă *or* roo-bē-**ō**´-lă
excise	ĕk-**sīz**´	sonographer	sō-**nŏg**´ră-fĕr
incise	ĭn-**sīz**´	tachycardia	tăk″ē-**kăr**´dē-ă

Communicating Through the Medical Record

The students in the lecture hall at Wyatt College moved on to a study of medical records. Students were reminded that the purpose of learning language is to communicate. Written communication includes medical documentation, most specifically, the medical record or chart. Charting is expected to be clear and concise. Sentences are very short, clear, and concise. As a result, word choice is critical to conveying specific detail and accurately reflecting a situation.

Today, medical records are increasingly becoming e-documents, and input is done electronically on computers. A patient's medical record includes all assessments, treatments, and interventions, as well as patient responses and outcomes. Charts are legal documents. For that reason, only qualified health professionals, and some allied health professionals, may record information on them.

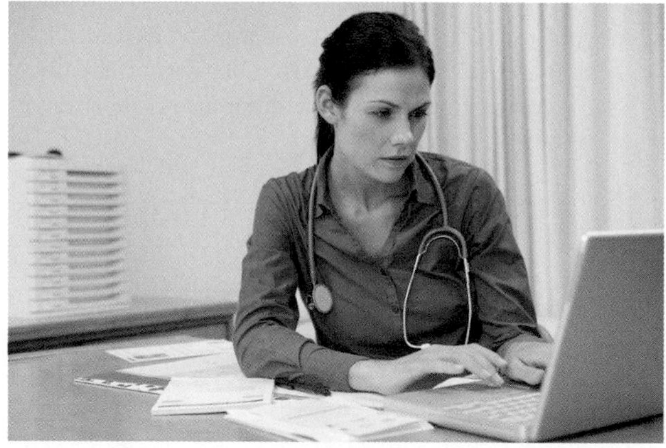

Figure 18.10: Documenting information in the e-medical record. (© Thinkstock.)

At various times in your career, you will be called to find information in a patient's medical record. Health and allied health professionals need to know where that information is located. There are a wide variety of reasons for locating information, the most important of which is to ensure that the patient is cared for safely, accurately, and in a timely manner. The medical record lets others know what was or was not done, when, and why. This information is enormously important in situations in which, for example, medication is to be administered or withheld.

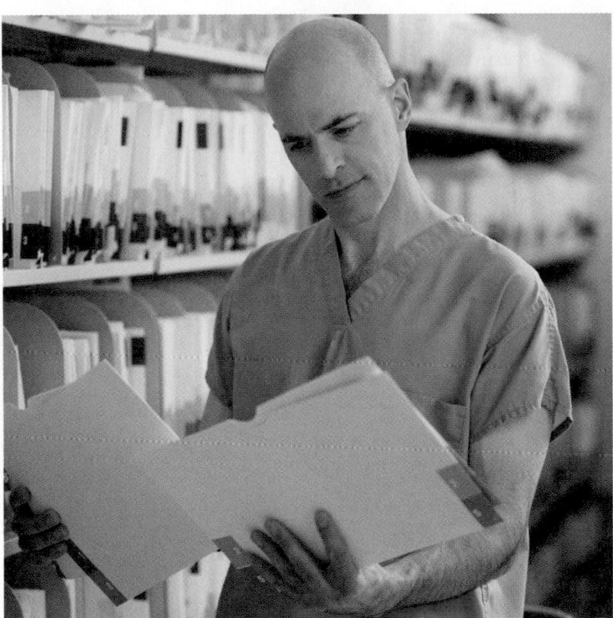

Figure 18.11: Searching for pertinent information in a medical record. (© Thinkstock/Medioimages/Photodisc.)

Patient medical records or patient care charts include assessment of the multiple domains of health: biological/physical, psychosocial, environmental, and spiritual health. They also include information about the patient's ability and motivation to care for self, any client teaching that occurs, and how discharge planning is designed with the care team and patient, collaboratively. Documentation must also include the patient's response to treatments and all other aspects of care provided. Additionally, the names and signatures of all persons recording in the chart will appear.

Legally, all assessment, care, and decisions regarding patient care *must* be documented in the patient's chart. When it is not, the nurse, doctor, or other care provider can be deemed negligent. This means that if something is not recorded in the patient chart, the courts can deem that the care was not provided. It does not matter if the care providers say that they did in fact complete assessments, treatments, and/or interventions. *If it is not recorded, it is not considered to be a fact.* It is also the legal and professional responsibility of all personnel granted charting privileges to ensure that documenting in the patient's record is done in a timely manner and per the policies and requirements of the care facility/employer and regulatory guidelines for the profession.

The sections of a medical record

Handwritten patient medical records (charts) are kept on clipboards at the bedside or in binders at the nursing station. These binders have multiple sections identified by tabs. Each section has a specific purpose, and only information related to that section should appear there. An e-medical record is organized into the same sections but is accessed via computer.

- The very first section will include the *Patient's Identifying Information* (name, date of birth, date of admission, and doctor's name) plus a notice of any allergies. This section is always at the beginning of the chart. It is a safety measure to protect the patient.
- This is followed by a *Physician's Orders* section. Here, the patient's doctor or doctors will write medication and treatment orders.
- Next, the *Physician's Notes* appear. Only doctors will make entries here. Sometimes this section is called *Progress Notes*. The first entry in this section will be the physician's admission note, which will provide a complete systems review and then assessment of the patient's injuries or conditions. The doctor may also make notes on an admission assessment form, which might appear here or at the end of the chart in the Admissions section.
- Nurses will enter data in the *Nurses' Notes* section. This section is often the largest in a patient's chart because nurses document assessments, treatments, vital signs, and other pertinent information on a 24-hour-a-day basis.

- The nurses' notes are most often followed by the *Medication Administration Records.*
- The *Patient History* section contains longer case summary reports from various health professionals who have been involved in the patient's care over time. These might include social workers, physiotherapists, family practice physicians, and so on. Collateral information gathered by these professionals from the patient's family members and significant others will also appear here.
- *Laboratory and Diagnostic Reports* may be found together or as separate sections further into the chart. *Reports of Surgical Procedures* may also appear there.
- There is usually a section at the back of the binder or end of the e-record for *Admission, Transfer, and Discharge Forms.* Admissions forms are completed by both nurses and doctors in the Emergency or Admissions departments of hospitals. Discharge forms are completed by the nurses in the hospital care unit (or ward) in which the patient was given care. The discharge form will include information regarding the patient's response to treatment, prognosis, and any referrals and follow-up care that have been recommended. A physician's discharge summary may appear here, too. If the patient has come to the hospital on transfer from another facility, a *transfer note* or *transfer summary* may also appear in this section. This section of the medical record will also contain completed forms for *billing and insurance*, as well as *signed consents* for treatment by the patient and any requisite *treatment authorizations.*

Critical Thinking: Medical Records

Think about all that you have learned to date about elements of the medical record as you answer these questions. They are all about one patient, Mrs. Williams. Mrs. Williams, a frail elderly woman, has just been admitted to your extended care facility from the local hospital.

1. You work in a medical billing office. Where would you find information about a patient's health insurance or whether the patient is able to self-pay for service?

   ____

2. Which form will accompany Mrs. Williams and will tell your care staff about her recent treatment at a hospital, her prognosis, the reason for her transfer to your facility, and recommendations for her follow-up care? Where is this form located in a medical record?

   ____

3. Now that your patient has settled into the new care facility, the doctor there has ordered some new blood work. When these results come back to you, where will you place them in the patient's chart? ______________________________

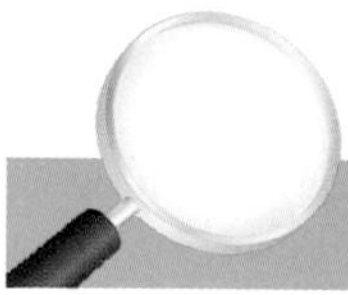

FOCUS POINT: Acute, Extended, and Long-Term Care

Acute care refers to a medical, mental health, or addictions facility in which patients are in need of active or immediate treatment for illnesses or injuries. The care provided is on a short-term basis. Acute care facilities include hospitals and walk-in clinics.

Extended care refers to a facility that provides a longer period of care for recovery and rehabilitation, when placement in an acute medical facility is no longer necessary or the best option for care. The focus of care is on working toward and achieving optimal health outcomes.

Long-term care refers to a facility that offers residential care for people with special health needs, disabilities, or chronic illnesses. The focus of care is on health promotion and maintenance, rather than recovery.

Decipher It

Once again, use your knowledge of medical terminology to decipher the following acronyms, abbreviations, and jargon in medical records. In this exercise, sentences appear directly from the case studies of the Loeppkys and Davises. Observe the term that is highlighted. If the term is an abbreviation, spell it out in long form. Then define each term.

1. We will use some lag screws and *k-wires* to hold the joint of the ankle together where the tibia, fibula, and talus meet.
   Term: ______________________ Meaning: ______________________
2. Your son is going to receive his nutrition by *NG tube* for about a week.
   Term: ______________________ Meaning: ______________________
3. He will be back in a little bit to apply a thumb *spica cast.*
   Term: ______________________ Meaning: ______________________
4. A *drug screen* and a *toxicology report* were ordered.
   Term: ______________________ Meaning: ______________________
   Term: ______________________ Meaning: ______________________
5. A *TENS unit* treats localized neuropathic pain, the result of disease, inflammation, and/or trauma to the peripheral nerves related to injury or surgery.
   Term: ______________________ Meaning: ______________________
6. "I'm going to start with a full chest exam. I'm going to *observe for symmetry.*"
   Term: ______________________ Meaning: ______________________
7. The *GAF* is by far the most commonly used test of overall (global) functioning by nurses, physicians, psychiatrists, occupational and physical therapists, medical social workers, and others.
   Term: ______________________ Meaning: ______________________
8. The *urine dip* is negative for everything.
   Term: ______________________ Meaning: ______________________
9. *Auscultation* of the thorax allows the physician to assess for symmetry of airflow bilaterally in the lungs.
   Term: ______________________ Meaning: ______________________
10. No *decels.*
   Term: ______________________ Meaning: ______________________

Decode It

Translate each question into plain English to demonstrate your level of comprehension. Spell out any abbreviations, acronyms, or jargon as well.

Then imagine that you have been asked to search through a file to find the answer to each question. Tell in which section of the patient's medical record you would find the answer.

1. Are the zygomatic arches intact?
   Translation: ______________________ Section ______________________
2. Did we get a panorex of the maxilla and the condyles?
   Translation: ______________________ Section ______________________
3. What was the name of the EMT on the scene who did the triage?
   Translation: ______________________ Section ______________________
4. Do you know if the MI patient was defibrillated in the ER or in the ambulance?
   Translation: ______________________ Section ______________________
5. What was the mechanism of injury for this abdominal wound?
   Translation: ______________________ Section ______________________
6. Did the patient have a surgical reduction to the hip last year?
   Translation: ______________________ Section ______________________

7. Is this patient on any antibiotics by intravenous at the moment?
   Translation: ______________________ Section ______________

8. Do we have a report confirming multiple facial fractures, particularly in the orbitonasal region?
   Translation: ______________________ Section ______________

9. Who made the final determination that injuries were sustained to the thoracic and abdominopelvic regions?
   Translation: ______________________ Section ______________

10. Do we have a report that says the bilateral scarring gives evidence of possible bilateral renal surgery?
    Translation: ______________________ Section ______________

Putting It All Together: Forensic Investigation of Case Studies

A great deal of patient information about five fictional patients is held within this book. These case studies could easily be transcribed into medical records. The following exercises ask you to search through the fictional records in this book to extract important data that helps build the case for care, treatment, admission, and discharge of specific patients.

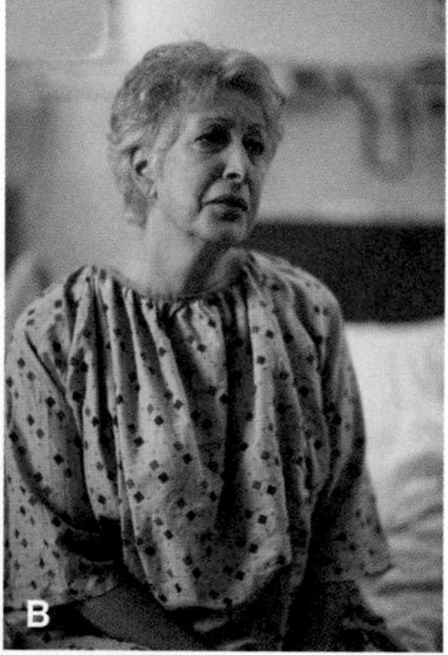

A

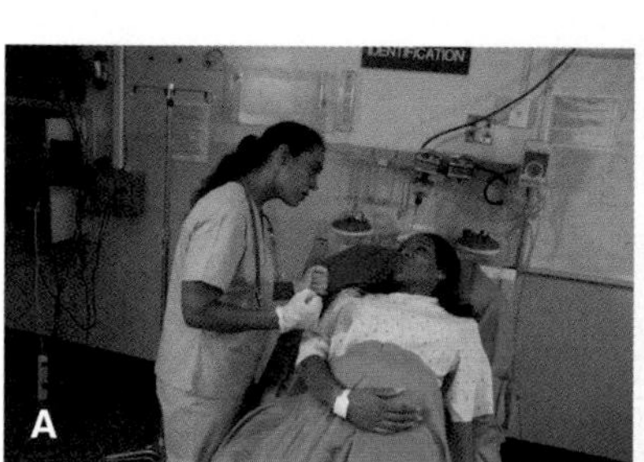

B

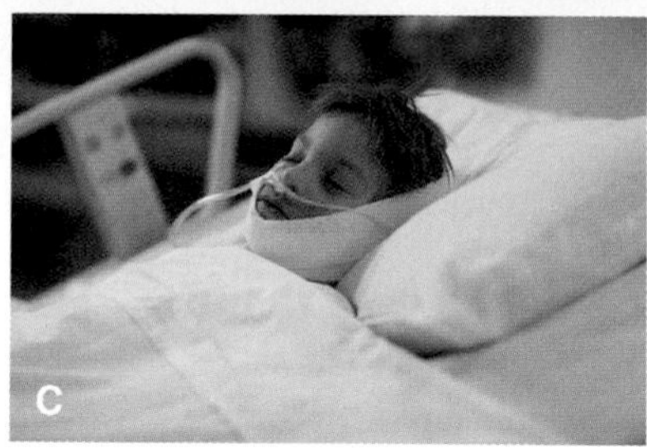

C

Dr. Haydel is continuing her session with the students at Wyatt College.

"Having warmed up by reviewing medical language and practicing with terminology, it is now time to apply that knowledge—and your new skills—to our case study patients, the Loeppkys and the Davises. If you look in the handouts I distributed as you came into the lecture hall today, you'll find the exercises we are about to do." She paused while people shuffled their papers, looking for the material. "Did everyone find them? Good."

"I understand that you've all been told to bring your textbook, *Medical Language: Terminology in Context*, with you to this meeting. You'll need to get those out now." She waited for them to do so. "Now, it has occurred to me that many students joined us today who are not taking medical terminology and don't have this book. So I'd like those of you with books, in the spirit of collegiality and cooperation, to invite a student without a book to join you." Students started looking about for partners, changing their seats and getting organized. Dr. Haydel smiled when she saw how some students were gathering in small clusters of three, four, and even five students. This, she thought, was a good idea.

When the noise and commotion died down, Dr. Haydel began again. She told them that, for these exercises, everyone would need to search through the patient scenarios in the textbook as if they were the patients' medical records. They would look for the specific information asked for and then complete their documentation accurately. She explained to them that this would help them all realize, not only how medical records were compiled, but also what kinds of information were found within them, scattered about in various sections, waiting to be located and used. She reinforced one more time that their ability to write a case summary or referral would depend on their ability to find such material.

"After each exercise, I'll pull up the answers on the screen here behind me and we can discuss your findings," concluded Dr. Haydel. "We can also discuss any insights you've gained through each exercise, as well as any frustrations you may have had. Let's begin."

Critical Thinking

Answer these questions based on what you know about the six patients in the case studies: Gil Loeppky, Glory Loeppky, Emily Grace Loeppky, Zane Davis, Stevie-Rose Davis, and Clay Davis.

1. Three patients have musculoskeletal injuries from the motor vehicle accident. Name each patient, and describe his or her injury or injuries.

   ____
   ____
   ____

2. One patient has symptoms that could be caused by psychological, neurological, or endocrine impairment or pathology. Who is this?

   ____

3. Three patients have respiratory challenges that need intervention, treatment, or continuing assessment. Who are they?

   ____________, ____________, and ____________

4. Clay Davis could not legally give consent for his own treatment. Why not?

   ____

Let's Practice

Practice the skill of searching through medical records to find pertinent information. At any time in your health care career you might be asked to do this. Find the following information in the medical records of your patients.

1. Who is/are Clay Davis's next of kin? (Chapter 6)

   ____

2. What kind of hospital ward (unit) was Glory Loeppky admitted to shortly after she was seen in the Emergency Department? (Chapter 8)

   ____

3. Which patients had CT scans taken and why? Which part or parts of the body were scanned? (Chapters 4, 5, 6, 10)

   ____
   ____
   ____

4. One of the patients had an injury to the knee. Who was it? What is the name of that injury? How did the injury occur? (Chapter 4)

5. Which patients are going to have some of their medical bills taken care of by Veterans Affairs? (Chapters 9, 16)

6. At one point in acute care, Glory Loeppky had a special type of belt, or strap, laid across her abdomen. What was that procedure called, and what was its purpose? (Chapter 8)

7. One of the patients gets a TAR completed. Who is it, and what is a TAR? Who took responsibility for ensuring that this document was completed? (Chapter 9)

8. Someone needed the immediate attention of a craniofacial surgeon. Who was it? What condition needed surgical treatment? (Chapter 6)

9. Stevie-Rose Davis does not have a functioning thyroid gland. What treatment is she on for that? (Chapter 7)

10. Gil Loeppky was placed in a cervical collar at the scene of the accident. What was the rationale for that? (Chapters 1, 4)

11. In the beginning, and for some time just after admission, both Gil Loeppky and Clay Davis were *NPO*. What does this mean, and why were they *NPO*? (Chapters 10, 11)

12. Which health professional was most focused on the recovery of a patient's ambulation and coordination? For which patient? (Chapter 15)

Investigating documentation and extracting pertinent information

Dr. Haydel continued working with the students who had come to hear her speak on matters of forensics. She directed them to the next set of learning activities that would help them develop their skills of inquiry, investigation, and research. She pointed out that the handouts contained two different types of forms to complete. Students were instructed to scour the textbook for the data each form requires.

Dr. Haydel highlighted a strict protocol: If someone does not think the information is provided in the textbook (the fictional medical record), then they must write the abbreviation for *n/a* for *not applicable* or *u/k* for *unknown* in the appropriate spaces. She stressed that under no circumstances should blank spaces be left in a medical record. She ended by reminding the students that medical records are legal documents and, as such, the forms must be completely filled out as a historical record.

Admission forms

Use all of the information you have learned about the patients at Oklahoma Trauma Center to complete the portions of the admissions forms (the admissions records) provided here.

1. Gil Loeppky (Chapters 4, 10, 15)

Okla Trauma

Okla Trauma Center - Admission Form

Hospital ID: AyZ29763

Patient name: ______________________ Patient DOB: ___/___/___ Date of admission: ___/___/___

Admitting diagnosis: ______________________

Attending physician: ______________________

Allergies: ______________________

____

Marital status: __ Married __ Single

Next of kin/significant other: ______________________

Contact number for next of kin/significant other: (___)-___-____

Emergency contact person (not living with patient): ______________________

Number for emergency contact: (___)-___-____

Relationship to patient: ______________________

Ambulatory: __ Yes __ No Conscious: __ Yes __ No

Medications prescribed or taken: __ Yes __ No

Provide details, including last dose: ______________________

____

Alcohol or substance use prior to admission: __ Yes __ No

Provide details: ______________________

____

Workplace accident: __ Yes __ No

Police involved: __ Yes __ No

Occupation: ______________________

Employer: ______________________

Health Insurance: __ Yes __ No

Provide billing details: ______________________

____

Hearing aids, glasses, or prosthetics: __ Yes __ No __ u/k

Provide details: ______________________

____

Wallet and ID taken for safekeeping by admitting clerk: __ Yes __ No __ u/k

Provide signature: ______________________

2. Zane Davis (Chapters 5, 9, 14)

Okla Trauma

Okla Trauma Center - Admission Form

Hospital ID: AyZ34293

Patient name: ____________________ Patient DOB: ____/____/____ Date of admission: ____/____/____

Admitting diagnosis: ____________________

Attending physician: ____________________

Allergies: ____________________

____

Marital status: __ Married __ Single

Next of kin/significant other: ____________________

Contact number for next of kin/significant other: (___)-___-____

Emergency contact person (not living with patient): ____________________

Number for emergency contact: (___)-___-____

Relationship to patient: ____________________

Ambulatory: __ Yes __ No Conscious: __ Yes __ No

Medications prescribed or taken: __ Yes __ No

Provide details, including last dose: ____________________

____

Alcohol or substance use prior to admission: __ Yes __ No

Provide details: ____________________

____

Workplace accident: __ Yes __ No

Police involved: __ Yes __ No

Occupation: ____________________

Employer: ____________________

Health Insurance: __ Yes __ No

Provide billing details: ____________________

____

Hearing aids, glasses, or prosthetics: __ Yes __ No __ u/k

Provide details: ____________________

____

Wallet and ID taken for safekeeping by admitting clerk: __ Yes __ No __ u/k

Provide signature: ____________________

3. Clay Davis (Chapters 6, 11, 13)

Okla Trauma

Okla Trauma Center - Admission Form

Hospital ID: Ay34256

Patient name: ______________________ Patient DOB: ____/____/____ Date of admission: ____/____/____

Admitting diagnosis: ______________________

Attending physician: ______________________

Allergies: ______________________

____

Marital status: __ Married __ Single

Next of kin/significant other: ______________________

Contact number for next of kin/significant other: (___)-___-____

Emergency contact person (not living with patient): ______________________

Number for emergency contact: (___)-___-____

Relationship to patient: ______________________

Ambulatory: __ Yes __ No Conscious: __ Yes __ No

Medications prescribed or taken: __ Yes __ No

Provide details, including last dose: ______________________

____

Alcohol or substance use prior to admission: __ Yes __ No

Provide details: ______________________

____

Workplace accident: __ Yes __ No

Police involved: __ Yes __ No

Occupation: ______________________

Employer: ______________________

Health Insurance: __ Yes __ No

Provide billing details: ______________________

____

Hearing aids, glasses, or prosthetics: __ Yes __ No __ u/k

Provide details: ______________________

____

Wallet and ID taken for safekeeping by admitting clerk: __ Yes __ No __ u/k

Provide signature: ______________________

Vital signs flowsheet on the e-medical record

For the next exercise, Dr. Haydel spoke to the audience about the importance of flowsheets and graphs on a medical record. She explained how this data provided a clinical snapshot of the patient's physical status at certain points in time. As an example, she mentioned that evidence of a patient's fever would appear in a *vital signs flowsheet*, and then again in the nurses' notes for the patient. These two documents, combined, provide evidence that assessment is occurring. Subsequent entries in the vital signs flowsheet may show that a high temperature has receded. Again, looking in the nurses' notes, the reason for this may become clear. It may be, for example, that the nurse administered an antipyretic medication that resulted in the lowering of the patient's temperature.

Complete the admission form provided by taking the information you have "on file" from previous chapters and entering it into the correct columns and spaces. *Do this only for the time of admission* for *Mrs. Stevie-Rose Davis at Fayette General Hospital.* Study this example first:

Okla Trauma Center

Clinical Documentation

Patient: Jane Doe | Unit/Bed: ICU/IC267A | Account #:

Age: 36 yrs | Gender: F | Height: | Weight: | Physician: Jones T.

Vital Sign Flowsheet

Date/Time			07/07 08:00	09:00	10:00	11:00	12:00	13:00	14:00	15:00	16:00
Temperature (TEMP)		°F	97.8 po				98.0 po				
		°C	36.6				36.7				
Heart Rate (HR)			70	69	76	70		77	75	71	80
Respiratory Rate (RESP)		br/min	25	27	21	14	17	19	15	14	23
Blood pressure (BP)	Manual	S/D (M) Source	/ ( )	/ ( )	/ ( )	/ ( )	/ ( )	/ ( )	/ ( )	/ ( )	/ ( )
	Noninvasive	S/D Measured Mean Source	/ ( )	137/59 (86)	/ ( )	122/56 (78)	122/46 (69)	115/58 (76)	96/82 (91)	99/65 (76)	/ ( )
Rhythm		Rhythm									
Ectopy		Frequency									
O_2 Therapy		L/min	3.0	3.0	3.0	3.0	3.0	3.0	3.0	3.0	3.0
		Device	NC	NC	NC	NC	NC	NC	NC	NC	NC
MONIT	O_2 sat	%									
MISC	Fingerstick Glucose	mg/dl		321							
	Glucose Interventions			Ins bolus 12 units							
Comments:											

Figure 18.12: Vital signs flowsheet on the e-medical record

Stevie-Rose Davis' vital signs on admission (Chapter 2)

Okla Trauma Center

Clinical Documentation

Patient: Unit/Bed: Account #:

Age: Gender: Height: Weight: Physician:

Vital Sign Flowsheet

Date/Time											
Temperature (TEMP)		°F °C									
Heart Rate (HR)											
Respiratory Rate (RESP)		br/min									
Blood pressure (BP)	Manual	S/D (M) Source									
	Noninvasive	S/D Measured Mean Source									
Rhythm		Rhythm									
Ectopy		Frequency									
O_2 Therapy		L/min									
		Device									
MONIT	O_2 sat	%									
MISC	Fingerstick Glucose	mg/dl									
	Glucose Interventions										

Comments:

Using diagrams to locate injuries and diseases

The students moved on to learn about *diagrams* in the medical record. Diagrams are certainly part of an emergency admission record. They are also included on first visits to physicians and other health specialists, such as physical therapists. They are used as quick references: maps of where injuries, disease, or symptoms lie. Diagrams must always be accompanied by words to describe them. These descriptive words may appear on a checklist or may be entered into the form by computer or by hand (see Figure 18-13).

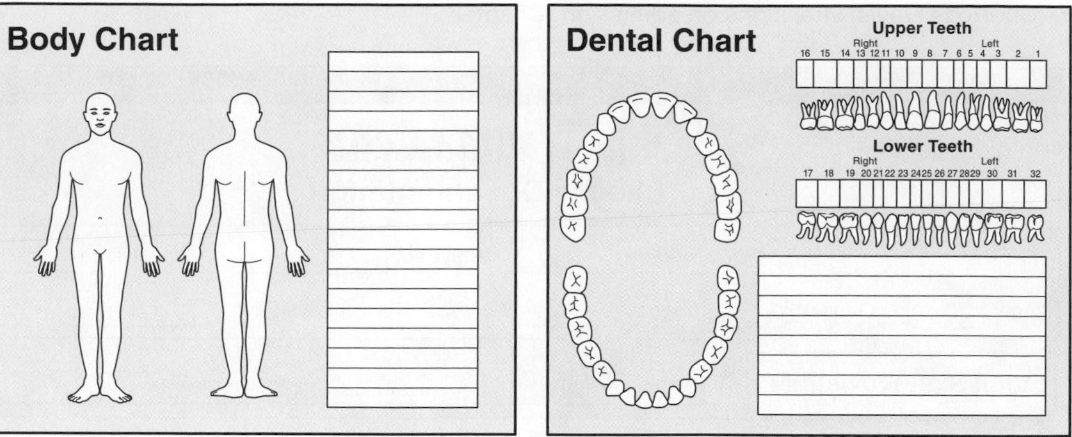

Figure 18.13: Diagrams found on medical records

Let's Practice

Complete each diagram by marking an X on the site of injury or disease for each patient. Be sure to place the X on at the correct location and on the correct side of the body. Then write the name of the injury or health concerns on the diagram. Follow the example shown in Figure 18-14.

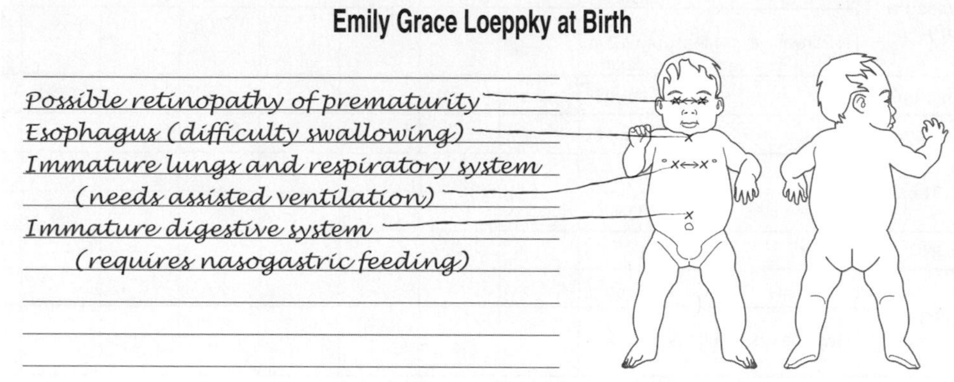

Figure 18.14: Injury diagram: Emily Grace Loeppky

1. Gil Loeppky

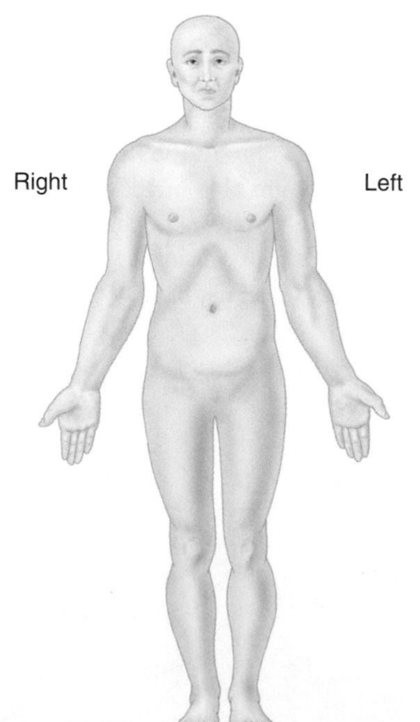

2. Glory Loeppky

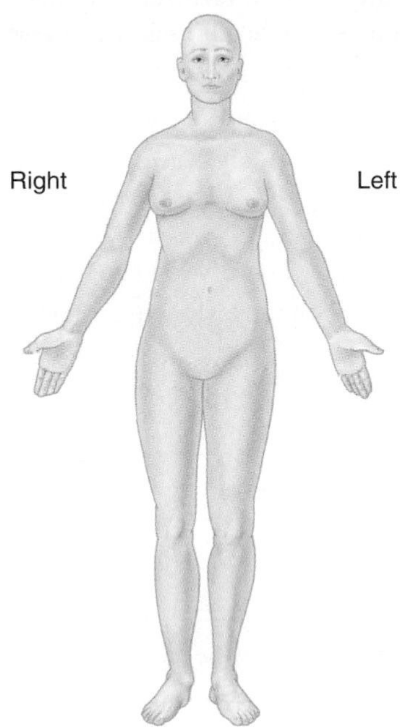

3. Clay Davis

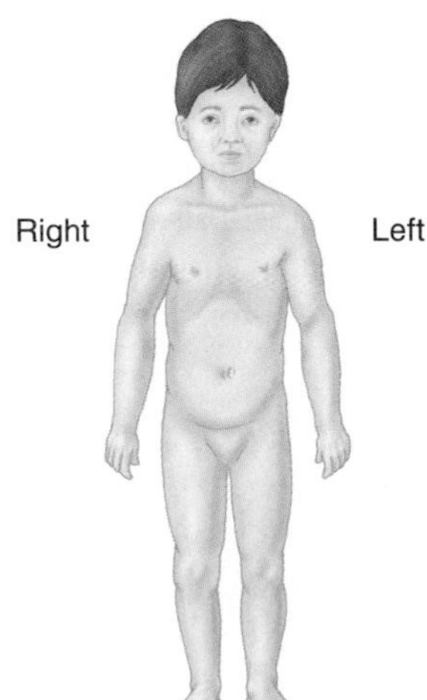

Investigating the mechanisms of injury

The **mechanisms of injury** in a motor vehicle accident are relevant to assessment of the direction and angle of injury, the degree of force exerted on the body, and other important factors. In this context, **mechanism** refers to the means or methods by which an injury occurs. For example, the mechanism of injury in a head trauma might be from the amount of force involved when the skull hit a windshield.

Awareness of the mechanism of injury also alerts the treatment team to the potential for complications. For example, in a head-on car crash, physicians will immediately look for frontal lobe and facial trauma, as well as fractured ribs (from the steering wheel) and leg fractures (from the front of the vehicle being pushed in on the people in the front seat). Spinal cord injuries may be possible from any sudden whipping of the head and neck back and forth.

Therefore, any facts collected from the patient, from emergency medical technicians, and from police officers involved at the scene are relevant to patient care. All of this data must be recorded in the medical record, and the source of each fact must be identified. For example, the physician in the emergency room may have made these admission and assessment notes when Gil Loeppky arrived in the trauma bay:

> *EMT Raybuck advised pt. was in the driver's seat. Found slumped over steering wheel, pinned in. May have struck head on windshield. Facial lacerations and unconscious. Cervical collar placed. Extracted from vehicle. Noticeable injuries to right leg.*

Let's Practice

For each injury described, search the chapter shown in parentheses to find the mechanism of injury.

1. Gil Loeppky's pilon fracture (Chapters 4, 10)

   ____

2. Glory Loeppky's ulnar collateral ligament injury to the thumb (Chapter 3)

   ____

3. Clay Davis's scald (Chapter 12)

   ____

4. Gil Loeppky's presentation of raccoon eyes (Chapter 4)

   ____

Incident reports

In Chapter 10, Gil Loeppky sustained a secondary injury as the result of a fall from his hospital bed. In a medical context, this fall is an example of an *adverse event, critical incident*, or *unusual occurrence*. Although Gil's example is of a physical injury, other incidents can include fires, medication errors, equipment failures, acts of violence or aggression, or the use of seclusion or restraint. When a critical incident occurs, the primary staff members involved in the patient's care are required to complete a specific form, often called an **incident report**. That document will contain a description of the incident, the suspected injury (if it has yet to be diagnosed by a doctor), and the mechanism of the injury. It will also include signs and symptoms that arise after the injury, as well as all immediate care interventions provided by those in attendance. A copy of this report will be sent to the hospital's administrators. An example of an incident report is provided in Figure 18-15.

Okla Trauma Center - Incident Report

Patient: *Gilbert Loeppky*	Date of incident: *June xx*	Date of birth/age: *36 years old*	ID #: *xxxxx*

Location of incident (unit, room, hallway, etc.; on the floor, bed,...).
Describe. *Room xxx, Surgical Unit. Found on the floor beside bed.*

Time of incident: *0200 hrs.* Patient's physician: *Dr. E. Karras*

Provide information for each of the following. Do not leave any blank spaces on this form.

REPORT OF FIRST RESPONDERS

Name and credentials of first responder: *Franklin xxxx, RN*

Type of Incident: ✓ physical injury - ✓ fall __ burn __ electrical __ other (describe) ________
__ aggression/violence (verbal or physical)
__ missing or A.W.O.L.
__ medication incident
__ other (describe) ________

Were ABCs assessed stat? ✓ yes __ no
Recorded? ✓ yes __ no

Was help called immediately to attend? ✓ yes __ no
Describe. *Called a code*

Identify all treatment interventions given stat:
ABCs, attempted to rouse pt, assessed neurological signs and level of consciousness (pt unconscious); cursory exam of skeletal system, particularly to the face and hips. Ensured IV line and urinary catheter were still in situ and patient. Assisted by team to place pt on backboard.

Was physician contacted? Whom? When? ✓ yes __ no
Physicians on call via Code. Drs. Swanson and Jensen attended

What time did physician arrive? *Within minutes. Time approx: xxxx hrs.*

REPORT OF FALL: INITIAL INCIDENT

Did hospital staff attempt to minimize the impact of the fall by **assisting** the patient's descent to the floor? __ yes ✓ no
Explain. *Did not witness fall.*

Was the fall **attended** by hospital staff? ✓ yes __ no
After the fall had occurred

Identify the **most significant** injury as a result of the fall. Describe mechanism of this injury.
Head injury and loss of consciousness. Fell onto floor from bed.
Mechanism: Frontal-temporal lobe impacted with floor.

Specify other injury:
No other new, overt injuries noted arising from this fall. Pt already has head injury and facial bruising. No new bruising noted. Pt has supports on right ankle and knee. These were in situ but needed slight adjustment.

FALL RISK RELATED DETAILS

Was the patient assessed previously for being at risk? ✓ yes __ no

Was the patient deemed to be at risk for falling according to the most recent risk assessment? ✓ yes __ no

Was a previous prevention/precautionary protocol implemented prior to the fall? ✓ yes __ no
Side rails up; frequent rounds; bathroom light left on for some illumination of the room.

Were there orders from the attending or consulting MD related to risks prior to the incident? ✓ yes __ no
Describe. *Use of side rails prn ordered; no walking or weight-bearing permitted.*

RESTRAINTS RELATED INFORMATION

Did the patient have restraint orders prior to the fall? __ yes ✓ no

Were restraints in use at the time of the fall? __ yes ✓ no

What types of restraints were in use? Describe. *N/A-not applicable*

Figure 18.15: Incident report for Gil Loeppky's fall from bed

Continued on next page

ETIOLOGY: FALL OR ACCIDENT CAUSE-RELATED INFORMATION

Provide medical status prior to fall or accident.
Pt pre-op for orthopedics: fracture and injuries to right leg. Nonambulant. Blunt-force injury to head and being assessed with Glasgow Coma Scale routinely. Analgesics administered Po/Lm q4h and prn. Anti-inflammatory meds given qbh. However, patient has been NPO since midnight.

Activity engaged in by the patient PRIOR to the fall/accident.
Describe. *Appeared to be sleeping on previous rounds, approximately 10 minutes prior to fall*

Other relevant patient activity.
Describe. *May have awoken and been disoriented to time and place; may not have been aware of his medical status/injuries and attempted to get out of bed*

FALL/ACCIDENT FACTORS & RELATIONSHIP INFORMATION

Identify environment of care factors that could have contributed to the fall/accident.
Possibly not enough lighting in room to cue or orient patient to his surroundings when he awoke. Call bell clipped to pillow but pt may not have known it was there.

Specify other environmental factors.
Side rails used to prevent a fall from bed did not prevent pt from trying to climb over them in an attempt to get out of bed.

What was the main patient factor associated with the fall/accident? Describe. Provide rationale.
Pt tried to get up on his own. ? confusion, disorientation; lack of awareness of injuries and nonambulant status; effects of analgesia; effect of brain injury from MVA clouding consciousness; side rails provided an additional obstacle to attempt to get up.

Other patient factors?
Unknown. Pt is unconscious and unable to provide details.

MEDICATIONS ADMINISTERED PRIOR TO FALL/ACCIDENT

Are there any medications the patient is taking that could have contributed to the fall/accident? ✓ yes __ no
Name them. *Morphine for analgesic effect can cloud consciousness and increase levels of confusion*

Were any of the following medications administered to the patient prior to the fall or accident? ✓ yes __ no

Specify time of last dose.
- ✓ analgesics/narcotics *2200 hrs, June xx*
- __ diuretics
- __ sedatives
- __ cardiac
- __ bowel prep
- __ other medication(s): Name it/them.

Were any other medications other than those specified above administered within 12 hours of the fall/accident? ✓ yes __ no
Name them. *The antibiotic cefalozin was given by IV in ER shortly after admission yesterday afternoon.*

NAME, CREDENTIALS, AND SIGNATURES OF FIRST RESPONDER AND A WITNESS

Franklin xxx, RN
FRANKLIN XXX, RN
June xx, xxxx

Lourdes xxx, LPN
Lourdes xxx, LPN
June xx, xxxx

Figure 18.15:—cont'd

Investigating medical histories

You may at some time in your career be asked to complete a medical history or to review a medical history form to ensure that it has been fully completed. If the history is not complete, you may need to search the patient's medical records for the missing information. Here is an example of a medical history form showing the types of data included.

CONFIDENTIAL PATIENT INFORMATION

BLUEVILLE FAMILY MEDICINE
15 MAIN STREET
BLUEVILLE, CT
860-555-3212

Name *Michelle Calabrese* Date of birth *6/21/1984* Full time student ☐ Yes ☒ No
Address *88 West Road* City *Presley, CT*
Home phone *123-9674* Cell phone *203-998-5633*
Insured name *self* Insured date of birth *01/11/1984* Relationship to patient *self*
Insured employer *Aloisio Advertising Associates* Employer address *33 Park Ave, Presley, CT*
Insurance carrier *United Health Systems* ID# *XGA00443* Group # *4488*

HEALTH HISTORY

Have you ever suffered from:

☐ Asthma	☐ Fainting	☐ Muscle weakness	☐ Lower back pain
☐ Diabetes	☐ Anxiety	☒ Difficulty sleeping	☐ Difficulty swallowing
☐ High blood pressure	☐ Bleeding disorder	☐ Allergies	☐ Neck pain or stiffness
☒ Migraine headaches	☐ Constipation	☒ Stomach upset	☐ Diarrhea
☐ Fatigue	☒ Stress	☐ Mental disorder	☐ Infection

☐ Cancer (If so, what kind?) *none* ☒ Chronic pain (If so, where?) *neck and right shoulder*

FAMILY HISTORY

☒ Cancer (Who?) *mother* What type? *breast cancer (died last year)*
☒ High blood pressure (Who?) *father, mother*
☒ Diabetes (Who?) *father, grandmother*

MEDICATIONS AND SUPPLEMENTS

Do you take any medications?
If so, please list (include dosages):
Tylenol for headaches
Synthroid - 5 mg a day

Do you take any nutritional supplements?
If so, please list:
none

REASON FOR TODAY'S VISIT

☒ Check up
☐ Physical for school, sports, or employment
☒ Other (please explain) *painful urination*

Women only

Date of last menstrual period *4/2/09*
Number of pregnancies *0* Miscarriages? *0*
Number of children *0* Difficult or painful menstruation? *sometimes*

Men only

Have you ever had erectile difficulty? ______ Prostate problems? ______
Do you get up at night frequently to urinate? ______

I understand that Blueville Family Medicine will file my insurance for payment of services rendered. I also understand that I am responsible for any amount due Blueville Family Medicine if my insurance is denied.

Signature of patient or guardian *Michelle Calabrese* Date *04/15/09*

Relationship to patient ______

Robert Greer, MD • Sharon Piecek, APRN • Hector Rodriguez, MD • Henry Lee, MD • Anne Wilson, MD

Figure 18.16: Medical History form. (From Eagle: *The Professional Medical Assistant*. Philadelphia: FA Davis, 2009, p 232. With permission.)

Complete the Form

Study the following example of a partially completed medical history form for Stevie-Rose Davis. Notice what information is included and what information still needs to be collected. Then, complete a similar form for her husband, Zane Davis, using as much information as you can find in Chapters 5, 9, and 14.

PATIENT MEDICAL HISTORY

Patient's Name *Stevie-Rose Davis* Date of Birth ____________

	Yes	No
1. Are you in good health *OK*	☐	☑
2. Have there been any changes in your general health within the past year	☑	☐
3. Date of your last physical exam ____________		
4. Physician's name ____________ Address ____________ Phone no. ____________		
5. Are you under the care of a physician	☑	☐
6. Have you ever been hospitalized for any surgical operation or serious illness Please explain: *Thyroidectomy*	☑	☐
7. Are you taking any medicine(s) including non-prescription medicine If yes, what medicines are you taking *Insulin, Levothyroxin, Ibuprofen, Glucosamine*	☑	☐
8. Have you had any abnormal bleeding	☐	☐
9. Do you bruise easily	☐	☐
10. Have you ever required a blood transfusion	☐	☐
11. Have you had a recent weight loss	☐	☐
12. Have you ever taken Fen-Phen or Redux	☐	☐
13. Do you use tobacco	☐	☑
14. Do you or have you used controlled substances	☐	☐
15. Are you wearing contact lenses	☐	☐
16. Do you have any disease, condition or problem not listed above that you think I should know about	☐	☐
Women Only:		
Are you pregnant or think you may be pregnant	☐	☑
Are you nursing	☐	☑
Are you taking birth control pills	☐	☑

	Yes	No
Are you allergic to or have you had reactions to:		
Local anesthetics like novocaine	☐	☐
Penicillin or other antibiotics	☐	☐
Sulfa drugs	☐	☐
Barbiturates, sedatives or sleeping pills	☐	☐
Aspirin	☐	☐
Iodine	☐	☐
Any metals (e.g., nickel, mercury, etc.)	☐	☐
Latex/rubber	☐	☐
Other (please list) ____________		
Do you have or have you ever had the following:		
Rheumatic heart disease or rheumatic fever	☐	☐
Scarlet fever	☐	☐
Heart defect or heart murmur	☐	☐
Heart trouble, heart attack, or angina	☐	☐
Chest pain	☐	☐
Shortness of breath	☐	☐
Pacemaker	☐	☐
Heart surgery	☐	☐
High/low blood pressure	☐	☐
Congenital heart problems	☐	☐
Swelling of feet, ankles, hands	☐	☐
Hepatitis, jaundice or liver disease	☐	☐
Stroke	☐	☐
Sinus trouble	☐	☐
Lung or breathing problems	☐	☐
Asthma or hay fever	☐	☐
Hives or skin rash	☐	☐
Fainting or dizzy spells	☐	☐
Diabetes	☐	☐
AIDS or HIV infection	☐	☐
Thyroid problems	☑	☐
Allergies	☐	☐
Arthritis or rheumatism	☑	☐
Joint replacement or implant	☐	☐
Stomach ulcer	☐	☐
Kidney trouble	☐	☐
Tuberculosis	☐	☐
Persistent cough	☐	☐
Cough that produces blood	☐	☐
Chemotherapy (Cancer, leukemia)	☐	☐
Sexually transmitted disease	☐	☐
Epilepsy or seizures	☐	☐
Anemia	☐	☐
Glaucoma	☐	☐
Nervousness	☑	☐
Tonsillitis	☐	☐
Tumors	☐	☐
Mental health care	☐	☐
Back problems	☐	☐
Chemical dependency	☐	☐
Mitral valve prolapse	☐	☐
Cortisone treatment	☐	☐
Cold sores/fever blisters	☐	☐
Hypoglycemia	☑	☐
Eating disorders	☐	☐

PATIENT NUMBER ____________

HEALTH HISTORY

Figure 18.17: Partially completed medical history form for Stevie-Rose Davis

Zane Davis's medical history

Medical History

Are you under a physician's care now? ○ Yes ○ No If yes
Have you ever been hospitalized or had a major operation? ○ Yes ○ No If yes
Have you ever had a serious head or neck injury? ○ Yes ○ No If yes
Are you taking any medications, pills, or drugs? ○ Yes ○ No If yes
Do you take, or have you taken, Phen-Fen or Redux? ○ Yes ○ No
Have you ever taken Fosamax, Boniva, Actonel or any other medications containing bisphosphonates? ○ Yes ○ No
Are you on a special diet? ○ Yes ○ No
Do you use tobacco? ○ Yes ○ No
Do you use controlled substances? ○ Yes ○ No

Women: Are you
☐ Pregnant/Trying to get pregnant? ☐ Nursing?
☐ Taking oral contraceptives?

Are you allergic to any of the following?
☐ Aspirin ☐ Penicillin ☐ Codeine ☐ Local Anesthetics ☐ Acrylic ☐ Metal ☐ Latex ☐ Sulfa Drugs
☐ Other

Do you have, or have you had, any of the following? [Select "No" for all]

						Radiation Treatments	○ Yes ○ No
AIDS /HIV Positive	○ Yes ○ No	Cortisone Medicine	○ Yes ○ No	Hemophilia	○ Yes ○ No	Recent Weight Loss	○ Yes ○ No
Alzheimer's Disease	○ Yes ○ No	Diabetes	○ Yes ○ No	Hepatitis A	○ Yes ○ No	Renal Dialysis	○ Yes ○ No
Anaphylaxis	○ Yes ○ No	Drug Addiction	○ Yes ○ No	Hepatitis B or C	○ Yes ○ No	Rheumatic Fever	○ Yes ○ No
Anemia	○ Yes ○ No	Easily Winded	○ Yes ○ No	Herpes	○ Yes ○ No	Rheumatism	○ Yes ○ No
Angina	○ Yes ○ No	Emphysema	○ Yes ○ No	High Blood Pressure	○ Yes ○ No	Scarlet Fever	○ Yes ○ No
Arthritis/Gout	○ Yes ○ No	Epilepsy or Seizures	○ Yes ○ No	High Cholesterol	○ Yes ○ No	Shingles	○ Yes ○ No
Artificial Heart Valve	○ Yes ○ No	Excessive Bleeding	○ Yes ○ No	Hives or Rash	○ Yes ○ No	Sickle Cell Disease	○ Yes ○ No
Artificial Joint	○ Yes ○ No	Excessive Thirst	○ Yes ○ No	Hypoglycemia	○ Yes ○ No	Sinus Trouble	○ Yes ○ No
Asthma	○ Yes ○ No	Fainting Spells/Dizziness	○ Yes ○ No	Irregular Heartbeat	○ Yes ○ No	Spina Bifida	○ Yes ○ No
Blood Disease	○ Yes ○ No	Frequent Cough	○ Yes ○ No	Kidney Problems	○ Yes ○ No	Stomach/Intestinal Disease	○ Yes ○ No
Blood Transfusion	○ Yes ○ No	Frequent Diarrhea	○ Yes ○ No	Leukemia	○ Yes ○ No	Stroke	○ Yes ○ No
Breathing Problem	○ Yes ○ No	Frequent Headaches	○ Yes ○ No	Liver Disease	○ Yes ○ No	Swelling of Limbs	○ Yes ○ No
Bruise Easily	○ Yes ○ No	Genital Herpes	○ Yes ○ No	Low Blood Pressure	○ Yes ○ No	Thyroid Disease	○ Yes ○ No
Cancer	○ Yes ○ No	Glaucoma	○ Yes ○ No	Lung Disease	○ Yes ○ No	Tonsillitis	○ Yes ○ No
Chemotherapy	○ Yes ○ No	Hay Fever	○ Yes ○ No	Mitral Valve Prolapse	○ Yes ○ No	Tuberculosis	○ Yes ○ No
Chest Pains	○ Yes ○ No	Heart Attack/Failure	○ Yes ○ No	Osteoporosis	○ Yes ○ No	Tumors or Growths	○ Yes ○ No
Cold Sores/Fever Blisters	○ Yes ○ No	Heart Murmur	○ Yes ○ No	Pain in Jaw Joints	○ Yes ○ No	Ulcers	○ Yes ○ No
Congenital Heart Disorder	○ Yes ○ No	Heart Pacemaker	○ Yes ○ No	Parathyroid Disease	○ Yes ○ No	Venereal Disease	○ Yes ○ No
Convulsions	○ Yes ○ No	Heart Trouble/Disease	○ Yes ○ No	Psychiatric Care	○ Yes ○ No	Yellow Jaundice	○ Yes ○ No

Have you ever had any seroius illness not listed above? ○ Yes ○ No

Birth Date:

[New Med Hx] [Comments] [View Previous] [View Form(s)] Print Y/N Form ☐ [Print Form] [Print Blank Form] [Print Answers] [Save] [Cancel]

A forensic investigation of the accident

Dr. Haydel told the students in the lecture hall that the session was about to wind up. She wanted to draw their attention back to her opening comments about forensic sciences, to complete the story of the motor vehicle accident, and to show them how much information had been provided to them throughout their studies. Again, she brought up PowerPoint slides. Each slide contained a critical thinking question. This time she invited everyone in the audience to suggest and share answers.

Critical Thinking About the Accident

Think back over all that you have heard and read in this book. Then answer each question. Support your answers with evidence from the patient scenarios, and explain which character in the scenarios provided this evidence.

1. What was the cause of the motor vehicle accident? Was it one thing or a combination of several circumstances occurring at the same time? How do you know? Which characters provided the evidence for your conclusions about what actually happened?

____

____

____

2. Who was driving the car involved in the accident? Did more than one person say this was so? If so, who were they?

____

____

Taking a Closer Look

Patient Update

"Okay, everyone, let's get back together now. Students, it has been my pleasure to speak to you today. I have been honored to work with you through your case studies. And I congratulate you on your ability to use medical language—terminology in context. You've done exceedingly well."

"I know you've been working very hard on researching patients, so I'd like to end our discussion with a little bit of trivia—a little test of your awareness about some subtle information I noticed in your textbook. It's not specifically about medical terminology or medical language, but I think it's quite interesting. I'm going to ask you two questions. Take a look at the screen again while I pull them up. Those of you who brought your laptops can search the Web for answers. Feel free to throw out the answers as we go."

Critical Thinking

1. Stevie-Rose Davis seeks medical and psychological help at the A. L. Murphy Clinic. Who is/was A. L. Murphy and why is this name appropriate for this facility?

   ____

2. Glory Loeppky's family physician, Dr. Antoine, works at the Mary Ezra Mahoney Clinic. Who was/is this Ms. Mahoney and why is the clinic named in her honor?

   ____

Moving On

You have now completed your course in medical language. The goal of this course has been to help you move beyond the boring memorization of terms. Instead, you were encouraged to read and listen to medical language as it is actually used in the context of the assessment, treatment, and rehabilitation of patients. By reading and listening to medical language in the context of five case studies, you have begun to understand the importance of using correct medical terminology in describing, explaining, and discussing the health challenges of real people. You have listened to the kind of language that doctors, nurses, and allied health professionals use among themselves and with their patients. And you have practiced applying that language in your own oral and written communication, in realistic "on the job" scenarios, especially in the documents that make up the medical records of patients' care.

Your learning of medical language in context has given you a strong foundation for communication in whatever medical or allied health profession you decide to pursue. And your memories of the fictional patients you have encountered in this book should help you in the months and years to come, as you begin to put your medical language to work in the service of real patients or clients in your chosen profession.

CHAPTER SUMMARY

In Chapter 18, you combined all of your new language skills and vocabulary and applied them in new ways to case studies. The chapter introduced the concepts of forensic science and forensic medicine. It demonstrated, through specific examples, the importance of attention to detail, specificity, and accuracy in all documentation and communication in health care. These concepts were linked to the clinical practices of completing forms and interpreting charts. The importance of formal and professional medical terminology as the basis for this communication was emphasized repeatedly.

For audio exercises, visit http://www.MedicalLanguageLab.com. 

Key Terms

cipher
ciphertext
code
composition
decomposition
electronic health records (EHRs)
electronic medical records (EMRs)
hospital code
incident report
jargon
mechanism
mechanisms of injury
medical code
user authentication protocol

CHAPTER REVIEW

Critical Thinking

As you answer these questions, think carefully about what Dr. Haydel said about the commonalities between the health sciences and forensic sciences.

1. If you choose a career in health or forensic sciences, what is the purpose of studying medical terminology?

____

2. If you worked in medical billing or for a health insurance provider, why might you study medical terminology? Provide an example of why medical terminology is important in each job setting.

____

Reflective Questions

1. In health care, what does *coded language* mean?

____

2. What is the difference between a medical *coder* and a medical *biller*?

____

Translate the Terminology

Imagine that you have come across the following summary reports written by the physicians caring for our patients, either at Okla Trauma Center or Fayette General Hospital. Use your cumulative knowledge of anatomy, physiology, medical terminology, and patient care to translate the following excerpts into everyday English.

1. Excerpt from the summary report by Dr. Hamidi, neurologist, regarding Gil Loeppky:

   Nursing staff are monitoring physical symptoms secondary to the injury, including impairment of balance and coordination and seizure activity. The extent of these may have residual effects on vocational potential.

____
____
____

2. Excerpt from the summary report by Dr. Bedard, obstetrician, regarding Glory Loeppky:

   Mrs. Loeppky underwent a Pfannenstiel incision during the C-section in which the peritoneal layers were sutured subsequent to having sutured the uterus in two layers.

____
____

3. Excerpt from summary report by Dr. Jasper, pediatrician, regarding Emily Grace Loeppky:

   Infant was removed from continuous oxygen prior to 32 wks gestation. This is a good predictor of normal respiratory outcomes.

   ____

   ____

4. Excerpt from consult report by Dr. Shawshank, endocrinologist, regarding Stevie-Rose Davis:

   Since hypothyroidism cannot be strictly ruled out for its contribution to significant neurocognitive deficits that may lead to a misdiagnosis of dementia, particularly in the elderly, periodic re-assessment of mental status (perhaps annually) should not be overlooked for its potential to determine possible endocrine involvement and provide early intervention.

   ____

   ____

   ____

Let's Practice

You have learned that the context in which words appear may determine how they should be interpreted. You have also learned that words are coded or encrypted for a wide variety of reasons. Complete the following table by writing the different meanings that the same abbreviation can have in different contexts.

Defining Abbreviations and Acronyms in Context

Abbreviation or Acronym	Medical Definition	Definition in Another Context (including text messaging)
PA		
Fx		
pc		
BR		
BS		
SOB		
NS		
OB		
K		

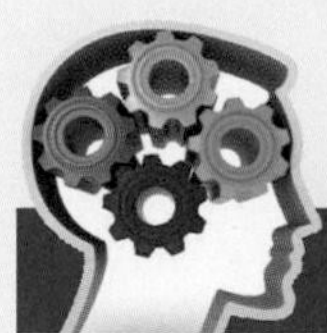

MEMORY MAGIC

To continue the work you have been doing with coded language, here are a few more mnemonics you might find helpful.

1. Completing a Glasgow Coma Scale: **MOVE**

   M = motor assessment

   O = open eyes

   V = verbal assessment

   E = estimate the score

2. Four Abdominal Muscles = **TIRE**

   T = transversus

   I = internal oblique

   R = rectus abdominus

   E = external oblique

3. Clinical manifestations of influenza = **FLU**

   F = fever

   L = lethargy

   U = upset stomach (nausea and/or vomiting)

APPENDIX

Answer Key

UNIT ONE

Introduction

Chapter 1: Context and Word Structure: The Keys to Learning Language

Reflective questions (p. 4)

1. *(Answers will vary.)*
2. *(Answers will vary.)*
3. *(Answers will vary.)*

Free writing (p. 7)

1. *Boat* and *house* are both root words.
2. Sample answers: *houses, housed, housing*
3. Sample answers: *boats, boated, boater, boating, boatful*
4. *(Answers will vary.)*
5. Some words are made up of two root words that are combined into one compound word.

Let's practice (p. 8)

1. pneum(o) - lungs; bio - life; ven(i/o) - vein or blood
2. esophagi - throat or gullet; hem(o/ato) - blood
   fract - break; orbi(to) - circular or around the eyes
3. myo - muscle; card(i) - heart
4. contra - against; nephron - kidneys

Break it down (p. 9)

1. root words: *thigh, bone*
2. root words: *collar, bone*
3. medical root: *fract*
4. medical root: *gastr*
5. medical root: *pneumo*

Let's practice (p. 10)

1. o
2. o
3. o
4. a
5. i

Break it down (p. 13)

1. ab-; away from
2. pre-; before
3. sang-; blood red
4. noct-; night
5. pre-; before
6. cyan-; blue
7. micro-; small

Build a word (p. 14)

1. e- (evacuate)
2. hypo- (hypoglycemia)
3. intra- (intravenous)
4. hyper- (hyperventilating)
5. hetero- (heterosexual)
6. leuko- (leukocyte)
7. epi- (epidermal)
8. sym- (symbiotic)

Mix and match: prefixes (p. 14)

1. hyperglycemia; high blood sugar levels
2. preoperative; occurring before surgery
3. atypical; not typical
4. polyuria; excessive production of urine
5. microorganism; a life form that is very small
6. disjointed; taken apart at the joints
7. semiconscious; half or partly conscious
8. postpartum; occurring after birth

Fill in the blanks (p. 15)

1. unconscious
2. blind
3. immobile
4. ill / unwell / sick
5. firm / rigid
6. loose
7. relaxed
8. relaxation / flexion / extension
9. grief / unhappiness
10. closing

Build a word (p. 15)

1. immobile
2. antibacterial
3. atypical
4. unmedicated
5. nonmedicinal
6. disequilibrium
7. unable
8. immobilize
9. noncompliant
10. misdiagnosed

Let's practice (p. 16)

1. balance
2. complete
3. operable
4. resectable
5. lodged

Mix and match: suffixes with roots (p. 22)

1. gynecology; the medical specialty that focuses on the female reproductive organs
2. orbital; related to the area around the eye
3. tonsillitis; inflammation of the tonsils *or* tonsillectomy; the surgical removal of the tonsils
4. appendicitis; inflammation of the appendix *or* appendectomy; the surgical removal of the appendix
5. carcinogen; a substance that causes cancer
6. sonogram; a diagnostic image produced with the use of sound waves
7. audible; able to be heard *or* audiology; the medical study of hearing
8. chemotherapy; treatment with the use of drugs
9. physician; a doctor
10. sarcoma; a tumor of the flesh

Break it down (p. 23)

1. -ed (dislocated); -ing (skiing); -ful (painful); -er (upper)
2. -pathy (neuropathy); -ed (generalized)
3. -ed (suffered); -ed (infected); -ectomy (tonsillectomy); -ed (resolved)
4. -ed (diagnosed); -ia (anemia); -ing (according)
5. -icians (Physicians); -ists (oncologists); -ed (registered)

Free writing (p. 23)

Sample answers

1. -itis; The patient with *dermatitis* had an itchy red rash on the skin of her swollen right hand.
2. -ian; The *physician* in the clinic examined the patient.
3. -algia; Walking is difficult for Brendan because he has *myalgia* and has pain in his legs.
4. -centesis; The pregnant woman was scheduled for *amniocentesis* to determine the health of her fetus.
5. -oma; People who work outdoors can develop *melanoma* or skin cancer as a result of exposure to the sun's ultraviolet rays.
6. -scope; A *gastroscope* is used to look inside the stomach.
7. -ory; The patient was experiencing *auditory* hallucinations or hearing voices that were not real.
8. -scopy; The doctor ordered a *colonoscopy* to view the patient's bowel.
9. -ician; A *pediatrician* is a doctor who works with children.

Let's practice (p. 24)

1. -pathy, -osis, -ia, -itis, -ism, -algia, -asthenia, -oma
2. -ment, -t/ion, -y
3. -ed
4. -er, -est
5. -algia
6. -centesis
7. -ist, -ician, -ian
8. -scope, -scopy
9. -ectasis

Let's practice (p. 25)

1. traumata
2. pelves
3. lumina
4. emboli
5. vertebrae
6. bacteria
7. diverticula
8. viscera
9. indices
10. appendices
11. thoraces
12. prognoses
13. diagnoses
14. neuroses
15. specialists
16. specialties
17. urologists
18. sciences
19. pharmacokinetics
20. pharynges

Right word or wrong word: ileo or ilio? (p. 26)
The combining form *ili/o/a* refers to a bone in the pelvis.

Right word or wrong word: dilation or dilatation? (p. 26)
Actually, they both mean the same thing (i.e., the process of expanding or widening), although *dilatation* is used more often for expansive discussions.

Right word or wrong word: diagnose, diagnosis, or diagnoses? (p. 26)
Q: *diagnosis* or *diagnoses:* Which word means more than one?

A: *Diagnoses* is the plural form of the noun *diagnosis.*

Q: *diagnoses:* Is it a verb or a noun?

A: It is both, although the noun and the verb have slightly different pronunciations. *Diagnoses* is used as a verb this sentence: "Dr. Smith diagnoses clients with skin rashes."

Diagnoses is used as noun in this sentence: "The frail elderly woman has multiple diagnoses that cause her to require home nursing care."

Chapter review

What do you know? (p. 27)
1. Body parts
2. In medicine, prefixes generally alert you to size, shape, color, and status.
3. Nouns that name pathologies, diagnostic or surgical procedures, and health professions or fields of medicine

Break it down (p. 27)
1. gynec/o = combining form of root; logy = root
2. post = prefix; operat = combining form of root; ive = suffix
3. anti = prefix; epilept = root; ic = suffix
4. contra = prefix; indica/t = combining form of root; ed = suffix
5. hema/t = root; ur = root; ia = suffix
6. thyroid = root; ectomy = suffix
7. pneumo = root; thorax = root
8. poly = prefix; un = prefix; saturat = combining form of root; ed = suffix
9. cerebro = combing form of root; spin = combining form of root; al = suffix
10. hyper = prefix; irrit = combining form of root; ability = suffix

Translate the terminology (p. 27)
Sample answers
1. The break in the shoulder blade is in the middle of the bone.
2. The client is breathing very, very quickly and in excess of what is normal or healthy.
3. The patient is having difficulty breathing.
4. Their patient has an abdominal injury that is causing bleeding inside of the abdominal cavity.
5. He would like to demonstrate a new instrument for measuring something about a patient's eyes (i.e., their refractive power).

Define the root (p. 28)
1. blood
2. blood sugars
3. feet
4. joints
5. muscles

Name the root (p. 28)
1. inert
2. tonsil
3. oste(o) / oss(a)
4. gastr/i/o
5. bio

Define the prefix (p. 28)

1. before
2. before
3. large or long
4. same or equal
5. outside of or without

Critical thinking (p. 28)

1. sciences
2. urologists
3. neurosis
4. appendix
5. vertebrae
6. bacteria
7. diagnoses
8. radiography

Chapter 2: Naming and Describing: Medical Language for the Body

Reflective questions (p. 32)

1. EMTs and at least 1 paramedic
2. She is confused about her whereabouts, why she is there, why her husband is nearby, and what has happened to her.
3. *(Answers will vary, but may include: shock, preliminary assessment, external injuries, ambulant, trauma, neurological assessment, fine tremor, disfigurement, palpate, cranium, cervical spine, proximal point, bilateral assessment, temporal pulses, mandible, clavicle, cardiovascular impairment, integumentary, circulatory, musculoskeletal, lower extremities.)*
4. *(Answers will vary.)*

Right word or wrong word: rescue unit or ambulance? (p. 34)

Rescue units generally belong to fire departments, but they contain all of the necessary equipment and supplies to rescue victims, as well as to treat them on the spot during an emergency. They are also equipped with the necessities for the administration of first aid. Ambulances do not contain rescue equipment, but they do have emergency medical equipment and first-aid capacities.

Build a word (p. 38)

1. skeletal system
2. respiratory system
3. reproductive system
4. gastrointestinal or digestive system
5. integumentary system

Mix and match (p. 38)

1. urinary system
2. respiratory system
3. muscular system
4. neurological system
5. immune system

Let's practice (p. 40)

1. cardiovascular / circulatory, muscular
2. urinary
3. gastrointestinal / digestive
4. neurological
5. integumentary
6. reproductive, endocrine
7. respiratory, muscular
8. muscular
9. gastrointestinal / digestive
10. respiratory
11. cardiovascular / circulatory
12. reproductive, endocrine
13. endocrine
14. endocrine
15. urinary
16. gastrointestinal / digestive

Critical thinking (p. 41)

1. Be careful. This question is not about sight; it is about a body part. The answer is yes, you can live without physically having an eyeball. However, if a sudden injury or a severe trauma was to occur to the eyeball in the form of an incoming projectile, the eyeball and the brain may both be pierced, thereby causing imminent if not immediate death.
2. Yes, it is possible to live without a stomach. In some cases, the stomach can be removed or bypassed; the esophagus will be connected directly to the intestines. The stomach is not essential or vital to life.
3. Yes, it is possible to live without your large intestine. For patients with certain disease states, the colon is removed and replaced with a colostomy bag that is worn outside of the body or with a small sac that is sutured inside the abdomen that functions as a pseudocolon.
4. No, having both kidneys is not vital; you can live quite well with only one kidney. In addition, with the help of a kidney dialysis machine, you can live without functional kidneys.

Right word or wrong word: colon or large intestine? (p. 41)

Yes, these terms can be used interchangeably. The colon consists of 5 anatomical divisions: the cecum, the ascending colon, the transverse colon, the descending colon, and the sigmoid colon. Together, these form the colon or the large intestine.

Build a word (p. 43)

1. peri + cardi + al = pericardial
2. periton + eal = peritoneal
3. pleur + al = pleural
4. peri + cardi+ um = (parietal) pericardium
5. periton + e (combining vowel) + um = visceral peritoneum

Fill in the blanks (p. 45)

1. cranial
2. pelvic
3. thoracic
4. abdominal
5. pelvic

Fill in the blanks (p. 47)

1. anterior / ventral
2. superior
3. proximal; distal
4. inferior / caudal
5. medial
6. lateral
7. distal
8. deep
9. superficial
10. dorsal / posterior

Mix and match (p. 47)

1. deep
2. posterior
3. ventral
4. superior
5. medial
6. distal

Let's practice (p. 49)

1. Rotation
2. To step up, the patient will have to flex and extend his knees; to flex, extend, and abduct his legs one at a time; and to use dorsiflexion and plantarflexion.
3. To put his hands together, the patients must extend both the hands and the fingers first. The thumbs will abduct radially away from the side of the hand and toward the radial bone. Then, as the hands come together, the patient will flex the fingers and adduct them inward toward the palm. Finally, the thumb will flex over the dorsal aspect of the hand.
4. Abduction of an arm, extension of an arm, extension of the fingers, and flexion of the fingers
5. Flexion of the knees and hips

Let's practice (p. 51)

1. horizontal
2. frontal
3. median

Fill in the blanks (p. 53)

1. cyano-
2. erythro-
3. micro-
4. macro-
5. hemi-
6. bi-

Chapter review

Critical thinking (p. 55)

1. Fowler's positions / Semi-Fowler's position
2. Transverse plane
3. Distal
4. Flexion

Break it down (p. 55)

1. ir (prefix)+ radi (root) + ate (suffix)
2. dis (prefix) + figur/e (combining form of root) + ment (suffix)
3. re (prefix) + product (root) + ive (suffix)

Translate the terminology (p. 56)

1. She felt the top of the patient's skull and the top of the patient's backbone, behind the neck.
2. Because the patient was able to move on her own and walk on her own, the EMT made a decision to keep walking with her over to the median.
3. She examined the facial bones beginning at a midway and central point of the nose, just at the top along the brow line. She then moved outward to examine the left and right sides of the face to get an assessment of both sides.

Label the body cavities (p. 56)

1. Cranial
2. Vertebral canal
3. Thoracic
4. Diaphragm
5. Abdominal
6. Pelvic
7. Ventral
8. Abdominopelvic

Name the root (p. 56)

1. circ (circulatory system)
2. crin/krin (endocrine system)
3. integ (integumentary system)
4. periton (peritoneum)

Name the prefix (p. 57)

1. erythro-, rubeo-, sangui-
2. ex-
3. ir-, in-, im-
4. multi-, poly-
5. uni-, mono-

Mix and match (p. 57)

1. adduct
2. extension
3. distal
4. median/medial
5. dorsal
6. posterior

UNIT TWO

The Language of Assessment

Chapter 3: Physical Assessment

Reflective questions (p. 62)

1. Fayette General Hospital
2. The status of the patient's fetus, the patient's wound and laceration status, and the possible fracture or dislocation of the patient's left thumb
3. No
4. Fetal monitor, CBC, hematocrit, HGB, ultrasound, and x-ray
5. Assisting the doctor with suturing the patient's leg wound

Let's practice (p. 67)

1. client / patient
2. triage
3. presents
4. circulation
5. registered

Fill in the blanks (p. 67)

1. emergency
2. urgently
3. presenting
4. urgent; emergent
5. presents

Right word or wrong word: oriented or orientated? (p. 68)

Answer: Yes and No. This is an interesting piece of trivia.

Orient is the root of both of these words. It is derived from Latin, and it means either *to rise* or *East* (because the sun rises in the East). As a noun, *Orient* refers to the Eastern part of the world: Asia. As a verb, *orient* means *to familiarize yourself or someone or something to a new situation* or *to align yourself.* Technically, *orientate* means *to turn your position to face the East,* whereas *orient* means *to familiarize.* The answers to the previous questions are both "yes" and "no" because, in the 21st century, these terms are often used interchangeably. However, if you wish to use proper terms and to improve your own language skills, you will want to use *orient* rather than *orientate*.

Free writing (p. 71)

Sample answers

1. The patient bleeds easily because he has *hemophilia* and his blood lacks the ability to clot.
2. If an artery is cut (severed), it is very likely that the patient will *hemorrhage* or bleed excessively.
3. The infant has a *hemangioma*, which is a temporary tumor on his or her skin.
4. The deep red color of the patient's blood indicated that it was rich in the pigment *hemoglobin*.
5. The doctor used a tool called a *hemostat* to compress the patient's blood vessel and stop the bleeding.

Right word or wrong word: hematocyturia or hematuria? (p. 71)

These words have the same meaning. Both refer to a condition in which there is blood in the urine.

Let's practice (p. 73)

1. sanguiferous
2. serosanguineous
3. sanguiferous
4. exsanguinate

Mix and match (p. 75)

1. red blood cells
2. respond to allergies or inflammation by releasing histamine
3. provide an immune defense
4. counter allergic reactions by releasing histamine
5. white blood cells

Critical thinking (p. 76)

1. a. Anemia; b. RBC and HGB to test for anemia
2. a. Eosinophils and basophils levels will be determined to ascertain whether the patient's condition is an allergic reaction or a parasitic invasion (although symptoms of parasites would not likely appear until some days later). The doctor may also order lymphocyte and leukocyte counts to see if the patient was infected with something.

Let's practice (p. 79)

1. tibialis anterior
2. vastus lateralis
3. trapezius
4. sartorius
5. flexor carpi radialis

Free writing (p. 83)

Sample answers

1. A diagnosis of *myasthenia* may be given to a person who has weakening of his or her muscles or whose muscles tire easily.
2. A *myovascular* condition is one in which there is an insufficiency of blood making it to the muscles.
3. When the bones and muscles work together, the *musculoskeletal* system gives us the ability to stand erect.
4. The name for diseases of the muscles is *myopathy*.
5. A condition in which there could be persistent twitching of the eye is *myokymia*.

Name the term and break it down (p. 83)

1. myalgia = my + algia: The word part *my* (combining form of root *my/o*) means *muscle;* the root *algia* means *pain*.
2. electromyography = electro + myo + graph + y: The root *electro* means *electricity*. The root *myo* means *muscle*. The root *graph* means *record* or *writing*. The suffix *-y* means *the act of.*
3. myo + kym + ia = myokymia: The root *myo* means *muscles*. The root *kym* means *wave*. The suffix *-ia* means *the state of.*
4. muscular = muscul + ar: *Muscul-* is the combining form of the root that means *muscle*. The suffix *-ar* means *pertaining to.*
5. polymyalgia = poly + my + algia: The prefix *poly* means *many*. The combining form *my* means *muscles*. The root *algia* means *pain*.

Fill in the blanks (p. 85)

1. Striae gravidarum
2. eviscerate
3. viscer/a/o

Name the term and break it down (p. 87)

1. tendoplasty = tendo + plasty: *Tendo* is the root of *tendon*. The suffix *-plasty* means *to mold.*
2. fibromyalgia = fibro + my + algia: The word part *fibro* is the root of *fiber*. The word part *my* is the combining form of *my/o,* which means *muscle*. The root *algia* means *pain.*
3. fasciitis = fasci + itis: The root *fasci* means *small bundle*. The suffix *-itis* means *inflammation.*
4. ligament = root word

Let's practice (p. 88)

1. muscles
2. musculoskeletal system
3. fascicules
4. tendon
5. fascia

Fill in the blanks (p. 89)

1. contracting / flexing
2. voluntary control
3. extending
4. opposition / opposing

Right word or wrong word: ligament or tendon? (p. 89)

No, they are not the same. Although they both consist of strong fibrous connective tissue, ligaments connect bones to bones, whereas tendons connect muscles to bones.

Fill in the blanks (p. 92)

1. temporalis
2. Gastrocnemius
3. rectus abdominus
4. erector spinae
5. quadriceps
6. frontalis
7. transverse abdominus
8. gluteus maximus
9. pectoralis major; pectoralis minor
10. trapezius

Mix and match (p. 94)

1. is
2. us
3. maximus
4. spinae
5. lateralis
6. viscerate
7. myopathy

Right word or wrong word: brachi/o or bracchi/o vs. brachy-? (p. 94)

No. *Brachys* means *slow*. It is the root of the combining form *brachy-*. *Brachium* means *arm*. It is the root of the combining forms *brachi/o* and *bracchi/o*.

Let's practice (p. 94)

1. temporalis
2. spinae
3. abdominus
4. trapezius
5. erector

Reflective questions (p. 96)

1. Glory has been sent to sonography for the assessment of her fetus and the assessment of the structures of her abdomen, because she has been in a motor vehicle accident.
2. No. Protocol demands that only the physician interpret the results of a sonogram to a patient.
3. Yes. The anesthetic will not harm the fetus.

Right word or wrong word: sonogram or ultrasound? (p. 97)

Not really, although this is very commonly done, and you should expect to hear it. However, if you want to build the best professional vocabulary possible, please choose to use the correct term. A *sonogram* is a graphical representation of a sound that is emitted by the ultrasound machine; it is a picture that is made of sound or echoes. The term *ultrasound* means *high-frequency sounds or sound waves that are used in medicine.* The word *ultrasound* is usually used to refer to the machine, the equipment, and the procedure but not the pictures that are made via the procedure.

Critical thinking (p. 97)

1. There is no exposure to x-ray radiation when using ultrasound. Radiation in any amount is considered a risk for harm in a developing fetus.
2. This is a procedure during which nothing physically enters or penetrates the body.
3. Abdominal sonography
4. Sonographer or ultrasound technician

Free writing (p. 98)

Sample answers

1. A *sonograph* is the record of pictures that are taken with the use of high-frequency sound waves.
2. A *sonographer* is a professional who examines people with the use of an ultrasound machine.

Fill in the blanks (p. 100)

1. protocol
2. triage
3. obstetrician
4. Gynecology
5. ER physician / attending physician

Critical thinking (p. 100)

1. A 3-month period of time
2. Three
3. During the first trimester

Let's practice (p. 101)

1. subjective
2. human chorionic gonadotropin (This is a blood test to determine pregnancy.)
3. pain or discomfort; the location of the fetus in the abdomen; the position of fetus, fetal movement
4. Vaginal

Chapter review

Critical thinking (p. 103)

1. Touch for assessment or examination purposes
2. A radiologist or a physician
3. The client or patient
4. Glory is in her third trimester. She informed the medical staff that she was 7 ½ months pregnant, which puts her in her third trimester of pregnancy.

Name the term (p. 103)

1. brachioradialis
2. pectoralis
3. femoris
4. trapezius

Break it down (p. 103)

1. hemat (combining form of the root that means *blood*) + ology (root meaning *study*)
2. sono (root meaning *sound*) + graph (root meaning *record*)
3. fibro (root for *fiber*) + *my* (combining form of *my/o,* meaning *muscle*) + *algia* (root for *pain*)

Translate the terminology (p. 104)

1. Dr. Abrams informed Glory Loeppky that it was safe to use something to numb her skin during the last third of her pregnancy (i.e., between weeks 29 and 40 of the pregnancy).
2. When she arrived at the emergency room, Glory was reported to be aware of what day it was, who she was, and where she was.
3. Dr. Abrams applied a tool to stop excessive bleeding from the cut on Glory's leg.
4. The medical professional used a device that emitted sound waves to view Glory's unborn child.

Fill in the blanks (p. 104)

1. gyne-: gynecology
2. hemo-: hemorrhage
3. quadri-: quadriceps
4. poly-: polymyalgia

Name the suffix (p. 104)

1. -ation / -tion
2. -plasty
3. -itis
4. -ency
5. -ous / -eous

Chapter 4: Diagnostic Imaging

Reflective questions (p. 108)

1. EMT Stanley is talking to the emergency physician, Dr. Raymond.
2. Professional protocol usually demands that you do not address an adult patient by his or her first name until he or she has given you permission to do so.
3. The phrase is *loss of consciousness*.
4. The term is created from *hemat* (combing form of root), which refers to blood, and *oma* (root), which usually refers to a tumor. *Orbit* (combining form of root) refers to a circle and the area around eye, and *-al* is a suffix that means *relating to*. In plain English, the EMT is reporting that the patient has an area of swelling and discoloration around his left eye that appears to be more significant than simple bruising. In this case, *oma* does not refer to a cancerous tumor but rather suggests a swollen mass of tissue under the skin.

Fill in the blanks (p. 112)

1. radiograph
2. radium; radioactive
3. radiation
4. radiology; radiologist

Let's practice (p. 112)

1. Radiologist, radiologic technologist (RT), and radiological nurse (R-RN)
2. The physician in the Emergency Department, Dr. Raymond
3. The physician in the Emergency Department, Dr. Raymond

Right word or wrong word: Ra or RA? (p. 113)

Ra is the chemical symbol for radium.

RA is an abbreviation for rheumatoid arthritis. Notice that RA is written with capital letters.

Fill in the blanks (p. 113)

1. radiologist
2. x-ray / radiography
3. radiological nurse
4. radiologist
5. medical imaging

Fill in the blanks (p. 115)

1. frontal
2. cranial
3. spinal
4. thoracic
5. cervical
6. pelvic

Right word or wrong word: radiology or medical imaging? (p. 115)

Radiology is the science and study of radiation and radioactive substances. *Medical imaging* is the process of taking images of the body with the use of radiation, as well as other means.

Let's practice (p. 117)

1. The cerebellum
2. The cranium
3. The cerebrum / the brain
4. Quadriplegia
5. Epilepsy

Right word or wrong word: contusion or concussion? (p. 117)

A *contusion* is a form of bruising. Contusions are localized to the area of injury, but the skin is not broken. Blood vessels near the surface are broken thereby causing temporary swelling, discoloration, and pain. Contusions can occur anywhere on or within the body; they are not always associated with a skull fracture or severe jostling of the brain. However, if either of these was to occur, then subdural and epidural hematomas that may arise from a contusion can lead to a seizure disorder or permanent brain injury.

A *concussion* is an injury to the brain, such as that which may occur as a result of a blow or a fall that has an impact on the head. Violent shaking can also cause a concussion if the brain is jarred against the skull. A concussion may cause partial or complete loss of function, as well as alterations in mental status Concussions are not localized to the area of injury but rather generalized to a greater area.

We'll learn more about concussions and contusions when we meet this patient again in Unit 10.

Break it down (p. 120)

1. neuro (root) + transmit (English root word meaning *send*) + er (suffix meaning *person or thing that does something*)
2. neuro (root) + path (root meaning *disease*) + y (suffix meaning *state or condition*)
3. neuro (root) + log (root or suffix meaning *study of*) + ical (suffix meaning *associated with or belonging to*))
4. neuro (root) + n (combining consonant) + al (suffix meaning *relating to*)
5. neur (root) + algia (suffix meaning *pain*)

Break it down (p. 121)

1. cerebro (root meaning *brain*) + physio (root meaning *nature*) + -logy (suffix or root meaning *study of*)
2. cerebro (root) + vasc/vascu/i (root meaning *blood vessel*) + -ar (suffix meaning *relating to*)
3. cerebr (root) + a (combining vowel) + -tion (suffix meaning *the state of something resulting from an action*)
4. cerebr (root) + otom (root meaning *incision*) + -y (suffix meaning *state or condition*)

Let's practice (p. 121)

1. cerebral
2. neurologist
3. cerebellum
4. neuron
5. neurotransmitter
6. neurosurgeon
7. cerebrum
8. neurosis
9. cerebrophysiology
10. neurological system

Critical thinking (p. 122)

1. Half of a sphere or half of a round object
2. Because of its spherical and divided shape
3. In the cerebrum
4. To control the pituitary gland and to regulate sleep, appetite, and emotions
5. The medulla oblongata
6. The pons and the medulla oblongata together

Let's practice (p. 123)

1. The pituitary gland
2. The mesencephalon or the midbrain
3. The medulla oblongata
4. The thalamus

Let's practice (p. 124)

1. The frontal lobe
2. The occipital lobe
3. The temporal lobe(s)

Fill in the blanks (p. 124)

1. anterior
2. caudal
3. superior; posterior
4. anterior

Critical thinking (p. 125)

1. Stupor
2. Glasgow Coma Scale
3. Neurovitals
4. A nurse
5. Coma
6. Dysfunction
7. Hypersomnia

Critical thinking (p. 127)

Sample answer

Mr. Loeppky's symptoms place him in the middle column. Working from top to bottom, the decision to place him there is based on what has already been shared about the patient: he has lost consciousness, but no one has ever mentioned a penetrating wound (although he does have a laceration near his eye). He is a medium risk and he has certainly been in a "dangerous situation": the motor vehicle accident.

Fill in the blanks (p. 127)

1. Blood
2. cerebrospinal
3. bilateral
4. Rhinorrhea
5. Otorrhea
6. periorbital hematoma

Break it down (p. 129)

1. rhino (root meaning *nose*) + -rrhea (suffix meaning *flow or discharge*)
2. peri- (prefix meaning *around*) + orbit (root meaning *circle*) + -al (suffix meaning *belonging to or related to*)
3. bi- (prefix meaning *two*) + lateral (root meaning *side*) + -ly (suffix meaning *in a certain way*)
4. uni- (prefix meaning *one*) + lateral (root meaning *side*) + -ly (suffix meaning *in a certain way*)
5. dys- (prefix meaning *not or difficult*) + arthr/ia/o (root meaning *joint or articulation*)

Let's practice (p. 129)

1. uni = one
2. un = not
3. dys = not or difficult
4. peri = around
5. dys = not or difficult
6. hyper = above or in excess of normal
7. hemi = half or partial
8. hypo = less than normal

Right word or wrong word: trauma or injury? (p. 129)

Trauma has a more specific meaning. A trauma is a severe and possibly life-threatening injury or wound that is often physical but may also be psychological. This root word originates in Greek. Plural forms are *traumas* or *traumata*.

Injury is a more general term. An injury may or may not be traumatic, but it does cause some form of damage to the body. In medicine, traumatic injuries can be amputations, burns, lacerations, or the result of penetration by an object.

Let's practice (p. 133)

1. mandible
2. vertebrae / spine
3. metacarpals
4. phalanges
5. metatarsals
6. ulna
7. coccyx
8. femur
9. patella
10. clavicle

Let's practice (p. 133)

1. vertebrae / spine
2. femur
3. mandible
4. metatarsals
5. radius
6. scapulae
7. pelvis
8. lumbar / lumbar spine
9. coccyx
10. rib / ribs / ribcage

Free writing (p. 135)

Sample answers

1. The elderly patient has swelling in the joints of his fingers, so the doctor may suspect that he has osteoarthritis.
2. The process of ossification must be proceeding too slowly in the child, because he has soft bones; they are not as hard or dense as they should be.
3. The doctors suspect that either the periosteum (the covering of the bones) is inflamed or that the patient has osteitis.

Critical thinking (p. 136)

1. Mr. Loeppky's femur, talus, and tibia are fractured.
2. The surgical treatment of fractures takes precedence because bones begin to repair themselves quickly. Osteoblasts or bone-forming cells immediately begin their healing work. In the case of a fracture, however, if the bones are not reset or realigned into their proper positions, then the injured person runs the risk of never being able to properly use or bear weight on them again.

Build a word (p. 138)

1. femorotibial
2. femoral
3. femora
4. tibial
5. tibiofemoral
6. tibiofibular
7. tibiotarsal
8. patellar
9. patellectomy
10. patellofemoral

Break it down (p. 139)

1. thorac/o + -ic
2. calvicul/o + -ar
3. cervic/o + -al
4. humer/o + -al
5. mandibul/o + -ar

Mix and match (p. 139)

1. shoulder, hip
2. wrist
3. elbow, knee
4. neck

Build a word (p. 140)

1. arthritis
2. articulate
3. bursitis

Mix and match (p. 141)

1. lumbar spine
2. coccyx
3. disc
4. cartilaginous joint
5. vertebrae
6. synovial fluid

Chapter review

Critical thinking (p. 143)

1. Mr. Loeppky's black eyes are the result of blunt force trauma to his brow and the top of his nose.
2. The nurse needs to monitor Mr. Loeppky's neurovital signs, because he may regain consciousness or slip deeper into unconsciousness and coma.
3. A CT scan and x-rays
4. A facial injury
5. A head-to-toe approach
6. A head-to-toe assessment begins at the head (i.e., the top of the body) and then proceeds right down to the toes.

Break it down (p. 144)

1. compound word: radi/o + graph (both roots)
2. vertebr (combining form of root) + -al (suffix)
3. cran/i (root) + -al (suffix)

Translate the terminology (p. 144)

Sample answers

1. Mrs. Davis is experiencing pain and stiffness in her joints as a result of swelling in these areas. The disease that she has is called *arthritis.*
2. Evan may have a nerve disease or condition that is causing his symptoms.

Fill in the blanks (p. 144)

1. Radi-
2. Neuro-

Name the root (p. 144)

1. oss/a
2. arthr
3. neuro

Name the suffix (p. 144)

1. -ic / -al
2. -t/ion
3. -algia
4. -itis
5. -ian / -cian / -ist

Chapter 5: Laboratory Diagnostics

Reflective questions (p. 148)

1. Mr. Zane Davis
2. Dr. Crowchild and EMT Orantes
3. Assessing for a cardiovascular accident (i.e., heart attack or myocardial infarction) or a cerebrovascular accident (i.e., stroke)
4. A blood test called a *complete blood count*
5. (1) Because he told the EMT that he has a history of a "bad heart"
   (2) Because he is elderly and elderly patients have the potential to deteriorate rapidly
6. An ECG is being done, and blood work has been ordered. The blood tests identified by the lab technician are CBC, platelets, PT, and PTT. A urinalysis and a CT scan have also been ordered.

Right word or wrong word: STAT or A.S.A.P.? (p. 151)

No and no.

STAT means *immediately* and does not leave room for hesitation or discussion: the situation is an absolute priority. In health care, the term *STAT* carries a sense of urgency, and all other work will be put on hold until the issue or task is addressed.

A.S.A.P. means *as soon as possible. A.S.A.P.* (or *a-sap,* as some people say) is a term that does not imply the same urgency or immediacy as *STAT.* A short lag time may be permitted. A.S.A.P. is sometimes seen in small font as a.s.a.p..

Critical thinking (p. 155)

Sample answer

In a hospital, lab techs move from patient to patient and run the risk of transmitting infection from patient to patient and to themselves. In the lab, careful attention to infection control protocol protects staff from the cross-contamination of specimens and decreases the likelihood that the lab tech and his or her colleagues will also become infected with one of the pathogens that is present in the specimens.

Build a word (p. 155)

1. pathogenic: producing disease or able to produce disease
2. pathophysiology: the science or study of the etiology (cause) and process of disease
3. bacteriotoxic: toxic to bacteria
4. bacteriosis: any disease that is caused by bacteria
5. colonoscopy: the examination of the colon
6. bacteremia: bacterial infection of the blood
7. gonorrheal: pertaining to the infection gonorrhea

Let's practice (p. 155)

1. *Candida albicans*
2. Herpes simplex virus type I
3. Trichophyton
4. *Staphylococcus aureus*
5. Tuberculosis
6. Diarrhea
7. Gastroenteritis
8. Colitis

Fill in the blanks (p. 157)

1. drawing it / venipuncture
2. venipuncture
3. phlebotomy
4. In the word *venipuncture*, the combining vowel is *i* rather than *a* or *o*.
5. Phlebitis, possibly leading to deep vein thrombosis
6. Venography / venogram

Critical thinking (p. 160)

1. She might want to find out if he has an unexplained internal bleed that may be causing stroke-like symptoms.
2. She may order a blood urea nitrogen test, because Mr. Davis may have some internal bleeding that could show up in his urine.
3. The oxygen that Mr. Davis is receiving may interfere with the results of the O_2SATs being taken by pulse oximeter, because the oximeter gets a reading from the skin. An ABG might be a better test, because it measures internal levels of oxyhemoglobin.
4. A blood gas analyzer, a coagulation analyzer, and a hematology analyzer

Mix and match (p. 161)

1. potassium
2. calcium
3. partial prothrombin time
4. blood urea nitrogen
5. complete blood count
6. fasting blood sugar
7. sodium

Critical thinking (p. 165)

1. *cerebro* (brain) + *vascular* (referring to blood vessels and circulation): Blood circulates in and out of the brain through blood vessels.
2. The blood vessels to the brain may be occluded (impeded); the patient may have a blood clot (thrombus) in the brain or circulatory system, which sometimes limits the amount of blood to the brain; or he may have a small bleed occurring in his brain (hemorrhage).

Right word or wrong word: arteritis or arthritis? (p. 169)

No, these two words are not the same.

Arteritis means *inflammation of an artery.*

Arthritis is a pathological condition of the joints.

Mix and match (p. 170)

1. arteriectomy
2. venipuncture
3. atypical
4. phleborrhaphy
5. phlebosclerosis
6. angiogram
7. phlebectomy
8. coronary artery disease
9. phlebectasia

Build a word (p. 170)

1. atherosclerosis
2. arteriorrhexis
3. arteriolonecrosis
4. perivenous
5. venesection
6. venoperitoneostomy
7. atheronecrosis
8. arteriotomy
9. arteriovenous
10. arteriolitis

Fill in the blanks (p. 170)

1. distributes
2. vessels / arteries / veins / capillaries
3. capillary
4. three
5. Arteries
6. Veins
7. Vena
8. lack of oxygen / anoxia

Let's practice (p. 174)

1. Valve
2. Tricuspid valve
3. Aortic valve
4. Pulmonary
5. Vena cava
6. Between the left atrium and the left ventricle
7. Pulmonary veins
8. Right atrium

Build a word (p. 176)

1. aortorrhaphy: suture of the aorta
2. aortosclerosis: hardening of the aorta
3. aortotomy: incision of the aorta
4. cardiogenic: originating in the heart
5. cardiologist: a medical doctor who is a specialist in the treatment of heart disease
6. cardiography: the study of the electrical activity of the heart
7. ventricular: pertaining to the ventricle(s)
8. ventriculotomy: surgical incision into a ventricle
9. valvuloplasty: surgery to restore a valve
10. valvectomy: surgical removal of a valve

Right word or wrong word: cardia or cardio? (p. 176)

Yes and no.

Although *cardia* means heart, it is also a term for the upper opening of the stomach where the stomach connects with the esophagus. Be very careful to always remember in which context you are reading, writing, listening, or speaking about terms with these roots. Ask yourself if the context is the heart and the cardiovascular system or the digestive system.

Fill in the blanks (p. 178)

1. receive and send forward electrical impulses initiated by the SA node
2. Purkinje fibers
3. SA node
4. bundle of His
5. SA node

Right word or wrong word: electrocardiogram or echocardiogram? (p. 181)

These words are related, because they both refer to a way of measuring cardiac conduction. However, they are *not* interchangeable, because they name two different ways of measuring that conduction:

The *electrocardiogram* does this through electrodes that are placed on the anterior surface of the chest.

An *echocardiogram* is a form of ultrasound technology in which the interior of the body is viewed with the use of Doppler echocardiography, which determines the velocity of blood flow within the heart and at the heart valves.

Free writing (p. 184)

Sample answers

1. An echocardiogram determines the velocity of blood flow within the heart and at the heart valves.
2. A Holter monitor is worn continuously over a period of time to monitor cardiac activity.
3. *Cardiac conduction* refers to the electrical activity of the heart.
4. A pulse is the result of the heartbeat and the pressure exerted on the arteries.
5. Purkinje fibers are found on the surface of the ventricles of the heart.

Critical thinking (p. 185)

1. Urinalysis
2. Patients are expected to arrive to the Emergency department momentarily.
3. He would have been notified by Emergency Medical Dispatch or directly by an EMT or a paramedic who was transporting the patient.
4. On the way
5. Fasting blood sugar (a type of blood test)

Build a word (p. 186)

1. cystogram: radiogram of the bladder
2. nephritis: inflammation of the kidney as a result of disease or infection
3. ureterocystoscope: a device inserted into the ureter to view the ureter and the bladder
4. nephralgia: kidney pain
5. urogenesis: the formation or creation of urine
6. urethrocystitis: inflammation of the urethra and bladder
7. renovascular: pertaining to the blood supply to the kidney
8. glomerulopathy: disease of the renal glomeruli
9. cystitis: inflammation of the bladder, usually as a result of a urinary tract infection
10. uretoeronephrectomy: the removal of a kidney and its ureter

Right word or wrong word: vesico, viscer/o, or vasculo? (p. 187)

No.

Vesico refers to a bladder, which could include a blister.

Viscer/o refers to *visceral*, meaning an internal organ.

Vasculo refers to the blood vessels.

Mix and match (p. 189)

1. the act of supplying or stimulating a body part
2. a circular band-shaped muscle at an orifice
3. urinate; to pass urine
4. loss of self-control over urination

Right word or wrong word: innervate or enervate? (p. 189)

No and no. These two words have very different meanings:

Innervate means *to supply nerves or stimulate a body organ or tissue.*

Enervate means *to weaken or lessen the strength of something.*

Reflective questions (p. 190)

1. Any two of these: to assess for a urinary tract infection or kidney disease, or for the presence of certain drugs, hormones, or alcohol
2. Visual inspection, chemical analysis, and microscopic analysis
3. Ketones, hemoglobin, leukocytes, and nitrates

Let's practice (p. 191)

1. Transparency
2. Ions
3. *nephr/o* and *ren/o*
4. Incontinence
5. Glomeruli

Reflective questions (p. 192)

1. She collected it from the urinary catheter bag, which is connected to the urinary catheter inside the patient.
2. He remembers that he has had a urinary catheter before.

Chapter review

Critical thinking (p. 195)

1. A Code Blue is a life-threatening emergency call in a hospital. It generally occurs when a patient is experiencing a cardiovascular or cerebrovascular event, and it requires all appropriate staff to attend.
2. Normal urine does not carry pathogens or other harmful or infectious elements. However, should these be present, it is impossible to see them during a visual inspection. Gloving protects against infection or contamination from all body fluids and substances.
3. Symptoms of urinary tract infection (UTI) and diabetes can cause confusion. The presence of pathogens or abnormal glucose levels in the urine can identify these conditions.

Name the term (p. 195)

1. Kidney
2. Urinary meatus / meatus
3. Thrombus
4. Thromboembolus
5. Phlebotomy

Break it down (p. 195)

1. cardio + vascul + -ar
2. phlebo + tom + -y
3. nephr + -itis

Right word or wrong word: ureters or uterus? (p. 195)

No.

Ureters are narrow tubes that take urea away from the bladder.

Uterus means *womb,* and it refers to an organ that is part of the female reproductive system.

Translate the terminology (p. 195)

Sample answers

1. Ask the laboratory to let us know the levels of ketones in the urine as soon as possible.
2. I'll have to collect the urine from the urinary catheter bag. He has a urinary catheter in place.
3. Let's begin an electrocardiogram on the patient and keep monitoring it continuously for now.
4. Take the pulses on both sides of the body at the wrist (radial pulse) and on the top of the foot.

Fill in the blanks (p. 196)

1. Ur-
2. nephr-
3. Cardi-

Name the prefix (p. 196)

1. glycol-
2. ket/o-
3. gluco- / glucos-

Chapter 6: Dental and Burn Assessment

Reflective questions (p. 200)

1. Two: the ER physician, Dr. Raymond, and the pediatrician, Dr. Lincoln
2. Dr. Sandor, the dental surgeon
3. A burn (or scald) and facial trauma, which appears to be a broken jaw
4. Airway, breathing, circulation, and spinal cord injury assessment
5. Mouth trauma and blood in the mouth; possible spinal cord injury causing cessation of breathing mechanisms; possible head injury to cerebrum impairing or causing cessation of breathing
6. Because the patient has a mouth injury and may gag on his own blood or teeth, suctioning must be readily available in case of such an emergency.
7. The cause of the injury

Let's practice (p. 203)

1. mandibular fracture
2. split lip
3. zygomatic arches
4. bimanually
5. aspirating
6. pretrauma
7. asymmetry
8. crepitus

Critical thinking (p. 203)

1. ABCs; level of consciousness; history of the dental injury and immediate care provided (before hospital admission); examination of the head and neck (extraoral wound assessment and just about to begin jaw assessment)
2. Examination of the head and neck: jaw examination, neurologic evaluation, oral examination of the hard and soft tissues, and ordering of the radiographic examination (followed by a review and assessment of the x-rays)
3. Medical and health history; radiographic examination (pretrauma dental records)

Fill in the blanks (p. 205)

1. inferior
2. superior
3. interior
4. anterior
5. superior; anterior
6. posterior
7. inferior
8. superior

Build a word (p. 206)

1. maxillodental: pertaining to both the upper jaw and the teeth together
2. maxillofacial: pertaining to both the face and the upper jaw together
3. faciocervical: pertaining to both the face and the neck together (*Cervic* is the combining form of *cervix*, meaning *neck* [see Chapter 3].)

Fill in the blanks (p. 206)

1. temporomandibular joint
2. maxillodental
3. faciolingual

Critical thinking (p. 206)

1. Tears

Right word or wrong word: turbinates or conchae? (p. 210)

Yes, these terms can be used interchangeably.

Build a word (p. 210)

1. nasolabial: pertaining to the nose and the lip
2. sinogram: a radiograph of the sinus(es)
3. paranasal: near or beside the nasal cavity
4. mucosanguineous: containing blood and mucus
5. septal: pertaining to a wall or a layer of tissue that separates two chambers or cavities
6. rhinolaryngitis: inflammation of both the nose and larynx at the same time
7. nasofrontal: pertaining to the frontal and nasal bones
8. rhinologist: a specialist in diseases of the nose
9. mucitis: inflammation of a mucous membrane
10. septotomy: incision of the nasal septum

Build a word (p. 212)

1. buccogingival: pertaining to the buccal and gingival surfaces of the teeth
2. pharyngoplasty: surgical repair of the pharynx
3. pharyngolaryngeal: concerning both the pharynx and the larynx
4. gingivoglossitis: inflammation of both the gums and the tongue (also called *stomatitis*)
5. laryngopharyngectomy: the removal of the larynx and the pharynx
6. linguogingival: concerning both the tongue and the gums
7. glossograph: an instrument that records the tongue's movement during speech
8. pharyngoglossal: concerning both the pharynx and the tongue
9. tonsillitis: inflammation of the tonsils
10. tonsillar: pertaining to the tonsils

Right word or wrong word: palate or pallet? (p. 212)

No, these are not interchangeable. They are homophones: they sound the same, but they have different meanings. A *palate* is natural structure that is found in the mouth. A *pallet* is a manmade structure that is used to transport and lift goods in industry.

Let's practice (p. 214)

1. Periodontal disease
2. Odontorrhagia
3. Dentalgia
4. Dentilabial
5. Dentist

Let's practice (p. 216)

1. Temporomandibular joint
2. Mandible
3. Coronoid process
4. Mental protuberance
5. Maxillomandibular fixation

Free writing (p. 216)

Sample answers

1. When I was 10 years old, I had a tonsillectomy.
2. My dentist says I have gingivitis, which is an inflammation of the gums.
3. It is possible to dislocate the jaw at the temporomandibular joints.
4. The medical term *bucca* means *cheek.*

Critical thinking (p. 220)

1. Cranial nerve V, trigeminal; cranial nerve VII, facial; cranial nerve IX, glossopharyngeal; cranial nerve X, vagus
2. A nerve that sends sensory messages to the brain through the spinal cord
3. Cranial nerve VIII, vestibulocochlear
4. To transmit motor or sensory messages
5. Because Mr. Loepkky, too, has had craniofacial trauma.

Mix and match (p. 221)

1. VIII. vestibulocochlear
2. VII. facial
3. III. oculomotor
4. II. optic
5. IX. glossopharyngeal
6. VII. facial
7. I. olfactory

Critical thinking (p. 222)

1. A mandibular fracture
2. Semi-Fowler's position
3. Any of the following: choking, aspiration, dehydration, pain, spinal cord injury, or infection or more trauma to his burn

Let's practice (p. 223)

1. Avulsion
2. Hemifacial
3. Extraoral wound
4. Subluxation
5. Malocclusion

Right word or wrong word: intra- or inter-? (p. 224)

No, they are not the same.

Intra- means *within*.

Inter- means *between* or *among*.

Mix and match (p. 224)

1. lingual
2. cranial
3. facial
4. ocular
5. maxillary

Build a word (p. 229)

1. epicranium: the skin that covers the head
2. submucosa: underneath or below the mucous
3. epidermitis: inflammation of the surface layer of the skin
4. dermavascular: concerning the skin and its blood vessels

Reflective questions (p. 233)

1. *(Answers will vary.)*
2. *(Answers will vary.)*

Chapter review

Critical thinking (p. 234)

1. The skin
2. It is a term used to identify the chin.
3. A nose
4. No; he may possibly need to have his jaw wired shut.
5. A standardized set of rules for estimating the total percentage of the body surface area that is affected by a burn.

True or false? (p. 234)

1. False
2. False
3. True
4. False
5. True

Fill in the blanks (p. 234)

1. sebaceous
2. lingu/a; gloss/a
3. palates
4. maxilla / maxillae
5. oral labia
6. brain / cranium

Mix and match (p. 235)

1. pharyngitis
2. laryngorhinology
3. second-degree burn
4. split lip
5. LeFort I, II, and III
6. avulsion

Identify the abbreviations (p. 235)

1. Temporomandibular joint
2. Body surface area
3. Posteroanterior (dental radiograph)
4. Ear, nose, and throat (specialist)
5. Nasogastric
6. Intravenous

Right word or wrong word: sublingual or subungual? (p. 235)

No; these are not the same words, and they do not sound the same, either.

Sublingual means *below the tongue* and is pronounced sŭb-**lĭng**′ gwăl.

Subungual means *below the nail(s) of the fingers or toes* and is pronounced sŭb-**ŭng**′ gwăl or sŭb-**ŭng**′ gwē-ăl.

Chapter 7: Mental Health, Drug Use, and Endocrine Assessment

Reflective questions (p. 238)

1. No; she is oriented to place and person but not to time.
2. The hospital social worker
3. Type 2 diabetes with low blood sugar; a problem with thyroid function (we do not know exactly what that is yet); the possibility of dementia; emotional trauma from the car accident; use of multiple medications to treat her thyroid condition and her arthritis; minor concussion
4. Emergency medical services
5. Possible answers: ongoing neurological and diabetic assessment; observation and/or mental health assessment related to her levels of confusion and disorientation
6. Mrs. Davis is 72 years old.

Critical thinking (p. 245)

1. Physical, psychological, socioeconomic, spiritual, and environmental
2. Resiliency
3. Flexibility
4. difficult; maintain
5. The expression of emotion and the emotional response

Critical thinking (p. 248)

1. Mental health is a subjective and objective sense of well-being that encompasses all dimensions of the self. Mental illness includes diseases, disorders, and other impairments that upset this state of mental well-being.
2. Resiliency
3. *Diagnostic and Statistical Manual*
4. No
5. Psychiatry

Build a word (p. 248)

1. phrenic: concerning the mind
2. psychopathology: the study of mental diseases and abnormal behavior, as well as their causes
3. psychogenic: related to the development of the mind

Right word or wrong word: schizophrenia or multiple personality disorder? (p. 251)

No; these conditions have very different symptoms.

Schizophrenia is a major thought disorder and does not involve a divided personality. This is a common mistake and misconception.

Right word or wrong word: psychotic or schizophrenic? (p. 252)

No.

Schizophrenia is a persistent mental illness. It can be treated, but it rarely if ever fully resolves.

Psychosis is a feature of schizophrenia. Psychosis is a state of mind in which reality is lost and there is a disruption of thinking, of the content of speech, and so on. Psychosis is generally temporary and can be treated to the point that it will resolve. It can be caused by various factors or present with other illnesses in addition to schizophrenia.

Let's practice (p. 253)

1. ADHD (attention deficit-hyperactivity disorder)
2. Seasonal affective disorder
3. Post-traumatic stress disorder
4. schiz/o
5. Anorexia
6. Bipolar disorder
7. Lability
8. Dementia
9. Dependence
10. Frustration intolerance or low frustration tolerance

Mix and match (p. 253)

1. lack of oxygen
2. thiamine
3. not otherwise specified
4. primary
5. expression of emotion
6. condition of the mind with a loss of contact with reality
7. phrenetic or excited
8. Alzheimer's dementia
9. denies self food
10. false perceptions of reality

Critical thinking (p. 254)

Anorexia is a symptom. *Anorexia nervosa* is a disorder. If you did experience a loss of appetite when you were physically ill, you simply had the symptom of anorexia and nothing more.

Right word or wrong word: psychiatrist or psychologist? (p. 254)

A *psychiatrist* sees clients in counseling and can also treat them in the hospital. A *psychologist* sees clients in counseling but cannot treat them in the hospital.

Build a word (p. 255)

1. abnormal: away from the norm or not normal
2. misdiagnosed: not diagnosed correctly or accurately
3. unimpaired: not impaired or not worse
4. misperception: a condition in which someone does not perceive a situation correctly
5. anorexigenic: causing a loss of appetite
6. euphoriant: something that causes euphoria; the agent or cause of euphoria
7. hypofunction: diminished or decreased function
8. hypomnesia: diminished memory
9. hypersensitivity: an abnormal or heightened sensitivity to stimuli
10. postexposure: occurring after exposure (contact) with a toxin or pathogen or with the root of a phobia

Critical thinking (p. 257)

1. No. She is not oriented to time (year), where she is, and who the people around her are.
2. They try to reorient her by telling her where she is, what year it is, and who they are.
3. A nurse in the armed forces
4. An auditory hallucination

Critical thinking (p. 257)

1. She continues to be disoriented; she has some degree of recent memory loss; and she has some ongoing confusion about why she is in hospital and what is going on. No one knows her at Fayette General Hospital; therefore, the treatment team cannot determine if she had these symptoms before the accident, if the symptoms are a result of the accident, or if they are the result of some other cause.
2. To be able to interview the client on a level that will be understood; to know where, when, and how to ask questions and to seek clarification appropriately and in a manner that will facilitate open communication with the client

Break it down (p. 258)

1. a. psycho + neuro + endo + crin/e + -ology
   b. psycho = psyche, psychological, or having to do with the mind; neuro = having to do with the brain or the nerves; endo = inside or within; crin/e = secretions; -ology = the study of, science of, or field of
   c. The study of hormones and how they affect the brain
2. a. psycho + endo + crin/e + -ology
   b. See previous entry
   c. The study of the interrelationship between mental states and endocrine function

Let's practice (p. 260)

1. Externally on the body
2. superior; posterior
3. medially; anterior
4. distal
5. anterior

Mix and match (p. 261)

1. adrenal glands
2. thyroid
3. pancreas
4. testes
5. pancreas
6. ovaries
7. hypothalamus

Free writing (p. 263)

Sample answers

1. A person's natural skin color is determined by cells called *melanocytes.*
2. The antidiuretic hormone stimulates the formation of urine.
3. TSH stimulates the thyroid gland to produce and secrete thyroid hormones.

Mix and match (p. 263)

1. decreases urine output
2. stimulates the uterus to contract during labor
3. growth
4. increases urine output

Critical thinking (p. 266)

1. Mrs. Davis has exhibited difficulty with concentration, muscle weakness, agitation, and nervousness.
2. She may be taking too much thyroid replacement medication, which could be causing her to have the symptoms of hyperthyroidism.

Critical thinking (p. 268)

1. A TSH test measures levels of thyroid-stimulating hormone (also known as *thyrotropin*) in the blood. A total T4 test measures levels of the hormone thyroxine in the blood. A total T4 test is not used to monitor thyroid replacement therapy.
2. Radioactive iodine treatment
3. Nodule
4. Thyroid-stimulating hormone
5. Calcitonin

Build a word (p. 268)

1. thyroidotoxin: toxic or poison to the thyroid gland
2. thyroidectomy: removal of the thyroid gland
3. thyrotome: an instrument that is used to cut the thyroid cartilage
4. calciuria: calcium in the urine

Let's practice (p. 268)

1. thyroid
2. parafollicular
3. formation
4. somatotropin
5. antidiuretic
6. hypophysis
7. luteinizing
8. iodine

Build a word (p. 273)

1. glycogenesis
2. glycopolyuria
3. glycometabolism
4. glucogenesis
5. pancreatopathy

Critical thinking (p. 275)

1. Difficulty paying attention; confusion; shakiness or trembling (see Chapter 2); dizziness (see Chapter 2); increased pulse rate; drowsiness (she takes a nap in the ER)
2. Glucopenia

Free writing (p. 275)

Sample answers

1. The organ that produces insulin and releases it into the blood is the pancreas.
2. Gestational diabetes is a temporary form of diabetes that can occur during pregnancy.
3. Glucocorticoids affect the metabolism, as well as blood glucose levels.
4. Subcutaneous injections of insulin are necessary for patients with type 1 diabetes.
5. The pancreas and the adrenal glands are both implicated in diabetes.

Right word or wrong word: abuse or misuse? (p. 279)

Yes and no; they are not the same in medicine and pharmacology.

Although *abuse* can mean *misuse,* it has a connotation of intent to use a drug improperly for a purpose that is not recommended.

Misuse can be the simple improper use of a medication or drug, such as taking an antihistamine (which is intended for allergies) to help get to sleep at night or taking three aspirins instead of two in the hopes that they will work more quickly that way. Drug misuse can turn into abuse.

Fill in the blanks (p. 280)

1. analgesic
2. Bipolar disorder
3. prescription
4. addiction
5. Dependency / Addiction
6. addicting
7. harmful / unfavorable / undesirable
8. Self-medicating
9. euphoria
10. hyperalertness / euphoria

Ruling out: complete the table (p. 281)

Overview of Mrs. Davis's symptoms by potential diagnosis

Minor Concussion	Mental Health or Illness	Hypoglycemia	Thyroid Disease	Polypharmacy
confusion	confusion	confusion	confusion	confusion
? anterograde amnesia	disorientation	disorientation	sudden moodiness or behavior change	disorientation
? retrograde amnesia	? amnesia or forgetfulness and memory loss or impairment	drowsiness		drowsiness
		difficulty paying attention or confusion		
		- shakiness or trembling		
		- dizziness		
		- increased pulse rate and blood pressure		
		sudden moodiness or behavior change		

Chapter review

Critical thinking (p. 283)

1. *Endocrine glands* empty into the bloodstream. *Exocrine glands* empty into ducts.
2. -crine
3. No. A large number of people abuse substances such as caffeine, sugar, tobacco, prescription drugs, over-the-counter drugs, and some illicit drugs, but these individuals may not become addicted. Addiction is the extreme end of substance abuse, when the individual has no choice but to take the substance or else risk serious withdrawal symptoms. Addiction is a disease.
4. Anti-
5. *Side effects* are common and not necessarily harmful. *Adverse effects* are harmful and can be permanently debilitating.

Right word or wrong word: disorder or disease? (p. 283)

Yes. Although you've learned that there are fine distinctions between *disorders* and *diseases*, these terms are generally used interchangeably, and many health professionals fail to make the distinction. Expect to hear both terms used as if they were synonymous.

Right word or wrong word: schizoid personality or multiple personality? (p. 283)

No, these terms have quite different meanings.

A *schizoid personality* involves a person who is quite withdrawn and introverted and who lacks the ability or capacity to be able to change this state.

Multiple personality is a diagnosis that is made when more than one actual personality exists within the mind of a person. It is a rare disorder.

Right word or wrong word: oxytocin or oxycontin? (p. 283)

No, these words are not the same.

Oxytocin is a hormone that is released by the pituitary gland during childbirth.

OxyContin is an opioid drug that is highly addictive.

Identify the abbreviations (p. 283)

1. Attention deficit disorder
2. Luteotropic hormone
3. Generalized anxiety disorder
4. Bipolar disorder

Fill in the blanks (p. 283)

1. Psych
2. Endocrin
3. Psychoendocrin

Name the prefix (p. 284)

1. eu-
2. post-

Break it down (p. 284)

1. para + follicul + -ar
2. anti + bodies
3. thyroid + -itis
4. melano + cyte
5. glyc + emia

Label the organs of the endocrine system (p. 284)

1. Pineal
2. Hypothalamus
3. Pituitary
4. Thyroid
5. Parathyroids
6. Thymus
7. Adrenals
8. Pancreas
9. Ovary (female diagram)

9\. Testes (male diagram)

UNIT THREE

The Language of Treatment

Chapter 8: Obstetrics, Labor, and Delivery

Reflective questions (p. 289)

1. Antepartum
2. The hospital social worker
3. A physician who specializes in all phases of care for pregnancy, delivery, and the period just after childbirth

Right word or wrong word: does msw mean medical social worker? (p. 291)

No. A medical social worker may sign his or her name in a patient record with the credential *SW* if the care facility or workplace requires this. However, if the person has a degree, he or she may be able to sign either *BSW* or *MSW* to indicate this. *MSW* refers to a university degree: a master's degree in social work. It does not mean *medical social worker*.

Let's practice (p. 291)

1. adrenal glands
2. hypothalamus
3. vagina
4. breasts
5. ovary

Name the suffix (p. 293)

1. -plasty
2. -itis
3. -algia
4. -ectomy
5. -ize
6. -ment
7. -ate
8. -ia

Fill in the blanks (p. 293)

1. uterus
2. -itis
3. hysterectomy
4. hypothalamus
5. Genitalia
6. perineum
7. cervix
8. ovaries
9. gynecologist

Let's practice (p. 296)

1. myometrium = myo- + metr + -ium
2. perimetrium = peri- + metr + -ium (This word breaks down to mean *surrounding tissues of the uterus.*)
3. endometrium = endo- + metr + -ium (This words breaks down to mean *the tissue within the uterus or the inner lining.)*

Fill in the blanks (p. 301)

1. Leopold's maneuvers
2. fetal
3. breech
4. antepartum
5. vertex
6. malpresentation

Right word or wrong word: hospital unit or hospital ward? (p. 301)

Yes, these two terms are synonymous.

The word *unit* means *a whole, a social unit, or a block of something specific* (i.e., the intensive care unit). *Unit* is currently the most up-to-date term to use.

The word *ward* means *a block of rooms or a division of a hospital shared by patients.* The term stems from the idea of someone being a "ward" or under the protection, care, or supervision of someone else. A ward generally has a supervisory nurse. The word *ward* is old, and it is being used less and less in official capacity. However, you can still expect to hear this term if you work in a hospital.

Name the term and break it down (p. 304)

1. embryopathy: embryo (product of conception) + pathy (disease)
2. periparturient: peri (around the time) + parturient (of birth)
3. uteralgia: uterus + algia (pain)
4. uterovaginal: uterus + vagina + suffix -al
5. intrapartal: intra (within; during) + part (combining form of parturient) + suffix -al
6. uteritis: uter/o (combining form) + -itis (suffix meaning *inflammation*)

Let's practice (p. 305)

1. no, non, or nil
2. many
3. one or first

Mix and match (p. 305)

1. labor
2. expands
3. afterbirth
4. pregnant
5. birth
6. motherhood
7. management of childbirth; pregnancy
8. apex
9. womb
10. after the birth

Let's practice (p. 306)

1. Hemoglobin
2. White blood cells / white blood cell count
3. International normalized ratio
4. Complete blood count
5. Red blood cells / red blood cell count
6. Partial thromboplastin time

Mix and match (p. 311)

1. antibodies screen
2. partial thromboplastin test
3. hemoglobin
4. arterial blood gases
5. a blood group system based on antigens, especially D
6. blood pressure
7. oxygen saturation level
8. fasting blood sugar

Free writing (p. 311)

Sample answers

1. To determine if the mother and child have compatible blood groups, Rh and ABO tests during pregnancy are important.
2. Antigens trigger antibodies.
3. Glucose and hemoglobin levels are measured in units of "g/dL."

Reflective questions (p. 313)

1. In the Antepartum Unit of Fayette General Hospital
2. A nonstress test
3. A placental tear and placental abruption
4. Learning about her husband's injuries

Critical thinking (p. 313)

1. She has a high-risk pregnancy because she was injured in an accident today so the doctor wanted to monitor the health status of her fetus.
2. Yes.
3. Yes; she's at risk for having the baby early. The doctor mentioned that a Cesarean section delivery may be required as a result of the placental tear.
4. It may put stress on the fetus, thereby causing the fetus's heart rate to go up and possibly increasing the fetus's movement. It could also lead to contractions.

Reflective questions (p. 317)

1. Hard
2. She has placental abruption.
3. Operating room
4. The unit clerk
5. A Cesarean section
6. She will deliver her child.

Critical thinking (p. 317)

No, she does not want to deliver today: she thinks it's too early, and she wants her husband by her side as they had planned.

Let's practice (p. 320)

1. Intraventricular hemorrhage
2. Hydrocephalus
3. Cystic fibrosis
4. Severe neonatal encephalopathy
5. Uterine contractions

Break it down (p. 320)

1. amnio + rrhexis: the rupture of the amnion or the amniotic sac
2. amnio + scopy: the visual examination of the fetus inside the womb through an endoscope

Fill in the blanks (p. 320)

1. severe neonatal encephalopathy; cerebral palsy; mental retardation
2. Cystic fibrosis
3. cerebral palsy
4. spina bifida
5. hypoxia
6. ischemia

Right word or wrong word: postpartal or postpartum? (p. 326)

No.

Postpartal refers to the period of 6 weeks directly after giving birth. During this time, the body is recuperating from the pregnancy and birth processes.

Postpartum refers to the period from 6 weeks to approximately 1 year after birth, during which the female reproductive cycle returns to normal. Hormones and mood may fluctuate as the mother comes to terms with physical and emotional changes related to caring for the new infant, as well as changes in her lifestyle patterns and habits.

Critical thinking (p. 330)

1. All of the indicators showed this. She had scores of less than 2 for everything.
2. There is some likelihood that the child will have long-term health problems. Her low scores at 1 minute improved to closer to normal by the 5-minute mark, but they never achieved a full normal as would be expected for a full-term neonate.
3. Approximately 1.6 kg
4. 40 weeks

Critical thinking (p. 332)

1. Retinopathy of prematurity (ROP)
2. Low risk; her birth weight is high, and she reached at least 30 weeks' gestation.
3. *Ductus* refers to a duct; *arteriosus* refers to an artery.

Let's practice (p. 333)

1. Bronchopulmonary dysplasia
2. Retinopathy of prematurity
3. Respiratory distress syndrome
4. Intraventricular hemorrhage
5. Patent ductus arteriosus

Break it down (p. 333)

1. retin + opathy: disease or damage to the retina
2. hypo + oxia: low or insufficient oxygen
3. pre + maturity: occurring before the expected time; born before full gestation; occurring before development is complete
4. intra + partal: during delivery or birth

Right word or wrong word: neonate or preemie? (p. 333)

All preemies are neonates, but not all neonates are preemies. The term *neonate* means *newborn* and refers to any newborn baby.

Chapter review

Critical thinking (p. 336)

1. *At risk* is a broad term that means *having the potential to come under threat of harm, danger, or loss.*
2. A vulnerable population is one that is underprivileged, underserved, disadvantaged, or at risk for exploitation or extinction.

Label the diagram (p. 337)

Working down from the top left:

1. Endometrium
2. Myometrium
3. Perimetrium
4. Cervix

Working down from the top right:

5. Fallopian tube
6. Ovary
7. Ova
8. Uterus
9. Vagina

Name the term (p. 337)

1. Perineum
2. Genitalia
3. Uterus
4. Cervix

Critical thinking (p. 337)

Possible responses include maternity, labor and delivery, and obstetrics.

True or false? (p. 337)

1. False. The assessment of color is performed to determine the infant's level of circulation and oxygenation.
2. True.
3. False. It's an English term for tube feeding.
4. False. It's a neurological condition.

Right word or wrong word: premature or preterm? (p. 337)

There is no difference in meaning. The two terms are synonymous.

Break it down (p. 338)

1. oro + gastr + ic = pertaining to the mouth and the stomach
2. naso + gastr + ic = pertaining to the nose and the stomach
3. ante + part + al = pertaining to the time before birth

Prefixes (p. 338)

1. none
2. before
3. during
4. after
5. new

True or false (p. 338)

1. False
2. False
3. False
4. True
5. True

Chapter 9: Medical Records, Test Results, and Referrals

Reflective questions (p. 342)

1. Victor is completing the patient care record (chart) for Mr. Davis in the ICU and specifically working on Mr. Davis's admission documents. He is also checking to confirm that the patient's billing information is correct.
2. The consent for treatment form
3. Transient ischemic attack, cerebrovascular accident, intensive care unit, and coronary artery disease

Critical thinking questions (p. 342)

1. The TAR is an approval provided by an insurance provider to pay for identified hospital services.
2. Veterans Affairs health care (U.S. Department of Veterans Affairs)

Right word or wrong word: diagnosis or diagnoses? (p. 345)

Yes, there is a difference. *Diagnosis* is singular, and *diagnoses* is plural.

Let's practice (p. 348)

1. The physician or the attending physician
2. A physician who works for the insurance company
3. All patient diagnoses, patient service and care needs, and expected duration of care
4. The consent for treatment form
5. The nursing assessment and admissions form
6. The consent form only

Let's practice (p. 348)

1. False
2. False
3. True

Critical thinking questions (p. 349)

1. Coughing
2. Sample answers: He is pale or ashen. His face exhibits pallor.
3. Anterograde amnesia
4. He ran into his grandmother when she had a coffee pot in her hand. The grandmother accidentally spilled the coffee on Clay, thereby scalding him.

Reflective questions (p. 351)

1. Stroke (cerebrovascular accident or TIA) and cardiac arrest
2. A urinary tract infection
3. His urinary catheter
4. Posteroanterior and lateral angles (see Chapter 2)
5. Mr. Davis's O_2SATs are low, he is experiencing shortness of breath, and he is coughing.

Let's practice (p. 354)

1. Troponin
2. AST/SGOT
3. ALT/SPGT
4. Fatigue
5. Antipyretic
6. Nitrates
7. Dipstick test (urine dipstick test)
8. High-density lipoprotein (HDL) cholesterol; also known as "good" cholesterol
9. Cardiac enzymes
10. Statins

Build a word (p. 358)

1. nephropyelography: radiography of the kidneys and the renal pelvis
2. nephrorrhaphy: suturing of the kidney(s)
3. nephrotoxin: a substance that is toxic (poisonous) to the kidney tissues
4. pyelotomy: an incision of the renal pelvis
5. nephrology: the study of the structure and function of the kidneys
6. nephrolithotomy: the surgical removal of kidney stones
7. nephropathy: disease of the nephrons

Mix and match (p. 358)

1. inflammation of the kidneys
2. bladder infection
3. surgical removal of a kidney
4. infection of the testes that affects the flow of urine
5. an x-ray or CT image of the renal pelvis and the ureters

Fill in the blanks (p. 361)

1. Andrology
2. Androsterone
3. andropathy

Critical thinking (p. 361)

1. The penis and the prostate
2. The prostate gland gradually enlarges, and urinary frequency increases.
3. The prostate gland

Fill in the blanks (p. 362)

1. epididymis
2. scrotum
3. vas deferens
4. urethra
5. testes

Build a word (p. 363)

1. epididymis
2. vas deferens
3. ductus deferens
4. seminal

Build a word (p. 365)

1. spermaturia: the release of semen with urine
2. spermatopathy: disease of the sperm cells or their associated glands
3. spermatogenesis: the creation of a mature and functional spermatozoon

Right word or wrong word: sperm or semen? (p. 366)

No, they are not synonymous.

Sperm are male reproductive cells. They are transported in semen.

Semen is the mix of secretions from the bulbourethral glands and the prostate gland plus spermatozoa produced by the testes.

Right word or wrong word: prostate or prostrate? (p. 366)

No, they are not the same. Check the spelling very carefully!

Prostate is the name of a gland in the male reproductive system.

Prostrate means the position of lying face down.

Fill in the blanks (p. 367)

1. erection
2. secrete
3. prostate gland
4. testes
5. urethra
6. androgens
7. penis
8. glans penis
9. prostatectomy
10. oncology

Let's practice (p. 368)

1. The prostate
2. The penis
3. hypothalamus
4. The testes

Reflective questions (p. 369)

1. Because he hears dry crackles in Mr. Davis's lungs and notices that the patient cannot fully expand his lungs during inhalation
2. The respiratory system

Critical thinking (p. 369)

He confirmed that the patient was Mr. Davis before beginning to discuss the patient's condition and before examining him. This protects the confidentiality of the patient and ensures that the physician does not treat the wrong patient.

Build a word (p. 373)

1. laryngitis: inflammation of the larynx or the voice box
2. laryngectomy: removal of the larynx
3. laryngopharyngitis: inflammation of both the pharynx and the larynx
4. laryngoscope: an instrument that is passed into the trachea (windpipe) to view the larynx

Build a word (p. 375)

1. bronchoedema: swelling of the bronchi
2. bronchorrhagia: a hemorrhage of or in the bronchi
3. bronchorraphy: the suturing of a bronchial wound
4. tracheolaryngotomy: an incision into both the larynx and the trachea
5. trachealgia: pain in the trachea

Let's practice (p. 375)

1. Bronchopneumonia
2. Bronchitis
3. Bronchiectasis
4. The lungs
5. The diaphragm
6. The oral and nasal cavities
7. The trachea
8. The larynx
9. The larynx
10. The nasal cavity

Build a word (p. 379)

1. pneumolithiasis: the formation of stones within the lungs
2. pneumonectomy: the removal of a lung
3. pneumonorrhapy: the suturing of a lung
4. pleuropericarditis: inflammation around and in the pleura at the same time that inflammation occurs around the heart (in the pericardium)
5. pleuropulmonary: concerning both the pleura and the lungs

Critical thinking (p. 382)

1. To perform gas exchange in the lungs
2. The alveoli and the pulmonary capillaries
3. Alveoli
4. The diaphragm
5. A mixture of gases
6. Apnea

Critical thinking (p. 384)

1. Pneumonomelanosis and pneumonoconiosis
2. Mesothelioma
3. dysfunction

Mix and match (p. 388)

1. a chronic condition that affects the bronchioles
2. a chronic condition that affects the alveoli
3. a malignant condition of cell membranes in the lung
4. a chronic condition of the bronchioles and the alveoli
5. any chronic pulmonary condition that adversely affects breathing

Let's practice (p. 388)

1. Dyspnea on exertion
2. Emphysema
3. Asthma

Critical thinking (p. 389)

1. Dr. Jackson is insistent because, if asbestosis is ruled in as a diagnosis, then there is an absolute need to rule out mesothelioma (a deadly cancer related to asbestosis).
2. Being *proactive* means taking the positive action of getting prostate checkups now, while the patient is healthy, which will allow the patient's doctor or another health-care provider to follow the health of his prostate gland and to monitor it for any changes. Being *reactive* means acting after the fact of a diagnosis of pathology, which perhaps could have been prevented.

Chapter review

What do you know? (p. 391)

1. eu-
2. Lung inflammation
3. Testosterone
4. -pnea

Label the diagram (p. 391)

Top left, downward:

1. Bladder
2. Pubic bone
3. Prostate gland
4. Penis
5. Urethra
6. Glans penis
7. Testes

Top right, downward:

8. Ureter from kidney
9. Seminal vesicle
10. Rectum
11. Bulbulourethral gland
12. Vas deferens
13. Epididymis
14. Scrotum

Name the term (p. 391)

1. The penis
2. Estrogen
3. Andrology
4. Pyelonephritis
5. Nephrolithiasis

Break it down (p. 392)

1. pneumo (combining form meaning *lung*) + thorax (root for *chest*)
2. cardio (root for heart) + pulmono (root meaning *air or breath*) + -ary (suffix meaning *concerning*)
3. lob/o (referring to the lobe of the lung) + -ectomy (suffix meaning *removal*)

Translate the terminology (p. 392)

Sample answers

1. Mr. Davis has some breathing difficulties.
2. Some people have a condition in which they stop breathing periodically during their sleep, and this condition can persist for a long period of time.
3. When you are running, you may start to breathe very quickly.

Mix and match (p. 392)

1. pyelonephrosis
2. trachea
3. tracheotomy
4. larynx
5. pharynx
6. pneumomelanosis
7. respiration
8. hydropneumothorax

Label the diagram (p. 392)

1. Nasal cavity
2. Oral cavity
3. Pharynx
4. Larynx
5. Trachea
6. Lung
7. Diaphragm
8. Mouth
9. Bronchial tree

Chapter 10: Orthopedics and Brain Injuries

Reflective questions (p. 397)

1. An orthopedic surgeon
2. Two: a fractured femur (femoral head) and a fractured tibia. The patient's knee is injured and also requires surgery, but it is not fractured.
3. The patient has to wait for two reasons: (1) it is risky to give anesthetics too soon to patients who have experienced a head injury or concussion, because the behaviors that they show as the anesthesia wears off may mimic the symptoms of worsening brain injury; and (2) under anesthesia, there is some risk that a patient with a head injury may develop hypoxia (decreased oxygen levels).
4. These movements will no longer be possible because the patient is having the ankle surgically fixated (i.e., fixed in place).

Critical thinking question (p. 397)

He is most worried about his ability to return to work so that he can financially support his wife and his new baby.

Right word or wrong word: orthopedic or orthopaedic? (p. 399)

The terms are the same; both are acceptable spellings of the same term. The version that includes the letter *a* is an older and more traditional form of the word.

Let's practice (p. 404)

1. Traction
2. Reduction
3. Intubate
4. Orthopedics

Mix and match (p. 404)

1. anteromedial
2. NPO
3. post-surgery
4. analgesic
5. mobilize
6. emerge from
7. fixate
8. arthrotomy
9. intubate

Reflective questions (p. 406)

1. The emergency occurs at night. The scenario states that both of the physicians who rush to the scene are on the night shift.
2. Subdural hematoma and second-impact syndrome
3. The physician palpates the patient's nose because Gil Loeppky's eyes are blackened, and the black eyes may be a symptom of a broken nose. When the patient fell out of bed, he may have fractured his nose when he made contact with the floor.

Critical thinking (p. 406)

1. The purpose of a code system is to protect patient confidentiality and to keep other patients at ease while alerting relevant medical personnel that they are immediately needed for an emergency (see Chapter 4).
2. He was dreaming about the motor vehicle accident and wanted to find and help his wife. He was not aware of where he really was or of his condition.

Critical reflection questions (p. 410)

1. Airway, breathing, and circulation
2. The nurses' notes say that Gil's head was stabilized between two pillows. This was done to prevent movement of and injury to the spinal cord. The notes also say that the team applied a backboard (i.e., inserted it underneath the patient). This was done for the same reason.

Mix and match (p. 410)

1. gurney
2. hematoma
3. intracranial
4. STAT
5. Code
6. cerebrospinal fluid
7. bagging

Let's practice (p. 413)

1. Viral meningitis
2. Meninges
3. Myelomeningocele

Name the term and break it down (p. 415)

1. meningitis = mening (root meaning *membrane*) + *-itis* (suffix meaning *inflammation*)
2. cerebrospinal = cerebro (combining form meaning *brain*) + spin (root for *spine*) + *-al* (suffix meaning *relating to*)

Mix and match (p. 415)

1. harmful
2. pachymeninx
3. stiff neck
4. meningomyelocele

Break it down (p. 416)

1. sub- (prefix meaning *below or under*) + dur (combining form meaning *hard*; in this case, referring to the dura mater) + -al (suffix meaning *relating to*)
2. hemat (combining form meaning *blood*) + oma (root meaning *tumor*)
3. intra- (prefix meaning *within*) + cerebr (combining form meaning *brain*) + -al (suffix that makes the word an adjective)
4. sub- (prefix meaning *below or under*) + arachnoid (root meaning *spider-like web*)

Right word or wrong word: paresis or paralysis? (p. 421)

Paresis refers to a reduced ability or a partial loss of motor function. Neurological or neuromuscular diseases, disorders, and conditions that cause the symptoms of paresis carry the risk of progressing to paralysis.

Paralysis refers to an inability to activate motor neurons when they are stimulated. The result is the complete loss of motor function. Paralysis is often described with the use of terms that end in the suffix *-plegia,* such as *paraplegia* and *quadriplegia* (see Chapter 4). Paralysis may be the result of neurological (central nervous system) trauma or disease.

Let's practice (p. 422)

1. epi-: on, over, on top of, or upon
2. intra-: inside or within
3. a-: without
4. para-: abnormal (in this context)
5. dys-: inability or lack of function
6. sub-: under, beneath, or below
7. hemi-: one half
8. leuk-: white
9. photo-: light
10. re-: again
11. neo-: new
12. entero-: intestines

Critical thinking (p. 423)

1. Anisocoria (unequal pupil sizes), muscles are pliant (not rigid), pupils sluggish, airway open, breathing shallow but regular, pulse thready and rapid at 150
2. He is showing symptoms of increased intracranial pressure (ICP), such as anisocoria, an altered level of consciousness (unconscious), and muscles that are pliant (not rigid).

Fill in the blanks (p. 423)

1. intracranial bleed
2. subdural hematoma
3. compressed
4. hemorrhaging
5. epidural hematoma
6. pressure
7. intracranial pressure
8. cranium

Mix and match (p. 423)

1. stiff neck
2. spider
3. cavity
4. sensitivity to light
5. three layers of mater
6. harmful

Let's practice (p. 423)

1. Aphasia
2. Paresis
3. Hemianesthesia
4. Dysarthria
5. Vertigo
6. Anisocoria

Right word or wrong word: intercranial or intracranial? (p. 423)

No, they are not the same.

Intercranial is not a word.

Intracranial means *within the cranium.*

Mix and match (p. 425)

1. normal
2. venous
3. dural
4. spinal
5. coccal
6. virus
7. anesthesia

Right word or wrong word: cerebro- or cephalo-? (p. 425)

The combining form *cephalo-* means *cranium.*

The combining form *cerebro-* means *brain.*

Let's practice (p. 429)

1. Neurons / nerve cells
2. Neuroglial cells
3. Dendrites
4. Nervous tissue
5. Nerves
6. Synapse
7. Myelin or myelin sheaths

Critical thinking (p. 430)

1. It will mean that he might be able to receive nerve impulses (stimuli) but that these impulses will not be conducted from the periphery into the central nervous system for processing and response. In other words, he will not be able to react to the stimulus.
2. Nothing will happen. He will not automatically lift his right leg to take the weight off of it and stop the pain. Instead, he will have to focus and find the site of the pain before voluntarily raising his leg.

Build a word (p. 430)

1. inoperable: not suitable for surgery = in- (not) + operar/ia (operate) + -able (worthy, capable)
2. encephalalgia: pain deep within the brain or head = en- (in) + cephal (cranium) + -algia (pain)
3. decompression: the removal of the pressure = de- (remove) + compress/i/o (compress) + -ion (condition, state, or process of)
4. cephalocele: protrusion of the brain from the cranial cavity = cephalo (cranium) + -cele (hernia)
5. demyelinate: to remove the myelin sheath around a nerve = de- (remove) + myelin (marrow) + -ate (to perform an action)

Right word or wrong word: nerve or nerve cell? (p. 430)

Yes, there is a difference in meaning.

A *nerve cell* (neuron) is the basic individual cell of the nervous system.

Numerous neurons working together form *nerves*.

Critical thinking (p. 433)

1. The autonomic nervous system
2. The peripheral nervous system

Build a word using suffixes (p. 433)

1. cytokinesis: the division of a cell during which the cytoplasm moves or separates into two parts
2. dysphasia: an impairment in the ability to use either written or spoken words
3. hemiparesis: half or partial paralysis
4. kinesthesia: self-awareness of the body's position and movement
5. analgesia: the absence of pain
6. epilepsy: a type of seizure disorder
7. ataxia: the loss of voluntary muscle control
8. neurasthenia: a lack of energy and motivation
9. quadriplegia: full paralysis of the body as a result of a spinal cord injury
10. anesthesia: the total or partial loss of sensation, which may include a loss of awareness

Fill in the blanks (p. 434)

1. central nervous system
2. denervation
3. sympathetic
4. central; peripheral
5. Innervation
6. afferent nerves
7. autonomic
8. parasympathetic
9. olfactory
10. gustatory

Mix and match (p. 434)

1. salty and sweet
2. blurry or clear
3. loud or soft
4. stinky or pleasant
5. soft or scratchy

Fill in the blanks (p. 435)

1. radio waves; a magnetic field
2. lie flat and still
3. meninges
4. musculoskeletal

Mix and match (p. 438)

1. collection of blood under the skin
2. beneath the dura mater
3. pertaining to the brain
4. incision into the skull
5. anticonvulsant
6. germ free

Build a word with the combining form crani/o (p. 438)

1. craniocerebral: referring to both the brain and the skull
2. craniocele: a protrusion of the brain through the skull
3. craniology: the scientific study of the skull

Critical reflection question (p. 441)

Gil's prognosis is good but guarded. Dr. Hamidi points out that there is no guarantee of a full recovery.

Chapter review

Critical thinking (p. 442)

1. An orthopedic surgeon
2. A neurosurgeon
3. An orthopedic technician
4. Meningitis

Prefixes (p. 442)

1. Within
2. Painful, difficulty, lack of function, or inability
3. On, above, or over
4. Spinal cord

Right word or wrong word: meningocele or myelomeningocele? (p. 443)

No, the conditions and their etiologies are not the same.

A *meningocele* does not involve spinal cord damage, but a *myelomeningocele* (spina bifida) does. *Meningocele* results when a vertebrae splits. *Myelomeningocele* occurs when the spine does not completely fuse closed during embryonic development.

Abbreviations (p. 443)

1. Cerebrospinal fluid
2. Subarachnoid hemorrhage
3. Central nervous system
4. Second-impact syndrome
5. Level of consciousness

Label the diagram (p. 443)

1. Synapse
2. Axon tip
3. Dendrites
4. Nucleus
5. Neuron cell body
6. Axon in myelin sheath

Sentence scramble (p. 444)

1. An MRI can detect minute abnormalities within the body, even within the bones.
2. MRI imaging is particularly useful for examining peripheral nerves and can help diagnose a broad range of nerve disorders.
3. The body contains nervous tissue, neurons, and neuroglial cells.
4. Neuroglial cells are not actually nerve cells but supporters of them.

Chapter 11: Postoperative Nutrition and Healing

Reflective questions (p. 448)

1. In PAR, recovering
2. To understand how Clay is going to be fed and how his nutrition is going to be supplied and to gain knowledge so that they can support their child through the process of being tube fed
3. The pediatric unit

Critical thinking question (p. 449)

To ensure that that the foods and nutrition are delivered in a manner that would not compromise the physical care and treatment of that patient (i.e., in the case of swallowing or digestion problems).

Right word or wrong word: dietician or dietitian? (p. 450)

They are two different spellings for the same term. The most common spelling is *dietician*, but *dietitian* is also correct. Professionals who work in the field of dietetics often prefer the spelling *dietitian*.

Right word or wrong word: esophagus or oesophagus? (p. 455)

They are the same word. *Oesophagus* is an archaic medical spelling for *esophagus*. It is rarely seen in the United States. However, you may occasionally come across it when working with hospital staff who have been trained in Britain or other countries in the United Kingdom, where *oesophagus* is somewhat more common.

Build a word (p. 460)

1. jejunocolostomy: the surgical formation of a passage between the jejunum and the colon
2. pylorectomy: surgical removal of the pylorus
3. enterocolitis: inflammation of the intestines (usually as a result of disease)
4. gastroduodenal: pertaining to the stomach and the duodenum
5. gastroenteritis: inflammation of the stomach and the intestines
6. colonopathy: any disease of the colon
7. sigmoidoscope: a tube-like device that is used to visualize the sigmoid colon and the rectum
8. rectosigmoid: pertaining to both the rectum and the sigmoid colon
9. gastrectomy: surgical removal of all or part of the stomach
10. anorectal: pertaining to both the anus and the rectum

Let's practice (p. 460)

1. Transverse
2. Ascending
3. Descending
4. Intra-
5. Retro-

Mix and match (p. 466)

1. inflammation of the liver
2. referring to the stomach and the liver
3. pertaining to the gallbladder and the liver
4. inflammation of the liver and kidneys
5. rupture of the liver
6. poisonous to the liver

Break it down (p. 466)

1. chole (gall or bile) + cyst (vessel or bladder) + -itis (inflammation): inflammation of the gallbladder
2. chole (gall or bile) + cysto (vessel or bladder) + pathy (disease) + -y (condition or state): disease of the gallbladder
3. cholangio (bile vessels or ducts) + graph (writing or record) + -y (condition or state) = an x-ray or radiograph of the bile ducts
4. cholangio (bile vessels or ducts) + -oma (tumor) = cancer of the bile ducts

Right word or wrong word: egestion, excretion, or elimination? (p. 467)

Egestion and *excretion* are both forms of *elimination*; however, *egestion* and *excretion* are not the same things.

Egestion is the elimination of undigested food matter.

Excretion is the elimination of waste products that are the result of digestion and the separating out of products of metabolism that are not or no longer required for bodily function. These include, for example, sweat and urine.

Elimination, in the medical sense, means the removal of waste products via the skin (i.e., sweat), lungs, kidneys (i.e., urine), and intestines.

Right word or wrong word: excretion or secretion? (p. 468)

They are different.

Excretion is the elimination of the waste byproducts of metabolism and digestion. This waste material is called *excreta*.

Secretion is the end product of a gland; it is a substance that is released by a gland or a cell.

Reflective question (p. 469)

Clay will likely be able to sit up in bed within 24 hours.

Let's practice (p. 470)

1. appendectomy
2. nasogastric tube
3. no history of fractures
4. in situ

Let's practice (p. 470)

1. The immobile child is incontinent of urine and needs to use an incontinence pad.
2. The admission record shows the patient has no known allergies.
3. Later, when the patient's mother arrived, she told the staff her child is allergic to shellfish.

Reflective questions (p. 472)

1. Via nasogastric tube, which is a form of enteral feeding
2. Through an intravenous line into a vein

Critical thinking questions (p. 475)

1. A urinary catheter and an intravenous catheter
2. The speech therapist is an expert in swallowing and will need to be with Clay when he first begins to take foods and fluids by mouth and as he progresses to more solid foods.

Break it down (p. 475)

1. *Par/a-* means *beside.*
2. *Intra-* means *within*
3. *In-* means *in or to place within.*
4. *Ex-* means *out or out of.*

Fill in the blanks (p. 475)

1. enteral
2. nasogastric tube
3. nasal cavity; esophagus; stomach
4. Parenteral nutrition; enteral nutrition

Let's practice (p. 478)

Sample answers

1. *Vitamins* are essential substances that promote growth, development, and normal cell function in the body. They boost the immune system. They are organic (i.e., from plants or animals).
2. The term *saccharide* refers to a category of carbohydrates that contain sugars.
3. *Compromised* is a medical term that means *impaired or complicated,* usually by a factor such as injury or disease. A compromised patient is unable to function normally or optimally.
4. A *polymer* is a chemical chain.
5. *Ascorbic acid* promotes the health of the gums and teeth, facilitates the absorption of iron, and promotes wound healing.

Mix and match (p. 478)

1. promotes the health of the gums and teeth
2. causes a cooling effect on the skin
3. assists with muscles, nerves, and heart rhythm
4. provide a cushion for some major organs
5. strengthens the teeth and bones

Build a word (p. 478)

1. hydration: a state of appropriate fluid or water balance or the action of providing water to achieve this state
2. dysphagia: difficulty eating (i.e., chewing and swallowing)
3. adipogenic: producing fat
4. liposuction: the surgical removal of subcutaneous fat by a process of suctioning
5. hidrotic: something that causes sweating

Let's practice (p. 478)

1. B_1
2. E
3. C
4. B_6
5. A

Reflective questions (p. 481)

1. To be proactive when setting up a nutritional plan for the future, after the NG tube is removed, so that she may begin to prepare the patient's parents for this eventuality
2. He will consume only liquids for a while, and then he will progress to more substantial or solid foods.
3. The function of the tongue and ability to swallow (i.e., a function of the muscles of the pharynx and the epiglottis)

Right word or wrong word: dietician or nutritionist? (p. 481)

Dieticians and *nutritionists* are similar, and the terms are often used interchangeably. However, they are not quite the same.

Licensing or other professional regulation may be used to protect the title of *dietician*. This ensures that the education and training of a dietician meets the standards that are acceptable to both the health-care profession and the public.

The title of *nutritionist* is not always protected. In many locales across the country, anyone can make the claim of being a nutritionist and go into business as such. However, in states and smaller jurisdictions in which the title of *nutritionist* is regulated, the distinction between the two professions narrows. This type of regulation sets standards for the education and training of nutritionists.

Critical thinking (p. 481)

1. He is at risk for choking because he is still producing saliva in his mouth. The saliva and mucous from the mouth and nasal cavities all flow back into the pharynx, and the patient can choke on these substances if the epiglottis does not function to promote swallowing into the esophagus. In addition, the epiglottis must recognize the difference between air and solids or liquids and open or close appropriately in response. Clay may be at risk for aspirating these substances into his lungs.
2. Gilbert Loeppky

Let's practice (p. 484)

1. nutritional treatment plans
2. fully functioning
3. aspirated
4. mechanism
5. gag reflex

Let's practice (p. 485)

1. Thickened fluid diet
2. Enteral nutrition / elemental formula
3. Clear fluids
4. Parenteral nutrition

Critical thinking questions (p. 486)

1. This patient should receive parenteral nutrition until he awakens from the medically induced coma, and this should be followed by clear or full fluids. He will progress to a soft diet and then to normal foods if there are no complications.
2. Diabetic diet; low calorie, restrictive
3. Cardiac diet; low sodium
4. This patient should receive a specialized enteral diet that is lactose free and allergen free. He will progress to clear fluids, a soft diet, and then to normal foods.
5. There are two possibilities for this patient. Enteral formula that may be specialized to include supplemental proteins and lipids for growth and development may be given. If the baby can breastfeed, then parenteral nutrition may be sufficient.
6. Diet as tolerated

Mix and match (p. 486)

1. eliminates possible sources of food allergies
2. promotes bowel elimination
3. for patients with liver, kidney, or heart disease
4. controls the levels of glucose and carbohydrate intake
5. restricts or eliminates spices and other irritants

Right word or wrong word: dysphagia or dysphasia? (p. 486)

These two words have totally different meanings:

Dysphagia means *difficulty eating or swallowing*. It is pronounced dĭs-fā´ jē-ă. The root *phagein* means *to eat*.

Dysphasia means *difficulty speaking or using words* (see Chapter 10). It is pronounced dĭs-fā´ zē-ă. The root *phasis* means *speech*.

Critical reflection questions (p. 488)

1. Miranda
2. Clay's pain assessment
3. She uses a pediatric pain scale and asks him to point to or mark his current level of pain.

Critical thinking questions (p. 489)

1. FLACC
2. Cry = 1 and Face = 1 for a total score of 2/10
3. It means *hurts a lot,* and it is rated as a 4 on a scale of 0 to 5.
4. It means *worst pain possible,* and it is rated as a 10 on a scale of 0 to 10.

Critical reflection questions (p. 491)

1. They are still intact.
2. The reduction and management of pain and the prevention of infection
3. No, probably not
4. Just another day or two at the most

Fill in the blanks (p. 493)

1. Blisters
2. Contracture
3. cutaneous
4. dermis
5. tissue; blisters
6. epidermis
7. fluid
8. regenerates

Chapter review

Critical thinking (p. 495)

Because a speech pathologist is concerned with the functioning of the organs and structures in the oral cavity that relate to speech but also to tongue and jaw movement, all of which are implicated in eating and swallowing safely

What do you know? (p. 495)

1. Laterally on the tongue
2. Cicatrix
3. Not known
4. Feces
5. The derma
6. Inferior to the ileum, in the lower right quadrant of the abdomen and at the beginning of, or the proximal end of, the ascending colon
7. Bulla or vesicle
8. The epidermis
9. Enteral nutrition occurs via feeding tubes placed directly into the stomach or intestines; parenteral nutrition occurs through the intravenous route and is supplied directly into the veins.
10. Enteral feeding / enteral nutrition

Label the diagram (p. 495)

1. Ascending colon
2. Transverse colon
3. Descending colon
4. Sigmoid colon
5. Rectum

Right word or wrong word: milk allergy or lactose intolerance? (p. 496)

No.

Lactose intolerance is the result of lactase in the digestive tract not being able to break down lactose.

Milk allergy is an immune response to milk proteins.

Mix and match (p. 496)

1. stool
2. large intestine
3. intestines
4. chain
5. nourishment
6. water
7. colonoscopy
8. ascorbic acid

Build a word (p. 496)

1. malnutrition
2. colonorrhagia
3. dermatopathology
4. fecaluria

True or false (p. 496)

1. F
2. T
3. F
4. T
5. F
6. T
7. F
8. T
9. T
10. F

Chapter 12: Diagnoses and Medication Administration

Reflective questions (p. 501)

1. Dr. Jensen
2. Endocrinology
3. No; her blood glucose levels have been erratic and often high.
4. An anti-anxiety medication

Critical thinking question (p. 501)

Angie reacted because she believes that her mother does have the symptoms of PTSD. However, she knows that this is a very contentious and difficult subject to broach with her mother.

Fill in the blanks (p. 504)

1. ketones
2. battery
3. void
4. bouts
5. confused
6. 2200
7. Per os
8. sedative

Build a word (p. 504)

1. ketonemia: the presence of acetones or ketones in the blood (This causes the symptom of fruity-smelling breath.)
2. acetonemia: large amounts or an excess of acetones in the blood
3. endocrinopathy: any disease that results from a disorder or disease of an endocrine gland (see Chapter 7)

Critical thinking questions (p. 507)

1. She is using denial. Even if she recognizes that she has some of the symptoms of PTSD, she is unwilling or psychologically unable to delve into the trauma that she has experienced.
2. A severe psychological trauma with which the individual is unable to cope
3. Medications (chemical substances) cause changes within the body by altering its chemistry and thus its functioning.

Let's practice (p. 507)

1. projection
2. rationalization
3. avoidance

Build a word (p. 508)

1. post-traumatic: pertaining to something that occurs after a trauma was incurred
2. traumatotherapy: the treatment of a wound or injury
3. traumatic: an adjective that describes the severity of an injury or wound
4. traumatopathy: a disease or state of suffering caused by a trauma

Right word or wrong word: pill, tablet, or capsule? (p. 512)

Pills include both tablets and capsules. A pill is any oral medication in solid form.

Let's practice (p. 516)

1. Dextromethorphan; no
2. Milligram; yes
3. Tablet; yes
4. Liquid; no
5. Medication administration record; yes

Critical reflection questions (p. 516)

1. A tablet is a solid. A capsule contains solids within a gelatinous container.
2. Topical
3. Enteral
4. The Institute for Safe Medication Practices or The Joint Commission will have such a list; alternatively, check directly with your employer.

Mix and match (p. 517)

1. depersonalization
2. a neurotransmitter
3. means
4. distribute or give
5. detachment from emotions

Right word or wrong word: mellitus or melitus? (p. 518)

They are not the same words.

Mellitus refers to something sweet or a characteristic of sweetness.

Melitus refers to the inflammation of the cheek.

Mix and match (p. 519)

1. excessive acetone in body; hyperglycemia
2. the presence of ketones in the urine
3. capacity to endure large amounts without adverse effects
4. sitting or minimal movement or activity
5. nerve damage or disease
6. sweating
7. results or outcomes
8. tendency or potential to develop a disease or medical condition

Build a word (p. 520)

1. Polyuria
2. Polyphagia
3. Polydipsia

Mix and match (p. 523)

1. blood glucose
2. assists
3. glycohemoglobin
4. controlled
5. hemoglobin A1C
6. inactive, sitting, or settled
7. breakfast or a small meal

Fill in the blanks (p. 523)

1. pricking; lancet; droplet
2. dipstick; ketones
3. glycohemoglobin
4. poorly managed diabetes
5. prandial
6. serum
7. fasting
8. self-monitoring blood glucose
9. glucometer
10. acetone breath; acetone; blood

Critical reflection questions (p. 523)

1. Blindness, heart disease, decreased circulation to the extremities, nerve damage, erectile dysfunction, and stroke
2. Type 2
3. No. She mentioned earlier that she has tried to control it with diet and exercise.
4. Glory Loeppky (see Chapters 3 and 8). It is important for pregnant women to be tested because a small percentage of women develop diabetes during pregnancy, and it may recur during the next pregnancy or later in life.

Let's practice (p. 526)

1. Oral glucose tolerance test
2. Fasting blood sugar test
3. Random blood sugar test
4. 2-hour postprandial blood glucose test

Mix and match (p. 527)

1. 2-hour postprandial blood glucose test
2. insulin-dependent diabetes mellitus
3. impaired glucose tolerance (test)
4. random blood sugar (test)
5. urine glucose test
6. non–insulin-dependent diabetes

Critical thinking questions (p. 527)

1. Type 1 diabetes
2. Type 2 diabetes

Critical reflection questions (p. 530)

1. Anti-anxiety medication
2. Scalding her grandson and causing his injuries in the motor vehicle accident
3. No

Critical thinking questions (p. 531)

1. The stress of finding out that her husband is seriously ill with a lung disease
2. It could trigger another hyperglycemic episode, a flashback, or a dissociative episode.
3. Insulin replacement therapy / insulin injections

Fill in the blanks (p. 534)

1. calibrated
2. insulin inhaler
3. pumps

Name the term (p. 534)

1. Inhale
2. Calibrations
3. Cartridge
4. Fluctuation
5. Infusion
6. Longevity
7. Peak
8. Syringe

Let's practice (p. 534)

1. syringe
2. insulin
3. preparation
4. humulin
5. reservoir

Critical reflection questions (p. 537)

1. Today / shortly
2. Glucophage and trazodone
3. She will see her own physician.
4. Diabetic diet

Fill in the blanks (p. 537)

1. Glucophage
2. antidepressant
3. addictive
4. sedative

Chapter review

Critical reflection questions (p. 538)

1. Stevie-Rose Davis
2. She is experiencing excessive stress that may lead to a physiological need for more energy; however, her pancreas cannot produce adequate insulin for this.
3. He is an endocrinologist. Yes, he is a physician.

Mix and match (p. 539)

1. serum glucose
2. by mouth
3. series
4. acetonuria
5. temporary
6. means
7. tingling

Build a word (p. 539)

1. neuropathy: nerve damage or disease
2. dysglycemia: disturbed or dysfunctional blood glucose regulation
3. glycosuria: glucose being present in the urine
4. tachypnea: rapid breathing
5. polyphagia: excessive hunger
6. retinopathy: a disease of the eye or worsening of eyesight

Critical thinking questions (p. 539)

1. Post-traumatic stress disorder
2. When she was a nurse in the military as part of a MASH unit in Vietnam

Name the prefix (p. 539)

1. Baro-
2. Post-
3. Hyper-
4. Hypo-
5. Poly-

Fill in the blanks (p. 539)

1. Insulin
2. droplet
3. capsule
4. PO
5. pill
6. defense mechanism
7. Flashbacks
8. therapy / counseling / psychotherapy

Name the device (p. 540)

1. Lancet
2. Continuous glucose monitor
3. Glucose monitor / glucometer
4. Urine dipstick / urine reagent strip / urine glucose test strip

True or false (p. 540)

1. F
2. T
3. F
4. F
5. F
6. T

UNIT FOUR

The Language of Reparative, Restorative, and Rehabilitative Care

Chapter 13: The Healing Process

Reflective questions (p. 546)

1. Tipping his head downward or tipping it backward too far or too quickly
2. *Ambulate*
3. The semispinalis capitis

Critical thinking (p. 547)

1. They are staying close to Clay for safety, in case his legs are weak from not walking much over the past week and in case the pressure in his face causes him any dizziness. They want to be very close so that he will not fall down and reinjure himself.
2. Clay's wide-eyed expression is one of fear, apprehension, and inquiry. On the basis of the traumas that this child has experienced during the past week and in the context of when this expression occurs, he is likely afraid of suffering more pain.
3. Exercise promotes health in general. For Clay, exercise will be important to stimulate his appetite, to improve his circulation (including at the wound sites), and to keep him alert and involved in life, thus promoting his mental health.

Right word or wrong word: mammillary or mamillary? (p. 550)

They are alternate spellings of the same word. They have the same meaning.

Right word or wrong word: carotene or keratin? (p. 550)

They are not the same. They are entirely different.

Carotene is a pigment that is found in plants. It is also the precursor of vitamin A (retinol).

Keratin is a type of protein that provides structural strength for the hair, nails, and skin.

Critical thinking (p. 552)

Yes. Edema will be part of the inflammatory response of the body to the trauma in combination with the loss of tissue fluid that occurs with a burn. The fluid loss occurs when the capillaries near the surface of the skin are damaged and leak into the tissues.

Let's practice (p. 553)

1. *Ambulate*
2. *Wound*
3. The semispinalis capitis muscle in his neck
4. *Residual scarring*
5. Clay is wearing a jaw wrap. It is a type of compression bandage that has been designed to keep the mandible fracture in alignment and to prevent movement, swelling, and pain at the site of the injury.

Right word or wrong word: postural hypotension or orthostatic hypotension? (p. 553)

Yes, these two terms are the same. *Orthostatic* means *standing upright.*

Build a word (p. 553)

1. hydrostatic: an adjective that describes water or other fluids being at rest, motionless, or not being caused by pressure or weight to move
2. semispinalis: pertaining to part of the spine; involving part of the spine rather than the whole spine
3. mammitis: inflammation or infection of the breast
4. concurrently: at the same time (con [together] + current [in progress])
5. hypertension: greater-than-normal tension; in medical terminology, this term usually refers to high blood pressure

Mix and match (p. 553)

1. jaw wrap
2. ambulant
3. healthful
4. ambulation
5. privileges
6. position or placement
7. enduring
8. abnormal pigmentation
9. disfigurement

Break it down (p. 553)

1. stern/o + -algia
2. mandibul/o + pharyng/e + -al
3. semi + spinal + -is
4. bar/o + -ethesia
5. stern/o + clavicul/o + ar

Right word or wrong word: ameliorate or meliorate? (p. 554)

They have the same meaning. They are synonyms.

Fill in the blanks (p. 555)

1. regenerate
2. recuperate / recover / convalesce
3. mitigate
4. alleviate
5. recover
6. aggravate / exacerbate

Mix and match (p. 556)

1. regenerate
2. recuperate
3. construct
4. recover
5. alleviate

Reflection question (p. 558)

Dr. Lincoln defers to Kuldeep Singh because Mr. Singh is a pediatric physician assistant who has special training and skills with regard to pediatric burns and because Mr. Singh has been attending to this aspect of the patient's care. (See the Career Spotlight at the beginning of chapter for more details about physician assistants.)

Critical thinking (p. 559)

1. The doctor is winking for two reasons: (1) because he has just advocated for the boy regarding the family stress between the boy's father and grandmother, and he showed Clay that he understood the boy's perspective; and (2) because he knows the boy wants to go home, and the wink shows that he also understands Clay's perspective regarding that issue.
2. When Clay and his grandparents were en route to the hospital because of Clay's burn injury, there was a bee in the vehicle, and Clay was afraid of it. The grandparents' attempt to calm Clay and to let the bee out of the car may have interfered with the driver's ability to pay attention to the road.

Fill in the blanks (p. 562)

1. occlusion
2. favoring
3. incremental steps
4. inflammatory
5. united
6. autonomic nervous
7. gloves; the patient's body / bodily fluids
8. Discharge planning

Critical thinking (p. 562)
1. Tachycardia
2. Tachypnea
3. Vasodilation

Reflective questions (p. 570)
1. The masseter and the lateral pterygoid
2. The medial pterygoid
3. The medial pterygoid and the temporalis

Let's practice (p. 570)
1. Protrusion
2. Protraction
3. Lateral movement
4. Protrusion
5. Protrusion
6. Lateral movement
7. Elevation
8. Depression

Break it down (p. 570)
1. di (two) + gastrics (belly): having two bellies; there are two parts or "bellies" to this muscle
2. pterygo (wing-shaped) + mandibul/o (referring to the lower jaw bone) + -ar (suffix that makes this word an adjective): referring to the pterygoid process of the sphenoid and mandible bones
3. mylo (myl) + o + hyoid (a "U"-shaped bone): pertaining to the molar teeth and the hyoid bone. (*Mylo* does not mean *muscle*. Rather, it means *mill* [as in grind], which is in reference to the molar teeth. You were not expected to know this. If you deconstructed this word by identifying *mylo-* as a term for muscle, you have still used excellent deciphering skills. After all, we are talking about muscles!)

Let's practice (p. 570)
1. Temporalis
2. Mylohyoid
3. Buccinators
4. Medial pterygoid
5. Orbicularis oris

Break it down (p. 575)
1. pre (before) + vertebr/a (a bone in the spinal column) + -al (regarding or in relation to)
2. stern/o (sternum) + algia (pain)
3. antero (anterior, front, or before) + lateral (side or beside)
4. supra (above, beyond, or on the top) + hyoid (bone in the neck)

Build a word (p. 575)
1. sternohyoid: pertaining to the sternum and the hyoid bone
2. sternovertebral: concerning both the sternum and the vertebrae
3. occipitotemporal: concerning both the occiput and the temporal bones of the skull
4. sternotomy: surgical incision or cutting through of the sternum
5. sternodynia: pain in the sternum; a synonym is *sternalgia*
6. occipitofrontal: concerning the forehead and the occiput

Let's practice (p. 575)
1. Suboccipital
2. Anterolateral
3. Suboccipital and prevertebral

Reflective questions (p. 577)
1. Physician assistant
2. The nerve endings at the burn site are damaged, and they trigger a pain response (see Chapters 10 and 11).
3. He can exercise the upper chest and neck muscles to promote circulation and healing across the burn site.
4. To prevent the infection of the raw, open skin

Critical thinking questions (p. 578)

1. Sample answers: trapezius, platysma, sternocleidomastoid, or any of the anterior or anterolateral neck muscles that connect into the proximal anterior of the torso
2. When tissue is regenerating, it heals from the outer boundary inward. The wound site will be dry rather than moist, as normal skin should be. This dryness causes a pull on the new skin as the wound site reduces in size over time (see Chapter 11 for more information about contractures and scars).

Build a word (p. 581)

1. myotropic: attached to muscle tissue (turning, rotating toward, or inserting)
2. dermatotropic: having an affinity for (preferring) or acting on the skin
3. creatinase: the enzyme that destroys or decomposes creatine
4. promonocyte: a precursor of the monocyte in white blood cell development
5. procephalic: pertaining to the front or anterior portion of the head

Fill in the blanks (p. 582)

1. don
2. Gauze
3. regenerate
4. pliable / flexible
5. collagen
6. Pigmentation
7. skin; contract
8. collagenase

Critical thinking (p. 587)

To protect it from infection

Build a word (p. 587)

1. staphylococcemia: the presence of staphylococci bacteria in the blood
2. staphylodermatitis: inflammation of the derma caused by staphylococci bacteria

Let's practice (p. 587)

1. Staphylococcus
2. Immunocompromised
3. Staphylococcal scalded skin syndrome
4. Bullae
5. Sterile burn sheet
6. Flaccid
7. Sloughing / sloughing off / casting off
8. Paraffin gauze dressing
9. Silver sulfadiazine cream / Flamazine 1% cream
10. Hypopigmentation

Mix and match (p. 588)

1. pliant
2. diminish
3. cotton dressing
4. casting off
5. bulla
6. everywhere

Critical thinking (p. 590)

The "3 Rs" of patient treatment are *restoration*, *rehabilitation*, and *recovery*.

Chapter review

Critical thinking (p. 592)

1. Sample answers: initially covering the burn with a sterile burn sheet; covering the burn and surgical wounds with gauze; applying antibiotic creams topically to the burn; wearing gloves when treating the patient.
2. Because he is growing, and the jaw needs to be free to expand with that growth

Right word or wrong word: physician's assistant or physician assistant? (p. 592)

The correct term is *physician assistant*. There is no apostrophe or letter "s" needed.

Label the diagram (p. 592)

Hyoid bone

Prefixes and suffixes (p. 592)

1. Enzyme
2. For or in front of
3. Cell
4. Dissolution
5. Anterior or front side
6. Again or back
7. Two, twice, or double
8. Above, beyond, or on top of

What do you know? (p. 592)

1. Macrophage
2. Inflammation, bone production, and bone remodeling
3. Intramembranous and endochondral
4. Collagenation, angiogenesis, proliferation, and remodeling

Mix and match (p. 593)

1. osteogenesis
2. mastitis
3. fight or flight response
4. injury
5. morphosis
6. unbearable
7. chew
8. mammary
9. lower
10. sternalgia

Define the Terms (p. 593)

1. Widespread
2. Only in a specific area or areas
3. Confined to a segment, portion, or certain area only
4. In the region of or pertaining to the sternum
5. In the region of or pertaining to the mandible
6. Having a darker color than normal

Chapter 14: Oncology and Cancer Care

Reflective questions (p. 599)

1. Certified nursing assistant
2. Tests done at Okla Trauma Center identified shadows on Zane Davis's lungs, so he needs to be assessed for the possibility of lung cancer (mesothelioma).

Critical thinking (p. 599)

Mesothelioma can be caused by prolonged exposure to asbestos.

Reflective questions (p. 600)

1. A medical e-scribe records the interaction between the physician, the patient or client, and the treatment team and records the doctor's orders. However, he or she does not participate in any way in the patient's treatment.
2. Although this may vary from State to State, generally the candidate requires a background in a health or allied-health profession. E-scribes can be students in these programs as well.
3. Mr. Davis is at the cancer care center for a more comprehensive assessment that is specifically focused on discovering whether he does or does not actually have cancer.

Free writing (p. 602)

Sample answers

1. Offering support programs for clients promotes optimal client outcomes.
2. Exposure to asbestos over a long period can cause mesothelioma.
3. Addiction to cigarettes is not atypical for smokers.
4. Asbestos in the environment can be a source of lung disease.
5. Without a full diagnostic workup, it would be premature to offer a diagnosis.

Right word or wrong word: oncology or cancer? (p. 604)

No, they are not exactly the same, but yes, they are sometimes used synonymously.

Notice that *oncology* does not mean *cancer* specifically, although the study of cancerous tumors is definitely included in oncology. *Onco-* means *tumor, swelling, or mass.*

Cancer, on the other hand, refers specifically to malignancy, malignant neoplasias (abnormal cells), or tumors marked by the uncontrolled growth of cells that may invade other healthy tissues.

Despite these differences, in most contexts, the terms *oncology* and *cancer* are used synonymously. It is quite correct to do so, but as a health or allied-health professional, awareness of the subtle differences can be important to know. It may be helpful to think of *oncology* as the science and branch of medicine and of *cancer* as the disease.

Build a word (p. 605)

1. oncology: the branch of medicine and science that deals with tumors and cancers
2. oncogenesis: the formation and development of tumors
3. oncovirus: any virus that causes malignant neoplasms
4. oncolysis: the dissolution or absorption of tumor cells
5. oncotherapy: the treatment of tumors
6. oncologist: someone who studies or treats tumors and cancers

Build a word (p. 605)

1. -therapy; psychotherapy
2. -plasm; endoplasm
3. -plasia; hypoplasia
4. -oma; endothelioma
5. -gen; allergen
6. -oma; melanoma
7. -gen; hallucinogen
8. -gen; non-carcinogen
9. -plasm; cytoplasm
10. -plasm; protoplasm

Break it down (p. 606)

1. cancer (root word) + -cidal (suffix): able to kill cancer
2. cancer (combining form) + o (combining vowel) + phobia (root word used as a suffix here): an uncontrollable and extreme fear of cancer
3. pre (prefix) + cancer (root word) + -ous (suffix): occurring before actual cancer appears

Right word or wrong word: hardiness or heartiness? (p. 608)

These two words do not mean the same thing.

Hardiness refers the ability to survive.

Heartiness refers to warm, heartfelt emotion.

Name the term (p. 609)

1. Carcinogens
2. Deoxyribonucleic acid (DNA) strand
3. Pesticides and asbestos
4. Chromosomes
5. Chromosomes
6. Resiliency

Critical thinking (p. 609)

1. Stevie-Rose Davis
2. Zane Davis
3. Zane Davis

Let's practice (p. 614)

1. Mutation
2. Chromosomes
3. Pathological hyperplasia
4. Leukemia
5. Congregate
6. Translocation
7. Differentiated

Build a word (p. 614)

1. translocation: the abnormal fusion of unrelated pieces of different chromosomes
2. leukemia: a disease of the white blood cells; a form of cancer of the blood
3. metaplasia: the alteration of tissue into an abnormal form
4. histoid: resembling normal tissue
5. cytoplasm: the contents or material of a cell (excluding the nucleus)
6. metainfective: occurring after an infection has occurred
7. hypoplasia: a decrease in the normal production of cells
8. leukocyte: a white blood cell

What do you know? (p. 614)

1. Nevus
2. Eu- (see Chapter 9)
3. Cell
4. White
5. A structure made up of DNA that carries genes
6. To provide instructions for the development of a person's (or other organism's) physical structures on the basis of inherited traits from both biological parents

Mix and match (p. 614)

1. acute myeloid leukemia
2. chronic myelogenous leukemia
3. multiple endocrine neoplasia, type 1
4. trisomy 21

Build a word (p. 619)

1. sarcolysis: the dissolution of soft tissues or flesh
2. carcinogen: any substance or agent that produces cancer or that increases the risk of developing cancer
3. teratocarcinoma: a cancer that develops from a teratoma
4. sarcocarcinoma: a malignant mixed tumor of both the epithelium and the soft tissues
5. oncotomy: surgical incision of a tumor, cyst, or abscess
6. carcinolysis: the destruction or dissolution of carcinoma cells
7. teratogenetic: pertaining to the development of abnormalities in an embryo
8. oncocidal: able to kill tumors

Break it down (p. 619)

1. carcin/o (combining form) + gen (combining form used here as a suffix)
2. sarco (combining form) + plasm (root word) + -tic (suffix)
3. adeno (combining form used as a prefix) + angio (combining form) + sarc/o (combining form) + -oma (suffix)
4. adeno (combining form used as a prefix) + carcin/o (combining form) + -oma (suffix)
5. hepat/o (combining form used as a prefix) + carcin/o (combining form) + gen (combining form used here as s suffix)
6. terat/o (combining form used as a prefix) + carcin/o (combining form) + -oma (suffix)
7. terat/o (combining form used as a prefix) + phobia (root word)
8. osteo (combining form used as a prefix) + carcin/o (combining form) + -oma (suffix)

Mix and match (p. 619)

1. germ
2. ulceration
3. histoid
4. germs
5. squamous
6. osteocarcinoma
7. teratism
8. Kaposi's disease

Critical thinking (p. 622)

1. *MAR* can refer to either bone marrow cancer or to a medical administration record (see Chapter 12).
2. *Noninvasive*
3. Bone or bony (see Chapter 4)
4. *Metastatic*
5. Yes. Metastatic tumors are malignant tumors and malignant tumors are a type of neoplasm

Fill in the blanks (p. 622)

1. blastoma
2. *Primary site*

Reflective questions (p. 624)

1. Neoplasms
2. The TNM (tumor, nodes, metastasis) system
3. The original tumor to show cancerous cells
4. Tis / TIS
5. Stage 0
6. Grade 4

Critical thinking (p. 624)

1. The distance of the new site of a tumor from the primary tumor site
2. No. Abnormal cells can be benign and cause no harm. They are not necessarily precursors to cancer.

Fill in the blanks (p. 624)

1. grade
2. Stage IV
3. staging

Right word or wrong word: staging or grading? (p. 625)

They are not the same things, although their descriptions sound quite similar.

Staging is concerned with measuring how much and how far a cancer has spread (i.e., its progression). It is an assessment of severity and extent.

Grading is concerned with the aggressiveness of a cancer. This is the cancer's likelihood of metastasizing, as well as the size and shape of the cancerous tumor.

Reflective questions (p. 626)

1. Zane Davis is afraid that he may have a malignant and metastasized type of cancer, specifically mesothelioma.
2. An oncology technician will be accompanying Zane Davis through his tests.

Critical thinking (p. 626)

1. Informed consumers of health care gather information about possible diagnoses for their condition so that they can ask intelligent questions and make good decisions about treatment possibilities. The Davises are informed consumers because they have researched cancer, mesothelioma, and asbestosis. They have arrived at the cancer center with some background knowledge of the diseases, the diagnostics, and the possible treatments. They will be able to ask questions on the basis of what they have learned through their research.
2.

Health Strengths	Health Weaknesses
• Physically active (i.e., square dances with his wife, walks his dog daily)	• Older adult: 74 years old • Chronic smoker
• Socially involved with family and friends (i.e., has a support network)	• Coronary artery disease • History of bronchitis
• In good mental health (alert, cognitively)	• History of pneumonia
• Eats healthy foods (related to his coronary artery disease)	• Possible prostate problems related to aging or illness

3. He is moderately resilient or slightly less so. Sample rationales for this belief include the following:
   - Age can adversely affect resiliency (although we cannot be absolutely sure that it will affect Zane's), and various organs may function at a reduced capacity.
   - Zane may also be suffering from benign prostate hypertrophy as part of aging, but this has not yet been clearly diagnosed.
   - Coronary artery disease and smoking over a lifetime have decreased his body's ability to cope with new threats (i.e., illnesses and diseases).
   - Aging has reduced the elasticity of the lungs, and years of smoking have likely caused some lung-tissue damage. This makes Zane's lungs very vulnerable to respiratory illnesses, and he thus has a reduced chance of recovering completely from such illnesses.
   - Mentally and emotionally, Zane seems able to cope. For example, he's researched possible illnesses and has come willingly for assessment.

Fill in the blanks (p. 627)

1. *symmetry*
2. diameter
3. terminal
4. auscultates

Right word or wrong word: metastasis, metastases, or metastasize? (p. 627)

The words are related, but they are not identical.

Metastasis is a singular noun. The last syllable has a short *i* sound.

Metastases is a plural noun. The last syllable has a long *e* sound.

Metastasize is a verb. The last syllable has a long *i* sound.

To hear the words pronounced correctly, go to the Audio Tutorial for Chapter 14.

Right word or wrong word: bacteria or bacterium? (p. 630)

Bacteria is the plural form of *bacterium*.

Right word or wrong word: lymphocyte or leukocyte? (p. 631)

No, they are not synonymous. There is a fine distinction between them.

The word *leukocytes* refers to all white blood cells.

The word *lymphocyte* refers to a particular kind of white blood cell.

Right word or wrong word: lymph nodes or lymph glands? (p. 632)

The two terms are not really interchangeable, but there is a good deal of confusion about this.

Glands are organs. They secrete. Only the thymus gland of the lymphatic system actually secretes.

Lymph nodes are tissues through which fluid material is transported. They do not secrete.

Even with this in mind, it is common to see the terms *lymph nodes* and *lymph glands* used synonymously, although the term *lymph gland* is now officially obsolete (i.e., it is no longer used).

Here's a challenge: ask a health professional you know what they think about these two terms. Enjoy a discussion about this medical terminology. Be sure to inquire about his or her reasoning, and share your own.

Reflective questions (p. 635)

1. B-cells
2. Lymph
3. A malignant tumor or cancer of the lymphatic system

Let's practice (p. 636)

1. Plasma cell
2. Bone marrow
3. Adenoid
4. Thymus

Fill in the blanks (p. 636)

1. masses / clusters
2. antibodies
3. suppressor T-cells
4. Antibodies; antigens

Build a word (p. 636)

1. lymphitis: inflammation of the lymphatic system
2. lymphadenogram: a radiograph of a lymph gland
3. lymphocytotoxin: any substance or agent that is toxic to lymphocytes and kills them

Reflective questions (p. 638)

1. The two exams were a computed tomography (CT) scan and a positron emission tomography (PET) scan.
2. Zane will be tested in the respiratory department. A more specific focus will be placed on his lungs (i.e., pulmonary assessment) to determine if he has mesothelioma or asbestosis.
3. Zane will get the results of his assessments as soon as today. Dr. Sweetgrass has said that he will see Zane after the tests to let Zane know the results.

Critical thinking (p. 638)

No, this is not the opportune time to talk to someone who is under a great deal of stress about his addiction. Zane is well aware of the implications of his lifelong smoking. He has said before (see Chapter 9) that he has tried to quit in the past and failed. He does not need to hear what he already knows from his wife at this moment; it would cause him more anxiety and possibly frustrate and anger him. The couple needs to work together to get through the day. Besides, as a nurse, Stevie-Rose is fully aware that this subject will be broached by Dr. Sweetgrass or another member of the treatment team as the day draws to an end. Zane may be more amenable to hearing about the need to stop smoking from Dr. Sweetgrass at the end of the day.

Reflective question (p. 643)

Zane has already had the following tests: a sputum specimen, a chest x-ray, a CT scan, and a PET scan.

Critical thinking (p. 643)

1. Gilbert Loeppky (see Chapter 4), Clay Davis (see Chapter 6), and Zane Davis (see Chapter 9)
2. Only Zane Davis (see Chapter 5) was clearly identified as having been assessed via pulse oximetry.
3. Stevie-Rose Davis may become a candidate for a PET scan because she has had changes in her diabetic status and is now taking anti-diabetic medication.
4. Zane Davis is likely to undergo all of the pulmonary function tests listed in Table 14-14. Of the tests in Table 14-15, he will not have a thoracoscopy, a thoracentesis, or a fluoroscopy because he is no longer NPO, there are not enough hours left in the day for some of the tests, and not all of the tests are relevant to his situation.

Free writing (p. 643)

Sample answer

An FEV is a measurement that is taken during the first second of expiration. An FEF is a measurement is taken midway through expiration. An FVC is a measurement that is taken at the end of the expiration, when lungs are cleared.

Let's practice (p. 644)

1. Excisional
2. Fine-needle aspiration
3. Biopsy
4. Cytogenic analyst
5. Immunohistochemistry
6. Protein markers

Critical thinking (p. 645)

1. The removal of a tissue sample from the body for microscopic analysis
2. An *excisional biopsy* removes an entire tumor or tissue mass; an *incisional biopsy* cuts out just a sample of the targeted tissue.

Let's practice (p. 647)

1. Surgery
2. Bone marrow transplantation
3. Chemotherapy
4. Radiation therapy
5. Chemotherapy

Fill in the blanks (p. 647)

1. antineoplastic
2. antidiarrheal
3. stimulate
4. bone marrow transplantation
5. alkylating
6. hyperthermia

Reflective questions (p. 650)

1. Dr. Sweetgrass heard late respiratory crackles over the lung fields.
2. The goal of respiratory therapy for Zane Davis will be the improvement and maintenance of optimal lung functioning.
3. Zane received four diagnoses: COPD (including chronic bronchitis and susceptibility to pneumonia), smoking addiction, asbestosis, and benign prostate hypertrophy.

Critical thinking (p. 650)

1. The words *health maintenance* were used because Zane cannot be cured of COPD or asbestosis, and his lungs cannot completely recover from damage incurred as a result of years of smoking.
2. He hesitates about stopping smoking.
3. Prostate cancer

Chapter review

Critical thinking (p. 652)

1. Zane is in the maintenance phase. He does require surgery or acute treatment, he is not recovering from COPD. He is maintaining his health for now.
2. Zane received another prostate-specific antigen test.
3. Ethan is an oncology technician.
4. Zane had a joint PET/CT scan.

Antonyms (p. 652)

1. Lymphocytopenia
2. Antibody
3. Fungal
4. Inhibiting / depressing
5. Anti-infective

Mix and match (p. 653)

1. terablastoma
2. sarcocarcinoma
3. trisomy 21
4. carcinomatosis
5. oncofetal
6. Wermer's syndrome

Translate the terminology (p. 653)

Sample answers

1. Insulinomas are rare tumors of the pancreas, so they are not as significant as other kinds of pancreatic cell tumors.
2. Scientists in the field of oncology study substances to identify whether they contain any carcinogens.
3. New capillary growth was influenced by a situation in which abnormal cell production was increasing and about to become uncontrolled cell production.

Synonyms (p. 653)

1. Curb / limit
2. B-lymphocytes
3. Immature T-cells
4. Helper T-cells
5. T-cells
6. Lymphocyte count
7. Sarcoadenoma
8. Celiothelioma
9. Pulmonary plethysmography
10. Leukocyte

Name the suffix (p. 654)

1. -plasia
2. -gen
3. -oma

Right word or wrong word: Wermer's syndrome or Werner syndrome? (p. 654)

Wermer's syndrome is multiple endocrine neoplasia.

Werner syndrome is adult progeria.

Chapter 15: Rehabilitation: Physical and Occupational Therapy

Reflective questions (p. 659)

1. 11 days
2. Nursing and physical therapy
3. He is recovering from traumatic injuries to the hip, knee, and tibia of that leg.
4. An orthopedic unit

Right word or wrong word: holism or -holism? (p. 661)

They are not the same.

Holism is a philosophy that involves a belief that a unit (human or otherwise) is the sum of all its parts.

The suffix *-holism* is a relatively new word construct. It refers to addiction, as seen in the word *alcoholism*.

The colloquial suffix *-aholic* is a similar type of construct that refers to addiction. Examples are *workaholic*, *alcoholic*, and *chocoholic*.

Critical thinking (p. 665)

1. Festinating gait
2. A wide base
3. Involuntary hastening
4. Gil may experience an antalgic gait because he may avoid putting weight on his injured leg to avoid pain, which may cause him to limp.

Fill in the blanks (p. 666)

1. hesitancy
2. presentation
3. tremors
4. sluggish
5. gait
6. quadriceps femoris

Right word or wrong word: hip or thigh? (p. 667)

They are not the same. The thigh joins the hip.

The hip is a bony structure. It consists of the pubis, the ischium, and the ilium bones. It sits laterally to the pelvic bone and distally on the torso. The anatomical term for hip is *coxa* (see Chapters 4 and 10).

The term *thigh* refers to the upper leg. It extends from the hip to the knee. The thigh bone is the femur.

Right word or wrong word: dorsal, posterior, or caudal? (p. 669)

These three words are synonyms in anatomy and medical terminology.

Define the term (p. 669)

1. Plantar - sole (of the foot)
2. Dorsal - back
3. Anterior - front
4. Lateral - side
5. Medial - middle

Let's practice (p. 670)

1. Extensor hallucis longus
2. Flexor hallucis longus
3. Biceps femoris, semimembranosus, and semitendinosus
4. Extensor digitorum longus, peroneus longus, and peroneus tertius
5. Biceps femoris, semimembranosus, semitendinosus, gracilis, sartorius, popliteus, and gastrocnemius
6. Biceps femoris and popliteus
7. Pectineus, rectus femoris, adductor brevis, adductor longus, and adductor magnus
8. Plantaris, soleus, flexor hallucis longus, gastrocnemius, and tibialis posterior

Fill in the blanks (p. 670)

1. extensor digitorum longus; extensor hallucis longus
2. adductor brevis; adductor longus; adductor magnus
3. biceps femoris; semimembranosus; semitendinosus
4. *digit*
5. popliteus

Label the diagram (p. 670)

1. Tensor fasciae latae
2. Rectus femoris
3. Vastus lateralis
4. Iliopsoas
5. Pectineus
6. Adductor longus
7. Sartorius
8. Gracilis
9. Vastus medialis

Right word or wrong word: myotonia or myotomy? (p. 674)

In a conversation, these two words may sound similar if you are not listening closely. The word endings are different and pronounced differently. The importance of attentive and accurate listening cannot be stressed enough for the health-care provider.

Myotonia refers to a muscle spasm (i.e., the tone is rigid) after use or stimulation. It is pronounced mī-ă-tō′ nē-ă.

Myotomy refers to the anatomical dissection or surgical incision or division of a muscle. It is pronounced mī-ŏt′ ō-mē.

Right word or wrong word: asthenia or anesthesia? (p. 677)

There is no spelling error.

Asthenia means *lack of strength.*

Anesthesia means *partial or complete loss of sensation or with or without loss of consciousness.*

Let's practice (p. 677)

1. Tonicity
2. Tone
3. Idiopathic
4. Hemidystonia
5. Tonic and clonic muscle spasms
6. Antagonist
7. Phasic
8. Sthenos or sthenia
9. Reciprocal innervation
10. Hypotonia

Build a word (p. 678)

1. neuromyotonia
2. innervation
3. calisthenics
4. hypersthenia
5. isometric

Reflective questions (p. 683)

1. TENS targets pain and provides pain relief. E-stim targets muscle activity and function.
2. No; isometric exercise does not involve resistance.
3. A morphine-like substance produced by the brain
4. *Analgesia*
5. The application of cold reduces inflammation.

Mix and match (p. 684)

1. The FIM Locomotion Scale
2. A goniometer
3. A myotonometer
4. The Walk Test
5. GARS
6. The Balance Test

Fill in the blanks (p. 684)

1. TENS
2. isometric
3. endurance
4. range-of-motion
5. functional balance
6. aquatherapy
7. massage
8. electrical stimulation
9. TENS
10. locomotor (functional independence measure)

Critical thinking (p. 684)

1. Electronic muscle stimulation
2. Emergency medical services

Critical thinking (p. 690)

1. No; it's not likely, because there has been no mention of him suffering from pain.
2. It was a good idea to involve Glory because she will be caring for Gil at home very shortly, and she needs to know how to help him. She may also need to know how to make the environment in the house more amenable to having a person with a wheelchair and crutches move about in it.
3. They both add weight (a form of resistance) to the muscles and joints of the injured leg in addition to the normal pull of gravity when a person stands or walks.

Reflective questions (p. 690)

1. Stitches
2. Sutures were removed from the site of the right hip incision and bilaterally along the incision sites at the distal portion of the tibia, where the pilon fracture was repaired.
3. Rehabilitation technician

Translate the terms (p. 691)

1. Point on the pelvic bone where the hip joint comes into contact with it
2. Repaired / realigned
3. Shin
4. A process of getting fit or well again
5. A protrusion or projection
6. Upright
7. Covering
8. Move / push forward
9. Farthest away from the center or a point of origin
10. Endure, tolerate, or withstand

Right word or wrong word: occupational therapist or physical therapist? (p. 692)

They are not the same.

Occupational therapists focus on activities of daily living and helping patients to strive for independence in that regard.

Physical therapists focus on muscle strength and the range of motion of joints to help patients achieve optimal functioning in these areas.

Reflective questions (p. 694)

1. His right hand
2. The brain
3. The OT assistant
4. A neurological assessment

Right word or wrong word: response time or reaction time? (p. 696)

These are not synonymous.

Reaction time is the period of time between the stimulus occurring and the reaction to it occurring.

Response time is the duration of a response or how long the response continues.

Fill in the blanks (p. 696)

1. contraindicated
2. impulse control center
3. reaction time
4. grasp response
5. fine motor
6. occupational therapy

Free writing (p. 696)

Sample answer

Gil Loeppky suffers from some short-term memory impairment that may be related to his minor concussion or his subsequent brain injury. He is being treated for this memory impairment in occupational therapy. He also suffers from distractibility and some irritability that the treatment team believes is a response to the pain that he feels in the pins and screws that have been surgically placed to repair and stabilize his right tibia. The patient also tires from prolonged activity. This lack of stamina may be in response to the fact he has recently been seriously injured and undergone surgery. Fatigue like this can also lead to some irritability. The treatment team is trying not to overload this patient's daily schedule and thus is providing him with ample time to rest between his treatments and activities.

Critical thinking (p. 701)

1. Retrospective memory deficit
2. An external memory strategy
3. The internal memory strategy of associating the smell of coffee with morning and the time to get up
4. Among the assessment tests that might be appropriate for Gil are the following:
   - Cognitive Assessment of Minnesota (CAM). This may be used because Gil has some problems with distractibility and attention span, as well as memory
   - Chessington Occupational Therapy Neurological Assessment Battery. This type of testing may be appropriate because Gil is somewhat unsteady on his feet, and this unsteadiness may be related to deficits in visual perception. The OT will also want to assess Gil's ability to follow directions, because the entire treatment team will be giving Gil directions for follow-up care and rehabilitation to prepare him for discharge. They will want to do so at a level that he is capable of comprehending at this point in time.
   - Loewenstein Occupational Therapy Assessment. Although Gil has not shown any significant neurological impairment, it is important to monitor his orientation to time, place, and person, as well as his ability to solve problem and apply skills, and this test will help with that monitoring.
   - Rivermead Behavioral Memory Test, third edition. Gil has an acquired brain injury. This test is an excellent choice for Gil and will provide the OT team with important information about how to proceed to rehabilitate his short-term memory.
   - Psychosocial Adjustment to Illness Scale. This test is appropriate for Gil because he has a number of situations to deal with now: a recovery period that will last an undetermined amount of time; job and income concerns; a new baby; a wife who was also injured; and even a potential court case related to the motor vehicle accident.

Let's practice (p. 702)

1. Kinetic Self-Image Test
2. Global Assessment of Functioning
3. Katz Index of Activities of Daily Living
4. Rancho Los Amigos Level of Cognitive Functioning Scale
5. Psychosocial Adjustment to Illness Scale / Derogatis Test

Critical thinking (p. 704)

Sample answers

1. This is another example of the mind-body connection, but now we see how this concept relates to healing. In previous chapters, we saw that Gil and his wife were both excited about the baby whom they were expecting. However, the baby came early and under difficult circumstances. Gil's wife, Glory, lamented that Gil could not be there for the birth as they had planned (see Chapter 8) because Gil was admitted to a different hospital at that time (see Chapter 10). Up to this point, Gil has been deprived of meeting and holding his baby, although he has received photos and updates daily. Psychologically, it is very healing for Gil to be able to see his baby at this time. The proof is certainly visible in his response to the offer of the visit and his reaction to finally meeting Emily Grace.
2. To prevent the spread of microorganisms in an intensive care unit for premature babies
3. She demonstrated the grasp response.

Chapter review

Critical thinking (p. 705)

1. A finger or toe
2. A number
3. Short-term memory deficit and distractibility / attention span deficits

Agonists and antagonists (p. 706)

1. Flexor digitorum longus
2. Hamstrings
3. Flexor hallucis longus
4. Soleus

Break it down (p. 706)

1. myo + tono + meter
2. loco + motion
3. dys + trophy
4. ant(i) + agonist
5. electr/o + encephal/o + gram
6. anti + convuls + ant

Right word or wrong word: self-esteem or self-image? (p. 706)

These are not the same.

Self-image is the view of the self that includes one's perceived attributes and personality traits but that does not necessarily include value judgments.

Self-esteem is the self-appraisal of one's own worth that does include many positive or negative value judgments about one's perceived attributes.

Label the muscles (p. 706)

1. Gastrocnemius
2. Peroneus longus
3. Soleus

Word accuracy (p. 707)

1. A spasm or a state of temporary rigidity after a muscle contraction
2. The state of lacking or being deficient in normal muscle tone (tonus)
3. Disordered tonicity of the muscles

Chapter 16: The Mind-Body Connection

Reflective questions (p. 711)

1. Stevie-Rose made the appointment because she does not think that she is coping well with her life right now. She wants some guidance for coping with stress, and she wants some lab tests to be taken to be sure that she is physically well.
2. The physical symptom of arthritis pain is causing some of Stevie-Rose's emotional challenges, such as her difficulties with concentrating and coping with stress.

Critical thinking (p. 712)

1. Post-traumatic stress disorder
2. She is considered a client because she is neither an inpatient nor an outpatient of the Sumac Veteran's Medical Center. Rather, she is a client of the clinic.

Right word or wrong word: counselor, therapist, or psychologist? (p. 713)

Although sometimes these words are used interchangeably, they are not synonyms.

A professional *counselor* is a practitioner who needs only a bachelor's degree. Counselors work with clients in short-term, solution-focused interactions. They cannot do not do the work of psychologists unless they achieve a PhD in counseling.

A *therapist* is a practitioner with a doctoral degree that prepares him or her to work over a long period of time and in great depth with clients. Professions that are qualified to enter into this work are psychotherapists, psychiatrists, and advanced-practice psychiatric nurses. Social workers with advanced training in this field may also do this work, but counselors may not.

Psychologists treat emotional and mental health challenges, including those with behavioral manifestations (i.e., demonstrations of ineffective, inappropriate, or dysfunctional behavior). Psychologists are licensed to conduct psychological tests and to determine appropriate courses of treatment that are based on the outcomes of these tests. Psychologists may do both counseling and therapy, as they so choose. They may also be involved in research.

Right word or wrong word: chronic or chorionic? (p. 717)

No, they are not the same. These are two separate and distinct words.

Chronic means *persisting over a long period of time.*

Chorionic means *pertaining to the chorion, the outer membrane covering an embryo.*

Critical thinking (p. 717)

A nurse practitioner is an advanced practicing nurse (APN) with a good deal of autonomy (independence) over clinical decision making and client care. Many nurse practitioners are able to prescribe medications (see Chapter 3).

Fill in the blanks (p. 717)

1. emotional / psychological
2. exhibiting
3. clinical
4. intake
5. disconnected
6. posture
7. open / open posture

Right word or wrong word: compensate or complement? (p. 720)

They are not the same.

Compensate means *to mitigate, counterbalance, or offset.*

Complement means *to enhance, accompany, bring balance, or match.*

Critical thinking (p. 721)

Flashbacks arise in the temporal lobe, particularly when they involve visual and emotional memory.

Let's practice (p. 721)

1. Mental math
2. Face memory, which is located in the temporal lobe
3. Impulsively
4. Frontal lobe / premotor region
5. In the parietal lobe
6. The temporal lobe / music memory

Let's practice (p. 723)

1. Endorphin
2. Sleep
3. Opium
4. Narcotic
5. Meditation
6. Therapeutic touch

Critical thinking (p. 723)

Sample answers

1. A lack of sleep influences physical health because the body does not have enough time to rest and repair any damage or physical stress. The immune system does not function at its optimal level, either. This can lead to feeling unwell during the waking hours, having difficulty concentrating, having a sense of low energy, and the inability to enjoy things or to participate in activities that are mentally stimulating or emotionally pleasing.
2. Lack of sleep influences mental health because there is no time for the mind to process the events of the day or to be calm and fully relaxed. It may be overstimulated for prolonged periods, and this can lead to frustration, moodiness, irritability, distractibility, and a sense of being unable to accomplish tasks. The more restless, unhappy, and fatigued the mind is, the more it is unable to release control to allow sleep. This can lead to insomnia and to physical exhaustion.

Right word or wrong word: domains or dimensions of health? (p. 724)

The terms *domains* and *dimensions* of health are often used synonymously in health care, although they do not have exactly the same meaning. The term *dimensions* more accurately refers to more than the five domains of health. For example, in Chapter 2, the dimensions of health included functional aspects of the patient that needed to be assessed and included on an admission chart. In Chapter 7, the dimensions of health included all factors that contribute to mental health and illness; these went above and beyond the five domains of health. In sum, the term *dimensions of health* can be used in a much a broader sense than the term *domains of health. Dimensions* can include the individual, family, group, community, and society, as well as their interrelationships with health, health care, and opportunities for a healthful life.

Critical thinking (p. 728)

- The amygdala: Stevie-Rose senses that she has lost her sense of humor for now; she does not seem to be upbeat or cheerful. She is also experiencing anxiety, and she may have some fear related to her husband's health and a pending court date.
- The hypothalamus: Stevie-Rose mentions her lack of energy, and this may have something to do with the adrenal glands or other hormone levels in her system.

Mix and match (p. 728)

1. hippocampus
2. thalamus
3. hypothalamus
4. cingulate gyrus
5. amygdala

Fill in the blanks (p. 729)

1. stressors
2. anxiety
3. preoccupation
4. disturbed thought process
5. limbic system
6. mind-body connection
7. hypothalamus
8. ruminating

Label the health assessment diagram (p. 729)

Sample answers

1. Psychological and emotional domain:
   - PTSD
   - may have either depression or anxiety, or these may be part of her PTSD
   - trying to cope with multiple stressors
   - currently taking an antidepressant to relieve insomnia (which may be physical or psychological in origin)
   - cognitively and intellectually high functioning (intact)
2. Physical domain
   - chronic illnesses present
   - experiencing some physical pain and discomfort
   - decreased activity and exercise
   - may have B_{12} deficiency, leading to what appears to be psychological / emotional challenges
   - currently taking an antidepressant to relieve insomnia (which may be physical or psychological in origin)
3. Social
   - square dances with a group
   - does not mention any friends
   - unsure about possible criminal actions against spouse (potential for social stigma and husband's loss of driver's license)
4. Family
   - family involvement that seems, for the most part, to be supportive
5. Environmental
   - drives a car, so is mobile and able to independently get to appointments and so on
   - details of housing not available but voices no concerns

Critical thinking (p. 730)

Stevie-Rose is not in an optimal state of physical or mental health. Her overall wellness is impaired: she is not functioning physically or mentally as well as she would like to be or as she would expect for herself. She needs medical and psychological or psychiatric assistance.

Reflective questions (p. 732)

1. Motor vehicle accident
2. Nurse practitioner
3. Temperature, pulse, and respiration
4. It's standard procedure in health care to assess the patient's physical body before assessing his or her mind. This point was addressed in Units 1 and 2.

Let's practice (p. 732)

1. F
2. F
3. F
4. F
5. T

Critical thinking (p. 733)

Counseling was called because, historically, this client would never accept or admit that she may have PTSD. In previous chapters, Stevie-Rose got angry each time this was suggested. Ophelia knows that this is often the way persons with PTSD react to their illness. Ophelia showed good clinical judgment by acting quickly on the client's admission that she has the disorder.

Right word or wrong word: phagocyte or phacocyst? (p. 737)

They are not the same with regard to spelling, pronunciation, or meaning. These are two very separate words. These two words illustrate just how important it is to listen carefully and to spell correctly.

A *phagocyte* is a white blood cell that ingests and destroys microorganisms and dead or dying cells.

A *phacocyst* is the capsule of the crystalline lens of the eye. The combining form *phaco-* means *lens.*

Critical reflection questions (p. 739)

1. Droplet
2. Vector borne
3. Macrophages
4. Basophils
5. Neutrophils
6. Interleukins

Critical thinking (p. 740)

Droplet via coughing

Break it down (p. 740)

1. phag/o + lysis = the dissolution or destruction of phagocytes (This is a synonym for *phagocytolysis.*)
2. eosin/o + penia = a small or low number of eosinophils in the bloodstream (The suffix *-penia* means *poverty of* or *lack of.)*
3. baso + philia = a condition of having a high number of basophils in the blood
4. neutr/o + penia = an abnormally small number of neutrophils in the blood

Let's practice (p. 740)

1. Necrophobia
2. Autophobia
3. Blogophobia
4. Homophobia
5. Coulrophilia
6. Agliophilia
7. Gerascophilia (gerontophilia)
8. Phalacophilia

Right word or wrong word: rubeola or rubella? (p. 743)

Rubeola is the medical term for measles.

Rubella is the medical term for German measles specifically.

Reflective questions (p. 745)

1. Exempt from or protected from
2. Eating, ingesting, or devouring
3. The process of dissolving, destroying, or disintegrating cells
4. Deficient, short of, lacking, or an insufficient quantity
5. Droplet contact
6. Innate immunity or acquired immunity (through immunization)
7. Innate or natural immunity (natural resistance)
8. Smallpox
9. Inoculation

Let's practice (p. 745)

1. Hepatitis A
2. Tetanus
3. Tuberculosis
4. German measles
5. Hepatitis B
6. Measles

Right word or wrong word: hives or rash? (p. 750)

No, they are not exactly the same. Although *hives* (urticaria) are a type of rash, they result only from exposure to allergens. There are many types of rashes, and most of them are not hives. Rashes can be caused by many things, such as heat, sunburn, friction / rubbing / irritation, disease (i.e., measles), or exposure of the skin to urine or feces over long periods (i.e., diaper rash).

Right word or wrong word: food allergy or food intolerance? (p. 750)

No, they are not the same. Most adverse reactions to food are intolerances and not specifically allergies. Diarrhea, vomiting, or stomach cramps may occur with both food allergies and food intolerance. These shared symptoms are what lead to the confusion about which term is correct to use. Food allergies bring on the additional (and often rapid) symptoms of tingling in the mouth; swelling of the lips, tongue, and throat; and difficulty breathing normally.

Let's practice (p. 752)

1. Pruritus
2. Epinephrine
3. Urticaria
4. Angioedema
5. Dyspnea
6. Smell
7. Laryngeal edema
8. Antigen desensitization
9. Symptomatic
10. Asymptomatic

Mix and match (p. 752)

1. egg allergy
2. cat allergy
3. peanut allergy
4. penicillin allergy
5. milk allergy

Build a word (p. 752)

1. autovaccine: a vaccine prepared from a virus in the person's own body
2. autohypnosis: self-hypnosis or self-induced hypnosis
3. autoantitoxin: an antitoxin (i.e., an antibody that opposes a toxin) that is produced in the body itself
4. autogenesis: self-generation
5. autohemolysin: an antibody that attacks or destroys a person's own blood
6. autophagia: biting or attempting to eat oneself (this term can be used to describe a disturbed behavior or the actions of cells)

Critical thinking (p. 752)

1. She has diabetes, and she has had it for some time.
2. Stevie-Rose has many health challenges that can cause or be caused by vitamin B_{12} deficiency. These include coping with significant stress, changes in appetite or nutrition, diabetes, and hypothyroidism.

Critical thinking (p. 756)

1. Pain and mood are both influenced by the limbic and immune systems. These systems have to decide where to spend their energy by determining which symptom requires more attention. This focus can deplete the ability to tolerate or cope with the other issue. In addition, pain makes people irritable and unhappy; they are restless and unable to eat and sleep adequately. Poor nutrition and lack of sleep also negatively affect mood.
2. Mood can be altered negatively because of immune and limbic system activity related to the disease but also because the person becomes increasingly aware of pending disability, an increase in pain, and so on. The person can become more irritable and frustrated. Self-efficacy and self-esteem may be affected, and a diagnosis of depression may occur.

Right word or wrong word: athero- or artho-? (p. 761)

No, they are not the same. They refer to different systems of the body.

Athero means *a deposit* and refers to the circulatory system (i.e., atherosclerosis).

Artho means *joint* and refers to the musculoskeletal system (i.e., arthritis).

Mix and match (p. 762)

1. thumb
2. neck
3. wrist
4. knee
5. skull sutures
6. hip

Let's practice (p. 762)

1. Revision arthroplasty
2. Amphiarthrosis
3. Gout
4. PQRST

Build a word (p. 762)

1. arthroscopy: the visual examination of a joint with the use of an arthroscope inserted into it
2. oligemia: too little blood in the system
3. arthrodynia: pain in a joint

Reflective questions (p. 762)

1. An established set of steps
2. The quality of pain (i.e., throbbing, stabbing)
3. A device that allows for patient-controlled analgesia
4. Five
5. Diarthrosis
6. *Convex* means *curving outward; concave* means *curving inward.*

Chapter review

Critical thinking (p. 767)

1. A group, cluster, or collection of symptoms
2. Stevie-Rose has a problem with being referred to as *elderly* because, to her, the word has connotations of someone frail who needs assistance with day-to-day living. She sees herself as younger, spry, mentally and cognitively well, and high functioning.
3. Arthritis is treated by rheumatologists because rheumatologists concern themselves with the pathology of the joints and connective tissues of the musculoskeletal system. Orthopedic surgeons also work with the musculoskeletal system, but they are more concerned with bones, trauma, infection, and congenital abnormalities.

Reflective questions (p. 767)

1. Hippocampi
2. T-cells
3. *Antigens* are pathogens or foreign invaders that trigger the immune response. *Antibodies* are the part of the immune system that responds to antigens.
4. A person becomes immune after exposure to an antigen, and the memory cell lymphocytes code for it or remember it to protect that individual from any future exposure to it.
5. No
6. Osteoarthritis

Translate the terminology (p. 767)

Sample translation

There are a number of groups of limbic nerve cells located deep within the brain. The limbic structures and the hypothalamus are found at the front of the brain, and they are crucial to survival. They stimulate the activities of finding food, protecting oneself, and adapting to the environment. There is also a link between the limbic system and motor function that helps a person to carry out these activities. Before the age of 3 years, the amygdala and the cingulate are involved in the creation of connections between nerve synapses. These connections lead to the ability to be social rather than withdrawn, the ability to bond with others, and the ability to respond with appropriate emotion. When these connections are not made, the opposite behaviors can occur.

Fill in the blanks (p. 768)

1. *fimbria*
2. short-term
3. gouty
4. Osteoarthritis
5. immune; limbic
6. Ageism

Break it down (p. 768)

1. gero + psych + iatr + y
2. rheuma + tic
3. arthro + scop + y
4. immuno + deficienc + y
5. phag/o + cyt/o + lysis

Right word or wrong word: osteo- or arthro-? (p. 768)

Osteo means *bone,* and *arthro* means *joint.*

Right word or wrong word: HPV or HBV? (p. 768)

No, they're not the same. *HPV* refers to human papillomavirus, and *HBV* refers to hepatitis B virus.

Word accuracy (p. 769)

1. A *therapist* can provide therapy. A *counselor* does not provide therapy, which is deeper, takes a long time, and requires more training and expertise than counseling.
2. *Active immunity* is dependent on exposure to an antigen and the ability of the immune-response lymphocytes to remember it. *Passive immunity* is the result of exposure to antibodies produced in one person's body and then acquired by another.
3. *Senior* is a term that refers to maturity or maturity of age. *Elderly* is an adjective that describes someone who is considered old.

Chapter 17: Reproductive and Family Health

Reflective questions (p. 772)

1. It has been 5 weeks since the accident.
2. It has healed, but it has left a scar.
3. It is healing well, but she wears a protective brace to support the injured site PRN.

Right word or wrong word: after birth or afterbirth? (p. 774)

No; it is not correct to write them as if they were the same word, because they are not.

After birth is the period of time that follows the birth of a child or the postpartum period. This is a descriptive term that describes when something has occurred.

Afterbirth is a noun that identifies the biological material that is expelled from the uterus immediately after the birth of a baby. It includes the placenta, the fetal membrane, and any debris. *Afterbirth* is sometimes used as a synonym for *placenta*, which is not completely accurate.

Right word or wrong word: postpartum or postnatal? (p. 774)

As a health professional, you will want to use the most appropriate term in your work.

These two words are technically not the same, although they are sometimes used interchangeably.

Postpartum refers to the mother after giving birth.

Postnatal refers to the infant after being born.

Reflective questions (p. 775)

1. Sutures
2. Frequency
3. Subcuticular

Critical thinking (p. 775)

Zane Davis went to a step-down unit.

Fill in the blanks (p. 776)

1. dissolve
2. pump
3. speculum

Reflective questions (p. 778)

1. Biological / physical, psychological, social (family, baby, supports), and environmental (managing in the home with someone with a temporary disability)
2. Because she is facing many stressors in her life right now in addition to being at risk for postpartum depression since she just had a baby

Critical thinking (p. 778)

1. Yes. She may be feeling some guilt for having taken Gil's hand off the steering wheel to feel her belly. This can be heard in her tone of voice and seen in her body language. She also mentions what she did by asking a question about it without seeking an answer. This behavior suggests that her actions just before the accident are weighing on her mind.
2. She feared losing her baby.
3. Because he wants to regain his independence
4. Dr. Antoine had this conversation because he understands the mind-body connection and the interplay of the domains of health. He has taken a more holistic approach to his patient as a unique individual in her own unique circumstances, and he wants to assess whether or not she has a healthy balance in her life right now. He also knows that, by engaging her in conversation, he can assess her mental health and her cognitive and emotional levels of functioning.

Right word or wrong word: bonding or attachment? (p. 779)

Bonding and attachment are not the same thing.

Bonding is a term often heard in maternal and child health care. It is also very common in psychiatry, psychology and social work. Under optimal circumstances parents bond with their children at the time of birth. However, there is good evidence that bonding can occur at any age when a core caregiver is present. Adult couples may bond with each other. It is possible for an adult to both bond and attach or simply achieve one or the other. People will bond under traumatic circumstances. After the event, the relationship is over. It is quite possible to feel bonded to someone and not have them reciprocate this feeling.

Attachment is a medical, psychological and sociological term that describes **the mutual** and emotionally positive relationship that occurs between infants and caregiver (i.e., parent(s) or others). Infants and children attach. A newborn baby attaches to the care-provider through the senses of touch, sound, sight, smell, as well as through a sense of safety, security and comfort.

Consider this, it is unlikely that a nanny or other childcare provider is bonded to the infant or child under her care. However in this instance, both adult and child can form very strong, loving attachments to each other, which provide comfort, joy and contentment for both. Parents, grandparents, relatives and/or significant others can also enjoy this attachment relationship.

Mix and match (p. 780)

1. sadness
2. tachypnea
3. unsure, undecided, or hesitant
4. tendency
5. passing, fleeting, temporary
6. panicky, hysterical, or desperate
7. distrustful, fearful, and suspicious

Let's practice (p. 780)

1. Postpartum
2. False beliefs
3. Murder of an infant

Reflective question (p. 781)

Two

Critical thinking (p. 782)

He means that Glory is physically able to have intercourse without risk of pain or injury, because she is no longer bleeding postpartum and she did not incur any injury to her vagina during the birth of her child.

Right word or wrong word: puberty or adolescence? (p. 784)

No, they do not describe the same thing.

Puberty is a biological period of sexual growth and development.

Adolescence is a period of psychosocial growth and development that occurs at approximately (but not exactly) the same time as puberty. Adolescence is a longer period of time.

Build a word (p. 787)

1. conceptive: capable of conceiving
2. infecundity: condition of not being fertile
3. impregnable: unable to become pregnant
4. preconception: in the context of this chapter, the timeframe of the female reproductive cycle that precedes pregnancy
5. puberulent: covered with fine, minute hairs

Let's practice (p. 787)

1. Prepubescence
2. Fertilization
3. Impregnation
4. Fecundation
5. Superfecundication

Free writing (p. 787)

Sample answers

1. Preconception health refers to the timeframe in the female reproductive cycle preceding pregnancy.
2. A prepubescent child is approximately 10 to 12 years of age.
3. Syphilis is a serious STD that requires early intervention with an intramuscular injection of penicillin.

Fill in the blanks (p. 787)

1. reproduce
2. *abortion*
3. Pregnancy / Conception
4. sexually transmitted disease
5. Bacterial
6. sexual transmission
7. dyspareunia

Let's practice (p. 787)

1. Impregnated / impregnation
2. Conception
3. Infertile

Mix and match (p. 788)

1. can lead to development of genital warts
2. can lead to blindness, deafness, heart disease
3. can lead to infertility if not treated
4. causes small blisters on the genitals
5. microscopic parasites infect urethra and vagina

Right word or wrong word: infertility or impotency? (p. 792)

No, they are not the same.

Impotency refers to a man's inability to have or maintain an erection, which has nothing to do with a man's *fertility* (i.e., the ability to produce viable sperm). *Infertile* males can certainly have erections. They may also be able to ejaculate, but they cannot produce an offspring. However, it is possible that a man can have both infertility and impotency at the same time. For example, in the case of a medical condition such as prostate cancer, the treatment may cause the patient to become both infertile and impotent.

Reflective questions (p. 793)

1. Hormones that are released to cause the onset of puberty (i.e., sexual and reproductive development)
2. Testicular teratoma
3. Cryptorchidism, testicular teratoma, testicular torsion, and varicocele can lead to infertility. Each of these conditions affects the testes, and sperm is produced in the testes.

Mix and match (p. 793)

1. azoospermia
2. ductus ejaculatori
3. motility
4. viscous
5. flagellum
6. agglutinated
7. libido
8. torsion

Let's practice (p. 794)

1. Infertility; impotency
2. Fertility
3. Vasography
4. Semen analysis
5. Erectile dysfunction / impotency
6. Cryptorchidism / cryptorchism

Fill in the blanks (p. 804)

1. infertility
2. *menses / menstruation*
3. follicular
4. *impregnated / impregnation*
5. oocyte
6. Estrogen
7. progesterone
8. estrogen; progesterone

Mix and match (p. 804)

1. zygote
2. womb
3. eggs
4. shedding
5. egg
6. menstrual period
7. ovigenesis
8. ovaries

Break it down (p. 804)

1. dysmenorrhea; dys-
2. menopause; men
3. endometrium; endo
4. menarche; men
5. fallotomy; -otomy

Build a word (p. 804)

1. ovariogenic: originating in the ovary
2. ovariotomy: the surgical incision of the ovary
3. ovariorrhexis: the rupture or hemorrhage of an ovary
4. oophorectomy: the surgical removal of an ovary

Critical thinking (p. 810)

1. Prolactin will be dominant, because she is breastfeeding.
2. Infection occurs when pathogens enter the body and cause symptoms or injury. Disease does not need an infection to begin (i.e., coronary artery disease, multiple sclerosis). However, some diseases can be transmitted to others; when this occurs, they are considered *infectious diseases* (i.e., syphilis, measles).

Reflective questions (p. 810)

1. Prolactin
2. Gynecomastia
3. Lobules
4. Phylloid tumors of the breast; galactorrhea
5. The shape, structure, and position of the breasts on the chest wall
6. The microscopic laboratory testing of tissue and blood

Build a word (p. 810)

1. lactogen: any substance that stimulates the production of milk (i.e., prolactin)
2. lactorrhea: the flow of milk (between nursings or feedings or after weaning the baby from the breast)
3. mammalgia: pain in the breast

Let's practice (p. 816)

1. Sample answers: sponge, diaphragm, condom, IUD
2. Conception
3. The client (i.e., the person who would have the child or not)
4. The uterus

Mix and match (p. 816)

1. spermicide
2. intrauterine device
3. coitus interruptus
4. abstention
5. birth control pills

Critical thinking (p. 821)

1. Because he or she is very likely to encounter these clients and their families throughout his or her career
2. infant
3. Poor motor coordination (Notice how many of the screening and diagnostic tests assess for motor coordination at this stage.)

Reflective questions (p. 821)

1. psychosocial
2. Through colostrum and breast milk
3. adolescence
4. Through the mother's bloodstream into the fetus's bloodstream (via the placenta) and then through colostrum and breast milk
5. Sucking at the breast by the baby
6. Toddler, preschooler, school-aged child, and preadolescent

Mix and match (p. 822)

1. respiratory, neuromuscular
2. severe dehydration and diarrhea
3. muscle fatigue and wasting; possible paralysis
4. pox (blisters; sores on the skin)

Let's practice (p. 822)

1. Wechsler Preschool and Primary Scale of Intelligence III
2. Developmental Indicators for the Assessment of Learning
3. Hawaii Early Learning Profile
4. Measles, mumps, and rubella (vaccine)
5. Diphtheria, tetanus, and pertussis (vaccine)
6. Early Screening Inventory, Revised
7. Pervasive developmental disorder
8. Denver Developmental Screening Test II
9. Peabody Picture Vocabulary Test 4 Public health nurse

Critical thinking (p. 825)

Biological: It provides a womb-like environment that is familiar to the newborn.

Psychological: The presence of another human being simulates what was experienced in the womb and also adds the comfort of knowing on a very deep level that one is not alone or unprotected and that one is safe and cared for. It enhances the bonding process.

Social: It introduces the baby to a variety of people, experiences, and sensation that stimulate growth and development while reinforcing a sense of belonging.

Chapter review

Critical thinking (p. 827)

1. *GRGH* refers to growth-releasing growth hormones, whereas *GRH* refers to gonadotropin-releasing hormone.
2. The childbearing years
3. The neonatal nursery is a step-down unit for the less critically ill or fragile neonate.
4. Roberta, the neonatal nurse, suggested that the Loeppkys visit the public health clinic, because it offers services and support for the parents of premature infants.

Right word or wrong word: oophorectomy or oophorocystectomy? (p. 827)

These are not the same, and there is no spelling error present.

Oophorectomy is the removal of an ovary.

Oophorocystectomy is the removal of an ovarian cyst.

Reflective questions (p. 828)

1. *Fecund* is the root, and it means *fruitfulness or fertility.*
2. A fertilized egg
3. *Cyst*
4. A liquid substance that contains antibodies that is first secreted by the mammary glands after childbirth
5. impregnate
6. abortion
7. human papillomavirus (HPV)

Mix and match (p. 828)

1. ovarian cyclicity
2. shedding
3. pouch
4. ovary
5. zygote

True or false (p. 828)

1. F
2. F
3. T
4. F
5. T
6. T
7. T
8. F
9. T
10. T

Translate the terminology (p. 828)

Sample answer

It may be possible that people who have had an STD are more susceptible to becoming infected with HIV. Science is researching this possibility. Researchers are also investigating whether the reverse might be true. Researchers are trying to discover if people who have open sores (ulcers) as a symptom of an STD are more vulnerable to HIV infection (or vice versa).

Fill in the blanks (p. 829)

1. The childbearing years
2. coitus
3. preschool-aged children
4. Infant / Sensory
5. Family
6. contagious / sexually transmitted

Label the diagram (p. 829)

1. seminal vesicle
2. ejaculatory ducts
3. bulbulourethral glan
4. penis
5. urethra
6. glans penis
7. ureter
8. bladder
9. prostate gland
10. vas deferens
11. epididymus

Chapter 18: Putting It All Together

Critical thinking (p. 833)

The Health Sciences department wants to present information about new career opportunities in forensic sciences and forensic medicine and to demonstrate how these fields can apply to courses that the students are now taking (i.e., medical terminology).

Critical thinking (p. 839)

1. Root / root word / combining form
2. Prefix
3. Suffix

Let's practice (p. 840)

1. crani/o (skull or cranium) + -tomy (incision)
2. radi/o (ray) + -graph (write or record)
3. leuk/o (white) + -cyte (cell)
4. micro- (small) + bio (life) + olog (science of) + -ist (suffix identifying a person)
5. glyc/o (sugars) + emia (blood)
6. sarco (flesh) + adeno (gland) + -oma (tumor)
7. keton/o (acetone) + ur (urine) + -ia (state or condition of)
8. sub- (under) + lingu/a (tongue) + -al (pertaining to or characteristic of)
9. dent/o/I (teeth) + -algia (pain)
10. odont/o (teeth/tooth) + -rrhagia (abnormal or excessive bleeding or flow)

Free writing (p. 840)

1. disoriented; b.
2. apnea / dyspnea; b.
3. non-ambulant; a.
4. postpartum; b.
5. hyperglycemic; a.
6. intra-oral; b.
7. non-cancerous; b.
8. immature; b.
9. tachycardic; b.
10. dysfunction; b.

Mix and match (p. 841)

1. dermis
2. therapy
3. -plasia
4. thermia
5. dontal
6. venous
7. arachnoid
8. oma

Decode it: anatomical terms (p. 843)

1. Bone(s)
2. Gland(s)
3. Structure in the uterus through which the fetus receives oxygen and nourishment
4. White blood cell
5. Jawbones
6. Cell
7. The structure in the brain that regulates hormone production
8. Nerve cell
9. A muscular structure that includes an orifice through which solid waste products are eliminated
10. Red blood cells that transport oxygen

Decipher it (p. 843)

1. Cerebrospinal fluid
2. Temporomandibular joint
3. Oxygen
4. Deoxyribonucleic acid
5. Tonsils and adenoids
6. Vastus lateralis (muscle)
7. Range of motion
8. Dorsal gluteal (muscle)
9. Cranial nerve
10. Autonomic nervous system

Decode it: pathology terms (p. 844)

1. A blood clot in the leg
2. A tear in the placenta; a detachment of the placenta from the uterus
3. A disease of the pancreas related to insulin production
4. A malignant or benign abnormal aggregate of cells
5. Chickenpox
6. A disease or disorder of the nervous system
7. A collection of blood outside of the blood vessels, in the surrounding tissue
8. Any pathology or disruption of the skin or the loss of function of a body part
9. Excessive fluid build up in the tissues that causes swelling
10. A condition that causes thin, brittle bones as a result of calcium loss
11. Bacterial, viral, fungal, or parasitic infection that causes inflammation of the meninges in the brain
12. A naturally occurring action taken by the body to defend injured, damaged, or infected tissue

Decipher it (p. 844)

1. Chronic obstructive pulmonary disease
2. Human immunodeficiency virus
3. Attention deficit-hyperactivity disorder
4. Mild traumatic brain injury
5. Insulin-dependent diabetes mellitus
6. Human papillomavirus
7. Ulnar collateral ligament
8. Fracture (it does not mean *number* in pathophysiology)
9. Acute myelogenous leukemia / acute myeloid leukemia
10. Metastases

Decipher it (p. 844)

1. Temperature, pulse, and respiration
2. Arterial blood gases
3. Prothrombin time (*not* physical therapy; the context of this question is diagnostics)
4. Blood urea nitrogen (test)
5. Magnetic resonance imaging
6. Human chorionic gonadotropin
7. Fine-needle aspiration biopsy
8. Positron emission tomography
9. Milligram
10. Deciliter

Identify the body system (p. 845)

1. Skeletal
2. Muscular
3. Circulatory
4. Neurological

Identify the body parts (p. 846)

1. Label the internal organs visible on this diagram.
   1. Trachea
   2. Lungs
   3. Esophagus
   4. Diaphragm
   5. Stomach

2. Label the craniofacial bones.
   1. Frontal
   2. Nasal
   3. Zygomatic
   4. Parietal
   5. Temporal
   6. Occipital

3. Label the organs of the digestive system.
   1. Mouth
   2. Liver
   3. Gallblader
   4. Large intestine
   5. Esophagus
   6. Stomach
   7. Small intestine
   8. Rectum

Let's practice (p. 849)

1. *-ectomy*: surgical removal or cutting out; *-otomy*: derived from *tome,* which means *an incision*

2. *incise*: to cut or slice into; *excise*: to remove

3. *sonographer:* a health professional who uses a sonogram (ultrasound) to see inside the body; *radiographer*: a health professional who uses an x-ray to see inside the body

4. *EEG*: electroencephalogram (of brain activity); *ECG*: electrocardiogram (of heart activity)

5. *edema*: tissue swelling caused by excessive fluids accumulated within the tissue; *adrenal*: pertaining to the adrenal glands and their secretions

6. *postnatal*: a period of time after birth for an infant; *postpartum*: the same period of time for the woman who gave birth

7. *tachycardia*: rapid heartbeat; *bradycardia*: slow heartbeat

8. *epithelia*: the plural form of *epithelium*, which is one of the connective tissues of the body that covers surfaces; *endothelia*: the plural form of *endothelium*, which is a layer of thin cells or tissues that line internal body cavities and vessels

9. *rubella*: German measles; *rubeola*: measles or red measles

10. *HIV*: human immunodeficiency virus; *AIDS*: acquired immunodeficiency syndrome, which is the disease that may result from HIV infection

Critical thinking: medical records (p. 852)

1. On the Admission Form and the Consent for Treatment Form

2. The Transfer Note or Transfer Summary. These forms are usually found in the Admission, Transfer, and Discharge section at the end of the patient's medical record.

3. In the section called Laboratory and Diagnostic Reports

Decipher it (p. 852)

1. Kirschner wires: sharp, stainless steel pins that are used to hold bone fragments in place
2. nasogastric tube: a tube that extends through the nose and the nasal cavity, down the esophagus, and into the stomach through which the patient will receive daily nutrition
3. spica cast: a type of splint that immobilizes and protects the bones and the adjacent joints, ligaments, and tendons so that they can heal
4. drug screen: a laboratory analysis of the types of drugs in the body toxicology report: a laboratory analysis of the levels of poisons (or substances deemed noxious or harmful) in the body
5. transcutaneous electrical nerve stimulation device: a device that transmits electrical impulses through the skin and on to nerve receptor sites to temporarily block a pain response
6. observe for symmetry: part of the physical assessment protocol; the thorax is examined visually from a number of angles to evaluate its evenness and proportions
7. Global Assessment of Functioning test: a test that evaluates the occupational, social, and psychological functioning of adults using a scale of 1 to 100
8. urine dipstick test: identifies any abnormal characteristics in the composition of the urine
9. auscultation: the act or process of listening to the internal body with a stethoscope
10. no decelerations: no slowing down is present in a fetal heart rate as compared with a baseline measure

Decode it (p. 853)

1. Are the cheekbones broken?
   Section: Physician's Admission Notes; Laboratory and Diagnostic Reports
2. Did we get a panoramic x-ray of the upper jaw and the rounded ends of the mandible bone where they form the joint with it?
   Section: Laboratory and Diagnostic Reports
3. Who was the emergency medical technician at the scene of the incident who assessed which victim needed treatment first?
   Section: Admission Forms
4. Do you know if the patient who had a heart attack (myocardial infarction) was treated in the emergency room or ambulance with a device that either restarted the heart or changed its rhythm?
   Section: Physician's Admission Notes and Admission Forms
5. What were the circumstances that caused the injury or trauma to the abdomen?
   Section: Admission Notes
6. Did the patient have a fractured femur or the femoral head of the bone straightened and returned to its natural state by way of surgical intervention last year?
   Section: Patient History
7. Is this patient receiving antibiotic medication by infusion or injection into his veins?
   Section: Medication Administration
8. Is there a report on file confirming that the patient has many broken bones, particularly around the nose and eyes?
   Section: Physician's Admission Notes and Laboratory and Diagnostic Reports
9. Which doctor diagnosed the injuries of the chest, abdomen, and pelvis?
   Section: Physician's Progress Notes and Physician's Admission Notes
10. Is there a report on the medical record that identifies or confirms that scars on both sides of the body show the patient possibly had surgery to both kidneys?
    Section: Physician's Admission Notes

Critical thinking (p. 855)

1. Gil Loeppky: acute patellar injury (L knee); pilon fracture (L ankle / tibia / fibula); spiral fracture of left femoral head
   Glory Loeppky: ulnar collateral ligament injury (L thumb); laceration to deep muscle tissue (L thigh)
   Clay Davis: fracture of the mandible at midline
2. Stevie-Rose Davis
3. Zane Davis, Clay Davis, and Emily Grace Loeppky
4. Clay Davis could not give consent because he is a child. To treat a minor, doctors need consent from the child's parents.

Let's practice (p. 855)

1. Steven Zane Davis and his wife, Mickey Davis
2. An antepartum unit
3. Gil Loeppky: CT scan of the head after blunt force head injury and then after secondary injury that potentiated an increase in intracranial pressure and hemorrhaging in the brain
   Zane Davis: CT scan of the head for possible TIA or CVA
   Clay Davis: CT scan of the face and skull to assess craniofacial trauma
4. Gil Loeppky; acute patellar injury as a result of force exerted on his knee during the accident as he was applying the brakes
5. Zane Davis and Stevie-Rose Davis
6. The procedure was a non-stress test (NST). It is a type of fetal monitor that electronically monitors the fetus's well-being byassessing fetal movement, heart rate, and reactivity.
7. Zane Davis. A TAR is a treatment authorization record. Victoria, the medical unit clerk in the ICU at Okla Trauma Center, was responsible for this document.
8. Clay Davis. He had a symphyseal fracture midline on the lower mandible.
9. Thyroid replacement therapy (she takes levothyroxine tablets)
10. The EMTs were unable to determine if he had a spinal cord injury and proactively placed the collar to prevent injury or further injury.
11. Gil was unconscious and semiconscious with a head injury, and the staff did not know if it would be safe or possible for him to swallow. Clay had a fractured jaw and would not be able to open his mouth to eat until at least a day or so after the fracture was reduced and stabilized.
12. The physical therapist was concerned with the recovery of Gil Loeppky.

Admission forms (p. 856)

1.

Okla Trauma

Okla Trauma Center - Admission Form

Hospital ID: AyZ29763

Patient name: *Gilbert Loeppky* Patient DOB: *U/K* Age: *36 Years* Date of admission: *xxx June 20xxx*

Admitting diagnosis: *Acute head injury: loss of consciousness, concussion, craniofacial or occipital injury fractured femur femoral head, Acute patellar knee injury, ankle fracture*

Attending physician: *Dr. Raymond*

Allergies: *N/K*

Marital status: ✓ Married __ Single

Next of kin/significant other: *Glory Loeppky, wife*

Contact number for next of kin/significant other: (*555*)-*xxx*-*xxxx*

Emergency contact person (not living with patient): *Pat and Pearl Loeppky*

Number for emergency contact: (*555*)-*xxx*-*xxxx*

Relationship to patient: *parents*

Ambulatory: __ Yes ✓ No Conscious: __ Yes ✓ No

Medications prescribed or taken: __ Yes __ No ✓ U/K

Provide details, including last dose: ____

Alcohol or substance use prior to admission: __ Yes ✓ No __ U/K

Provide details: ____

Workplace accident: ✓ Yes __ No __

Police involved: ✓ Yes __ No

Occupation: *delivery truck driver*

Employer: *Hull Transport and Delivery*

Health Insurance: ✓ Yes __ No

Provide billing details: *per employer*

Hearing aids, glasses, or prosthetics: __ Yes ✓ No

Provide details: ____

Wallet and ID taken for safekeeping by admitting clerk: ✓ Yes __ No __ U/K

Provide signature: *D. Daboczi*

2.

Okla Trauma

Okla Trauma Center - Admission Form

Hospital ID: AyZ34293

Patient name: *Zane Davis* Patient DOB: *U/K* Age: *74 Years* Date of admission: *xxx June 20xxx*

Admitting diagnosis: *TIA, concussion, CVA*

Attending physician: *Dr. Crowchild*

Allergies: *N/K*

Marital status: ✓ Married __ Single

Next of kin/significant other: *Stevie-Rose Davis, wife*

Contact number for next of kin/significant other: (*555*)-*xxx*-*xxxx*

Emergency contact person (not living with patient): *Quincy Davis*

Number for emergency contact: (*555*)-*xxx*-*xxxx*

Relationship to patient: *eldest son*

Ambulatory: ✓ Yes __ No Conscious: ✓ Yes __ No

Medications prescribed or taken: __ Yes __ No ✓ U/K

Provide details, including last dose:

Alcohol or substance use prior to admission: __ Yes ✓ No __ U/K

Provide details:

Workplace accident: __ Yes ✓ No

Police involved: ✓ Yes __ No

Occupation: *telecommunications technician*

Employer: *retired from U.S. Navy*

Health Insurance: ✓ Yes __ No

Provide billing details: *Department of Veterans Affairs*

Hearing aids, glasses, or prosthetics: ✓ Yes __ No __ U/K

Provide details: *Wears glasses*

Wallet and ID taken for safekeeping by admitting clerk: __ Yes __ No ✓ U/K

Provide signature: *D. Daboczi*

3.

Okla Trauma

Okla Trauma Center - Admission Form

Hospital ID: Ay34256

Patient name: Clay Davis Patient DOB: U/K Age: 7 Years Date of admission: xxx June 20xxx

Admitting diagnosis: Mandibular Fracture - symphyseal plus other craniofacial trauma. Partial thickness burn (L) upper torso scald

Attending physician: Dr. Raymond, ER; Dr. Lincoln, Pediatrics; Dr. R. Sandor, Dental/craniofacial surgeon

Allergies: Unknown at this time.

Marital status: __ Married ✓ Single

Next of kin/significant other: Steven Zane Davis and Mickey Davis

Contact number for next of kin/significant other: (555)-xxx-xxxx

Emergency contact person (not living with patient): Zane and Stevie-Rose Davis

Number for emergency contact: (555)-xxx-xxxx

Relationship to patient: grandparents

Ambulatory: __ Yes ✓ No Conscious: ✓ Yes __ No

Medications prescribed or taken: __ Yes __ No ✓ U/K

Provide details, including last dose:

Alcohol or substance use prior to admission: __ Yes ✓ No __ U/K

Provide details: young child

Workplace accident: __ Yes ✓ No

Police involved: ✓ Yes __ No

Occupation: N/A

Employer: N/A

Health Insurance: ✓ Yes __ No

Provide billing details: per parents HMO xxxxxxxxxx

Hearing aids, glasses, or prosthetics: __ Yes __ No ✓ U/K

Provide details:

Wallet and ID taken for safekeeping by admitting clerk: __ Yes __ No ✓ U/K

Provide signature: D. Daboczi

Vital signs flowsheet on the e-medical record

FAYETTE GENERAL HOSPITAL

Clinical Documentation

Patient: STEVIE-ROSE DAVIS Unit/Bed: ER Account #:

Age: 72 Gender: F Height: Weight: Admit Physician: JENSEN

Status: ALERT & CONFUSED Attend Physician: JENSEN

Vital Sign Flowsheet

Date/Time			06/xx 2 PM	06/xx 3 PM	06/xx 4 PM	5 PM					
Temperature (TEMP)		°F °C	98°								
Heart Rate (HR)/Pulse			100 bpm								
Respiratory Rate (RESP)		br/min	18								
Blood pressure (BP)	Manual	S/D (M) Source	130/88 Ⓛarm								
	Noninvasive	S/D Measured Mean Source									
Rhythm		Rhythm									
Ectopy		Frequency									
O_2 Therapy		L/min									
		Device									
MONIT	O_2 sat	%									
MISC	Fingerstick Glucose	mg/dl	55								
	Glucose Interventions		orange juice 4 oz stat								

Comments:

Let's practice (p. 862)

1.

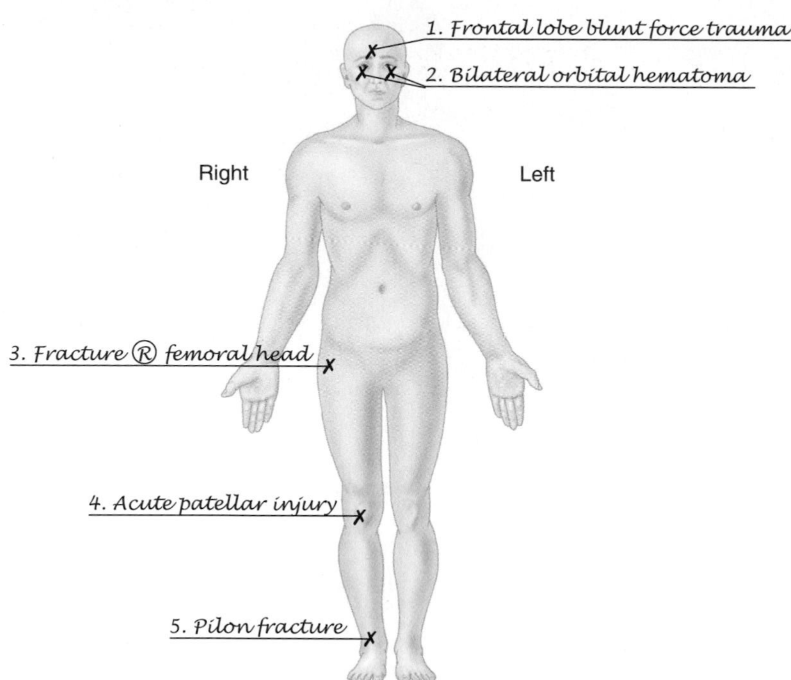

Gilbert Loeppky's Injuries on Admission

2.

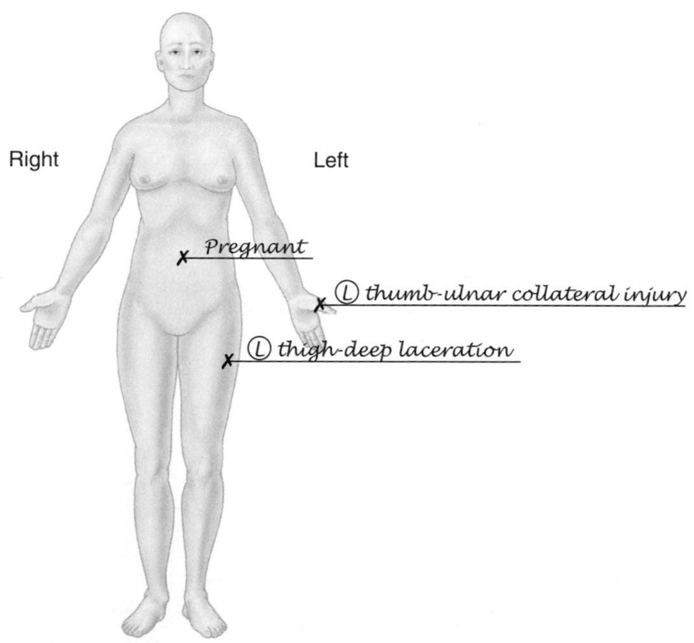

Glory Loeppky's Injuries on Admission

3.

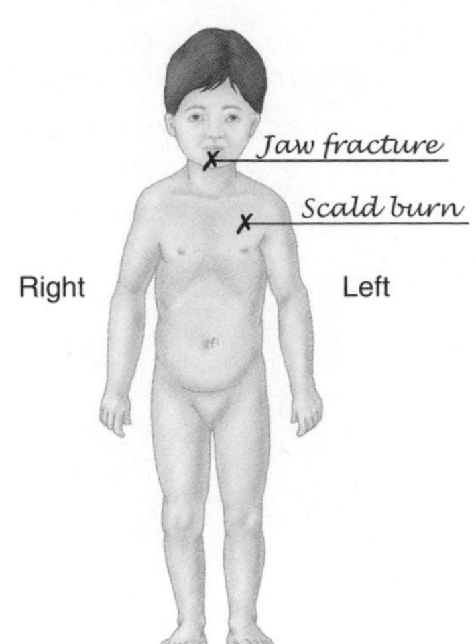

Clay Davis's Injuries on Admission

Let's practice (p. 864)

1. A high-energy, high-impact fracture sustained from trying to brake to prevent a motor vehicle accident
2. She had her thumb hooked into her seatbelt while riding in the truck with her husband. It was hooked there when Gil hit the brakes and the accident occurred. The force against her thumb caused the injury.
3. Clay's grandmother, Stevie-Rose, accidentally spilled hot coffee on him, thereby causing his skin to scald.
4. This may be the result of a skull fracture from blunt force trauma to the head when Gil hit the windshield of his truck.

Complete the form (p. 868)

Medical History for ZANE DAVIS

Are you under a physician's care now?	○ Yes ⦿ No	If yes
Have you ever been hospitalized or had a major operation?	○ Yes ⦿ No	If yes
Have you ever had a serious head or neck injury?	○ Yes ⦿ No	If yes
Are you taking any medications, pills, or drugs?	○ Yes ⦿ No	If yes
Do you take, or have you taken, Phen-Fen or Redux?	○ Yes ⦿ No	
Have you ever taken Fosamax, Boniva, Actonel or any other medications containing bisphosphonates?	○ Yes ⦿ No	
Are you on a special diet?	○ Yes ⦿ No	
Do you use tobacco?	⦿ Yes ○ No	
Do you use controlled substances?	○ Yes ⦿ No	

Women: Are you
☐ Pregnant/Trying to get pregnant? ☐ Nursing?
☐ Taking oral contraceptives?

Are you allergic to any of the following?
☐ Aspirin ☐ Penicillin ☐ Codeine ☐ Local Anesthetics ☐ Acrylic ☐ Metal ☐ Latex ☐ Sulfa Drugs
☐ Other

Do you have, or have you had, any of the following? [Select "No" for all]

						Radiation Treatments	○ Yes ⦿ No
AIDS /HIV Positive	○ Yes ⦿ No	Cortisone Medicine	○ Yes ⦿ No	Hemophilia	○ Yes ⦿ No	Recent Weight Loss	○ Yes ⦿ No
Alzheimer's Disease	○ Yes ⦿ No	Diabetes	○ Yes ⦿ No	Hepatitis A	○ Yes ⦿ No	Renal Dialysis	○ Yes ⦿ No
Anaphylaxis	○ Yes ⦿ No	Drug Addiction	○ Yes ⦿ No	Hepatitis B or C	○ Yes ⦿ No	Rheumatic Fever	○ Yes ⦿ No
Anemia	○ Yes ⦿ No	Easily Winded	⦿ Yes ○ No	Herpes	○ Yes ⦿ No	Rheumatism	○ Yes ⦿ No
Angina	⦿ Yes ○ No	Emphysema	○ Yes ⦿ No	High Blood Pressure	○ Yes ⦿ No	Scarlet Fever	○ Yes ⦿ No
Arthritis/Gout	○ Yes ⦿ No	Epilepsy or Seizures	○ Yes ⦿ No	High Cholesterol	○ Yes ⦿ No	Shingles	○ Yes ⦿ No
Artificial Heart Valve	○ Yes ⦿ No	Excessive Bleeding	○ Yes ⦿ No	Hives or Rash	○ Yes ⦿ No	Sickle Cell Disease	○ Yes ⦿ No
Artificial Joint	○ Yes ⦿ No	Excessive Thirst	○ Yes ⦿ No	Hypoglycemia	○ Yes ⦿ No	Sinus Trouble	○ Yes ⦿ No
Asthma	○ Yes ⦿ No	Fainting Spells/Dizziness	⦿ Yes ○ No	Irregular Heartbeat	○ Yes ⦿ No	Spina Bifida	○ Yes ⦿ No
Blood Disease	○ Yes ⦿ No	Frequent Cough	⦿ Yes ○ No	Kidney Problems	○ Yes ⦿ No	Stomach/Intestinal Disease	○ Yes ⦿ No
Blood Transfusion	○ Yes ⦿ No	Frequent Diarrhea	○ Yes ⦿ No	Leukemia	○ Yes ⦿ No	Stroke	○ Yes ⦿ No
Breathing Problem	⦿ Yes ○ No	Frequent Headaches	○ Yes ⦿ No	Liver Disease	○ Yes ⦿ No	Swelling of Limbs	○ Yes ⦿ No
Bruise Easily	○ Yes ⦿ No	Genital Herpes	○ Yes ⦿ No	Low Blood Pressure	○ Yes ⦿ No	Thyroid Disease	○ Yes ⦿ No
Cancer	○ Yes ⦿ No	Glaucoma	○ Yes ⦿ No	Lung Disease	⦿ Yes ○ No	Tonsillitis	○ Yes ⦿ No
Chemotherapy	○ Yes ⦿ No	Hay Fever	○ Yes ⦿ No	Mitral Valve Prolapse	○ Yes ⦿ No	Tuberculosis	○ Yes ⦿ No
Chest Pains	⦿ Yes ○ No	Heart Attack/Failure	○ Yes ⦿ No	Osteoporosis	○ Yes ⦿ No	Tumors or Growths	○ Yes ⦿ No
Cold Sores/Fever Blisters	○ Yes ⦿ No	Heart Murmur	○ Yes ⦿ No	Pain in Jaw Joints	○ Yes ⦿ No	Ulcers	○ Yes ⦿ No
Congenital Heart Disorder	○ Yes ⦿ No	Heart Pacemaker	○ Yes ⦿ No	Parathyroid Disease	○ Yes ⦿ No	Venereal Disease	○ Yes ⦿ No
Convulsions	○ Yes ⦿ No	Heart Trouble/Disease	⦿ Yes ○ No	Psychiatric Care	○ Yes ⦿ No	Yellow Jaundice	○ Yes ⦿ No

Have you ever had any seroius illness not listed above? ○ Yes ⦿ No

Birth Date:

[New Med Hx] [Comments] [View Previous] [View Form(s)] Print Y/N Form ✓ [Print Form] [Print Blank Form] [Print Answers] [Save] [Cancel]

Critical thinking about the accident (p. 869)

1. A cyclist pulled out and crossed in front of Gil's vehicle, cutting him off. Gil swerved to miss the cyclist and ended up in the line of the oncoming vehicle driven by Zane. Glory explained this. Many circumstances contributed to the possibility that both Gil and Zane were not fully attentive to their driving at that exact moment. According to Glory, Gil did not have both hands on the wheel, and she was distracting him. Then, a man on a bicycle suddenly got in the way and cut Gil off just as he was entering the intersection. According to Zane, Stevie-Rose was shouting and leaning between the two front seats swatting at a bee, trying to protect their grandson in the backseat. Zane himself said that he was coughing during this commotion.
2. Zane was driving. Both he and Stevie-Rose mention this.

Critical thinking (p. 870)

1. A.L. Murphy (Audie Murphy) was the most decorated U.S. war hero of all time. He fought in World War II. This is why his name is appropriate for a veterans' clinic. He was also a very famous movie star in the 1940s and 1950s.
2. Mary Ezra Mahoney (1845–1926) was the first African-American registered nurse in the United States. She went on to cofound the National Association of Colored Graduate Nurses, which eventually merged with the American Association of Nurses in the 1950s. She was a leader, a role model, and an advocate for African-American nurses and nursing students.

Chapter review

Critical thinking questions (p. 871)

1. The purpose of studying medical terminology is to learn a standard form of communication that you will need to work with others in the same or similar disciplines. This is a language that others in these fields will understand and will expect you to understand.
2. You would want to be able to find and extract specific information that is relevant to your work. For example, in medical billing, you might be asked to find the final diagnosis for a patient so that your company may better prepare for what the next medical steps or treatments may entail. Working for a health insurance provider, you might be asked to consider the options for treatment for a specified diagnosis. You would have to understand the terminology that is inherent to that diagnosis.

Reflective questions (p. 871)

1. It means language that is meant to be understood only by (or mostly by) those who are working in the field of health care and not by everyone else.
2. Not all medical coders work in billing. Coders do not necessarily attach costs to the items that they are coding. Medical billers may use the same codes as medical coders, but they affix a price to items.

Translate the terminology (p. 871)

Sample answers

1. Nurses are monitoring the patient's level of physical functioning to identify impairments or dysfunction and to note any changes. The results may indicate whether the patient will be able to return to work, whether he will need to change the type of work that he does, or whether he will not be able to work again.
2. After her Cesarean section, Mrs. Loeppky received sutures to two layers of uterine tissue before having the peritoneal incision sutured closed.
3. The baby no longer needed assistance with breathing via forced ventilation by the time she was 32 weeks gestational age. As a result, it is expected that she will be able to continue to breathe on her own and that her respiratory system will continue to develop normally.
4. Because hypothyroidism can cause signs of neurological and cognitive (thinking) losses or impairments, it is sometimes misdiagnosed in older adults as dementia. An annual mental status exam would be a good strategy to assess this patient's mental functioning and help identify any problems before they become too severe. A further assessment could then be made for endocrine system involvement that may be causing her symptoms.

Let's practice (p. 872)

Defining Abbreviations and Acronyms in Context

Abbreviation or Acronym	Medical Definition	Other Definitions (Including in Text Messaging)
PA	physician assistant pulmonary artery	public address system
Fx	fracture	effects (a term from media referring to special visual effects in a film or video)
pc	after eating or after meals	personal computer player character (text messaging)
BS	blood sugar breath sounds bowel sounds	*bulls*— (This is a term that means that what has been said or done is not correct or honest. This is a common expression that is also a profanity and that should not be used in any health-care setting.)
BR	bathroom bed rest breathing rate breech bronchitis	best regards (text messaging)
SOB	shortness of breath	*son of a b*— (This is a colloquialism used as an expression. It is a profanity that should not be used in any health-care setting.)
NS	normal saline	no show (text messaging) nice score (text messaging)
OB	obstetrics	oh baby (text messaging) oh brother (text messaging)
K	potassium	okay (text messaging)
GAS	general adaptation syndrome	greetings and salutations (text messaging)

Medical Word Elements

Medical Word Elements

Element	Meaning
A	
a-	lacking, without, negation; absence; absence of; not
ab-	not
ab/s-	away from
-able	describes a capacity; what can be done or accomplished
aborto	to miscarry
ad-	toward, near
adeno	pertaining to the adrenal glands
adren/o	pertaining to the adrenal glands
adreno	of or pertaining to the endocrine system
adrenal/o	pertaining to the adrenal glands
-ae	plural form
aer/i/o	air
-age	suffix that changes a verb to a noun
-al	refers to a characteristic; related to
albu-	white
algesi	pain
-algia	pain
-algesia	pain or sensitivity
ambul-	to move about
amni/o	the thin, transparent sac holding a fetus in utero
ampl-	breadth or width
an-	lacking, without, negation; absence; absence of; not
ana-	upward, backward
andr/o/os	male
angio-	vessel
ante-	before, prior
anter/o	front, anterior, ahead of, before, or in front of
anti-	against
antr	cavity
aort/o	aorta
append	appendix
-ar	referring to
arch/e/i-	original, first, beginning
-aris	pertaining to
arteri/a/o	artery
arteriol/o	arteriole; small artery
arthr	of or pertaining to the skeletal system
arthr/o	joint
-ase	enzyme
-asthenia	loss of strength
-ate	action, use, possession, having the form of, undergo a process
ather/o	fatty plaque or patch
-ation	indicating an action, process, state, condition, or result
aud/i	hear
audi/it	hearing
auto-	self
azo/t-	nitrogenous waste or compounds
B	
balan/o	penis
baro-	weight or pressure (atmospheric)
bas	step
bi-	two, twice, or double
bio	life
-blast	newly created cell, immature cell, embryonic cell, germ cell
botul	botulinum, a neotoxin
brach-	short, small, or brief
brady-	slow rate of
brevis-	short, small, or brief
brochiol/o/io	air passage
bronch/i/io/o	windpipe
bucco/o	check
C	
carcin/o	cancer
cardi/io/iolog	heart; of or pertaining to the circulatory system
caud/o	lower; below other structures or parts; pertaining to the tail of the tail end
cent/i	one hundredth
-centesis	puncture or aspirate
cephalo-	cranium
cerebr/o	brain
cerebro	of or pertaining to the nervous system
cervic/o	neck
chemo	drug
chlor/chloro-	green
cholangi/o	bile duct
cholecyst/o	gallbladder
choledoch/o	bile duct
chron/o	over a long period of time
circ	to go around as in a circuit
circum	surrounding, around
cirrho-	orange-yellow; reddish-yellow
-clasia	break, breaking or crushing
-clast	to break
clastic	broken or divided into pieces
calvicul/o	related to the clavicle
clini	medical practice
clit-	clitoris
co-	with

Medical Word Elements—cont'd

Element	Meaning	Element	Meaning
co/n-	together	-en	made of; consisting of
coagul	congealing or solidifying	-ence	the act, state, or condition of
cocc	berry	encephala/o	brain
col/o	colon	encephalo	of or pertaining to the nervous system
colp/o	vagina	-ency	the state or condition of
colon/o	colon	end/o	within or inside
concha	shell or shell-shaped	-ent	having the characteristics of
consc	aware	enter/o	intestine
contra-	opposite or against	-eous	full of
cortico	cortex; outer surface of an organ or structure	epi-	on, upon, in addition
cran	head	ephitheli/o	tissue that forms skin or a protective surface
crin-	to secrete	equi-	equal, same
cutane/o	both the epidermis and dermis layers of the skin tissue	-er	compares two persons or things; the person who is doing something
cyano-	blue	erect/o	to stand
cycl/e/o	circle, cycle	erythr/o-	red
cyst/o/i	bladder	es-	into
cyt/o	cell, of or pertaining to the integumentary system	-es	more than one
D		esophagi/o	throat, gullet, esophagus
de-	down, away, or from	-est	compares three or more persons or things
deca-	ten	esthesi/o	feeling or sensation
deci-	one tenth	-esthesia	feeling or sensation
demi-	one half	eu-	well, health, or normal
dent/o/i	teeth	ex-	out, off, former, without, outside of
-desis	binding	extra-	in addition to; outside
derm/a/o	skin, of or pertaining to the integumentary system	*F*	
dext-	right	faci/o	face or surface of something
di-	two, twice, or double	fer	to carry
dia-	across, through	fibra	fiber
digest/i/o	to break down or chemically alter	flay-	yellow
dis-	not, the opposite of; to separate or take apart	fluor/o	luminous or fluorescent
dist/o	further from the center or point of attachment	fract	break
dors/a/o	back	-ful	full of;/ able to be; identifies an amount
duc/t	lead	-fy	to make or to cause to become
dys-	painful, difficult, impaired; lack of, inability, or bad	*G*	
E		gaster/o	stomach
e-	out of, out from, outside	gastr/i/o	stomach; of or pertaining to the digestive system
-eal	relating to	-gen	formation, produce
ectas	dilation	gestio-	digestion
-ectasia	distention, swelling, enlargement	gingiv/o	gum
-ectasis	dilation, dilation, distension, stretching	glan/s	gland
-ectomy	to remove	glomerul/o	ball-shaped mass in the kidneys
-ed	past tense	gloss/o	tongue
-emia	blood	gluc/o	sugar, sweetness
en-	in, on		

Continued

Medical Word Elements—cont'd

Element	Meaning
glucose/o	sugar, sweetness
glyc-/o-	sugar and/or glycerin
glycol	sugar
glycos/o	sugar, sweetness
gono	genitals
-gram	photographic or pictorial representation; record, weight
-graphy	field or science of taking photographs or creating, developing, and interpreting pictorial representations
gyn-	gyne
gyne	woman, female; of or pertaining to the reproductive system
gynec/o	gyne
gyno-	gyne
H	
halit	breath
hect/o	hundred
hem/o/ato	blood; of or pertaining to the circulatory system
hemi-	one half
hep/at/ato	liver
heter/o	different, other
hist/o/io	tissue
hol-	whole, complete, holistic, or entire
hom/eo/o	alike, same, unchanged
hydro-	water
hymen/o	skin or membrane
hyper-	over, above, excessive
hypo-	under, decreased below
hyster/o	womb; of or pertaining to the womb (uterus)
I	
-i/ty	identifies a quality or condition
-ia	condition that is usually but not always abnormal; the state of
-ial	refers to a characteristic
-ian	doctor specializing in
-iatry	field of medicine dealing with the treatment of
-ible	describes a capacity; what can be done or accomplished
-ic	having a characteristic or property of
-ician	doctor specializing in
-icle	very small
icter-	orange-yellow; reddish-yellow
-ific	to produce or to become
-ify	to make or cause to become
-ile	relating to
ile/o	ileum
ileu	intestine
ili/o	ilium
im-	not; causing
immune/o/e	protected from or resistant to disease or infection from a pathogen
in-	not or in
inert	not active
infer/o	lower; below other structures or parts; pertaining to the tail of the tail end
-ing	present participle; happening now; ongoing action
integ	to make whole or cover
inter-	between
intesti	pertaining to the intestine
intra-	within
-ion	action or condition
ir-	against, toward, into or not
-ism	state or condition
-ismos	condition
-ismus	condition
-ist	physician specializing in the health and function of
-it is	inflammation
-iton	the act of; process of; state of
-ium	tissue or structure
-ive	nature of, quality of
-iz/e	to make
iejun/o	the second portion of the small intestine
J, K	
juncto/io	place where two things come together
ket/o	acids and acetone
kilo-	one thousand
kines	motion
kinesi/o	movement
-kinesia	movement
krin-	to secrete
L	
labia	lips or fleshy border
laryng/o	upper windpipe
later/o	toward the side
latero-	side or to the side
-lepsy	seizure
-leptic	seizure
-less	without
leuco/leuko-	white
lingu/o	tongue
-lithiasis	condition of having a stone
liv-	blue
lob	a well-defined part of an organ

Medical Word Elements—cont'd

Element	Meaning
loc/a	place
-logy	the study of
-ly	describing how something occurs
lymphat/o	lymph
lymph/o	lymph
-lysis	separation, breakdown, loosening, dissolution, destruction
-lytic	dissolution
M	
macr/o-	long or large, inclusive
major/a	greater or larger
mal-	bad; not good; poor or abnormal
mal/o	black
mamm/a/o	breast
man/u	manual
mano	thin
mast/o	breast
maxillo-	upper jawbone
meatu/o	referring to the meatus
medi/o	toward the center
meg/a/alo-	large
melan/o	black
men/o	month
mening/o	membrane
-ment	the end result of an action
ment/o	the mind
met/er/r	measure
metro/o	womb; of or pertaining to the womb (uterus)
micro/o	small or very small
mid-	middle
mil/e/i/o-	one thousandth
min-	small or lesser
minor/a	smaller or lesser
mis-	wrongly
mobile	moveable
mon/a/er/o-	only, sole, or singular
muc/o/i	mucus
muscul/o	muscle
multi-	many
my/a	muscle
myc	fungus
myelo-	spinal cord
myo/mylo	muscle; of or pertaining to the muscular system
N	
nas/o	nose
nausea/a	nausea
neo-	new
nephr/o	of or pertaining to the kidneys or urinary system
-ness	the state of or condition of
neur/o	nerve, brain, or mind
neuro	of or pertaining to the nervous system
nitr-	salt
noct/i/o-	night
non-	not
nucle/o	pertaining to the nucleus
nulli-	no
O	
obstetr/i	pregnancy, childbirth
obstetr/o	midwife
occipit/o	related to the occiput
odont/o	teeth
-oid	shape or form
-ole	small
oligo-	few, scant, or not many
-ologist	doctor who assesses, diagnoses, and treats diseases and conditions of
-ology	the study of
-oma	tumor
onco-	tumor, swelling, or mass
oophor/o	ovary
-opsy	view of something
optham/olog	eye, vision
orbi/t/to	circular or around the eye
orch/o	testes
orchid/o	testes
oro-	pertaining to the mouth
orth/o-	correct, straight, or in proper order
-ory	pertaining to; relating to
-osis	condition, disease, or increase
oste/o	bone; of or pertaining to the skeletal system
-ostomy	creating an opening or mouth
-otics	of, affecting with, or producing
-otomy	cutting
-ous	having the quality of
ova/i/ri/io	eggs
ovari/o	ovary
over-	above or excessive
ox	oxygen
P, Q	
pall-	pale, sallow, ashen
pan-	all
pancret/o	pertaining to the pancreas
par/a-	beside, at or to one side, by, near, beyond, or passing; resembling apart from, or abnormal
-para	birth
parathyroid/o	parathyroid glands

Continued

Medical Word Elements—cont'd

Element	Meaning
-paresis	weakness
parturi	to be in labor or to give birth
path/o	disease
-pathy	disease or suffering
ped/i/o	child
pedi/atr	child
pen/o	penis
-penia	lack of, decreased level of
per/i-	surrounding, though, around, or by means of
pertion	the peritoneum or the lining of the abdominal cavity
-pexia	fixation
phag/o	eating, ingesting, or devouring
pharyng/o	throat
-phasia	speech
phren/o	the mind
-phila	tendency toward
phleb/o	veins, blood vessels
phor	to bear
physic/o	body
-phyte	plant
pineal/o	pineal gland or epiphysis
pituitary/o	pituitary gland or hypophysis
placent/a	placenta
-plasia	growth or formation
-plasm	form or mold; growth or formation
-plasty	remolding or reshaping surgically
-plegia	paralysis; loss of movement
pleur/o/a	side, rib, pleura; of or pertaining to the respiratory system
-pnea	breathing
pneum/a/ato	air or breath
pneumo	lungs; of or pertaining to the respiratory system
pneumono	air or breath
pod	foot
polio-	gray; ash-colored
poly-	many
-porosis	porous
porphyry-	purple
post-	behind, backward, after
poster/o	back
postero-	after
pre-	anterior, ahead of, before, or in front of
pregn	before giving birth
primi-	first
pro-	anterior, ahead of, before, or in front of
product/i/o	to produce
prostat/e/o	prostate
proxim/o	nearer the center or point of attachment
psych/o	the mind or the soul
pulmo	lung
pulmon/o	lung
punctur/a	point, prick, or pierce
purpr/purpureo-	purple
pyelo-	of or pertaining to the pelvis, renal pelvis
R	
-r	related to
Ra-	relates to the element radium
radi/o	*radiation*
re-	again or back
ren/o	of or pertaining to the kidney
respir	to breathe; breathing
retro-	behind, backward, after
rheum/a	flowing, watery, or running
rheumat/a	flowing, watery, or running
rhin/o	nose
rrhag	burst, rupture, or discharge
-rrhea	flow, discharge
rub/e/o-	red
rubr-	blood red
S	
-s	more than one
sang/ui	blood red
sarco-	flesh or muscle
scapula/o	scapula
schiz/o/a	division or divided
scler	hard
-scope	to view
-scopy	field or science of viewing and interpreting same
script	write
sebo-	grease
semi-	partial or half, on half (amount)
sero	serum
skeleton	a dried or dry body; bones
somat/o	body
somia	sleep
son/o	sound
sperma/to	seed
sphere	ball
staphylo-	clump, irregular-shaped mass
sterno-	pertaining to the sternum
sthen/i/ia	strength or unusual strength (over all)
-sthenia	strength (overall)
sten/o	strength (musculoskeletal)
stria	striped or furrowed

Medical Word Elements—cont'd

Element	Meaning
sub-	below or beneath; underneath
super/o	upper; above other structures or parts
superfic/i	near the surface
supra-	over, above
susceptibil/i	having the capability of being affected by or receiving something
sym-	joined, together, with, alongside
syn-	joined, together, with, alongside
T	
-t/ion	the state resulting from an action
-t/ive	having the nature or tendency of
tachy-	rapid rate of
tard-	late, tardy, slow
-taxia	muscle coordination
terat/o	inherited deformity or abnormal development
terti-	third
test/o	testes; testicles
testicul/o	testes
-theraphy	treatment
thorac	thorax
thym/o	testes
-therapy	treatment
thorac	thorax
thym/o	thymus gland
thyr/o	thyroid
tom/e/i/a	incision or cutting
-tome	incision
-tomy	incision
ton/o	tension
-tonia	the degree or state of muscle tension
tonsil/a	tonsil
trache/o	windpipe
trachelo-	neck
trans-	across, through, over
traumato/o	wound
trop/o/e	turn or turning
-tropic	having the ability to influence
tropin	effect of a substance
tubercul	a little swelling
turb/o/i	a child's top (top)
typic	the original form
U	
-ule	little, small
un-	not
under-	under or beneath the surface
unguia	nail
uni-	one or single
ur/o	urinary; of or pertaining to urine, the urinary system
-ure	changes word to a noun
ureter/o	ureters
urethra/o	urethra
uria	urine
uter/o	womb; of or pertaining to the womb (uterus)
V, W	
vac	empty
vagin	vagina
vagin/o	vagina
valv/ul/o	valve
vas/o	vascular; fluid-carrying vessel or duct
vascu	small vessels
ven/ai/o/e	blood, veins
ventr/o	front
ventricul/o	ventricle
vesic/o	bladder
vesicul/o	bladder or bladder-shaped container; a vesicle
viscer/o	internal organ
volu-	rolled
X, Y, Z	
xatho-	yellow
-y	having the quality of, apt or inclined to; the act of
zyg/o/us-	joined, together, with, alongside

GLOSSARY TWO

Common Abbreviations

Common Abbreviations

Abbreviations	Meanings
Symbols and Numbers	
ψ	Psychiatry or psychology
μg	Micrograms
5-HT	Serotonin
A	
ABC	Airway, breathing, and circulation
ABGs	Arterial blood gases
ABO	Antibody screen
ac	Antes comer or before meals
ACTH	Adrenocorticotropic hormone
AD	Alzheimer's disease
ADD	Attention deficit disorder
ADH	Antidiuretic hormone
ADHD	Attention deficit-hyperactivity disorder
ADR	Adverse drug reaction
AIDS	Acquired immunodeficiency syndrome
ALT	Alanine aminotransferase
AMBU	Air-shields manual breathing unit
AML	Acute myelogenous leukemia; acute myeloid leukemia
ANS	Autonomic nervous system
AP view	Anteroposterior view; Towne's view
AS	Ankylosing spondylitis
A.S.A.P.	As soon as possible
ASD	Autism spectrum disorder
AST	Aspartate aminotransferase
ATA	Anterograde amnesia
AV	Atrioventricular
B	
BaFPE	Bay area functional performance evaluation
BCG	Bacille Calmette-Guérin (tuberculosis vaccine)
BGT	Blood glucose level
BMD	Becker's muscular dystrophy
BP	Blood pressure
BPD	Bipolar disorder
BPD	Bronchopulmonary dyplasia
BPH	Benign prostatic hyperplasia
BPMD	Benign pseudohypertrophic muscular dystrophy
BR	Bed rest
BS	Breath sounds
BSA	Body surface area
BSW	Bachelor of social work (degree)
BUN	Blood urea nitrogen
C	
Ca	Cancer
Ca	Chemical symbol for *calcium*
CA	Cancer
CA	Cancer antigen
CA	Cardiac arrest
CA	Chronological age
CA	Cytosine arabinoside
CAD	Coronary artery disease
CAM	Cognitive assessment of Minnesota
CAT	Computed axial tomography
CBC	Complete blood count
CEA	Carcinoembryonic antigen
CF	Cold formula
Cl	Chloride
CIS	Cancer in situ
CK	Symbol for *creatinine*
CK	Total creatinine kinase
CML	Chronic myelogenous leukemia; chronic myeloid leukemia
CNA	Certified nursing assistant
CNS	Central nervous system
CO_2	Carbon dioxide
COPD	Chronic obstructive pulmonary disease
COTNAB	Chessington occupational therapy neurological assessment battery
CPAP	Continuous positive airway pressure
CPK	Creatinine phosphokinase
CPK-MD	Creatinine kinase
CPU	Central processing unit
CRT	Certified respiratory technician
CSF	Cerebrospinal fluid
CT	Computer axial tomography
CV	Cardiovascular
CVA	Cerebrovascular accident
D	
DAI	Diffuse axonal injury
DAT	Dementia of the Alzheimer's type
DDM	Doctor of dental medicine
DDS	Doctor of dental surgery
DDST-II	Denver developmental screening test II
DI	Diagnostic imaging
DIAL3	Developmental indicators for the assessment of learning
DID	Dissociative identity disorder
dL	Deciliter
DM	Dextromethorphan
DM	Diabetes mellitus
DNA	Deoxyribonucleic acid

Common Abbreviations—cont'd

Abbreviations	Meanings
E	
E. coli	*Escherichia coli*
ECG	Electrocardiogram
ED	Erectile dysfunction
ED	Emergency department
EDH	Epidural hematoma
EEG	Electroencephalogram
EMD	Emergency medical dispatcher
EMT	Emergency medical technician
ER	Emergency room
ER	Extended release
ESI-R	Early screening inventory-revised
ETA	Estimated time of arrival
ETOH abuse	Alcoholism
F	
FASIAR	Follicle aspiration, sperm injection, and assisted follicular rupture
FBS	Fasting blood sugar (test)
FHM	Fetal heart monitor
FHR	Fetal heart rate
FIM	Functional independence measure
FNA	Fine-needle aspiration biopsy
FNAC	Fine-needle aspiration cytology
FSH	Follicle-stimulating hormone
G	
GAD	Generalized anxiety disorder
GAF	Global assessment of functioning
GARS	Gait assessment rating score
GCS	Glasgow Coma Scale
GHRF	Growth hormone-releasing factor
GIFT	Gamete intrafallopian tube transfer
gm	gram
GRGH	Growth-releasing growth hormone
GRH	Gonadotropin-releasing hormone
GYN	Gynecology
H	
H_2O	Water
HBV	Hepatitis B virus
hCG	Human chorionic gonadotropin
HCL	Hydrochloride
HCT	Hematocrit
HCT	Hydrochlorothiazide
HELP	Hawaii early learning profile
HGB	Hemoglobin
HGH	Human growth hormone
HHV-8	Human herpes virus (herpesvirus) 8
HIV	Human immunodeficiency virus
HL	Hodgkin's lymphoma
HMO	Health maintenance organization
HPV	Human papillomavirus
hr	Hour
HSV-1	Herpes simplex virus type I
HSV-2	Herpes simplex virus type II
I	
ICH	Immunohistochemistry
ICP	Intracranial pressure
ICSI	Intracytoplasmic sperm insertion
ICU	Intensive care unit
ID	Identification
IDDM	Insulin-dependent diabetes mellitus
Ig	Immunoglobin
IGT	Impaired glucose tolerance (test)
ILs	Interleukins
INR	International normalized ratio
IQ	Intelligence quotient
IUD	Intrauterine device
IUI	Intrauterine insemination
IV	Intravenous
IVF	In-vitro fertilization
J, K	
JDM	Juvenile dermatomyositis
K	Chemical symbol for *potassium*
K-ABC	Kaufman assessment battery
kg	kilogram
KS	Kaposi's sarcoma
KVO	Keep vein open
L	
LA	Long acting
lb(s)	pound(s)
LH	Luteinizing hormone
Li	Chemical symbol for *lithium*
LOTCA	Loewenstein occupational therapy assessment
LPM	Lateral pterygoid muscle
LPN	Licensed practical nurse
LQ	Liquid
LSD	Lysergic acid diethylamide (acid)
LVN	Licensed vocational nurse
M	
MASH	Mobile Army Surgical Hospital
MCV	Mean corpuscular volume
MCHC	Mean corpuscular hemoglobin concentration
MCP	Metacarpal phalangeal
MDMA	Methylenedioxymethamphetamine (ecstasy)
mets	Metastases
mg	Milligram
MG	Myasthenia gravis
MHNP	Mental health nurse practitioner

Continued

Common Abbreviations—cont'd

Abbreviations	Meanings
MI	Myocardial infarction
MMR	Measles, mumps, and rubella (vaccine)
MMRV	Measles, mumps, rubella, and varicella (vaccine)
MPD	Multiple personality disorder
MRSA	Methicillin-resistant *Staphylococcus aureus*
MTBI	Mild traumatic brain injury (mild concussion)
MTS	Musculotendinous stiffness
MVA	Motor vehicle accident
N	
Na	Chemical symbol for *sodium*
NB	Newborn
NG	Nasogastric
NHL	Non-Hodgkin's lymphoma
NICU	Neonatal intensive care unit
NIDDM	Non-insulin-dependent diabetes mellitus
NKO	No known allergies
NO_3	Chemical symbol for *nitrogen*
NPO	Nothing by mouth
NRT	Nicotine replacement therapy
NS	Nasal spray
NS	Normal saline
NST	Nonstress test
O	
O_2	Chemical symbol for *oxygen*
O_2SATs	Oxygen saturation
OB	Obstetrician
OB	Obstetrics
OCI	Occipitocervical injury
OSD	Occupational stress disorder
OT	Occupational therapist
OT	Occupational therapy
OTC	Over-the-counter (when referring to medications)
oz	Ounce
P	
PA	Physician assistant
PA	Posteroanterior view
PAIS	Psychosocial adjustment to illness scale
panorex	Panoramic topographic
PAR	Post-anesthetic recovery room
pc	Post comer or after meals
PCOS	Polycystic ovarian syndrome
Peds	Pediatrics
PEOP	People-environment-occupational-performance
PET	Positron emission tomography
pH	Parts hydrogen; hydrogen ion concentration
PID	Pelvic inflammatory disease
PIH	Pregnancy-induced hypertension
PLT	Platelet count
PNS	Peripheral nervous system
PO	Per os (by mouth)
PPA	Pediatric physician assistant
PPGT	Postprandial glucose testing
PPVT-4	Peabody picture vocabulary test (4)
PQRST	Heart waves
PRN	As needed
PSA	Prostate-specific antigen
PT	Prothrombin time
PT	Physical therapist
PT	Physical therapy
PTSD	Post-traumatic stress disorder
PTT	Partial thrombopastin time
R	
Ra	Chemical symbol for *radium*
RA	Radiologic technologist or radiological technician
RAI	Radioactive iodine
RAIU	Radioactive iodine uptake
RBMT-3	Rivermead behavioural memory test, third edition
RBS	Random blood sugar (test)
RCDW	Red cell distribution width
RDS	Respiratory distress syndrome
resps	Respirations
reqs	Requisitions
Rh	Rhesus factor in the blood
RHIT	Registered health information technician
RN	Registered nurse
RNA	Ribonucleic acid
RRT	Registered respiratory therapist
RT	Respiratory technician
RT	Recreational therapist
S	
SA	Semen analysis
SA	Sinoatrial
SAD	Seasonal affective disorder
SAH	Subarachnoid hemorrhage
schiz	Schizophrenia
SCMs	Sternocleidomastoid muscles
SDH	Subdural hemotoma
SGOT	Serum glutamic oxaloacetic transaminase (cardiac enzyme)
SIRS	Systemic inflammatory response syndrome

Common Abbreviations—cont'd

Abbreviations	Meanings
SIS	Second-impact syndrome (of a concussion)
SMBG	Self-monitor blood glucose
SOB	Shortness of breath
SR	Sustained release
SSRIs	Selective serotonin reuptake inhibitors
SSSS	Staphylococcal scalded skin syndrome
St	Stage
STAT	Statim; immediately
STD	Sexually transmitted disease
STI	Sexually transmitted infection
STS	Soft-tissue sarcoma
SW	Social worker
T	
T	Topical
T	Symbol for *troponin*
T and A	Tonsils and adenoids
T3	Tri-iodothyronine
T4	Thryoxin
TAR	Treatment authorization request
TB	Tuberculosis
TBIL	Total bilirubin test
TENS	Transcutaneous electrical nerve stimulator
TIA	Transient ischemic attack
tid	Three times a day
Tis	Tumor in situ
TnI	Troponin T (cardiac enzyme)
TnT	Troponin T (cardiac enzyme)
TPN	Total parenteral nutrition
TRUS	Transrectal ultrasound
TSH	Thyroid-stimulating hormone
TT	Tetanus toxiod
U, V,	
UA or U/A	Urinalysis
UC	Unit clerk
UC	Uterine contractions
UCL	Ulnar collateral ligament
UGT	Urine glucose test
VD	Venereal disease
W	
WBC	White blood cell
WBC-Diff	White blood cell differential
WOW	Workstation on wheels
WPPSI-III	Wechsler preschool and primary scale of intelligence III
X, Y, Z	
XL	Extended release
ZIFT	Zygote intrafallopian transfer

Key Terms

A

ABCs A quick overall assessment completed by emergency responders on the scene of an accident or medical emergencies that focuses on the **a**irway, **b**reathing, and **c**irculation of a patient.

Absorption In the context of digestion, the movement of products of digestion into the circulatory and lymphatic systems. This occurs through the process of diffusion through the membranes of the intestines.

Accelerations (accels) Increases in the fetal heart rate as compared with the baseline. This normally occurs when the fetus moves, and it is to be expected.

Accompanied by A medical expression that is used to describe how one symptom, illness, or process often includes or goes along with another; they are found together.

Acetabulum The part of the pelvic bone that is shaped like a saucer and that provides a socket for the head of the femur.

Acinar cells Exocrine cells that secrete enzymes.

Active immunity A state of immunity that does not come naturally, also known as acquired or adaptive immunity.

Acute appendicitis A life-threatening emergency situation in which the appendix is inflamed and may burst.

Addiction A physical or emotional dependence on a harmful or toxic drug, substance, person, or behavior.

Adenoids A mass of lymphoid tissue that sits at the nasopharynx, near the uvula at the back of the oral cavity.

Admission record A patient's biographical information, as well as his or her immediate assessment and treatment at the time of admission to hospital.

Adverse effects In the context of pharmacology, side effects that are actually harmful, even when a drug is taken in its normal, appropriate dose.

Affect The expression of emotions, emotional response, and mood.

Ageism Discrimination against, stereotyping of, or stigmatization of older adults.

Agent Term meaning *the means or the cause of something*.

Aging The natural process of growing older.

Air-shields manual breathing unit (AMBU) A bag that forces air into a patient's lungs to sustain brain vitality (life) by compressing and decompressing the AMBU bag that is attached to an airway valve placed over the patient's nose and mouth.

Alae nasi The fleshy external structures that flare open for breathing and that close to protect the nasal cavity.

Albumin A protein found in blood that helps to maintain blood pressure and blood volume.

Alimentrary Descriptor meaning *food, nutrition, or the digestive tract itself.*

Allergen Any substance that triggers an allergy response.

Allergy An immune response to a foreign antigen that leads to inflammation, organ dysfunction, or both; a hypersensitivity or an inability to tolerate exposure to an allergen.

Allergy response A hypersensitive reaction or an abnormal immune response caused by an allergen.

Altered levels of consciousness In and out of consciousness; sometimes alert and aware and other times semi-stuporous or completely unaware.

Alveoli Tiny air sacs in the lungs with structures that accommodate gas exchange.

Alveoli pulmonis The air sacs of the lungs.

Ambivalent Unsure, undecided, or hesitant.

Ambulate To walk.

Amnesia Loss of memory.

Amniotic fluid A fluid that gathers in the amniotic sac that surrounds the fetus, particularly by the second trimester. The fetus floats in this fluid, and he or she breathes and swallows it. The amniotic fluid provides a cushioning function, helps with the development of the lungs, prevents fetal heat loss, and allows for movement that enhances bone growth. Amniotic fluid is released just before birth, when the amniotic sac bursts and is commonly referred to as "the water breaking."

Amphetamines Stimulants, which are medications that promote wakefulness.

Amyotony A condition in which a person lacks or is deficient in normal muscle tone (tonus) as the result of a disease or severe brain or spinal cord injury. An alternative name is amyotonia.

Analgesic A pain-relief medication.

Anaphylaxis An acute and potentially life-threatening allergy response resulting from an extreme sensitivity to an allergen; emergency situation during which airways close as they swell in response to an allergen.

Anaplastic Descriptor meaning reverted to a state of being undifferentiated rather than differentiated by function and size.

Anatomy The study of the body's structures.

Androgens Hormones produced in the testes and adrenal glands.

Andrology The field of science and medicine involved in male reproductive health.

Anemia of prematurity A condition that occurs because the premature neonate lacks the appropriate number of red blood cells necessary to carry adequate oxygen to the body.

Anesthesia A total or partial loss of the sensation of pain; causing numbness.

Anesthetic A type of medication that is used to induce a loss of sensation and thereby reduce or eliminate a sense of pain.

Aneurysm A balloon-like widening or bulge in an artery, which can occur in the chest, the brain, and other parts of the body.

Antepartum Term meaning *before birth*.

Antepartum unit Part of a hospital's obstetrical unit designed specifically for expectant mothers who are experiencing high-risk complications.

Anterograde Memory loss of events that occurred after a traumatic event.

Anteromedial Term meaning *in front and toward the center*.

Anti-depressant Drug that influences the production, uptake, or reuptake of serotonin in the body to treat depression.

Antibodies Specialized proteins produced in response to foreign antigens being introduced into the body; they detect, trap, and neutralize foreign antigens.

Antibody Screen (ABO) A blood test performed during the last trimester of pregnancy. The ABO identifies antibodies in the mother's blood that reacts with antigens in the fetus's blood.

Anticoagulant A medication that prevents blood from clotting and is often referred to as a *blood thinner*.

Anticonvulsive A medication that is used to prevent seizures.

Antigens Proteins, glycoproteins, carbohydrates, or glycolipids found on red blood cells that provoke an immune response (antibody reaction); usually the core of allergic responses.

Antipyretic A medication used to clear a fever.

Antonyms Words opposite in meaning, such as *good* and *bad* or *happy* and *sad*.

Anxiety disorder Any mental disorder that involves recurring feelings of uneasiness and dread when no real danger exists.

Apgar test A screening tool that is used to determine whether or not a newborn (NB) requires medical attention to stabilize his or her heart and his or her breathing functions.

Apnea Term meaning *without breath*.

Apnea of prematurity A generally non-life-threatening condition affecting preterm babies that is the result of neurological immaturity in which preterm babies will have brief pauses in breathing.

Appendectomy The surgical removal of the appendix.

Appendix A tube-like structure that is attached to the cecum; it is more formally known as the *vermiform appendix* or the *cecal appendix*. The appendix seems to serve no known purpose in the human body, although pathology of the appendix can be life threatening.

Approximated Medical term meaning *come together in close proximity, in a manner that closes the wound or incision*.

Arachnoid mater A loose, sac-like membrane with a web-like appearance located between the dura mater and the pia mater that covers the brain.

Arrhythmias Abnormal heart rhythms.

Arterial blood gases (ABGs) Gases normally present in hemoglobin that can be tested to determine kidney failure, diabetes, lung disorders, and other diseases.

Arterial ischemic stroke A rare event, life-threatening complication seen most often seen in premature babies who are born before 31 weeks' gestation that can lead to brain damage during which a stroke and arterial bleeding occur in the brain.

Arteries Blood vessels that circulate blood *away* from the heart.

Arterioles Smaller arteries further away from the heart that are narrow and regulate blood pressure.

Arthritis Name given to autoimmune diseases affecting the joints and movement.

Arthroplasty A surgical procedure to remove bone or to replace tissue to facilitate the function and stability of a joint.

Arthrotomy Term meaning *cutting into a joint*.

Articulation The place where movement occurs; the joint.

Asbestosis A chronic disease of the lungs that stems from exposure over time to asbestos particles; when it is inhaled, asbestos penetrates the bronchioles and the alveoli and causes inflammation.

Asepsis Prevention of or being free from pathological microorganisms, disease, infection, or putrefaction achieved through rigorous cleanliness and good hygiene practices.

Aspect (1) part or area; (2) facet; (3) viewpoint.

Aspirating Medical term meaning *inhaling an object* or drawing up a substance into a syringe.

Aspiration A situation in which a foreign material or substance has been sucked or drawn into the lungs.

Assisted feeding A common term in health care that implies that the patient needs help to eat and cannot feed himself or herself.

Assisted reproduction A variety of techniques now available to aid in fertilization through intrauterine insemination (IUI).

Asthma A chronic inflammatory disease of the airways in which they are particularly sensitive to irritants and allergens; the bronchi and the bronchioles become inflamed and mucous production increases. The muscles that permit the passage of air into the lungs can narrow or close.

Asymmetry not evenly shaped.

Atrioventricular (AV) node Conducts stimuli from the sinoatrial node onward to the bundle branches and Purkinje fibers during the cardiac conduction system process.

Atrophy Wasting, weakening, or degenerating of, generally, muscular tissue.

Atypical Unusual.

Auscultate To listen to with a stethoscope.

Autoimmunity A state that occurs when the immune system produces antibodies that are directed against the self.

Autonomic nervous system (ANS) Subsystem of the peripheral nervous system, the ANS functions without our conscious awareness or control to monitor conditions in the body and help the body to keep functioning; examples of functions are the fight-or-flight response, the rest-and-digest response function, and homeostasis.

Autoregulation The body's ability to keep blood flow constant, even though blood pressure may vary; autoregulation can happen at the level of the organs and tissues, which are able to autoregulate their required levels of blood supply.

Axon The long projection that stems from a neuron that functions to conduct nerve impulses away from the cell body and outward to the next receptor.

B

B-lymphocytes (B-cells) Antibodies formed in bone marrow that are fundamental to the immune system. Each individual B-cell can uniquely recognize and target a specific foreign antigen. When a B-cell recognizes a particular antigen, it rapidly divides and differentiates into plasma cells or B-memory cells to combat that antigen.

B_{12} A vitamin that assists with the maintenance of the central nervous system and that facilitates metabolism and the formation of red blood cells.

Backboard A protective and supportive device that is placed under a patient or an accident victim to prevent the movement of the spine.

Barbiturates Medications that produce sleep; designed to calm and promote a sense of tranquility.

Baresthesia Term meaning *a sense of weight or pressure.*

Bartholin's glands Mucous glands located near the vaginal opening at the base of the labia majora that keep the vagina lubricated.

Baseline(s) In the context of maternity and obstetrics, this term refers to the baseline fetal heart rate. In the context of vital signs in general, this term refers to the usual, expected, or so-called normal vital signs for a patient.

Bathroom privileges Medical permission given to a patient who is deemed medically well enough to get up to use the toilet and sink. Full bathroom privileges would mean that the patient can also shower on his or her own without supervision.

Benign prostatic hyperplasia (BPH) The technical term for an enlarged prostate, a natural occurrence in the male body that results from the presence of testosterone, which triggers the prostate's growth over a man's life span.

Beta hCG A test that measures the presence of the hormone human chorionic gonadotropin (hCG) in a patient's blood.

Bile A thick, yellow-green substance that is stored in the gallbladder and used to digest fats.

Bilirubin The yellowish pigment found in bile that is the result of the natural breakdown of red blood cells over time and does not indicate infection.

Biopsy A tissue sample removed from the body and examined microscopically.

Biotechnology The analysis of specimens from the human body, such as blood, body fluids, and tissue.

Birth The act of being born; medically, birth occurs when the child passes through the uterus into the world.

Blastoma An immature tumor that develops or arises in tissue that forms part or all of an organ.

Blister a bubble-like skin formation containing serous fluid formed as part of the body's reaction to heat and nerve damage.

Blood gas analyzer A device for measuring the pH of blood and the amount of oxygen and carbon dioxide in the blood.

Blood glucose testing Measurements of the concentration of glucose in the bloodstream that under normal circumstances, when a specimen is tested before a meal, it provides a measure that is low; when it is tested after a meal, it provides a measure that is higher.

Blood pressure (BP) The amount of force that blood is actually exerting on blood vessels as it passes through them.

Bolus A small, round, soft mass.

Bonding The innate, natural proclivity to attach ourselves to others to meet biological, psychosocial, and even spiritual needs.

Bone healing A 6- to 8-week process during which a fracture goes through the three phases of healing: inflammation, production, and remodeling.

Bony prominences Places on the body where a bone is near the surface of the skin, such as the hip, the elbow, or the ankle.

Brainstem The pons, the medulla, and the midbrain together; the function of the brainstem is vital to sustain life because it regulates the constriction and dilation of blood vessels and automatically regulates heart rate and breathing.

Breakthrough pain Pain that breaks through the barrier imposed by analgesic medication or other pain-reducing and pain-numbing treatments. This is usually a sign that the medication or treatment is wearing off or the situation is worsening.

Bronchi Two bronchial tubes that branch off from the trachea as it reaches the lungs, which transport air directly into the lungs.

Bronchioles The smaller secondary bronchi that branch off from the two main bronchi.

Bronchitis The inflammation of the bronchi.

Bronchopulmonary dysplasia (BPND) A chronic lung disease that is caused by injury to the immature lungs. It is more common in very premature babies (i.e., 24 to 26 weeks' gestation and weighing < 2 pounds).

Buccinators Cheek muscles involved in chewing.

Bulbourethral glands (Cowper's glands) Two small glands on either side of the prostate that are similar in function to Bartholin's glands in females by secreting a substance called *pre-ejaculate* to help lubricate the urethra.

Bundle branches Very fine branches off the bundle of His that ensure the heart actually pumps and that the contraction and relaxation of the heart muscle actually occur.

Bundle of His Specialized heart muscle cells that transmit electrical stimuli to the bundle branches and Purkinje fibers as the atria begin to fill during the cardiac cycle.

Burn A type of tissue injury that can be caused by chemicals, electricity, radioactive agents, or exposure to temperatures of more than 120°F.

Bursa A sac-like membrane that contains and secretes fluid to facilitate joint movement.

C

Calcification Process of cartilage hardening to become bone.

Call bell A device found in hospitals and care facilities that is used to summon the care staff to the patient's bedside.

Cancer The growth of abnormal cells that eventually overtake and destroy healthy, normal cells. A disease.

Cannula A fine, soft, plastic needle or piece of tubing (as in nasal cannula).

Capillaries Very thin, tiny, tubular extensions that branch off of arterioles that serve to diffuse (deliver) essential nutrients and other matter into the cells of the body.

Capillary puncture The process of drawing blood from a capillary.

Capillary tube A device that is usually used for the accurate measurement of small amounts of liquid.

Capsule A small soluble container of medicine. A capsule is usually made of gelatinous material.

Carbohydrates Organic compounds consisting of starches, fiber, and sugars and functioning as sources of energy, particularly for the neurological system. Carbohydrates are classified as *simple* or *complex,* depending on their chemical makeup and how quickly they can be digested and absorbed by the body.

Carcinogens Environmental toxins that produce cancer.

Carcinomas Cancerous tumors of the epithelium that either infiltrate local tissues or metastasize via their own extensions, annexing or taking over nearby cells of the bloodstream or the lymphatic system.

Cardiac conduction system Process of electrical conduction that causes the contraction and expansion of the heart.

Cardiac cycle The sequence of steps in the cardiac conduction system that consist of a continuous rhythm of alternating contraction and relaxation of the heart muscle, which is coordinated by the actions of the five parts of the heart.

Cardiac enzymes Essential proteins released by the heart muscles into the bloodstream that are essential to the healthy functioning of the heart and also serve as biochemical markers of heart disease, malfunction, or injury.

Cardiac muscle A specific type of involuntary muscle found in the heart that functions like other smooth muscles but has the appearance and strength of striated muscles.

Cardiac wave A series of events that occur in a heartbeat when the heart first contacts.

Cartilage A type of dense, strong connective tissue that can withstand physical pressure, exertion, and tension. It is found in the joints between vertebrae and between any bones that articulate.

Catalysts Chemicals that regulate most of the biochemical reactions in the body.

Catheter A hollow, flexible tube that is inserted into the body either to keep a passage open or to administer or withdraw fluids.

Cavity A hollow space within the body.

Cecum A pouch-like structure that is located at the very beginning of the large intestine, in the lower right quadrant of the abdomen, that functions as a receptacle for liquids and for the salts and electrolytes that are contained within liquids. It then absorbs these materials through its membranes to replenish the body. It also targets plant material (cellulose fibers) and completes their digestion.

Celiothelioma See *Mesothelioma.*

Cell The smallest unit of life.

Cell differentiation The process of creating cells that are different in function from each other.

Cell membrane Cell part that protects the cell while allowing for the transportation of nutrients into it and the secretion of waste products outward.

Central nervous system Subsystem of the neurological system that consists of the brain and spinal cord.

Centrifuge A device that is used to separate components of a substance such as blood.

Cerebellum Posterior portion of the brain located at the superior end of the spinal cord, and is responsible for coordination of voluntary movements such as walking. Injury here could lead to the paralysis of the arms and legs.

Cerebral herniation A downward displacement of the brain into the brainstem.

Cerebrospinal fluid (CSF) A clear, colorless liquid that circulates in the ventricles and the spaces around the brain and spinal cord.

Cerebrovascular accident (CVA) See *stroke.*

Cerebrum Anterior portion and largest part of the brain; commonly referred to simply as "the brain." The cerebrum is responsible for higher-level functions such as judgment, reasoning, problem solving, learning, memory, and sensations. It is divided into two hemispheres or halves: the left hemisphere and the right hemisphere.

Cervical collar A protective and supportive device that encircles the neck to prevent the movement of the head and neck and that also helps to support the weight of the head. This device is most often used at the scene of an accident when there is a potential risk of spinal injury.

Cervical spine (neck) This region, consisting of seven vertebrae, begins at the base of the skull and extends to the thoracic spine. Unlike other vertebrae, these contain a small opening through which blood vessels bring blood to the brain. The atlas and axis vertebrae of the cervical spine are designed specifically to accommodate the rotation of the head.

Cervix The narrow passage that leads from the uterus into the vagina.

Cesarean section A surgical procedure in which the birth occurs through an abdominal and uterine incision.

Challenge Medical jargon substituted for *problem* or *issues* during consultations with clients.

Chemical dependency The persistent use of a certain drug or drugs. Lack of the drug can cause withdrawal symptoms.

Chemistry analyzer A device that measures sugars, salts, and other small molecules and ions in body fluids.

Chemotherapy The systemic treatment of cancer with use of chemical compounds that target pathogens. The goal is to destroy the cancer cells or to prevent their proliferation.

Chlamydia A bacterial infection of the urethra and reproductive system treated and resolved with the use of antibiotics.

Choking A blocking of the airways to the lungs.

Chromosomes The structures that carry genes and that determine the characteristics and sex of an organism.

Chronic Descriptor meaning *lasts for a long period of time.*

Chronic obstructive pulmonary disease (COPD) A group of disorders that include asthma, chronic bronchitis, emphysema, and others in which the lungs are the focus of the illness.

Chyle A fluid product of the intestines transported by the lymphatic system.

Cilia Fine, hair-like projections that trap dust, allergens, and other foreign particles and prevent them from entering the respiratory system.

Cipher A type of written code that conceals data to prevent access by others.

Ciphertext Letters transformed into systems of numbers, binary codes.

Clear fluids Liquids that leave no gastric residue (leftovers) and that are not likely to cause nausea and vomiting postoperatively; a type of diet that is ordered preoperatively.

Clubbing Descriptive term referring to club-shaped fingers that can be a sign of chronic hypoxemia

Coagulation analyzer A device that measures the time that it takes for a sample of blood to clot.

Coccyx (tailbone) A small bone at the very end of the spinal column.

Code (1) A system of numbers, letters, or symbols used to hide information so that only those authorized will be able to read it. (2) Medical jargon that refers to a protocol and policy for responding to an emergency.

Code team In a large medical center, this is a group of doctors and nurses who are designated responders to any Code alert that occurs during a specific work shift. In smaller facilities, a Code Team may include all available nurses and doctors on site, as well as laboratory, respiratory, and electrocardiology staff members.

Cognition Thought processes that include thinking, knowing, reasoning, learning, applying what is learned, deciding, judging, remembering, language, awareness, imagination, problem solving, and more.

Cognitively Involving the mental processes of thinking, judging, imagining, reasoning, and so on.

Coitus Penetration of a vagina by a penis.

Collagen A major protein in the body found in connective tissue, cartilage, tendons, and bone that connects the cells of the body.

Colon This organ completes the digestion and elimination process, with a particular focus on the extraction and absorption of water and electrolytes. Formal name for the large intestine.

Colostrum A liquid substance, secreted by the mammary glands, produced by the female body to prepare for lactation. The substance contains a large number of antibodies that are able to enter the infant's bloodstream and, by doing so, provide another level of naturally acquired immunity.

Coma A condition in which a patient cannot be roused by any stimuli whatsoever.

Combining forms The combination of a medical roots and a vowels.

Commode Any portable chair equipped with a container that can be used as a toilet.

Compensate A common term in medicine that means to counterbalance, to offset, or to oppose or lessen the effects of something.

Complete blood count (CBC) See *Hemogram.*

Composition Arrangement or construction; in medicine, it can refer to how cells, tissues, and organs are put together. In linguistics, composition refers to word formation: how words are formed from their pieces or parts.

Compromised Medical term meaning *impaired or complicated by a factor such as injury or disease.*

Computed tomography (CT or CAT) A test that provides highly detailed image scans of the body's internal organs and structures.

Concussion A temporary impairment of mental functioning, the result of a blow to the head.

Condylar region The area at and around the temporomandibular joint in the mouth.

Condyle A rounded, knuckle-like process (i.e., not a true, separate bone) at the end of any bone that becomes part of a moving ball-and-socket joint. Condyles are found in the hip and the shoulder. The jaw consists of one condyle on each side or end of the mandible that fits into the joints.

Confabulate To make up stories to fill in gaps in memory.

Congenital Term meaning *present at birth.*

Connective tissues These tissues connect organs and other tissues; they consist of a variety of different cell types like bone marrow, cartilage, tendons, ligaments, blood vessels, nerves, and organs.

Conscious A person's state when he or she is fully alert and aware of his or her surroundings. This person can interpret what is happening and is oriented to persons, places, and things (i.e., the person can name what he or she is seeing).

Consents Signed legal documents in which the patient or next of kin gives approval for specific diagnostic tests, treatments, and health-care interventions that must be part of every medical record.

Context The circumstances that form the setting for an event, statement, or idea, and in terms of which it can be fully understood and assessed.

Continuous positive airway pressure (CPAP) A machine that blows oxygenated air into the patient at a prescribed pressure through nasal prongs.

Contraception A term that generally refers to a pharmaceutical preparation or a technique that prevents pregnancy; however, people use natural forms of contraception as well.

Contraction The shortening or bending of muscles; also referred to as *flexion.*

Contraindicated A term that indicates an action is not advisable, not warranted, or not necessary.

Controlled cord traction The placenta (including the umbilical cord) is removed from the mother through a controlled procedure.

Copulation See *coitus.*

Cord gases A blood test performed on specimens that are taken from the umbilical cord that helps to identify the newborn's pH balance and also detects neurological complications and hypoxia at birth.

Coronal plane Also called the *frontal plane*, divides the body into front and back (anterior and posterior).

Coronoid process Triangular area of the distal end of the mandible that connects a muscle of mastication (chewing) with the bone.

Cotton gauze A type of dressing or material that is used in wound care because it is highly effective for the promotion of skin healing.

Crackles A crackling sound that occurs within the lungs when the lungs are inflamed or congested with mucous or other fluids.

Cramps Painful muscular contractions that last much longer than muscle spasms.

Cranial (cranial cavity) A division of the dorsal cavity that houses the brain.

Cranial vault The portion of the skull that houses and protects the brain.

Craniectomy A procedure in which a section of the skull is actually removed to expose the brain and relieve pressure.

Craniofacial complex The dental, oral, and craniofacial tissues that house the sense organs.

Craniofacial examination An examination of the head and face.

Craniotomy A procedure in which an incision is made in the skull through which blood can exit.

Cranium The skull.

Crash cart A portable trolley that includes medication and equipment for the treatment of cardiac arrest, injury, and other emergencies.

Crepitus Medical term for a crackling or rattling sound.

Crown The top, the uppermost part, or the highest point.

Culture In the context of laboratory diagnostics, a culture is the organic result of reproduction of microorganisms or cells in an environmental medium such as a laboratory Petri dish.

Cyst A membrane-covered growth consisting of fluid or semi-solid substances, such as pus, or a cyst could also simply be filled with air. Although the majority of cysts are harmless, some are not and may need antibiotic therapy and/or surgical removal. All cysts have the potential to become painful.

Cytoplasm The gel-like substance in the cell, which contains organelles.

D

Decelerations (decels) A slowing of the fetal heart rate as compared with the baseline rate that occurs in relation to contractions. They are not norm in a non-laboring patient.

Decerebrate rigidity An abnormal posture in which there is a rigid extension of the extremities.

Decomposition Breakdown; in medicine, it can refer to the decay and putrefaction of living matter such as cells and tissues. In linguistics, the word refers to the deconstruction of words, phrases, paragraphs, and so on.

Deep laceration A cut or incision that goes beyond the skin and into the musculature or organs.

Deep muscles The muscles farthest from the surface of the skin.

Defense mechanism A psychological defense mechanism is a method of coping that is unconscious in origin and that alleviates feelings of unbearable anxiety, fear, or other stress.

Defibrillator A device that is used to send an electrical impulse into the heart to either restart it or to change a life-threatening arrhythmia (abnormal rhythm).

Degenerative Term meaning that symptoms of a disease or disorders may not be present at birth, but develop or worsen over time.

Deglutition The act of swallowing.

Degrade To diminish, reduce, or corrupt.

Dehydration A serious condition involving increased fluid loss, which results in a water and sodium deficit caused by trauma, fever, blood loss, infection, or disease.

Delivery The end point of labor, including expulsion of the placenta and its membranes.

Dementia A type of mental disorder that primarily affects cognition and results in the death of neurons in the brain.

Dendrite An extension of a nerve cell, it is the first part to receive electrical or chemical stimuli during the process of nerve conduction. It is also referred to as a *sensory receptor*.

Denial A defense mechanism in which a person denies a painful truth that would cause anxiety if it was admitted to himself or herself.

Deoxyribonucleic acid (DNA) The primary carrier of genetic information found in the chromosomes of almost all organisms composed of genes. The entwined double structure allows the chromosomes to be copied exactly during cell division.

Depigmented When skin becomes lighter than it should be.

Derma or dermis The thick layer of skin just under the epidermis.

Descriptor Term used to identify descriptive words that can be adjectives, adverbs, or phrases.

Despondency Feeling discouraged and sad.

Diabetes Term that is used for a group of medical conditions in which both the pancreas and the adrenal glands are implicated.

Diabetes mellitus Formal medical name for diabetes.

Diabetic ketoacidosis State during which too little insulin can lead to hyperglycemia, and acute hyperglycemia can be life threatening. Cardinal symptoms are fruity-smelling breath, tachypnea, flushed face, nausea, and vomiting.

Diaphragm A dome-shaped muscle that sits inferior to the lungs that contracts, flattens, and pulls downward toward the abdomen during inhalation and expands to reduce the amount of space that is available to the lungs during exhalation.

Diastole The relaxation phase of the heart muscle's during the cardiac cycle.

Dictation The transcription of spoken words into a print document.

Dietetics The dissemination of nutritional information through teaching and learning strategies that enables individuals to make healthy nutritional choices.

Diffuse axonal injury (DAI) A common condition when cerebral trauma is involved that contributes to loss of consciousness and can be the cause of profound coma and brain damage.

Diffuse interstitial fibrosis Irreversible deep scarring of the lungs caused by the body's defensive reaction to asbestos.

Digestion The conversion of substances in the stomach and intestines into soluble or diffusible (able to pass through membranes) products that can be absorbed into the bloodstream.

Diploid Type of fertilized egg containing a full set of chromosomes, half from each donor.

Dipstick test A biochemical test that uses a reagent strip to identify the following elements and characteristics of urine.

Discs Soft pads of tissue that prevent the vertebrae from exerting pressure on each other. This tissue can be injured, inflamed, pinched by imposing vertebrae, or displaced, thereby causing pain and limited movement of the spine.

Dislocated In the context of joints, a dislocation means that the ends of the bones in the joint are no longer articulating or connecting with each other and that movement is either impaired or impossible until this condition is corrected.

Dissociative states Experiences during which a person feels disconnected from himself or herself or from his or her surroundings, as if watching or dreaming his or her experiences. The person usually has no memories of what occurs around him or her during a dissociative state.

Distorted In a surgical sense, this term refers to an alteration in shape as a result of surgery or injury and the companying inflammation.

Disturbed Word meaning *showing signs of mental illness or disorder.*

Disturbed thought process A broad term referring to alterations in cognition or thinking. These can be minor or major, depending on the wellness or illness of the patient.

Diuretic A medication that increases urine output to prevent the buildup of excess fluid in the body.

Dorsal A medical and anatomical term that is derived from the root *dorso,* meaning *the back or posterior.*

Drape A sterile sheet made of fabric or paper draped onto the patient that provides a sterile surface next to the patient.

Drug chemical agent A chemical agent that affects the functioning of a living organism; medications are drug chemical agents.

Drug screen A laboratory analysis of the types of drugs in the body.

Drugs of choice The best or preferred drug chemical agents for a particular condition or disease. The chosen drug will generally offer the best therapeutic outcomes with the lowest range and rate of side effects or risk of toxicity.

Duct Special openings through which chemicals are secreted.

Duodenum The first part of the small intestine; as partially digested matter and fluids are released intermittently into the duodenum from the stomach, digestive enzymes from the liver and pancreas are also released into the duodenum by way of the common bile duct.

Dura mater The outermost membrane of the meninges that supports the larger blood vessels of the brain.

Dyspareunia Painful intercourse; pain during intercourse.

Dystonia Term meaning disordered tonicity of the muscles used to identify a group of neurological disorders of movement.

E

Ejaculatory duct The duct that conveys sperm from the vas deferens into the urethra.

Electocardiogram (ECG) A device that monitors and records the electrical activity of the heart.

Electrical stimulation of muscles (E-stim, EMS) Using specialized equipment, electricity is passed through muscles to elicit contractions to strengthen the affected muscles, to prevent atrophy, and to force non-functioning muscles to function until they can do so on their own again.

Electroencephalogram (EEG) A recording of the electrical activity of the brain achieved by placing electrodes on the surface of the skull and recording brain-wave patterns on a computer-like monitoring device called an electroencephalograph.

Electroencephalograph Computer-like monitoring device that produces records of brain-wave patterns called electroencephalograms.

Electrolyte analyzer A device for measuring and comparing the amounts of ions such as Na, K, Cl, Ca, Li, and phosphate in the serum, plasma, and urine.

Electrolytes Ions immersed in fluids that gain the ability to conduct electrical impulses.

Electronic health records (EHRs) See *Electronic medical records (EMRs).*

Electronic medical records (EMRs) Electronic documentation of patients health records that are encrypted with ciphers to protect patient identity security and unauthorized access to their medical and billing details.

Element (1) basic or fundamental part; (2) part of a process.

Elimination In the context of anatomy, the removal of solid wastes through the process of defecation and the removal of fluids through the kidneys, the lungs, and the skin.

Emboli Large masses of material that block blood vessels, the trachea, or esophagus.

Emotional numbing Protective mechanism that is adopted to avoid experiencing emotional pain. This numbing process is not a conscious decision; rather, it is a form of self-protection that is frequently found among patients with PTSD. A synonym for *emotional numbing* is *emotional detachment.*

Emotionally Pertaining to feelings and the ability to express or respond with emotion.

Emphysema A chronic disease of the lungs that is related to smoking and chronic bronchitis; the lungs are unable to expel air and impair participation in gas exchange as a result of progressive inflammation, damage, or death of alveoli.

Endocrine A term that pertains to secretions that are directed within the body.

Endorphin A substance that is produced in the brain, a neurotransmitter that has an opioid or analgesic effect.

Endorphin theory According to this theory, endorphins (natural morphine-like substances) are released by the brain when the nerves are stimulated by certain frequencies, thereby providing analgesia.

Enteral Descriptor meaning *into the digestive/GI tract.*

Environment Environmental factors that may influence a patient's health. Although these factors are often thought of as elements in the physical environment, they can also include psychological environmental factors.

Environmental toxins Chemicals that adversely affect physical well-being and that may be disease producing.

Enzymes Catalysts that allow cells to carry out chemical reactions.

Epidermis The top or outer layer of the skin.

Epididymis The internal tube-like structure that contains sperm.

Epididymitis An inflammation and infection of the epididymis, which can be caused by urinary infections, as well as by mumps, syphilis, or tuberculosis.

Epidural hematoma (EDH) A buildup of blood between the dura mater and the bone in the brain or the spinal cord, an extremely serious condition that requires immediate surgery.

Epithelial tissues Two main types: (1) *Covering and lining epithelia* cover and protect internal organs, cavities, and the external surface of the body, (2) *Glandular epithelia* form glands, which are structures that secrete chemicals that promote important processes in the body.

Erythrocytes Red blood cells; they provide oxygen to the cells of the body and partially remove carbon dioxide.

Estrogens Female sex hormones; their purpose in males has not been determined.

Evacuate Medical term for *remove.*

Excruciating pain Pain that is unbearable and requires medical or pharmacological intervention.

Exocrine Secretions that are directed externally, toward the outside of the body.

Exposure The general meaning is *the process of revealing something.* However, in the context of imaging, the term derives from the field of photography. An image is exposed in its negative form onto film to create an image.

Extension The opening, lengthening, straightening, or expanding of a muscle.

Extracellular matrix A substance that surrounds all cells found within the tissue for structural support.

Extubation The opposite of *intubation* meaning *the removal of a tube;* this term is rarely used.

F

Facet joints Synovial joints that link vertebrae and provide flexibility in the spine.

Family practice medicine Medical specialty, providing continuing, comprehensive health care, concerned with the health, growth, and development of families as a whole and with the individual members making up a family unit. This field of health care integrates a number of other fields, including the biological, psychological, and behavioral sciences, making it more holistic in its approach.

Fascia A fibrous membrane that covers, supports, and separates the muscles internally; it also exists just below the surface of the skin, where it connects the skin with the muscles.

Fascicules Long muscle fibers that form bundles and that are joined by connective tissue; they help to give shape to muscles and to protect them.

Feces Fecal matter.

Fecundity Term that refers to the ability to produce offspring, but it more specifically refers to the ability to produce many offspring and to do so frequently.

Feeding tube Latex or plastic tubing through which liquid nutrition is delivered.

Femur The longest and strongest bone in the body, located in the upper leg. The top or proximal head of the femur forms part of the ball-and-socket joint, which is commonly referred to as the *hip.* The femur itself is most commonly referred to as the *thighbone.* The distal or lower end of the femur articulates with the patella.

Fertility The medical term for the ability to conceive children: the ability to become pregnant naturally.

Fetal attitude The posture of the fetus in utero during the last months of pregnancy.

Fetal heart monitor (FHM) A machine designed to monitor the fetus's heartbeat in utero or the fetal heart rate (FHR). The FHM is composed of two sensitive electrodes that are placed on the abdomen; the FHM also detects the presence and duration of uterine contractions.

Fetal position The relationship of the fetus's bony landmarks (which are found through palpation) with their location or position within the woman's abdomen.

Fetal presentation The determination of which part of the fetus is entering the birth canal first discovered through vaginal inspection.

Fetus The medical term for the stage of human development from 8 gestational weeks until birth.

Fibroblasts Specialized cells that are capable of producing collagen and that are critical for wound healing and skin repair.

Fibrous Composed of thin, threadlike structures or fibers.

Fibrous joints A joint consisting of fibrous connective tissue. It is formed from connective tissue that may eventually harden. Movement is possible in this type of joint, but it is not freely occurring.

Fibula The smaller bone of the lower leg. It lies posterior to the tibia. The fibula is one of the thinnest and longest bones in the human body, and it articulates with the tibia and the talus.

First-degree burns (superficial burns) Limited to the epidermis, these burns heal themselves within days and do not leave a scar. There is mild pain and discomfort associated with this burn.

Fissures Gaps that divide the lungs into portions.

Fixation A state of being held firmly in place to prevent movement.

Fixed Descriptor meaning *held firmly in place to prevent movement.*

FLACC A mnemonic for the elements of behavioral assessment related to a pain response in children: F = face, L = legs, A = activity, C = crying, and C = consolability. Each of these areas is given a score of 0, 1, or 2. Pain is rated by scoring each criterion, finding the total, and then multiplying it by 10. The higher the number, the more severe the pain.

Flaccid Loose, limp, drooping, or not firm.

Flashbacks Unexpected recurrences of images or sensations specific to a traumatic event that may occur as the result of a mental disorder or from the use of a hallucinogenic drug.

Flat affect A lack of emotional response.

Flat bones Provide protection for the body and function as attachment sites for muscles (i.e., the sternum, scapula, and ribs).

Fracture A break or a broken bone.

Fracture fragments Bone chips that are the result of injury rather than of bone pathology.

Frail elderly A classification of older adults who are unable to manage or care for themselves. They may have physical or mental health challenges.

Frontal lobe One of the four lobes of the cerebral hemisphere that is involved with reasoning, judgment, emotions, planning, and strategizing, as well as some memory and speech functions.

Frontotemporal Term meaning *the front and side (near the temple) of the skull.*

Functional capacity The ability or potential ability to function.

G

Gag reflex An automatic response to the presence of matter touching the soft palate at the back of the mouth. This reflex is not under voluntary control.

Gait A person's style or manner of walking.

Gallbladder A small, sac-like structure that is located on the underside of the liver and on the right side of the abdomen that functions as a reservoir and stores bile that is produced by the liver

Gamete(s) A reproductive cell containing half the genes of a parent that fuses with one of the opposite sex to form a zygote, or fertilized egg.

Gate theory A theory which asserts that only one message can be carried along a nerve at a time.

Gavage Nutrients are administered either through nasogastric (nose to stomach) or orogastric (mouth to stomach) tubes when digesting, sucking, and swallowing are difficult for preterm babies.

General anesthetic A drug that causes a complete lack of consciousness.

Genes Molecules are contained within every living cell that function as a set of instructions for the physical structure and function of organisms.

Genetics The study of heredity.

Genital herpes A very common viral STD transmitted through direct, person-to-person contact only through body fluids (blood, saliva), vaginal, oral, and anal sex and contact with the blisters.

Genitalia The reproductive organs and the structures located in the lower abdomen and pelvis.

Gestation The length of time from conception to birth. The average *gestational period* for humans is 40 weeks.

Gestational diabetes A temporary type of diabetes that only occurs during pregnancy for some women.

Glands Tissues that work together to synthesize or produce substances to be secreted within the body.

Glans penis The distal end of the penis.

Glasgow Coma Scale (GCS) An internationally recognized scale that assesses neurological functions such as reflexes and responses to sound and touch, including shaking, pinching, and attempts to elicit a pain response.

Glia Early Greek term meaning *glue.*

Global Assessment of Functioning (GAF) Scale Most commonly used test of overall (global) functioning that evaluates the occupational, social, and psychological functioning of adults. It also assesses how well an individual is coping with or adapting to the challenges that they meet during their lives. The patient is given a score from 1 to 100 to evaluate his or her overall level of occupational, social, and psychological functioning.

Glomeruli Small balls or bundles of capillaries inside each nephron.

Glucocorticoid Type of hormone that affects the metabolism and facilitates an increase in the level of blood glucose.

Glucometer A glucose-monitoring device that uses a droplet of blood from the fingertip.

Glucosamine An over-the counter substance that is used to treat the pain of arthritis; a health-food supplement.

Glucose The medical term for sugar; glucose is a type of sugar that is used by the body for energy.

Glycemia levels The levels of blood glucose that a person with diabetes must manage.

Gonorrhea A bacterial infection of the urethra, cervix, rectum, anus, and/or throat that can be well treated with antibiotics.

Grasp response A reflexive action that occurs when the fingers or interior surface of the hand (the palm) are stimulated and they immediately begin to close around the stimulus.

Gravid Adjective meaning pregnant; heavy with child.

Gravida A pregnant woman; a woman's status regarding pregnancy.

Gurney A synonym for *stretcher.*

Gustatory Medical term for *sense of taste.*

Gynecology (GYN) A field of medicine that treats women only, and is particularly focused on reproductive health.

H

Hallucinations Sensations and images that are either not based on reality or that are the result of a sensory misperception of reality.

Haploid Type of gamete containing half the genes of the parent.

Hard callus Hard bone that over time replaces soft callus.

Hard palate The roof of the mouth.

Hardiness The vitality of a person; it can also be thought of as his or her strength, energy, and drive.

Healing process A natural process by which the body (or mind) heals or restores itself to health.

Hematic cells See *Hemocytes.*

Hematology analyzer An instrument that is used to count the different kinds of cells found in blood.

Hematoma Swelling and an accumulation of blood that is caused by a break in a blood vessel.

Hemiplegia Weakness on one side of the body.

Hemocytes A term that refers to erythrocytes and leukocytes only.

Hemoglobin A1C Term referring to hemoglobin A cells, which are the blood cells to which glucose binds.

Hemogram Series of tests pertaining the blood and the circulatory system; also called a complete blood count (CBC).

Hemorrhagic stroke This condition is the result of a broken blood vessel caused by an aneurysm, a break in the thin, brittle arteries as a result of atherosclerosis causing bleeding into the brain via an intracerebral or subarachnoid hemorrhage.

Herniation A term derived from *hernia,* meaning *the protrusion of a bodily structure through a wall that normally contains it.*

Hesitancy An involuntary delay in action, the cause of which may be physiological or psychological. The term is frequently used to refer to urination and the inability to initiate a urine stream, but it can be used in a musculoskeletal context as well.

Hirsutism Growth of facial hair.

Histogenesis A microscopic process that is capable of identifying cells that produce tumors.

Histopathology The microscopic, laboratory testing of tissue and blood.

Homeostasis The maintenance of a constant balanced internal environment necessary for the body to function normally achieved through structural, functional, and behavioral activities that are both voluntary and involuntary.

Homographs Words that are spelled alike but that have different meanings and, often, different pronunciations

Homonyms Words that sound alike but that have different meanings.

Hormones Chemically regulatory substances that regulate the internal body.

Hospital code Codes called over the intercom or public address system to communicate specific messages to hospital staff, but not to other people in the hospital. These codes are most often used only for emergency situations.

Human papillomavirus (HPV) A viral infection of the genital tract contracted by skin-to-skin, genital contact that cannot be treated, only prevented.

Hyoid Term meaning *u-shaped.*

Hyoid bone A bone that sits at the anterior midline of the neck and functions to anchor the tongue.

Hyperglycemia An excess level of glucose in the blood, which is the prime symptom of diabetes

Hyperpigmented When skin becomes darker than it normally should be.

Hypersomnia Similar to a very deep sleep, patients only awaken from hypersomnia by shaking or other strong stimuli such as pain. Even so, these patients may not completely awaken. If they do, they will be confused and only partially alert before drifting back into hypersomnia.

Hypertension of pregnancy (preeclampsia) A condition of abnormally high blood pressure that only occurs for some women during pregnancy.

Hypnotics See *Barbiturates.*

Hypodermis A thin layer of tissue under the dermis that contains nerve cells and tiny blood vessels; sometimes referred to as the subcutaneous layer.

Hypophysis See *Pituitary gland.*

Hypopigmented See *Depigmented.*

Hypothalamic-pituitary-adrenal (HPA) pathway A process initiated when a stressor is perceived, and the limbic system is activated. The amygdala triggers a response in the hypothalamus, which triggers the pituitary gland, which in turn triggers the adrenal glands to release adrenaline and cortisol.

Hypothalamus A smaller structure located within the thalamus that controls the pituitary gland, regulates sleep, appetite, and emotions, and is responsible for the release of a number of growth hormones that lead to the development of the genital organs and the functioning of the reproductive system.

Hypothyroidism A condition of low levels of thyroid hormones in the body.

Hypoxemia Low levels of oxygen present in the blood over a long period.

Hypoxia Term meaning *lack of oxygen.*

I

Ibuprofen An anti-inflammatory analgesic (pain-relieving) medication.

Ileocecal valve Valve, situated at the base of the ileum, where it meets the cecum of the large intestine that prevents the contents of the ileum from passing into the cecum too rapidly. It also prevents any backflow from the cecum into the ileum.

Immune response A series of steps that occur when the body perceives a threat from pathogens. It may take as many as 2 or 3 weeks to produce sufficient numbers of antibodies to fight the infection or disease. A successful immune response is one in which the foreign pathogens are eradicated or depleted to the extent that they are no longer viable and thus can no longer harm the body.

Immunity Protection from disease and infection; the body's mechanism for defending itself and the capability or capacity to do so successfully. Immunity is also a process: it is the result of the activities of antibodies that are specific to certain types of antigens binding to those antigens to destroy or inactivate them. Immunity can be acquired or innate (inborn).

Immunization The process of converting an individual who is not immune to a pathogen(s) or toxin(s) to a state of immunity against that pathogen or toxin. Artificial immunization is achieved through vaccinations.

Immunoglobulins (Ig) Glycoprotein molecules, antibodies that have a distinct "Y" shape, whose function is to identify foreign invaders in the body, to attach to the invaded cells, and to create an immune complex. Immunoglobulins do not destory cells on their own. Instead they trap the antigen, and T-cells assist in destroying the invaders.

Immunology analyzer A device that identifies and measures molecules such as antibodies, hormones, and drugs.

Immunosuppression A state in which an immune response has been diminished or turned off altogether as a result of exposure to disease, certain types of drugs, radiation, or deterioration of the immune system over long periods of illness.

Impulse control center Area of the brain located in the frontal lobe that affects how reactions occur (i.e., whether with thought and judgment or impulsively). Impulse control can be a challenge for patients who have experienced frontal head injuries. It is also a factor in decision making during adolescence, this part of the brain is not fully developed until the early because 20s.

Incident report Document created by the primary staff members involved in a patient's care when a critical incident occurs containing a description of the incident, the suspected injury (if it has yet to be diagnosed by a doctor), and the mechanism of the injury. It will also include signs and symptoms that arise after the injury, as well as all immediate care interventions provided by those in attendance.

Incision line The line on the skin where two sides of an incision have now come together.

Incisor One of the teeth at the front of the mouth.

Incontinence pad A hygiene product designed to catch any substances or liquids voided from the body. It is made of multiple layers of material that are permeable to liquids and that trap and hold liquids to prevent leakage beyond the pad.

Incontinent Involuntarily emptying of the bladder.

Increased intracranial pressure A rise in the normal pressure exerted within the cranium.

Incremental steps A process in which a goal is achieved one step at a time. Healing occurs in incremental steps.

Indwelling catheter A urinary catheter inserted through the urinary meatus into the bladder.

Inextricably Two or more things are so intricately enmeshed or combined that one of them cannot be separated from the other.

Infancy The period from birth to the end of the child's first year of life.

Infection The result of the transmission of infectious agents or microorganisms.

Infection control A policy and protocol adhered to by all health professionals and facilities to prevent the spread of infection by limiting the potential for contamination and containing the spread of infection should one occur.

Infectious agents Organisms that cause communicable (contagious) diseases (i.e., bacteria, viruses, fungi, and protozoa).

Inflammatory response The automatic defense process that begins when tissue is attacked or damaged with the goal to protect the body.

Ingestion The action of taking in a substance by mouth and then swallowing it; oral consumption.

Innate immunity A state of natural immunity to some pathogens, that with which humans are born.

Innervation Process initiated when a muscle fiber is stimulated by electrical impulses that are interpreted by the neurological system. Segments of the spinal cord then conduct these impulses to specific motor and sensory regions of the body. For example, when the bladder is nearly full, the brain sends nerve impulses that cause the bladder muscles to tighten.

Innominate bones The ilium, the ischium, and the pubis form the pelvis.

Inoculations Injections containing small doses of an antigen, which stimulate the primary response to the antigen without causing the illness, causing memory cells to develop the ability to detect and intervene in cases of future exposure to the pathogen. This process provides active, ongoing immunity.

Inpatient A label given to patients who are admitted to and staying in a hospital.

Insoluble Descriptor meaning *does not dissolve or break down.*

Insomnia The inability to fall asleep or the inability to stay asleep for a sufficient period to attain necessary rest for the mind and the body.

Insulin A naturally occurring pancreatic hormone and a protein that functions to lower blood glucose levels by allowing glucose to leave the bloodstream and enter the cells of the body, where it becomes an essential source of energy.

Insulin inhaler A device that involves the use of a powdered form of insulin, which is inhaled before meals. Insulin inhalers are very new to the market and offer an alternative form of treatment for diabetics.

Insulin pen A pen-like device into which an insulin-filled cartridge is placed for administration. At one end is a calibrated dial that can be rotated to the correct dosage; at the other end is a fine syringe (a pen needle) that delivers the dose when the apparatus on the pen is pushed to release it. Cartridges are removed and replaced after each use.

Insulin pump A continuous subcutaneous insulin infusion device. The release of insulin is controlled by a computer chip to ensure a steady rate of flow. Short-acting insulin is used in the pump.

Insulin-dependent diabetes mellitus (IDDM) An autoimmune disease in which the pancreas does not produce insulin or does not produce enough insulin to control and maintain healthy blood glucose levels. The beta cells of the pancreas are eventually completely destroyed, and insulin production ceases.

Intact Medical jargon meaning *undamaged* or *unharmed*; whole; not compromised; fully functioning.

Integument A root word meaning *covering*.

Intercellular fluid Fluid that surrounds cells and is found between cells, which allows nutrients to enter the cells, absorbs metabolic wastes from the cells, and transports this waste away; also known as interstitial fluid.

Intercostal muscles Muscles located around the chest wall and between the ribs that assist with the breathing process by allowing the rib cage to expand as the lungs take in air.

Intercostal spaces The spaces between the ribs.

Intercourse A term literally meaning "to run between." When used in the context of sexuality it means *coitus*.

Interleukins Proteins that are naturally secreted when the presence of a foreign invader is detected, triggering the immune response by alerting lymphocytes and antibodies and then stimulating them into action.

Internal bleeding Bleeding that occurs within the body as a result of damage to an artery or vein and generally cannot be seen.

Internal fixation The use of pins and screws to fixate or hold bone segments together.

International normalized ratio (INR) A test that measures the level of coagulation in the blood.

Interstitial fluid See *Intercellular fluid*.

Interval The time lapse between cardiac waves or heartbeats.

Intestine An organ divided into two distinct parts, the small intestine and the large intestine. It plays an essential role in digestion by distinguishing the nutrients and water needed by the body and absorbing them, and identifies the wastes products of digestion and propels them along so they can be expelled from the body.

Intracerebral hematoma (ICH) An emergency situation, usually the result of severe head injury wherein fluid accumulates in the brain, causing death or irreversible brain damage.

Intracranial hemorrhage A medical condition wherein there is bleeding within the cranium as a result of head injury that caused a jostling and tearing of the brain and its blood vessels. ICP can also be the result of blood disorders, blood clots, or other factors.

Intracranial pressure (ICP) The pressure level of cerebrospinal fluid within the skull that remains constant and unchanging; increased intracranial pressure compresses the brain, and brain damage or death may be the result.

Intraoral space Within the mouth.

Intravenous (IV) Term meaning *within a vein*; A needle attached to a tube inserted into a patient's vein through which qualified health professionals can rapidly dispense blood transfusions, IV solutions, and medications.

Intraventricular hemorrhage (IVH) An acute, critical event during which a blood vessel in the brain bursts and floods the ventricles of the brain, as well as the surrounding tissues.

Intubation The condition of having a tube inserted and in place in the body.

Involuntary A term that means not controllable.

Involuntary control A term that indicates control by will or thought is not possible. For example, some muscles like the heart cannot be stopped voluntarily.

Iodine A non-metallic chemical element; it is a natural element in digestion, and it occurs in low doses in the human body.

Ischemic stroke A medical condition that is the result of a blood clot (thrombus) impeding circulation and cutting off blood supply to the brain.

Islets of Langerhans Endocrine cells that produce the pancreatic hormones insulin and glucagon, which help with the maintenance of normal glucose levels in the blood.

Isometric A specific type of strength-training exercise that is common for muscle rehabilitation: the muscle is required to push against something (i.e., the physical therapist's hand) for short intervals of time. At no time does the muscle lengthen or do any joints move. The goal is to maintain muscle strength while a patient is bedridden or chair bound.

J

Jargon A set of words and phrases that is recognized and used by only a select group of people.

Jaundice A yellowing of the skin and of the sclera of the eyes caused by bile backing up into the bloodstream.

Jaw wrap A type of compression bandage that fits over the head and under the jaw to reduce swelling, pain, and movement.

Jejunum The second section of the small intestine. It is partially responsible for the absorption of nutrients such as carbohydrates, fats, proteins, and vitamins A and D into the bloodstream.

Joint A point of connection or articulation between two or more bones.

Joint stamina The resiliency or strength of a joint.

K

Ketones Water-soluble compounds in the body that are byproducts of the breakdown of fatty acids.

Kidney Sitting just below the ribs and closer to the back in the abdomen, this organ functions as a filter for the blood—removing urea and other nonessential or harmful soluble and liquid waste from the blood.

Kirschner wires (K-wires) Sharp, stainless steel pins that are used to hold bone fragments in place.

Knee support A pull-on or wraparound orthotic device designed to provide medial and lateral stabilization of the knee. Some include bilateral hinges to help support movement. All prevent hyperextension of the knee.

L

Lab work Results and requisitions pending for any laboratory tests ordered by the physician.

Labor The process of giving birth that begins when uterine contractions are repetitious and become more frequent and forceful as birth becomes imminent.

Lacrimal The smallest bones in the face situated at the inner corners of the eyes, which form part of the orbits.

Lactiferous ducts Ducts capable of lactation organized into clusters of ducts called lobules. There are approximately 15 to 20 lobules in one breast that transport breast milk from the ducts to the nipple.

Lactivorous Descriptor meaning "living on milk;" usually describes newborns receiving all nourishment from breast mil.

Lactose A sugary product that is found in milk and milk products.

Lactose intolerant Not having the ability to digest lactose or digesting it only with difficulty.

Lag screws Specific types of stainless steel screws that are used in orthopedic surgery that can be tightened to keep pressure on the bone to stabilize and support it.

Lancet A sharp, pin-like device that punctures the skin no deeper than 0.75 mm used for diabetic testing.

Larynx The voice box; an organ of muscle and cartilage at the upper end of the trachea (windpipe) that is involved in the production of sound (the voice) and that protects the entrance to the main respiratory tract.

Lead An electrocardiographic conductor or electrode.

Lead time Time before an event during which to prepare.

Left lateral tilt A position in which the patient's right hip is slightly elevated on the operating table.

Leopold's maneuvers Methodical movements used in the processes of palpation and evaluation of the position of the fetus in utero (in the uterus).

Leukocytes White blood cells; they function as part of the body's autoimmune system defending against invaders in the form of bacteria, infection, allergy, and disease.

Levels of consciousness (LOC) Four stages of unconsciousness in which a patient's awareness ranges from drowsy and confused to completely unresponsive.

Levothyroxine A thyroid preparation given to supplement low thyroid levels.

Libido A medical term commonly understood to mean *sex drive*. A term from psychology and psychoanalysis that refers to the innate psychological and emotional energy involved in striving for sexual activity and sexual intimacy (the sex drive).

Lifecycles Stages of growth and development.

Lifestyle A way of life that reflects a person's life choices, circumstances, and behaviors. It includes a person's attitudes and beliefs about life, as well as that person's attitudes and beliefs about health and illness.

Ligaments A type of fibrous connective tissue that connects the articulating ends of bones (i.e., the joints) and binds them together.

Lipids Molecules that consist of fats, oils, and waxes.

Liquid diet A diet of fluids only.

Liver A major organ located in the upper right quadrant of the abdomen that removes toxins from the blood.

Lobes Sections of the brain or lungs.

Localized Appearing in only one specific area or location.

Locomotion The ability to move oneself from one place to another. Walking is a form of locomotion and so is using a wheelchair, driving, or even riding a bus or train.

Locus of control Term borrowed from psychology to describe how a person perceives the events of his or her life. It reflects personal attitudes and beliefs about one's own power to influence life events.

Long bones Bones providing the core support for the body. They link with one another to allow for movement. These bones (i.e., humerus, femur, tibia, and metatarsals) are longer than they are wide.

Lorazepam A common anti-anxiety medication of the benzodiazepine family of drugs. This quick-acting medication is highly effective, but it should be used sparingly, because it is highly addictive.

Lumbar spine (lower back) This region, consisting of five vertebrae that eventually connect the spine to the pelvis, bears most of our weight. It is the site of a great deal of body movement, such as bending and turning.

Lungs Cone-shaped organs that sit lateral to the heart in the pleural cavity of the thorax. The lungs are the core of the respiratory system's gas exchange process of inhalation and exhalation.

Lymph The clear, watery component of blood plasma, which contains oxygen, glucose, proteins, and white blood cells. It transports and removes any perceived harmful or unwanted matter within it.

Lymph nodes Clusters of lymphatic tissue; within each node are lymphocytes (B-cells and T-cells), macrophages, and dendritic cells.

Lymphangiogenesis A medical term that describes how cancer cells influence the development of any new lymphatic vessels or channels by influencing where, how, and by which route cancer cells are able to metastasize.

Lymphocyte count (WBC-diff) A diagnostic measure; a blood test that measures or estimates the number of white blood cells in the body. Also known as a white blood cell differential test.

Lymphocytes Lymph cells, a type of leukocyte produced in bone marrow that responds to antigens by producing antibodies to fight them.

Lymphocytopenia A decrease in the number of lymphocytes that can occur in cases of starvation, malnutrition, lupus, and acquired immunodeficiency syndrome.

Lymphocytosis An increase in the number of lymphocytes, particularly seen in cases of viral infection, tuberculosis, bone marrow cancer, and leukemia.

Lymphoma A malignant tumor that is a cancer of the lymphatic system.

Lysis The process of dissolving, destroying, or disintegrating cells.

M

Macrophage A scavenger cell that hunts for, detects, and then ingests foreign matter, dead cells, or other cell debris. Macrophages are found in abundance in the tissues of the skin, the digestive tract, the lungs, the spleen, and some blood vessels; they play an important role in the initiation of some immune responses.

Mammillary line An imaginary vertical line that crosses through the center of a nipple used to pinpoint locations on the patient's chest.

Mammograms Noninvasive radiographs of the breast/breast tissues used to detect cysts, tumors, and other changes in breast tissues; excellent diagnostic tool for the screening of breast cancer.

Mammology The medical field specializing in the breast; synonymous with *mastology*.

Manageable In medical context, this word is used to determine if the pain is controlled enough for the patient to be able to tolerate or manage it.

Mandible The lower jaw bone; it is the strongest bone of the face, and it also forms the chin (mental tuberosity) and the sides of the face. This bone has a horseshoe shape.

Mandibular alignment Correct positioning of the two parts of the mandible (the lower jaw) on either side of the fracture line. When a mandibular fracture is reduced, the bones are realigned in their proper position.

Mast cells A type of immune cell found in connective tissue.

Mastication Medical terminology for *chewing*.

Mastoid hematoma Swelling or bruising around the ears.

Mastology The medical field specializing in the breast; synonymous with *mammology*.

Maternal health The health of the mother during pregnancy, childbirth, and the postpartum period.

Maternity Term meaning motherhood. This is also the typical name for the obstetrical unit in a hospital.

Maxillae The largest bones of the face fused together to form part of the orbits (eye sockets), the hard palate (roof of the mouth), the base of the nose, and the tooth sockets.

Maxillomandibular Descriptor meaning *pertaining to both the maxilla and the mandible*.

Mechanism(s) The means or methods by which an injury occurs.

Mechanisms of injury The means or methods by which an injury occurs.

Medical code A system of communication known to certain health care agencies, workers compensation organizations, and private insurance companies that takes a medical description, diagnosis, or procedure and transforms it into a standardized code number.

Medical terminology The specialized vocabulary that medical professionals use to identify human anatomy (structures) and physiology (functions), as well as words that indicate location, direction, planes of the body, medical status, and instructions for administering medication.

Medication administration record (MAR) The general name of a form, paper or electronic, on which medication administration must be documented including the name of the patient, the name of the drug, the amount of drug, the route by which it was given, and the time that it was given. After the medication is actually administered, the person who has administered in must sign his or her name on the MAR.

Medulla Connects the spinal cord to the brain; part of the brainstem.

Medulla oblongata Proper name of "the medulla."

Membranes Thin layers of tissue that surround organs and cells.

Memory A complex phenomenon with many different aspects that can be separated into two basic types: retrospective memory, how to do things; and prospective memory, what to do and when.

Meninges Specialized membranous connective tissues that surround the brain and the attached spinal cord.

Meningitis An inflammation of the meninges, either infectious or non-infectious, that can cause brain damage or even death.

Menopause The cessation of menstruation and, therefore, female reproductive ability.

Menses A root word meaning *month;* name for the physiological processes between days 21 and 28 of the menstrual cycle.

Mental health A state of mental well-being that allows a person to cope with life, to function effectively to take care of himself or herself, and to achieve a sense of wellness, satisfaction, or contentment.

Mental illness A broad range of psychiatric and emotional disorders.

Mental status examination An examination of an individual's mental state, which includes a number of target areas from which diagnostic criteria can be identified.

Mesencephalon Formal name of "the midbrain."

Mesenchyme cells Cells found within the mesoderm, which eventually develop into connective tissues of either bone or blood.

Mesothelial cells Cells that form the surface layer of the pleura, the peritoneum, or the pericardium.

Mesothelioma A malignant and untreatable form of lung cancer that affects the mesothelial cells which derives from asbestosis, the worst form that this disease can take.

Metabolism The chemical activity within the cells during which energy is released from nutrients or energy is used to create other substances (i.e., proteins).

Metastasis (mets) The spread of cancer cells through a process of invasion, which involves the moving into and taking over of other cells.

Metastasized Term meaning *spread to the rest of the body.*

mg/dL Symbol for milligrams per deciliter unit of measurement.

Micrograms (mcg, µg) Unit of measurement where 1 mcg = .000001 g.

Midbrain A part of the brainstem responsible for embryonic brain development and the creation and maintenance of motor (movement) pathways in the developed brain.

Midline shift Shifting of the brain's position to make way from a hematoma, bleeding, or swelling.

Mild-traumatic brain injury (MTBI) See *Concussion.*

Mind-body connection A term derived from holistic health care that reflects an understanding of how the mind influences the body in all aspects of functioning and vice versa.

Minerals Inorganic compounds from soil and water that are eaten or absorbed by plants and animals and essential to growth and development. Minerals play key roles in regulating the permeability of the cell membranes and the capillaries, allowing muscle contraction, and facilitating the metabolism of water to regulate blood volume.

Mitosis The process of cell division.

mm^3 (µL) Symbol for cubic millimeter unit of measurement; synonymous with microliters, µL.

Mobile army surgical hospital (MASH) A combat support unit in the field whose main purpose is to provide emergency medical, trauma, and surgical care for military personnel.

Mobilize To move or put into action so that muscle atrophy (wasting) does not occur and so that healthy circulation is maintained to tissues and bone.

Morbid Root word that means *diseased or sick.* In health care, the term is used widely to describe many conditions or situations that require intervention or treatment.

Motility The capacity for movement.

Motor functioning The ability to use and control muscles to achieve movement.

Muscle Tissue composed of contractile cells and fibers that permit movement.

Muscle tension The continuous partial contraction of a muscle (i.e., when the arm is naturally bent at the elbow).

Muscle tissues Tissues designed to flex, contract, or move. There are three categories of muscle tissue: visceral, cardiac, and striated.

Muscle tone The amount of tension or resistance present in a muscle at any given time. The natural or normal firmness of a muscle and its functionality.

Musculature The arrangement of muscles in the body.

Mutagen See *Tetragen*.

Mutation Any change or alteration of the genetic material.

Mycoplasma An infection of the urethra and the reproductive system that causes painful inflammation of the urethra and other genital areas.

Myocardial infarction (MI) A heart attack.

Myocardium The medical term for the heart muscle.

Myotonia Tonic spasm or a state of temporary rigidity after a muscle contraction.

N

Nailbeds The parts of the fingers that are covered by fingernails. By examining their color, physicians can diagnose a patient's cardiac output if the patient is suffering from hypoxia or has cyanosis, is experiencing of poor circulation, or difficulties with capillary refill.

Nares The medical term for the nostrils.

Nasal The oblong-shaped bones that form the bridge of the nose.

Nasal septum The fleshy part of the nose.

Nasoethmoid A descriptor referring to the upper portion of the face.

Nasogastric Descriptor meaning *from the nose to the stomach or intestines*.

Neo-natal intensive care unit (NICU) Specialized unit of a hospital that treats newborn babies with life-threatening conditions such as premature birth, underdeveloped internal organs, or respiratory failure.

Neoplasia An uncontrolled proliferation of cells, generally the spread of malignancies and the invasion of the lymphatic system by cancer cells.

Neoplasm An abnormal formation of tissues that may be malignant or benign, which serves no function, and it takes over space where healthy, normal tissues should exist at the expense of those healthy tissues.

Nephrons Fine filters in the kidneys that sift urea, liquid waste, nonessentials, and harmful soluble from the blood.

Nerves Bundles of axons and dendrites that communicate stimulus to the brain.

Nervous tissues Tissues specifically responsible for sensing stimuli and transmitting impulses about stimuli to appropriate parts of the body.

Neuro Combining form meaning *nerve*.

Neuroglial cells Cells that do not have synapses or dendrites but support neurons and function to preserve the electrochemical balance of the nerve cells and to form the myelin sheaths that protect neurons.

Neuron The basic unit of nervous tissue consisting of consists of a nucleus, an axon, and dendrites.

Neurons Nerve cells that receive stimuli or impulses in an action-reaction response.

Neuropathways Routes throughout the body that lead to and from the neurons that carry impulses and neurotransmitters.

Neurotransmitters Chemicals that allow a stimulus to be transported across neurons to eventually stimulate muscles, glands, hormones, and other bodily responses. Examples of neurotransmitters include dopamine, serotonin, acetylcholine, and epinephrine (adrenalin).

Next of kin A patient's closest family member who is legally entitled to give permission for the treatment of a patient who is unconscious or otherwise incapacitated.

Nipple line An imaginary horizontal line that crosses the chest through the center of both nipples.

Nitrates (NO_3) Inorganic compounds that are composed of nitrogen and oxygen, which inhibit the ability of hemoglobin to carry oxygen, and are, therefore, detrimental to health.

Nocturia The need to urinate during the night.

Nonstress test (NST) An external and noninvasive method of monitoring the fetus, not usually performed until after the 27th week of pregnancy, used to assess fetal heart rate and movement.

Normal dental occlusion A normal bite.

Normal saline A type of sterile intravenous solution that consists of sodium chloride (NaCl) and water that is hydrating and mirrors the body's own fluids; medications can be added to it through a port in the intravenous line.

Nose (proboscis) The organ of inspiration, expiration, and smell that sits externally and medially on the face.

Nucleotides The four bases of DNA: cystosine, guanine, adenine, and thymine.

Nucleus Part of a cell that contains the genetic information of the cell, including its deoxyribonucleic acid (DNA) and ribonucleic acid (RNA).

Nullipara Term describing a woman who has never given birth before.

Nutrients Substances that provide nourishment for the body.

Nutrition The study of the nutrients in food and of how the body makes use of those nutrients. This field includes the research and study of the relationships among health, illness, and diet.

Nutritional status The balance between the intake of nutrients and the expenditure of energy from nutrients; the extent to which the nutrients available are able to meet a person's metabolic needs.

O

Obstetrics (OB) The medical field that specializes in pregnancy and childbirth.

Obtundation The drowsy state of consciousness when alertness is reduced and the patient acts confused when aroused. Also called *semiconscious.*

Occipital lobe One of the four lobes of the cerebral hemisphere; responsible for vision and the ability to recognize objects.

Occlusion The relationship between the upper and lower teeth when the jaw is closed.

Occupational stress disorder (OSD) A name for post-traumatic stress disorder used in reference to workers in police, emergency, and military occupations.

Occupational therapy (OT) A branch of health care that focuses on self-care activities and the promotion of independent functioning. It is concerned with the maintenance and restoration of fine-motor functioning and coordination, particularly those of the upper limbs. OT also concerns itself with an individual's ability to perform an occupation, or goal-directed activity, at home or at work.

Oncology The branch of medicine that deals with potentially cancerous swollen tissue, tumors, and masses, as well as with cancer research, care, and treatment.

Oocyte Term for immature ovum.

Oogenesis A process in the ovaries of the female body that eventually produces a mature ovum, beginning soon after conception in the female embryo and continuing from puberty to menopause.

Opiate A drug that contains opium.

Opioids Synthetic narcotics or opium-like substances designed to alleviate pain and are highly addictive.

Opposes/opposing (in muscles) Works or stands against; also referred to as *agonists* and *antagonists.*

Optimal patient outcomes The best possible results of care and treatment.

Oral cavity The inside of the mouth, including the hard and soft palates, pharynx, tonsils, associated muscles, salivary glands, teeth, gums, uvula, and tongue.

Oral labia The lips.

Oral mucosa A mucous barrier in the mouth that protects against temperature, irritants, and trauma.

Orbital rims The eye sockets.

Orchitis An inflammation or infection of the testes, which can be caused by the mumps but it may also result from a bacterium, virus, or trauma.

Organ systems Groups of organs that work together to carry out the body's essential functions.

Organelles Cell parts responsible for the cell's reproduction and survival.

Organs Groups of tissues that perform specific tasks or functions in the body.

Orogastric A term that means from mouth to stomach.

Orthopedics The field of medicine that deals with the musculoskeletal structures of bones, ligaments, muscles, and joints.

Ossa The anatomical term for a bone.

Ossification The medical term for the process of bone creation.

Osteoblasts Primitive cells that make bones.

Osteophytes Swellings on the bone that are eventually seen as knobby, gnarled, or disfigured joints.

Otorrhea Cerebrospinal fluid leaking from the ears.

Outpatient A label given to patients who do not require full admission to a hospital but who still need medical treatment or follow-up care. These patients are ambulatory. They come and go to outpatient appointments on their own.

Ova Eggs produced by the female reproductive system; plural of ovum.

Overtax Descriptor meaning to overwhelm or exhaust.

Ovulation The ripening and release of an egg from an ovary approximately 2 weeks after the onset of menstruation.

Ovum The female gamete; egg.

Oxygen saturation (O_2SATS) A diagnostic measure of the amount of oxygen that is bound to hemoglobin in the blood (oxyhemoglobin); normal saturation is recorded as 95% to 100%.

P

Padded dressings Coverings for a wound that provide some form of cushioning to protect it from further injury. The cushioning may be cotton, a cotton-like fabric, or foam.

Pain management A broad medical term that pertains to how individuals perceive and cope with pain when they experience it: In a hospital or clinical setting, nurses and doctors help patients to manage their pain. During outpatient or home care, patients and clients manage their pain independently, with the guidance of a care provider.

Pain scale A common system of pain measurement in which the patient rates the intensity of his or her pain on a scale of 1 to 10, with 1 being pain free and 10 being very bad or unbearable.

Pain-scale diagram a cartoon-like depiction of pain rated from 1 (very bad and intolerable) to 10 (not evident or not discomforting) used in pediatric care.

Palates Structures that separate the nasal cavity from the mouth: the *hard palate* forms the anterior portion of the roof of the mouth; the *soft palate* lies posterior to the hard palate.

Palatines These bones are situated behind the maxillae and form part of the hard palate at the back and base of the nose.

Palliative care unit A highly specialized unit that provides comfort and quality of life for patients with serious, often (but not always) terminal, life-ending medical challenges.

Palpated bimanually Medical term meaning the health provider used both hands to touch and assess both sides of the patient at the same time.

Palpation A technique used in physical examination in which the examiner feels the texture, size, consistency, and location of certain body parts with the hands.

Pancreas An endocrine and exocrine gland located deep within the abdomen, between the stomach and the spine, and adjacent to the duodenum that is integral to the digestive and to system the maintenance of appropriate blood glucose or sugar levels in the body.

Parallel bars An apparatus that consists of two bars that are side by side between which a person can walk while holding onto one bar with each hand. In physical therapy and rehabilitation programs, parallel bars are used for gait training (walking).

Paranasal A position located bilaterally to the nose.

Parenteral Descriptor for a tube *inside the body but bypassing the digestive tract.*

Paresthesias Tingling of the extremities.

Pareunia Penetration of a vagina by a penis; synonym for *coitus.*

Parietal Layer of a membrane that faces outward.

Parietal lobe One of the four lobes of the cerebral hemisphere that has the ability to distinguish the five senses and control some language functions.

Partial thromboblastin time (PTT) A test that evaluates the function of all coagulation factors, usually ordered in cases of unexplained bleeding, bruising, or recurrent miscarriage. This test is also ordered as a safety precaution prior to surgery.

Passive immunity The result of exposure to antibodies that are produced in one person's body and then acquired by another.

Passive range-of-motion exercises Exercises that involve moving parts of the body without causing the muscles to contract or relax.

Patella A sesamoid bone situated in tendon that is located at the front (anterior aspect) of the knee. It is commonly referred to as the *kneecap.*

Patency of the nares A medical term referring to whether or not the nasal airways are open and whether air is able to travel in and out of the nares.

Patent ductus arteriousus (PDA) A condition in which a short blood vessel that connects the main blood vessels that support the lungs and the aorta has not closed during fetal development.

Pathogen A term that refers to a germ, parasite, bacteria, pollution, viruse, fungus, toxin, or carcinogen that are disease producing.

Pathological processes The progression and effects of a disease or illness.

Patient complaint A patient's subjective, personal report of why he or she is seeking medical attention.

Pelvic girdle The structure of bones that attach the upper parts of the skeleton (i.e., the head and the trunk) to the lower parts. It is commonly referred to as the *pelvis.*

Pelvis Part of the skeleton in the lower abdominal area that gives shape, protection, and support to the organs and structures located within.

Pericardial membranes Membranes that surround the heart and the roots of the large blood vessels that originate within the heart.

Perineum The external area between the vulva and the anus for women, and between the scrotum and anus for men.

Periorbital hematoma Swelling or bruising around the eyes.

Peripheral nervous system Subsystem of the neurological system consisting of the network of nerves that carry messages to and from the CNS to the rest of the body.

Peristalsis A naturally occurring wavelike motion caused by the muscular contractions of the digestive tract. Peristalsis is critical to a well-functioning digestive system.

Peritoneal membranes Membranes that surround and line the abdominal cavity.

Pervasive Persistent and all-encompassing; developmental delays encompass all aspects of the person's life: activity, relationships, experiences, and so on.

Pervasive development disorders (PDD) A syndrome of multiple developmental delays occurring together, which leads to disabilities in function, cognition, social ability, and communication. It may also include the absence of imagination.

PET scan A machine that is an extremely sensitive device. That can pick up and measure even the tiniest amounts of radioactive matter in the body. It also uses trace amounts of glucose—the cells of which begin to metabolize quickly—to detect tumors. Also known as positron emission tomography.

Pfannenstiel incision An incision that transverses the lower abdomen, including the rectus abdominis muscle, and takes a semicircular shape just above the mons pubis.

Phagocytes Leukocytes that attract and engulf harmful foreign bodies and dead or dying cells and kill them by ingestion.

Phagocytosis Ingestion process used by phagocytes to kill harmful foreign bodies and dead or dying cells; plays a significant role in fighting infection and providing immunity.

Pharmacokinetics A field that focuses specifically on the metabolism of drugs, how they are absorbed and distributed, how the body excretes them, how long it takes for them to achieve a therapeutic effect, and the duration of the desired effect.

Pharmacology The study of the science of drugs, including how they work and interact with the body, as well as with other drugs.

Pharyngeal reflex See *Gag reflex.*

Pharynx The throat; sits posterior to the oral and nasal cavities and is connected to both.

Phlebotomist A technician with specialized training and certification that permits him or her to take blood from a vein or capillary for the purpose of blood donation or diagnostic testing.

Phlebotomy The process of puncturing or cutting into a vein.

Physical therapy A health-care discipline that is concerned with the care, treatment, maintenance, and rehabilitation of injuries and pathologies that affect the musculoskeletal system.

Physiology The study of how the body's structures interact and function.

Pia mater The meningeal membrane permeated by blood vessels that adheres to the brain and the spinal cord.

Pin A retrograde nail (screw) or a K-wire that has threads that help to ease it into a bone to fixate the bone.

Pipette or pipettor A device that is used to measure liquid. The word *pipette* is more often used to describe a device that is operated by hand. The word *pipettor,* however, is more often used to describe a device that operates with the assistance of electricity or that is automated.

Pituitary gland (hypophysis) A gland housed in the brain that is responsible for the growth of bone. The pituitary also contributes to metabolism and homeostasis, and it activates sexual growth and development through the release of hormones. It exerts control over the most of the endocrine system.

Placenta An organ of reproduction that attaches the embryo or fetus to the inside of the uterine wall and, by doing so, is able to provide nutrients, remove waste products, and provide vital gas exchanges that promote healthy growth.

Placental abruption A detachment of the placenta from the uterus that occurs when blood collects between the placenta and the uterus; as the pressure and volume of blood increase, the placenta eventually tears away from the uterus.

Plate A steel plate that is embedded in person's body to help support and restructure an injured area that has been fractured during bone healing. These plates can be permanent or temporary depending on the fractured area and the extent of the fracture.

Platelets Clear or colorless thrombocytes (particles in blood) that clot blood.

Plethysmograph Device used during pulmonary plethysmography. This device is actually a small chamber in which the client sits for the test. The client's nose will be plugged, and he or she will breathe into a mouthpiece.

Pleura A type of serous membrane that protects the lungs from coming into direct contact with the thoracic wall and the diaphragm.

Pleural membranes Membranes that surround the lungs by lining the pleural cavity.

Pliability Flexibility or suppleness.

Pliant Descriptor meaning moveable, flaccid (not rigid), flexible, and bendable.

Point of insertion The end of a muscle's attachment to bones at a moveable bone (i.e., the ulna and humerus at the elbow joint).

Point of origin The beginning of a muscle's attachment to bones at a stationary bone, which is a bone that does not move (i.e., the tibia or shin bone).

Polycystic ovarian syndrome (PCOS) Term for a number of co-occurring pathological conditions developed when ovulation fails to occur, the primary one of which is multiple cysts on the ovaries. The other conditions might include acne, obesity, anovulation, hirsutism, baldness, low bone density, and menstrual irregularities.

Polydipsia Excessive thirst, a cardinal symptom of diabetes.

Polymers Material that consists of chains of chemicals.

Polyphagia Excessive hunger, a cardinal symptom of diabetes.

Polypharmacy A situation in which many medications are being taken at the same time.

Polyuria Excessive urination, a cardinal symptom of diabetes.

Pons Structure in the brain that contains the cerebrum and cerebellum with other parts of the brain.

Pool To collect.

Positive pressure Forcing air into the lungs.

Post-traumatic stress disorder (PTSD) Disorder caused by a severe psychological trauma with which the individual is unable to cope. This disorder can occur immediately, shortly after the event, or years later and includes flashbacks or nightmares of the event, insomnia, withdrawal from friends or family, as well as the avoidance of incidents that remind the person of the traumatic event and that may trigger a dissociative state.

Postoperatively Term meaning *after surgery.*

Postpartum depression A serious type of major clinical depression that can occur within the first 6 months after delivery during which the new mother becomes preoccupied with thoughts of worthlessness, inadequacy to the tasks of motherhood, and lack of self-confidence in her ability to care for and protect her baby. Symptoms of the illness include persistent anxiety and fatigue.

Postpartum psychosis A rare mental illness that almost always requires hospitalization because it can lead to suicide and infanticide. Symptoms include extreme states of erratic or disorganized behavior, confusion, agitation, and lability of mood. These symptoms may be accompanied by rapid speech, manic behaviors, fatigue, and feelings of hopelessness and possibly shame. The woman experiencing postpartum psychosis may also become frantic and paranoid.

Postprandial Term meaning *after a meal.*

Postural alignment The proper placement of the bones of the skeleton related to the posture. Ideal postural alignment involves standing up straight.

Prefix A word part made up of a syllable or syllables that appear at the beginning of many words.

Pregnancy A 9-month process that begins with conception and ends with birth; the period in between these two events in termed pregnancy and is divided into three trimesters, three 3-month periods of time.

Pregnancy-induced hypertension (PIH) See *Hypertension of pregnancy (preeclampsia).*

Premature Too early or ahead of time.

Premorbid Term meaning *occurring before the medical incident, trauma, or disease.*

Preoccupation A state of being fully absorbed in one's own thoughts to the exclusion of the external world.

Presenting condition See *patient complaint.*

Primagravida Term that describes a woman who is pregnant for the first time.

Primary site Term meaning the first or original location of the cancer cells, where the primary tumor first appears.

Proliferate To grow by the rapid production of new cells.

Prostate gland A gland in the human male anatomy that secretes a substance that forms part of the semen.

Prostheses Artificial limbs or organs.

Protein A naturally occurring compound of amino acids.

Proteins Organic compounds that provide nourishment and energy composed of amino acids and are essential elements at all levels of the body.

Prothrombin time (PT) A test to determine the time that it takes for the blood to thicken and clot, usually ordered to identify the cause of unexplained bleeding, the status of the liver, and the effectiveness of anticoagulant medication such as warfarin (Coumadin) or heparin.

Pruritus The medical term for itchiness.

Psych assessment Medical jargon referring to a mental health assessment. *Psych* can refer to psychiatry or psychology.

Psychiatry The field of medicine concerned with the diagnosis, treatment, and prevention of mental illness.

Psychopathology A medical condition in which there is a pattern of psychological and behavioral disruption that involves alterations in mood, cognition, and behavior.

Puberty The period of growth and development in which a person reaches biological, reproductive maturity. In other words, gamete production occurs, and fertility and impregnation become possible: the reproductive system of both males and females becomes functional.

Puerperal Term meaning *occurring during or immediately after childbirth.*

Pulmonary circulation A subsystem of the cardiovascular system concerned with the oxygenation of blood in the lungs.

Pulmonary plethysmography The measure of how much air can be held in the lungs during times of rest. It can help to determine if there is structural damage to the lungs or if they have lost the ability to expand properly as the patient inhales.

Pulmonologist A medical internist with advanced training in pulmonology.

Pulmonology The branch of science and medicine that is concerned with pathologies of the lungs, the bronchioles, and the upper respiratory tract.

Pulse oximeter A device that measures any changes in blood volume in the skin and oxygen saturation, and it also measures the patient's pulse.

Pulse rate The number of times that the heart beats per minute at a pulse site located a distance away from the heart itself.

Purkinje fibers Specialized conductive fibers that lie within the ventricular walls and conduct electrical impulses throughout the cells of the ventricles, causing them to contract and empty.

Pursed lips Term meaning *puckered lips.*

Pyelonephritis An infection of the kidneys that includes inflammation of the kidney and renal pelvis, which can result if cystitis is not treated promptly

Pyretic Term meaning *fever.*

Q

Quadriceps Four specific muscles that sit on the anterior aspect of the thigh: the *rectus femoris,* the *vastus intermedius,* the *vastus lateralis,* and the *vastus medialis.* They work cooperatively to extend to straighten the leg and to contract to bend the knee.

Quadriceps femoris A group of muscles in the upper leg.

Quantitative blood serum See *Beta hCG.*

R

Reaction times The amount of time that elapses (the interval) between a stimulus occurring and a response to it.

Readout (trace) The written record of the data (either printed out or on a screen) acquired by a computer or a computer-assisted device.

Reagent strip A dry, plastic strip with tiny microfiber pads attached, used in laboratory and diagnostic testing.

Reciprocal innervation A simultaneous process that happens when the innervation of an agonist muscle occurs. The reciprocal innervation stimulates the antagonist muscle response. For example, when a skeletal muscle is innervated to contract, the antagonist muscle simultaneously relaxes.

Rectum A repository for feces spanning the sigmoid colon to the anus. When feces enter the rectum, they are held until sensors within the tissue alert the brain that the rectum and bowels need to be evacuated.

Reflex irritability Measure of infant who grimaces, coughs, sneezes, or cries vigorously in response to an irritant.

Rehabilitation (rehab.) The process of recovering function and as much self-sufficiency and independence as possible after a physical or psychological trauma, injury, or disease.

Rehabilitation counseling A service that helps people to deal with disabilities of a personal, social, or vocational nature. It can include assistance with recovery from accidents, dealing with diseases, and living with congenital or acquired disabilities (i.e., amputation).

Relax/relaxes In the context of muscles, the term describes the state of the muscles at ease; resting in a straighter or more open position; sometimes also referred to as *extension,* although a relaxed muscle is not always fully or rigidly straight.

Removable brace In the context of orthopedics, this is an orthotic device made of lightweight plastics or polymers that protects and stabilizes fractures and joints after injury. These braces are often held in place by Velcro strips or straps and can be removed at night for some relief and to protect the skin from breakdown.

Repetitions Tasks that are repeated for a set number of times.

Residual Descriptor meaning *remaining, lingering, or left over.*

Residual effects in the context of healthcare, these are the aftereffects of a treatment, medication, procedure, or other medical action.

Resiliency A person's ability to bounce back or to recover quickly from an unfavorable circumstance or situation.

Respiration Term meaning *the act of breathing.*

Respiratory Term meaning *related to breathing.*

Respiratory distress syndrome (RDS) When the lungs lack the ability to produce surfactant, a substance needed for the lungs to expand properly after birth, the lungs stop functioning. It is one of the most common problems that affects preterm infants, and its onset can be immediate and life threatening.

Respiratory effort Breathing effort.

Respiratory failure The cessation of breathing, which occurs when the respiratory center in the cerebellum has ceased to function.

Respire A root word meaning *to breathe oxygen and expel carbon dioxide.*

Resps Respirations per minute.

Resuscitation Process of reviving or bringing to life by providing air.

Retina The organ in the back of the eye that senses light and sends impulses to the brain that enable humans to see.

Retinopathy of prematurity (ROP) A condition in which the eyes of premature infants are vulnerable to injury after birth as a result of the incomplete or abnormal growth of the blood vessels in the fetus' or newborn's eyes, particularly those blood vessels that feed the retina.

Retrograde A term meaning prior to. In the context of memory, the term describes loss of memory related to the events that occurred just before an injury.

Review of systems (ROS) A series of questions that ask about each of the patient's body systems to provide a comprehensive overview of the patient's health history.

Rh Type of antigen (protein) found on the membranous surface of red blood cells.

Rh factor A classification system used to type blood for transfusion purposes.

Rheuma The fluid within the joint spaces inside the body.

Rheumatology The field of medicine that specializes in disorders of the joints, muscles, and bones as well as the diagnosis and treatment of arthritis.

Rhinorrhea The condition of cerebrospinal fluid leaking from the nose.

Ribonucleic acid (RNA) Any of a group of nucleic acids, present in all living cells, that play an essential role in the synthesis of proteins.

Right-hand dominant Medical term for being right-handed.

Rights of medication administration Term used in medicine to identify safe practices for administering medications. Each right is checked before giving the patient the medicine.

Rigid fixation A surgical technique in which tiny screws or plates are attached directly onto the fractured section of the jawbone.

Ritter von Ritterschein disease A type of staphylococcal infection that is seen in newborn babies that has the appearance of a severe burn and can be life threatening if not treated promptly and effectively.

Root word A term referring to that part of the word that can stand alone as its own word.

Rounds The term *rounds* refers to a routine inspection of the unit, when a nurse or other health care provider sees all of his or her assigned patients.

Route of administration Term referring to how the medication is actually taken into or applied to the body (i.e., oral, topical, inhalation).

Rule of Nines for Burns A universally accepted tool used to assess the extent of burns, calculate safe and appropriate medication dosages and amounts of IV fluids to be administered, and identify the total body surface area (BSA) affected by the burn.

Rumination Repeatedly and deeply going over and over a subject of concern or an anxiety-producing subject to the point that normal daily functioning is impaired.

Rupture A term meaning burst or to burst.

S

Saccharides A category of carbohydrates that contain sugars.

Sacrum A triangular-shaped structure found at the base of the spine.

Sagittal plane Also called the *median plane,* the directional line runs lengthwise, and it divides the body into two parts: the left and right lateral planes.

Salient Significant, relevant, or noteworthy.

Saliva The substance produced by the salivary glands near the oral cavity with the purpose to keep the oral cavity moist and to assist with the transport of food by moistening it. Saliva (spit) also carries digestive enzymes and actually initiates digestion.

Sarcomas Cancers of the soft tissues of the body. They most notably arise from the mesenchymal tissues of the bones and muscles and the glial cells of the brain.

Scalded skin syndrome A type of staphylococcal infection that is seen in newborn babies and young children, particularly among those who are younger than 6 years old, as well as in adults who are challenged by renal failure or immune deficiency disorders and who have become immunocompromised. It has the appearance of a severe burn and can be life threatening if not treated promptly and effectively.

Scars A type of fibrous tissue that has replaced injured tissue. It is initially red and swollen. Over time, scar tissue shrinks, and it may disappear almost entirely from view.

Sebum A fatty, grease-like secretion that originates in the sebaceous glands of the skin.

Second-degree burns (partial thickness burns) Burns that extend into the dermis but do not injure or destroy all of the dermis and cause the skin to appear swollen and red. Blisters form. There is a good deal of pain involved during the acute phase of this type of burn, and medical treatment may be required.

Second-impact syndrome An injury to the brain that happens after an initial, primary brain or head injury and increases intracranial pressure.

Sedation The result of medicating a patient to induce a state of calm or relaxation.

Sedative A medication with the primary purpose of calming a patient.

Seizure A medical condition in which the electro-conductivity of the brain is abnormal, causing the brain to temporarily dysfunction. There may be some degree of loss of consciousness of one's surroundings.

Selective serotonin reuptake inhibitors (SSRIs) A class of drugs that inhibit or block the reuptake of serotonin in the brain. By doing so, they leave the serotonin circulating in the nervous system, thus maintaining a more stable and appropriate level for functioning.

Self-medicating An individual takes medications or drugs in a manner that he or she thinks is appropriate to achieve a desired effect.

Self-monitor blood glucose (SMBG) Patients are given instruction with regard to how to operate a glucose monitoring device, and they are able to follow a set routine for self-testing on their own.

Semen A viscous fluid secretion containing sperm that is discharged through the urethra of a male at the time of ejaculation.

Semiconscious See *Obtundation*.

Seminal vesicles Two sac-like glands that sit below the bladder in males. They produce a substance that enhances the viability and motility (movement) of sperm.

Semispinalis capitis A longitudinal and deep skeletal muscle that is located in the posterior portion of the neck and that originates in the cervical spine and the thoracic spine. It sits just under the trapezius muscle, and its movement allows for the rotation and extension of the head.

Sepsis A medical term meaning *decay, putrefaction, or the decomposition of animal matter;* a serious medical condition that can occur as a result of uncontrolled infection and it can lead to blood clots, organ failure, and gangrene. Another name for sepsis is systemic inflammatory response syndrome (SIRS).

Serotonin A neurotransmitter whose natural function is to control mood. It also affects bodily functions such as appetite and sleep.

Serous membrane A membrane supplied by blood.

Sesamoid bones Type of short bones that function to modify the angle of bone where it is inserted into a muscle; embedded within tendons or joint capsules (i.e., the patella or kneecap.)

Sexual function A term that refers to the ability of a male or female to engage in a complete sexual activity.

Sexually transmitted A term identifying the mode of infection by pathogens from one carrier to another. In this case, the mode of infection is person-to-person, skin-to-skin sexual contact: intimate sexual relations of intercourse and/or oral sex.

Sexually transmitted diseases (STD) More enduring and often much harder to treat than infections, STDs can cause damage to organs and systems; they can even be life-threatening. If the cause of the sexually transmitted disease is viral, then the disease is untreatable and will stay in the body forever, sometimes dormant and sometimes active, producing acute symptoms and/or injury to organs and cells.

Sexually transmitted infections (STIs) Infections transmitted through sexual contact with an infected person that can be treated by various anti-infective medications and antibiotics.

Short bones These bones are less dense than the long bones. Their internal consistency is spongier than that of most other bones, and, as a protective measure, they are covered with a thin layer of compact bone (i.e., the carpal and tarsal bones). Short bones provide for movement, flexibility of the body, shock absorption, and elasticity.

Side effects Any effects other than the intended ones that a drug may cause, either temporary or permanent, mild or severe.

Sinoatrial (SA) node A mass of cardiac muscle cells in the right atrium that serves as the natural pacemaker of the heart by releasing electrical stimuli at regular intervals (beats) causing a wave of contraction to occur in both atria of the heart.

Sinuses Small air pockets lined in mucus within the craniofacial complex that are connected to the nasal cavity by small tubes, which permit airflow into the nasal passages and allow for the drainage of mucous.

Skeletal muscles Muscles that permit movement and support the skeleton.

Skin breakdown A process during which the integrity of the surface of the skin is broken and the underlying tissue is exposed to the air. This situation can result from long periods of immobility, allergies, exposure to the sun, wounds, and other causes.

Skin discoloration In the context of a burn, this term refers to a change in skin color that is the natural result of a burn; it may be bright red (as a result of the inflammatory process) that lessens to pink and that eventually turns back to the patient's normal skin tone.

Slough off The casting off of dead skin to make way for new skin that is developing underneath it.

Sluggish Term meaning slow.

Soft callus A thickened area of skin that results in clotted blood is replaced with fibrous tissue and cartilage.

Soluble Descriptor meaning *able to pass through membranes.*

Solutes A term referring to any substance or compounds found in liquids. In the context of the urinary systems, solutes are waste products found in urine (i.e., creatinine, uric acid, and enzymes).

Sonogram The image produced on the computer monitor during an ultrasound examination.

Sonograph Term referring to the examination record of an ultrasound.

Spasms Brief involuntary muscle contractions that can happen anywhere in the body, with or without pain.

Specific gravity A measurement that identifies how concentrated a sample of urine is by measuring against a standard volume of water.

Speculum A plastic or metal device used for internal exams for women to dilate the vaginal canal for examination.

Sperm The male reproductive cell, or gamete, containing half of the parent's genetic code.

Spermatogenesis The production of fully mature, functional spermatozoa that occurs in the testes, more specifically in the seminiferous tubules of the testes.

Spermatozoa The plural form of *spermatozoon,* meaning *a mature male sex cell,* which are produced in the testicles and stored in the seminal vesicles.

Sphincters Circular bands of muscle that control the flow of matter (liquids or solids) through body orifices or openings.

Spinal (spinal cavity) Another name for the vertebral canal, a division of the dorsal cavity.

Spinal column Structure made from the 24 vertebrae that form the spine.

Spinal cord A column of nerve fibers and neuropathways that extends from the brain to the end of the first lumbar vertebra of the spine through a hole in the center of each vertebra.

Spirometer A device that measures flow rates and the amount of air is moving through the lungs.

Spirometry A pulmonary function test or a series of breathing tests that ascertain and monitor lung capacity and function.

Spleen A lymphoid organ located on the left of the abdominal cavity, just below the diaphragm and posterior to the stomach. It is a reservoir for blood that makes blood available when it is needed. The spleen contains lymphocytes and macrophages that trap and destroy foreign bodies that enter it.

Split lip A trauma to the lip in which the skin is broken.

Stage theory A number of commonly used theories that group people of certain ages (i.e., children, adults, elderly) and then identify specific physical and psychosocial developmental tasks that each age group should or will complete.

Staphylococcal scalded skin syndrome (SSSS) See *Scalded skin syndrome.*

Statin A type of medication proven to reduce levels of low-density cholesterol and to lower the risk of heart attack.

Status Condition.

Stave off Term meaning *to ward off or prevent the occurrence of.*

Sterile burn sheet A light, non-woven sheet of synthetic material that can be used on either wet or dry to cover burns.

Sterile prep Preparation of the patient for surgery with the use of disinfecting agents and the creation of a sterile environment or sterile field from which to work.

Sternoclavicular joint An anatomical point between the sternum (the breastbone) and the medial extremity of the clavicle bone; at the end of the clavicle, where it sits at a near mid-torso point.

Stiff Descriptor meaning *inflexible or difficult to flex.*

Stigma The shame attached to negative labels. This may be shame feel for oneself or demonstrated by others who feel shamed or ashamed. It is usually caused by misunderstanding or a lack of knowledge about a condition.

Stimulus A motivator, something that causes a response.

Stirrups An apparatus attached to an examining table in which the heels of the feet are placed; the knees are bent, much like placing feet in the stirrups of a saddle.

Stoma An opening made from outside the body to a desired organ or region of the body.

Stomach A temporary storage unit for solids and fluids during the process of digestion that sits inferior to the esophagus and on the left side of the abdomen.

Stress A descriptive term that explains a myriad of experiences during which demands are placed on the individual to cope or act.

Stressors Demands placed on the individual to cope or act.

Striated A type of muscle that appears striped or striated.

Stroke A sudden loss of brain function caused by interruption of blood flow or excessive blood flow to the brain.

Structure (1) composition or makeup; (2) organization or arrangement.

Stupor State of deep unconsciousness from which a person cannot be awakened or aroused without a stimulus such as a very loud noise or strong pain. Even then, he or she may only awaken briefly before slipping back into this level of unconsciousness.

Subcuticular sutures Sutures located below the epidermis.

Subdural Below the dura mater, this is a layer of tissue that covers and protects the brain.

Subdural hematoma (SDH) A collection of blood that occurs between the brain tissue and the dura mater caused by a stretching or tearing of the veins that bridge between the dura mater and the brain.

Substance abuse A use pattern of drugs, alcohol, or other substances (i.e., glue) that are harmful to the body or mind and that have the potential to adversely affect all dimensions of health. Substance abuse does not necessarily connote addition.

Suffix Word part added to the end of a root word to change its meaning or its part of speech.

Superficial muscles The muscles that lies closest to the skin.

Support In the context of orthopedics and medicine, this term refers to a type of brace, wrap, or other device that provides stabilization and that may also enhance circulation surrounding a joint or a moveable body part.

Support groups Groups of patients, family members, friends, significant others, or coworkers who come together voluntarily to seek emotional support and information about specific issues.

Support program Any type of program that is designed to offer encouragement, education, comfort, and help to people and family of people with illnesses, injuries, addictions, and psychological or psychiatric needs.

Surfactant A substance that allow the lungs to expand properly after birth.

Surgical asepsis The sterile protocols required before entering the operating room or performing any sterile procedure such as when caring for specific types of wounds or working in some fields of oncology and chemotherapy.

Surgical prep A preoperative meeting between patient and physician during which the physician discusses the upcoming surgery with the patient.

Surgical reduction A term referring to the process of when a fractured bone is straightened and returned to its natural state by way of surgical intervention.

Suture line A row of stitches (sutures) over an incision line.

Suture lines The points where the dura mater attaches itself to the bones of the skull at the places where the bones meet.

Swallow To pass ingested material from the mouth to the esophagus.

Sweat (perspiration) An emission of clear, odorous moisture that originates in the sudoriferous (sweat) glands within the skin and subcutaneous tissues, through the pores of the skin, with the purpose of cooling the skin and the body as it evaporates off the surface of the skin.

Synapse Any place where an axon of one neuron comes into contact with a dendrite from another neuron.

Synovial fluid A viscous (thick and sticky) fluid found in joints that helps them to move smoothly.

Synovial membrane A layer of connective tissue that lines the cavities of joints.

Syphilis A bacterial infection disease that proceeds through a number of worsening stages and takes a great toll on body systems, organs, and the mind. Long-term effects can include blindness, sores on the genitals and other body parts, deafness, heart disease, and insanity. Syphilis can be contracted only by person-to-person contact with a syphilitic sore. Treatment is simple: penicillin by intramuscular injection.

Systemic Term meaning symptoms that cause reactions in other systems of the body besides the original infected system as the immune system mobilizes to defend the body against the infection.

Systemic circulation A subsystem of the cardiovascular system concerned with the circulation of oxygenated blood.

Systemic inflammatory response syndrome (SIRS) See *Sepsis (medical condition)*.

Systole The contraction phase of the heart muscles during the cardiac cycle.

T

T-stem cells The precursors of T-cells produced in bone marrow. T-cells regulate the immune system by turning the immune response on or off. More importantly, these cells directly attack and destroy infectious agents.

Tablet A solid substance that contains medicinal compounds.

Tachycardic Referring to a faster-than-usual pulse rate or heart rate, which is measured in beats per minute.

Tactile Medical term for *sense of touch.*

Talus The ankle bone that articulates with the tibia and fibula, as well as with other bones of the ankle.

Tarsus The combination of all seven small bones that make up the ankle: the talus, the calcaneus, the navicular, the cuboid (outer bone of the instep), and three cuneiform bones (small internal, external, and middle). Together, these seven bones are generally referred to as the *ankle.*

Taste receptors Medical term for *taste buds.*

Temporal lobe One of the four lobes of the cerebral hemisphere that is divided into two parts, one for each side of the brain. The temporal lobes are responsible for speech, making meaning from sensory input, and hearing.

Temporomandibular joints (TMJs) Bilateral hinge joints that connect the mandible to the upper facial skeleton near the ears.

Tender to the touch An assessment term that describes a hypersensitivity of the skin or its underlying structures. When touched even lightly, the skin feels sore.

Tendons A type of fibrous tissue that forms into strong cords, which connect muscles to bones, also referred to as *sinew.*

Teratogen Anything that can adversely affect the normal cell development of an embryo or fetus.

Teratoma A cancerous tumor in an embryo or a tumor that has extraembryonic features.

Terminal Term meaning *incurable*; *dying.* Terminal does not necessarily mean a quick death.

Testes Reproductive organs that not only produce sperm and testosterone but also function as endocrine glands.

Testosterone A specific androgen related to the sex drive and hormone important to the development of secondary sex characteristics produced in the interstitial cells of the testes.

Thalamus Part of the brain responsible for sensations (i.e., pain, pleasure).

Thermoregulation Temperature regulation.

Third-degree burns (full-thickness burns) Burns involving the destruction of the dermis, and leave subcutaneous tissue exposed. There is no pain involved because the nerve endings have been destroyed. Visually, these burns look leathery and dry, and may be white in color. Medical treatment is absolutely required.

Thoracic Adjective describing the thorax, the chest, or the upper part of the torso, both internally and externally.

Thoracic spine (mid back) This region of the body consists of 12 vertebrae that connect to the ribs and form the back.

Thready A commonly used descriptor for a pulse that is fine or barely perceptible.

Thrombin An enzyme that is the basis of a blood clot.

Thromboemboli Blood clots.

Thromboplastin A substance in the blood and tissues that increases clotting time.

Thrombosis The presence of a blood clot in the circulatory system.

Thrombus A blood clot that adheres to the wall of a blood vessel.

Thymus A lymphoid organ that is also a gland. It sits near the lower posterior portion of the neck, behind the sternum. The thymus contains lymphocytes and epithelial cells. Its main function is the production of T-lymphocytes (T-cells), which it secretes into the body to mature and circulate when stimulated by a hormone. During the early years of life, the thymus is instrumental to the development of the body's immune system. The thymus becomes inactive after childhood.

Thyroid A gland that is located internally just below the larynx and on the anterior surface of the throat that produces and secretes thyroid hormone.

Tibia The largest bone of the lower leg, the tibia is situated between the knee and the ankle, anterior to the fibula. The tibia actually articulates with the femur (above it) through the process of the knee joint, as well as with the talus in the ankle. The tibia is commonly referred to as the *shinbone.*

Tissues Groups of cells that are similar in structure and function.

Titanium mini-plates Small strips of titanium metal that are placed along a fracture with screws to support bone healing. This allows the two sides of the fracture to come together and to remain in exceptionally close proximity until new tissues and bone are able to fill the gaps caused by the break.

TNM staging system A system used to identify the presence or absence of tumors. This system classifies cancers by assessing the **t**umor, the **l**ymph node involvement, and the degree of metastasis.

Toddler Referring to children ages 1 to 3; the term is indicative of the developmental task of learning to walk. The toddler is able to be away for his or her parent or caregiver for longer and longer periods. He or she is very curious and experiences life by touching, tasting, and asking why.

Tolerance In regard to medications or other drugs or alcohol, tolerance occurs when the user needs ever-increasing doses of the substance to achieve the same effects that smaller doses initially provided.

Tolerate Term meaning *endure* or *withstand.*

Tone A medical synonym for *tension* or the partial contraction of a muscle.

Tongue A large mass of muscular tissue situated on the floor of the mouth that extends into the upper pharynx with the purpose to assist with speech and to move food and fluids backward through the mouth to the esophagus for digestion. The tongue is also the primary organ of taste; the taste buds are located on the tongue.

Tonsils Two small masses of lymphoid tissue found at the base of the tongue located in the mucous membranes of the pharynx.

Torso The trunk or main part of the body.

Total parenteral nutrition (TPN) The administration of all nutrition through an intravenous line into the vena cava and the bloodstream.

Tourniquet A device or tool such as a long strip of elastic or cloth that is used to staunch or stop bleeding. a temporary tourniquet is used to impede circulation when blood needs to be drawn for diagnostic purposes. It may be made of rubber, latex or other material with elastic properties.

Toxic *Lethal, noxious,* or *poisonous.*

Toxicology report A laboratory analysis of the levels of poisons or of substances deemed noxious or harmful in the body.

Toxicology screens Technical analyses of urine, hair, blood, sweat, and tissue to determine if toxins are present.

Trachea (windpipe) A cartilaginous organ situated in the neck that permits the flow of air into and out of the respiratory system and connects the oral and nasal cavities to the lungs.

Tract Word meaning *pathway.*

Traction In the context of orthopedics, a medical procedure in which a device called an *orthosis* is used to apply a pulling force on a bone to maintain its alignment that helps to reduce pain and prevents the formation of a hematoma. A small degree of temporary intermittent traction can be used in physical therapy.

Trade name Name given to a medication by a pharmaceutical company to brand or identify its product.

Transcutaneous electrical nerve stimulation (TENS) An electrical technique that targets pain and the peripheral nerves rather than the muscles; a TENS unit treats localized neuropathic pain that is the result of disease, inflammation, or trauma to the peripheral nerves caused by injury or surgery.

Transient Term meaning *temporary or fleeting.*

Transient dissociative states Periods of re-living or re-experiencing an event as if it were still occurring. As this happens, the person is not connected to the present reality but is dissociated from it (unaware of it).

Transient ischemic attack (TIA) A temporary interruption in the blood flow to the brain.

Translocation In the context of biochemistry or molecular biology, an abnormal fusion or merging of two separate regions of chromosomes on the DNA strand.

Transverse plane Also called the *horizontal plane,* divides the body crosswise into upper and lower (superior and inferior) halves horizontally at an invisible line at the middle of the body.

Treatment authorization request (TAR) A request that an insurance company or health maintenance organization (HMO) make payment for the tests, procedures, or other care identified by the health-care provider.

Tremors A type of continuous, involuntary muscle activity that causes the movement of a limb.

Triage Process by which patients are accessed to determine treatment priorities.

Trichomoniasis (trich) A common parasitic infection of the urethra and vagina by the protozoa *Trichomonas vaginalis.*

Trimesters In pregnancy, a period of 3 months in a series of three to total 9 months.

Turbinators (inferior nasal conchae) Thin bones that form the sides of the nasal cavity.

Type 1 diabetes See *Insulin-dependent Diabetes Mellitus (IDDM).*

Type 2 diabetes Once referred to as non-insulin-dependent diabetes mellitus, type 2 diabetics are unable to accept or unable to use naturally produced insulin in the body.

U

Ultrasound A machine that provides a view of the internal organs by emitting a high-pitched sound through the transducer wand and into the body; these sound waves echo off of dense or solid masses to produce an image on an attached monitor.

Unconsciousness A term meaning not conscious; not alert to or aware of the external world. Usually a sign of neurological dysfunction, unconsciousness has four stages: obtundation, hypersomnia, stupor, and coma.

Unguis The nail of the finger or toe.

United fracture A fracture in which the broken bone is healing.

Urea Substance produced when foods that contain protein are metabolized in the body and transported via the bloodstream into the kidneys, where it is filtered out.

Urethra A tubelike structure that extends from the bladder to the outside of the body.

Urinalysis (UA or U/A) A biochemical analysis of a patient's urine.

Urinary incontinence A person's ability to exert self-control over emptying his or her bladder is diminished and the person cannot control where or when he or she will void.

Urine Liquid composed of urea and other soluble substances that have been filtered through the kidneys.

Urine analyzer A device that identifies and measures molecules in urine.

Urine dip A urine test in which a dipstick is inserted into the patient's urine. The stick, which is usually made of plastic, is coated with a number of colored patches. When this stick is exposed to the various composites of urine, the colors brighten or change. This test is a quick way to assess the patient's condition.

Urine glucose test strips Paper strips that have been specially designed with small embedded pads that are glucose sensitive. When dipped in urine, these pads change color in the presence of glucose.

Urine hat A plastic receptacle that has the appearance of a white hat used to collect urine for testing.

User authentication protocol A protocol process required to access electronic medical records that could include a user-specific password and identification.

Uterine activity Contractions and any changes in the sound and frequency of the fetal heartbeat.

Uterine pressure Pressure exerted onto the pelvis by the expanding uterus. When uterine contractions occur, they push or exert force on the fetus.

Uterine wall The outer edge of the uterus that separates it from the other organs in the abdomen (i.e., bladder, rectum).

Uterus The female reproductive organ that provides a safe, protective, and nourishing environment for the growing embryo and fetus; also known as the *womb*.

Uvula The fleshy appendage (attachment) of tissue that appears at the posterior of the mouth, above the tongue, that closes the nasal fossa (cavity) during swallowing.

V

Vaccination See *Inoculation*.

Vaccine A biological substance; a biological preparation used to promote immunization.

Vaginal bleeding In the context of maternity and obstertics, a type of bleeding that is not expected in a pregnant woman. During the first trimester, it may indicate miscarriage. Throughout the rest of the term, it can indicate placentae previa (i.e., the cervix or opening to the womb is blocked by the placenta, and some placental blood vessels may rupture) or abruptio placentae. In the context of female sexuality, the term can refer to menses or symptoms of certain conditions such as endometriosis.

Vaginal discharge Secretions from the vagina.

Variability (baseline) In the context of maternity and obstetrics, this is a measure of the difference in the beat-to-beat intervals of the fetal heart rate. Normal variability in a term fetus is 6 to 25 beats per minute. This indicates a normally functioning central nervous system.

Vas deferens A duct or a narrow channel or tube-shaped vessel that carries sperm from the epididymis to the ejaculatory duct in the urethra.

Veins Blood vessels that carry blood *to* the heart.

Venipuncture The process of drawing blood from a vein.

Ventilation In a medical context, means the use of a ventilator machine that pumps continuous oxygenated air for a patient who cannot breathe on his or her own.

Ventral A term derived from the Latin *ventro*, meaning *the belly*.

Ventricle (brain) The four main cavities of the brain filled with cerebrospinal fluid that connect to the canal of the spinal cord.

Venules Tiny veins that function with capillaries to receive waste materials from the blood.

Vertebrae Bones, stacked one on top of the other, somewhat visible through the skin, connected by ligaments, and separated by discs, which protect and support the spinal cord as it extends through the spinal canal, the hollow center of the vertebra.

Vertebral (vertebral canal) A division of the dorsal cavity, also called the spinal cavity, that houses the spine and vertebre.

Vertex The normal presentation for a fetus, with the head tucked down on the chest and the crown of the head facing the birth canal.

Vertigo Dizziness; a sense of whirling and loss of balance.

Visceral A term referring to the internal organs of the body.

Visceral muscles Also known as smooth muscles, visceral muscles are involuntary and are found in hollow organs such as the lungs, the gastrointestinal tract, and the blood vessels.

Vital A term derived from a Latin root meaning *life.*

Vitals A medical reference to the vital signs: temperature, pulse, respirations, and blood pressure (TPR and BP).

Vitamin E cream An antioxidant topical cream that enhances production of collagen.

Vitamins Essential organic substances that promote growth, development, and normal cell function in the body and boost the immune system.

Voided Emptied the bladder; urinated.

Volume calibration Markings that indicate standardized measurements of liquid.

Voluntary control Muscles under conscious control and moving as a person chooses to move them.

Vomer Plow-shaped bone that forms part of the floor of the nasal cavity and part of the nasal septum.

Vulva The external genital organs of a female.

W

Water An essential nutrient made of two parts hydrogen and one part oxygen that affects the natural pH balance of the body; also a natural solvent for other nutrients. Water provides the means of delivery of these nutrients throughout the body.

Wave Any rhythmic motion with a defined amplitude and frequency.

Weight bearing The ability to carry the load of one's own weight on a bone or joint.

Wellness The absence of disease and a subjective sense of mental and physical well-being.

Wires Stainless steel wires used in dentistry to hold the jaws in place.

XYZ

X-ray A form of electromagnetic radiation that involves the use of photons. Another term that is sometimes used for this is *ionizing radiation.* The term *x-ray* also refers to a type of image that is produced on radiographic film by exposing the body to x-rays.

Zygote Fertilized egg formed from two haploid gametes.

Zygomatic arches The cheekbones.

Zygomatic bones (malar bones) Pair of bones that forms the cheekbones and part of the orbits.

Index

Note: Page numbers followed by f indicate figures; t, tables.

B

C

D

E

G

H

I

J

K

P

Q

R

S

T

U

V